Perioperative Transesophageal Echocardiography

PERIOPERATIVE TRANSESOPHAGEAL ECHOCARDIOGRAPHY

A companion to Kaplan's Cardiac Anesthesia

David L. Reich, MD
Horace W. Goldsmith Professor and Chair of Anesthesiology
Mount Sinai School of Medicine
New York, New York

Gregory W. Fischer, MD
Associate Professor of Anesthesiology and Cardiothoracic Surgery
Director of Adult Cardiothoracic Anesthesia
Department of Anesthesiology
Mount Sinai School of Medicine
New York, New York

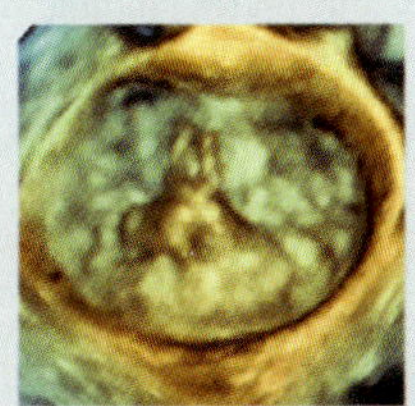

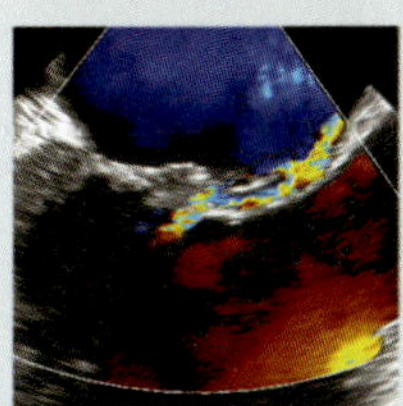

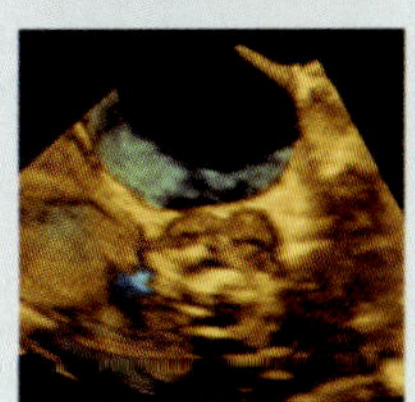

ELSEVIER
SAUNDERS

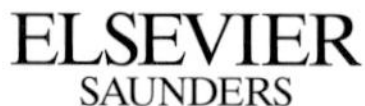

ELSEVIER
SAUNDERS

1600 John F. Kennedy Blvd.
Ste 1800
Philadelphia, PA 19103-2899

PERIOPERATIVE TRANSESOPHAGEAL ECHOCARDIOGRAPHY:
A COMPANION TO KAPLAN'S CARDIAC ANESTHESIA   ISBN: 978-1-4557-0761-4
Copyright © 2014 by Saunders, an imprint of Elsevier Inc.

Notices

Knowledge and best practice in this field are constantly changing. As new research and experience broaden our understanding, changes in research methods, professional practices, or medical treatment may become necessary.

Practitioners and researchers must always rely on their own experience and knowledge in evaluating and using any information, methods, compounds, or experiments described herein. In using such information or methods they should be mindful of their own safety and the safety of others, including parties for whom they have a professional responsibility.

With respect to any drug or pharmaceutical products identified, readers are advised to check the most current information provided (i) on procedures featured or (ii) by the manufacturer of each product to be administered, to verify the recommended dose or formula, the method and duration of administration, and contraindications. It is the responsibility of practitioners, relying on their own experience and knowledge of their patients, to make diagnoses, to determine dosages and the best treatment for each individual patient, and to take all appropriate safety precautions.

To the fullest extent of the law, neither the Publisher nor the authors, contributors, or editors assume any liability for any injury and/or damage to persons or property as a matter of products liability, negligence or otherwise, or from any use or operation of any methods, products, instructions, or ideas contained in the material herein.

Library of Congress Cataloging-in-Publication Data

Perioperative transesophageal echocardiography : a companion to Kaplan's
cardiac anesthesia/[edited by] David L. Reich, Gregory W. Fischer.
    p. ; cm.
  Complemented by: Kaplan's cardiac anesthesia/editor, Joel A. Kaplan. 6th ed. c2011.
  Includes bibliographical references and index.
  ISBN 978-1-4557-0761-4 (hardcover : alk. paper)
  I. Reich, David L. (David Louis), 1960-, editor of compilation. II.
Fischer, Gregory W., editor of compilation III. Kaplan's cardiac anesthesia.
Complemented by (work):
  [DNLM: 1. Echocardiography, Transesophageal. 2. Heart-physiology.
  3. Heart Diseases--surgery. 4. Perioperative Care. WG 141.5.E2]
  RC683.5.U5
  616.1'207543--dc23   2013019956

Acquisitions Editor: William Schmitt
Developmental Editor: Andrea Vosburgh
Publishing Services Manager: Anne Altepeter
Project Manager: Jennifer Nemec
Design Direction: Steven Stave
Illustration Specialist: Karen Giacomucci

Printed in China

Last digit is the print number: 9 8 7 6 5 4 3 2 1

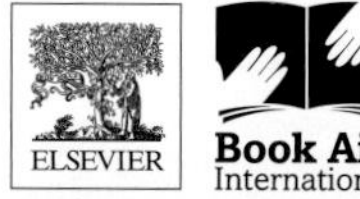
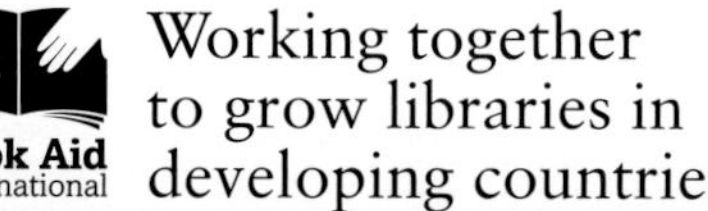

To our loved ones and our mentors:
We gain strength and inspiration from you.

Jafer Ali, MD
Assistant Professor
Department of Anesthesiology and Perioperative Medicine
Case Western Reserve University School of Medicine
Cleveland, Ohio

Diana Anca, MD
Assistant Professor of Clinical Anesthesiology
Columbia University College of Physicians and Surgeons;
Division of Cardiothoracic Anesthesia, Department
   of Anesthesiology
St. Luke's Roosevelt Hospital Center
New York, New York

Patricia M. Applegate, MD
Director, Echocardiography
Department of Cardiology
Jerry L. Pettis Loma Linda VA Hospital;
Associate Professor of Medicine
Department of Cardiology
Loma Linda University School of Medicine
Loma Linda, California

Richard L. Applegate II, MD
Professor and Vice Chair
Department of Anesthesiology
Loma Linda University School of Medicine
Loma Linda, California

John G. Augoustides, MD, FASE, FAHA
Associate Professor
Cardiothoracic and Vascular Section
Department of Anesthesiology and Critical Care
Perelman School of Medicine
University of Pennsylvania
Philadelphia, Pennsylvania

Edwin G. Avery IV, MD
Chief, Division of Cardiac Anesthesia
Vice Chairman, Director of Research
Department of Anesthesiology and Perioperative Medicine
University Hospitals, Case Medical Center
Associate Professor of Anesthesiology
Case Western Reserve University School of Medicine
Cleveland, Ohio

Dalia A. Banks, MD, FASE
Associate Clinical Professor
Medical Director for Procedural Treatment Unit/Cardiovascular
   Anesthesia Sulpizio Cardiovascular Center
Director of CT Anesthesia Fellowship
University of California San Diego Medical Center
San Diego, California

Manish Bansal, MD
Consultant
Department of Cardiology
Medanta-The Medicity
Gurgaon, Haryana, India

Dominique A. Bettex, MD
Associate Professor
Department of Anesthesiology
University Hospital Zurich
Zurich, Switzerland

Puneet Bhatla, MD
Noninvasive Imaging Fellow
Division of Pediatric Cardiology
Mount Sinai Medical Center
New York, New York

Marco Bosshart, MD
Institute of Anesthesiology
University Hospital Zurich
Zurich, Switzerland

Mary W. Brandon, DO
Fellow
Division of Cardiothoracic Anesthesiology and Critical Care
   Medicine, Department of Anesthesiology
Duke University Health System
Durham, North Carolina

Albert T. Cheung, MD
Professor
Department of Anesthesiology and Critical Care
Perelman School of Medicine
University of Pennsylvania
Philadelphia, Pennsylvania

Joanna Chikwe, MD, FRCS
Department of Cardiothoracic Surgery
Mount Sinai Medical Center
New York, New York

Pierre Couture, MD, FRCPC
Associate Professor of Anesthesiology
Montreal Heart Institute
Montreal, Quebec, Canada

André Y. Denault, MD, FRCP(C), PhD
Clinical Associate Professor
Department of Anesthesiology
University of Montreal;
Anesthesiologist, Intensivist
Department of Anesthesiology
Montreal Heart Institute
Anesthesiologist, Intensivist
Department of Anesthesiology and Intensive Care
Centre Hospitalier de L'Universite de Montreal
Montreal, Quebec, Canada

Alain Deschamps, MD, FRCPC
Associate Professor of Anesthesiology
University of Montreal
Associate Professor of Anesthesiology
Montreal Heart Institute
Montreal, Quebec, Canada

Stephen A. Esper, MD, MBA
Fellow
Division of Cardiothoracic Anesthesiology and Critical Care
    Medicine, Department of Anesthesiology
Duke University Health System
Durham, North Carolina

Renata G. Ferreira, MD
Fellow
Division of Cardiothoracic Anesthesiology and Critical Care
    Medicine, Department of Anesthesiology
Duke University Health System
Durham, North Carolina

Gregory W. Fischer, MD
Associate Professor of Anesthesiology and Cardiothoracic Surgery
Director of Adult Cardiothoracic Anesthesia
Department of Anesthesiology
Mount Sinai School of Medicine
New York, New York

Jonathan K. Frogel, MD
Assistant Professor
Department of Anesthesiology and Critical Care
Hospital of the University of Pennsylvania
Philadelphia, Pennsylvania

Maria Galati, MBA
Vice Chair, Administration
Department of Anesthesiology
Mount Sinai School of Medicine
New York, New York

Martin E. Goldman, MD
Director of the Echocardiography Laboratory
Mount Sinai Medical Center
Professor of Cardiology
Mount Sinai School of Medicine
New York, New York

Matthias Greutmann, MD
Head, Congenital Heart Disease
Department of Cardiology
University Hospital Zurich
Zurich, Switzerland

Jacob T. Gutsche, MD
Assistant Professor
Department of Anesthesiology and Critical Care
University of Pennsylvania
Philadelphia, Pennsylvania

Rafael Honikman, MD
Assistant Professor
Department of Anesthesiology
Mount Sinai School of Medicine
New York, New York

Gregory M. Janelle, MD
Associate Professor of Anesthesiology and Surgery
Chief, Division of Cardiovascular Anesthesiology
Department of Anesthesiology
University of Florida College of Medicine
Gainesville, Florida

Ronald A. Kahn, MD
Professor of Anesthesiology and Surgery
Mount Sinai Medical Center
New York, New York

Marc S. Kanchuger, MD
Associate Professor and Vice Chair of Performance
    Improvement and Risk Management
Department of Anesthsiology
New York University School of Medicine
Attending
Department of Anesthesiology
New York University Langone Medical Center
New York, New York

John C. Klick, MD
Assistant Professor
Department of Anesthesiology and Perioperative Medicine
Case Western Reserve University School of Medicine
Cleveland, Ohio

Sandeep Krishnan, MD
Assistant Professor of Anesthesiology
New York University Langone Medical Center
New York, New York

Michelle M. Liao, MD
Chief Resident
Department of Anesthesiology
Columbia University College of Physicians and Surgeons
New York, New York

Sanford M. Littwin, MD
Assistant Professor of Clinical Anesthesiology
Columbia University College of Physicians and Surgeons
Director, Clinical Anesthesia (CA I) Education
Division of Cardiothoracic and Pediatric Anesthesia,
    Department of Anesthesiology
St. Luke's Roosevelt Hospital Center
New York, New York

Sansan S. Lo, MD
Assistant Professor
Division of Cardiothoracic Anesthesiology
Department of Anesthesiology
Columbia University
New York Presbyterian Hospital
New York, New York

William J. Mauermann, MD
Assistant Professor of Anesthesiology
Department of Anesthesiology
Mayo Clinic College of Medicine
Rochester, Minnesota

Timothy Maus, MD, FASE
Assistant Clinical Professor
Department of Anesthesiology
University of California San Diego Medical Center
San Diego, California

Teresa A. Mulaikal, MD
Cardiothoracic and Critical Care Fellow
Department of Anesthesiology
Columbia University
New York Presbyterian Hospital
New York, New York

Jagat Narula, MD, PhD
Zena and Michael A. Wiener Cardiovascular Institute
Mount Sinai School of Medicine
New York, New York

Jennie Y. Ngai, MD
Assistant Professor
Department of Anesthesiology
New York University Langone Medical Center
New York, New York

Gregory A. Nuttall, MD
Professor of Anesthesiology
Department of Anesthesiology
Mayo Clinic College of Medicine
Rochester, Minnesota

William C. Oliver, Jr., MD
Professor of Anesthesiology
Department of Anesthesiology
Mayo Clinic College of Medicine
Rochester, Minnesota

Jeremy S. Poppers, MD, PhD
Assistant Professor of Anesthesiology
Division of Cardiothoracic Anesthesiology
Columbia University College of Physicians and Surgeons
New York, New York

Kent H. Rehfeldt, MD
Assistant Professor of Anesthesiology
Department of Anesthesiology
Mayo Clinic College of Medicine
Rochester, Minnesota

David L. Reich, MD
Horace W. Goldsmith Professor and Chair of Anesthesiology
Mount Sinai School of Medicine
New York, New York

Amanda J. Rhee, MD
Assistant Professor
Department of Anesthesiology
Mount Sinai Medical Center
New York, New York

Antoine G. Rochon, MD, FRCPC
Assistant Professor of Anesthesiology
Montreal Heart Institute
Montreal, Quebec, Canada

Cesar Rodriguez-Diaz, MD
Assistant Professor
Department of Anesthesiology
Mount Sinai School of Medicine
New York, New York

Ivan S. Salgo, MD, MS
Senior Director, Global Cardiology
Philips Ultrasound
Andover, Massachusetts

Joseph S. Savino, MD
Professor and Vice Chairman
Department of Anesthesiology and Critical Care
University of Pennsylvania Perelman School of Medicine
Hospital of the University of Pennsylvania
Philadelphia, Pennsylvania

Barry J. Segal, MD
Associate Professor
Department of Anesthesiology
Mount Sinai School of Medicine
New York, New York

Partho P. Sengupta, MD, DM, FASE
Zena and Michael A. Wiener Cardiovascular Institute
Mount Sinai School of Medicine
New York, New York

Jack S. Shanewise, MD
Professor of Clinical Anesthesiology
Columbia University College of Physicians and Surgeons;
Director, Division of Cardiothoracic Anesthesiology
Columbia University Medical Center
New York, New York

W. Brit Smith, MD
Fellow, Adult Cardiothoracic Anesthesiology
Department of Anesthesiology
University of Florida College of Medicine
Gainesville, Florida

Shubhika Srivastava, MBBS
Associate Professor of Pediatrics
Director, Pediatric and Fetal Echocardiography
Division of Pediatric Cardiology
Mount Sinai Medical Center
New York, New York

Marc E. Stone, MD
Associate Professor
Program Director, Fellowship in Cardiothoracic Anesthesiology
Department of Anesthesiology
Mount Sinai School of Medicine
New York, New York

Madhav Swaminathan, MD, FASE, FAHA, MBBS
Associate Professor
Division of Cardiothoracic Anesthesiology and Critical Care
  Medicine, Department of Anesthesiology
Duke University Health System
Durham, North Carolina

James E. Szalados, MD, MBA, MHA, JD, FCCP, FCLM, FCCM, Esq.
Professor of Anesthesiology and Medicine
University of Rochester;
Director, Surgical Critical Care, SICU, and Critical
    Care Telemedicine
Rochester General Hospital;
Critical Care, Medicine, and Anesthesiology
Unity Health System
Rochester, New York;
Vice President for Medical Affairs
Chief Medical Officer
Lakeside Health System
Brockport, New York;
Principal, Counselor, and Attorney at Law
The Szalados Law Firm
Hilton, New York

Daniel M. Thys, MD
Professor Emeritus of Anesthesiology
Columbia University College of Physicians and Surgeons;
Chairman Emeritus
Department of Anesthesiology
St. Luke's Roosevelt Hospital Center
New York, New York

Paula Trigo, MD
Former Cardiothoracic Anesthesiology Fellow
Icahn School of Medicine
Mount Sinai Medical Center
New York, New York

William J. Vernick, MD
Assistant Professor
Department of Anesthesiology and Critical Care
Hospital of the University of Pennsylvania
University of Pennsylvania;
Director of Cardiac Anesthesia
Department of Anesthesia and Critical Care
Penn-Presbyterian Medical Center
Philadelphia, Pennsylvania

David J. West, MD
Attending Anesthesiologist
TeamHealth Anesthesia at Palm Beach Gardens
    Medical Center
Palm Beach Gardens, Florida

Robert Williams, MBA, RRT
Director, Clinical Operations
Department of Anesthesiology
Mount Sinai Medical Center
New York, New York

PREFACE

Over the past three decades, perioperative echocardiography has become an indispensable tool in the perioperative care of the cardiac surgical patient. Beyond the published evidence and professional practice parameters, the utility of perioperative echocardiography is perhaps best demonstrated by the insistence of surgeons that complex surgery be performed with the assistance of qualified echocardiographers. Consequently, the subspecialty of cardiac anesthesia has embraced perioperative echocardiography as one of the cornerstones of modern-day practice, and the cardiac anesthesiologist has assumed a unique position within the specialty of anesthesiology. Anesthesiologist-guided assessment of perioperative anatomy and physiology not only leads to optimal anesthetic and surgical management but also has fully integrated the cardiac anesthesiologist as a member of the surgical team.

Despite its importance, perioperative echocardiography is only a portion of the skill set and science of cardiac anesthesia. Although perioperative echocardiography enhances perioperative care, it must be considered in the context of a thorough understanding of patient history, as well as the goals and objectives of the planned surgical procedure. The primary aim of this textbook is to provide echocardiographic insight as a component of a holistic approach to the cardiac surgical patient. Hence, several chapters reflect the expertise of cardiologists and cardiac surgeons.

Although multiple authors have contributed to this textbook, we have endeavored to create consistency in the content and the editorial voice. The book is divided into four major sections:

1. Basic principles and normal cardiac anatomy and physiology;
2. Understanding how echocardiography demonstrates cardiovascular pathology;
3. Maintaining quality of perioperative echocardiography; and
4. Oversight and administration.

Many fine textbooks exist pertaining to perioperative echocardiography. The current one continues in the tradition of these texts, while providing unique insight into newer modalities of echocardiography, such as three-dimensional TEE, speckle tracking, and flow visualization. Additionally, the editors have included nonclinical chapters, such as "Equipment, Infection Control, and Safety" and "Regulatory, Legal, and Liability Issues Pertaining to Transesophageal Ecocardiography," as complementary elements to the classic chapters on physics, valvular pathophysiology, and so on.

We express our sincere gratitude to all authors of the individual chapters. Without their hard work and dedication, this textbook could not have been completed. We would also like to acknowledge the professionalism and talent of Andrea Vosburgh of Elsevier.

David L. Reich, MD

Gregory W. Fischer, MD

CONTENTS

VIDEO CONTENTS

Video 19-2. Aortic arch dissection. High esophageal long-axis view of aortic arch. Note complex fenestrated intimal flap in aortic arch. Intimal flap is highly mobile and a risk factor for brachiocephalic malperfusion at various stages during cardiopulmonary bypass when blood flow direction, pressure, and pulsatility change significantly.

Video 19-3. Three-dimensional (3D) imaging of intimal flap in Stanford type A dissection. This is a 3D image of ascending aorta at a multiplane angle of 115 degrees. Ascending aorta is dissected. Image has been rotated to focus on intimal flap, which has highly mobile components and static components with fenestrations evident in foreground.

Video 19-4. Descending thoracic aortic dissection. Midesophageal short-axis view of descending thoracic aorta. Note intimal flap, confirming that dissection extends from ascending aorta beyond arch. Taken together, this dissection can be classified as a DeBakey type I aortic dissection. True lumen is compressed by larger false lumen. This echocardiographic finding prompted decision to avoid femoral arterial cannulation for cardiopulmonary bypass.

Video 19-5. Three-dimensional (3D) imaging of intimal flap in descending thoracic aortic dissection. This 3D color imaging shows intimal flap in descending thoracic aorta at a multiplane angle of zero degrees. Image has been rotated to depict blood flow from true lumen into false lumen across an intimal fenestration.

Video 19-6. Cannulation of dissected aortic arch: true lumen confirmation. Intraoperative transesophageal echocardiography (TEE) was initially used to identify true lumen in descending thoracic aorta, then to track position of true lumen into aortic arch. Under TEE imaging guidance, direct arterial cannulation of true lumen in friable aortic arch was completed successfully with a Seldinger technique.

Video 19-7. Cannulation of dissected aortic arch: wire guidance. Upper esophageal long-axis image of aortic arch. This view was chosen to confirm that cannulation guidewire was positioned within true lumen of aortic arch prior to insertion of arterial cannula.

Video 19-8. Cannulation of dissected aortic arch: cannula confirmation. Withdrawal of transesophageal echocardiography probe from midesophageal short-axis view of descending aorta to reveal upper esophageal long-axis aortic arch view. This imaging technique demonstrates that arterial cannula for cardiopulmonary bypass has been correctly positioned in true lumen of dissected aorta.

Video 19-9. Monitoring status of true lumen in aortic dissection. Short-axis views of dissected descending thoracic aorta with color flow imaging after initiation of cardiopulmonary bypass (CPB) via arterial cannulation of aortic arch (see Videos 19-6 to 19-8). True lumen has significantly expanded in distal descending thoracic aorta. Blood flow from true lumen into false is evident through fenestrations in intimal flap. This case confirms that intraoperative transesophageal echocardiography can guide aortic cannulation for surgical repair of aortic dissection to decrease risk of malperfusion during CPB.

Video 19-10. Imaging artifact in ascending aorta: color Doppler imaging. Midesophageal ascending aorta long-axis in two-dimensional imaging (left panel) and color Doppler imaging (right panel). Note linear ultrasound imaging artifact within lumen of ascending aorta caused by side lobes as a consequence of pulmonary artery catheter in right pulmonary artery. In contrast to a true intimal flap within ascending aorta, color Doppler imaging demonstrates no blood flow disturbance associated with this linear imaging artifact.

Video 19-11. Imaging artifact in ascending aorta: anatomic boundaries. Midesophageal ascending aorta long-axis view. Left panel depicts a linear ultrasound imaging artifact within ascending aortic lumen caused by side lobes as a consequence of a pulmonary artery catheter (PAC) in right pulmonary artery. Right panel depicts how manual inflation of balloon on tip of PAC causes side lobe artifact to change appearance and cross boundaries of aorta.

Video 19-12. Compression of pulmonary artery by giant aortic aneurysm. Midesophageal ascending aortic short-axis view at level of right pulmonary artery (RPA) in patient with a 7.5-cm-diameter ascending thoracic aortic aneurysm. Left panel depicts compression of RPA between aneurysm and transesophageal echocardiography probe in esophagus. Color flow Doppler imaging depicts antegrade flow within compressed RPA (right panel).

Video 19-13. Three-dimensional (3D) transesophageal echocardiographic analysis of left ventricular (LV) morphology: true aneurysm. Full-volume 3D midesophageal LV long-axis view of patient with large posterior-lateral LV aneurysm extending from LV base to papillary muscle level; 3D quantification using endocardial border detection permitted measurement of ventricular volume and left ventricular ejection fraction (LVEF) without geometric assumptions. In this patient, LV end-diastolic volume was 304 mL, end-systolic volume was 257 mL, and LVEF was 16%.

20 Transesophageal Echocardiography in the Diagnosis and Management of Endocarditis 218
MARTIN E. GOLDMAN

Video 20-1. Four-chamber view showing vegetations on both anterior and posterior leaflets.

Video 20-2. Three-dimensional en face view of same valve seen in Video 20-1. Vegetations seen in both commissures and at A2.

Video 20-3. PM wires with vegetations.

Video 20-4. Commissure view showing aneurysm and perforation of anterior leaflet.

Video 20-5, A. Tricuspid valve endocarditis.

Video 20-5, B. Tricuspid valve endocarditis.

Video 20-6, A. Long-axis view of bioprosthetic aortic valve endocarditis with annular abscess. Note rocking motion of valve during cardiac cycle.

Video 20-6, B. Short-axis view showing annular abscess.

Video 20-7. Three-dimensional (3D) view from left atrial perspective, looking at a mitral valve prosthesis from anterior to posterior. Exact anatomic localization of the paravalvular leaks can easily be seen with 3D transesophageal echocardiography.

21 Imaging of Cardiac Tumors and Solid and Gaseous Materials 224
PATRICIA M. APPLEGATE | RICHARD L. APPLEGATE II

Video 21-1. Modified midesophageal bicaval view evaluation of the atrial septum. Lipomatous atrial septal hypertrophy (LASH) is present along with a redundant fossa ovalis. A central venous catheter is also noted in superior vena cava.

Video 21-2. Midesophageal four-chamber evaluation of the aortic and tricuspid valves. Mobile cystic mass is noted moving between right atrium and right ventricle.

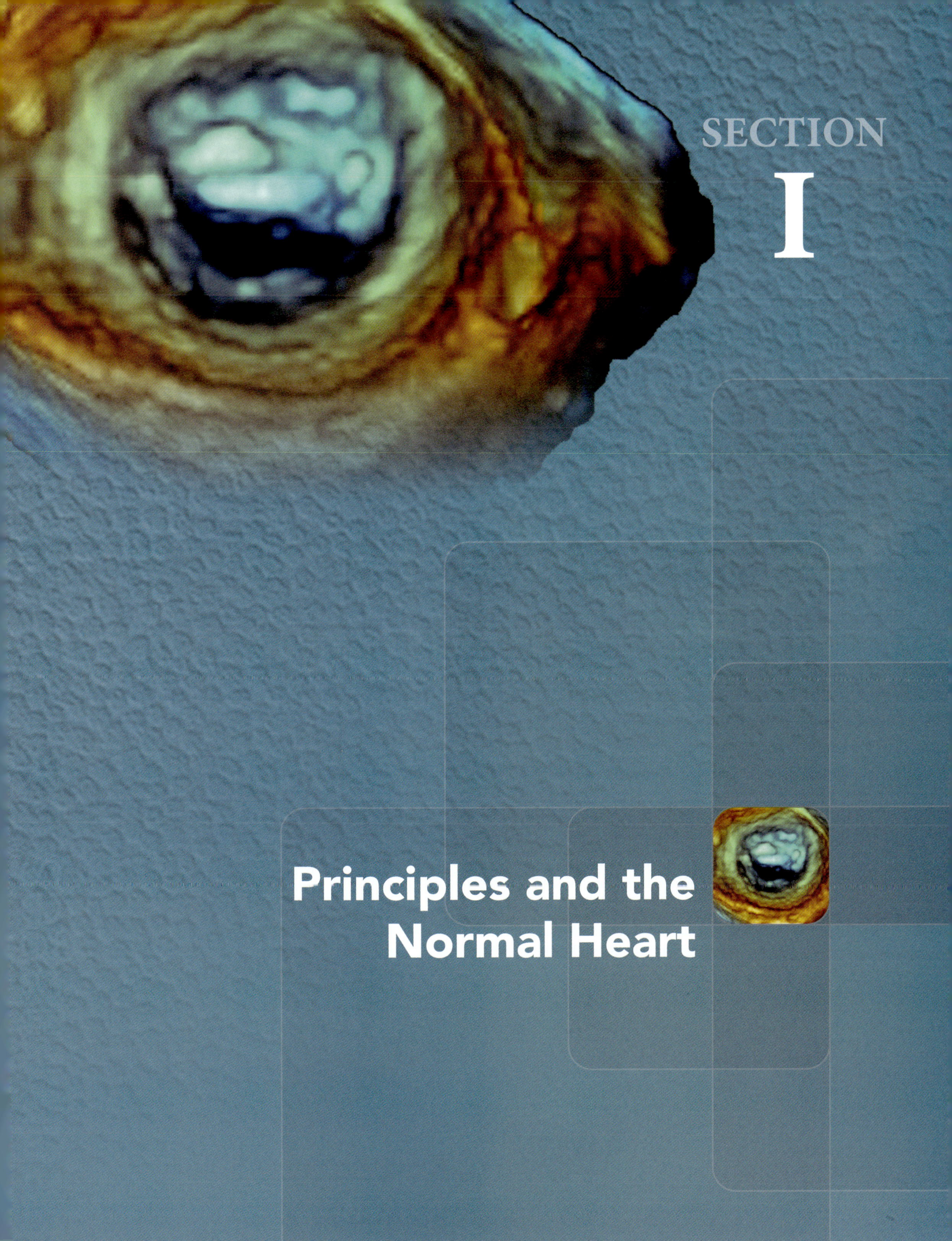

Principles and the Normal Heart

Getting Started with Echocardiography: The Twenty Standard Views

SANSAN S. LO | JEREMY S. POPPERS | TERESA A. MULAIKAL | DAVID J. WEST
MICHELLE M. LIAO | JACK S. SHANEWISE

TEE: Indications, Complications, Probe Insertion, and Manipulation

The clinical utility of transesophageal echocardiography (TEE) has expanded since its introduction into the perioperative setting in the 1980s. TEE is a versatile tool that can be used to assess cardiac function and diagnose unanticipated problems. The American Society of Anesthesiologists (ASA) and the Society of Cardiovascular Anesthesiologists (SCA) issued guidelines for the intraoperative use of TEE in 1996 in which indications for intraoperative TEE fall under three categories.[1] Category A includes clinical scenarios for which supportive literature suggests that TEE is strongly beneficial for clinical evaluation. Examples include valve repair, congenital heart defects, hypertrophic obstructive cardiomyopathy, aortic dissection, infective endocarditis, and unstable hemodynamics. Category B indications for TEE are those for which there is suggestive evidence for a benefit, and include myocardial ischemia, valve replacement, cardiac aneurysms, and intracardiac tumors. Category C indications are those for which there is equivocal literature, and include myocardial perfusion, monitoring for emboli during orthopedic procedures, and placement of intraaortic balloon pumps and pulmonary artery catheters. These guidelines were revised in 2010 and now state that in adult patients without contraindications, TEE should be used in all open (e.g., valvular) heart and thoracic aortic surgical procedures and should be considered for coronary artery bypass graft surgeries to: (1) confirm and refine the preoperative diagnosis, (2) detect new or unsuspected pathology, (3) adjust the anesthetic and surgical plan accordingly, and (4) assess the results of surgical intervention.[2]

Although TEE is considered relatively safe and noninvasive, the TEE probe may cause oropharyngeal, esophageal, or gastric trauma. Other TEE complications may include dental trauma, laryngeal dysfunction, postoperative aspiration, endotracheal tube displacement, and upper gastrointestinal bleeding. In infants, bronchial and aortic compression are also possible. Therefore, prior to TEE, the medical history should be aimed at eliciting a history of esophageal disease, dysphagia, and hematemesis. Past medical history should be reviewed as well. Relative contraindications to TEE include a history of dysphagia, odynophagia, mediastinal radiation, recent upper gastrointestinal surgery, recent upper gastrointestinal bleeding, thoracic aortic aneurysm, esophageal stricture/tumor/diverticula/varices, esophagitis, and recent chest trauma. In patients with distal esophageal or gastric pathology, efforts should be made to obtain needed information without advancing the TEE probe into the distal esophagus. Preoperative esophagoscopy can also be considered when risk of TEE is unclear.

Prior to TEE probe insertion, it may be useful to suction esophageal and gastric air through an orogastric tube. Then, using the left hand to perform a jaw thrust, the mandible is displaced anteriorly, and the right hand is used to insert a lubricated TEE probe toward the posterior pharynx along a midline axis and advanced into the esophagus. Although a mild degree of resistance is frequently experienced as the probe passes the upper esophageal sphincter, probe insertion and manipulation should always be performed gently, and excessive force should never be used. If necessary, laryngoscopy can be performed to displace the mandible and better visualize the esophageal opening.

Flexion of the neck may facilitate insertion of the TEE probe, whereas extension may make it more difficult. Once the probe reaches the level of the thoracic esophagus (≈30 cm from incisors), the heart should come into view on the screen. On the rare occasion that the probe cannot be placed into the esophagus despite multiple attempts by qualified practitioners, TEE placement should be abandoned to avoid harm to the patient.

When imaging the heart with TEE, the structure visualized depends on the probe's position between the upper esophagus and stomach and the direction of the ultrasound beam. For example, in the upper esophagus, midesophagus, and transgastric positions, the structures closest to the TEE probe are the great vessels, left atrium, and left ventricle, respectively, and will be displayed at the top, or vertex, of the imaging sector.

The TEE probe can be manipulated and adjusted to optimize visualization of cardiac anatomy (Fig. 1-1). The wheels of the probe should be unlocked and in neutral position prior to movement to prevent trauma. The probe can be advanced or withdrawn within the esophagus, and the orientation of the ultrasound beam can be manipulated by rotating the probe to the patient's left (counterclockwise) or right (clockwise). Turning the large control wheel clockwise will anteflex the probe (flex the tip anteriorly), whereas counterclockwise turning will retroflex (flex posteriorly) it. The small knob will flex the probe

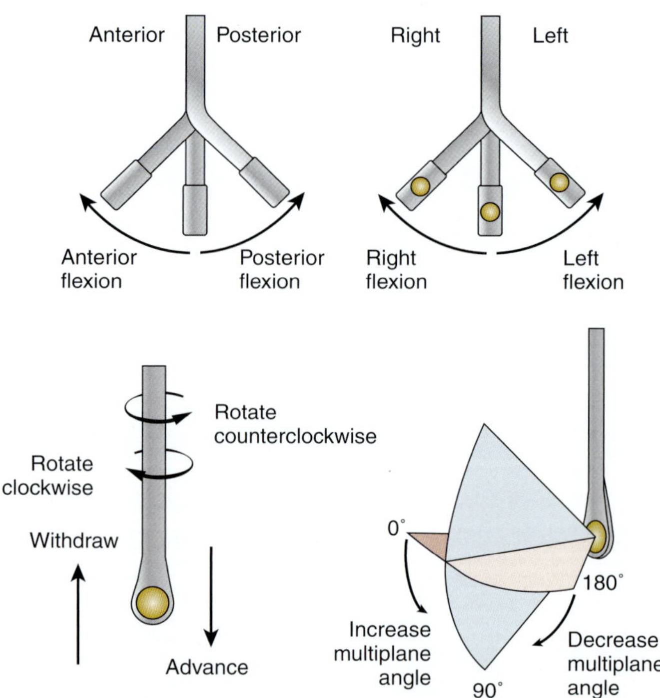

Figure 1-1 Terminology used to describe manipulations of the transesophageal echocardiography probe and transducer.

leftward or rightward. With a multiplane TEE probe, the transducer angle can be rotated axially from 0 (horizontal) to 90 (vertical) to 180 degrees (mirror image of 0 degrees horizontal plane) while the tip remains in a fixed position. Orienting oneself with respect to the ultrasound beam and the image displayed on the screen may be a source of confusion. An easy method often employed to orient the echocardiographer utilizes the right hand, with its thumb pointing to the left and palm facing the floor. With the patient in supine position, the operator stands at the head, facing the patient's feet. In this position, the fingers represent the ultrasound beams as they extend perpendicularly from the head of the probe, and the thumb will point toward the left-sided structures that appear on the right side of the screen at 0 degrees. As the multiplane angle is increased to 90 degrees, the right hand is rotated clockwise until the thumb points toward the ceiling and now demonstrates anterior structures of the heart on the right side of the screen; inferior structures are displayed on the left side of the screen.

The Twenty Standard Views

In 1999 the American Society of Echocardiography (ASE) and SCA published guidelines for performing a comprehensive intraoperative TEE examination that described and named 20 TEE views that comprise a complete routine examination.[3] These 20 views are summarized in Table 1-1 and described in the sections that follow.

TABLE 1-1	Standard Transesophageal Echocardiography Views		
Standard Views	*Multiplane Angle (Degrees)*	*Depth of Probe Insertion*	*Structures Visualized*
ME four-chamber view	0-20	ME 30-40 cm from incisors	LA RA LV RV TV MV Left and right pulmonary veins
ME mitral commisural view	50-80	ME 30-40 cm from incisors	LA LV Anterolateral PPM Posteromedial PPM P1-A2-P3 scallops of MV
ME two-chamber view	90	ME 30-40 cm from incisors	LA LAA MV Anterior wall LV Inferior wall LV Circumflex artery in SAX Coronary sinus in SAX Left pulmonary veins
ME LAX view	110-160	ME 30-40 cm from incisors	LA A2-P2 scallops of MV Anteroseptal wall LV Inferolateral wall LV AV in LAX Right coronary artery
ME AV SAX view	30-60	ME 30-40 cm from incisors	LA Interatrial septum RA RVOT PV AV in SAX Left coronary artery
ME AV LAX view	110-160	ME 30-40 cm from incisors	AV in LAX AV annulus Sinus of Valsalva Sinotubular junction MV LA LV Right coronary artery
ME RV inflow-outflow view	60-90	ME 30-40 cm from incisors	LA Interatrial septum RA TV RV RVOT PV Main PA AV in SAX Left coronary artery
ME bicaval view	90-110	ME 30-40 cm from incisors	RA SVC in LAX IVC in LAX LA RUPV
ME ascending aortic SAX view	0	ME 30-40 cm from incisors	Ascending aorta in SAX Main PA in LAX Right PA in LAX SVC in SAX

Continued on following page

TABLE 1-1   Standard Transesophageal Echocardiography Views (Continued)

Standard Views	Multiplane Angle (Degrees)	Depth of Probe Insertion	Structures Visualized
ME ascending aortic LAX view	90	ME 30-40 cm from incisors	Ascending aorta in LAX Right PA in SAX
TG mid-papillary SAX view	0	TG 40-45 cm from incisors	Anterolateral & posteromedial PPM Anterior, lateral, inferior, & septal walls of LV
TG two-chamber view	90	TG 40-45 cm from incisors	Anterior wall LV Inferior wall LV Sub-MV apparatus
TG LAX view	110-140	TG 40-45 cm from incisors	Anteroseptal wall LV Inferolateral wall LV LVOT AV in LAX
TG RV inflow view	90-120	TG 40-45 cm from incisors	RA RV TV Sub-TV apparatus RV PPM
TG basal SAX view	0	TG 40-45 cm from incisors	Basal LV wall Anterior & posterior MV leaflets
Deep TG LAX view	0	Deep TG 45-50 cm from incisors	LA MV LV LVOT Aortic valve in LAX
Desc aortic SAX view	0	ME 30-40 cm from incisors	Descending aorta in SAX Left pleural space
Desc aortic LAX view	90	ME 30-40 cm from incisors	Descending in LAX Left pleural space
UE aortic arch LAX view	0	Upper esophageal 20-25 cm from incisors	Aortic arch in LAX Left SCA
UE aortic arch SAX view	70-90	Upper esophageal 20-25 cm from incisors	Aortic arch in SAX PV in LAX RVOT Left SCA

AV, Aortic valve; *Desc*, descending; *IVC*, inferior vena cava; *LA*, left atrium; *LAA*, left atrial appendage; *LAX*, long axis; *LUPV*, left upper pulmonary vein; *LV*, left ventricle; *LVOT*, left ventricular outflow tract; *ME*, midesophageal; *MV*, mitral valve; *PA*, pulmonary artery; *PPM*, papillary muscle; *PV*, pulmonic valve; *RA*, right atrium; *RUPV*, right upper pulmonary vein; *RV*, right ventricle; *RVOT*, right ventricular outflow tract; *SAX*, short axis; *SCA*, subclavian artery; *SVC*, superior vena cava; *TG*, transgastric; *TV*, tricuspid valve; *UE*, upper esophageal.

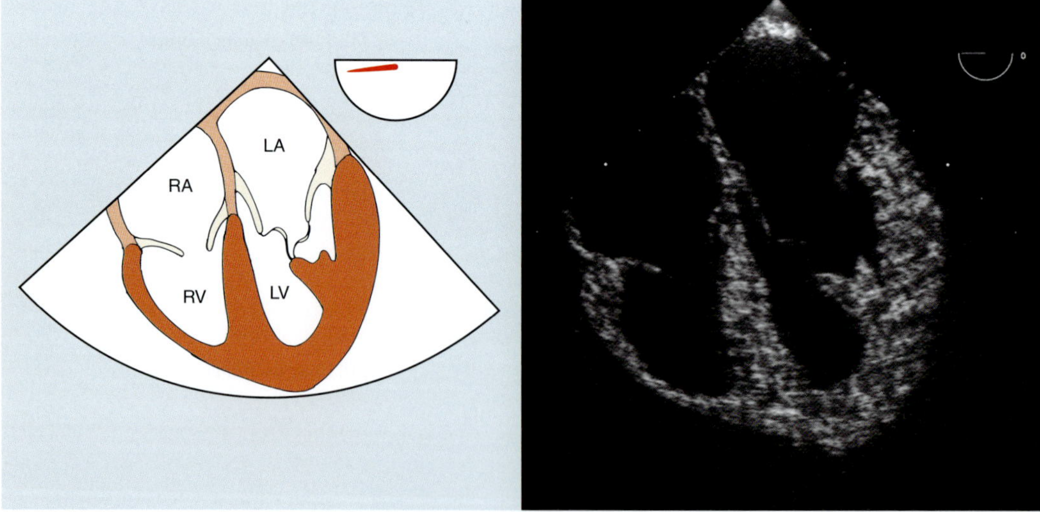

Figure 1-2   Midesophageal four-chamber view. *LA,* Left atrium; *LV,* left ventricle; *RA,* right atrium; *RV,* right ventricle. *(Two-dimensional TEE images generated using software developed by Heartworks, Inventive Medical Ltd., London, UK.)*

Midesophageal Four-Chamber (ME Four-Chamber)

The midesophageal (ME) views (Fig. 1-2) are typically located at a probe depth of about 30 to 40 cm from the incisors. The ME four-chamber view is often the first one that appears upon probe insertion with a multiplane angle of 0 to 20 degrees. Both atria, both ventricles, and the mitral and tricuspid valves are visualized. Much like a chest x-ray, structures on the left side of the patient appear as images on the right side of the screen and vice versa. The septal and anterior or posterior leaflets of the tricuspid valve, as well as the anterior and posterior mitral valve leaflets, are visualized in the central portion of the image sector. Either the anterior or posterior tricuspid valve leaflet appears on the left side of the image sector, depending on the degree of anteflexion.

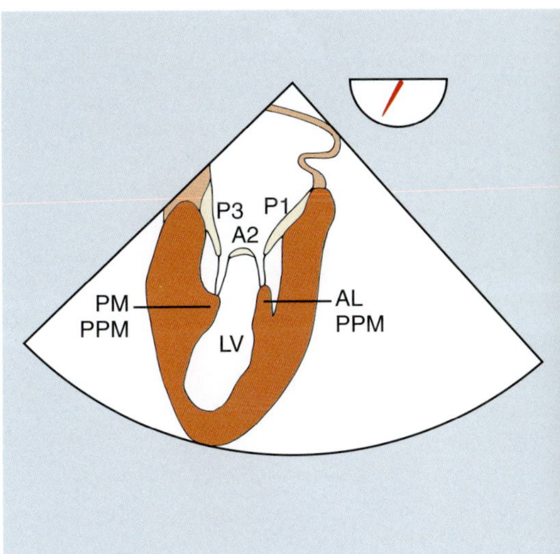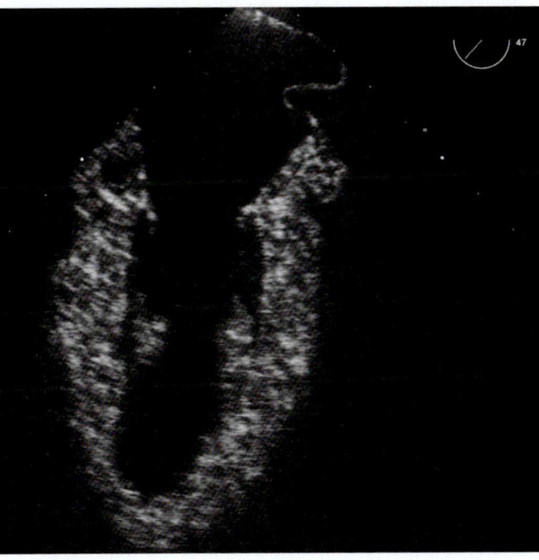

Figure 1-3 Midesophageal mitral commissural view. Mitral valve (P3, A2, P1 segments). *AL PPM,* Anterolateral papillary muscle; *LV,* left ventricle; *PM PPM,* posteromedial papillary muscle. *(Two-dimensional TEE images generated using software developed by Heartworks, Inventive Medical Ltd., London, UK.)*

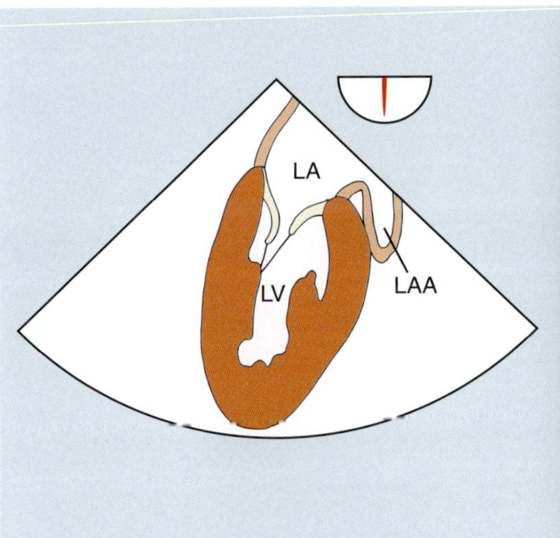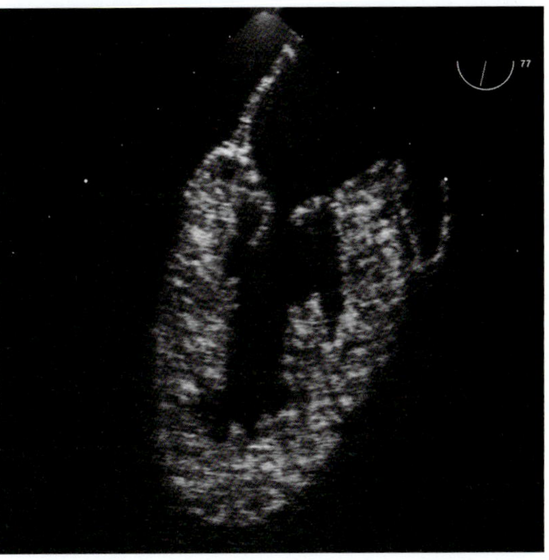

Figure 1-4 Midesophageal two-chamber view. *LA,* Left atrium; *LAA,* left atrial appendage; *LV,* left ventricle. *(Two-dimensional TEE images generated using software developed by Heartworks, Inventive Medical Ltd., London, UK.)*

Midesophageal Mitral Commissural (ME Mitral Commissural)

From the ME four-chamber view, the multiplane angle is rotated to 50 to 80 degrees to obtain the mitral commissural view (Fig. 1-3). In a neutral position, the P1-A2-P3 segments of the mitral leaflets are visualized. Chordae from the anterolateral papillary muscle, which appears on the right side of the image sector, attach to P1 and the lateral side of A2. Chordae from the posteromedial papillary muscle, which appears on the left side of the image sector, attach to P3 and the medial side of A2.

Midesophageal Two-Chamber (ME Two-Chamber)

From the ME mitral commissural, continue rotation of the multiplane angle to 90 degrees to obtain the ME two-chamber view of the left atrium and left ventricle (Fig. 1-4). The anterior and inferior walls of the left ventricle lie to the right and left sides of the imaging sector, respectively. The left atrial appendage appears on the right upper portion of the image plane. The circumflex artery and coronary sinus are often visualized as well to the right and left of the image, respectively.

Midesophageal Long Axis (ME LAX)

From the ME two-chamber view, rotate the multiplane angle to 110 to 160 degrees. The left atrium, located at the apex of the image sector, mitral valve, left ventricle, left ventricular outflow tract (LVOT), aortic valve, and aortic root are all visualized (Fig. 1-5). Frequently the right coronary artery may be seen originating from the sinus of Valsalva toward the bottom of the image. The A2 and P2 segments of the mitral valve are illustrated, with the anterior mitral leaflet comprising the superior portion of the LVOT. The anteroseptal and inferolateral walls of the left ventricle are pictured on the right and left sides of the image plane, respectively.

Midesophageal Aortic Valve Short Axis (ME AV SAX)

This view is developed by starting with the ME four-chamber view and withdrawing the probe until the aortic valve is in the middle of the image sector, then the multiplane is increased to 30 to 60 degrees until the aortic valve and all of its leaflets come into view (Fig. 1-6). The structure located at the apex of the image sector is the left atrium. The structure located at the bottom left of the image sector is the right

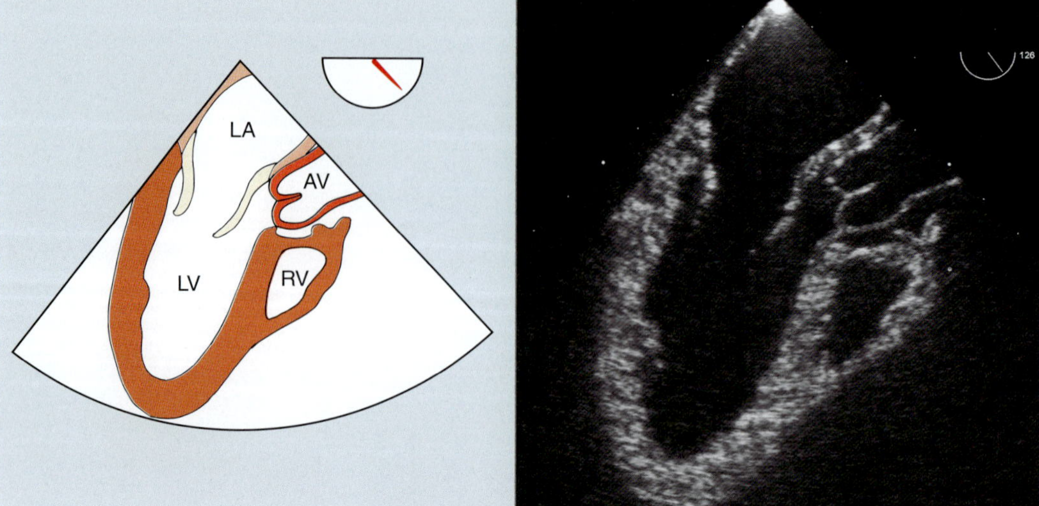

Figure 1-5 Midesophageal long-axis view. *AV,* Aortic valve; *LA,* left atrium; *LV,* left ventricle; *RV,* right ventricle. *(Two-dimensional TEE images generated using software developed by Heartworks, Inventive Medical Ltd., London, UK.)*

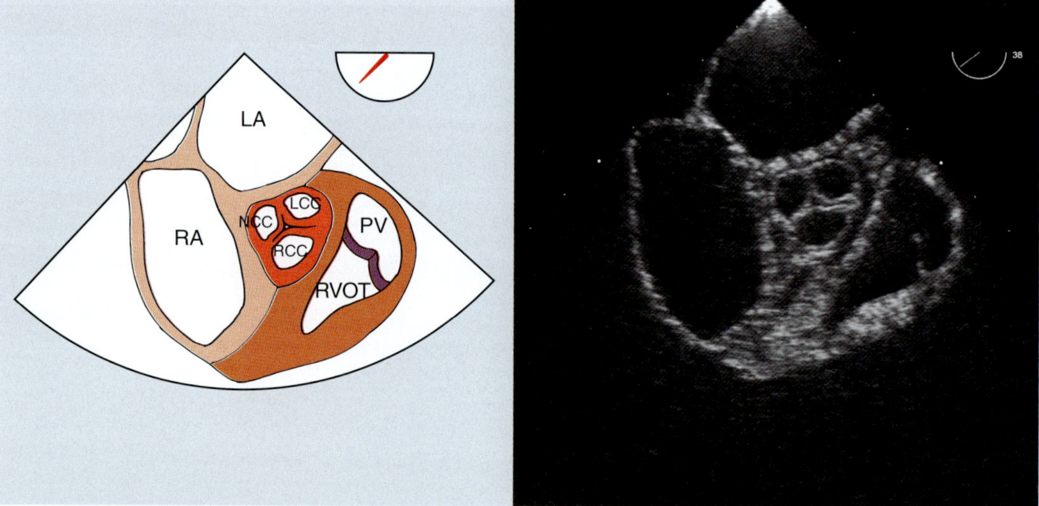

Figure 1-6 Midesophageal aortic valve short-axis view. *LA,* Left atrium; *LCC,* left coronary cusp of aortic valve; *NCC,* noncoronary cusp of aortic valve; *PV,* pulmonary valve; *RA,* right atrium; *RCC,* right coronary cusp of aortic valve; *RVOT,* right ventricle outflow tract. *(Two-dimensional TEE images generated using software developed by Heartworks, Inventive Medical Ltd., London, UK.)*

atrium. The interatrial septum separates the left from the right atrium. In the middle of the image is the aortic valve in short axis. The noncoronary cusp of the aortic valve is located adjacent to the interatrial septum. Just to the right of the noncoronary cusp in the image sector is the left coronary cusp, and the cusp closest to the bottom of the image sector is the right coronary cusp. Frequently the left coronary artery is visualized to the right of the left coronary cusp of the aortic valve.

Midesophageal Aortic Valve Long Axis (ME AV LAX)

To obtain this view, the multiplane angle is increased by 90 degrees from the angle required to obtain the ME aortic valve short-axis view (Fig. 1-7). This is usually accomplished using angles between 110 to 160 degrees. Slight rotation of the probe to the right may be necessary to obtain the LVOT, the aortic valve, and the proximal ascending aorta all in the same image. The left atrium is located at the apex of the image sector. At the bottom of the left atrium is the mitral valve leading into the left ventricle. Exiting from the left ventricle is the LVOT, which leads to the aortic valve, and finally the sinuses of Valsalva, sinotubular junction, and the proximal ascending aorta. Frequently the right coronary artery may be seen originating from the sinus of Valsalva toward the bottom of the image.

Midesophageal Right Ventricular Inflow-Outflow (ME RV Inflow-Outflow)

From the ME four-chamber view, the multiplane angle is increased, usually to 60 to 90 degrees (Fig. 1-8). As the multiplane angle is increased, the right ventricle will open up at the bottom portion of the image sector. The aortic valve should remain in the middle of the image. Frequently the left coronary artery is visualized to the right of the left coronary cusp of the aortic valve. Starting at the apex of the image sector and traveling counterclockwise, the structures encountered include the left atrium, interatrial septum, right atrium, tricuspid valve, right ventricle, right ventricular outflow tract (RVOT), pulmonic valve, and main pulmonary artery.

Midesophageal Bicaval (ME Bicaval)

The ME bicaval view is developed by turning the probe to the right from the ME four-chamber view and increasing the multiplane to about 90 to 110 degrees (Fig. 1-9). In this view, the left atrium is located toward the apex of the image sector and the right atrium just beneath the left atrium in the image sector. The interatrial septum separates the atria. The superior vena cava is located toward the right side of the image sector and the inferior vena cava toward the left side of the image sector.

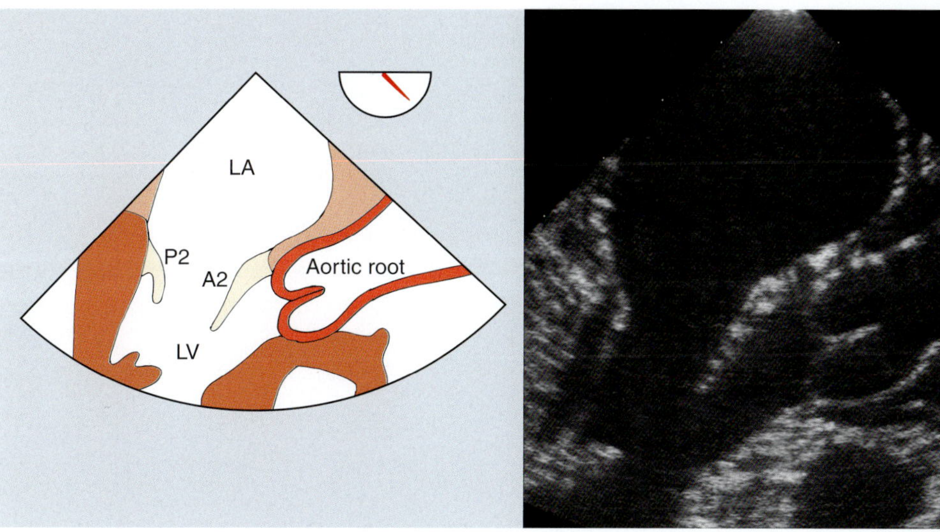

Figure 1-7 Midesophageal aortic valve long-axis view. *LA,* Left atrium, mitral valve [P2, A2 segments]; *LV,* left ventricle. *(Two-dimensional TEE images generated using software developed by Heartworks, Inventive Medical Ltd., London, UK.)*

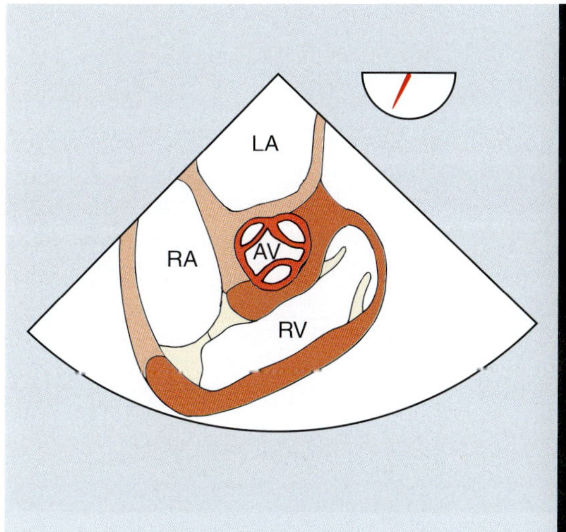

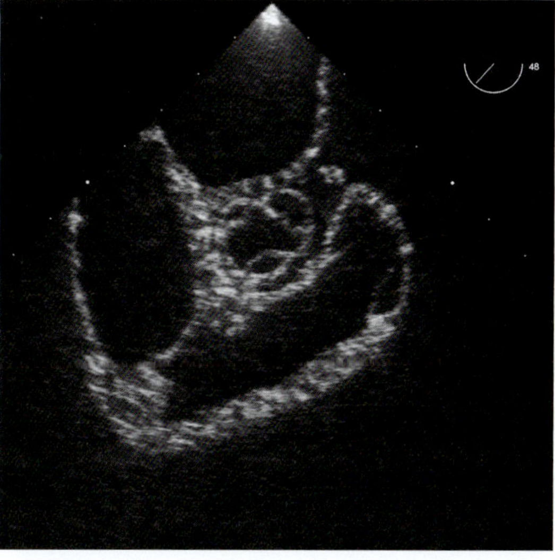

Figure 1-8 Midesophageal right ventricle inflow-outflow view. *AV,* Aortic valve; *LA,* left atrium; *RA,* right atrium; *RV,* right ventricle. *(Two-dimensional TEE images generated using software developed by Heartworks, Inventive Medical Ltd., London, UK.)*

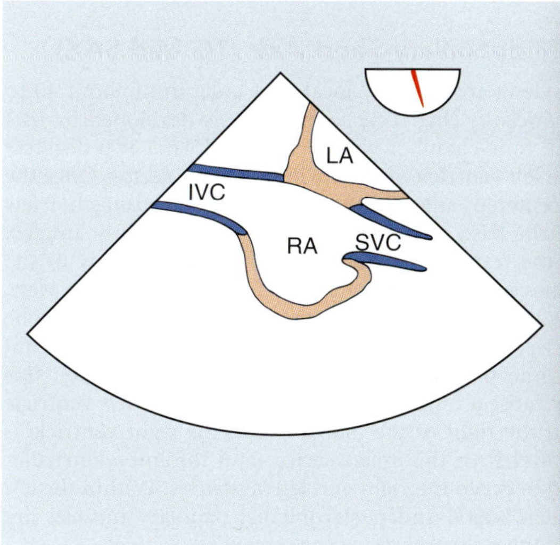

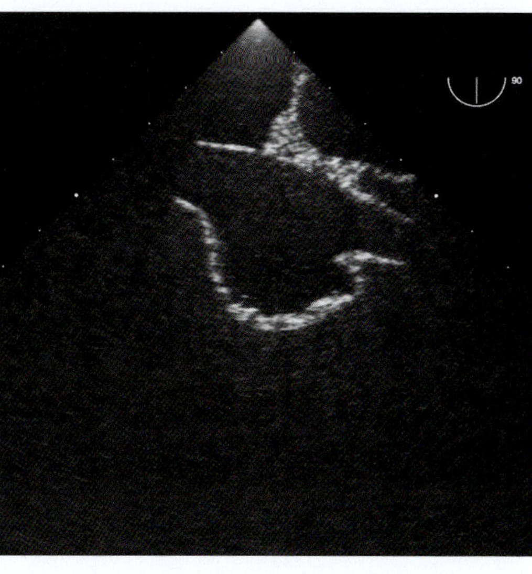

Figure 1-9 Midesophageal bicaval view. *IVC,* Inferior vena cava; *LA,* left atrium; *RA,* right atrium; *SVC,* superior vena cava. *(Two-dimensional TEE images generated using software developed by Heartworks, Inventive Medical Ltd., London, UK.)*

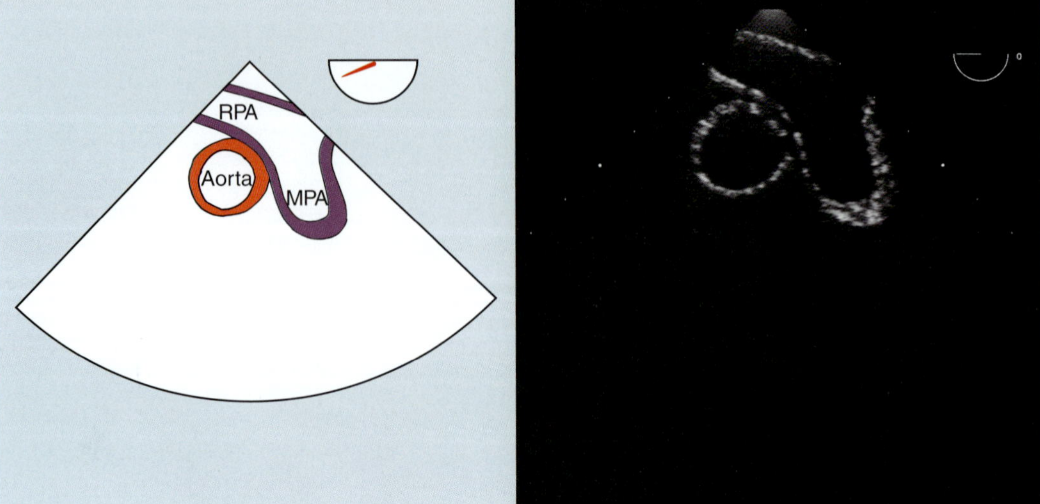

Figure 1-10 Midesophageal ascending aortic short-axis view. *MPA,* Main pulmonary artery; *RPA,* right pulmonary artery. *(Two-dimensional TEE images generated using software developed by Heartworks, Inventive Medical Ltd., London, UK.)*

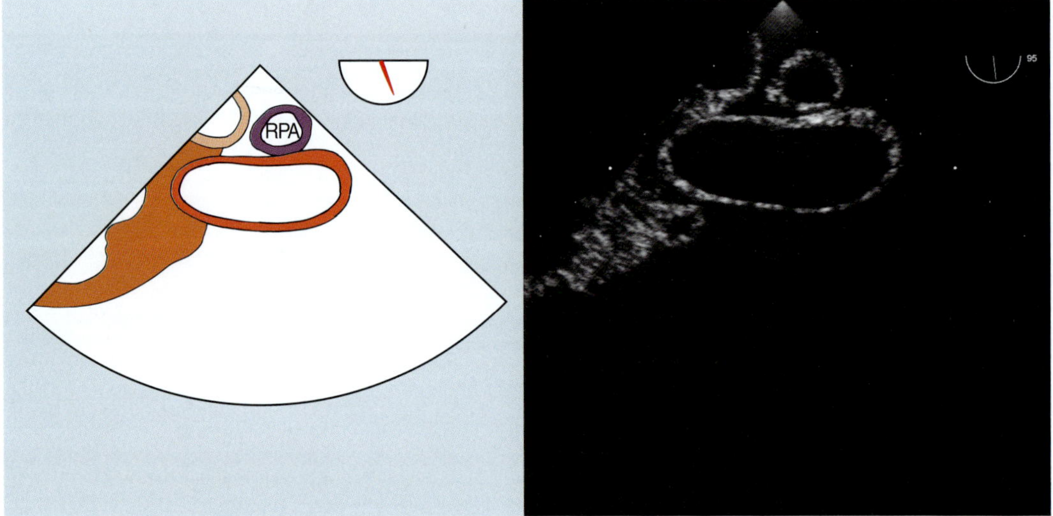

Figure 1-11 Midesophageal ascending aortic long-axis view. *RPA,* Right pulmonary artery. *(Two-dimensional TEE images generated using software developed by Heartworks, Inventive Medical Ltd., London, UK.)*

Midesophageal Ascending Aortic Short Axis (ME Asc Aortic SAX)

The ME ascending aortic short-axis view is developed by withdrawing the probe from the midesophageal four-chamber view until the aortic valve is no longer in view and then anteflexing the probe (Fig. 1-10). In this view, the main pulmonary artery and its bifurcation are seen leading to the right and left pulmonary arteries. The right pulmonary artery is closest to the probe and is therefore located closest to the apex of the image. Just anterior (toward screen bottom) to the right pulmonary artery is the ascending aorta in short axis. On the display, the superior vena cava is located just to the left (patient's right) of the ascending aorta.

Midesophageal Ascending Aortic Long Axis (ME Asc Aortic LAX)

From the ME ascending aortic short-axis view, the multiplane is increased an additional 90 degrees (usually to a multiplane angle of 90 degrees [Fig. 1-11]). In this view, the right pulmonary artery is seen in short axis and is the structure located closest to the apex of the image sector. The ascending aorta is seen in long axis and is located just anterior to the right pulmonary (toward screen bottom).

Transgastric Midpapillary Short Axis (TG Mid SAX)

The transgastric views are typically located at a depth of about 40 to 45 cm from the incisors (Fig. 1-12). This view is developed by first obtaining the ME four-chamber view (with multiplane at 0 degrees) and centering the left ventricle vertically in the image sector. Once the left ventricle is centered, advance the probe into the stomach a few centimeters past the base of the left ventricle. Then slightly anteflex the probe until the transgastric midpapillary short-axis view of the left ventricle comes into view. If the image does not come into view, slightly withdraw the probe to make better contact between the probe and the stomach wall (DO NOT advance or withdraw the probe within the esophagus while the probe is not in the neutral position; this could potentially cause a mucosal tear). In this view, the left ventricle is located toward the right of the image sector, the right ventricle is located toward the left of the image sector, and the interventricular septum is located between the right and left ventricles. Within the left ventricle, the anterolateral and posteromedial papillary muscles are visualized toward the right and top of the screen, respectively.

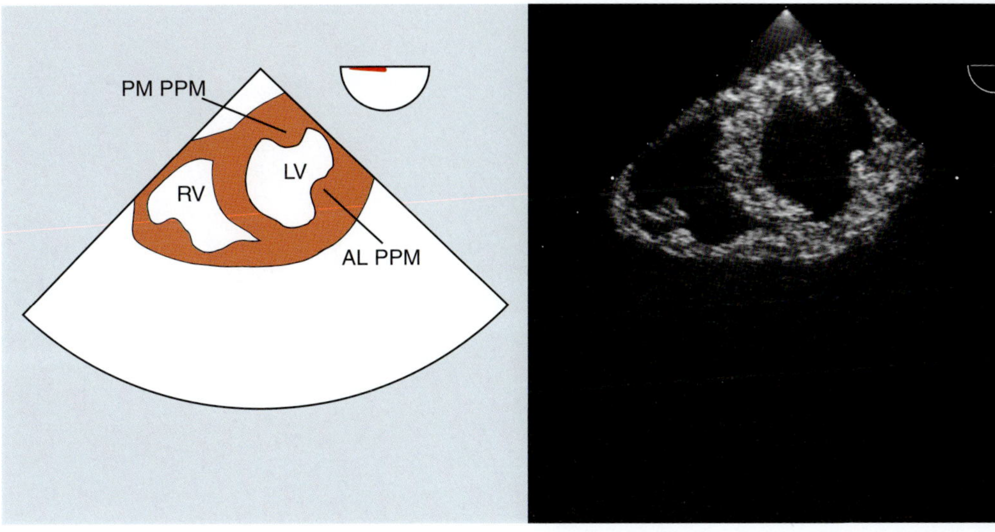

Figure 1-12 Transgastric mid-papillary short-axis view. *AL PPM,* Anterolateral papillary muscle; *LV,* left ventricle; *PM PPM,* postero-medial papillary muscle; *RV,* right ventricle. *(Two-dimensional TEE images generated using software developed by Heartworks, Inventive Medical Ltd., London, UK.)*

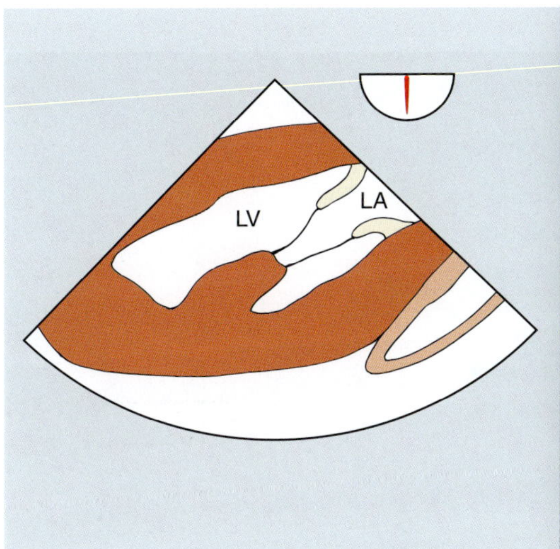
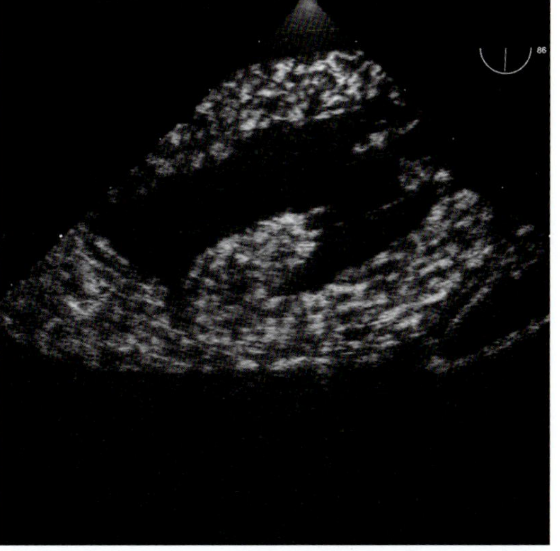

Figure 1-13 Transgastric two-chamber view. *LA,* Left atrium; *LV,* left ventricle. *(Two-dimensional TEE images generated using software developed by Heartworks, Inventive Medical Ltd., London, UK.)*

Transgastric Two-Chamber (TG Two-Chamber)

From the transgastric midpapillary short-axis view, the multiplane angle is increased to 90 degrees (Fig. 1-13). In this view, the left atrium is visualized to the far right of the image sector, and the left ventricle is to the far left of the image sector. Between the left atrium and left ventricle is the mitral valve apparatus, including portions of the valve leaflets and the subvalvular chordae tendinae.

Transgastric Long Axis (TG LAX)

From the transgastric two-chamber view, rotate the multiplane angle to 110 to 130 degrees to obtain the transgastric long-axis view of the left ventricle (Fig. 1-14). The anteroseptal wall of the left ventricle is visualized at the bottom of the image sector, with the inferolateral wall at the top, as well as components of the mitral subvalvular apparatus. The LVOT and aortic valve are illustrated toward the bottom right of the image.

Transgastric Right Ventricular Inflow
(TG RV Inflow)

This view is obtained by starting with the transgastric midpapillary short-axis view and then rotating the probe slightly to the patient's

right until the right ventricle comes into view (Fig. 1-15). The multiplane angle is then increased until the apex of the right ventricle comes into view in the left side of the image, usually at 90 to 120 degrees. The right atrium is located to the right side of the image sector, and the right ventricle is located toward the left of the image sector. The tricuspid valve chordae tendinae are visible interior to the tricuspid valve.

Transgastric Basal Short Axis (TG Basal SAX)

From the transgastric mid–short axis, the probe is withdrawn slightly and anteflexed (Fig. 1-16). In this view, the posterior mitral leaflet is located at the upper portion of the image sector, and the anterior mitral leaflet is directly opposite toward the center of the image. Likewise, the posteromedial mitral valve commissure is closest to the interventricular septum, usually toward the top of the screen, while the anterolateral mitral valve commissure is directly opposite near the right side of the view.

Deep Transgastric Long Axis (Deep TG LAX)

This view is obtained by starting from the transgastric mid–short-axis view and then further advancing the probe into the stomach toward the apex of the left ventricle (Fig. 1-17). Anteflexion and leftward

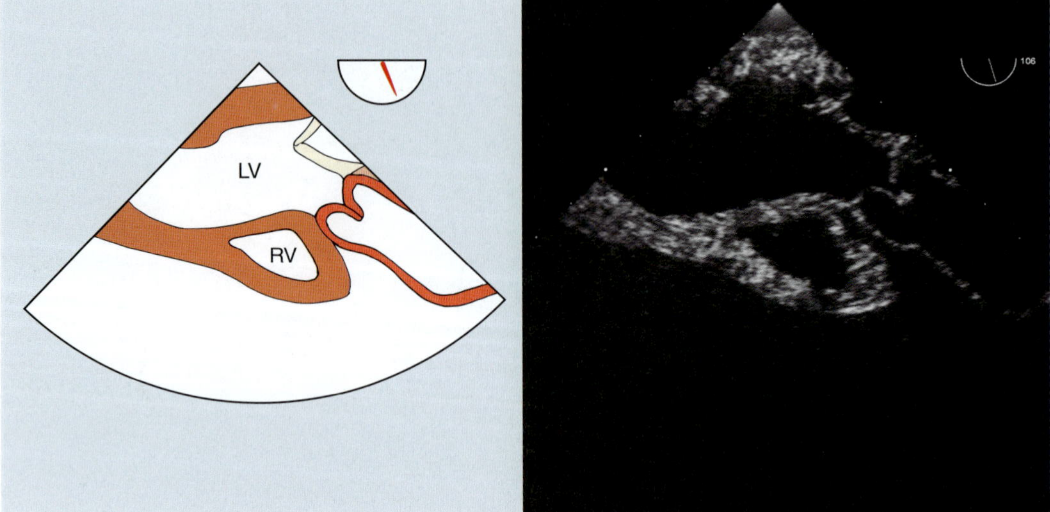

Figure 1-14 Transgastric long-axis view. *LV,* Left ventricle; *RV,* right ventricle. *(Two-dimensional TEE images generated using software developed by Heartworks, Inventive Medical Ltd., London, UK.)*

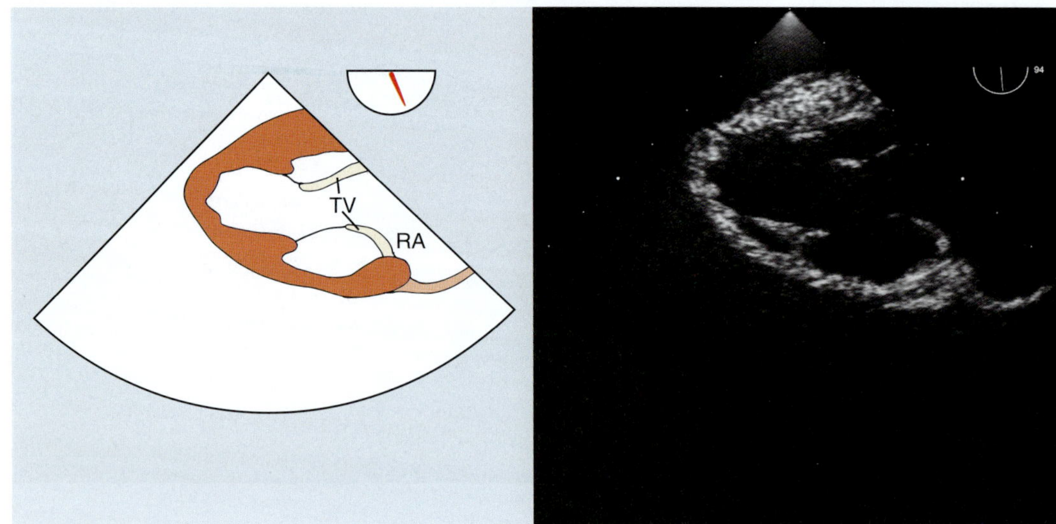

Figure 1-15 Transgastric right ventricle inflow view. *RA,* Right atrium; *TV,* tricuspid valve. *(Two-dimensional TEE images generated using software developed by Heartworks, Inventive Medical Ltd., London, UK.)*

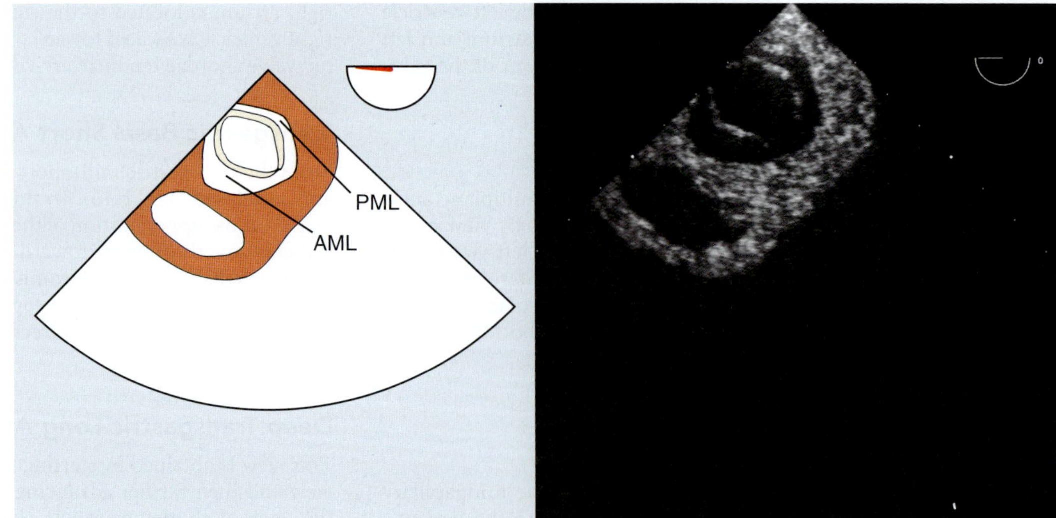

Figure 1-16 Transgastric basal short-axis view. *AML,* Anterior mitral leaflet; *PML,* posterior mitral leaflet. *(Two-dimensional TEE images generated using software developed by Heartworks, Inventive Medical Ltd., London, UK.)*

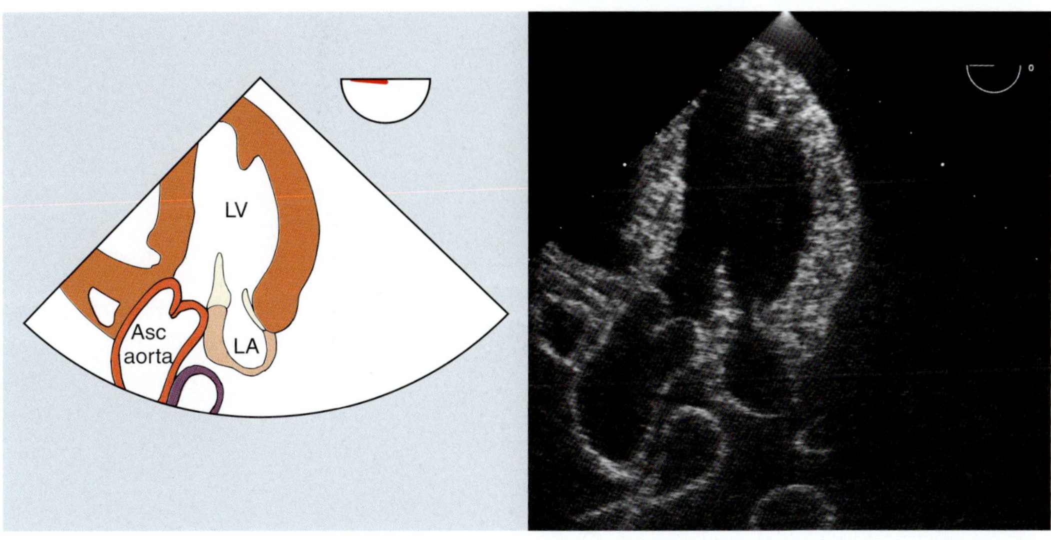

Figure 1-17 Deep transgastric long-axis view. *Asc aorta,* Ascending aorta; *LA,* left atrium; *LV,* left ventricle. *(Two-dimensional TEE images generated using software developed by Heartworks, Inventive Medical Ltd., London, UK.)*

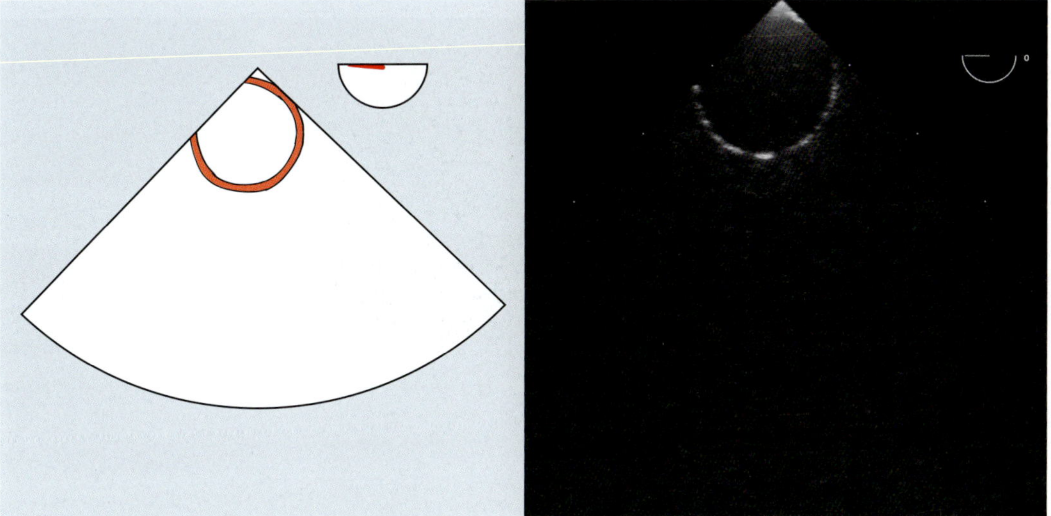

Figure 1-18 Descending aortic short-axis view. *(Two-dimensional TEE images generated using software developed by Heartworks, Inventive Medical Ltd., London, UK.)*

flexion optimizes the image by creating better contact with the cardiac structures of interest. Counterclockwise, starting from the right side of the image sector, are the left atrium, mitral valve with its associated submitral apparatus, left ventricle, LVOT, and aortic valve. Occasionally the right ventricle comes into view adjacent to the left ventricle on the left side of the image sector.

Descending Aortic Short Axis (Desc Aortic SAX)

From the deep transgastric long-axis view, relax the anteflexion and rotate the probe to the patient's left to image the descending aorta in short axis (Fig. 1-18). Decrease the image depth to about 8 cm and increase the time-gain compensation at the top of the sector for optimal image quality. Withdraw the probe slowly while rotating as necessary to maintain the aorta in the center of the image sector for its entire length.

Descending Aortic Long Axis (Desc Aortic LAX)

Repeating the maneuvers for the descending aortic short-axis view at a multiplane angle of 90 degrees will yield the descending aortic long-axis images (Fig. 1-19). Increase the multiplane angle to 90 degrees for a long-axis image of the descending aorta. The newer TEE machines

with 3D technology will allow for simultaneous imaging of both short and long axes (X plane function).

Upper Esophageal Aortic Arch Long Axis (UE Aortic Arch LAX)

As the probe is withdrawn further from the descending aortic short-axis view and turned slightly to the patient's right, the long axis of the aortic arch comes into view (Fig. 1-20). The left subclavian artery may often be seen as it branches from the aortic arch at the top right of image sector. The trachea obscures the proximal aortic arch, thereby making visualization of the innominate and left carotid arteries difficult with TEE.

Upper Esophageal Aortic Arch Short Axis (UE Aortic Arch SAX)

From the upper esophageal aortic arch long axis, increase the multiplane angle to 70 to 90 degrees for a view of the aortic arch in short axis (Fig. 1-21). Occasionally the left subclavian artery appears at the top right of the image as it branches from the aorta. The left side of the image sector shows the right ventricular outflow tract, pulmonary valve, and pulmonary artery in some patients.

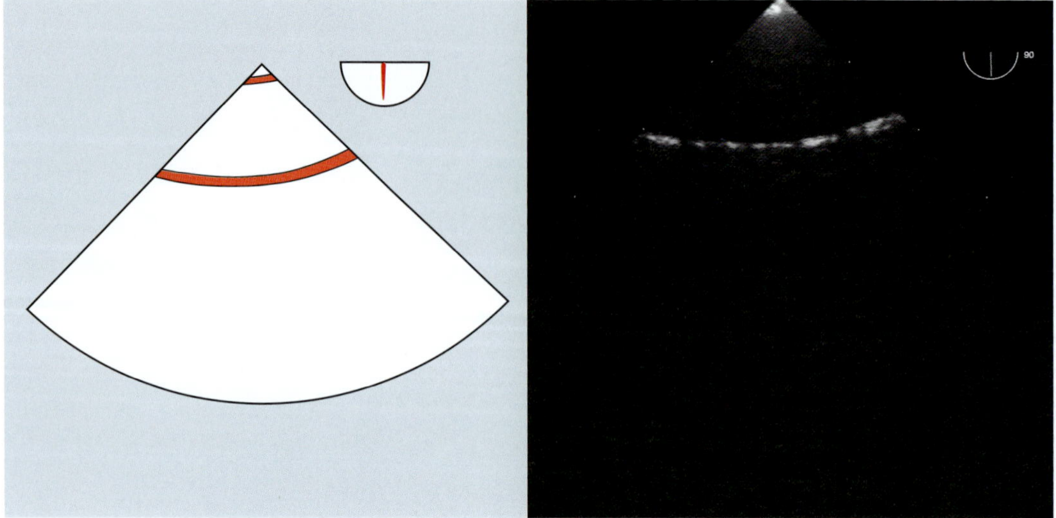

Figure 1-19 Descending aortic long-axis view. *(Two-dimensional TEE images generated using software developed by Heartworks, Inventive Medical Ltd., London, UK.)*

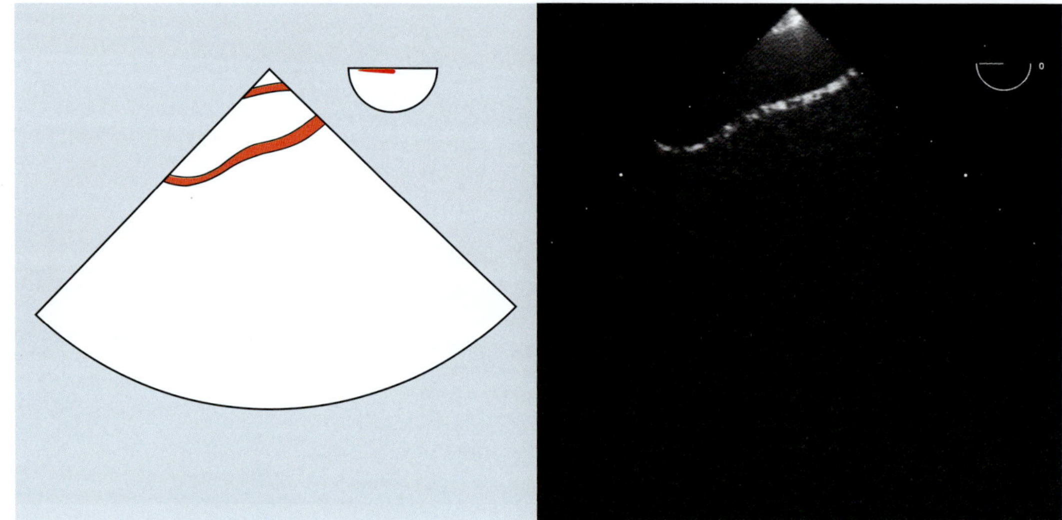

Figure 1-20 Upper esophageal aortic arch long-axis view. *(Two-dimensional TEE images generated using software developed by Heartworks, Inventive Medical Ltd., London, UK.)*

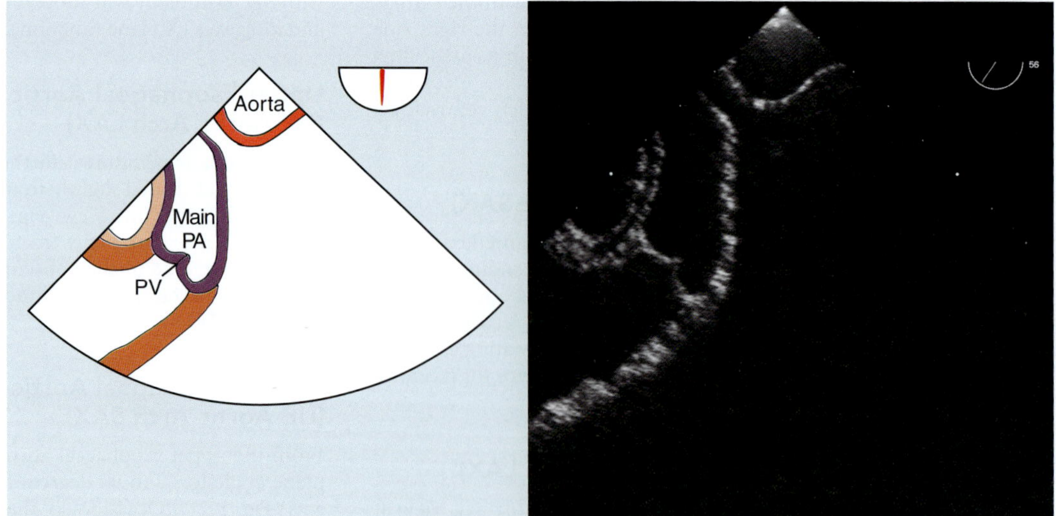

Figure 1-21 Upper esophageal aortic arch short-axis view. *PA,* Pulmonary artery; *PV,* pulmonic valve. *(Two-dimensional TEE images generated using software developed by Heartworks, Inventive Medical Ltd., London, UK.)*

REFERENCES

1. Practice guidelines for perioperative transesophageal echocardiography: a report by the American Society of Anesthesiologists and the Society of Cardiovascular Anesthesiologists Task Force on Transesophageal Echocardiography. *Anesthesiology*. 1996;84:985-1006.
2. Practice guidelines for perioperative transesophageal echocardiography: an updated report by the American Society of Anesthesiologists and the Society of Cardiovascular Anesthesiologists Task Force on Transesophageal Echocardiography. *Anesthesiology*. 2010;112:1084-1096.
3. Shanewise JS, Cheung AT, Aronson S, et al. ASE/SCA guidelines for performing a comprehensive intraoperative multiplane transesophageal echocardiography examination: recommendations of the American Society of Echocardiography Council for Intraoperative Echocardiography and the Society of Cardiovascular Anesthesiologists Task Force for Certification in Perioperative Transesophageal Echocardiography. *Anesth Analg*. 1999;89:870-884.

2

Principles and Physics: Principles of Ultrasound

RONALD A. KAHN | IVAN S. SALGO

An ultrasound beam is a continuous or intermittent train of mechanical or pressure waves emitted by a transducer or wave generator. These waves can exist in any solid medium (i.e., not in a vacuum.) As the waves travel past any fixed point along an ultrasound beam, the pressure cycles regularly and continuously between a high and a low value. The number of cycles per second (Hertz [Hz]) is called the *frequency* of the wave. Perceptible sound waves have frequencies from 20 to 20,000 Hz. Ultrasound is sound with frequencies above 20 kilohertz (kHz), while medical ultrasound often uses frequencies between 2 and 12 megahertz (MHz). In addition to frequency, ultrasound waves are characterized by their wavelength and velocity.[1] *Wavelength* is the distance between the two nearest points of equal pressure or density along an ultrasound beam, and *velocity* is the speed at which the waves propagate through a medium. The relationship among the frequency (f), wavelength (λ), and velocity (v) of an ultrasound wave is defined by the formula:

$$v = f \times \lambda$$

The velocity of ultrasound waves varies with the properties of the medium it travels through. In low-density gases, molecules must traverse long distances before encountering the adjacent molecules, so ultrasound velocity is relatively slow. In air, the velocity of ultrasound is 330 m/sec. In contrast, molecules are constrained in solids, and ultrasound velocity is relatively high. For soft tissues, this velocity is approximates 1540 m/sec, but varies from 1475 to 1620 m/sec and approaches 3360 m/sec in bone. Because the frequency of an ultrasound beam is determined by the properties of the emitting transducer, and the velocity through soft tissue is approximately constant, wavelengths are inversely proportional to the ultrasound frequency.

Ultrasound waves transport energy through a given medium; the rate of energy transported per time is expressed as "power" (P), which is expressed in joules per second or watts.[1] Since medical ultrasound is normally concentrated in a small area, the strength of the beam is usually expressed as power per unit area or "intensity" (W/m²). In most circumstances, intensity is expressed with respect to a standard intensity. For example, the intensity of the original ultrasound signal may be compared with the reflected signal. Since ultrasound amplitudes may vary by a factor of 10^5 or greater, amplitudes are expressed using a logarithmic scale, the decibel, which is defined as:

$$\text{decibel (dB)} = 10 \bullet \log (P_1/P_{ref})$$

where P_1 is the power of the wave to be compared, and P_{ref} is the power of the reference waves.

Since this is a logarithmic scale, positive values imply a wave of greater intensity than the reference wave, and negative values indicate a lower intensity. Increasing the wave's intensity by a factor of 100 yields 20 dB. Increasing by a factor of 10 yields 10 dB. Doubling the intensity yields 3 dB.

Ultrasound Beam

In physics, *transduction* is the conversion of one form of energy to another. A heating element is a transducer that converts electrical energy into heat energy. Piezoelectric crystals convert between ultrasound (pressure) and electrical signals. When presented with a high-frequency electrical signal (pulse), the crystals oscillate to produce ultrasound energy; when they are presented with an ultrasonic vibration, they produce an electrical alternating current signal. Most piezoelectric crystals used in clinical applications are manufactured ceramic ferroelectrics, the most common of which are barium titanate, lead metaniobate, and lead zirconate titanate. Some modern piezoelectric materials are more homogeneous in the solid state and hence are more efficient at generating broader bandwidth pulses (i.e., with more high- and low-frequency content). Pulses with a broader bandwidth have a broad spectrum in the frequency domain and are shorter pulses in the time domain. During most ultrasound applications, a brief ultrasound signal is emitted from the piezoelectric crystal, which is directed toward the areas to be imaged. This pulse duration is typically 1 to 2 microseconds. After this ultrasound burst emission, the crystal "listens" for the returning echoes for a given period of time and then pauses prior to repeating this cycle. This cycle length is known as the *pulse repetition frequency* (PRF) and must be of sufficient duration to allow a signal to travel to and return from a given object of interest. Typically, PRF varies from 1 to 10 kHz, which results in 0.1 to 1 milliseconds between pulses. When reflected ultrasound waves return to these piezoelectric crystals, they are converted into electrical signals that may be appropriately processed and displayed. Electronic circuits measure the time delay between the ultrasound emissions and their echoes. Since the speed of ultrasound through tissue is a constant, this time delay may be converted into the precise distance between the transducer and tissue. The amplitude or strength of the returning ultrasound signal provides information about the characteristics of the insonated tissues.

The three-dimensional shape of the ultrasound beam is dependent upon both the physical aspects of the ultrasound signal and the design of the transducer, especially its aperture. Further details of ultrasound transducers will be discussed in Chapter 5. An unfocused ultrasound beam may be thought of as an inverted funnel where the initial straight columnar area is known as the "near field" (also known as the *Fresnel zone*), followed by a conical divergent area known as the "far field" (also known as the *Fraunhofer zone*) (Fig. 2-1). The length of the near field is directly proportional to the square of the transducer diameter and inversely proportional to the wavelength; specifically:

$$F_n = D^2/4\lambda$$

where F_n is the near-field length, D is the diameter of the transducer, and λ is the ultrasound wavelength.

Increasing the frequency of the ultrasound increases the length of the near field. In this near field, most energy is confined to a beam width no greater than the transducer diameter. Long Fresnel zones are preferred with medical ultrasonography, which may be achieved with large-diameter transducers and high-frequency ultrasound. The angle of the far-field convergence (θ) is directly proportional to the wavelength and inversely proportional to the diameter of the transducer, and is expressed by the equation:

$$\sin \theta = 1.22\lambda/D$$

where D is the diameter of the transducer.

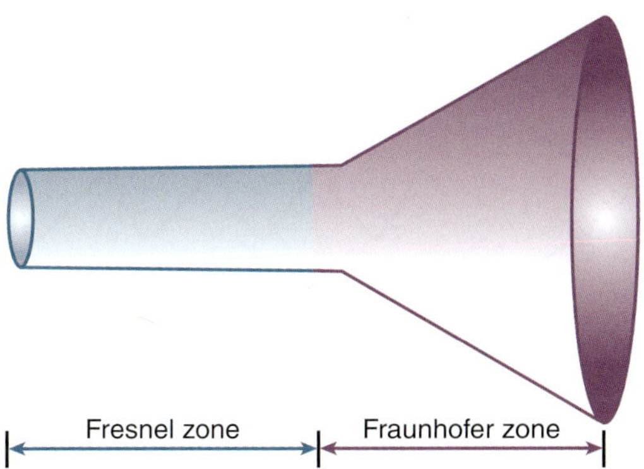

Figure 2-1 Shape of a focused ultrasound beam. Near and far fields are illustrated.

Further shaping of the beam geometry may be adjusted using acoustic lenses or the shaping of the piezoelectric crystal. Ideally, imaging should be performed within the near-field or focused aspect of the ultrasound beam, since the ultrasound beam is most parallel and of greatest intensity, and the tissue interfaces are most perpendicular to these ultrasound beams.

Attenuation, Reflection, and Scatter

Waves interact with the medium they travel in and with one another. Interaction among waves is called *interference*. The manner in which waves interact with a medium is determined by its density and homogeneity. When a wave is propagated through an inhomogeneous medium, it is partly reflected, partially absorbed, and partly scattered.

For a given object to be visualized by ultrasonography, the ultrasound waves must be accurately reflected and return to the transducer from the object of interest. Ultrasound waves are reflected when the presenting surface of the reflecting object is larger than one fourth of the ultrasound wavelength. Because of the relatively constant velocity of ultrasound in soft tissue, shorter wavelengths may be obtained by increasing the frequency of the ultrasound beam. Large objects may be visualized using low frequencies (i.e., long wavelengths), but smaller objects require higher frequencies (i.e., short wavelengths) for visualization. Additionally, the object's ultrasonic impedance (Z) must be significantly different from the ultrasonic impedance of the adjacent soft tissue such that the ultrasound will "bounce off" the object. The ultrasonic impedance of a given medium is equal to its density multiplied by its ultrasound propagation velocity. Air has a low density and low propagation velocity, so it has low ultrasound impedance. Bone has a high density and high propagation velocity, so it has high ultrasound impedance. For normal incidence, the fraction of the reflected pulse compared with the incidence pulse is:

$$I_r = (Z_2 - Z_1)^2/(Z_2 + Z_1)^2$$

where I_r is the intensity reflection coefficient, and Z_1 and Z_2 are the acoustical impedances of the two media.

The greater the differences in ultrasound impedance between two objects at a given interface, the greater the ultrasound reflection. Because the ultrasound impedances of air or bone are significantly different from blood, ultrasound is strongly reflected from these interfaces, limiting the availability of ultrasound to interrogate deeper structures. Reflected echoes, also called "specular echoes," are usually much stronger than scattered echoes. Specular reflection occurs where the ultrasound wave is much smaller than the spatial characteristic of the material being interrogated. A grossly inhomogeneous medium, such as a cardiac valve in a blood-filled heart chamber, produces strong specular reflections at the blood/valve interface because of their significant differences in ultrasonic impedance. Furthermore, if the interface between the two objects is not perpendicular to the ultrasound beam, the reflected signal may be deflected at an angle and may not return to the transducer for construction of an image.

If objects are small compared with the ultrasound wavelength or the difference in acoustic impedances at the interface is small, the ultrasound wave will be scattered in many directions—not just 180 degrees. For example, muscle is inhomogeneous at the microscopic level and produces more scatter than specular reflection, since the differences in adjacent ultrasound impedances are low and the objects are small. These small objects produce echoes that reflect through a large range of angles with only a small percentage of the original signal reaching the ultrasound transducer. Scattered ultrasound waves will combine in constructive and destructive fashions with other scattered waves, producing an interference pattern known as "speckle." The speckle pattern is a direct consequence of tissue structure. Compared with specular echoes, the returning ultrasound signal amplitude will be lower and displayed as a darker signal. Although smaller objects can be visualized with higher frequencies (i.e., short wavelengths), these higher frequencies result in greater signal attenuation, limiting the depth of ultrasound penetration through tissues.

Attenuation refers to loss of ultrasound power as it transverses tissue. Tissue attenuation is dependent on ultrasound reflection, scattering, and absorption. The greater the ultrasound reflection and scattering, the less ultrasound energy is available for penetration and insonation of deeper structures; this effect is especially important during scanning with higher frequencies. In normal circumstances, however, absorption is the most significant factor in ultrasound attenuation.[2] Absorption occurs as a result of the oscillation of tissue caused by the transit of the ultrasound wave. These tissue oscillations result in friction, with the conversion of ultrasound energy into heat. The transit of an ultrasound wave through a medium causes molecular displacement, which requires the conversion of kinetic energy into potential energy as the molecules are compressed. At the time of maximal compression, the kinetic energy is minimized and the potential energy maximized. The movement of molecules from compressed locations to their original locations requires conversion of this potential energy back into kinetic energy, after which the process is repeated. In most cases, this energy conversion (either kinetic into potential energy or vice versa) is not 100% efficient and results in energy loss as heat.[1]

Absorption is dependent upon both the material the ultrasound is passing through and the ultrasound frequency. The degree of attenuation through a given thickness of material may be described by:

$$\text{Attenuation (dB)} = a \bullet \text{freq} \bullet x$$

where *a* is the attenuation coefficient in dB/cm at 1 MHz, *freq* is the ultrasound frequency in MHz, and *x* is the thickness of the tissue in centimeters.

Whereas water, blood, and muscle have low ultrasound attenuation, air and bone have very high tissue ultrasound attenuation, limiting the ability of ultrasound to transverse these structures.

Imaging Techniques

As already discussed, in echocardiography the heart and great vessels are insonated with ultrasound, which is sound above the human audible range. The ultrasound is sent into the thoracic cavity and is partially reflected by the cardiac structures. From these reflections, distance, velocity, and density of objects within the chest are derived.

M-Mode

The most basic form of ultrasound imaging is M-mode echocardiography. In this mode, the density and position of all tissues in the path of a narrow ultrasound beam (i.e., *along a single line*) are displayed as a function of time (Fig. 2-2). This modality produces an updated, continuously changing time plot of the studied tissue section of several seconds in duration. Since this is a timed *motion display* (normal cardiac tissue is always in motion), it is called "M-mode." Because only a very limited part of the heart is being observed at any one time, and because the image requires considerable interpretation, M-mode is not currently used as a primary imaging technique. This mode is,

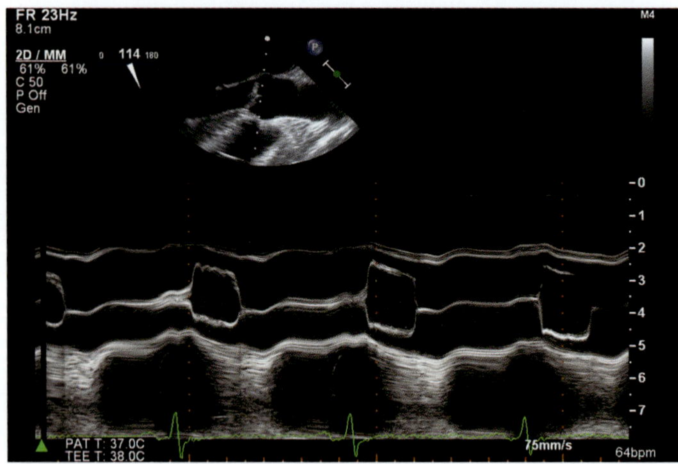

Figure 2-2 M-mode imaging. Density and position of all tissues in the path of a narrow ultrasound beam (i.e., along a single line) are displayed as a function of time. In this image, ultrasound beam insonates the line from left atrium through posterior and then anterior aspect of ascending aorta. Excursion of aortic valve cusps may be measured with great accuracy during systole.

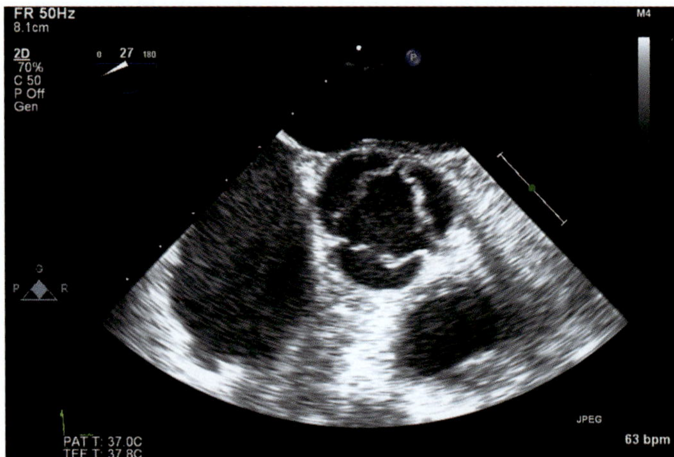

Figure 2-3 B-mode or two-dimensional (2D) imaging. By rapid, repetitive scanning along many different radii within an area in the shape of a fan (sector), a 2D image of a section of heart is generated. The midesophageal aortic valve short axis view is illustrated.

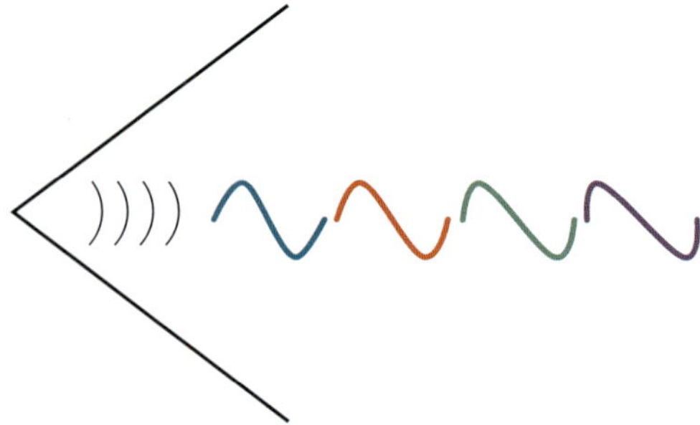

Figure 2-4 Harmonic imaging. Velocity of ultrasound transit is directly proportional to density, so peak amplitudes will travel slightly faster than trough. With time, this differential velocity transit of peak with trough wave results in distortion of propagated sine wave, resulting in a more peaked wave. (*From Kahn RA, Skubas N, Fischer G, et al. Intraoperative transesophageal echocardiography. In: Kaplan JA, Reich DL, Savino J, eds. Cardiac Anesthesia. 6th ed. Elsevier: St. Louis; 2011.*)

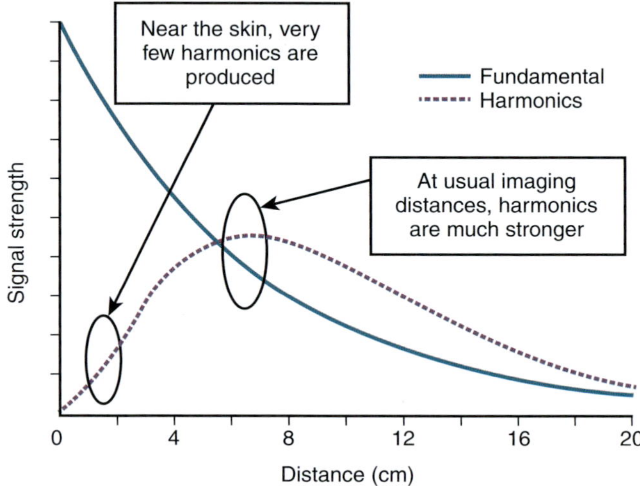

Figure 2-5 Relation between imaging distance and strength of fundamental and harmonic frequencies. As ultrasound pulse propagates, strength of fundamental frequency declines while strength of harmonic frequency increases. At usual imaging distances for cardiac structures, strength of harmonic frequency is maximized. Note: Harmonic frequency strength is exaggerated in this schematic. Harmonic frequency signal strength is much lower than fundamental frequency signal strength. (*From Thomas JD, Rubin DN. Tissue harmonic imaging: why does it work? J Am Soc Echocardiogr 1998;11:803-808.*)

however, useful for the precise timing of events within the cardiac cycle and is often used in combination with color flow Doppler for the timing of abnormal flows. Because M-mode images are updated 1000 times per second, they provide greater temporal resolution than two-dimensional (2D) echocardiography; thus, more subtle changes in motion or dimension can be appreciated.

B-Mode

The different reflectivities of various cardiac structures result in variations of the returning ultrasound wave. The detected ultrasound signals are translated from the amplitude of the reflected signal to luminance and displayed as a brightness-mode (B-mode) image. By rapid, repetitive scanning along many different radii within an area in the shape of a fan (sector), a 2D image of a section of the heart is generated. Information on structures and motion in the plane of a 2D scan is updated 20 to 40 times per second. This repetitive update produces a "live" (real-time) image of the heart (Fig. 2-3).

Harmonic Imaging

Harmonic frequencies are ultrasound transmissions of integer multiples of the original frequency. For example, if the fundamental frequency is 4 MHz, the second harmonic is 8 MHz, the third fundamental is 12 MHz, and so on. *Harmonic imaging* refers to a technique of B-mode imaging in which an ultrasound signal is transmitted at a given frequency but will "listen" at one of its harmonic frequencies.[3,4] As ultrasound is transmitted through a tissue, the tissue undergoes slight compressions and expansions that correspond to the ultrasound wave temporarily changing the local tissue density. Since the velocity of ultrasound transit is directly proportional to density, the peak amplitudes will travel slightly faster than the trough. This differential velocity transit of the peak versus the trough wave results in distortion of the propagated sine wave, resulting in a more peaked wave (Fig. 2-4). This peaked wave will contain frequencies of the fundamental frequency as well as the harmonic frequencies. Very little distortion of the ultrasound wave occurs in the near field, and the amount of energy contained within these harmonics is minimal close to the transducer (Fig. 2-5). As the distance traversed by the ultrasound increases, the ultrasound wave becomes more peaked, with greater energies in the harmonic frequencies. Eventually the effects of attenuation will be more pronounced on these harmonic waves, with a subsequent decrease in harmonic amplitude. Because the effects of attenuation are greatest with high-frequency ultrasound, the second harmonic usually is used.

The use of tissue harmonic imaging is associated with improved B-mode imaging. Near-field scatter is common with fundamental imaging. Since the ultrasound wave has not yet been distorted, very little harmonic energy is generated in the near field, minimizing near-field scatter when harmonic imaging is used. Since higher frequencies are used, greater resolution may be obtained. Finally, with tissue harmonic imaging, side-lobe artifacts are substantially reduced and lateral resolution is increased (see Chap. 6)

Resolution

An ultrasound image may be described by its axial, lateral, and elevational resolution. *Axial resolution* is the minimum separation between two objects located along the beam so that they can be imaged as two different interfaces. The most precise image resolution is along this axial plane. The higher the frequency of the ultrasound signal, the greater the axial resolution, since ultrasound waves of shorter wavelengths may be used. Shorter bursts of ultrasound waves (i.e., short pulse length) provide greater axial resolution. Pulse length should be no more than two or three cycles. The range of frequencies contained within a given ultrasound transmission is referred to as the *frequency bandwidth*. Generally, the shorter the pulse of the ultrasound produced, the greater the frequency bandwidth. Because of the relationship between short pulse lengths and high bandwidths, high bandwidths are associated with better axial resolution. High transducer bandwidths also allow for better resolution of deeper structures.

Lateral resolution is the minimum separation of two interfaces aligned along a direction perpendicular to the ultrasound beam. The most important determinant of lateral resolution is the ultrasound beam width or ultrasound beam focusing; the narrower the beam, the better the lateral resolution. If a small object appears within the near field, it can be resolved accurately laterally; however, if it appears within the far field, the size of this small object will appear to increase with the increase in the width of the ultrasound beam. This increase in size associated with object resolution in the far field results in blurring of deeper structures. *Elevational resolution* refers to the ability to determine differences in the thickness of the imaging plane. The thickness of the ultrasound beam is a major determinant of elevational resolution.

REFERENCES

1. Hendee WR, Ritenour ER. *Medical Imaging Physics.* 4th Ed. New York: Wiley-Liss; 2002.
2. Hangiandreou NJ. AAPM/RSNA Physics Tutorial for Residents: Topics in US. B-mode US: Basic Concepts and New Technology. *Radiographics.* 2003;23:1019-1033.
3. Kerut EK, McIlwain EF, Plotnick GD. *Handbook of Echo-Doppler Interpretation.* 2nd ed. Blackwell Futura: New York; 2004.
4. Thomas JD, Rubin DN. Tissue harmonic imaging: why does it work? *J Am Soc Echocardiogr.* 1998;11:803-808.

3

Principles and Physics: Principles of Doppler Ultrasound

RONALD A. KAHN | IVAN S. SALGO

The Doppler Principle

When a wave is reflected from a moving object, the frequency of the wave will be different from the original emitted wave. This frequency change is known as the *Doppler principle*. The magnitude and direction of the frequency shift are related to the velocity and direction of the moving target. The velocity of the target may be calculated with the Doppler equation:

$$v = (cf_d)/(2f_0 \cos \theta)$$

where

v = the target velocity (blood flow velocity)
c = the speed of sound in tissue
f_d = the Doppler frequency shift
f_0 = the frequency of the emitted ultrasound from the ultrasound probe
θ = the angle between the ultrasound beam and the direction of the target velocity (blood flow).

Rearranging the terms,

$$f_d = v \, (2f_0 \cos \theta)/c$$

As is evident in the second equation, the greater the velocity of the object of interest, the greater the Doppler frequency shift (Fig. 3-1). Additionally, the magnitude of the frequency shift is directly proportional to the initial emitted frequency. Lower emitted frequencies produce low Doppler frequency shifts, while higher emitted frequencies produce greater Doppler frequency shifts. This phenomenon becomes important with aliasing, as will be discussed later. Furthermore, the only ambiguity in the second equation is that the direction of the ultrasonic signal could refer to either the transmitted or the received beam. By convention, Doppler displays are made with reference to the received beam, however, so if the blood flow and the reflected beam travel in the same direction, the angle of incidence is zero degrees and the cosine is +1. As a result, the frequency of the reflected signal will be higher than the frequency of the emitted signal.

Most modern echo scanners combine Doppler capabilities with their two-dimensional (2D) imaging capabilities. Information on blood flow dynamics can be obtained by applying Doppler frequency shift analysis to echoes reflected by the moving red blood cells.[1,2] Blood flow velocity, direction, and acceleration can be instantaneously determined. After the desired view of the heart has been obtained by 2D echocardiography, the Doppler beam, represented by a cursor, is superimposed on the 2D image. The operator positions the cursor as parallel as possible to the assumed direction of blood flow, and then empirically adjusts the direction of the beam to optimize the audio and visual representations of the reflected Doppler signal. At the present time, Doppler technology can be utilized in at least four different ways to measure blood velocities: pulsed, high repetition frequency, continuous wave, and color flow.

Equipment currently used in clinical practice displays most Doppler blood flow velocities as waveforms. The waveforms consist of a spectral analysis of velocities on the ordinate and time on the abscissa. By convention, blood flow toward the transducer is represented above the baseline, and blood flow away from the transducer below the baseline. When the blood flow is perpendicular to the ultrasonic beam, no blood flow will be detected. Since the cosine of the angle of incidence is a variable in the Doppler equation, blood flow velocity is measured most accurately when the ultrasound beam is parallel or antiparallel to the direction of blood flow. In clinical practice, a deviation from parallel of up to 20 degrees can be tolerated, because this only results in an error of 6% or less.

Pulsed Wave Doppler (PWD)

In pulsed wave Doppler (PWD), blood flow parameters can be determined at precise locations by emitting repetitive short bursts of ultrasound at a specific frequency (pulse repetition frequency, or PRF) and analyzing the frequency shift of the reflected echoes at an identical sampling frequency (f_s) (Fig. 3-2). A time delay between emission of the ultrasound signal burst and sampling of the reflected signal determines the depth at which the velocities are sampled; the delay is proportional to the distance between the transducer and the location of the velocity measurements. To sample at a given depth (D), sufficient time must be allowed for the signal to travel a distance of $2 \times D$ (from the transducer to the sample volume and back).

The operator varies the depth of sampling by varying the time delay between emission of the ultrasonic signal and sampling of the reflected wave. In practice, the sampling location or *sample volume* is represented by a small marker that can be positioned at any point along the Doppler beam by moving it up or down the Doppler cursor. On some devices, it is also possible to vary the width and height of the sample volume.

The inherent limitation to measurement of flows at precise locations is that ambiguous information is obtained when flow velocity is very high. Information theory suggests that an unknown periodic signal must be sampled at least twice per cycle to determine even rudimentary information such as the fundamental frequency; therefore, the rate of PRF of PWD must be at least twice the Doppler shift frequency produced by flow.[3] If not, the frequency shift is "undersampled." In other words, this frequency shift is sampled so infrequently, the frequency reported by the instrument is erroneously low.[4]

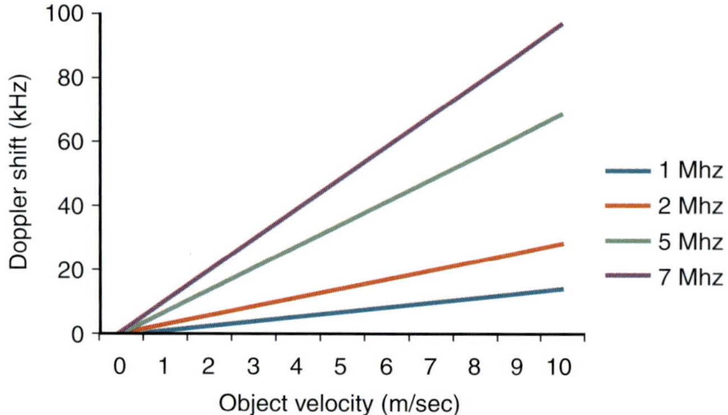

Figure 3-1 Graph of Doppler shift frequency versus velocity for various emitted ultrasound frequencies. A lower emitted ultrasound frequency will produce a lower Doppler frequency shift for a given velocity. This lower Doppler frequency shift will allow for a higher-velocity measurement before aliasing occurs. (*From Kahn RA, Skubas N, Fischer G, et al. Intraoperative transesophageal echocardiography. In: Kaplan JA, Reich DL, Savino J, eds. Cardiac Anesthesia. 6th ed. St. Louis: Elsevier; 2011.*)

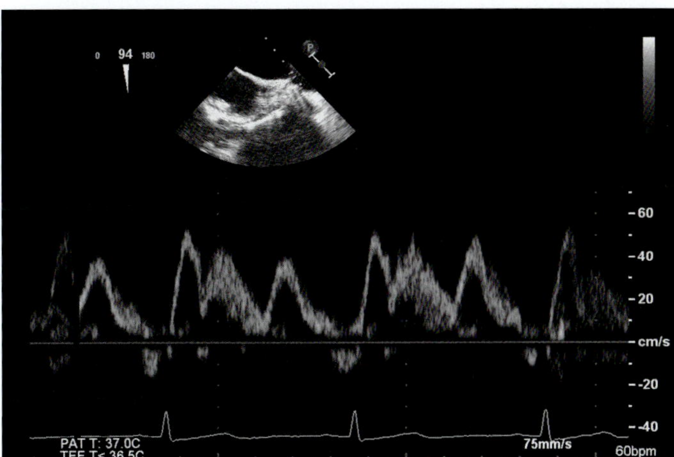

Figure 3-2 Example of pulse wave Doppler. Blood flow parameters can be determined at precise locations within heart by emitting repetitive short bursts of ultrasound at a specific frequency and analyzing frequency shift of reflected echoes at an identical sampling frequency. This example shows blood flow velocity spectrum of right upper pulmonary vein.

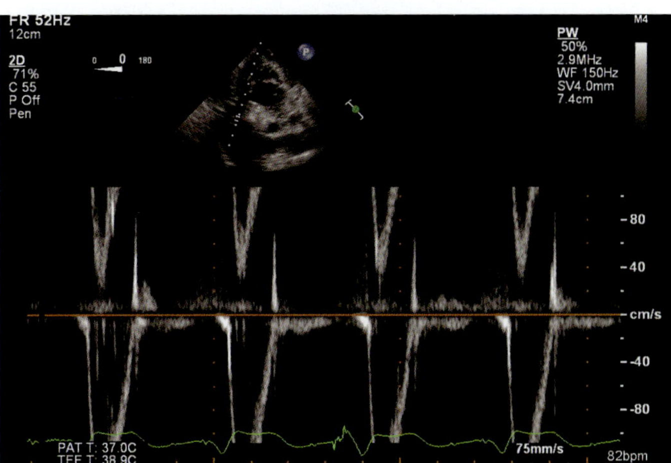

Figure 3-3 Example of aliasing. When Doppler shift becomes close to pulse repetition frequency, artifacts described as "aliasing" or "wraparound" are created. Blood flow velocities will appear in a direction opposite to conventional one.

A simple reference to Western movies will clearly illustrate this point. When a stagecoach gets underway, its wheel spokes are observed as rotating in the correct direction. As the speed of the spokes approach the frequency of the camera frame rate, the spokes appear to rotate in the reverse direction. In PWD, the ambiguity exists because the measured Doppler frequency shift (f_d) and the sampling frequency (f_s) are in the same frequency range. Ambiguity will be avoided if the f_D is less than half the sampling frequency:

$$f_d < f_s/2$$

The expression $f_s/2$ is also known as the *Nyquist limit*. Doppler shifts above the Nyquist limit will create artifacts described as "*aliasing*" or "*wraparound*," and blood flow velocities will appear in a direction opposite to the conventional one (Fig. 3-3). Blood flowing with high velocity toward the transducer will result in a display of velocities above and below the baseline. The maximum velocity that can be detected without aliasing is dictated by:

$$V_m = c^2/8\,R\,f_0$$

where
V_m = the maximal velocity that can be unambiguously measured
c = the speed of sound in tissue
R = the range or distance from the transducer at which the measurement is to be made
f_0 = the frequency of emitted ultrasound

Based on this equation, this "aliasing" artifact can be avoided by either minimizing R or f_0. Decreasing the depth of the sample volume in essence increases f_s. This higher sampling frequency allows for the more accurate determination of higher Doppler shift frequencies (i.e., higher velocities). Furthermore, since f_0 is directly related to f_d (see equation 2), a lower emitted ultrasound frequency will produce a lower Doppler frequency shift for a given velocity (see Fig. 3-1). This lower Doppler frequency shift will allow for a higher-velocity measurement before aliasing occurs.

High Pulse Repetition Frequency Doppler (HPRF)

On some instruments, PWD can be modified to high pulse repetition frequency (HPRF) mode. Whereas in conventional PWD only a single burst of ultrasound is considered to be in the body at any given time, in HPRF Doppler, two to five sample volumes are simultaneously presented. Information coming back to the transducer may be coming back from depths of either two, three, or four times the initial sample volume depth. The returning signals can be a mix of signals that have been emitted previously and have traveled to distant gates and other signals that were just sent and returned from the first range gate.

The HPRF mode allows an increase in the sampling frequency because the scanner does not wait for return of information from distant gates; nonetheless, it receives information back within the specified time gate period. Since higher sampling frequencies are used, higher velocities can be measured with this method than with PWD, but because the exact gate the ultrasound signals are reflected from is unknown, there is range ambiguity with HPRF.

Color Flow Doppler (CFD)

Advances in technology have allowed the display of real-time blood flow within the heart as colors, while also showing 2D images in black and white. In addition to showing the location, direction, and velocity of cardiac blood flow, images produced by these devices allow estimation of flow acceleration and differentiation of laminar and turbulent blood flow. CFD echocardiography is based on the principle of multigated PWD, in which blood flow velocities are sampled at many locations along many lines covering the entire imaging sector.[5] At the same time, the sector also is scanned to generate a 2D image.

Flow toward the transducer (top of image sector) is commonly assigned the color red and flow away from the transducer is assigned the color blue (Fig. 3-4). This color assignment is arbitrary and determined by the equipment's manufacturer and the user's color mapping. In the most common color flow coding scheme, the faster the blood flow velocity (up to a limit), the more intense the color displayed. Flow velocities that change by more than a preset value within a brief time interval (flow variance or acceleration) may have an additional hue added. Both rapidly accelerating laminar flow (change in flow speed) and turbulent flow (change in flow direction) satisfy the criteria for rapid changes in velocity.

Continuous Wave Doppler (CWD)

The continuous wave Doppler (CWD) technique uses continuous rather than discrete pulses of ultrasound waves (Fig. 3-5). During CW ultrasound, waves are continuously being both transmitted and received by separate transducers. As a result, the region in which flow dynamics are measured cannot be localized precisely. Because of the large range of depths being simultaneously insonated, a large range of frequencies is returned to the transducer. This large frequency range corresponds to a large range of blood flow velocities known as *spectral broadening*. Spectral broadening during CWD interrogation contrasts

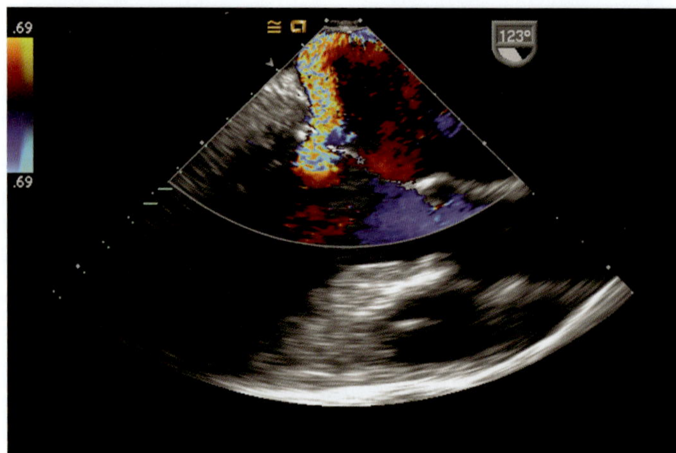

Figure 3-4 Color flow Doppler. Flow toward transducer is assigned the color red, and flow away from transducer is assigned the color blue. Flow variance or acceleration is represented by an additional hue. This example shows a mid-esophageal long-axis view; regurgitant flow through mitral valve can be seen.

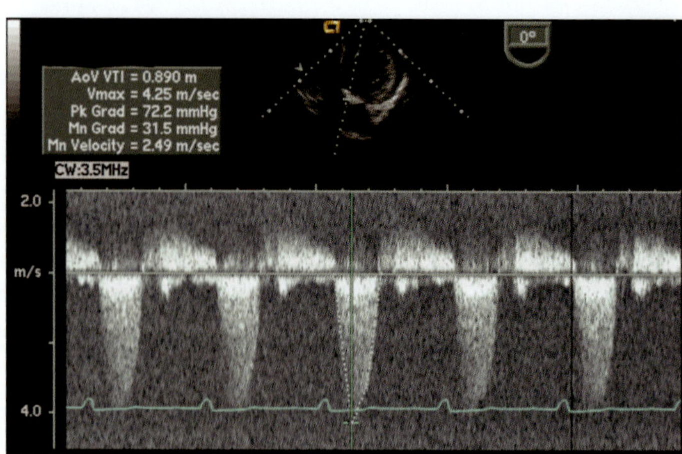

Figure 3-5 During continuous wave Doppler ultrasound, waves are continuously being both transmitted and received by separate transducers, allowing for measurement of high-velocity blood flow (at the expense of spatial specificity). In this example, a deep transgastric view is used to insonate high-velocity blood flow through aortic valve in patient with aortic stenosis.

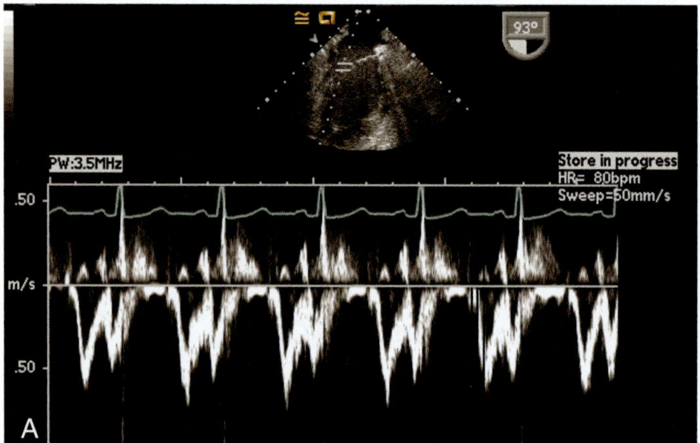

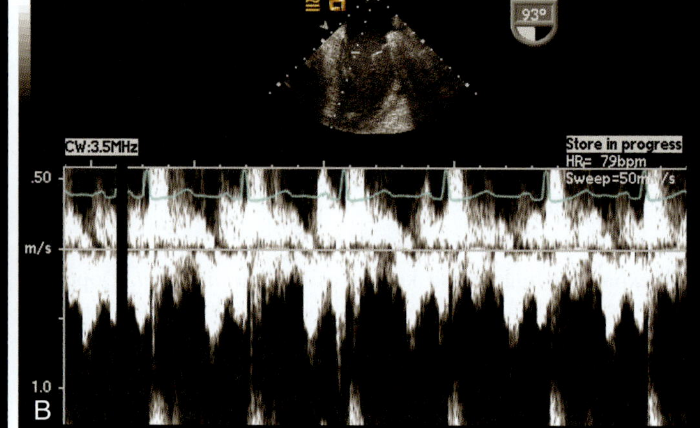

Figure 3-6 Spectral broadening. Pulse wave Doppler (PWD) versus continuous wave Doppler (CWD). Both images are Doppler spectra through mitral valve. **A,** PWD. Since a specific region of interest is defined by the Doppler gate, a clean envelope of transmitral flow is displayed. **B,** CWD. Since spatial specificity is lost, spectral broadening of velocities is displayed.

the homogenous envelope obtained with PWD (Fig. 3-6). Since the sampling frequency is very high, blood flow velocity is measured with great accuracy even at high flows. CWD is particularly useful for evaluating patients with stenotic valvular lesions or congenital heart disease, in whom high-pressure/high-velocity signals are anticipated. It also is the preferred technique when attempting to derive hemodynamic information from Doppler signals.

Determination of Tissue Movement: Tissue Doppler and Speckle Analysis

Spectral Doppler is commonly used to determine blood flow velocities. Because these velocities are relatively high and the amplitude of the Doppler signal is low, high-amplitude/low-velocity ultrasound signals usually are ignored. In contrast, during tissue Doppler examination, the primary interest is in the high-amplitude/low-velocity ultrasound signals created by the myocardium; low-amplitude/high-velocity signals are ignored. Doppler tissue imaging (DTI) of the mitral valve annulus may be used to judge diastolic function.[6] Most modern ultrasound machines have presets optimized for tissue Doppler analysis to include the high-amplitude/low-velocity signals that normally are excluded.

The major limitation of tissue Doppler analysis is the need to align tissue movement with the ultrasound beam. If tissue movements occur at right angles to the projected beam, determination of DTI is impossible. An alternative for measuring tissue movements that are independent of the ultrasound beam direction is utilizing *speckle analysis*. Interactions of ultrasound with myocardium result in reflection and scattering, which generate a finely gray-shaded, speckled pattern. This speckled pattern is unique for each myocardial region and relatively stable throughout the cardiac cycle. The speckles function as markers; they are equally distributed within the myocardium and change their position from frame to frame in accordance with the surrounding tissue motion. In speckle track imaging, the speckles within a predefined region of interest are followed automatically frame by frame, and the change in their geometric position (which corresponds to local tissue movement) is used to extract information about its movement. Because these acoustic markers can be followed in any direction, speckle tracking is a non-Doppler, angle-independent technique for calculating cardiac deformation along two dimensions.

REFERENCES

1. Hatle L, Angelsen B. *Doppler Ultrasound in Cardiology.* 2nd ed. Philadelphia: Lea & Febiger; 1984.
2. Kisslo J, Adams D, Mark DB. *Basic Doppler Echocardiography.* New York: Churchill Livingstone; 1986.
3. Evans DH, McDicken WN, Skidmore R, et al. *Doppler Ultrasound: Physics Instrumentation and Clinical Applications.* New York: John Wiley & Sons; 1989.
4. Hendee WR, Ritenour ER. *Medical Imaging Physics Fourth Edition.* New York: Wiley-Liss; 2002.
5. Kisslo J, Adams DB, Belkin RN. *Doppler ColorFlow Imaging.* New York: Churchill Livingstone; 1988.
6. Ommen SR, Nishimura RA. A clinical approach to the assessment of left ventricular diastolic function by Doppler echocardiography: Update 2003. *Heart.* 2003;89(Suppl III):iii18-iii23.

Principles and Physics: Equations to Remember (the Bernoulli Equation, Velocity-Time Integrals, and the Continuity Equation)

RONALD A. KAHN | IVAN S. SALGO

The Bernoulli Equation

Echocardiographic techniques may be used to estimate intracardiac and intravascular gradients and flows. Newton's conservation of energy states that the energy within a closed system must remain the same. If blood passes through an area of stenosis, the potential energy (as represented by a high pressure) must be converted into kinetic energy, as seen as high blood flow velocities. Additionally, some energy will be expended for blood acceleration and deceleration in pulsatile systems. Finally, some energy will be lost as heat by the viscous forces generated by friction.

These relationships have been described by Bernoulli as:

$$p_1 - p_2 = 0.5\,\rho(v_2{}^2 - v_1{}^2) + \rho \int (dv/dt)ds + R(\mu) \qquad \text{(Equation 4-1)}$$

where
p_1 = the pressure proximal to the obstruction
p_2 = the pressure distal to the obstruction
$p_1 - p_2$ = the pressure difference over the obstruction
v_1 = the velocity proximal to the obstruction
v_2 = the velocity distal to the obstruction
ρ = the density of blood, which is equal to approximately 1060 kg/m^3
$\int (dv/dt)ds$ = the integral of the blood flow acceleration over a given distance
$R(\mu)$ = the resistance, R, as a function of blood viscosity, μ

The first term represents the kinetic energy expenditure that results in acceleration of blood over the obstruction. The second term of the equation represents unsteady acceleration and deceleration of pumping blood. These are "inertial" terms. The final term represents kinetic energy loss due to viscous friction. The Bernoulli equation uses the assumption that blood is incompressible. During clinical application, the energy expended due to the cyclic acceleration and deceleration, as well as the energy loss due to viscous forces, are negligible and may be ignored, leaving just the first term. Since both velocities are squared, and v_2 is significantly larger than v_1 ($v_2 \gg v_1$), v_1 may be ignored as well. Thus, the equation may be simplified to: $p_1 - p_2 = 0.5\,\rho(v_2{}^2)$.

For clinical echocardiography, the simplified Bernoulli equation may be modified further to convert SI units (Pascals, kg/m^2) to mm Hg. Since 1 mm Hg is equal to 133.3 Pa:

$$p_1 - p_2 \times 133.3 = 0.5 \times 1060 \times v_2{}^2$$

Thus, $p_1 - p_2 = 3.976\, v_2{}^2$, and the clinically relevant simplified Bernoulli equation is:

$$p_1 - p_2 = 4v_2{}^2 \qquad \text{(Equation 4-2)}$$

With this formula, the pressure gradient across a fixed orifice can be approximated. It may be applied to the measurement of intravascular pressures as well as the gradient across a stenotic orifice.

Determination of Intravascular Pressures

The Bernoulli equation may be used to estimate intracardiac pressures. By measuring retrograde flow velocity through a regurgitant valve, transvalvular pressures during systole may be determined, allowing for estimation of intracardiac pressures. For example, the maximum velocity of the tricuspid regurgitation (TR) jet reflects the pressure drop across a regurgitant tricuspid valve (P_{TR}), which is the systolic pressure difference between the right ventricle (RV) and right atrium (RA). RV systolic pressure can be obtained by adding an estimated or measured RA pressure (RAP) to the systolic pressure gradient across the tricuspid valve during systole. Assuming there is some degree of tricuspid regurgitation (TR), the peak blood flow velocity during systole across the tricuspid valve may be measured using continuous wave Doppler (CWD), as described in Chapter 3. The pressure gradient across the tricuspid valve may be calculated using the simplified Bernoulli equation (Equation 4-2). If this value is added to the estimated or measured RA pressure, the RV end-systolic pressure (RVESP) may be measured. In the absence of right ventricular outflow tract obstruction, pulmonary artery (PA) systolic pressure will be the same as RVESP. For example,

$$P_{RV} = P_{TR} + P_{RA}$$

If TR velocity = 3.0 m/s and RAP = 8 mm Hg, then:

$$RVESP = (TR\ maximum\ velocity)^2 \times 4 + RAP$$
$$RVESP = (3)^2 4 + 8$$
$$RVESP = PA\ systolic = 44\ mm\ Hg$$

Similarly, pulmonary regurgitation (PR) velocity represents the diastolic pressure difference between the PA and the RV. Therefore, PA diastolic pressure = RV end-diastolic pressure (RVEDP) + 4 × (PR end-diastolic velocity)^2, assuming that RVEDP is equal to RAP (estimated or measured). Similarly, mitral regurgitation (MR) jet velocity represents the systolic pressure difference between the left ventricle (LV) and the left atrium (LA). In patients without LVOT obstruction or aortic stenosis, systolic blood pressure (SBP) is essentially equal to LV systolic pressure; therefore, LAP is equal to SBP $- 4 \cdot \times (MR)^2$. Finally, aortic regurgitation (AR) velocity reflects the diastolic pressure gradient between the aorta and the LV. In summary:

$$PAP\ systolic = RVESP = 4 \times (TR)^2 + RAP$$
$$PAP\ diastolic = 4 \times (PR)^2 + RAP$$
$$LAP = SBP - 4 \cdot \times (MR)^2$$
$$LVEDP = DBP - 4 \cdot \times (AR)^2$$

Stevenson compared six different echocardiographic techniques to measure PA pressure.[1] When compared with direct measurements, some of these techniques yielded highly accurate correlations ($r = 0.97$), but they were not applicable in all patients.

Doppler Measurements of Flow: Velocity-Time Integral (VTI)

In addition to measuring gradients, the measurements of blood flow velocity may be used to estimate flow within a given structure. The derivative of a function is the slope of the curve at a given point, while an integral of a function is the area under the curve between two points along its x-axis. Given an equation that would describe distance transversed, the time derivative or slope at any given point would represent its velocity; the time derivative of the velocity at any given point would be its acceleration (Fig. 4-1). Similarly, given a graph of acceleration versus time, the integral would yield a velocity measurement; the integral of a velocity-versus-time graph would yield a distance traversed. A CWD velocity profile is a display of velocity versus time. If one integrates this velocity profile between two time points (i.e., calculates the area under the curve), the distance traversed of "a region of blood" flowing during this period may be estimated. Since flow velocity is not constant throughout a flow cycle, all of the flow velocities during the entire ejection period is integrated to measure "distance traversed" of this "region of blood." This integration of flow velocities in a given period of time is called the *velocity-time integral* (VTI) and yields length or distance (in centimeters [cm] or meters [m]). When flows at a particular location along the LVOT or aorta are required (i.e., spacial specificity is necessary), PWD should be used, provided the velocity does not exceed the PW Nyquist limit. High pulse repetition frequency (HPRF) may also be used. Multiple "ROI" points may be seen indicating range ambiguity of the cursor. If the velocities are too high, it is not possible to localize the jet without assumptions.

VTI may be used to calculate flow. The cross-sectional area (CSA) for a circular orifice such as the LVOT is:

$$CSA = \pi \, (D/2)^2 \qquad \text{(Equation 4-3)}$$

where D represents the diameter obtained by two-dimensional (2D) imaging. Flow across a given orifice is equal to the product of the CSA of the orifice and distance transversed during a single cardiac cycle, as calculated by the VTI. This is the formula for a "cylinder" of blood: exactly what would fill a cylindrical container of area CSA and height VTI. Stroke volume (SV) and cardiac output (CO) may thus be calculated as:

$$SV = CSA \times VTI \qquad \text{(Equation 4-4)}$$

$$CO = SV \times HR \qquad \text{(Equation 4-5)}$$

Use of these equations entails a number of assumptions, including (1) laminar blood flow in the area interrogated, (2) a flat or blunt flow velocity profile such that the flow across the entire CSA interrogated is relatively uniform, and (3) Doppler angle of incidence between the Doppler beam and the main direction of blood flow is less than 20 degrees, so that the underestimation of the flow velocity is less than 6%.

A number of Doppler methods have been attempted to calculate SV. Probably the most popular and accepted utilizes the left ventricular outflow tract (LVOT) approach. Other methods using the mitral, tricuspid, and pulmonic orifices have been attempted with variable results. Their respective accuracy is dependent upon the angle between the insonated Doppler signal and blood flow. It should be noted, however, that the major determinant of variability in estimating SV by any technique is the accuracy of the CSA measurement. As described by Equation 4-3, the measurement of the CSA is directly proportional to the square of the radius; therefore, any error in diameter measurement would be squared in the final results.

A second source of variability in measuring flow involves proper recording of reproducible Doppler signals. If the LVOT is chosen as the CSA, the VTI should be obtained from the Doppler signal at this level. For this purpose, the systolic forward flow must be obtained from either a deep transgastric or transgastric long-axis view. The sample volume of the pulsed Doppler should be placed in the high portion of the LVOT *exactly* at the same level where the diameter was measured. Occasionally the Doppler signal is difficult to obtain, and

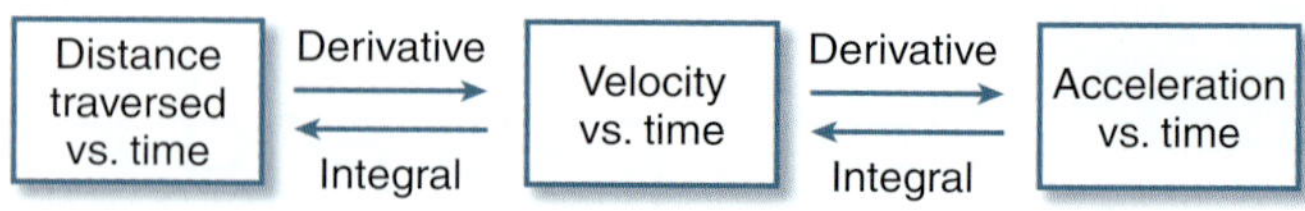

Figure 4-1 Relationship among distance, velocity, and acceleration. Derivative of function of position versus time results in its velocity; derivative of velocity at any given point would be its acceleration. Conversely, the integral of acceleration over time is velocity, and the integral of velocity over time is distance traversed. This is a Doppler spectral display of velocity versus time. Integrating this spectrum between two time points (i.e., calculating the area under the curve), distance traversed during this period may be calculated.

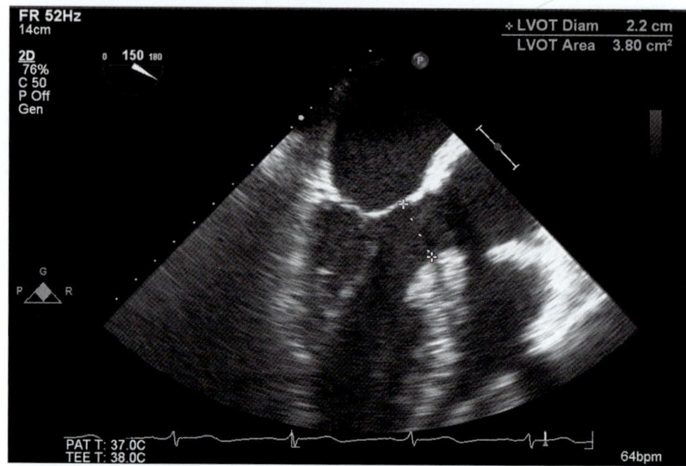

Figure 4-2 Mid-esophageal long-axis view. Diameter of left ventricular outflow tract is measured.

the morphology of the spectrum may be similar to a triangle with a spike at the peak velocity rather than a round "bell-shaped" flow signal. Under such circumstances, it is inappropriate to estimate the VTI because under- or overestimations are likely to result. If attention is given to proper recording techniques, interobserver variability in measuring the aortic VTI in normal subjects should be less than 5%.

An example of the use of PWD to measure stroke volume is illustrated in Figure 4-2, where the mid-esophageal long-axis view is used to image the LVOT. The diameter of the LVOT is 2.2 cm, which corresponds to a radius of 1.1 cm. As described earlier:

$$\begin{aligned} CSA &= \pi \, r^2 \\ &= 3.14 \, (1.1)^2 \\ &= 3.80 \text{ cm}^2 \end{aligned}$$

In Figure 4-3, a PWD spectrum is measured through the LVOT as imaged in the deep transgastric view, and the VTI is calculated as 19 cm. The stroke volume is:

$$\begin{aligned} SV &= CSA * VTI \\ &= 3.8 * (19) \\ &= 72 \text{ cm}^3 \end{aligned}$$

Three-dimensional (3D) echocardiography may increase the accuracy of CO measurements. Since geometric variability is more easily compensated in these measurements, end-systolic and end-diastolic volumes may be calculated and CO determined. Culp et al. compared 3D echocardiographic determinations of CO with thermodilution during the pre-cardiopulmonary bypass period in 20 patients undergoing cardiac surgery.[2] In their study, the mean bias was 0.27 L/min with ±35% limits of agreement. They observed good correlation between these two measurements, but there were both significant bias and wide

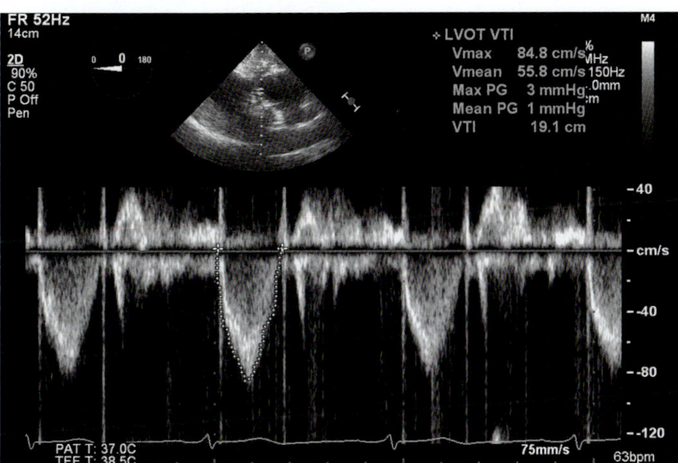

Figure 4-3 Velocity-time integral through left ventricular outflow tract. Since spatial specificity is necessary, a pulse wave Doppler spectrum is used.

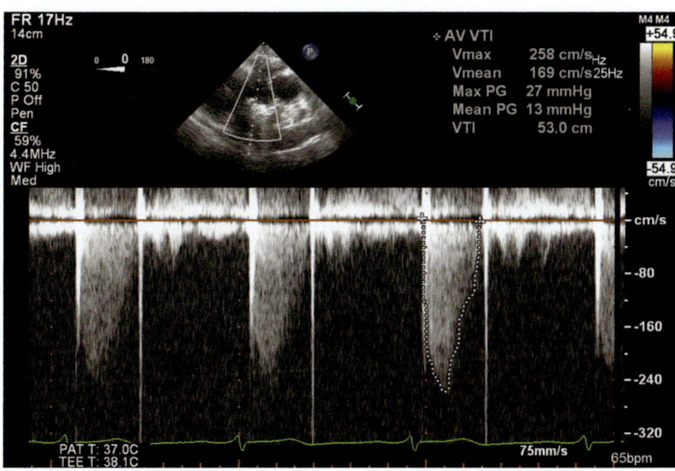

Figure 4-4 Velocity-time integral through aortic valve. Since high velocities through stenotic aortic valve are expected, continuous wave Doppler is used.

limits of agreement between the measurements. Off-line analysis of 3D echocardiographic images may be used to estimate CO. In a study of 40 patients undergoing heart transplantation, 3D echocardiographic reconstruction of LV end-diastolic and end-systolic volumes were estimated, allowing for calculation of SV and CO.[3] These CO measurements were correlated closely with thermodilution-derived measures, with a mean bias of 0.06 L/min and a standard deviation of 0.4 L/min. It should be noted, however, that each measurement required approximately 3 minutes per case, and poor image quality precluded analysis in four patients. Transthoracic 3D echocardiographic determination of SV was highly correlated to catheterization data.[4] These 3D data sets tended to underestimate the SV by 7.5 mL or 17%.

As already noted, homogenous laminar flow and a cylindrical outlet are assumed during Doppler measurements, but unfortunately this may not be the case. Here, 3D color Doppler echocardiography may be used to more accurately define the CSA of either the LVOT or mitral valve, as well as more accurately describe blood flow through these areas. In 3D color Doppler determination of CO, multiple 2D echocardiographic slices with their associated Doppler data are obtained through a particular surface. Flow data may be computed by summing of all velocity components normal to the surface.

Continuity Equation

The continuity equation describes the conservation of a physical quantity, such as energy and mass. In clinical echocardiography, this implies that blood flow in one portion of the heart must be equal to the blood flow in another portion. Assuming there are no intracardiac shunts, blood passes through atria to ventricles to arteries. In simple terms, what goes in must come out.

This application of the continuity equation is commonly used to calculate the aortic valve area (AVA). For AVA calculation, it is assumed that blood flow (stroke volume) at the level of the LVOT must be equal to blood flow through the aortic valve. As discussed earlier, SV may be estimated by multiplying the CSA of a particular orifice by the VTI over one cardiac cycle through that orifice. When estimating the severity of aortic stenosis, SV through the LVOT is measured to calculate the unknown CSA of the aortic valve.

Using either the deep transgastric or transgastric long-axis view, the Doppler spectra of the aortic valve and LVOT are displayed. Since spatial specificity is necessary for the LVOT measurement, PWD is used. The high velocities detected across the stenotic AV usually preclude use of PWD because of aliasing (i.e., exceeding the Nyquist limit), so CWD is used. The loss of special specificity with CWD is not important, since physiologically the highest-velocity flows **must** be across the stenotic aortic valve **if** that is the smallest orifice. Once these Doppler spectra

have been obtained, the VTI over one cardiac cycle through each of these structures is calculated. The diameter of the LVOT is then measured in a mid-esophageal long-axis view.

The continuity equation states that the SV through the LVOT must equal the SV through the AV, or:

$$SV_{LVOT} = SV_{AV} \qquad \text{(Equation 4-6)}$$

Substituting the stroke volume equation into the continuity equation,

$$CSA_{LVOT} \times VTI_{LVOT} = AVA \times VTI_{AV} \qquad \text{(Equation 4-7)}$$

Re-arranging the terms,

$$AVA = CSA_{LVOT} \times VTI_{LVOT}/VTI_{AV} \qquad \text{(Equation 4-8)}$$

Since the LVOT is essentially cylindrical, the CSA_{LVOT} may be estimated by:

$$CSA_{LVOT} = \pi \, (radius_{LVOT})^2 = \pi \, (diameter_{LVOT}/2)^2$$
$$\text{(Equation 4-9)}$$

The CWD spectrum through the aortic valve of the above patient is illustrated in Figure 4-4. In this case, the peak velocity is approximately 2.6 m/sec, which corresponds to a peak gradient of 27 mm Hg. The VTI through the AV is 53 cm. Using Equation 4-8 and the values obtained in the above illustration from Figures 4-1 and 4-2:

$$AVA = CSA_{LVOT} * VTI_{LVOT}/VTI_{AV}$$
$$= 3.8 \text{ cm}^2 * 19 \text{ cm}/53 \text{ cm}$$
$$= 1.36 \text{ cm}^2$$

Multiple sources of error may affect the calculation of AVA using the continuity equation.[5] LVOT measurements may vary from 5% to 8%, so when it is squared in the continuity equation, this may become a large source of error. Since the accuracy of the SV measurement through the LVOT assumes laminar flow, any sources of turbulence will affect results. In the presence of aortic insufficiency, compensatory increases in systolic velocities may result in a skewed velocity profile.

Although multiplane transesophageal echocardiography (TEE) planimetric estimations of AVA may be flawed by heavy aortic valvular calcification, measurements using the continuity equation are accurate compared with Gorlin-derived values.[6,7] In a study using TEE, Stoddard et al. reported good correlation between AVA measurements using the continuity equation and planimetry; however, they reported a steep learning curve for the acquisition of a suitable transgastric long-axis view that adequately aligns flow through the aortic valve with the ultrasound beam.[8]

Proximal Isovelocity Surface Area (PISA)

Another application of the conservation of mass and energy may be used to quantify the severity of valvular regurgitation, most commonly mitral regurgitation (MR), using proximal isovelocity surface area (PISA). Quantification of MR by PISA assumes that as blood flows toward a regurgitant lesion, flow converges radially and accelerates.[9] This convergence occurs along increasing isovelocity hemispheres that converge on the regurgitant lesion (Fig. 4-5). The flow through any of these shells must be equal to the flow through any of the other shells as well as the regurgitant valve orifice. Color flow Doppler (CFD) may be used to identify these hemispheres of increasing velocity proximal to the lesion (identified by aliasing), and flow may be determined. Prior to performing the PISA calculations, a well-defined hemisphere must be imaged at the point of CFD aliasing (see Fig. 4-5). This may be performed by either reducing the Nyquist limits or by shifting the CFD mapping baseline toward the direction of flow.

Flow at a given point in time may be calculated as:

$$\text{Flow} = (\text{velocity}) \times (\text{area}) \qquad \text{(Equation 4-10)}$$

It should be noted that this calculation of flow is an instantaneous flow measurement and must be differentiated from the SV and CO measurements (of volume) discussed earlier.

Applying Equation 4-10, the flow through a well-defined hemisphere is:

$$\text{Flow} = (\text{velocity at hemisphere}) \, (\text{surface area of hemisphere})$$

$$\text{(Equation 4-11)}$$

$$\text{The surface area of a hemisphere} = 2 \pi r^2$$

$$\text{(Equation 4-12)}$$

where r is the radius of the hemisphere. Then flow through a hemisphere at the point of aliasing at a given time is:

$$\text{Flow through ``PISA shell}= 2 \pi r^2 \, v_n$$

$$\text{(Equation 4-13)}$$

where v_n is the Nyquist limit.

Similarly, applying Equation 4-10 to the regurgitant mitral valve,

$$\text{Flow through the regurgitant mitral valve} = (\text{ROA}) \, (V_o)$$

$$\text{(Equation 4-14)}$$

where *ROA* is the area of the regurgitant orifice area, and V_o is the maximal regurgitant velocity.

Applying the continuity equation, flow through these isovelocity spheres equals flow through the regurgitant lesion, and Equations 4-13 and 4-14 may be combined to:

$$2 \pi r^2 \, v_n = \text{ROA} \, V_o \qquad \text{(Equation 4-15)}$$

Solving for ROA yields:

$$\text{ROA} = 2 \pi r^2 \, v_n/V_o \qquad \text{(Equation 4-16)}$$

For example, in Figure 4-5, the radius of the PISA shell is 0.48 cm when the Nyquist limits are set at 39 cm/sec. Figure 4-6 is the CWD spectrum through the regurgitant mitral valve. The maximum velocity is 471 cm/sec. Applying Equation 4-16,

$$\begin{aligned}
\text{ROA} &= 2 \pi r^2 \, v_n/V_o \\
&= 2 \pi \, (0.48)^2 (39)/471 \\
&= 0.12 \text{ cm}^2
\end{aligned}$$

Once the ROA is calculated, regurgitant volume may be determined. Applying the principle in Equation 4-4 that states that volume is the product of cross-sectional area VTI, the regurgitant volume may be determined by multiplying the area of the regurgitant lesion (ROA) by the velocity-time integral of the regurgitant velocity (VTI_{regurg}):

$$\text{Regurgitant volume} = \text{VTI}_{regurg}(\text{ROA}) = \text{VTI}_{regurg}(2 \pi r^2 v_n/V_o)$$

$$\text{(Equation 4-17)}$$

Applying the VTI calculated in Figure 4-6, the regurgitant volume is 18 mL. The PISA method of determining MR is time-consuming, but it has been validated as a method of identifying patients with severe MR.[10] Generally, it is more accurate for a central jet compared with an eccentric one.[9] Since the hemispheric radius is squared, care must be taken to ensure and measure a well-defined shell.

If the Nyquist limits are set for 40 cm/sec, and assuming the patient has "normal" systolic blood pressures (difference between systolic LV pressure and LA pressure is $\approx$ 100 mm Hg, corresponding to a Doppler velocity of 5 m/sec [500 cm/sec]), the calculation of ROA may be estimated to be:

$$\begin{aligned}
\text{ROA} &= 2 \pi r^2 v_n/V_o \\
&= 2 \pi r^2 (40)/500 \\
\text{ROA} &= r^2/2 \qquad \text{(Equation 4-18)}
\end{aligned}$$

where r is the radius of the PISA shell in centimeters.[11]

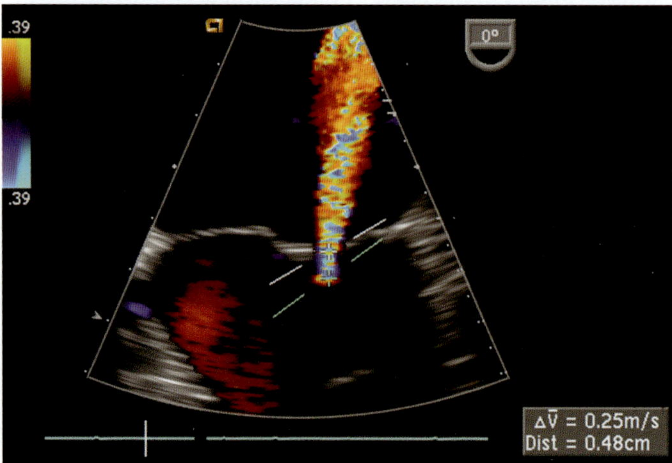

Figure 4-5 Proximal isovelocity surface area (PISA) illustration. As blood flows toward a regurgitant lesion, flow converges radially, which occurs along increasing isovelocity hemispheres.

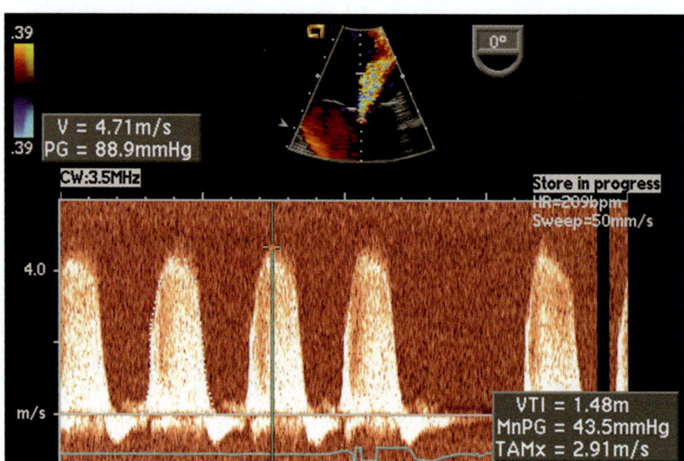

Figure 4-6 Continuous wave Doppler spectrum through mitral valve during systole.

REFERENCES

1. Stevenson JG. Comparison of several noninvasive methods for estimation of pulmonary artery pressure. *J Am Soc Echocardiogr.* 1989;2:157.
2. Culp Jr WC, Ball TR, Burnett CJ. Validation and feasibility of intraoperative three-dimensional transesophageal echocardiographic cardiac output. *Anesth Analg.* 2007 Nov;105(5):1219-1223.
3. Hoole SP, Boyd J, Ninios V, Parameshwar J, Rusk RA. Measurement of cardiac output by real-time 3D echocardiography in patients undergoing assessment for cardiac transplantation. *Eur J Echocardiogr.* 2008 May;9(3):334-337.
4. Fleming SM, Cumberledge B, Kiesewetter C, Parry G, Kenny A. Usefulness of real-time three-dimensional echocardiography for reliable measurement of cardiac output in patients with ischemic or idiopathic dilated cardiomyopathy. *Am J Cardiol.* 2005 Jan 15;95(2):308-310.
5. Baumgartner H, Hung J, Bermejo J, et al. Echocardiographic assessment of valve stenosis: EAE/ASE recommendations for clinical practice. *J Am Soc Echocardiogr.* 2009;22:1-23.
6. Cormier B, Iung B, Porte JM, et al. Value of multiplane transesophageal echocardiography in determining aortic valve area in aortic stenosis. *Am J Cardiol.* 1996;15:882.
7. Hoffmann R, Flachskampf FA, Hanrath P. Planimetry of orifice area in aortic stenosis using multiplane transesophageal echocardiography. *J Am Coll Cardiol.* 1993;22:529.
8. Stoddard MF, Hammons RT, Longaker RA. Doppler transesophageal echocardiographic determination of aortic valve area in adults with aortic stenosis. *Am Heart J.* 1996;132:337.
9. Chandra S, Salgo IS, Sugeng L, et al. A three-dimensional insight into the complexity of flow convergence in mitral regurgitation: adjunctive benefit of anatomic regurgitant orifice area *Am J Physiol Heart Circ Physiol.* 2011 Sep;301(3):H1015-H1024:Epub 2011 Jun 10.
10. Xie G, Berk MR, Hixson CS, et al. Quantification of mitral regurgitant volume by the color Doppler proximal isovelocity surface area method: a clinical study. *J Am Soc Echocardiogr.* 1995;8:48.
11. Lambert AS. Proximal isovelocity surface area should be routinely measured in evaluating mitral regurgitation: a core review. *Anesth Analg.* 2007;105:940-943.

$$\text{Figure MVA 1st} \longrightarrow SV_{MVA} \; \underline{\text{NO PISA}} \qquad (\text{Figure RgVol 1st}) \longrightarrow EROA$$

$$RgVol \quad S_{MV} - SV_{LVOT}$$

$$S_{MV} = MVA \times TVI\,mrjet$$

$$SV_{LVOT} = CSA_{LVOT} \times TVI_{LVOT}$$

$$MVA = 220/PHT \quad \begin{array}{l}CE\\ PISA\end{array}$$
$$760/OT$$

$$EROA = RgVol / VTI\,mrjet$$

$$R\% = RgVol / SV_{MV}$$

$$\underline{PISA} \qquad (\text{Figure } EROA \; 1st \longrightarrow RgVol)$$

$$EROA = PISA / Vpeak\,mrjet$$

$$RgVol = EROA \times VTI\,mrjet$$

$$PISA = 2 \times \pi \times r^2 \times Va \times \alpha/180$$
$$6.28 \times r^2 \times Va \times \alpha/180$$
$$\alpha\,(\approx 120 - 130)$$

$$\text{If Nyquist} = 40 \; + pt \; has \; norm \; BP \quad SBP - LAP => 100$$
$$\text{then } EROA = r^2/2$$

$$\underline{\text{For AI}}$$

$$RgVol = SV_{LVOT}\,(AV) - SV_{MV}\,(or\,RVOT)$$

$$EROA = RgVol / VTI\,AIjet$$

$$Reg\% = RgVol / SV_{LVOT}$$

$$RgVol = EROA \times VTI_{AIjet}$$

$$LV\,Inflow < LV\,Outflow \; \bar{c}\,AI$$

$$LV\,inflow > LV\,outflow \; \bar{c}\,MR$$

Principles and Physics: Transducer Characteristics

IVAN S. SALGO | RONALD A. KAHN

Transducers

As discussed in Chapter 2, piezoelectric crystals convert ultrasound (pressure waves) into electrical signals and vice versa. Specifically, when presented with high-frequency electrical signals, these crystals produce ultrasound energy and, conversely, produce electrical alternating current signal from ultrasound energy. During most ultrasound applications, a 1- to 2-microsecond ultrasound pulse is emitted from the piezoelectric crystal, which is directed toward the areas to be imaged, after which the crystal "listens" for the returning echoes for a given period of time. The time delay between the pulse emission and its detection is proportional to the distance of the objects of interest, which allows image display (Fig. 5-1).

Current two-dimensional (2D) systems transmit and receive acoustic beams in a 2D scanning plane. Typically, a conventional transducer consists of 64 to 128 elements spaced according to the ultimate frequency (and hence wavelength) of the acoustic vibrations; these propagate radially along the direction of the scanline. This array of elements steers the outward ultrasound beam by utilizing interference patterns generated by varying the spatiotemporal phase of each element's transmit event (Fig. 5-2). More simply stated, if all of the crystals are stimulated simultaneously, the summated beam is steered directly forward; if the crystals are stimulated sequentially from right to left, the summated beam is steered leftward. As opposed to M-mode (one spatial and one temporal dimension), 2D scanning systems sweep a scanline within this 2D imaging plane; the angular position of the beam is said to vary in the "azimuthal" dimension. Even though traditional 2D scanning consists of two spatial dimensions plus one temporal dimension, we do not call this "three-dimensional (3D) imaging." These principles are common to any phased array system.[1]

Resolution is the ability to distinguish two point targets as distinct. A scanline is not a perfectly "thin" line but actually has width or "fuzziness." The thickness of the line varies with depth, focus, and other physical parameters.[2] Physicists call this the *point spread function*. *Focus* is the act of bringing the point spread function as finely as possible on a target. If targets are in the near field, the focus must be adjusted to the near field. Increasing the size of the aperture improves the ability to focus. However, the physical aperture cannot be too large or the probe tip cannot be placed within the esophagus. Radiology probes used to scan the liver have much larger apertures and ability to focus.

A conventional transesophageal probe consists of a handle, insertion tube, bending neck, and tip. Conventional probes for 2D imaging have 64 elements mounted on a "stack" (Fig. 5-3). The electrical pulses can have a driving potential of 50 volts or greater, so electrical isolation is important. The spacing of the elements (known as *pitch*) determines the limits of resolution. Modern systems typically use a pitch of a quarter wavelength. As higher ultrasound frequencies are used, the wavelength increases and approaches this distance between elements. When the element spacing is greater than one half a wavelength ($\lambda/2$), relatively large-magnitude angular grating lobes occur. In practice, grating lobes are not seen, since modern systems do not exceed the frequency limit whereby the ultrasound wavelength is greater than the pitch.

The stack also contains a lens and backing. The lens couples the acoustic wave to the esophagus. The backing limits the return of ultrasound pulses reflected from the back of the tip to the lens. A row of 64 elements are mounted on a turntable that rotates from 0 to 180 degrees. This rotation allows multiplane capability by rotating this turntable during 2D imaging. These probes only generate a relatively "flat" beam that interrogates a 2D slice. Modern 2D transducers therefore consist of thousands of electrically active elements that steer a scanline "left and right" as well as "up and down." Newer materials that allow more bandwidth (i.e., simultaneous high and low frequencies) allow these matrix array transducers to produce images with both higher penetration and resolution.[3]

True 3D ultrasound steering has been the subject of much academic and industrial research that began in the 1980s. To steer an ultrasound beam, a 2D matrix array comprising equal elements in the elevational and azimuthal dimension were fabricated by "dicing" a block of transducer material with a diamond-tipped saw to create each element (Fig. 5-4). Today's 3D imaging matrix array transducers comprise thousands of elements and can have over 60 rows and columns. Note that this is a "2D matrix array" that generates "3D images." Electrical independence of the individual elements makes steering possible. This steering allows both azimuthal and elevational independence, thus allowing for a true 3D scanline. Although possessing electrically independent rows, early transducers did not have every element electrically active; the technology to connect such a dense array was not yet developed. Newer types of electrical circuitry independently connecting each element were first commercialized in 2002.

Three-dimensional imaging transesophageal probes are more complex but have no moving parts at the imaging tip other than the ability to flex the bending neck (Fig. 5-5). Currently, miniaturization has allowed the fitting of thousands of fully sampled elements into the tip of a transesophageal ultrasound transducer. The physical aperture has to be designed for the application. The wider the aperture in each dimension, the better the scanline can be focused. To steer the beam in the left-right and up-down directions, 3D matrix array transesophageal echocardiography (TEE) probes use temporal variation in the stimulation sequence of the elements (in the "checkerboard").

Beamforming

Beamforming constitutes the steering and focusing of transmitted and received scanlines. Each element must have independent electrical control by the ultrasound system; a conventional cable that would be used to connect each element would make the transducer cable unwieldy. To reduce both the size of the cable and power consumption, a significant portion of the beam steering is performed within the transducer in highly specialized integrated circuits. The main system steers at coarse angles, but the transducer circuits steer in fine increments in a process termed *micro-beamforming*. This creates a 3D spherical wedge of acoustic information that is subsequently processed.

The resonance frequency (RF) data is summed and processed using various signal techniques and finally converted into rectangular (Cartesian) space by a 3D scan converter in circuitry and software; this

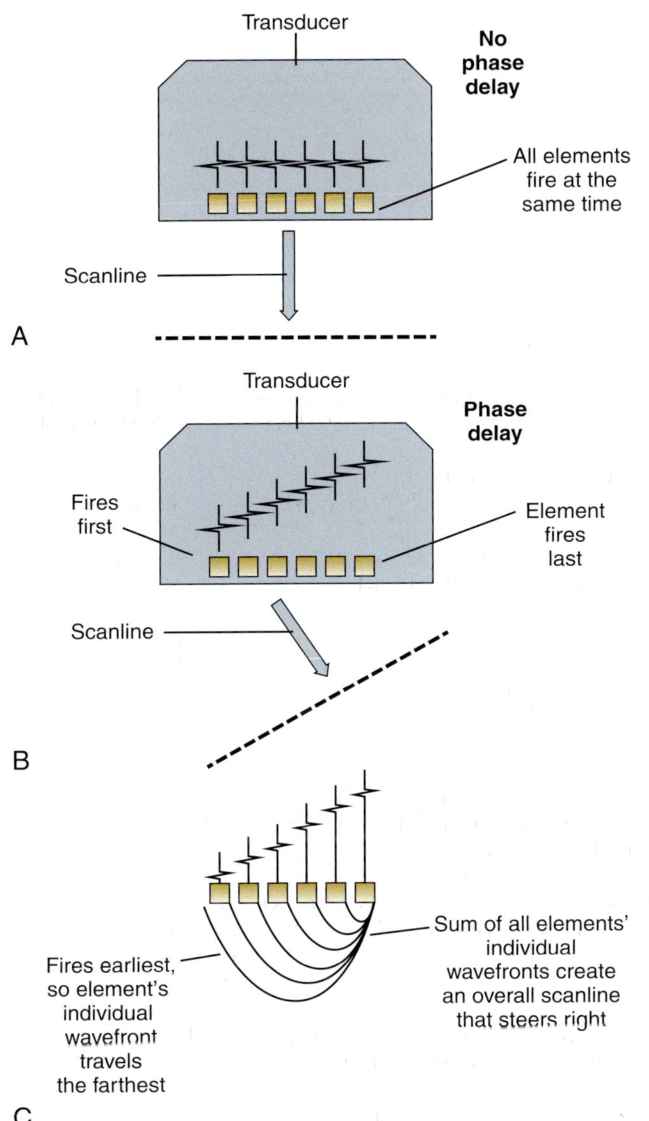

Figure 5-1 Beamforming controls delay of transmit events and creates scanlines. If all elements fire at the same time, the effective wavefront travels straight ahead of the elements. The sum of each element's wavefront creates a scanline. If elements to one side are phase delayed, beam steers in that direction. **A,** Scanline steers straight ahead. **B,** Scanline steers to right, since element on figure's right are delayed the longest. **C,** Effective summation of elements' individual wavefronts create an effective overall wave called a *scanline*.

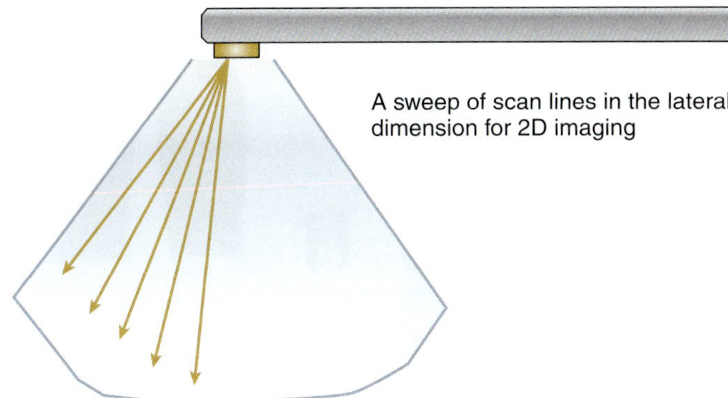

Figure 5-2 A two-dimensional image is created by sweeping ultrasound scanlines at an angular line spacing; the less the spacing, the higher the resolution. However, firing more scanlines per frame (for constant depth) lowers frame rate, so frame rate must be balanced against resolution.

1st TEE generation

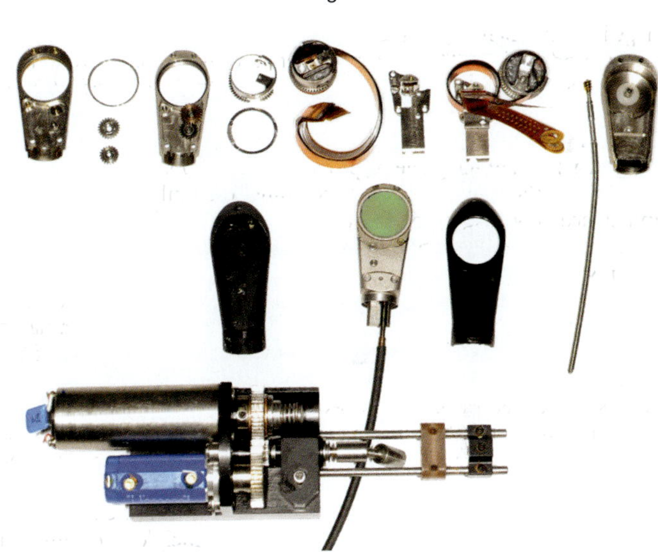

Figure 5-3 A multiplane transducer consists of a "stack" of ultrasound elements, lens, and window, shown in green. Motor below (located in handle) rotates a cable that moves turntable from 0 to 180 degrees; gears used in assembly are shown. Electrical connections to elements (under green lens) are shown at top, as well as flexible bands. Typically, potentials of 50 to 100 V are used to fire elements; housing is therefore electrically isolated.

is an extension of the traditional phased array approach. Older 3D techniques used in the 1990s did not steer electronically, but rather involved combining 45 to 100 cardiac loops and recombining them to create a 3D data set. This works for static structures, but irregular rhythms limited gated reconstruction of many beats. Any transducer movement during acquisition of these many gates created artifacts and required a significant amount of smoothing of the data. While this reduced attention to "slippage" or misalignment, it reduced the overall image quality if significant stitching was required.

There are two major black-and-white modes in an electronically steered 3D system. The first is a "live" mode where the system scans in real time in 3D; if the transducer is removed, the image disappears. As with sector scanning, the volume pyramid may be reduced to a wide sector–focused mode. With current computer and

beamforming processing power, the speed of sound within tissue is the limiting factor. Larger-volume pyramids at greater distances from the element matrix result in very low frame rates in which the temporal resolution limits the diagnostic value. Gating as few as 4 to 8 cardiac cycles facilitates the generation of wider-volume pyramids while maintaining the frame rate. This is performed by "stitching" four or more gates together in a large-sector mode. This can generate greater than 90-degree scanning volumes at frame rates greater than 30 cycles/sec (Hz). In patients with arrhythmias, RR intervals that fall out of a set range result in the discarding of the errant subvolume, and the system scans again until all subvolumes are generated from suitable beat intervals. Thus, in patients with irregular intervals, so long as the average RR rate falls within a reasonable range, a full volume can be reconstructed.

4th TEE generation

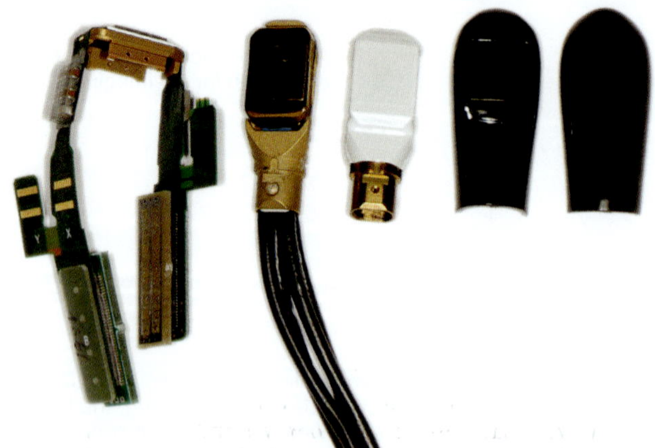

Figure 5-4 Modern two-dimensional (2D) matrix array of a three-dimensional transesophageal echocardiography (TEE) probe has no moving parts in probe tip (i.e., no gears, cables, etc.). The 2D matrix array is shown under foil on left.

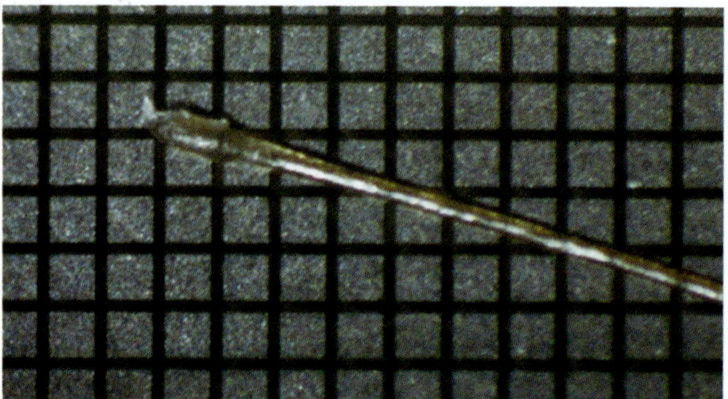

Figure 5-5 A two-dimensional matrix array comprising equal elements in elevational and azimuthal dimension are fabricated by "dicing" a block of transducer material with a diamond-tipped saw to create each element. A human hair is shown.

REFERENCES

1. Blackstock DT. Fundamentals of Physical Acoustics. *John Wiley Interscience.* 2000.
2. Kinsler LE, Frey AR, Coppens AB, Sander JV. *Fundamentals of Acoustics.* 4th ed. John Wiley; 2000.
3. Szabo TL. *Diagnostic Ultrasound Imaging: Inside Out.* Academic Press; 2004.

6

Principles and Physics: Imaging Artifacts and Pitfalls

IVAN S. SALGO | RONALD A. KAHN

Ultrasound travels as transverse waves in the direction of propagation, with compression and expansion of tissue occurring in the direction of travel. Because both light and ultrasound are wave phenomena, wave physics have a large role in image generation. Understanding wave physics is essential to correctly interpret artifacts that do not represent pathologic structures. Furthermore, it is essential to understand the limitations of ultrasound so the underlying anatomy and pathology are assessed correctly.

Ultrasound imaging consists of transduction, beamforming, and image presentation. To create the best possible image, each of these processes should be optimized by adjusting the transmission frequency, gain, image brightness, and contrast. The transducer should use a transmission frequency appropriate for the sector length. Higher frequencies will result in the best resolution of a given object of interest, but they are attenuated more than lower frequencies, limiting their penetration. *Gain* may be thought of as a volume control. Adjusting the overall and sector time gain compensation does not affect the magnitude of the transmitted ultrasound but changes the manner of its display. System processing, such as "smoothing," can average out small structures like small plaques or vegetations. Finally, image brightness and contrast should be optimized for faint structures. Altogether these adjustments are known as *optimizing signal-to-noise ratio*.

Reflection and Multipath

The ultrasound beamformer assumes a direct line of travel to and from a target. Specular targets, such as prosthetic valves, can cause ultrasound waves to "veer off." This mirroring can cause ultrasound energy to be reflected in other directions. In Figure 6-1, there are two targets; the ultrasound beam is directed toward target 1. Most of the energy is reflected from this target to the transducer and is accurately imaged. A portion of the energy is reflected from target 1 to target 2 and returns to the transducer after following a circuitous path. Since "time-of-flight" is equivalent to depth, the longer length of the multipath transmission will be interpreted as a deeper target along the original axis (i.e., in the axis of target 1), resulting in artifact production.

Refraction

Refraction artifact is similar to a multipath artifact. In a multipath artifact, the echo lines are reflected between two targets. In a refraction artifact, the ultrasound beam is bent by a refractor (Fig. 6-2). Ultrasound scanlines are all directed in a straight path. During their transit, however, some may be refracted (steered off at an angle). These refracted beams may then be reflected back toward the transducer. The machine measures both the refracted and non-refracted echoes, but assumes that all the returned echoes traveled along a straight path. Thus, two images are seen: the true image of the target formed by the straight path echoes, and a false double image seen in line with the refracted beams.

Ringing, Rattling, and Reverberation

Structures of interest are usually imaged by assuming an ultrasound pulse is reflected once by an object of interest. The dimensions of the

object are generally determined by the duration between the emitted and received signal. Certain targets of high acoustical impedance, however, may trap ultrasound waves and result in a to-and-fro reflection of ultrasound energy within it. This reverberation may be seen as either a mirror artifact or as a linear reverberation ("ringdown"). For example, when one attempts to image a beaker, one beaker wall will be closer to the transducer and one farther away. If ultrasound energy is reflected *once* from each beaker wall, the object will be accurately imaged, but it is possible for an ultrasound wave to continue to be reflected between the beaker walls, thus delaying return of this ultrasound energy to the transducer. Since the ultrasound transducer has no means of differentiating a singly reflected wave from a wave that has been reflected multiple times, a copy of the image appears in the far field (Fig. 6-3 and Video 6-1). Alternatively, ultrasound energy may be trapped within a very thin object. This trapping of ultrasound energy in this small space may result in a continuous return of ultrasound energy to the transducer, which will be displayed as an echogenic line called *linear reverberation* or "ring-down." This vibration or rattling of the target causes bright targets to appear but limits interrogation in the far field beyond the reverberating target.

Attenuation

As discussed in Chapter 2, ultrasound energy may be absorbed (converted to heat) and reflected by tissues and other targets. As ultrasound is propagated through tissues, these interactions cause ultrasound to lose signal strength, making images appear faint and bright tissues appear dark in the far field. This phenomenon is known as *attenuation*. There are several determinants of these interactions (as previously discussed), but the major factor that may be easily controlled is the ultrasound frequency. Higher frequencies afford greater resolution but attenuate more rapidly than lower frequencies. In contrast, lower frequencies are better at far-field imaging. Systems typically have settings that allow adjustment of frequency.

Reflective Shadowing

The degree of reflection of ultrasound images is primarily determined by the difference in acoustic impedances of structures. There may be an interface with a structure of low acoustic impedance (e.g., air) or, more commonly, a structure of high acoustic impedance, such as a prosthetic valve or calcium. When these structures are encountered, most if not all of the ultrasound energy is reflected back to the transducer. The object itself will appear to be very echogenic (Fig. 6-4 and Video 6-2). These strong reflectors can also prevent further transmission of ultrasound energy, causing echolucent streaks known as "shadows." These shadows appear as "black" flashlight patterns originating from the reflecting echogenic structure. For example, flecks of calcium on a highly calcified aortic valve can prevent imaging beyond or "below" the valve. If the entire valve is heavily calcified, it will be impossible to image beyond it. Where far-field imaging is limited by a physical phenomenon, other views and windows must be employed to accurately image the structures of interest.

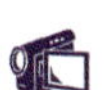

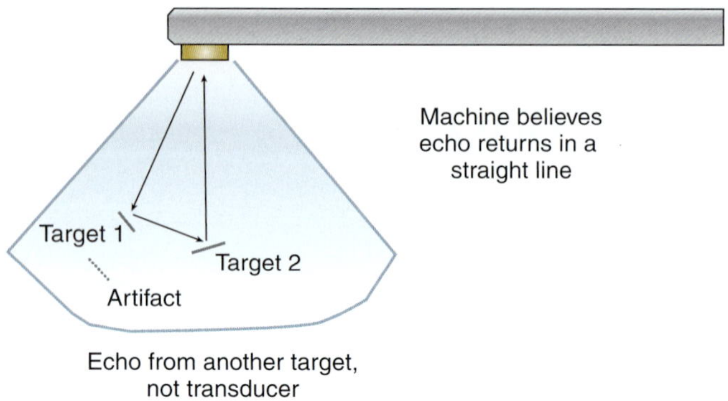

Figure 6-1   Multipath artifacts are caused by echoes striking two targets. Internal reflection between targets within the scanning field can cause this artifact.

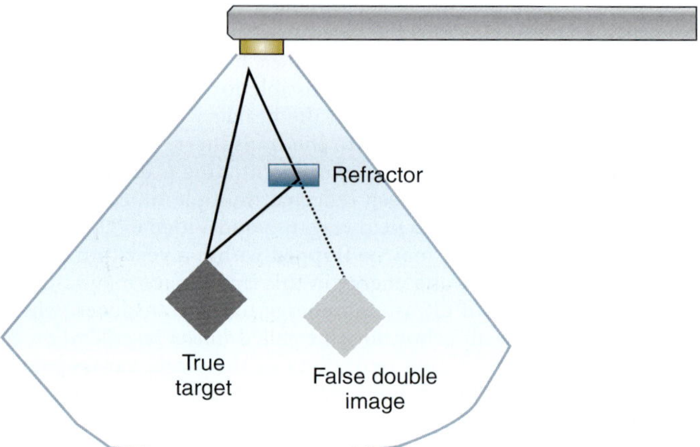

Figure 6-2   Refraction can bend ultrasound energy away from a straight path. These bent lines appear "straight" to the beamformer, so a double image is created. The beam is first transmitted to the true target. Some energy returns back on axis. However, some off axis energy travels back to a refractor which steers the energy back to the transducer for receive. Since the received energy is at a different angle from the true target, a false double image appears.

Near-Field Clutter

To produce ultrasound signals, the piezoelectric crystals vibrate at a high frequency. Although this is a necessary component of ultrasound wave generation, the vibrations of the crystals may interfere with image formation close to the transducer, resulting in near-field clutter. This artifact is commonly seen during epiaortic ultrasonography when the probe is held on the anterior surface of the ascending aorta. The near-field clutter limits anterior wall imaging. This clutter may be eliminated by using an echogenic spacer between the transducer and the object of interest so the objects are physically removed from the very near field of the transducer.

Side Lobes

During image formation, the software assumes the ultrasound beams originate and are transmitted from the center of the transducer;

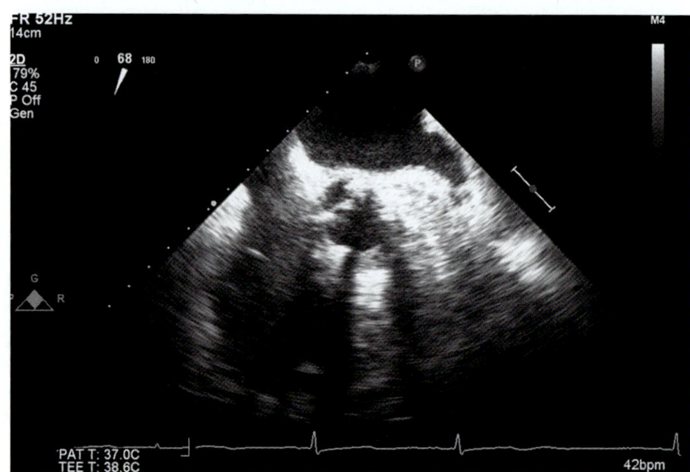

Figure 6-4   Reflective shadowing. Dark lines extending downward in image are created by early reflections of transmitted ultrasound energy. No more energy can penetrate into far field, so shadows appear where there is no acoustic energy "seen" by the beamformer (see Video 6-2). 

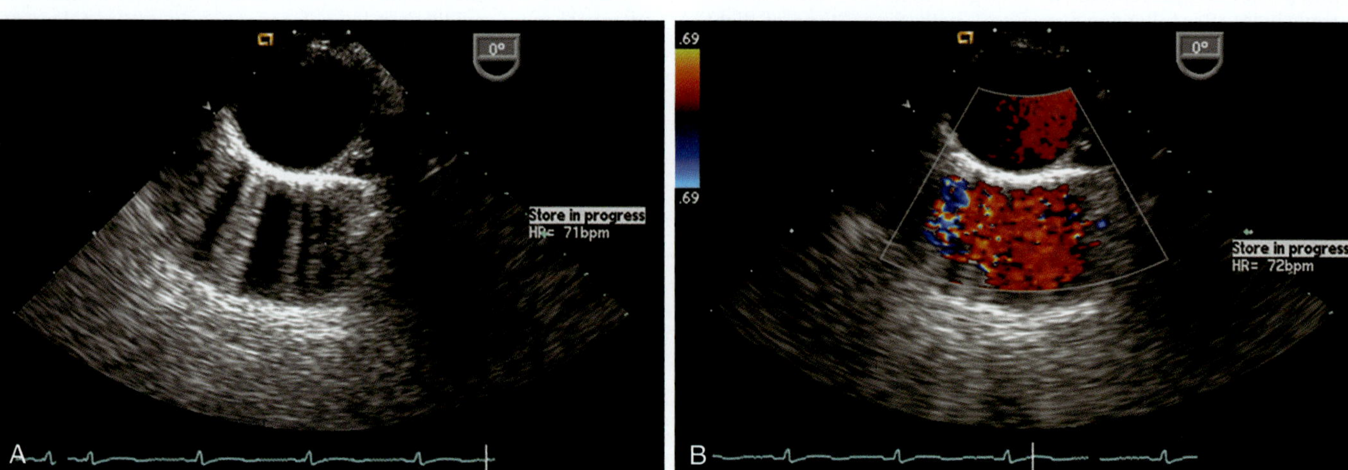

Figure 6-3   Reverberation. **A,** Two examples of reverberation in descending aorta in cross-section. Aortic calcification resulted in "rattling" of acoustic energy, or internal reflections. These internal excitations result in linear reverberations or "ring-down," resulting in bright "flashlight" artifacts. Second, while aorta is clearly imaged in near field, an additional mirror image of aorta is seen in far field as well (see Video 6-1). **B,** Application of color flow Doppler reveals flow in both true aortic lumen and reverberation.

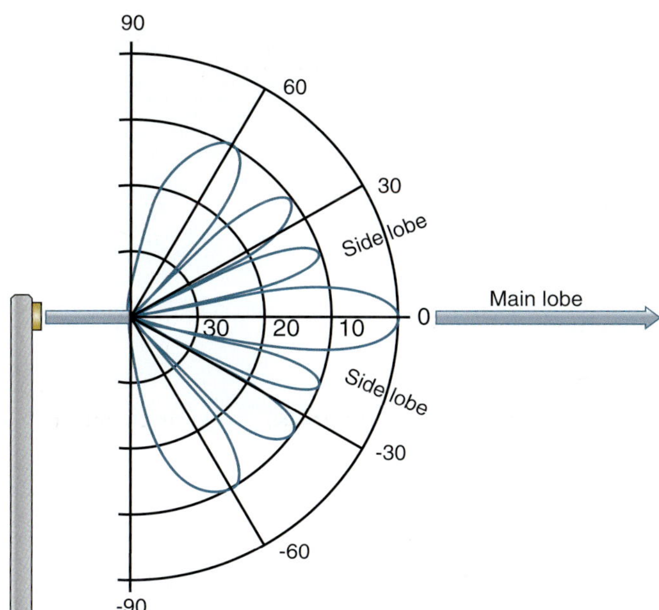

Figure 6-5 Ultrasound energy is not transmitted in a perfectly straight line but is the summation of excitations from multiple elements. These create a main lobe of energy (transmit line), but energy gets created on sides of main lobe. Side lobes are exaggerated here for illustrative purposes.

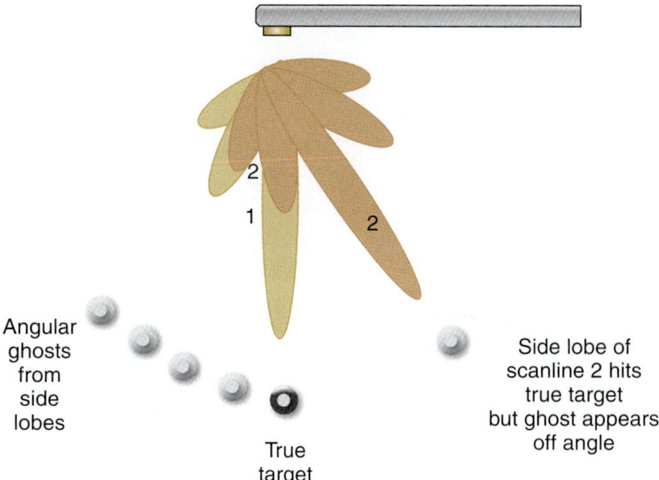

Figure 6-6 Side lobes create an "angular smear" of a target image even though there is only one target.

unfortunately, this is not always the case. Instead of producing a narrow beam of ultrasound, the ultrasound signal is emitted as multiple radiation lobes at various angles. Energy generated from the probe's aperture is summed as a constructive and destructive interference pattern. The best "construction" forms the main lobe of energy. However, smaller lobes of energy can be transmitted off the side of the transducer as well (Fig. 6-5). The intensity of the side lobe energy decreases with the increasing angle of production. When reflections return from these side lobes, the software cannot differentiate these signals from those received from the main lobe. Side lobes superimpose echoes of structures located to the side of the target with echoes from the target itself, so structures to the side of the main transducer beam appear to be more centrally located (Fig. 6-6). Generally these side lobes produce images that are not anatomically accurate; structures may appear in large echolucent areas such as the left atrium or descending aorta (Fig. 6-7 and Video 6-3). Since the ratio of main to side lobe energy is quite large, these side lobe artifacts are usually not as echogenic as the centrally imaged structures. Production of these echoes generally increases the noise in the image, but a bright metal reflector (e.g., prosthetic valve) can transmit significant side lobe energies.

Grating Lobes

A grating lobe is a type of side lobe. It is created by multiple elements in a phased array probe or antenna. When the element spacing is greater than one half a wavelength ($\lambda/2$), relatively large-magnitude angular lobes occur, which tend to be significantly larger than side lobes. Since manufacturers ensure that the elemental spacing remains lower than this wavelength threshold, grating lobes do not normally occur in practice.

Suboptimal Focusing and Lateral Resolution

As noted, the transmit beam is not "perfectly thin." As discussed in Chapter 2, an unfocused ultrasound beam contains a near field and a far field. The near field is usually characterized by a relatively parallel set of ultrasound waves, whereas the far field contains divergent waves similar to an inverted funnel (Fig. 6-8). The width and divergence of the main lobe affects resolution. As targets lie farther than the focal zone, the beam width or point spread function gets larger. This means that point-like structures in the focal zone start to appear flatter farther away from the focus. This divergence reduces lateral resolution, or the ability to resolve objects perpendicular to the direction of the ultrasound wave. Although ultrasound beams may be focused using acoustic lenses, thus increasing lateral resolution, the length of the near field continues to be dictated by the ultrasound frequency and transducer diameter.

Range Ambiguity

During image generation, the piezoelectric crystal emits a short ultrasound burst, after which it "listens" for the returning signals. Most of the time the ultrasound machine is listening for the returning signal. As with sonar in submarines, ultrasound systems calculate the target distance by measuring the amount of time required for the emitted ultrasound signal to return to the crystal. Whereas the velocity of sound is roughly a constant, the distance of an object may be easily calculated:

Length from tip = (Speed of sound in tissue)/(Round trip time/2)

This assumption will work assuming that all returning echoes originated from the original emitted ultrasound burst. However, it may be possible that ultrasound waves from a previous duty cycle were reflected from a very deep structure and may be returning late (Fig. 6-9). In this case, the deep structure may appear to be more superficial. For example, if a target from a previous emitted pulse travels a long way and hits a very deep target at 30 cm, it can return on the next duty cycle and appear within the image, for example, at 15 cm. This is because the system "stopwatch" has confused the prior transmit event with the one it has just fired.

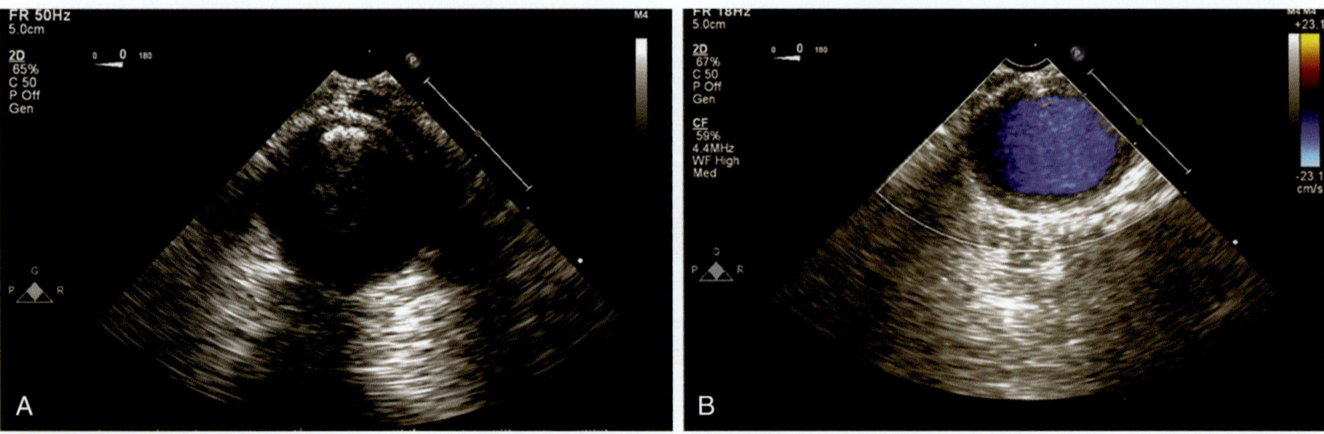

Figure 6-7   Side lobes. Descending aorta is imaged in cross-section. **A,** Central portion of aorta is usually echogenic, but in this example contains a fluffy echogenic side lobe artifact (see Video 6-3). **B,** Color Doppler spectrum is superimposed on image. Laminar flow is seen throughout entire lumen. If this side lobe artifact were a true structure in lumen, aortic blood flow would have been affected.

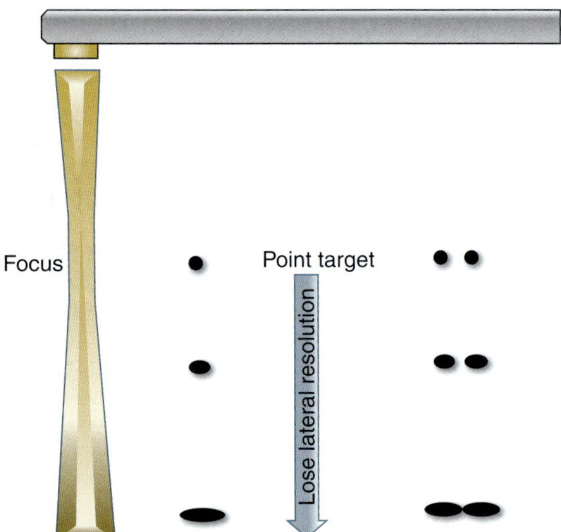

Figure 6-8   Targets do not appear point-like as the ultrasound beam spreads out.

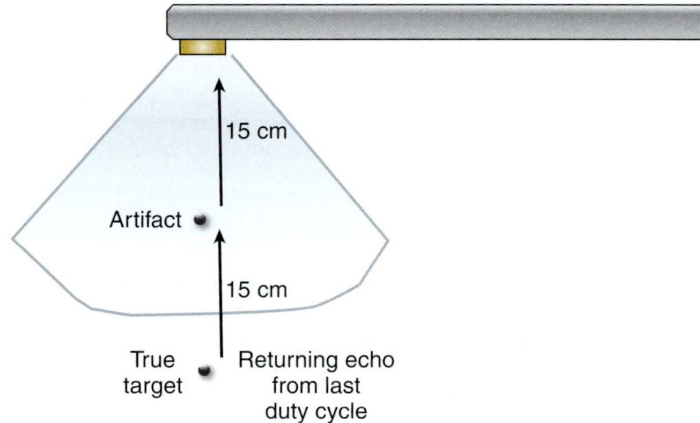

Figure 6-9   Range ambiguity artifacts from an earlier returning signal. The machine assumes an echo from a far target is from the current duty cycle. A target 30 cm away from the transducer appears to be 15 cm deep.

REFERENCES

1. Blackstock DT. *Fundamentals of Physical Acoustics.* New York: Wiley-Interscience; 2000.
2. Kinsler Lawrence E, Frey Austin R, Coppens Alan B, James V. *Fundamentals of Acoustics.* 4th ed. Sanders, John Wiley; 2000.
3. Szabo Thomas L, Lewin. *Diagnostic Ultrasound Imaging: Inside Out.* Academic Press; 2004.

Normal Anatomy and Flow During the Complete Examination: Components of the Complete Examination

JEREMY S. POPPERS | SANSAN S. LO | DAVID J. WEST | TERESA A. MULAIKAL | MICHELLE M. LIAO | JACK S. SHANEWISE

Introduction

Each clinician develops his or her own systematic approach to the assessment of valvular pathology and biventricular function. In this chapter, we discuss a structure-based approach to the normal transesophageal echocardiography (TEE) exam (Table 7-1). In the operating room, it may be prudent to first obtain the Doppler and three-dimensional (3D) full-volume images, since the use of electrocautery will interfere with image acquisition using these modalities.

Left Atrium, Pulmonary Veins, and Left Atrial Appendage

The left atrium (LA) lies directly anterior to the esophagus and is the structure in closest proximity to the TEE probe. It appears at the apex of the image sector and is the receiving chamber for pulmonary venous inflow. The left atrial appendage (LAA) is imaged within the LA. The coronary sinus runs posterior to the LA in the atrioventricular groove, returning deoxygenated blood to the right atrium. The circumflex artery branches from the left main coronary artery and runs in the anterior portion of the left atrioventricular groove lateral and inferior to the LA.

The pulmonary veins are often imaged in conjunction with the LA and mitral valve because of both anatomic proximity and physiologic relevance in the assessment of mitral regurgitation and diastolic function. The left pulmonary veins can be imaged in the midesophageal (ME) two-chamber (Fig. 7-1, Video 7-1) and four-chamber (Fig. 7-2, Video 7-2) views. From the ME two-chamber view, the left upper pulmonary vein can be seen above the level of the LAA on the right side of the image sector by withdrawing the probe slightly along with leftward rotation. The ideal multiplane angle to view the left upper pulmonary vein will vary and may be found anywhere from 0 (ME four-chamber) to 90 degrees (ME two-chamber). Once the upper pulmonary vein has been identified, slightly advancing the probe further will occasionally bring the left lower pulmonary vein into focus as it converges with the left upper pulmonary vein.

The right upper and lower pulmonary veins may be imaged by starting with the ME four-chamber view. Slight rightward rotation while slowly withdrawing the probe will reveal the veins as they merge and drain into the LA. Alternatively, the right upper pulmonary vein may be located by first finding an ME long-axis view (Fig. 7-3, Video 7-3) and then rotating the probe to the right. The vein will appear at the right lower portion of the image sector as it passes posterior to the superior vena cava (SVC) into the LA.

There are four phases to the normal pulmonary venous Doppler flow velocity profile (Fig. 7-4). Place the pulsed wave Doppler gate 1 cm into the pulmonary vein to assess the inflow patterns. There is an antegrade systolic component, or S wave, composed of two phases, S1 and S2, but frequently seen as a single peak. S1 represents LA relaxation during systole, and S2 represents the effects of left ventricular contraction and mitral regurgitation if present. The third phase of the pulmonary venous Doppler flow velocity profile, the D wave, corresponds to the antegrade flow seen in early diastole. The A_r wave is the final phase, in which there is retrograde flow into the pulmonary veins during late diastole as a result of atrial contraction.[1,2]

Left Ventricle

A comprehensive evaluation of the left ventricle (LV) includes an assessment of its chamber size, wall thickness, and function. LV function is assessed both qualitatively and quantitatively. Qualitative assessment of LV function is a skill developed over time and should frequently be checked against accepted quantitative measures of LV function (e.g., endocardial fractional shortening, fractional area change, method of disks, full-volume 3D, etc.). Segmental wall motion is assessed by analyzing each segment for endocardial excursion (movement of endocardium toward center of LV) and wall thickening. Normal endocardial excursion is greater than 30%, and normal wall thickening is 30% to 50%.[3]

To assist in describing LV function and regional wall motion abnormalities, the LV is described using a 17-segment model[4] in which the LV is divided into four levels from base to apex: basal, mid-, apical, and apical cap (Fig. 7-5). The basal level is divided circumferentially into six segments: basal anteroseptal, basal anterior, basal anterolateral, basal inferolateral, basal inferior, and basal inferoseptal. The mid-level is also divided circumferentially into six segments: mid-anteroseptal, mid-anterior, mid-anterolateral, mid-inferolateral, mid-inferior, and mid-inferoseptal. The apical level is divided circumferentially into four segments: apical anterior, apical lateral, apical inferior, and apical septal. The apical cap consists of the tip of the LV apex beyond the end of the LV cavity. When describing LV function, it is recommended that each segment of the 17-segment model be analyzed individually and in more than one view. A numeric scoring system is used to classify LV function of each segment based qualitatively on each segment's motion and systolic thickening: normal or hyperkinesis = 1, hypokinesis = 2, akinesis (negligible thickening) = 3, dyskinesis (paradoxical systolic motion) = 4, and aneurysmal (diastolic deformation) = 5.[4]

At least three views are required to evaluate all segments of the LV. Use of all six views described provides some redundancy (segments seen in more than one view) and may improve the accuracy of regional wall motion assessment. Examination of LV function begins with the ME four-chamber view (see Fig. 7-2, Video 7-2). Slight retroflexion in this view may help avoid foreshortening of the LV during its assessment. Each segment of the LV is examined for regional wall motion abnormalities. In the ME four-chamber view, the following segments of the LV are evaluated: inferoseptal (basal, mid-, and apical), anterolateral (basal, mid-, and apical), and the apical cap. Next, the multiplane angle is increased until the ME two-chamber view (see Fig. 7-1, Video 7-1) is obtained; the following segments of the LV are evaluated: anterior (basal, mid-, and apical), inferior (basal, mid-, and apical), and

TABLE 7-1	Structure-Based TEE Exam	
Structure	**View**	**Diagnostic Utility**
LA	ME four-chamber	LA size; integrity of interatrial septum
	ME two-chamber	LA size; LAA morphology; left upper pulmonary vein inflow (with slight probe manipulation)
	ME bicaval	LA size; integrity of interatrial septum; bubble study
	ME LAX	Right upper pulmonary vein inflow
LV	ME four-chamber	LV function; LV size
	ME two-chamber	LV function
	ME LAX	LV function
	TG basal SAX	LV function
	TG mid SAX	LV function; LVEDD; LV wall thickness
	TG two-chamber	LV function
MV	ME four-chamber	MV morphology; MV pathology; transmitral inflow
	ME mitral commissural	MV morphology; MV pathology; MV medial-lateral annular diameter; transmitral inflow
	ME two-chamber	MV morphology; MV pathology; transmitral inflow
	ME LAX	MV morphology; MV pathology; MV anterior-posterior annular diameter
	TG basal SAX	MV morphology; MV pathology
	TG two-chamber	Subvalvular apparatus
	Deep TG LAX	Subvalvular apparatus
AV	ME AV SAX	AV leaflet morphology; AV pathology
	ME AV LAX	AV pathology; measurements of LVOT, AV annulus, SV, STJ, and ascending aorta
	TG LAX	AV pathology; LVOT VTI; AV VTI
	Deep TG LAX	AV pathology; LVOT VTI; AV VTI; calculation of left ventricular stroke volume
RA	ME four-chamber	RA size; coronary sinus; integrity of interatrial septum
	ME bicaval	RA size; integrity of interatrial septum; bubble study; presence of foreign bodies in RA (e.g., wire for central venous line/cannula, pacemaker leads, etc.)
RV	ME four-chamber	RV function; RV size; TAPSE
	ME RV inflow-outflow	RV function
	TG mid SAX	RV function; RV size
	TG RV inflow	RV function; subvalvular apparatus
TV	ME four-chamber	TV leaflet morphology; TV pathology
	ME RV inflow-outflow	TV leaflet morphology; TV pathology; estimation of PASP
	TG RV inflow	TV morphology; TV subvalvular apparatus
	TG mid SAX	TV morphology; TV pathology
PV	ME AV SAX	PV morphology; PV pathology
	ME RV inflow-outflow	PV morphology; PV pathology
	UE aortic arch SAX	Main PA diameter; PA VTI; calculation of right ventricular stroke volume
Ao	Descending aortic SAX	Size, shape, and integrity of descending Ao; atherosclerosis
	Descending aortic LAX	Size, shape, and integrity of descending Ao; atherosclerosis
	UE aortic arch LAX	Size, shape, and integrity of aortic arch; atherosclerosis
	UE aortic arch SAX	Main PA diameter; PA VTI; calculation of right ventricular stroke volume
	ME ascending aortic SAX	Size, shape, and integrity of ascending Ao; atherosclerosis; main PA diameter
	ME ascending aortic LAX	Size, shape, and integrity of ascending Ao at level of right PA; atherosclerosis; right PA diameter

Ao, Aorta; *AV*, aortic valve; *LA*, left atrium; *LAA*, left atrial appendage; *LAX*, long axis; *LV*, left ventricle; *LVEDD*, left ventricular end-diastolic dimension; *LVOT*, left ventricular outflow tract; *ME*, midesophageal; *MV*, mitral valve; *PA*, pulmonary artery; *PASP*, pulmonary artery systolic pressure; *PV*, pulmonic valve; *RA*, right atrium; *RV*, right ventricle; *SAX*, short axis; *STJ*, sinotubular junction; *SV*, sinuses of Valsalva; *TAPSE*, tricuspid annular plane systolic excursion; *TG*, transgastric; *TV*, tricuspid valve; *UE*, upper esophageal; *VTI*, velocity-time integral.

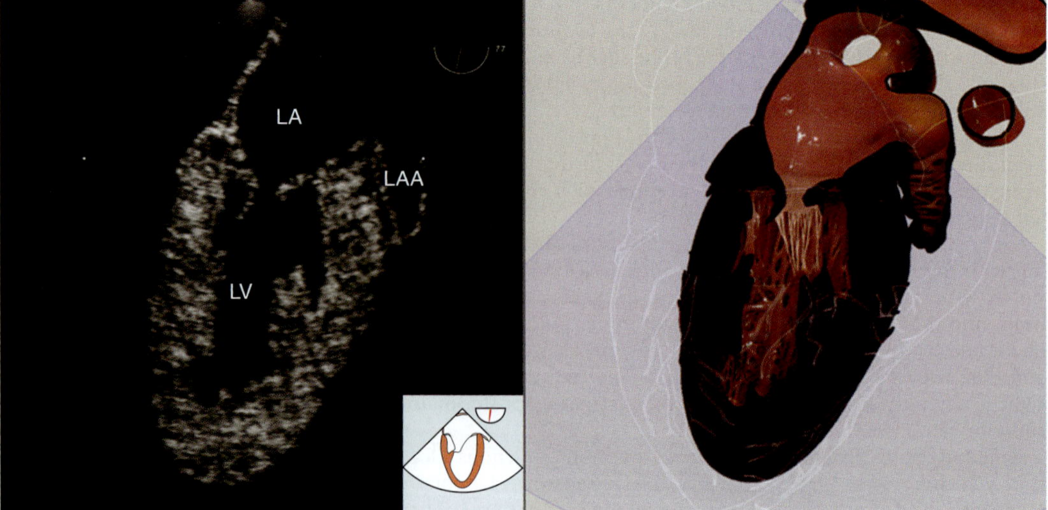

Figure 7-1 Midesophageal two-chamber view. *LA,* Left atrium; *LAA,* left atrial appendage; *LV,* left ventricle. *(Two-dimensional TEE images and three-dimensional pictures generated using software developed by Heartworks, Inventive Medical Ltd., London, UK.)*

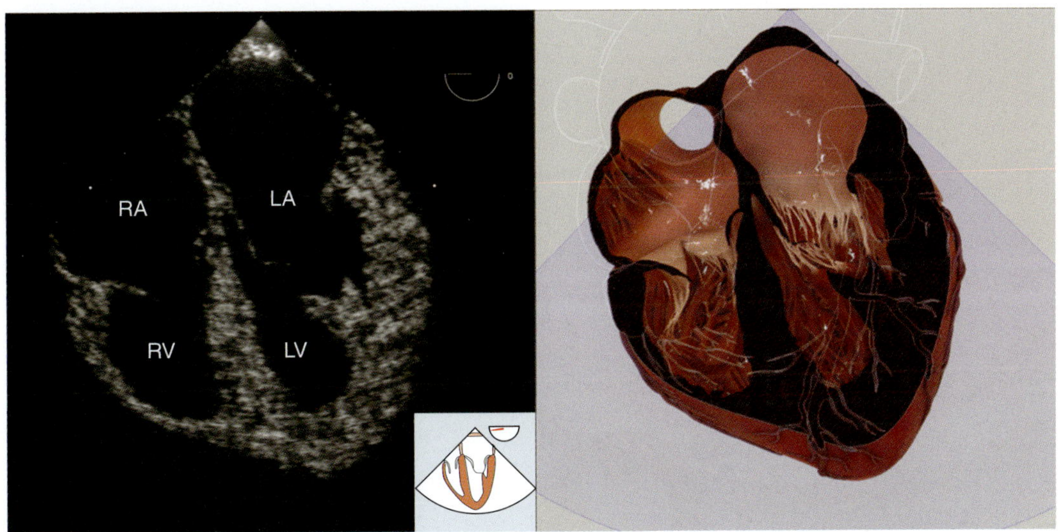

Figure 7-2 Midesophageal four-chamber view. *LA*, Left atrium; *LV*, left ventricle; *RA*, right atrium; *RV*, right ventricle. *(Two-dimensional TEE images and three-dimensional pictures generated using software developed by Heartworks, Inventive Medical Ltd., London, UK.)*

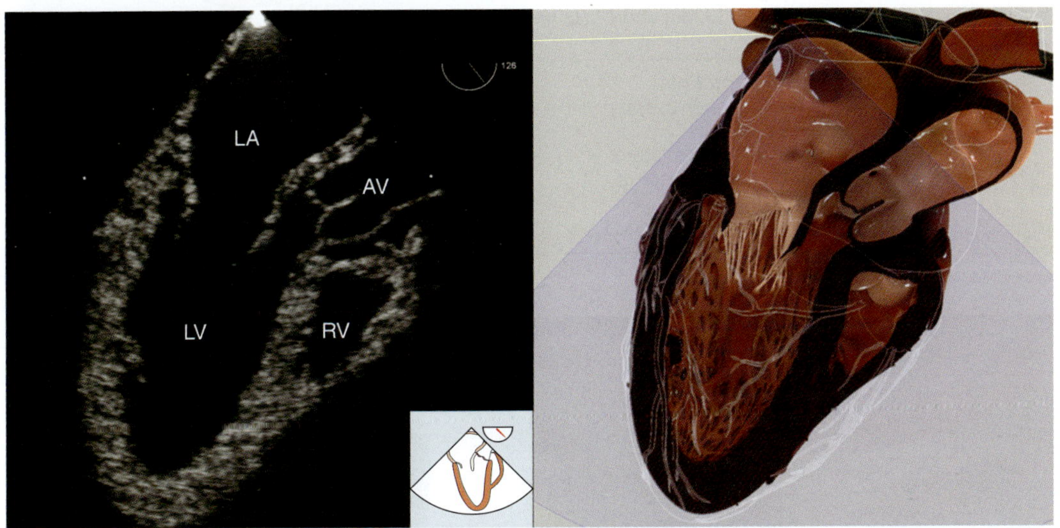

Figure 7-3 Midesophageal long-axis view. *AV*, Aortic valve; *LA*, left atrium; *LV*, left ventricle, *RV*, right ventricle. *(Two-dimensional TEE images and three-dimensional pictures generated using software developed by Heartworks, Inventive Medical Ltd., London, UK.)*

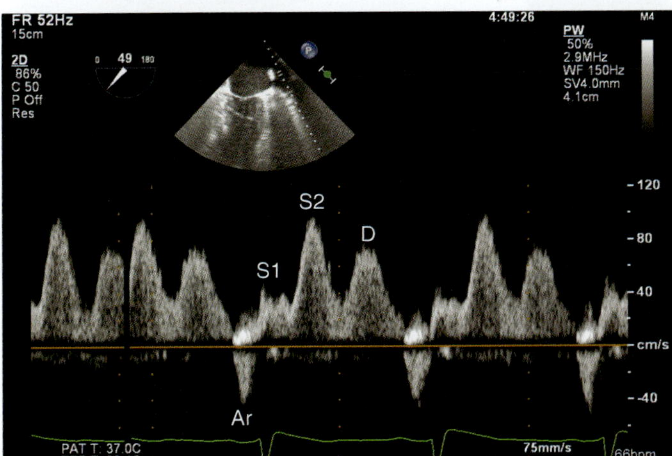

Figure 7-4 Normal pulse wave Doppler velocity profile of left upper pulmonary vein (LUPV) inflow. S1 corresponds to left atrial relaxation during systole. S2 represents effects of right ventricular contraction and mitral regurgitation during ventricular systole. D wave depicts antegrade blood flow from LUPV into left atrium in early diastole. A$_r$ wave is retrograde flow into LUPV during late diastole as a result of atrial contraction.

the apical cap. Next, the multiplane angle is increased to obtain the ME long-axis view (see Fig. 7-3, Video 7-3); the following LV segments are evaluated: anteroseptal (basal, mid-, and apical), inferolateral (basal, mid-, and apical), and the apical cap. Next, the probe is advanced into the stomach to obtain the transgastric (TG) basal short-axis view (Fig. 7-6, Video 7-4) to evaluate the following segments: basal anterior, basal anterolateral, basal inferolateral, basal inferior, basal inferoseptal and basal anteroseptal. Then the TG midpapillary short-axis view (Fig. 7-7, Video 7-5) is obtained to evaluate the following segments: mid-anterior, mid-anterolateral, mid-inferolateral, mid-inferior, mid-inferoseptal and mid-anteroseptal. The probe is then advanced slightly to evaluate the apex in short axis. Finally, increasing the multiplane angle to 90 degrees from the TG midpapillary short-axis image brings the TG two-chamber (Fig. 7-8, Video 7-6) into view. Here, the inferior wall is toward the top of the image sector, and the anterior wall lies at the bottom of the screen.

Determination of LV chamber size and wall thickness is most easily accomplished in the TG mid–short-axis view. Normal LV septal and inferolateral wall thicknesses are 0.6 to 0.9 cm for women and 0.6 to 1 cm for men. Normal LV end-diastolic diameter is 3.9 to 5.3 cm for women and 4.2 to 5.9 cm for men.[4] The electrocardiogram tracing should be used to ensure that measurements are made during the corresponding period of the cardiac cycle.

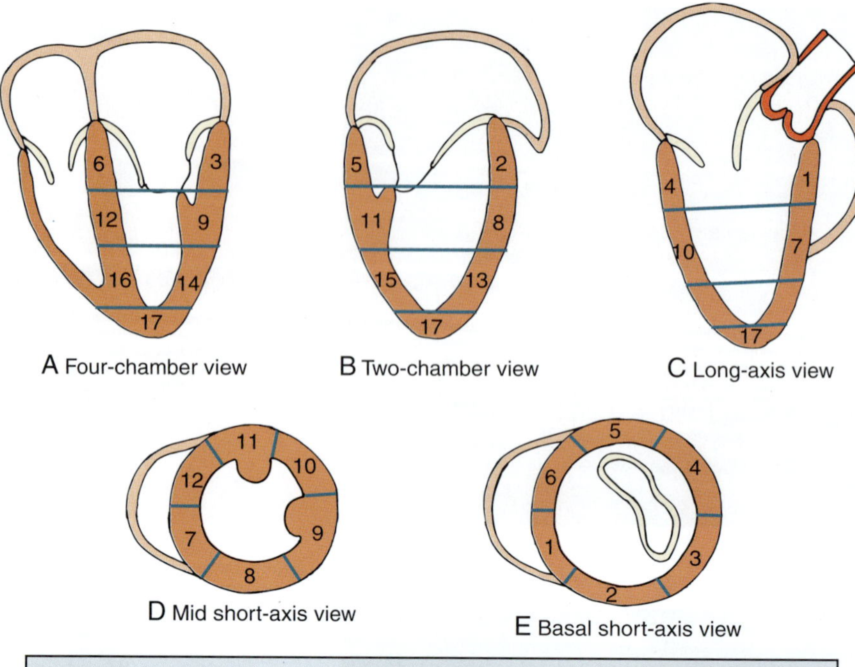

Basal Segments	Mid Segments	Apical Segments
1 = Basal anteroseptal	7 = Mid-anteroseptal	13 = Apical anterior
2 = Basal anterior	8 = Mid-anterior	14 = Apical lateral
3 = Basal anterolateral	9 = Mid-anterolateral	15 = Apical inferior
4 = Basal inferolateral	10 = Mid-inferolateral	16 = Apical septal
5 = Basal inferior	11 = Mid-inferior	17 = Apical cap
6 = Basal inferoseptal	12 = Mid-inferoseptal	

Figure 7-5   Left ventricular 17-segment model.

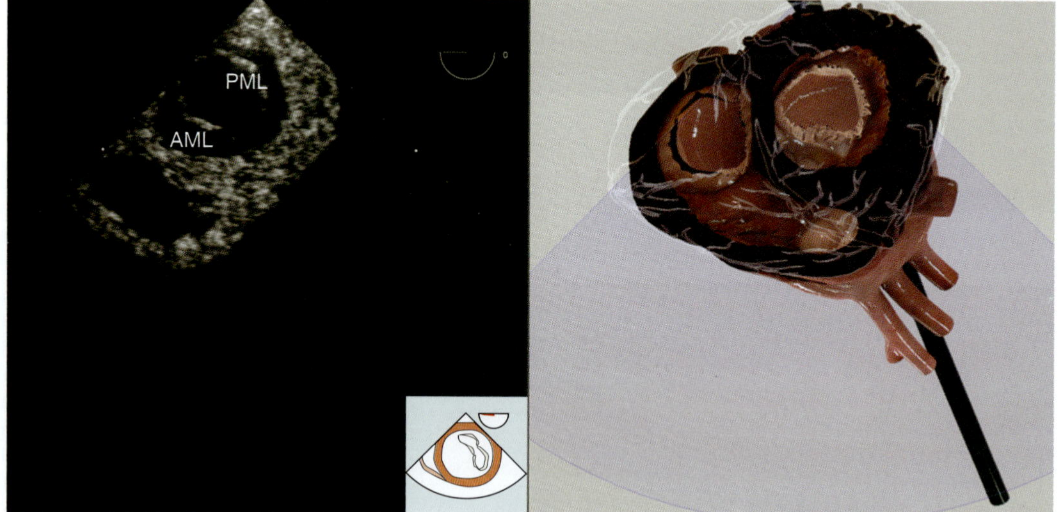

Figure 7-6 Transgastric basal short-axis view. *AML,* Anterior mitral leaflet; *PML,* posterior mitral leaflet. *(Two-dimensional TEE images and three-dimensional pictures generated using software developed by Heartworks, Inventive Medical Ltd., London, UK.)*

Mitral Valve

The bileaflet mitral valve is the conduit through which blood travels from the LA to the LV. The larger anterior leaflet comprises two thirds of the entire valve surface but is attached to only one third of the annular circumference.[5] The anterior mitral valve leaflet is adjacent to the left and noncoronary aortic valve cusps. The posterior leaflet is smaller and scalloped and makes up two thirds of the annular circumference. The nomenclature described by Carpentier is most commonly used to identify the multiple anatomic segments of the mitral valve leaflet (Fig. 7-9). From lateral to medial, the anterior leaflet is divided into the A1, A2, and A3 segments that are opposed by P1, P2, and P3 scallops of the posterior leaflet. The anterolateral and posteromedial commissures are the convergence points of A1 and P1, and A3 and P3, respectively. The anterolateral and posteromedial papillary muscles support the mitral valve leaflets and are associated with the similarly named commissure. Three orders of chordae attach the mitral valve to these papillary muscles. Primary chordae attach to the free edge of the mitral leaflets. Secondary chordae attach to the middle, or body, of the leaflets. Tertiary chordae attach only the posterior leaflet to the posteromedial papillary muscle. The mitral valve is in close proximity to the circumflex artery, coronary sinus, right fibrous trigone, and bundle of His, making these structures susceptible to injury during mitral valve surgery.[5]

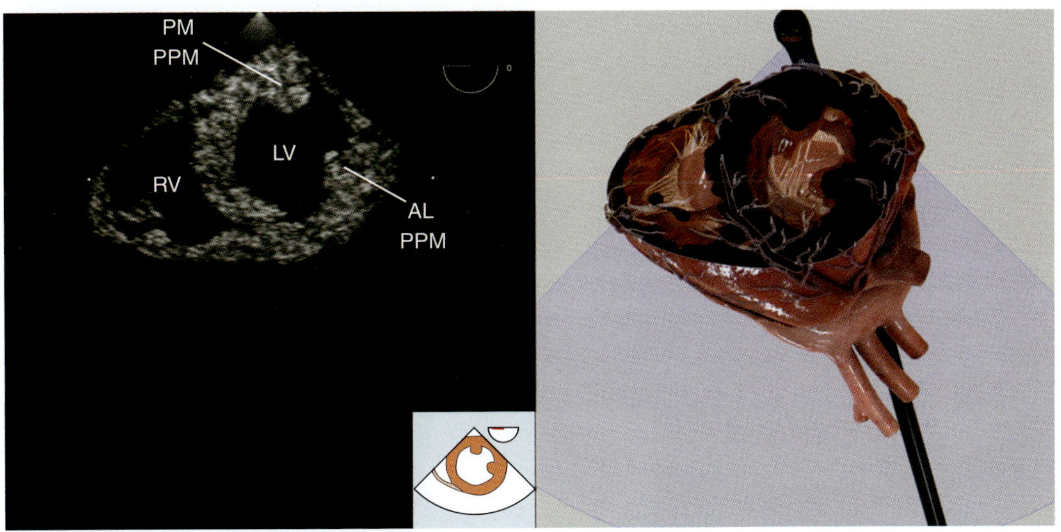

Figure 7-7 Transgastric midpapillary short-axis view. *AL PPM,* Anterolateral papillary muscle; *LV,* left ventricle; *PM PPM,* posteromedial papillary muscle; *RV,* right ventricle. *(Two-dimensional TEE images and three-dimensional pictures generated using software developed by Heartworks, Inventive Medical Ltd., London, UK.)*

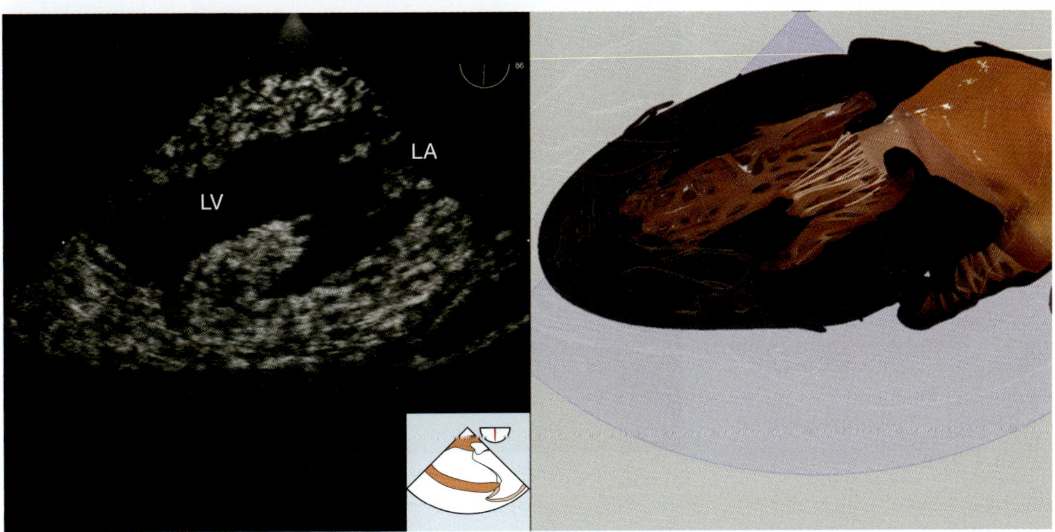

Figure 7-8 Transgastric two-chamber view. *LA,* Left atrium; *LV,* left ventricle. *(Two-dimensional TEE images and three-dimensional pictures generated using software developed by Heartworks, Inventive Medical Ltd., London, UK.)*

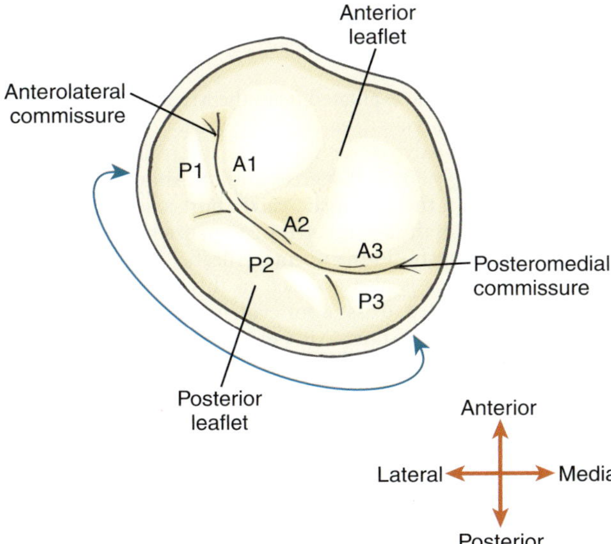

Figure 7-9 Mitral valve, depicting nomenclature used by Carpentier to describe the three scallops of posterior mitral leaflet and three segments of anterior mitral leaflet.

The mitral valve can be evaluated using the ME as well as TG views. In the ME four-chamber view (see Fig. 7-2, Video 7-2), the anterior leaflet will appear in the center of the image sector and the posterior mitral leaflet to the right of the image. Any abnormalities of the mitral apparatus such as excessive or restricted leaflet motion, annular or subvalvular calcification, or redundant or myxomatous leaflet tissue should be noted. Color flow Doppler (CFD) is useful to assess for mitral stenosis or regurgitation.

From the ME four-chamber view, rotate the multiplane angle to about 60 degrees for an ME mitral commissural view (Fig. 7-10, Video 7-7). The exact angle depends on the individual's anatomy and usually varies from 50 to 80 degrees. In a neutral position, the P3-A2-P1 segments of the mitral leaflets are visualized from the middle to right of the image sector. Chordae from the anterolateral papillary muscle, which appears on the right side of the image sector, attach to P1 and the lateral side of A2. Chordae emanating from P3 and the medial side of A2 insert into the posteromedial papillary muscle, which appears on the left side of the image sector. CFD is again used to document the presence of regurgitation or stenosis. The medial-lateral mitral annular diameter is measured from the ME commissural view. Finally, by rotating the probe to the left (counterclockwise), all three scallops of the posterior mitral leaflet may be inspected, whereas rightward (clockwise) rotation brings the segments of the anterior leaflet into view. Further rightward rotation will reveal the aortic valve in the middle of the image sector,

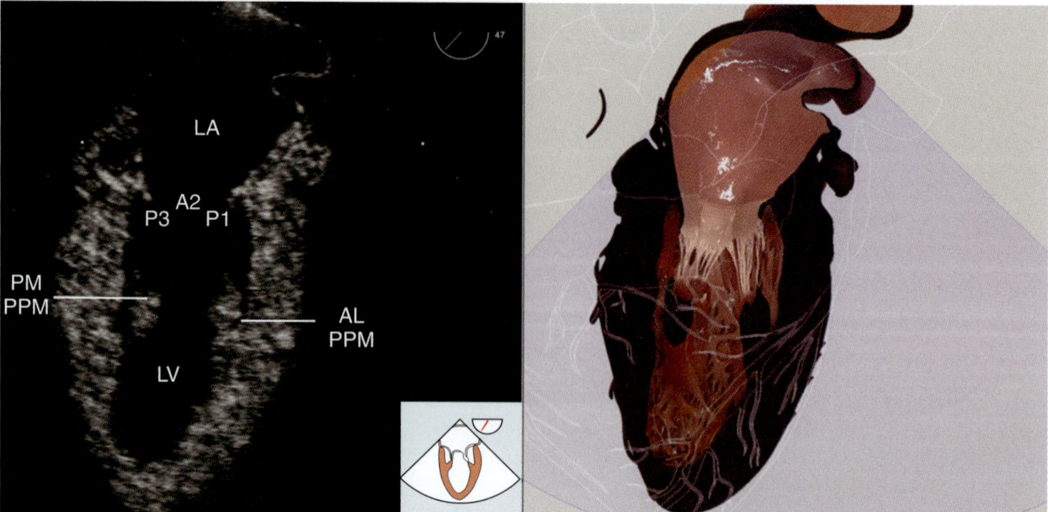

Figure 7-10 Midesophageal mitral commissural view. Mitral valve (P3, A2, P1 scallops). *AL PPM,* Anterolateral papillary muscle; *LA,* left atrium; *LV,* left ventricle; *PM PPM,* posteromedial papillary muscle. *(Two-dimensional TEE images and three-dimensional pictures generated using software developed by Heartworks, Inventive Medical Ltd., London, UK.)*

emphasizing its anatomic relationship to the mitral valve, lying just anterior.

The ME two-chamber view (see Fig. 7-1, Video 7-1) is obtained by continuing to advance the multiplane angle to 90 degrees. The anterior leaflet is located to the right of the image sector near the LAA, and the posterior leaflet is visualized to the left of the image sector. By further increasing the multiplane angle to 110 to 160 degrees, the mitral valve can now be seen in the ME long-axis view (see Fig. 7-3, Video 7-3). In this view, the P2 scallop is seen in the middle of the image sector, whereas A2 is seen to the right. It also becomes evident that the anterior mitral leaflet forms the superior posterior portion of the left ventricular outflow tract (LVOT). The anterior-posterior mitral annular diameter is measured in this view, and CFD is again used to document the presence of regurgitation or stenosis. By rotating the probe from left to right, a sweeping motion across the valve can be created, enabling the echocardiographer to inspect the A1-P1 and A3-P3 scallops of the mitral valve, respectively. The anterolateral commissure (A1-P1) is seen by rotating the probe to the left, and the posteromedial commissure (A3-P3) is seen by rotating the probe to the right.

The transmitral inflow velocity profile may be obtained in the ME four-chamber, mitral commissural, or two-chamber views. Choose the image that best aligns the Doppler beam parallel to the transmitral inflow, and place the pulsed wave Doppler sample gate over the coaptation point of the mitral valve leaflets to optimize the velocity profile (Fig. 7-11). Recall that there are four phases of diastole: isovolumic relaxation, early diastolic filling, diastasis, and late diastole or atrial contraction. The transmitral E wave represents filling of the LV during early diastole. Atrial contraction, occurring during late diastole, is marked by the transmitral A wave. The interval between the two is referred to as *diastasis.* The normal mitral inflow patterns are affected by a number of factors, including preload, afterload, diastolic function, and cardiac rhythm.[6]

Transgastric views are also useful to assess the mitral valve. The TG basal short-axis view (see Fig. 7-6, Video 7-4), or "fish-mouth" view, offers a perspective from the ventricular underside of the valve. The larger anterior leaflet is noted at the center of the image, with the posterior leaflet at the right side of the image. The coaptation of the leaflets can be assessed here, as well as any defects in the mitral leaflets themselves. CFD is particularly useful in this view because it occasionally will precisely identify the origin of a regurgitant lesion. Finally, the mitral subvalvular apparatus may be examined for chordal thickening and calcification with the TG two-chamber (see Fig. 7-8, Video 7-6) and deep TG long-axis (Fig. 7-12, Video 7-8) views.

Aortic Valve

The aortic valve is a trileaflet semilunar valve that consists of right, left, and noncoronary cusps. The aortic valve sits within the aortic root.

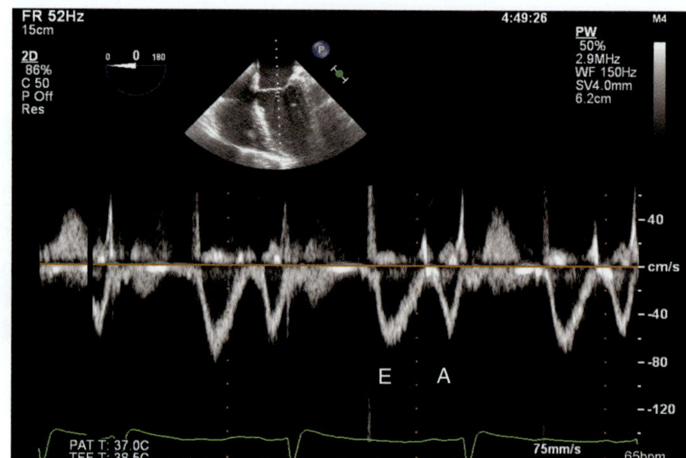

Figure 7-11 Normal pulse wave Doppler velocity profile of transmitral inflow. E wave corresponds to early diastolic filling of left ventricle; A wave represents atrial contraction during late diastole.

The aortic root, which lies between the anterior mitral valve leaflet and interventricular septum, extends from the aortic valve to the sinotubular junction. The right and left coronary arteries arise from their corresponding sinuses of Valsalva.[7]

The aortic valve can be evaluated from the ME and TG views. From the ME four-chamber view (see Fig. 7-2, Video 7-2), withdraw the probe until the aortic valve comes into view, and rotate the multiplane angle to approximately 30 to 60 degrees until the short-axis view of the valve is seen. Here in the ME aortic valve short-axis view (Fig. 7-13, Video 7-9), all cusps of the aortic valve are visualized, and their appearance in systole demonstrates the normal trileaflet valve. Mobility and coaptation of all cusps is also assessed in this imaging plane. Place CFD over the aortic valve to assess for evidence of aortic insufficiency. From the ME aortic valve short-axis view, rotate the multiplane angle to 110 to 160 degrees for a long-axis view of the aortic valve. Here in the ME aortic valve long-axis view (Fig. 7-14, Video 7-10), measurements of the LVOT, annulus, sinuses of Valsalva, sinotubular junction, and ascending aorta are made during mid-systole. Two-dimensional (2D) quantification of annular size is obtained from the hinge points of the aortic valve leaflets. Place CFD over the aortic valve, focusing on the LVOT, to appreciate the presence of regurgitation. Turbulent color flow in the LVOT or ascending aorta during systole is suggestive of obstruction of the LVOT or stenosis of the aortic valve, respectively.

Quantification of the pressure gradient across the aortic valve, calculating the valve area by the continuity equation, and estimation of

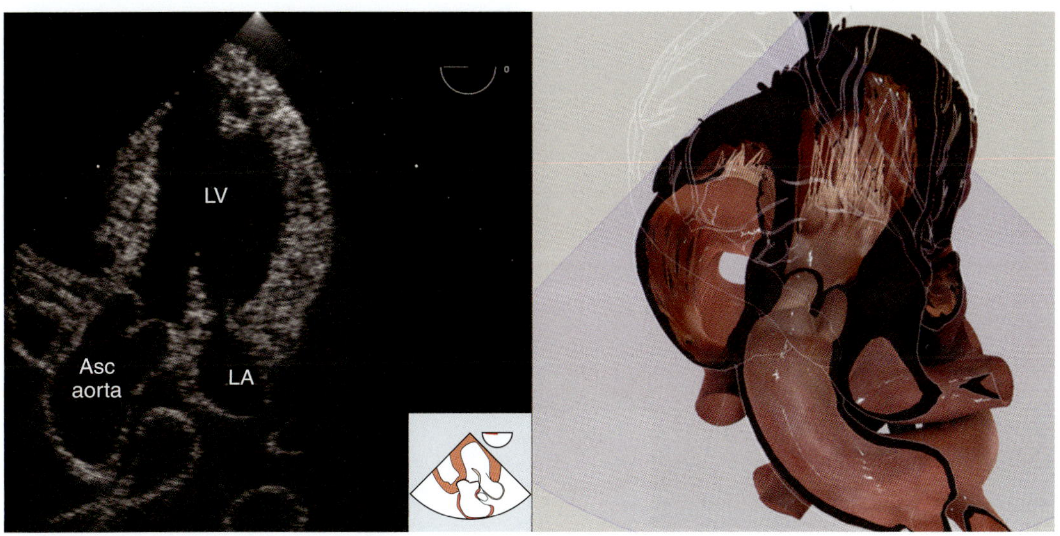

Figure 7-12 Deep transgastric long-axis view. *Asc aorta,* Ascending aorta; *LA,* left atrium; *LV,* left ventricle. *(Two-dimensional TEE images and three-dimensional pictures generated using software developed by Heartworks, Inventive Medical Ltd., London, UK.)*

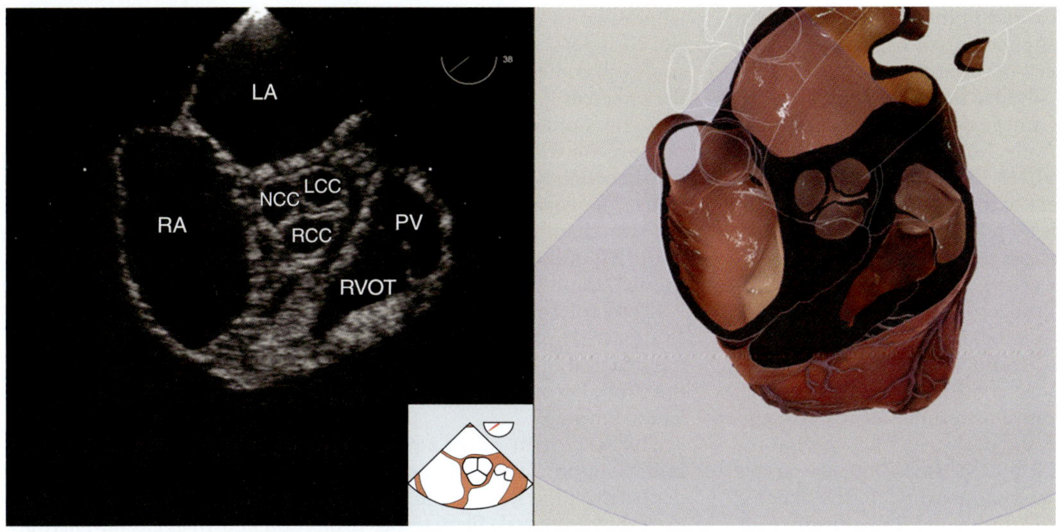

Figure   7-13 Midesophageal aortic valve short-axis view. *LA,* Left atrium; *LCC,* left coronary cusp; *NCC,* noncoronary cusp; *RA,* right atrium; *RCC,* right coronary cusp; *RVOT,* right ventricle outflow tract. *(Two-dimensional TEE images and three-dimensional pictures generated using software developed by Heartworks, Inventive Medical Ltd., London, UK.)*

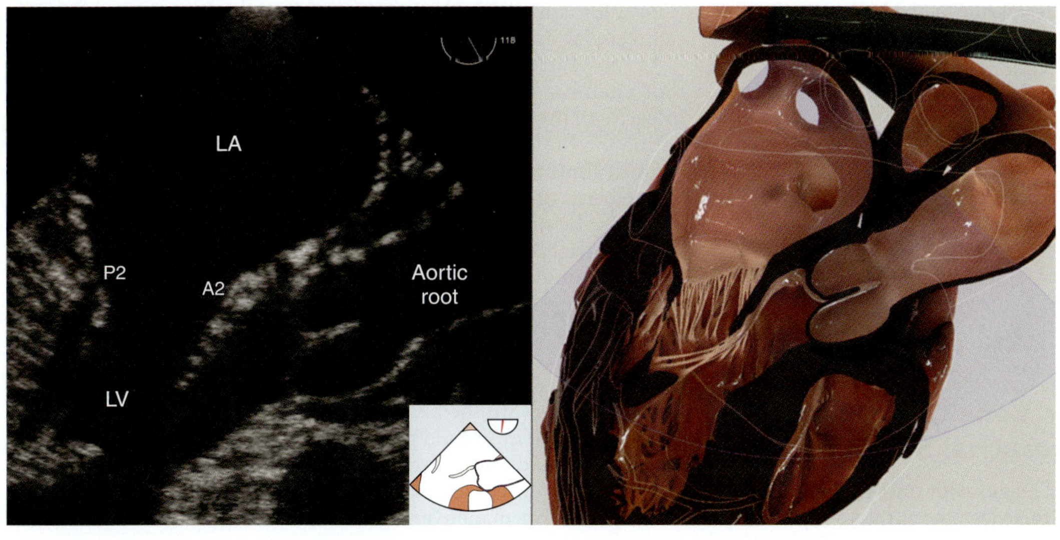

Figure   7-14 Midesophageal aortic valve long-axis view. *LA,* Left atrium; *LV,* left ventricle; mitral valve (P2 scallop, A2 segment). *(Two-dimensional TEE images and three-dimensional pictures generated using software developed by Heartworks, Inventive Medical Ltd., London, UK.)*

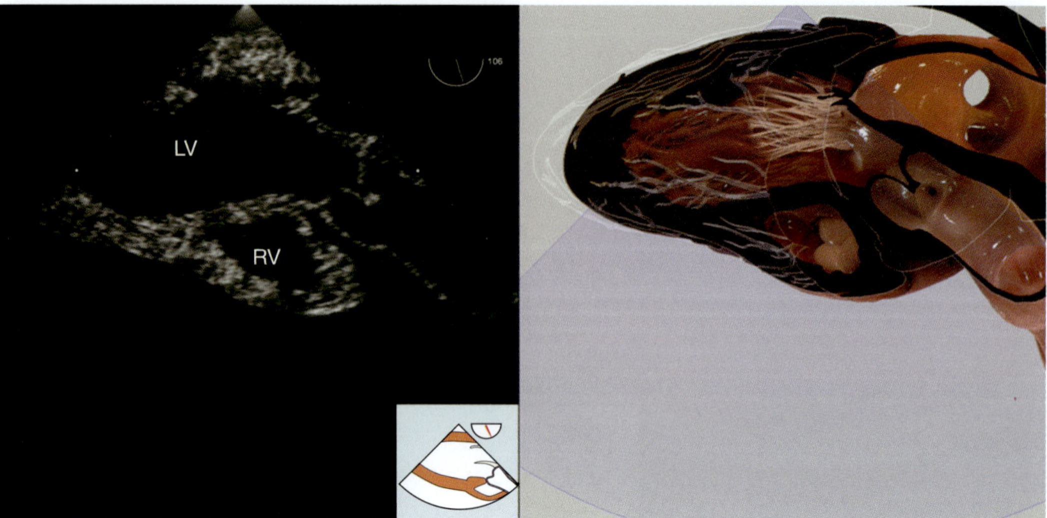

Figure 7-15 Transgastric long-axis view. *LV,* Left ventricle; *RV,* right ventricle. *(Two-dimensional TEE images and three-dimensional pictures generated using software developed by Heartworks, Inventive Medical Ltd., London, UK.)*

left-sided cardiac output can be made in either the deep TG long-axis (see Fig. 7-12, Video 7-8) or the TG long-axis (Fig. 7-15, Video 7-11) views, depending on which image provides optimal alignment of the Doppler beam parallel to the flow being measured. Begin by inserting the probe into the stomach for TG views of the aortic valve. Rotate the multiplane angle to zero degrees and advance the probe for a deep TG long-axis view. Develop the image by anteflexion and leftward flexion until the aortic valve appears. Alternatively, withdraw the probe slightly and increase the multiplane angle to 110 to 130 degrees for a TG long-axis view of the aortic valve. Assessment of the aortic valve for regurgitation or stenosis by CFD can be made as described earlier. Next, place the continuous wave Doppler beam across the aortic valve and LVOT, parallel to the direction of blood flow (Fig. 7-16, *A*). In this view, flow above the baseline or toward the transducer in diastole is regurgitant flow into the LVOT, whereas systolic flow below the baseline is indicative of forward flow through the LVOT and valve. The image yields a pair of parabolic envelopes, one above and one below the baseline, which can be traced, yielding quantitative assessment of the velocity-time integral (VTI) of the aortic valve, the peak velocity, as well as the peak and mean gradients. Similarly, a pulsed wave Doppler sample volume placed within the LVOT 0.5 to 1 cm proximal to the opening of the aortic valve yields the LVOT VTI and blood flow velocity (Fig. 7-16, *B*). Next, calculate the area of the LVOT by measuring its diameter (d) (Fig. 7-16, *C*) and multiplying $(d/2)^2$ by pi (π). The aortic valve area (AVA) is calculated by dividing the LVOT stroke volume (SV) by the VTI of the aortic valve. Left-sided cardiac output (CO) can be estimated by multiplying the LVOT stroke volume by the heart rate (HR).

$$AVA = (Area_{LVOT} \times VTI_{LVOT})/VTI_{AV}$$

therefore,

$$AVA = \pi \, (d_{LVOT}/2)^2 \times VTI_{LVOT}) \, / \, VTI_{AV}$$

$$CO_{LV} = SV_{LVOT} \times HR$$

where

$$SV_{LVOT} = \pi \, (d_{LVOT}/2)^2 \times VTI_{LVOT}$$

therefore,

$$CO_{LV} = \pi \, (d_{LVOT}/2)^2 \times VTI_{LVOT} \times HR$$

Right Atrium, Inferior Vena Cava, Superior Vena Cava, Interatrial Septum

Examination of the right atrium (RA) begins with the ME four-chamber view (see Fig. 7-2, Video 7-2). In this view, the absolute size of the

RA can be measured using the calipers on the TEE machine. Then the RA should be centered in the image sector and the probe inserted and withdrawn to examine as much of the RA as possible from its inferior to superior borders. As the probe is inserted deeper, the coronary sinus will come into view diagonally at the mid–upper-right portion of the screen as it drains into the posteroinferior portion of the RA. This view, in conjunction with 3D echocardiography, is ideal for assisting the surgeon with placement of coronary sinus catheters. Occasionally the thebesian valve may be visualized at the entrance of the coronary sinus. The coronary sinus may also be visualized in short axis in the ME two-chamber view (see Fig. 7-1, Video 7-1) because it appears just to the left of the atrioventricular groove on the image sector.

Next, the RA is examined in the ME bicaval view (Fig. 7-17, Video 7-12) by rotating the probe to the right and increasing the multiplane to about 90 to 110 degrees. Here, the SVC appears on the right side of the image sector and the inferior vena cava (IVC) on the left. Finally, the probe is rotated left and right to image the RA from its medial to lateral borders.

The eustachian valve (not a true valve in the adult) may be visualized as a thin ridge of tissue of varying size located at the lower border between the RA and the IVC on the image sector. Occasionally, an even thinner mobile filamentous projection known as a *Chiari network* may be seen emanating from the eustachian valve. Like the eustachian valve, a Chiari network is considered a normal variant and a vestigial remnant. Also, a ridge-like projection called the *crista terminalis* may be seen at the junction between the RA and SVC. The ME bicaval view is ideal for confirming the location of the wire during central venous catheter placement via the internal jugular or subclavian veins.

The interatrial septum (IAS) should be evaluated in both the ME four-chamber view and the ME bicaval view. In both these views, the integrity of the IAS is evaluated first by 2D then by CFD. When evaluating for the presence of a patent foramen ovale (PFO), the CFD Nyquist limit should be decreased to about 20 to 30 cm/s, because the velocity of blood flow across a PFO is usually low and might otherwise be missed at a higher Nyquist limit (Video 7-13, A). If no PFO or atrial septal defect is appreciated with CFD, the integrity of the IAS should be evaluated by a saline contrast study. To perform this study, approximately 10 mL of agitated saline or blood containing less than 0.5 mL of air is readied for injection. Next, enough positive airway pressure (PAP) is instituted, held, and then released in an intubated patient to increase central venous pressure (CVP) to shift the IAS toward the LA. One must be vigilant at this time, taking note of the patient's blood pressure; excessive or prolonged PAP will decrease preload and cause a significant drop in blood pressure. In an awake and/or sedated patient, this increase in CVP may be generated by Valsalva maneuvers such as coughing. The PAP is released

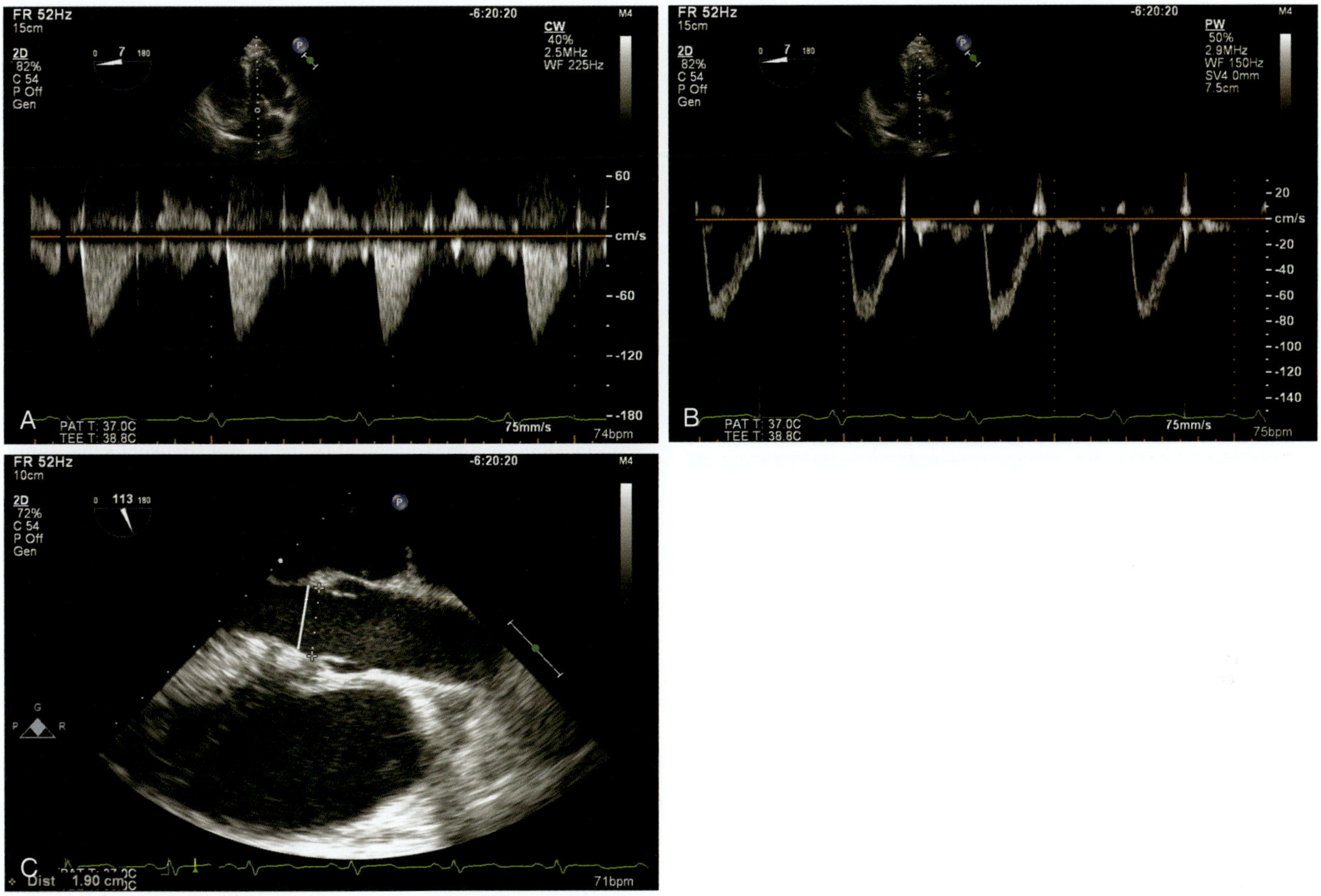

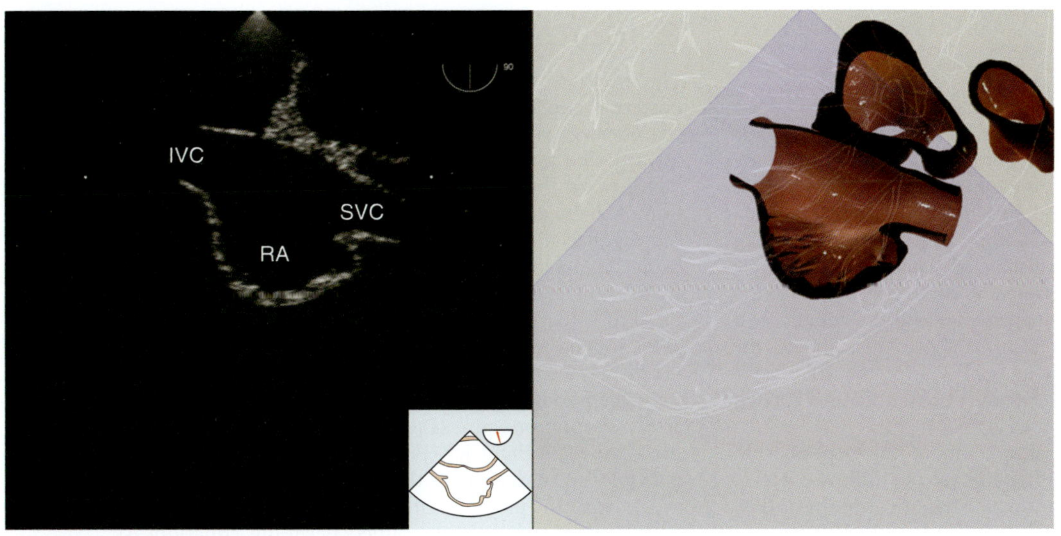

Figure 7-16 **A,** Continuous wave Doppler velocity profile of aortic valve with associated velocity-time integral (VTI) tracing. **B,** Pulse wave Doppler velocity profile of left ventricular outflow tract (LVOT) with associated VTI tracing. **C,** LVOT diameter; measurement should be made 0.5 to 1 cm proximal to aortic valve *(solid line).* Annular measurement also shown *(dashed line).*

Figure 7-17 Midesophageal bi-caval view. *IVC,* Inferior vena cava; *RA,* right atrium; *SVC,* superior vena cava. *(Two-dimensional TEE images and three-dimensional pictures generated using software developed by Heartworks, Inventive Medical Ltd., London, UK.)*

just prior to rapid injection of the blood or saline. A bubble study is considered positive for a defect in the IAS if air bubbles are noted in the LA in fewer than five cardiac cycles, to distinguish it from bubbles that may be seen later coming through the pulmonary veins  (Video 7-13, B).

Hepatic Veins

The liver receives approximately 1500 mL of blood per minute or 20% to 25% of cardiac output, of which three fourths is from the portal vein and one fourth from the hepatic artery.[8-10] Blood flows from the portal

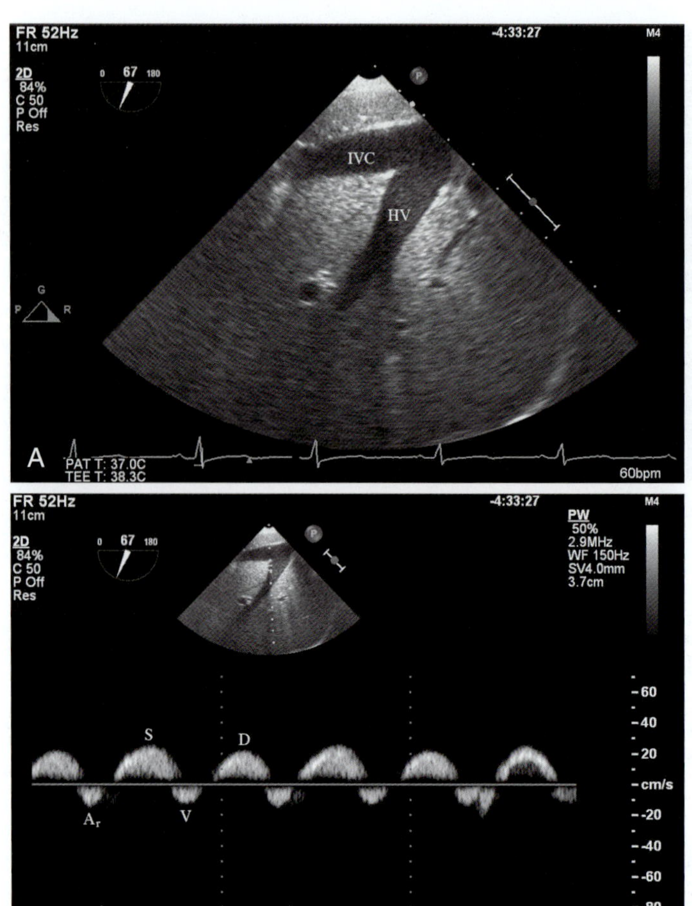

Figure 7-18   *A,* Hepatic vein *(HV)* as it diverges from inferior vena cava *(IVC)*. *B,* Pulse wave Doppler velocity profile of HV. S wave represents antegrade flow to right atrium and corresponds to atrial relaxation as well as ventricular systole. V wave is a period of brief reversal of blood flow occurring toward end of ventricular systole. D wave is a period of antegrade blood flow during diastole. A_r represents retrograde blood flow during atrial contraction in late diastole.

vein through this low-resistance system to the hepatic sinusoids, hepatic veins, vena cava, and finally to the RA. The pressure is highest in the portal vein and lowest in the RA, favoring forward flow to the heart.

The hepatic veins may be imaged by starting at the ME four-chamber view (see Fig. 7-2, Video 7-2) while advancing and turning the probe rightward until the liver is visualized. The multiplane angle should then be increased, usually between 50 to 90 degrees, until the IVC is almost horizontal across the image sector and the hepatic vein is seen as it converges with the IVC (Fig. 7-18, *A*). Alternatively, the hepatic veins may be located by following the IVC from the ME bicaval view (see Fig. 7-17, Video 7-12) as the probe is advanced and rotated rightward.

Place the pulsed wave Doppler gate 1 cm in the hepatic vein adjacent to the IVC to examine the hepatic venous inflow pattern. There are four components of the normal hepatic venous inflow (Fig. 7-18, *B*). First, the S wave, which represents antegrade flow to the RA, corresponds to atrial relaxation and ventricular systole, during which time the right ventricle (RV) pulls the tricuspid annulus in the apical direction during contraction. The S wave appears above baseline. Next is a period of physiologic systolic reversal referred to as the *V wave*. This is followed by the D wave or antegrade flow during diastole, corresponding to early ventricular filling. Finally, the retrograde A wave (A_r) represents atrial contraction during late diastole.[11]

Right Ventricle

The RV serves as an important conduit for the systemic venous return to be pumped through the pulmonary circulation. In the ME four-chamber view (see Fig. 7-2, Video 7-2), the basal anterior free wall of the RV is located toward the left side of the image sector, and the apical portion of the RV anterior free wall is located toward the center of the image sector. This view is useful for qualitative assessment of RV size and function. Compared to the LV, the RV has a thinner wall and comprises approximately one third of the total ventricular size in this view. Normally, only the LV forms the apex of the heart, so an RV that contributes to part of the apex is considered enlarged. An RV more than two thirds the size of the LV is also considered enlarged. The moderator band is a rim of specialized trabeculation that may be seen in the RV, extending from the RV free wall to the septum.

Movement of the RV free wall and tricuspid annulus are examined to determine RV function. The tricuspid annular plane systolic excursion (TAPSE) is a measurement of the lateral tricuspid valve annulus as it moves toward the cardiac apex during systole; in a normal heart, it measures approximately 20 to 25 mm.[12] If regional wall motion abnormalities exist remote to the tricuspid annulus, RV systolic performance may be overestimated using TAPSE alone. It is therefore imperative to always evaluate any structure using more than one method or view prior to making any diagnostic conclusions. Increasing the multiplane to 60 to 90 degrees reveals the ME RV inflow-outflow view (Fig. 7-19, Video 7-14). The right ventricular outflow tract is visualized toward the right side of the image sector, and the diaphragmatic portion of the RV free wall is seen toward the bottom of the image sector. This view is ideal for assessing RV function as well as RV wall thickness.

Finally, RV function is inspected from TG views. In the TG mid-papillary short-axis view (see Fig. 7-7, Video 7-5), the RV is observed in short axis toward the left side of the image sector and appears as a crescent-shaped (rightward concavity) structure. RV wall thickness and function are again noted. From the TG mid–short-axis image, the multiplane angle is increased to 90 to 120 degrees and the probe turned to the patient's right to reveal the TG RV inflow view (Fig. 7-20, Video 7-15). Here, the apex of the RV is seen toward the left side of the image sector and the RV segment closest to the diaphragm is located toward the top of the image sector.

Tricuspid Valve

The tricuspid valve (TV) is a trileaflet structure comprised of anterior, posterior, and septal leaflets. The TV is examined first in the ME four-chamber view (see Fig. 7-2, Video 7-2), where the septal leaflet is seen toward the right side of the RV and the anterior or posterior leaflet is seen toward the left side of the image sector, depending on the rotation of the heart. In this view, it can be seen that the TV is more apically displaced in comparison to the MV. The TV should be examined using 2D imaging for normal leaflet motion and morphology, as well as stenosis or regurgitation by CFD. As the multiplane angle is increased to 60 to 90 degrees to reveal the ME RV inflow-outflow view (see Fig. 7-19, Video 7-14), the posterior leaflet of the TV is seen on the left of the display and the anterior leaflet sits more medially.

In the ME RV inflow-outflow view, an estimate of the pulmonary artery systolic pressure (PASP) can be made if there is an adequate tricuspid regurgitant jet (Fig. 7-21). First, continuous wave Doppler is employed to determine the velocity of the tricuspid regurgitant jet (v_{TR}). Next, the pressure differential (ΔP) between the RV and RA can be calculated using the simplified Bernoulli equation, $\Delta P = 4(v_{TR})^2$. The PASP can then be calculated by adding the right atrial pressure (CVP) to the calculated pressure differential between the RV and the RA during ventricular systole:

$$PASP = CVP + \Delta P$$

where

$$\Delta P = 4(v_{TR})^2$$

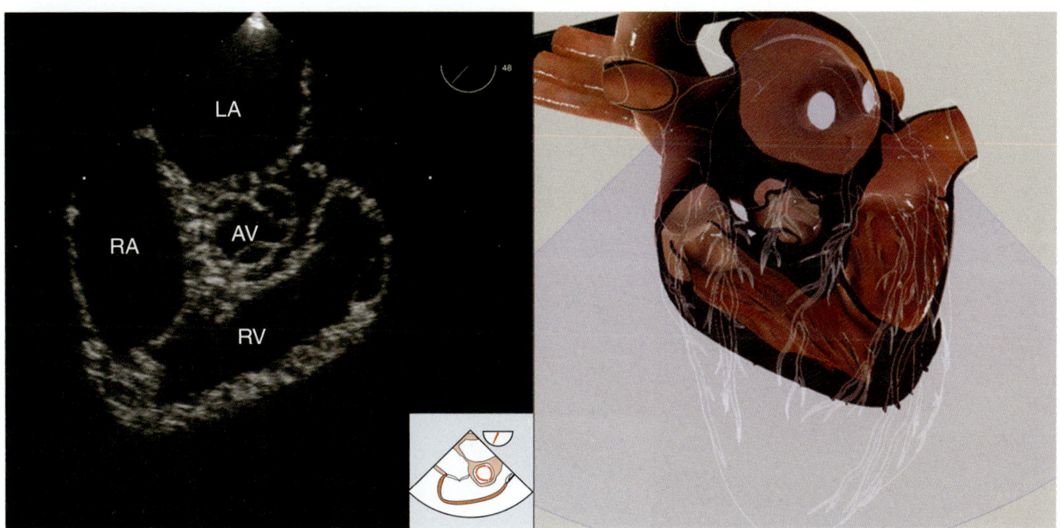

Figure 7-19 Midesophageal right ventricle inflow-outflow view. *AV,* Aortic valve; *LA,* left atrium; *RA,* right atrium; *RV,* right ventricle. *(Two-dimensional TEE images and three-dimensional pictures generated using software developed by Heartworks, Inventive Medical Ltd., London, UK.)*

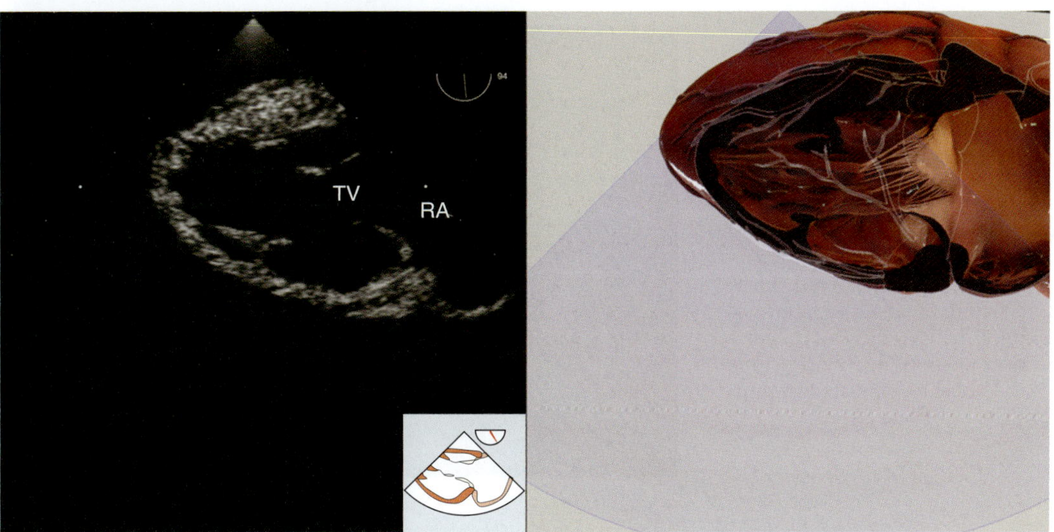

Figure 7-20 Transgastric right ventricle inflow view. *RA,* Right atrium; *TV,* tricuspid valve. *(Two-dimensional TEE images and three-dimensional pictures generated using software developed by Heartworks, Inventive Medical Ltd., London, UK.)*

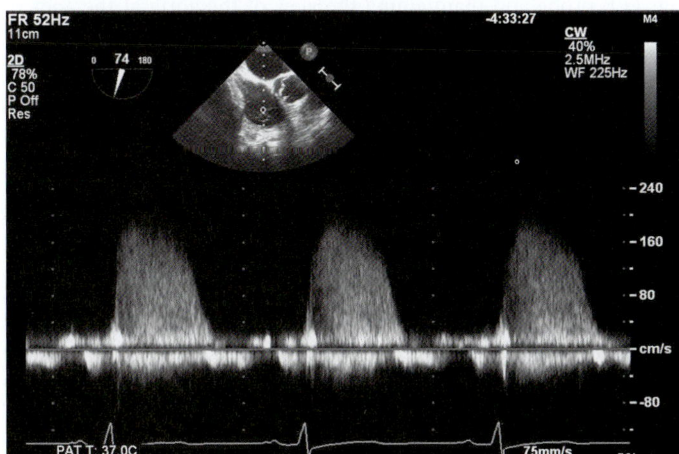

Figure 7-21 Continuous wave Doppler velocity profile of tricuspid regurgitation jet, with associated velocity-time integral tracing.

therefore,

$$PASP = CVP + 4(v_{TR})^2$$

This calculation assumes there is no pulmonic valve stenosis.

Next, the TV is examined from the TG RV inflow view (see Fig. 7-20, Video 7-15), where the TV is visualized in the middle of the image sector. This view is ideal for assessing the integrity of the chordae tendinae and three papillary muscles of the TV subvalvular apparatus.

Finally, from the TG midpapillary short-axis view (see Fig. 7-7, Video 7-5), slight anteflexion of the probe will reveal the tricuspid valve and all three of its leaflets on the left side of the image sector. The anterior leaflet is located toward the bottom of the RV in the image sector, the septal leaflet is located toward the right side of the RV in the image sector (near septum), and the posterior leaflet is located toward the top of the image sector.

Pulmonic Valve

The pulmonic valve (PV) has three cusps: anterior, left, and right. This semilunar valve connects the RV to the pulmonary artery (PA). It is often difficult to image the PV with TEE owing to its thin leaflet structure, its location farther from the esophagus than any of the other cardiac valves, and potential dropout due to shadowing distal to the aortic valve. The PV should be examined for normal leaflet motion, normal leaflet morphology, stenosis, and regurgitation. The PV is orthogonal

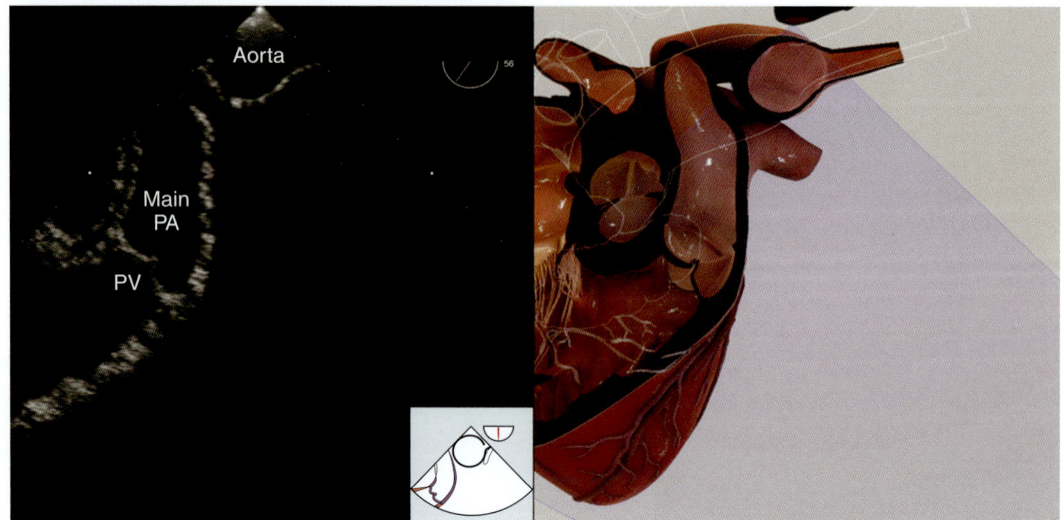

Figure 7-22 Upper esophageal aortic arch short-axis view. *PA,* Pulmonary artery; *PV,* pulmonary vein. *(Two-dimensional TEE images and three-dimensional pictures generated using software developed by Heartworks, Inventive Medical Ltd., London, UK.)*

to the aortic valve within the heart. In the ME aortic valve short-axis (see Fig. 7-13, Video 7-9) and RV inflow-outflow (see Fig. 7-19, Video 7-14) views, the PV is visualized toward the right side of the screen immediately below and to the right of the aortic valve on the image display. Additionally, the PV may be examined in some patients from the upper esophageal aortic arch short-axis view (Fig. 7-22, Video 7-16), where the PV and the main PA are seen on the left side of the image sector. This view is ideal for estimating the right ventricular cardiac output (CO_{RV}). First, calculate the area of the main PA by measuring its diameter (d_{PA}) and multiplying ($d_{PA}/2$)^2 by pi (π). Next, place the pulsed wave Doppler sample volume within the main PA approximately 0.5 to 1 cm distal to the opening of the PV (Fig. 7-23). Trace this spectral Doppler envelope for a measurement of the velocity-time integral (VTI) of the main PA (VTI_{PA}). CO_{RV} can be estimated by multiplying the PA stroke volume (SV_{PA}) by the heart rate (HR):

$$CO_{RV} = SV_{PA} \times HR$$

where

$$SV_{PA} = \pi \, (d_{PA}/2)^2 \times VTI_{PA}$$

therefore,

$$CO_{RV} = \pi \, (d_{PA}/2)^2 \times VTI_{PA} \times HR$$

Aorta

The ascending aorta, aortic arch, and descending aorta can all be visualized with TEE. However, portions of the distal ascending aorta and the proximal aortic arch are typically obstructed by the left mainstem bronchus and therefore not accessible with TEE. The aorta can be evaluated for dilation, aneurysms, dissection, and atherosclerosis.

Begin by advancing the TEE probe into the stomach. Rotate the probe to the patient's left until the descending aortic short-axis view is obtained (Fig. 7-24, Video 7-17). Increasing the multiplane angle to 90 degrees will demonstrate the descending aortic long-axis view (Fig. 7-25, Video 7-18). If the probe has 3D capabilities, the X-plane function can be used to simultaneously assess the short-axis and long-axis views. In these views, the size, shape, integrity, and degree of atherosclerosis of the descending aorta can be assessed while withdrawing

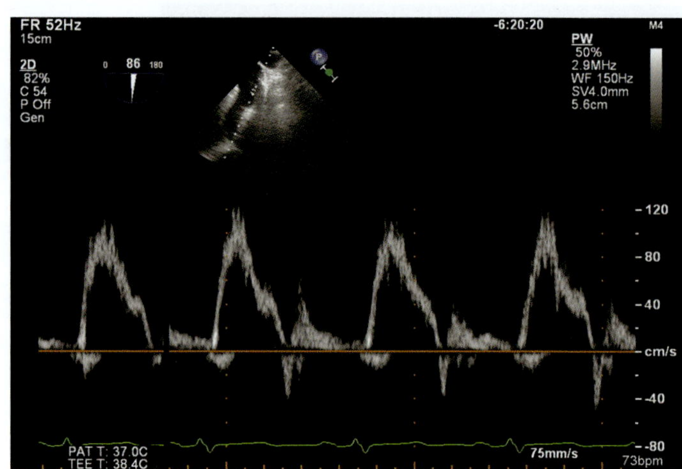

Figure 7-23 Pulse wave Doppler velocity profile of pulmonary artery, with associated velocity-time integral tracing.

the TEE probe and maintaining the view of the aorta at the apex of the sector. When the level of the aortic arch is reached, the probe will have to be slightly rotated to the patient's right to maintain the view of the aorta. This is the upper esophageal aortic arch long-axis view (Fig. 7-26, Video 7-19). Increasing the multiplane angle to approximately 70 to 90 degrees reveals the upper esophageal aortic arch short-axis view (see Fig. 7-22, Video 7-16). The main PA and the pulmonic valve may be seen toward the lower left portion of the image sector.

Next, return to the ME four-chamber view and slightly withdraw the probe such that the aortic valve begins to appear in the middle of the imaging screen. Anteflexion of the probe will demonstrate the ME ascending aortic short-axis view (Fig. 7-27, Video 7-20). Here, both the ascending aorta and the smaller SVC to its left on screen can be evaluated in short axis and their respective diameters measured. In this view, the main, right, and proximal portion of the left PAs are also visualized in long axis. Advancing the multiplane angle to 90 degrees will develop the ME ascending aortic long-axis view (Fig. 7-28, Video 7-21). The mid-ascending aorta lies approximately at the level of the right PA in this view.

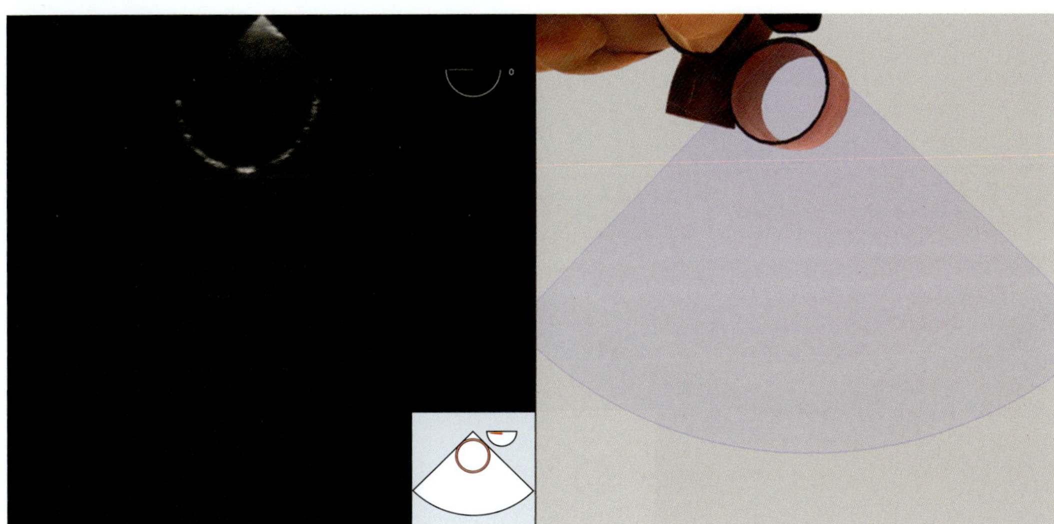

Figure 7-24 Descending aortic short-axis view. *(Two-dimensional TEE images and three-dimensional pictures generated using software developed by Heartworks, Inventive Medical Ltd., London, UK.)*

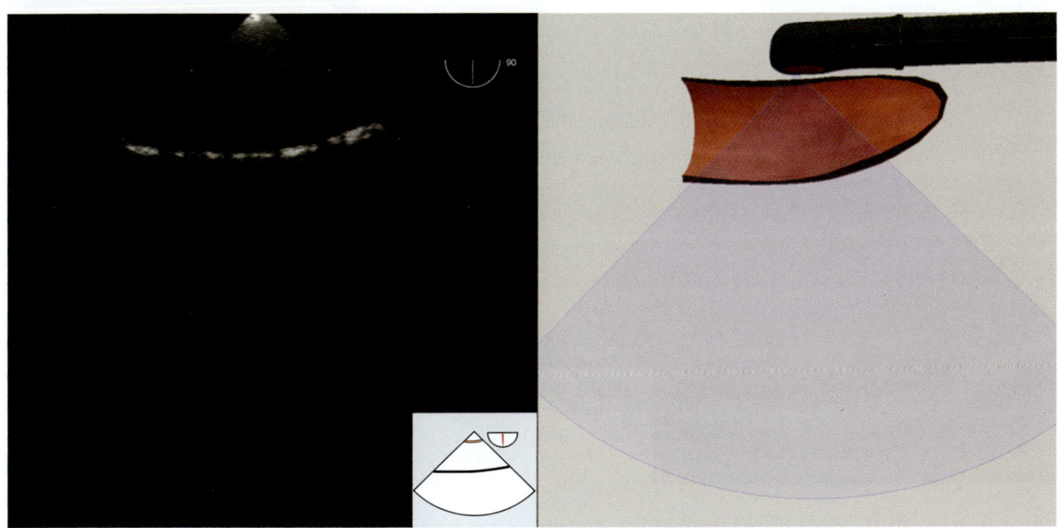

Figure 7-25 Descending aortic long-axis view. *(Two-dimensional TEE images and three-dimensional pictures generated using software developed by Heartworks, Inventive Medical Ltd., London, UK.)*

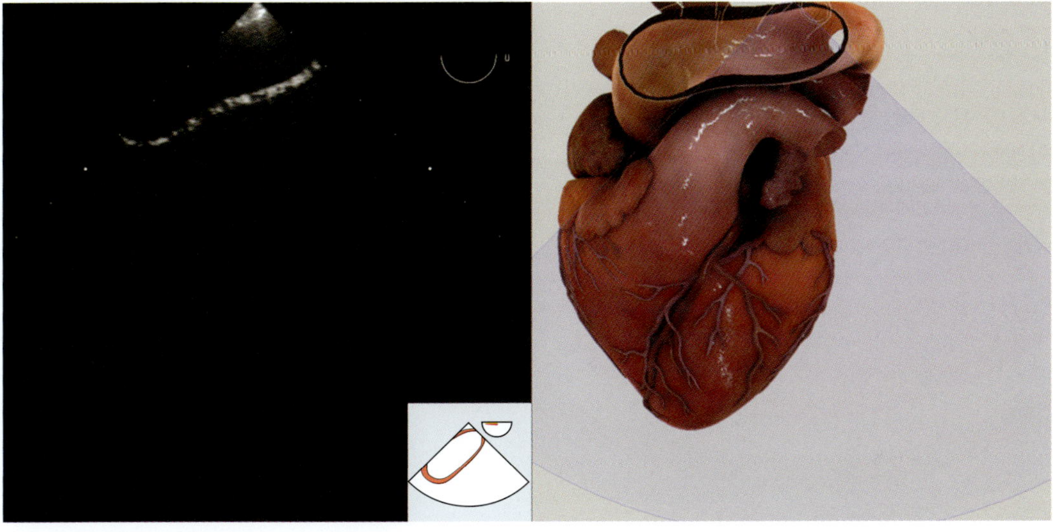

Figure 7-26 Upper esophageal aortic arch long-axis view. *(Two-dimensional TEE images and three-dimensional pictures generated using software developed by Heartworks, Inventive Medical Ltd., London, UK.)*

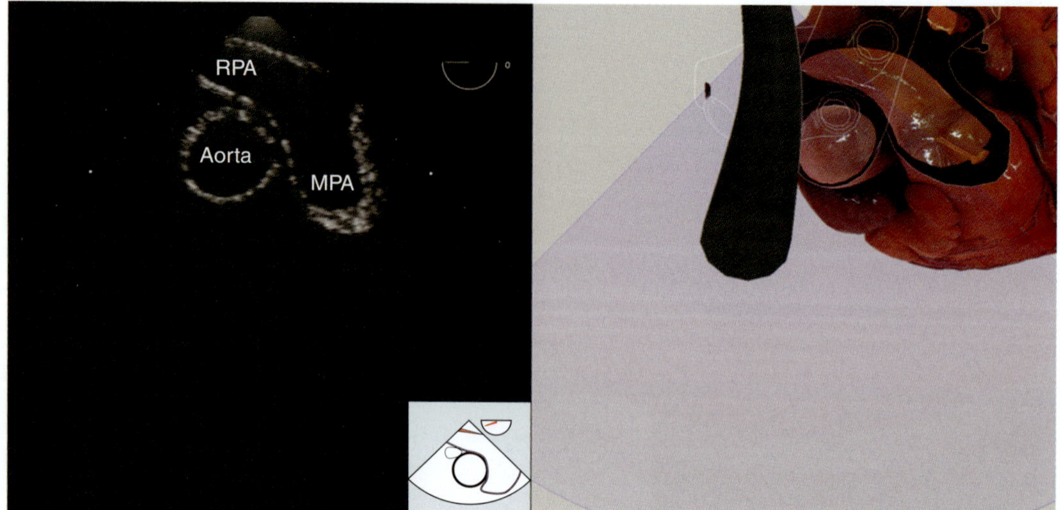

Figure 7-27 Midesophageal ascending aortic short-axis view. *MPA,* Main pulmonary artery; *RPA,* right pulmonary artery. *(Two-dimensional TEE images and three-dimensional pictures generated using software developed by Heartworks, Inventive Medical Ltd., London, UK.)*

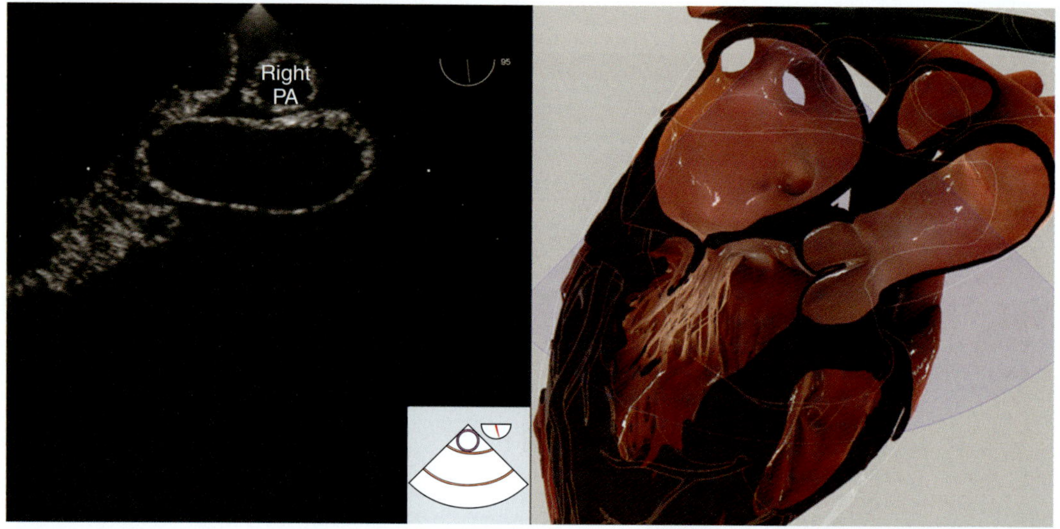

Figure 7-28 Midesophageal ascending aortic long-axis view. *PA,* Pulmonary artery. *(Two-dimensional TEE images and three-dimensional pictures generated using software developed by Heartworks, Inventive Medical Ltd., London, UK.)*

REFERENCES

1. Shernan SK. A Practical Approach to the Echocardiographic Evaluation of Ventricular Diastolic Function. In: Perrino AC, Reeves ST, eds. *A Practical Approach to Transesophageal Echocardiography.* 2nd ed. Philadelphia: Lippincott Williams & Wilkins; 2008:153-155.

2. Troianos CA, Konstadt S. Evaluation of mitral regurgitation. *Semin Cardiothorac Vasc Anesth.* 2006;10(1):67-71.

3. London MJ. Diagnosis of Myocardial Ischemia. In: Perrino AC, Reeves ST, eds. *A Practical Approach to Transesophageal Echocardiography.* 2nd ed. Philadelphia: Lippincott Williams & Wilkins; 2008:87-92.

4. Lang RM, Bierig M, Devereux RB, Flachskampf FA, Foster E, Pellikka PA, et al. Recommendations for chamber quantification: a report from the American Society of Echocardiography's Guidelines and Standards Committee and the Chamber Quantification Writing Group, developed in conjunction with the European Association of Echocardiography, a branch of the European Society of Cardiology. *J Am Soc Echocardiogr.* 2005;18:1440-1463.

5. Doty JR, Timek T. Mitral Valve Disease. In: Yuh DD, Vricella LA, Baumgartner WA, eds. *The Johns Hopkins Manual of Cardiothoracic Surgery.* 1st ed. New York: McGraw-Hill Medical; 2007:607-622.

6. Khouri SJ, Maly GT, Suh DD, Walsh TE. A practical approach to the echocardiographic evaluation of diastolic function. *J Am Soc Echocardiogr.* 2004;17(3):290-297.

7. Piazza N, de Jaegere P, Schultz C, Becker AE, Serruys PW, Anderson RH. Anatomy of the aortic valvular complex and its implications for transcatheter implantation of the aortic valve. *Circ Cardiovasc Interv.* 2008;1(1):74-81.

8. Lautt WW. Regulatory processes interacting to maintain hepatic blood flow constancy: Vascular compliance, hepatic arterial buffer response, hepatorenal reflex, liver regeneration, escape from vasoconstriction. *Hepatol Res.* 2007;37(11):891-903.

9. Reynaert H, Thompson MG, Thomas T, Geerts A. Hepatic stellate cells: role in microcirculation and pathophysiology of portal hypertension. *Gut.* 2002;50(4):571-581.

10. Sheth K, Bankey P. The liver as an immune organ. *Curr Opin Crit Care.* 2001;7(2):99-104.

11. Abu-Yousef MM. Duplex Doppler sonography of the hepatic vein in tricuspid regurgitation. *AJR Am J Roentgenol.* 1991;156(1):79-83.

12. Rudski LG, Lai WW, Afilalo J, Hua L, Handschumacher MD, Chandrasekaran K, et al. Guidelines for the Echocardiographic Assessment of the Right Heart in Adults: A Report from the American Society of Echocardiography Endorsed by the European Association of Echocardiography, a registered branch of the European Society of Cardiology, and the Canadian Society of Echocardiography. *J Am Soc Echocardiogr.* 2010;23:685-713.

Normal Anatomy and Flow During the Complete Examination: Epiaortic Imaging

RAFAEL HONIKMAN | AMANDA J. RHEE

Introduction

Epiaortic ultrasound (EAU) is an imaging modality whereby a hand-held transducer is placed directly upon a surgically exposed aorta. EAU provides high-quality sonographic data depicting aortic anatomy and pathology. The use of ultrasound imaging directly applied to the surgical field predates the introduction of intraoperative transesophageal echocardiography (TEE).[1,2] Epicardial ultrasound was used in the 1980s at The Mount Sinai Medical Center and at Columbia University College of Physicians and Surgeons in New York City to assess left ventricular function,[3] myocardial perfusion,[4] the presence of intracardiac air,[5] and mitral valve function after mitral valve repair.[6] In addition to epicardial ultrasound, EAU is a useful tool in the echocardiographer's armamentarium to address clinical situations such as evaluating a diseased aorta in the face of aortic manipulation or instrumentation.

The most recent guidelines by the American Society of Echocardiography (ASE) and the Society of Cardiovascular Anesthesiologists (SCA) recommend five standard views.[7] Its ease of use, minimal time to perform, negligible complication rate, and high accuracy has made EAU an appealing tool. The guidelines recommend its use in patients at high risk for embolic events, but also speculated on more widespread use of EAU, given its favorable risk/benefit ratio.

This chapter will discuss the indications and theoretic underpinnings for EAU use, as well as technical aspects for optimizing image acquisition. The chapter will then present standard sonographic views and normal aortic anatomy. Finally, important pathologic findings will be reviewed, including grading aortic atherosclerosis, to enable effective communication and decision making among practitioners.

Indications

The initial impetus for the use of EAU stemmed from attempts to reduce the rate of perioperative stroke during cardiac surgery. The 2008 ASE/SCA guidelines for comprehensive intraoperative ultrasonographic examination recommend the use of EAU in patients with increased risk for embolic stroke, history of cerebrovascular disease, peripheral vascular disease, and patients in whom other imaging modalities demonstrate the presence of aortic atherosclerotic disease.[7] Risk factors for stroke in cardiac surgery include advanced age, female gender, proximal aortic atherosclerosis, calcified aorta, history of cerebrovascular disease, peripheral vascular disease, diabetes, hypertension, prior cardiac surgery, preoperative infection (including endocarditis), urgent surgery, greater than 2-hour cardiopulmonary bypass (CPB) time, intraoperative hemofiltration, and transfusion. EAU can identify diseased aortic segments containing atherosclerotic plaque, calcification, or thrombus that are at high risk for distal embolization.[8] Once these areas are identified, the surgical approach to the aorta may be altered or aborted to reduce this risk.[9] In addition to possible alterations in surgical strategy, the examination can provide information for stratification of a patient's risk of complication from distal embolization.

Stroke

Stroke (cerebrovascular accident) is a potentially devastating complication of an otherwise successful cardiac operation. Although there are many types of cerebral injury after CPB, such as transient ischemic attack, delirium, and cognitive dysfunction, this chapter will focus on stroke. Stroke is defined by the World Health Organization as a "neurological deficit of cerebrovascular cause that persists beyond 24 hours or is interrupted by death within 24 hours." Neurologic complications are the second most common causes of morbidity and mortality after cardiac surgery, second only to heart failure. Stroke can lead to delayed discharge from a long-term care facility, increased hospital stay, and increased mortality.[10,11] The incidence of perioperative stroke varies in the literature, based on study design and the population examined.[12-14] The stroke rate clearly increases with age, cardiovascular comorbidities, CPB time, and the complexity of the operation. In a published review of the Society of Thoracic Surgeons (STS) database from 2002 to 2006 examining over 700,000 CABG operations and over 100,000 mitral valve surgeries, the stroke rates were most common in combined mitral valve and coronary artery bypass grafting (CABG) and least common in isolated CABG (Table 8-1).[15-17]

Additional risk factors are similar to those encountered for stroke in the general population. These include prior stroke, diabetes, female gender, renal failure, hypertension, atrial fibrillation, peripheral vascular disease, and others.[18-22] Most relevant for our discussion is the risk of stroke conferred by severe atherosclerotic disease of the thoracic aorta, as screened by ultrasound as discussed earlier. Although there has been controversy regarding the importance of aortic atherosclerosis as a risk factor for primary strokes in the general population,[23-34] it has now been strongly established in the cardiac surgery population that aortic plaque correlates with postoperative stroke incidence.[9,35-42] The more extensive and complex the plaque burden, the higher the risk of postoperative stroke.

Possible mechanisms of stroke include arterial-to-arterial embolization of plaque or thrombus, embolization from intracardiac sources, or paradoxical embolization from venous to arterial circulations across intra- or extracardiac shunts.[43-48] Other etiologic pathways include in situ arterial thrombosis that leads to critical obstruction of brain perfusion, as well as a low-flow state causing ischemic injury due to hypotension and reduced cardiac output. Air entrainment from open cardiovascular structures has been implicated in both stroke and more subtle neurologic impairments after cardiac surgery.[49] Stroke may also be caused by cerebral hemorrhage, decreased cerebral venous drainage, and as a sequela of prolonged seizure activity. Based on radiographic studies, it appears that embolization to the cerebral arterial system is the most common cause of stroke after cardiac surgery.[50,51]

Three common types of matter that embolize to cause neurologic injury are cholesterol-laden atheromas, particles of embolized thrombus, and entrained air. It is likely that the larger the embolic particle and the more frequent the occurrence of embolic events, the greater the risk and severity of neurologic injury.[52,53] It is also thought that low-flow states augment the ischemic injury from embolized particles by failing to "wash out" the cerebral circulation of these obstructing particles.[54-56]

TABLE 8-1	Society of Thoracic Surgeons Stroke Rates for Coronary Artery Bypass Graft and Valve Surgery (2002-2006)*	
Type of Procedure		*Stroke Rate*
CABG		1.4%
Aortic valve replacement (only)		1.5%
Mitral valve repair (only)		1.4%
Mitral valve replacement (only)		2.1%
Valve and CABG		2.9%
Mitral valve and CABG		3.9%

*Stroke rates as described by 2002-2006 Society of Thoracic Surgeons database. Most frequent cohort of patients to suffer stroke is the group that received mitral valve and coronary artery bypass graft (CABG) surgery. Smallest stroke risk was in the isolated CABG surgery group.

Data from Shahian DM, et al. The Society of Thoracic Surgeons 2008 cardiac surgery risk models: part 1—coronary artery bypass grafting surgery. *Ann Thorac Surg.* 2009;88:S2; O'Brien SM, et al. The Society of Thoracic Surgeons 2008 cardiac surgery risk models: part 2—isolated valve surgery. *Ann Thorac Surg.* 2009;88:S23; Shahian DM, et al. The Society of Thoracic Surgeons 2008 cardiac surgery risk models: part 3—valve plus coronary artery bypass graft surgery. *Ann Thorac Surg.* 2009;88:S43.

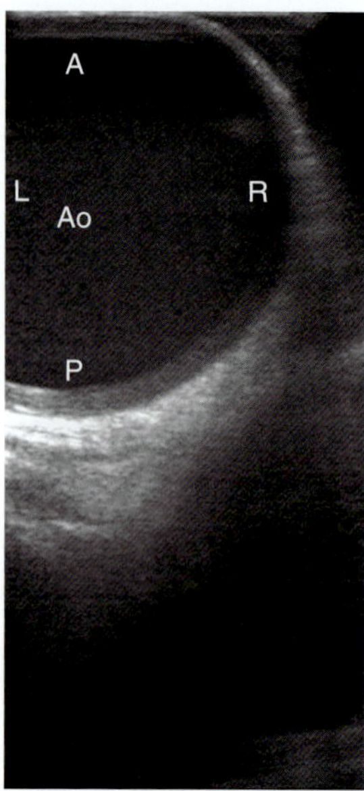

Figure 8-1 Epiaortic ultrasound image of tubular ascending aorta (*Ao*) using linear probe. *A,* Anterior; *L,* left lateral wall; *P,* posterior; *R,* right lateral wall.

During cardiac surgery, the aorta is manipulated in several ways that may lead to plaque disruption and embolization. These include aortic clamp placement and removal, insertion of the aortic cannula, the antegrade cardioplegia vent, the proximal anastomosis of coronary grafts, as well as the aortotomy itself. Flow from the aortic cannula while on CPB may cause a "sandblasting effect" that may disrupt plaque downstream from the cannula.[57,58]

Several methods are used to detect and characterize the patient's atheromatous burden within the ascending aorta. Preoperatively, plaque and calcification may be detected by means of radiologic scanning with computed tomography (CT) or magnetic resonance imaging (MRI). Intraoperatively, three methods are currently employed: direct surgical palpation of the aorta to feel for the hardness of calcification, TEE, and EAU. Several studies clearly demonstrate the superiority of TEE and EAU over surgical palpation. Surgical palpation is much less sensitive than ultrasound, considerably underestimating the atherosclerotic burden; EAU has the greatest sensitivity.[59-67] In one study, Linden et al. examined 921 consecutive cardiac surgery patients. EAU revealed that 26% had plaque on the ascending aorta measuring more than 5 mm thick, but surgical palpation only detected 40% of these lesions.[30] Calcified areas the surgeon is able to feel may be stable plaques with a lower risk for embolization than the soft atheromas that may only be detectable by ultrasound.[68]

Although the TEE probe may already be in place and its use does not interrupt the surgical flow, EAU offers several advantages over TEE for characterizing aortic plaque. Most surgical manipulation occurs in the region of the ascending aorta considered to be the "blind spot" of TEE. This is where the trachea and left mainstem bronchus interpose between the esophagus and aorta, causing disruption of ultrasound transmission. Thus, although parts of the ascending aorta can be visualized by TEE,[69] Konstadt et al. have shown that TEE is frequently unable to image the region of greatest interest of the ascending aorta.[70] Since EAU is placed closer to the area of interest, enabling higher transducer frequencies to be used, higher-quality images with fewer artifacts are possible.

Well-designed trials demonstrating a morbidity or mortality benefit to EAU are lacking, but an accumulating body of data indicates that in high-risk patients the use of EAU alters surgical management and that these changes may be beneficial.[56,71-78] Some examples of modifications of surgical technique are off-pump (as opposed to on-pump) CABG, "no-touch" techniques, and alterations in the site of aortic manipulation and instrumentation (e.g., axillary cannulation).[79-82] More radical surgical approaches may include aortic endarterectomy or aortic arch replacement, although these approaches may produce worse outcomes.[83]

There are very few disadvantages of using EAU. These include the need for sterility when placing the transducer on the surgical field, with the potential for surgical field contamination, as well as the potential to cause arrhythmia as the transducer contacts cardiac structures.

Probes and Technique

An EAU exam is simple to perform. After surgical exposure of the aorta, the handheld transducer, sheathed in a sterile covering, is placed directly upon the ascending aorta, with or without a sonographic "standoff." *Standoff* refers to the distance between the probe and the object of interest, discussed later. Sonographic views are then captured for analysis and storage.

The first step in a direct ultrasonographic evaluation of the aorta is to expose the ascending aorta. The surgeon will open the chest via sternotomy, then incise and retract the pericardium, exposing the entire ascending aorta from root to arch. The sonographer and surgeon then prepare the ultrasound probe for use in the sterile surgical field by placing the probe in one or two sterile sheaths. There are three different types of probes available for acquiring EAU images: a linear probe that produces a rectangular image, and phased and matrix array probes that both produce wedge-shaped windows. All these probes may be used with good results, although each offer specific advantages and disadvantages.

The linear probe scans both the anterior aortic wall (near field) and the posterior aortic wall (far field) without the need for a transducer standoff. One drawback is that linear probes tend to have a large "footprint," which refers to the large surface area of the probe itself. Thus, a linear probe may be difficult to maneuver in a small surgical field. Second, the entire left-to-right dimensions of the aorta may not fit in a single ultrasonographic window, creating a "tunneled" view, and the transducer may have to be repositioned rightward and leftward to acquire the entire cross-sectional picture of the aorta (Fig. 8-1).

The wedge-shaped images of the phased and matrix array transducers enable simultaneous imaging of the right and left aortic walls, and they also tend to have a smaller footprint, enabling greater maneuverability within the surgical field. The drawback of phased or matrix array transducers is the need for a standoff. Because of the wedge shape of the image, if the transducer is placed directly on the aorta, the anterior aortic wall (near field) will not be completely imaged; only a small section will be displayed while the rest will be outside the sector. To capture the near field in its entirety, the transducer is held at some distance away from the aorta (the standoff) (Fig. 8-2). This

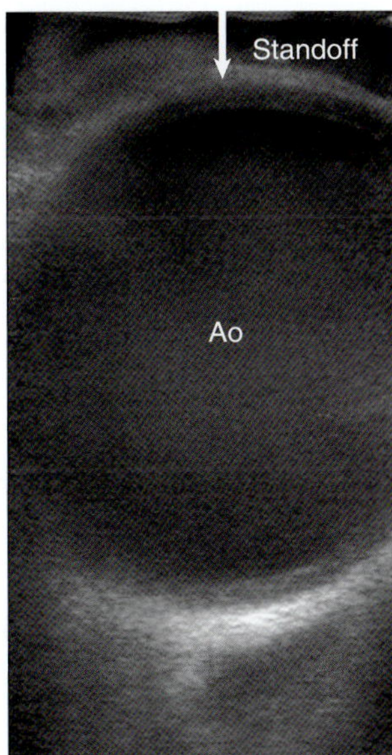

Figure 8-2 Epiaortic ultrasound of ascending aorta *(Ao)* with "stand-off," the distance held off image being interrogated by probe.

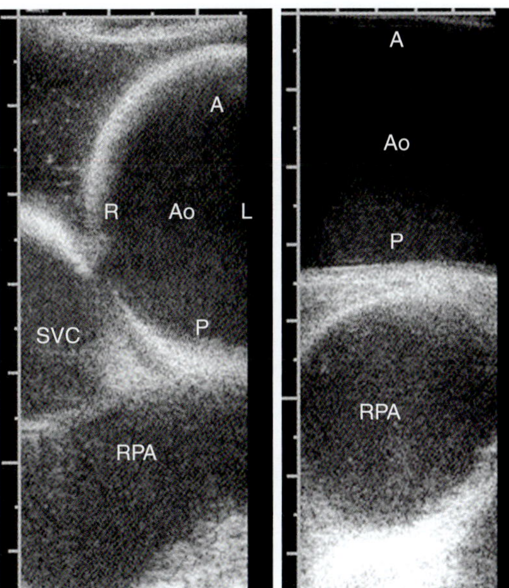

Figure 8-3 *Left,* Epiaortic ultrasound (EAU) using linear probe of mid–ascending aorta *(Ao)* in short axis. *Right,* EAU using linear probe of mid–ascending aorta *(Ao)* in long axis. *A,* Anterior wall of aorta; *L,* left lateral wall of aorta; *P,* posterior wall of aorta; *R,* right lateral wall of aorta; *RPA,* right pulmonary artery; *SVC,* superior vena cava.

requires addition of a medium that conducts ultrasound waves. Air cannot be used because it is a poor acoustic conductor. The standoff may be provided by a gel that can either be purchased as a pad or as gel already incorporated into the sterile cover wrapping surrounding the transducer tip. Another simple approach is to fill the sterile condom sheath with a column of saline, enabling the transducer to be held away from the aorta while transmitting ultrasound waves though the saline to the aorta. At our institution, we place sterile gel within the sterile sheath, fill the pericardial well with warm sterile saline, and hold the transducer immersed in the saline at a distance from the aortic wall so that the anterior wall of the aorta can be visualized in its entirety.

It is of great importance to maintain sterility when introducing the handheld transducer onto the surgical field. The probe is passed from the nonsterile area into a sterile condom sheath on the surgical field. Some institutions place a double sheath, exercising extra precaution. At our institution, we disinfect the transducers between cases and pass these probes into a sterile sheath from the field. It is important to note that different manufacturers recommend specific disinfection techniques for their probes; one must check with the manufacturer to identify the appropriate cleaning technique (see Chapter 29).

When scanning, one must establish correct orientation with the probe handle to ensure a proper exam and effectively communicate with the surgeon. Transducers usually have a marker for orientation on one side of the probe. The marker should correspond to the dot on the display screen. Another approach for establishing "sidedness" is to touch a finger to the probe while observing movement on the display. In echocardiography, it is standard to have the patient's left side displayed on the right side of the screen. If this convention is not observed, the images should be labeled to indicate the orientation for accurate interpretation of saved images at a later time.

Imaging Planes

The ascending aorta and arch should be systematically scanned throughout their entirety, paying particular attention to the sites of proposed aortic manipulation. Several papers have proposed standardized schemes for aortic scanning.[7,84,85] To complete a comprehensive EAU examination from the sinotubular junction to the innominate artery and aortic arch, a minimum of five views are recommended. Usually, TEE allows for visualization of the proximal ascending aorta and distal aortic arch.[86]

The ascending aorta is divided into proximal, mid-, and distal segments. Each segment of the ascending aorta can be described as having four walls: anterior (near field), posterior (far field), right, and left. This leaves 12 total wall segments of the ascending aorta to characterize. The location of the trachea and left mainstem bronchus can interrupt ultrasound waves, preventing adequate imaging of the distal ascending aorta and proximal aortic arch. Therefore, if indicated, it is recommended that these areas be visualized by EAU.

The ascending aorta should be evaluated in short and long axis in each of the proximal, mid-, and distal segments. In short axis with the ultrasound probe perpendicular to the aorta, the aorta should be measured from the near-field inner edge to the far-field inner edge of the aorta in each segment. Manipulation of the probe in perpendicular orientation as the probe is moved from proximal to distal allows for evaluation of all three portions of the ascending aorta. The proximal ascending aorta is demarcated by the beginning of the sinotubular junction, where it is common to see the aortic valve and right pulmonary artery. The mid–ascending aorta is defined by the part of the aorta that is juxtaposed with the right pulmonary artery (Fig. 8-3). The distal ascending aorta is from the distal right pulmonary artery to the innominate artery. Movement farther distally will allow for examination of the proximal aortic arch, which is necessary if not clearly seen on TEE (Fig. 8-4).

The long-axis views are obtained at 90 degrees from the short-axis views, in plane with the direction of blood flow within the ascending aorta. The proximal long-axis view should provide visualization of the sinus of Valsalva, sinotubular junction, and aortic valve. Continuation of the examination distally allows for examination of the mid–ascending aorta. Finally, the distal ascending aorta includes locating the innominate artery. The aortic arch, with origins of the left common carotid and left subclavian artery, should be located as a final part of the examination (see Fig. 8-4, *B*).

During the examination, atherosclerotic grading and diameter measurements should be performed. Particular attention should be paid to regions of the aorta likely to be manipulated by the surgeon. Abnormal pathology at risk for embolization (e.g., areas of atherosclerosis, mobile plaque, ulcerated plaque) should be communicated to the surgeon, which may alter the surgical plan. Other aortic pathology such as dissection flaps and intramural hematoma should be ruled out and,

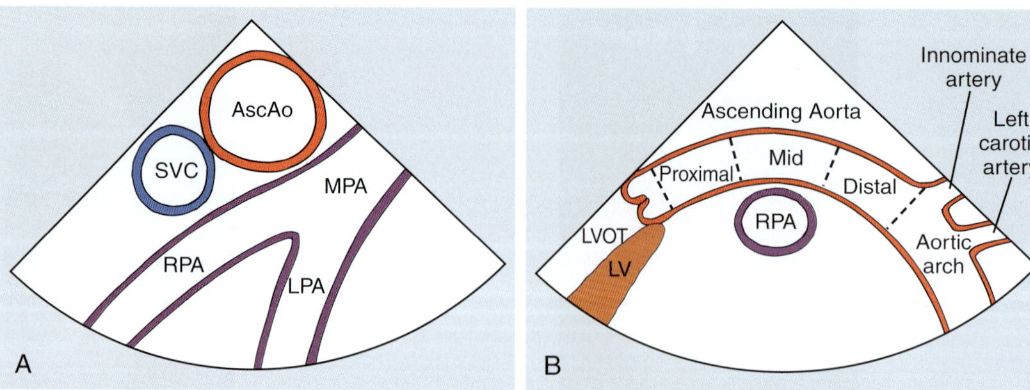

Figure 8-4 Epiaortic ultrasound diagram of short-axis view (**A**) and long-axis view (**B**) of ascending aorta *(AscAo)* and surrounding structures. *LPA,* Left pulmonary artery; *LV,* left ventricle; *LVOT,* left ventricular outflow tract; *MPA,* main pulmonary artery; *RPA,* right pulmonary artery; *SVC,* superior vena cava.

if present, communicated as well. Video clips and still images of the complete examination should be stored for future referral as dictated by institutional protocol.

Atherosclerotic Plaque Grading

It is useful to have a grading system for atherosclerotic plaques that conveys plaque severity and extent of aortic disease. Having a standardized grading system offers several advantages. First, it provides a common language that can be understood across disciplines to accurately describe disease. This allows practitioners to clearly communicate informed decisions on how to best proceed with aortic manipulation or to argue against any manipulation at all. Second, it provides a descriptive platform of categorization for research purposes. Unfortunately, there is no current consensus on which grading system should be employed. The ASE/SCA guidelines for EAU examination list eight of many potential grading systems, which range in complexity from a two-grade scale up to a five-grade scale; all have much in common. They emerged from the use of grading in studies attempting to correlate plaque features with stroke risk. Some studies examined the perioperative period of cardiac surgery while others looked at the general stroke population. A scale may include a grade for a normal aorta or a minimally diseased low-risk aorta. Most scales define a size cutoff that defines a larger protruding plaque that indicates a substantially higher risk of stroke; this size definition has varied among different studies. Plaques with 5-mm-thick focal hyperechoic regions of the aortic layers intima to media and/or lesions with ulcerations, mobile structures, or lumen irregularities are defined as high-risk plaques.[87] In all studies, regardless of which size was used, the larger plaques above the cutoff were associated with higher stroke rates. The highest-risk lesions were "complex plaques," features of which include ulcerations, heavy calcifications, adherent thrombus, and any plaque with a mobile component. Our institution uses the five-point grading system described by Katz et al. (Table 8-2). However, until any one grading system is shown to be superior, any grading system is acceptable assuming it relates the important risk factors for plaques (Fig. 8-5).

In addition to atheroma characteristics described earlier, the spatial extent of the disease in the aorta may also be characterized. The ascending aorta is divided into three segments: proximal, mid-, and distal. Each of these three segments has four walls which are graded separately. These four walls are the anterior (near field), posterior (far field), right, and left aortic walls. This leads to 12 wall segments that may be reported separately to better describe the exact location of disease within the ascending aorta.

Investigation into the use of various alternative descriptive means of classifying aortic atherosclerotic burden has been undertaken. One paper looked at the image frame in each segment with the greatest burden of atherosclerotic disease. They compared the plaque area by planimetry to the total aortic cross-sectional area. They then calculated the ratio of the two areas as an indicator of atherosclerotic burden.[88]

TABLE 8-2	Katz Grading System for Aortic Atheroma
Grade	**Description**
1	Normal aorta to mild intimal thickening
2	Severe intimal thickening without protruding atheroma
3	Protruding atheroma <5 mm into lumen
4	Protruding atheroma ≥5 mm into lumen
5	Mobile atheroma

From Katz ES, Tunick PA, Rusinek H, Ribakove G, Spencer FC, Kronzon I. Protruding aortic atheromas predict stroke in elderly patients undergoing cardiopulmonary bypass: experience with intraoperative transesophageal echocardiography. *J Am Coll Cardiol.* 1992;20:70-7.

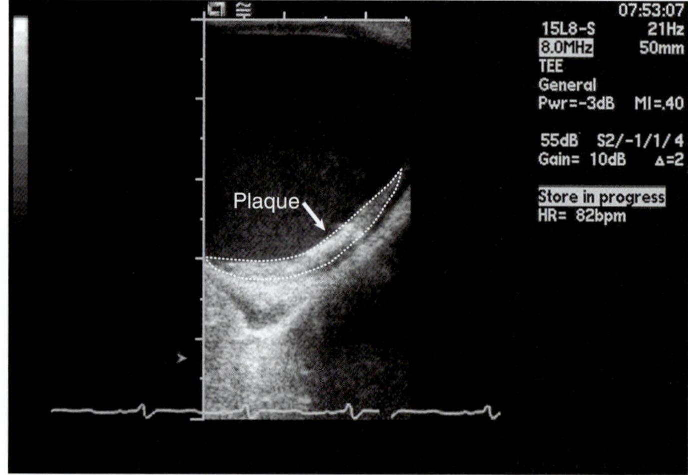

Figure 8-5 Epiaortic ultrasound image of ascending aorta with grade 3 atheroma.

Other groups have studied plaque echodensity through postprocessing analysis, attempting to discern its histopathology as fatty, fibrous, or calcific, followed by correlating their findings with thromboembolic outcomes.[89,90] With the introduction of live three-dimensional (3D) ultrasound probes, there is potential to evaluate the true extent of atherosclerotic disease.[91,92]

Normal Dimensions

Normal ascending aortic dimensions have been obtained from a compilation of data across gender, body surface area, height, and age. These dimensions are measured by MRI, CT, helical CT, invasive angiography, and echocardiography.[93-97] Although some papers show no association, most studies have found ascending aorta diameter to increase with increasing age.[93-97] The Framingham Heart Study showed that age was the most important determinant in aortic root size in men and women. This study found a cumulative aortic root measurement to vary widely with age, gender, and body size of individuals.[97-100]

According to the ASE recommendations for chamber quantification, the ascending aorta should be examined with two-dimensional (2D) echocardiography using four measurements.[101] These recommendations were written for TEE and transthoracic echocardiography, but they are applicable to epiaortic echocardiography as well. Although some clinicians use inner edge–to–inner edge techniques, normative data for echocardiography were obtained using leading edge to leading edge and thus should be favored. Measurements that should be taken are the aortic valve annulus, sinus of Valsalva, and sinotubular junction. A short-axis dimension of the ascending aorta may be useful for surgical planning as well. The measurement should be taken at the largest diameter, that is, during systole and as perpendicular to the aorta as possible. Biaggi et al. used echocardiography to determine normal ascending aortic dimensions in 64,686 patients. Using the leading edge–to–leading edge technique acquired at end-systole, the mean sinus of Valsalva measurement was 3.4 cm in men and 3.1 cm in women. The mean ascending aortic values using the right pulmonary artery as a landmark were 3.2 cm for men and 3.0 cm for women.[96] The aortic annulus is normally 2.2 cm in diameter (Fig. 8-6).[102]

Aortic root dilation at the sinuses of Valsalva is defined by an aortic root diameter greater than the 95% confidence interval based on body surface area by age (Fig. 8-7).[97] Roman et al. looked at 135 normal adults and found the absolute upper limits of normal for the sinus of Valsalva to be 4.0 cm for men and 3.6 cm for women, and the supra-aortic ridge was 3.5 cm for men and 3.2 cm for women. A leading edge–to–leading edge technique at end-diastole was used.[97]

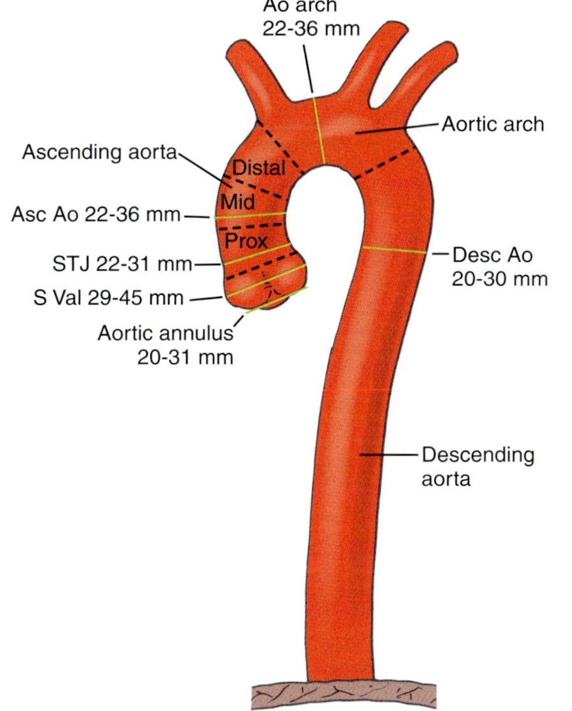

Figure 8-6 Diagram of normal aortic anatomy and dimensions from aortic valve to diaphragm. Ascending aorta *(Asc Ao)* is divided into three segments: proximal ascending aorta is from sinus of Valsalva *(S Val)* to pulmonary artery, mid–ascending aorta is demarcated by the part of aorta adjacent to pulmonary artery, distal ascending aorta is from pulmonary artery to innominate artery. Aortic arch *(Ao arch)* is from innominate artery to left subclavian artery, and descending aorta *(Desc Ao)* extends distal to subclavian artery to iliac bifurcation below diaphragm. Relevant dimensions provided on diagram. *STJ,* Sinotubular junction.

Doppler Interrogation of Ascending Aorta and Aortic Valve

Use of EAU for Doppler interrogation of the aortic valve is limited. In some cases, color Doppler may be useful to diagnose the presence or absence of dissections and hematomas.[103] EAU has been used to guide aortic cannulation of patients with type A aortic dissections. In these cases, use of 2D EAU and color Doppler EAU helped identify true and false channels for successful arterial cannulation of the true lumen.[104,105] One case report described the use of EAU to measure the gradient across a stenotic aortic valve when the Doppler insonation angle was unacceptable using TEE.[106]

There are currently no guidelines recommending how to perform an EAU Doppler exam. It is difficult to obtain Doppler beam orientation parallel to aortic flow in many parts of the ascending aorta, because more frequently than not, the orientation of the ultrasound probe to flow in the aorta will be perpendicular (Fig. 8-8). One must be careful to recognize that there is an element of error when the Doppler beam is not parallel to the direction of flow. The angle between the Doppler

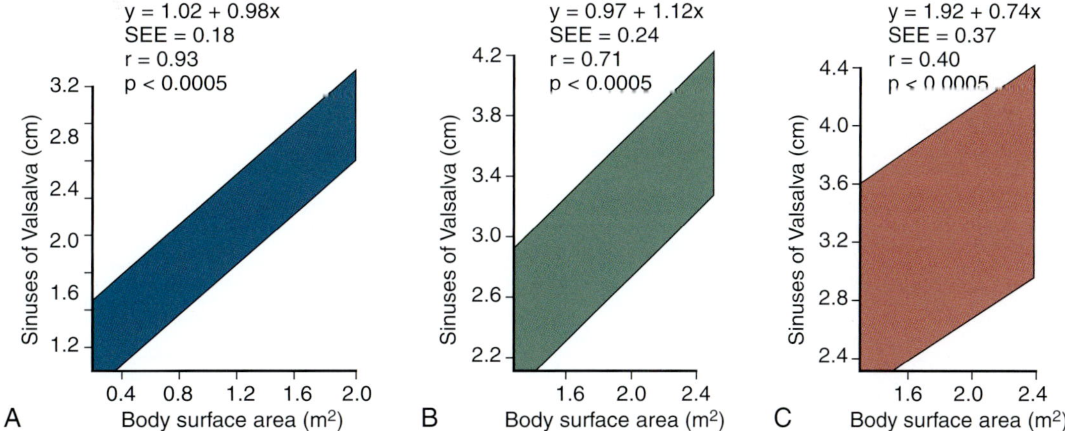

Figure 8-7 The 95% confidence interval to signify sinus of Valsalva dilation in **(A)** children and adolescents, **(B)** adults aged 20 to 39 years, and **(C)** adults aged 40 years or older. Figure depicts relationship of sinus of Valsalva to body surface area and age. *(From Lang RM, Bierig M, Devereux RV, et al. Recommendations for chamber quantification: a report from the American Society of Echocardiography's Guidelines and Standards Committee and the Chamber Quantification Writing Group, developed in conjunction with the European Association of Echocardiography, a branch of the European Society of Cardiology. J Am Soc Echocardiogr. 2005;18:1440-1463.)*

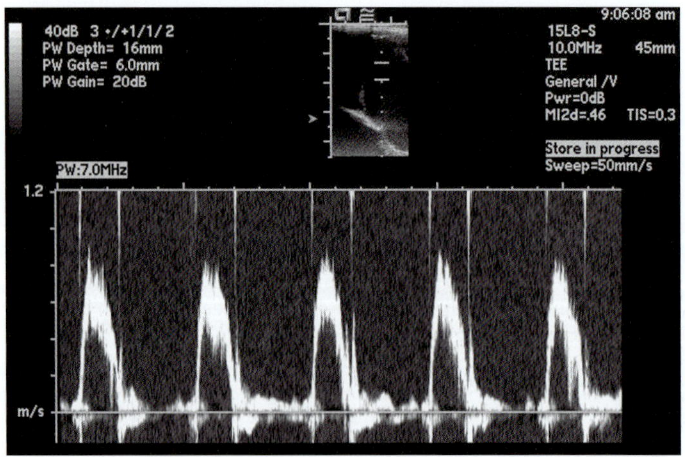

Figure 8-8   Pulsed wave Doppler interrogation of ascending aorta using linear epiaortic ultrasound probe.

beam and the direction of flow within the aorta is called the *insonation angle*. It should be less than 30 degrees to maintain an error less than 15%.

Summary

EAU offers a useful tool to evaluate the ascending aorta to allow for informed decision making regarding management of the ascending aorta during cardiac surgery. It offers advantages over TEE and surgeon palpation, with few risks. Pathology such as atherosclerosis, dilation, and dissection can be identified, graded, and localized. Future and alternative directions include better description through 3D rendering with matrix array probes and the possible use of plaque planimetry.

REFERENCES

1. Wild JJ, Crawford HD, Reid JM. Visualization of the excised human heart by means of reflected ultrasound of echography; preliminary report. *Am Heart J.* 1957;54:903-906.
2. Johnson ML, Holmes JH, Spangler RD, Paton BC. Usefulness of echocardiography in patients undergoing mitral valve surgery. *J Thorac Cardiovasc Surg.* 1972;64:922-934.
3. Dubroff JM, Wong CY, et al. Left ventricular ejection fraction during cardiac surgery: A two-dimensional echocardiographic study. *Circulation.* 1983;68:95-103.
4. Goldman ME, Mindich BP. Intraoperative cardioplegic contrast echocardiography for assessing myocardial perfusion during open heart surgery. *J Am Coll Cardiol.* 1984;4:1029-1034.
5. Rodigas PC, Meyer FJ, Haasler GB, et al. Intraoperative 2-dimensional echocardiography: ejection of microbubbles from the left ventricle after cardiac surgery. *Am J Cardiol.* 1982;50:1130-1132.
6. Goldman ME, Mindich BP, Teichholz LE, et al. Intraoperative contrast echocardiography to evaluate mitral valve operations. *J Am Coll Cardiol.* 1984;4:1035-1040.
7. Glas KE, et al. Guidelines for the performance of a comprehensive intraoperative epiaortic ultrasonographic examination: recommendations of the American Society of Echocardiography and the Society of Cardiovascular Anesthesiologists; endorsed by the Society of Thoracic Surgeons. *J Am Soc Echocardiogr.* 2007;20:1227-1235.
8. Bucerius J, Gummert JF, Borger MA, et al. Stroke after cardiac surgery: a risk factor analysis of 16.184 consecutive adult patients. *Ann Thorac Surg.* 2003;75:472-478.
9. Djaiai G, Ali M, Borger MA, et al. Epiaortic scanning modified planned intraoperative surgical management but not cerebral embolic load during coronary artery bypass surgery. *Anesth Analg.* 2008;106:1611-1618.
10. Roach GW, Kanchuger M, Mangano CM, et al. Adverse cerebral outcomes after coronary bypass surgery. *N Engl J Med.* 1996;335:1857-1863.
11. McKhann GM, et al. Encephalopathy and stroke after coronary artery bypass grafting; incidence, consequences, and prediction. *Arch Neurol.* 2002;59:1422-1428.
12. Anyanwu AC, Filsoufi F, Salzberg SP, Bronster DJ, Adams DH. Epidemiology of stroke after cardiac surgery in the current era. *J Thorac Cardiovasc Surg.* 2007;134:1121-1127.
13. Coffey CE, Massey EW, Roberts KB, Curtis S, Jones RH, Pryor DB. Natural history of cerebral complications of coronary artery bypass graft surgery. *Neurology.* 1983;33(11):1416-1421.
14. Breuer AC, et al. Central nervous system complications of coronary artery bypass graft surgery: prospective analysis of 421 patients. *Stroke.* 1983;14(5):682-687.
15. Shahian DM, et al. The Society of Thoracic Surgeons 2008 cardiac surgery risk models: part 1–coronary artery bypass grafting surgery. *Ann Thorac Surg.* 2009;88:S2.
16. O'Brien SM, et al. The Society of Thoracic Surgeons 2008 cardiac surgery risk models: part 2–isolated valve surgery. *Ann Thorac Surg.* 2009;88:S23.
17. Shahian DM, et al. The Society of Thoracic Surgeons 2008 cardiac surgery risk models: part 3–valve plus coronary artery bypass graft surgery. *Ann Thorac Surg.* 2009;88:S43.
18. Stamou SC, Hill PC, Dangas G, et al. Stroke after coronary artery bypass; incidence, predictors, and clinical outcomes. *Stroke.* 2001;32:1508-1513.
19. Hogue Jr CW, Barzilai B, Pieper KS, et al. Sex differences in neurological outcomes and mortality after cardiac surgery; a Society of Thoracic Surgery National Database report. *Circulation.* 2001;103:2133-2137.
20. Charlesworth DC, Likosky DS, Marrin CAS, et al. Development and validation of a prediction model for strokes after coronary artery bypass grafting. *Ann Thorac Surg.* 2003;76:436-443.
21. Puskas JD, Winston AD, Wright CE. Stroke after coronary artery operation: incidence, correlates, outcome, and cost. *Ann Thorac Surg.* 2000;69:1053-1056.
22. McKhann GM, Goldsborough MA, Borowicz Jr LM. Predictors of stroke risk in coronary artery bypass patients. *Ann Thorac Surgery.* 1997;63:516-521.
23. Amarenco P, Duyckaerts C, Tzourio C, Henin D, Bousser MG, Hauw JJ. The prevalence of ulcerated plaques in the aortic arch in patients with stroke. *N Engl J Med.* 1992;326:221-225.
24. Amarenco P, Cohen A, Tzourio C, et al. Atherosclerotic disease of the aortic arch and the risk of ischemic stroke. *N Engl J Med.* 1994;331:1474-1479.
25. Amarenco P, Hienzlef O, Lucas C, et al. The French Study of the Aortic Plaques in Stroke Group. Atherosclerotic disease of the aortic arch as a risk factor for recurrent ischemic stroke. *N Engl J Med.* 1996;334:1216-1221.
26. Di Tullio MR, Russo C, Jin Z, Sacco RL, Mohr JP, Homma S. Aortic arch plaques and risk of recurrent stroke and death. *Circulation.* 2009;119:2376-2382.
27. Tunick PA, Perez JL, Kronzon I. Protruding atheromas in the thoracic aorta and systemic embolization. *Ann Intern Med.* 1991;115:423-427.
28. Karalis DG, Chandrasekaran K, Victor MF, Ross JJ, Mintz GS. Recognition and embolic potential of intraaortic atherosclerotic debris. *J Am Coll Cardiol.* 1991;17:73-78.
29. Tunick PA, Rosenzweig BP, Katz ES, Freedberg RS, Perez JL, Kronzon I. High risk for vascular events in patients with protruding aortic atheromas: a prospective study. *J Am Coll Cardiol.* 1994;23:1085-1090.
30. Ferrari E, Vidal R, Chevallier T, Baudouy M. Atherosclerosis of the aorta and aortic debris as a marker of poor prognosis: benefit of oral anticoagulants. *J Am Coll Cardiol.* 1999;33:1317-1322.
31. Tunick PA, Ambika CN, Goodkin GM, et al. Effect of treatment on the incidence of stroke and other emboli in 519 patients with severe thoracic aortic plaque. *Am J Cardiol.* 2002;90:1320-1325.
32. Russo C. Kin z, Rundek T, Homma S, Sacco RL, Di Tullio MR. Atherosclerotic Disease of the Proximal Aorta and the Risk of Vascular Events in a Population-Based Cohort; The Aortic Plaques and Risk of Ischemic Stroke (APRIS) Study. *Stroke.* 2009;40:2313-2318.
33. Petty GW, Khandheria BK, Meissner I, et al. Population-Based Study of the Relationship Between Atherosclerotic Aortic Debris and Cerebrovascular Ischemic Events. *Mayo Clin Proc.* 2006;81(5):609-614.
34. Meissner I, Khandheria BK, Sheps SG, et al. Atherosclerosis of the Aorta: Risk Factor, Risk Marker, or Innocent Bystander; A Prospective Population-Based Transesophageal Echocardiography Study. *J Am Coll Cardiol.* 2004;44:1018-1024.
35. Wolman RL, Nussmeier NA, Aggarwal A, et al. Cerebral Injury after Cardiac Surgery; Identification of a Group at Extraordinary Risk. *Stroke.* 1999;30:514-522.
36. Hartman GS, Yao FSF, Bruefach III M, et al. Severity of Aortic Atheromatous Disease Diagnosed by Transesophageal Echocardiography Predicts Stroke and Other Outcomes Associated With Coronary Artery Surgery: A prospective Study. *Anesth Analg.* 1996;83:701-708.
37. Linden JVD, Hadjinikolaou L, Bergman P, Lindblom D. Postoperative Stroke in Cardiac Surgery Is Related to the Location and Extent of Atherosclerotic Disease in the Ascending Aorta. *J Am Coll Cardiol.* 2001;38:131-135.
38. Katz ES, Tunick PA, Rusinek H, Ribakove G, Spencer FC, Kronzon I. Protruding Aortic Atheromas Predict Stroke in Elderly Patient's Undergoing Cardiopulmonary Bypass: Experience With Intraoperative Transesophageal Echocardiography. *J Am Coll Cardiol.* 1992;20:70-77.
39. Davila-Roman VG, Murphy SF, Nickerson NJ, Kouchoukos NT, Schechtman KB, Barzilai B. Atherosclerosis of the Ascending Aorta Is an Independent Predictor of Long-Tern Neurologic Events and Mortality. *J Am Coll Cardiol.* 1999;33:1308-1316.
40. John R, Choudhri AF, Weinberg AD. Ting w, Rose EAU, Smith CR, OZ MC. Multicenter Review of Preoperative Risk Factors for Stroke After Coronary Bypass Grafting. *Ann Thorac Surg.* 2000;69:30-36.
41. Hogue Jr CW, Murphy SF, Schechtman KB, Davila-Roman VG. Risk Factors For Early Or Delayed Stroke After Cardiac Surgery. *Circulation.* 1999;100:642-647.
42. Gardner TJ, Horneffer PJ, Manolio TA, et al. Stroke following coronary artery bypass grafting: a ten-year study. *Ann Thorac Surg.* 1985;40(6):574-581.
43. Doty JR, Wilentz RE, Salazar JD, Hruban RH, Cameron DE. Atheroembolism in Cardiac Surgery. *Ann Thorac Surg.* 2003;75(4):1221-1226.
44. Thurlbeck WM, Castleman B. Atheromatous emboli to the kidneys after aortic surgery. *N Engl J Med.* 1957;257(10):442-447.
45. Freedberg RS, Tunick PA, Kronzon I. Emboli in transit: the missing link. *J Am Soc Echocardiogr.* 1998;11(8):826-828.
46. Ezzeddine MA, Primavera JM, Rosand J, Hedley-Whyte ET, Rordorf G. Clinical characteristics of pathologically proved cholesterol emboli to the brain. *Neurology.* 2000;54:1681-1683.
47. Cross SS. How common is cholesterol embolism? *J Clin Pathol.* 1991;44:859-861.
48. Fukumoto Y, Tsutsui H, Tsuchihashi M, Masunoto A, Takeshita A. Cholesterol Embolism Study (Chest) Investigators: The Incidence and Risk Factors of Cholesterol Embolization, A Complication of Cardiac Catheterization: A Prospective Study. *J Am Coll Cardiol.* 2003;42:211-216.
49. Hammon Jr JW, Stump DA, Kon ND, et al. Risk factors and Solutions for the Development of Neurobehavioral Changes after Coronary Bypass Grafting. *Ann Thorac Surg.* 1997;63(6):1613-1618.
50. Ascione R, Reeves BC, Chamberlain MH, Ghosh AK, Lim KH, Angelini GD. Predictors of Stroke in the Modern Era of Coronary Artery Bypass Grafting: A Case Control Study. *Ann Thorac Surg.* 2002;74(2):474-480.
51. Likosky DS, Marrin CAS, Caplan LR, et al. Determination of Etiologic Mechanism of Strokes Secondary to Coronary Artery Bypass Graft Surgery. *Stroke.* 2003;34:2830-2834.
52. Blauth CI. Macroemboli and Microemboli During Cardiopulmonary Bypass. *Ann Thorac Surg.* 1995;59:1300-1303.
53. Abu-Omar Y, Balacumaraswami L, Matthews PM, Taggart Solid DP, Cerebral Gaseous. Microembolization during Off-Pump, On-Pump, and Open Cardiac Surgery Procedures. *J Thorac Cardiovasc Surg.* 2004;127:1759-1765.
54. Schreiber S, Serdaroglu M, Schreiber F, Skalej M, Heinze HJ, Goertler M. Simultaneous Occurrence and Interaction of Hypoperfusion and Embolism in a Patient with Severe Middle Cerebral Artery Stenosis*Stroke.* 2009;40(7):e478-e480 (epub).
55. Sedlaczek O, Caplan L, Hennerici M. Impaired Washout—Embolism and Ischemic Stroke: Further Examples and Proof of Concept. *Cerebrovasc Dis.* 2005;19(6):396-401.
56. Caplan LR, Hennerici M. Impaired Clearance of Emboli (Washout) is an Important Link Between Hypoperfusion, Embolism, and Ischemic Stroke. *Arch Neurol.* 1998;55(11):1475-1482.
57. Swaminathan M, Grocott HP, Mackensen GB, Podgoreanu MV, Glower DD, Matthew JP. The "Sandblasting Effect of Aortic Cannula on Arch Atheroma During Cardiopulmonary Bypass. *Anesth Analg.* 2007;104(6):1350-1351.
58. Hamano K, Ikeda Y, Okada H, et al. Atheromatous Plaque in the Distal Aortic Arch Creating the Potential for Cerebral Embolism During Cardiopulmonary bypass. *Jpn Circ J.* 2001;65(3):161-164.
59. Mackensen GB, Ti LK, Phillips-Bute BG, et al. Cerebral embolization during cardiac surgery: Impact of aortic atheroma burden. *Br J Anaesth.* 2003;91:656.
60. Sharony R, Bizekis CS, Kanchuger M, et al. Off-pump coronary artery bypass grafting reduces mortality and stroke in patients with atheromatous aortas: A case control study*Circulation.* 2003;9(suppl I):II-115.
61. Arrowsmith JE, Grocott HP, Reves JG, et al. Central nervous system complications of cardiac surgery. *Br J Anaesth.* 2000;84:378.
62. Davila-Roman VG, Phillips KJ, Daily BB, Davila RM, Kouchoukos NT, Barzilai B. Intraoperative Transesophageal Echocardiography and Epiaortic Ultrasound for Assessment of Atherosclerosis of the Thoracic Aorta. *J Am Coll Cardiol.* 1996;28:942-947.

63. Marshall Jr WG, Barzilai B, Kouchoukos NT, Saffitz J. Intraoperative Ultrasonic Imaging of the Ascending Aorta. *Ann Thorac Surg.* 1989;48(3):339-344.
64. Royse C, Royse A, Blake D, Grigg L. Screening the Thoracic Aorta for Atheroma: A Comparison of Manual Palpation, Transesophageal and Epiaortic Ultrasonography. *Ann Thorac Cardiovasc Surg.* 1998;4(6):347-350.
65. Ohteki H, Itoh T, Natsuaki M, Minato N, Suda H. Intraoperative Ultrasonic Imaging of the Ascending Aorta in Ischemic Heart Disease. *Ann Thorac Surg.* 1990;50(4):539-542.
66. Wareing TH, Davila-Roman VG, Barzilai B, Murphy SF, Kouchoukos NT. Management of the severely atherosclerotic ascending aorta during cardiac operations. a strategy for detection and treatment. *J Thorac Cardiovasc Surg.* 1992;103(3):453-462.
67. St Amand MA, Murkin JM, Menkis AH, et al. Aortic atherosclerotic plaque identified by epiaortic scanning predicts cerebral embolic load in cardiac surgery. *Can J Anaesth.* 1997;44:A7.
68. Cohen A, Tzourio C, Bertran B, Chauvel C, Bousser MG, Amarenco Aortic Plaque Morphology P, Events Vascular. A Follow-Up Study in Patients With Ischemic Stroke; FAPS Investigators. French Study of Aortic Plaques in Stroke. *Circulation.* 1997;96:3838-3841.
69. Konstadt SN, Reich DL, Kahn R, et al. Transesophageal echocardiography can be used to screen for ascending aortic atherosclerosis. *Anesth Analg.* 1995;81:225-228.
70. Konstadt SN, Reich DL, Quintana C, Levy M. The ascending aorta: how much does transesophageal echocardiography see? *Anesth Analg.* 1994;78:240-244.
71. Hangler BH, Nagele G, Danzmayr M, et al. Modification of surgical technique for ascending aortic atherosclerosis: impact on stroke reduction in coronary artery bypass grafting. *J Thorac Cardiovasc Surg.* 2003;126:391-400.
72. Barzilai B, Marshall Jr WG, Saffitz JE, Kouchoukos N. Avoidance of embolic complications by ultrasonic characterization of the ascending aorta. *Circulation.* 1989;80(3 Pt 1):1275-1279.
73. Trehan N, Mishra M, Kasliwal R, Mishra A. Reduced neurological injury during CABG in patients with mobile aortic atheromas: a five-year follow-up study. *Ann Thorac Surg.* 2000;70:1558-1564.
74. Djaiani G, Ali M, Borger MA, et al. Epiaortic Scanning Modifies planned Intraoperative Surgical Management But Not Cerebral Embolic Load During Coronary Artery Bypass Surgery. *Anesth Analg.* 2008;106:1611-1618.
75. Gold JP, Torres KE, Maldarelli W, Zhuravlev I, Condit D, Wasnick J. Improving Outcomes in Coronary Surgery: The Impact of Echo-Directed Aortic Cannulation and Perioperative Hemodynamic Management in 500 Patients. *Ann Thorac Surg.* 2004;78:579-585.
76. Davila-Roman VG, Barzilai B, Wareing TH, Murphy SF, Kouchoukos NT. Intraoperative Ultrasonographic Evaluation of the ascending aorta in 100 Consecutive Patients Undergoing Cardiac Surgery. *Circulation.* 1991;84(suppl 5):11147-11153.
77. Ribakove GH, Katz ES, Galloway AC, et al. Surgical Implications of Transesophageal Echocardiography to Grade the Atheromatous Aortic Arch. *Ann Thorac Surg.* 1992;53(3):758-761.
78. Trehan N, Mishra M, Dhole S, Mishra A, Karlekar A, Kohli VN. Significantly Reduced Incidence of Stroke During Coronary Artery Bypass Grafting Using Transesophageal Echocardiography. *Eur J Cardiothorac Surg.* 1997;11(2):234-242.
79. Kapetanakis EI, Stamou S, Dullum MKC, et al. The Impact of Aortic Manipulation on Neurologic Outcomes After Coronary Artery Bypass Surgery: A Risk-Adjusted Study. *Ann Thorac Surg.* 2004;78:1564-1571.
80. Royse AG, Royse CF, Ajani AE. Reduced Neuropsychological Dysfunction Using Epiaortic Echocardiography and the Exclusive Y. Graft. *Ann Thorac Surg.* 2000;69:1431-1438.
81. Dijk DV, Jansen EWL, Hijman R, et al. Cognitive Outcome After Off-Pump and On-Pump Coronary Artery Bypass Graft Surgery. *JAMA.* 2002;287:1405-1412.
82. Cleveland Jr JC, Shroyer ALW, Chen AY, Peterson E, Grover FL. Off-Pump Coronary Artery Bypass Grafting Decreases Risk-Adjusted Mortality and Morbidity. *Ann Thorac Surg.* 2001;72:1282-1289.
83. Stern A, Tunick PA, Culliford AT, et al. Protruding aortic arch atheromas: risk of stroke during heart surgery with and without aortic arch endarterectomy. *Am Heart J.* 1999;138(4 Pt 1):746-752.
84. Eltzschig HK, Kallmeyer IJ, Mihaljevic T, Alapati S, Shernan SK. A practical approach to a comprehensive epicardial and epiaortic echocardiographic examination *J Cardiothorac Vasc Anesth.* 2003;17(4):442-429.
85. Royse A, Royse C. A Standardized intraoperative Ultrasound Examination of the Aorta and Proximal Coronary Arteries. *Interact Cardiovasc Thorac Surg.* 2006;5:701-704.
86. Glas K, Swaminathan M, Reeves S, et al. Guidelines for the performance of a comprehensive intraoperative epiaortic ultrasonographic examination: recommendations of the American Society of Echocardiography and the Society of Cardiovascular Anesthesiologists; Endorsed by the Society of Thoracic Surgeons. *Anesth Analg.* 2008;106:1376-1384.
87. Sekoranja L, Vuille C, Bianchi-Demicheli F, et al. Thoracic aortic plaques, transesophageal echocardiography and coronary artery disease. *Swiss Med Wkly.* 2004;134:75-78.
88. MacKenson GB, et al. The Perioperative Outcomes Research Group and Cardiothoracic Anesthesiology Research Endeavors (C.A.R.E.) Investigators of the Duke Heart Center. Preliminary report on the interaction of apolipoprotein E polymorphism with aortic atherosclerosis and acute nephropathy after CABG. *Ann Thorac Surg.* 2004;78:520-526.
89. Barzilai B, Saffitz JE, Miller JG, Sobel BE. Quantitative Ultrasound Characterization of the Nature of Atherosclerotic Plaques in Human Aorta. *Circ Res.* 1987;60:459-463.
90. Nohara H, Shida T, Mukohara N, Obo H, Higami T. Ultrasonic Plaque Density of Aortic Atheroma and Stroke in Patients Undergoing On-Pump Coronary Bypass Surgery. *Ann Thorac Cardiovasc Surg.* 2004;10:235-240.
91. Bainbridge DT, Murkin JM, Menkis A, Kiaii B. The Use of 3D Epiaortic Scanning to Enhance Evaluation of Atherosclerotic Plaque in the Ascending Aorta: A Case Series. *Heart Surg Forum.* 2004;7(6):E636-E639.
92. Bainbridge D. 3-D Imaging for Aortic Plaque Assessment. *Semin Cardiothorac Vasc Anesth.* 2005;9(2):163-165.
93. Hager A, Kaemmerer H, Rapp-Bernhardt U, et al. Diameters of the thoracic aorta throughout life as measured with helical computed tomography. J Thorac Cardiovasc Surg 123(6): 1060–1066.
94. Wolak A, Gransar H, Thomson EJ, Friedman JD, et al. Aortic size assessment by noncontrast cardiac computed tomography: normal limits by age, gender, and body surface area. *JACC Cardiovasc Imaging.* 2008;1(2):200-209.
95. O'Rourke M, Farnsworth A, O'Rourke J. Aortic dimensions and stiffness in normal adults. *JACC Cardiovasc Imaging.* 2008;1(6):749-751.
96. Biaggi P, Matthews F, Braun J, Rousson V, Kaufmann PA, Jenni R. Gender, age, and body surface area are the major determinants of ascending aorta dimensions in subjects with apparently normal echocardiograms. *J Am Soc Echocardiogr.* 2009;22:720-725.
97. Roman MJ, Devereux RB, Kramer-Fox R, O'Loughlin J. Two-dimensional echocardiographic aortic root dimensions in normal children and adults. *Am J Cardiol.* 1989;64:507-512.
98. Vasan RS, Larson MG, Benjamin EJ, Levy D. Echocardiographic reference values for aortic root size: the Framingham Heart Study. *J Am Soc Echocardiogr.* 1995;8(6):793-800.
99. Vasan RS, Mg Larson, Levy D. Determinants of echocardiographic aortic root size. The Framingham Study. *Circulation.* 1995;91(3):734-30.
100. Erbel R, Alfonso F, Boileau C, et al. Diagnosis and management of aortic dissection. *Eur Heart J.* 2001;22:1642-1681.
101. Lang RM, Bierig M, Devereux RV, et al. Recommendations for chamber quantification: a report from the American Society of Echocardiography's Guidelines and Standards Committee and the Chamber Quantification Writing Group, developed in conjunction with the European Association of Echocardiography, a branch of the European Society of Cardiology. *J Am Soc Echocardiogr.* 2005;18:1440-1463.
102. Kazui R, Izumoto H, Yoshioka K, et al. Dynamic morphologic changes in the normal aortic annulus during systole and diastole. *J Heart Valve Dis.* 2006;15:617-621.
103. Demertzis S, Casso G, Torre T, et al. Direct epiaortic ultrasound scanning for the rapid confirmation of intraoperative aortic dissection. *Interact Cardiovasc Thorac Surg.* 2008;7:725-726.
104. Inoue Y, Takahashi R, Ueda T, et al. Synchronized epiaortic two-dimensional and color Doppler echocardiographic guidance enables routine ascending aortic cannulation in type A acute aortic dissection. *J Thorac Cardiovasc Surg.* 2011;141:354-360.
105. Seki T, Maruyama R, Inoue Y, et al. Ascending aorta cannulation in Stanford type a acute aortic dissection. *Kyobu Geka.* 2012;65:184-188.
106. Edrich T, Shernan SK, Smith B, et al. Usefulness of intraoperative epiaortic echocardiography to resolve discrepancy between transthoracic and transesophageal measurements of aortic valve gradient—a case report. *Can J Anesth.* 2003;50:293-296.

Normal Anatomy and Flow During the Complete Examination: Three-Dimensional Views: Replicating the Surgeon's View

GREGORY W. FISCHER

Noninvasive cardiac imaging centers on the ability to visualize and quantitate cardiac structure and function. To perform these tasks, there are currently multiple modalities at the clinician's disposal (e.g., magnetic resonance imaging [MRI], computed tomography [CT], and nuclear medicine). Although CT and MRI technology provide the imager with excellent image resolution and three-dimensional (3D) volumetric quantification capabilities, these imaging modalities entail space and infrastructure requirements that render them impractical for the operating room environment. Conversely, echocardiography is highly mobile and easily integrated into the operating room environment. Recently, technological advances enabling real-time 3D imaging have made echocardiography competitive with these more expensive and operationally intensive modalities. The introduction of real-time 3D transesophageal echocardiography (TEE) into clinical practice within the last several years offers the perioperative team new qualitative and quantitative imaging capabilities.

For two-dimensional (2D) TEE, the landmark paper published by Shanewise et al.[1] is considered the definitive standard for a complete perioperative TEE exam. This complete exam consists of 20 views (see Chapter 1). The orientation of these views is determined by the anatomic relationship of the esophagus to the heart (transesophageal views) or the stomach to the heart (transgastric views). Unfortunately, because of this orientation and the 2D nature of the display on screen, interpretation is rarely intuitive, and months of dedicated training are required to master the skill of 2D echocardiography. An experienced echocardiographer creates a "mental" reconstruction of a 3D image of cardiac structures of interest by assimilating information from multiple 2D views, but less experienced imagers or non-echocardiographers find interpreting 2D views challenging, and this impairs transfer of information in the perioperative setting.

A major advantage of 3D echocardiography is the ability to spatially orient and crop the acquired data block at the discretion of the echocardiographer. Consequently, image orientation and 3D structure should facilitate communication between surgeon and echocardiographer, especially if the image is displayed in an orientation that replicates the surgeon's view intraoperatively. This chapter will provide an overview of 3D echocardiography and demonstrate image orientations that best simulate the views of cardiac structures seen by surgeons in the most common surgical approaches.

Transducer Design

The foundation of echocardiography revolves around the transduction of electrical energy into mechanical energy (i.e., vibrational waves) and vice versa. The parameters that constrain echocardiography (the "acoustic triangle of constraint") are: (1) frame rate, (2) sector/volume size, and (3) imaging resolution. In general, increasing the requirement of one of these causes a drop in either or both of the other two, assuming other parameters are maintained constant, such as the number of transmit events (Fig. 9-1). While clinicians who are inexperienced in echocardiography often believe 3D TEE will provide images

of superior quality when compared to 2D TEE, it is important to note that 3D echocardiography is subject to the same laws of acoustic physics as 2D echocardiography. Artifacts such as ringing, reverberations, shadowing, and attenuation occur in 3D as well as 2D and M-mode.

Conventional 2D imaging transducers transmit and receive acoustic beams in a flat scanning plane. The to-and-fro sweeping action of a scanline enables a sector to be imaged. Typically, a modern-day conventional 2D imaging transducer consists of 128 linear (1D) "elements" that are interconnected electronically to sum radiofrequency (RF) scanlines. By varying the spatiotemporal phase of initiating each element's transmit event, the ultrasound beam can be steered. These principles represent the basis for any phased array system (Fig. 9-2; also see Chapter 6).

In contrast to 2D imaging transducers, 3D imaging matrix arrays have both columns and rows of elements. Instead of a single dimension (column) of 128 elements, a matrix array comprises more than 50 rows and 50 columns of elements. As described in Chapter 6, the 2D block of approximately 2500 elements is created by "dicing" a block of transducer material by a diamond-tipped saw to create each element (Fig. 9-3). This 2D block allows for 3D scanning and forms the foundation of a matrix array transducer (Fig. 9-4). Additional innovations, such as incorporation of materials that allow more acoustic bandwidth (simultaneous high and low frequencies), enable matrix array transducers to enhance both tissue penetration and image resolution.

Display of Three-Dimensional Images

Electronically steered matrix transducers have additional modes of operation when compared to conventional 2D phased array transducers. Owing to the ability of matrix transducers to capture a data block of information, two 2D images at different imaging angles can be displayed on screen simultaneously as two real-time images. The software allows the imager to adjust the angle of one image while comparing it to the other, enabling a complete 180-degree sweep around an area of interest. This mode of operation is called the *simultaneous multiplane mode* and is unique to matrix array transducers (Fig. 9-5 and Video 9-1).

The major technological advance of the matrix transducer is its ability to render 3D images. There are two different modes of operation in 3D echocardiography. The first is a "live" mode where the system scans in real-time 3D. The second integrates two to six gated beats, which enables wider volumes to be generated while maintaining frame rate and resolution. This is achieved by acquiring multiple narrow-volume data sets and subsequently stitching them together to create a single large volumetric data block. This technique, however, is subject to a consistent R-R interval in the electrocardiogram (ECG) and lack of respiratory movement, otherwise imaging artifacts will occur (Fig. 9-6 and Video 9-2).

Live 3D: Real-Time

In this mode, a 3D volume pyramid is obtained. The image shown in this mode is real-time. The 3D image changes as the transducer is moved, just as in the live 2D imaging case. Manipulations of the TEE

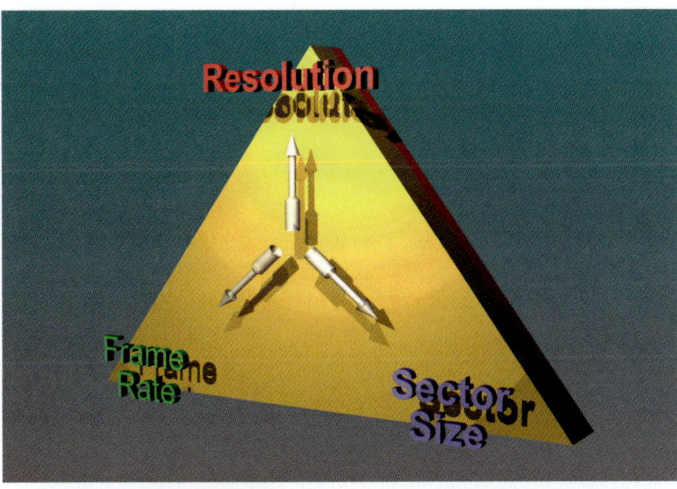

Figure 9-1   Triangle of constraint.

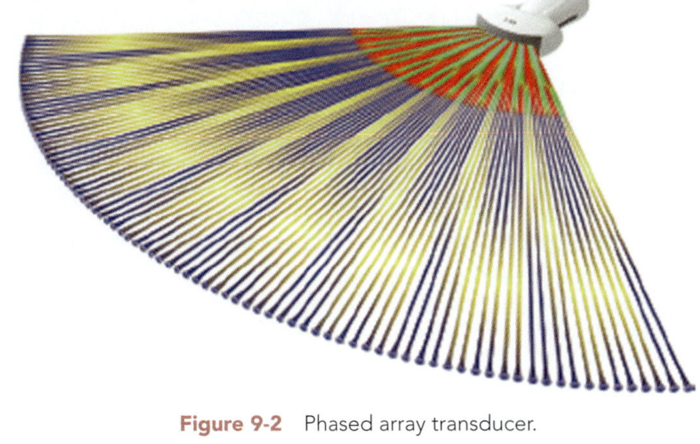

Figure 9-2   Phased array transducer.

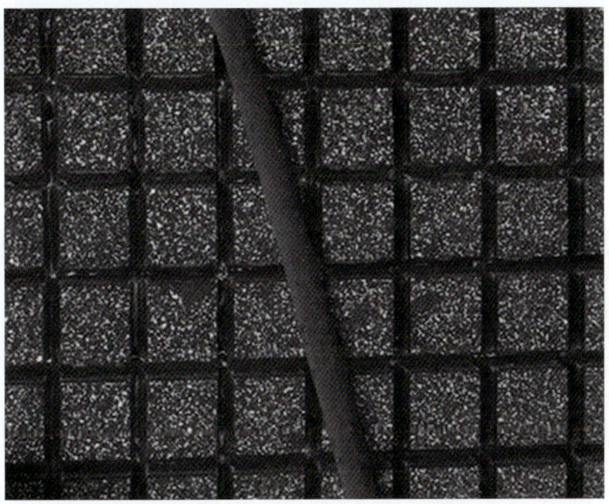

Figure 9-3   Matrix transducer consisting of 2500 piezoelectric crystals. Human hair is shown to demonstrate size of each element.

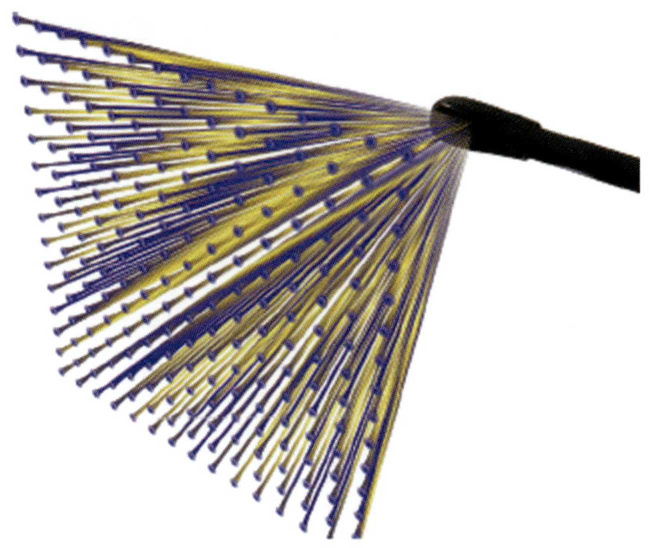

Figure 9-4   Matrix transducer producing a three-dimensional scanning beam.

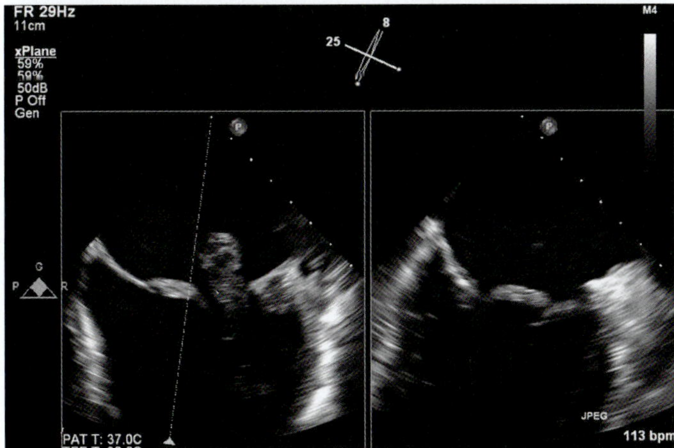

Figure 9-5   Simultaneous multiplane mode. Echocardiographer has the ability to scan around region of interest while comparing image on right with original image on left.

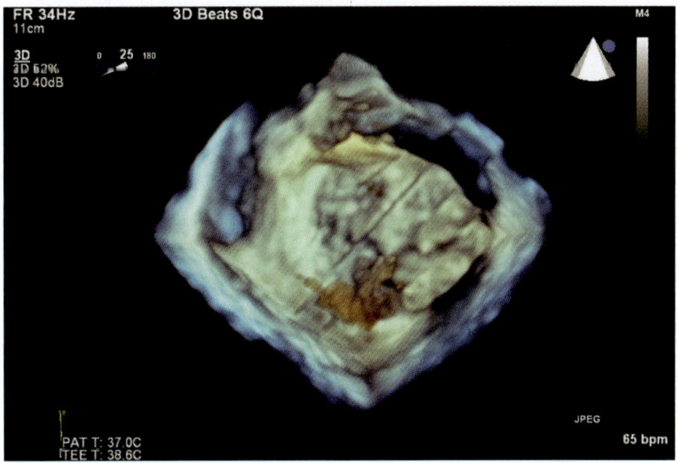

Figure 9-6   Stitch artifacts seen in full-volume mode.

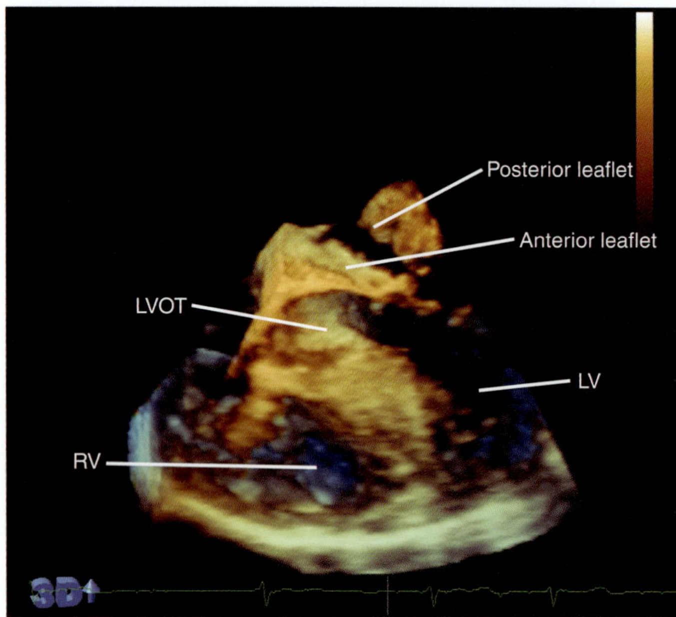

Figure 9-7   Live three-dimensional mode. *LV,* Left ventricle; *LVOT,* left ventricular outflow tract; *RV,* right ventricle.

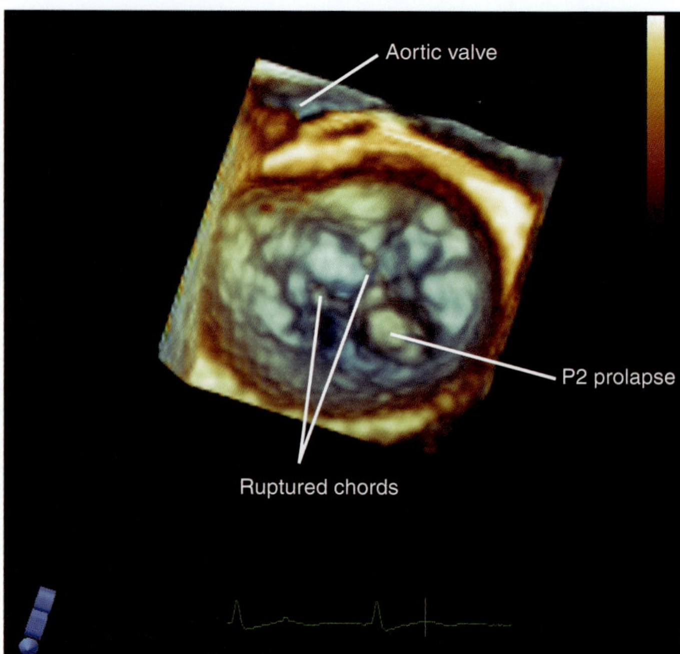

Figure 9-8   Three-dimensional zoom mode. *P2,* Mitral valve posterior leaflet P2 scallop.

 probe (e.g., rotation, change in position) lead to instantaneous changes in the image seen on the monitor (Fig. 9-7 and Video 9-3).

3D Zoom: Real-Time

This mode displays a small, magnified pyramidal volume that may vary from 20 × 20 degrees up to 90 × 90 degrees, depending on the density setting. This small data set can be spatially oriented at the discretion of the echocardiographer, enabling views of the mitral valve from both the left atrial and left ventricular perspectives. The real-time 3D images are devoid of rotational artifacts, as are commonly encountered with  ECG-gated 3D acquisitions (Fig. 9-8 and Video 9-4).

Full Volume: Gated

The image quality of 3D echocardiography is not limited by computer and circuit processing power but by the speed of sound. There is insufficient time for sound to travel back and forth in large volumes while maintaining a frame rate of over 20 Hz and reasonable resolution in live scanning modes. One maneuver to overcome this entails stitching two to six gates together to create a "full-volume" mode. These gated "slabs" or "subvolumes" represent a pyramidal 3D data set as would be acquired in the live 3D mode. This technique can generate greater than 90-degree scanning volumes at frame rates above 30 Hz. Increasing the gates from two to six creates smaller 3D slabs. As explained earlier, the acoustic triangle of constraint principle is partially overcome by 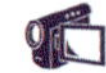 gating so as to maintain frame rates and/or resolution as the volumes (pyramids) become larger (Video 9-5).

The acquired real-time 3D data set can subsequently be cropped, analyzed, and quantified using postprocessing software (Figs. 9-9 and 9-10).

3D Color Doppler: Gated

Color flow Doppler (CFD) requires obtaining multiple samples along a common scanline. Unfortunately, firing more events along a stationary scanline degrades the frame rate because of limitations imposed by the underlying physics. To increase the frame rate, a gating method must be used. As opposed to 2D echocardiography, the 3D image allows the echocardiographer to appreciate jet direction, extent, and geometry. Reports started emerging a decade ago showing that the strength of this

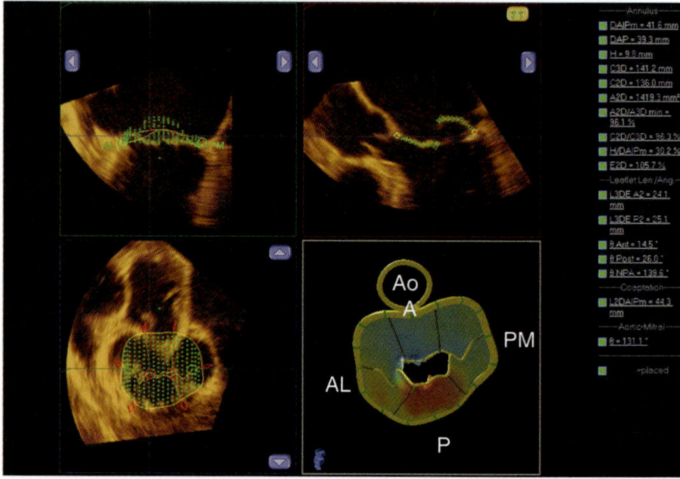

Figure 9-9   Mitral valve quantification (MVQ) in QLAB. *A,* Anterior; *AL,* anterolateral commissure; *Ao,* aorta; *P,* posterior; *PM,* posteromedial commissure.

methodology lies in its ability to quantitate; 3D quantification of mitral regurgitation correlates better than 2D imaging when using angiography as the gold standard.[2,3] In an experimental setting, 3D quantification was more accurate (2.6% underestimation) than 2D or M-mode methods, which had the tendency to underestimate regurgitant volumes (44.2% and 32.1%, respectively) (Fig. 9-11 and Video 9-6).[4] 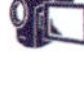

Mitral Valve

Intraoperative TEE represents a class I indication for perioperative management of mitral valve surgery.

The mitral valve is a complex 3D structure that can be visualized with either the 3D zoom or full-volume mode. The advantage of the zoom mode is the ability to quickly obtain an image immune to ECG, respiratory, or electrocautery artifacts (Video 9-7). The disadvantage 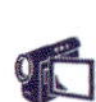

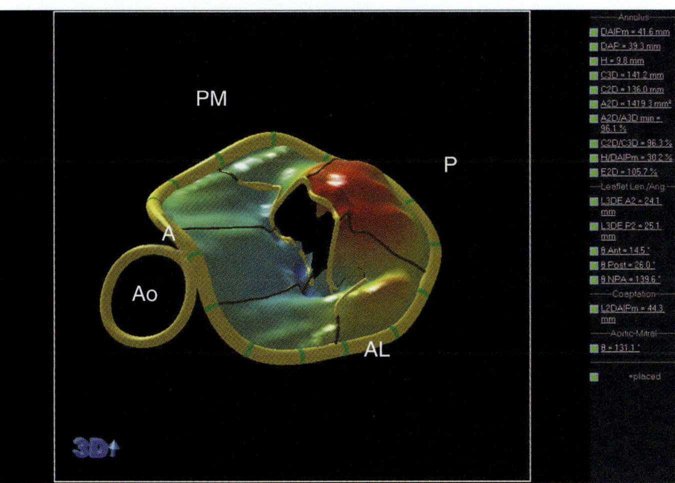

Figure 9-10   Mitral valve quantification (MVQ) model of mitral valve. *A,* Anterior; *AL,* anterolateral commissure; *Ao,* aorta; *P,* posterior; *PM,* posteromedial commissure.

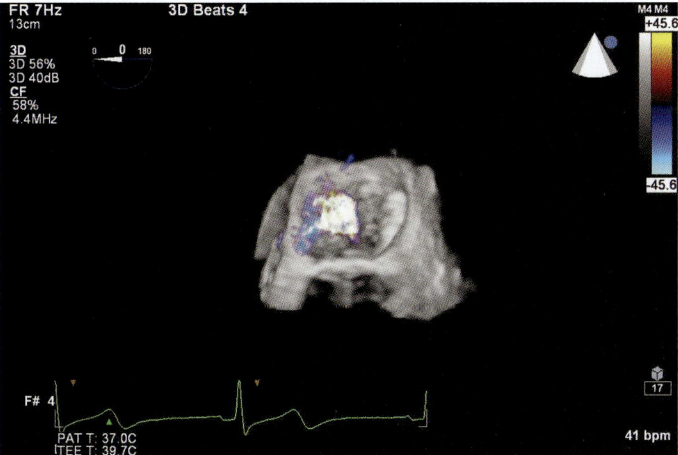

Figure 9-11   Three-dimensional color flow Doppler image of mitral valve.

of this mode is found in the constraints of echocardiography. Larger valves (e.g., Barlow disease) can only be imaged in their entirety by sacrificing temporal and spatial resolution. In these cases, the author recommends full-volume acquisition (Video 9-8). Regardless of which mode is used, it is imperative that the 3D image be optimized by adjusting gain and compression (Fig. 9-12 and Video 9-9). Subsequently, the image is spatially rotated and cropped such that the data set is displayed to reflect the surgeon's view (i.e., the view the surgeon has when positioned on the patient's right side and examining the mitral valve through the opened left atrium). The anterior leaflet is seen on the top and the posterior leaflet at the bottom of the screen. The anterolateral commissure is to the left and the posteromedial commissure to the right of the screen. Image resolution is so remarkable that topographical structures within the leaflet's anatomy (e.g., indentations and clefts) can easily be viewed. Pathologic processes (e.g., chordal rupture with segmental flail, billowing, or leaflet restriction) are quickly identified and precisely localized. The ability to rotate the data set freely in all axes enables the imager to view the mitral valve apparatus from all clinically relevant angles (e.g., left atrial or left ventricular perspective) (Video 9-10).

The strength of 3D echocardiography lies not only in the qualitative analysis of the images but also in the ability to quantitate in three dimensions. This is performed by the postprocessing of acquired images utilizing 3D software such as QLAB or TomTec. Measurements that can be obtained include:

1. The major anatomically oriented 3D axes of the annulus, anteroposterior (A-P) and anterolateral-posteromedial (AL-PM) diameters, and annular height
2. 3D curvilinear leaflet lengths and areas of all segments (A1, A2, A3, P1, P2, P3)
3. Total and functional anterior and posterior leaflet surface areas
4. The angle between the aortic valve annulus and mitral valve annulus (aortomitral angle). A narrow angle should alert the imager to the possibility of systolic anterior motion (SAM) during the postrepair period (see Figs. 9-9 and 9-10).

Imaging the Aortic and Tricuspid Valves

Unlike the mitral valve, acquiring high-quality images of the aortic and tricuspid valves represents a more difficult undertaking. The explanation lies in the thinner leaflet tissue both the aortic and tricuspid valves are generally composed of and the orientation of the tissue as a reflector. Since these factors result in weaker acoustic signal strength, the 3D volume renderer is more apt to tag these as transparent and render the voxels as blood—meaning invisible.

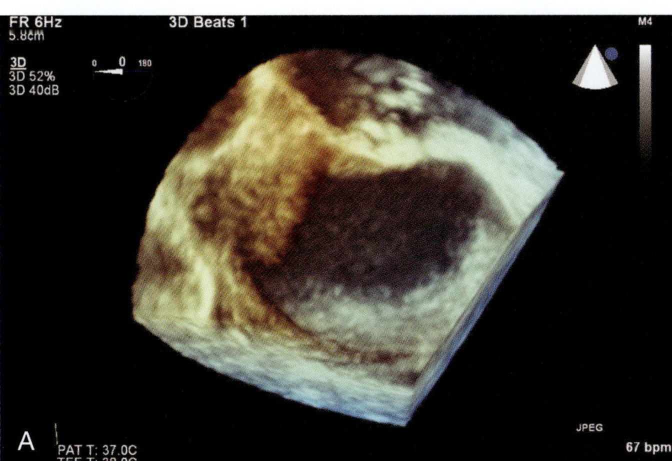

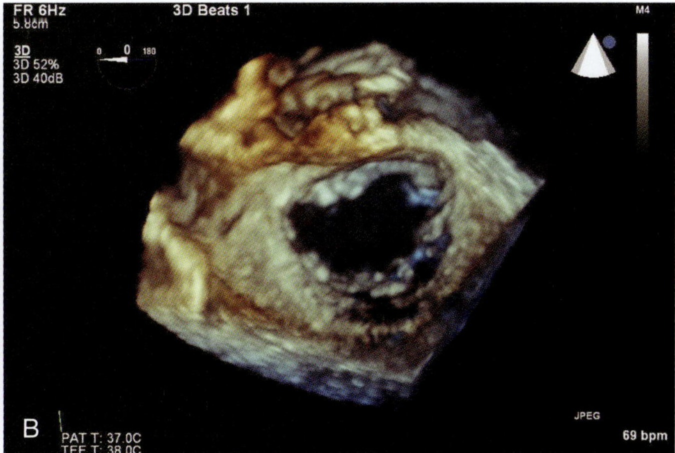

Figure 9-12   **A,** Three-dimensional image with excessive gain. **B,** Same image after correction of gain.

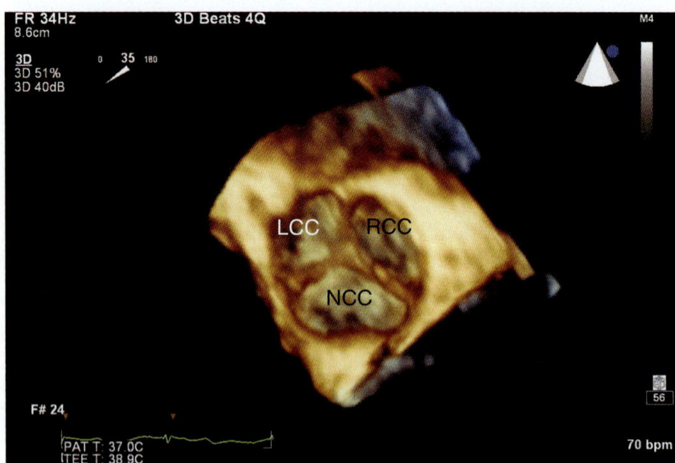

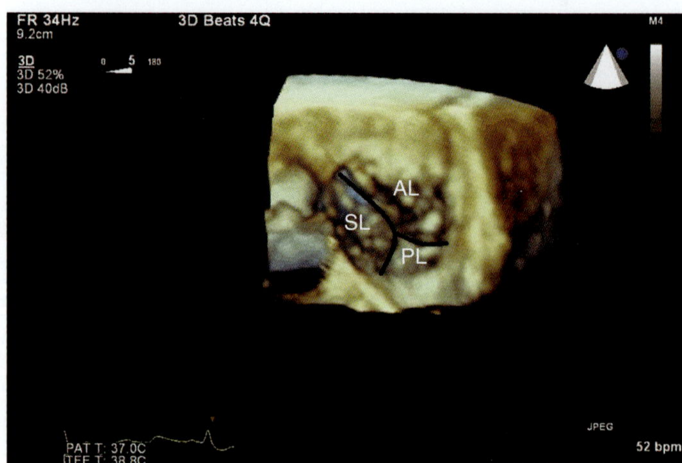

Figure 9-13   Aortic valve (AV) "surgeon's view." Note that as opposed to two-dimensional echocardiography, AV is displayed as would be seen by surgeon. *LCC,* Left coronary cusp; *NCC,* non-coronary cusp; *RCC,* right coronary cusp.

Figure 9-14   Tricuspid valve (TV) "surgeon's view." TV is rotated to be seen as encountered by surgeon after right atriotomy. *AL,* Anterior leaflet; *PL,* posterior leaflet; *SL,* septal leaflet.

As recommended with the mitral valve apparatus, the author performs the same maneuver and spatially orients the 3D image of the aortic valve in a similar fashion to simulate the view as seen by the surgeon after aortotomy. This view is different from the views echocardiographers are accustomed to seeing with 2D TEE. The right-left commissure is at the top of the screen in the 12 o'clock position, the left non-coronary "anterior" commissure is seen at 4 o'clock, and the right non-coronary "posterior" commissure can be found at 8 o'clock. The right coronary cusp lies between the right-left commissure and the anterior commissure, the non-coronary cusp is found between the anterior and posterior commissure, and the remaining cusp is the left coronary cusp (Fig. 9-13 and Video 9-11).

In a similar fashion, the tricuspid valve should be oriented such that the position of the leaflets are quickly recognized by a surgeon after opening the right atrium. In the surgeon's view, the septal leaflet lies medially, and the posterior leaflet will be found at the bottom lateralmost aspect of the valve. The anterior leaflet will be seen at the top portion of the screen. Unfortunately, the tricuspid valve rarely provides the imager with leaflets of adequate quality for diagnostic interpretation (Fig. 9-14 and Video 9-12).

Summary

As the field of echocardiography continues to make great advances, it is imperative that echocardiographers learn to make optimal use of new technologies such as 3D imaging. Not only does 3D imaging improve diagnostic precision, it also improves the echocardiographer's ability to communicate normal anatomy, pathology, and pathophysiology with greater comprehension on the part of surgeons and other physicians. The promise of 3D imaging is improved information transfer to all members of the perioperative team.

REFERENCES

1. Shanewise JS, Cheung AT, Aronson S, et al. ASE/SCA guidelines for performing a comprehensive intraoperative multiplane transesophageal echocardiography examination: recommendations of the American Society of Echocardiography Council for Intraoperative Echocardiography and the Society of Cardiovascular Anesthesiologists Task Force for Certification in Perioperative Transesophageal Echocardiography. *J Am Soc Echocardiogr.* 1999 Oct;12(10):884-900.
2. De Simone R, Glombitza G, Vahl CF, et al. Three-dimensional color Doppler: a clinical study in patients with mitral regurgitation. *J Am Coll Cardiol.* 1999;33:1646-1654.
3. De Simone R, Glombitza G, Vahl CF, et al. Three-dimensional Doppler. Techniques and clinical applications. *Eur Heart J.* 1999;20:619-627.
4. Coisne D, Erwan D, Christiaens L, et al. Quantitative assessment of regurgitant flow with total digital three-dimensional reconstruction of color Doppler flow in the convergent region: in vitro validation. *J Am Soc Echocardiogr.* 2002;15:233-240.

10

Normal Anatomy and Flow During the Complete Examination: Extracardiac Anatomy

BARRY J. SEGAL

Introduction

Although the primary indication for transesophageal echocardiography (TEE) lies in the assessment of cardiac anatomy and function, the experienced transesophageal echocardiographer can acquire a wealth of additional information when examining structures adjacent to the heart and great vessels, which in turn can be used to further optimize perioperative care. By extending the routine "20 view" TEE examination beyond the heart, two-dimensional (2D), and Doppler flow patterns, the imager can visualize the lungs and pleural spaces above the diaphragm, as well as the liver, stomach, spleen, kidneys, and peritoneal space below it.

Anatomic Relationships

The esophagus extends from the oropharynx to the cardia of the stomach, transversing the chest and abdomen. It is anatomically situated posterior to the heart and trachea, running alongside the descending aorta, and then passing anterior to it as it crosses the diaphragm to enter the stomach. Therefore, as the TEE probe is placed through the esophagus and into the stomach to obtain upper-esophageal (UE) and midesophageal (ME) views, the imager will view the great vessels, heart, lungs, and pleural spaces on either side. As the probe then enters the stomach, the transgastric (TG) views are obtained. Using these views as a starting point, the imager can also evaluate the peritoneal space, liver, spleen, stomach, and kidneys. These topographical relationships are appreciated in Figures 10-1 through 10-7.[1]

Lungs and Pleural Spaces

Because of their close proximity to the heart, the lungs should be easily viewed by turning the TEE probe either to the left (counterclockwise) or right (clockwise) from a standard ME four-chamber view. However, in its normal physiologic state, the lung is difficult to image sonographically because of the aerated nature of the organ, preventing penetration of acoustic energy. Low density and stiffness result in low acoustic impedance as well as a high attenuation coefficient, which in turn make acoustic imaging of this organ impractical.[2-5]

This stands in contrast to imaging capabilities under pathologic conditions. In the presence of lung collapse or consolidation, which results in loss of aeration, excellent visualization of the lungs and pleural spaces by TEE can be achieved.[5,6] Ultrasonic air bronchograms and blood vessels are seen, along with relatively uniform tissue, producing a mosaic of echo images (Fig. 10-8).[7] Therefore, the ability to obtain TEE images of the lung means, by definition, there is at least partial lung collapse.

The left lung may be imaged by turning the probe to the left, or counterclockwise, from the standard ME four-chamber view and is seen in the area adjacent to the region of the descending aorta. Advancing the probe more distal into the stomach and withdrawing it will allow imaging along the length of the lung. A pneumothorax can be

diagnosed by seeing an echo-free area next to a bright edge of the associated collapsed lung. Pleural effusion and hemothorax are visualized in the same area, often with associated septations, denoting fluid with a high protein content, blood, or blood clots, which appear as more highly echogenic images (Fig. 10-9 and Video 10-1).[5,7] 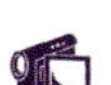

By rotating the probe to the right, or clockwise, from the ME four-chamber view, the right lung and pleural space can be imaged. It is often more difficult to visualize this space unless there is a large accumulation of air and/or fluid (see Figs. 10-8 and 10-9).

In contrast to transesophageal imaging, B-mode imaging obtained by transthoracic sonography provides the imager with reverberation artifacts that are produced by the interface of the chest wall and the pleural surface of the lung. M-mode imaging may produce a "sliding lung" or lung movement images in the normal lung and be absent with a pneumothorax.[6-8]

Intraabdominal Fluid and Organs

As the probe is further advanced into the stomach, the diaphragm and peritoneal space will appear on the monitor screen, posterior to the inferior wall of the left ventricle. Rotating the probe clockwise and counterclockwise will allow the echocardiographer to sweep across the abdominal cavity, investigating for any accumulation of fluid (ascites) or blood. The intraabdominal organs that can be visualized include the liver, stomach, spleen, and often the kidneys, assuming the patient is not too tall.

Practice guidelines have been established for transabdominal ultrasonography of the abdomen and retroperitoneum, but these have not yet been transferred into the practice of TEE.[9]

Peritoneum

Physiologically the peritoneal space usually contains only a small amount of fluid, creating a virtual space allowing the intraabdominal organs to seamlessly glide past each other during movement. Owing to the close anatomic relationship of the intra- and retroperitoneal organs and the fact that they have similar acoustic impedances, it can become challenging to differentiate where one organ starts and the other one ends. Accumulation of ascites or blood will produce a greater (and potentially enlarging) space within the abdominal cavity, making identification of the organs easier (Fig. 10-10).

Differentiation between an exudate and transudate of peritoneal fluid has been described using transabdominal ultrasound.[10,11] Similar images may be obtained by TEE. Septations in the peritoneal fluid may represent fluid with a higher protein content, infected fluid, or blood, which in turn would be more indicative of an exudate.[12,13]

Hemoperitoneum may show septations in the peritoneal fluid and blood clots. If there is ongoing bleeding, as encountered with a ruptured viscus or vascular injury, a dynamic increase in the size of the peritoneal cavity can be appreciated sonographically and quantitatively documented by placing calipers (Figs. 10-11 to 10-13).[14-16]

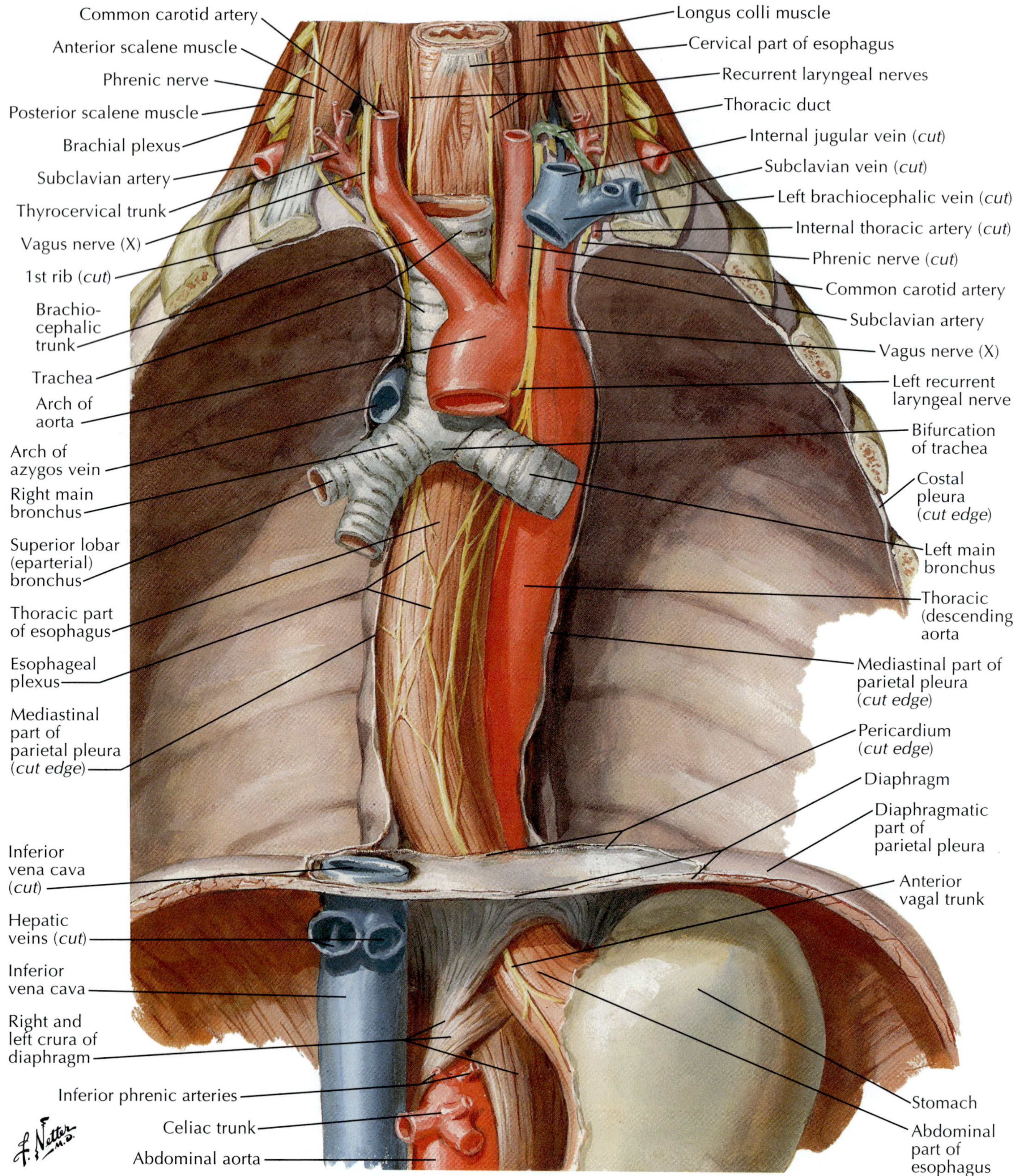

Figure 10-1   Esophagus as it courses through chest to abdomen. (*Netter illustration from www.netterimages.com. © Elsevier Inc. All rights reserved.*)

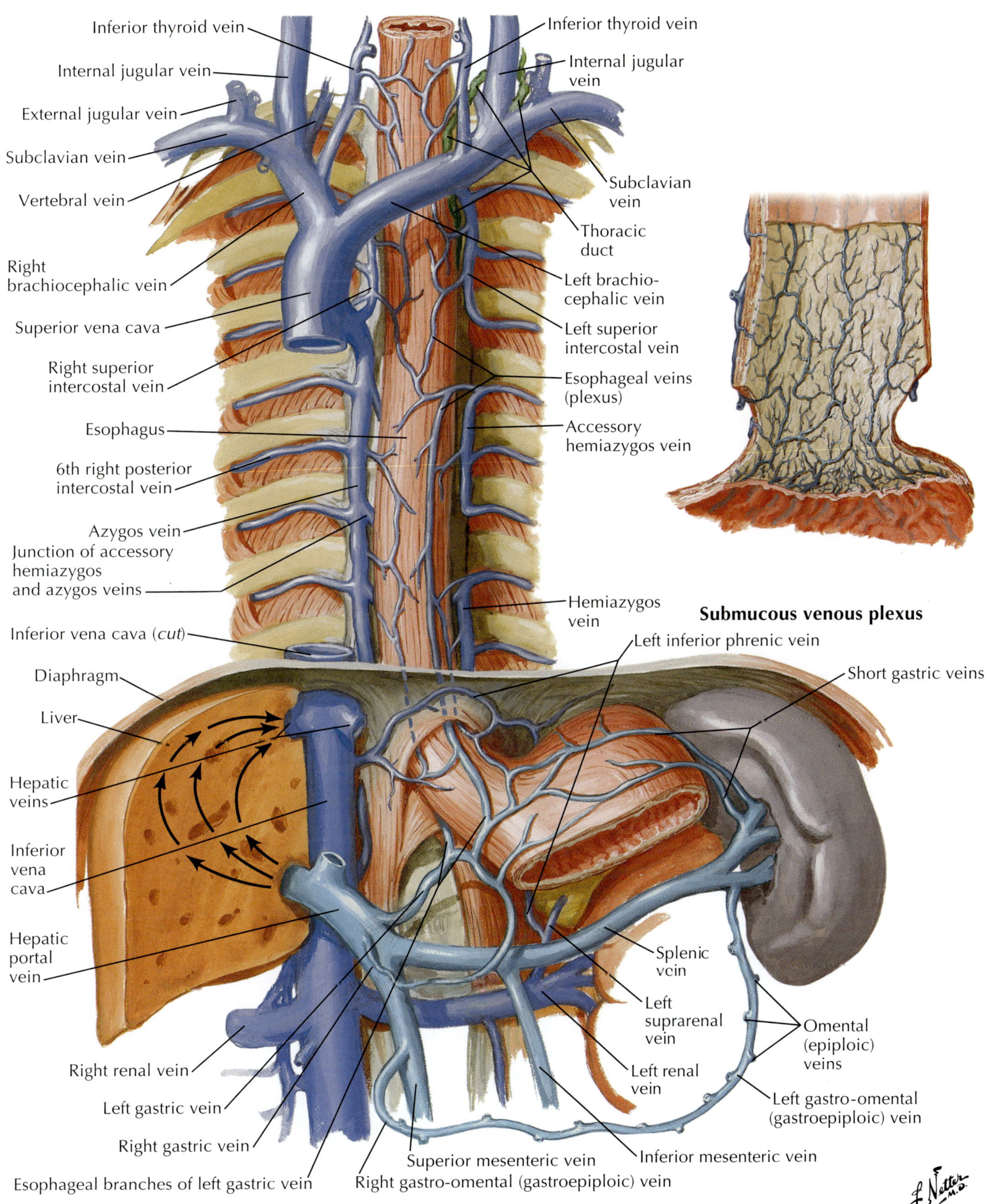

Figure 10-2   Esophagus, great veins in chest and upper abdomen, stomach, liver, and spleen. (*Netter illustration from* www.netterimages.com. © Elsevier Inc. All rights reserved.)

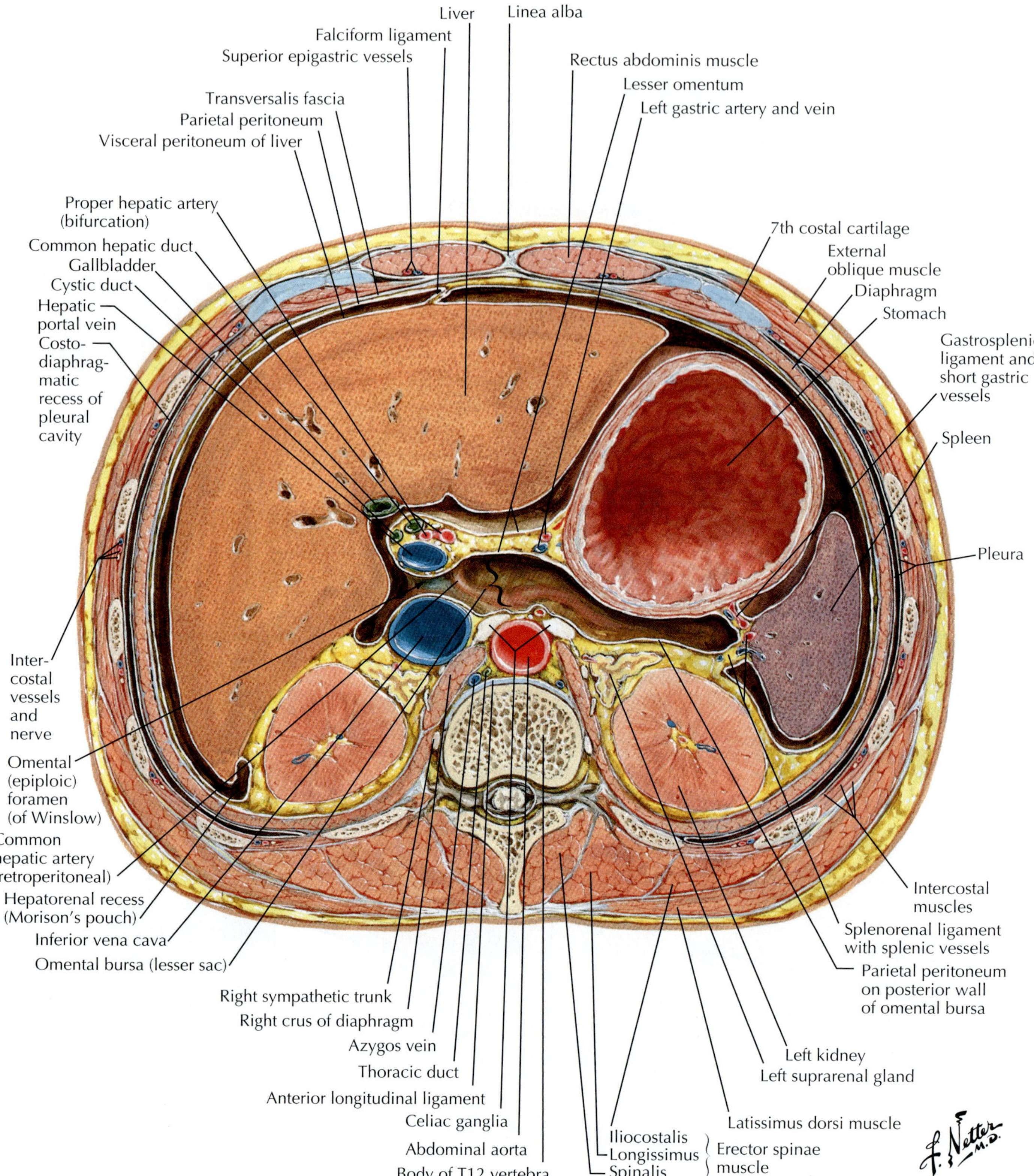

Figure 10-3 Cross-sectional view of upper abdomen, revealing stomach, liver, spleen, kidneys, and great vessels. (*Netter illustration from www.netterimages.com. © Elsevier Inc. All rights reserved.*)

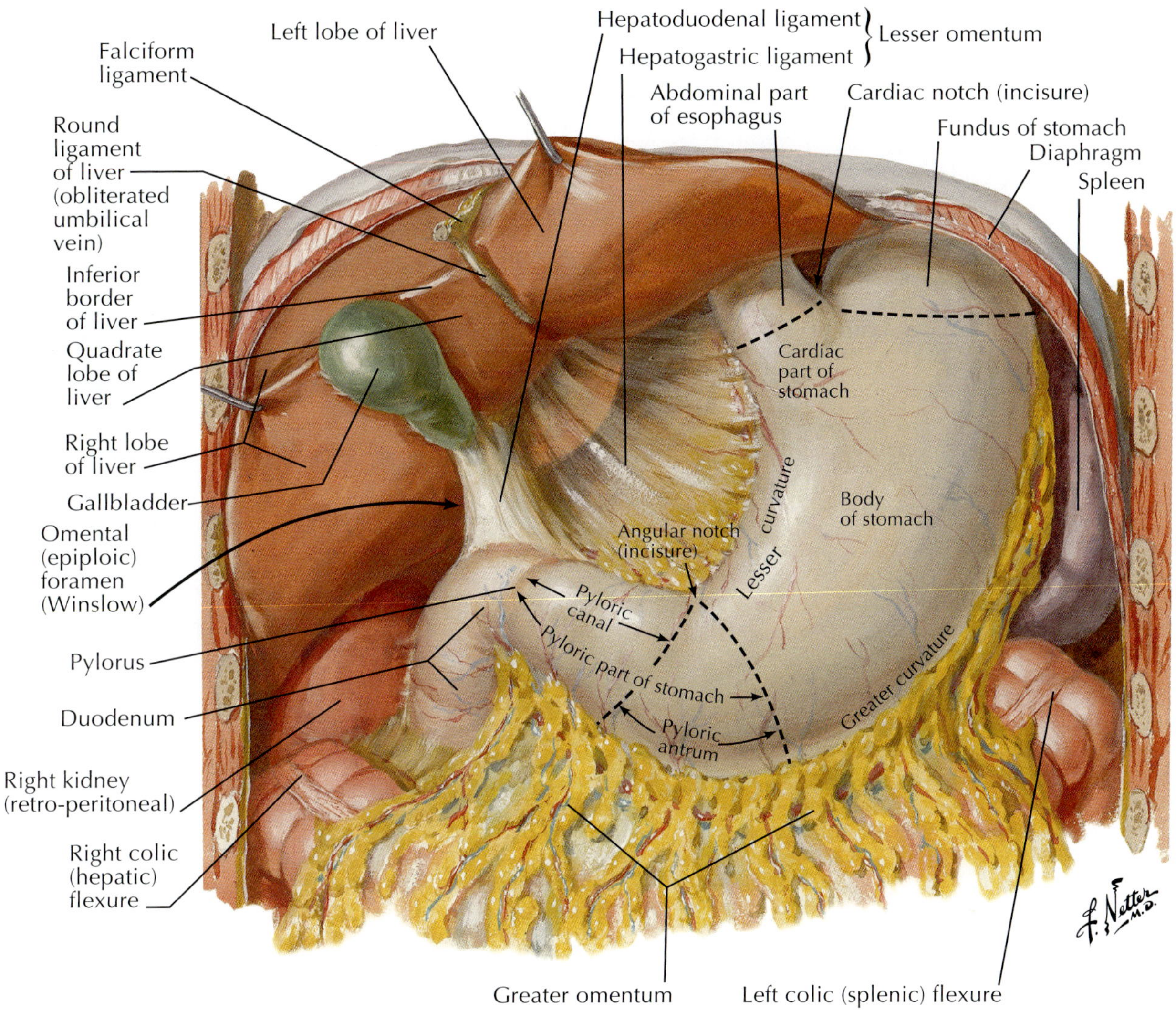

Figure 10-4 Stomach, its anatomy, and its relationship to liver and spleen. *(Netter illustration from www.netterimages.com. © Elsevier Inc. All rights reserved.)*

Liver

In gross anatomic terms, the liver comprises four distinct lobes: the larger right, the left, the caudate, and the quadrate lobes. In practice, however, liver anatomy has been described in terms of its vascular supply. Sir James Cantlie described the division of the liver into right and left lobes, determined by the right and left portal venous blood supply along a line running from the fundus of the gallbladder to the center of the inferior vena cava (IVC).[17] Couinaud proposed a model that divides the liver into eight functional segments, and this model has been adopted by current liver surgical practice. This allows for resection of segments of the liver with their own blood supply while sparing the remaining segments.[18,19]

The liver may easily be imaged below the diaphragm by turning the probe to the right from the TG position. The right lobe is most easily visualized. The lobes appear as somewhat homogenous gray parenchymal tissue interposed with more echogenic vascular and ductal elements. Cysts of the liver are visualized as lucent round or elliptical areas within the parenchyma that do not show any flow pattern when a color Doppler field is superimposed.

Tumors of the liver are usually more echogenic than the surrounding liver tissue, appearing as brighter (whiter), denser, and usually circular objects within the liver, occasionally with lucent areas within them representing cystic or infarcted portions of the tumor (Figs. 10-14 and 10-15; Video 10-2).

Normally about 25% of the cardiac output is distributed to the liver. Some 75% of blood flow to the liver is from the portal venous system, draining from the gastrointestinal tract to the liver via the confluence of the superior mesenteric, inferior mesenteric, and splenic veins. The other 25% is from the hepatic arteries after they branch from the celiac artery.

Venous drainage of blood from the liver is by means of the right, middle, and left hepatic veins, emptying into the IVC shortly before it merges into the right atrium (RA). The thin-walled IVC and the right hepatic vein and its branches that empty into it are readily seen by TEE. Color Doppler imaging can be used to determine flow within these structures. Pulsed wave Doppler (PWD) allows for flow assessment and any changes that occur with increased right-sided heart pressures, including tricuspid regurgitation, pulmonary hypertension, and changes in the systolic and diastolic function of the heart.[20]

Correct placement of venous cannulae in preparation for extracorporeal circulation can also be verified by TEE. Especially in the setting of bicaval cannulation, imaging of the liver can rule out inadvertent placement of the IVC cannula into a hepatic vein.

TEE is very useful in the anesthetic management of patients undergoing liver transplantation. Pre-anhepatic assessment of heart function, the presence of valvular abnormalities, patent foramen ovale, atrial or ventricular septal defects, and existence of aortic abnormalities

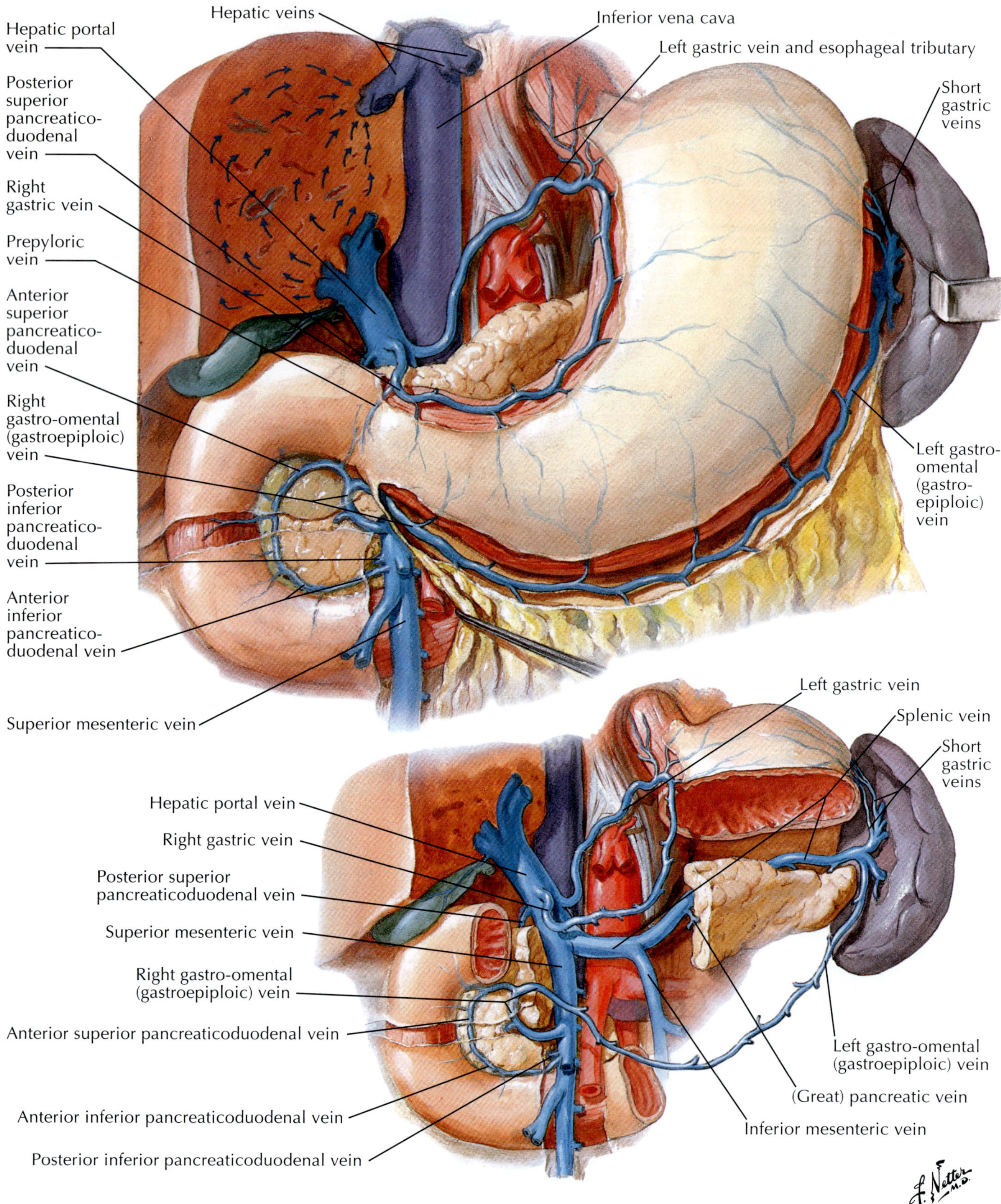

Figure 10-5   Stomach, spleen, and liver and their venous drainage. *(Netter illustration from www.netterimages.com.* © *Elsevier Inc. All rights reserved.)*

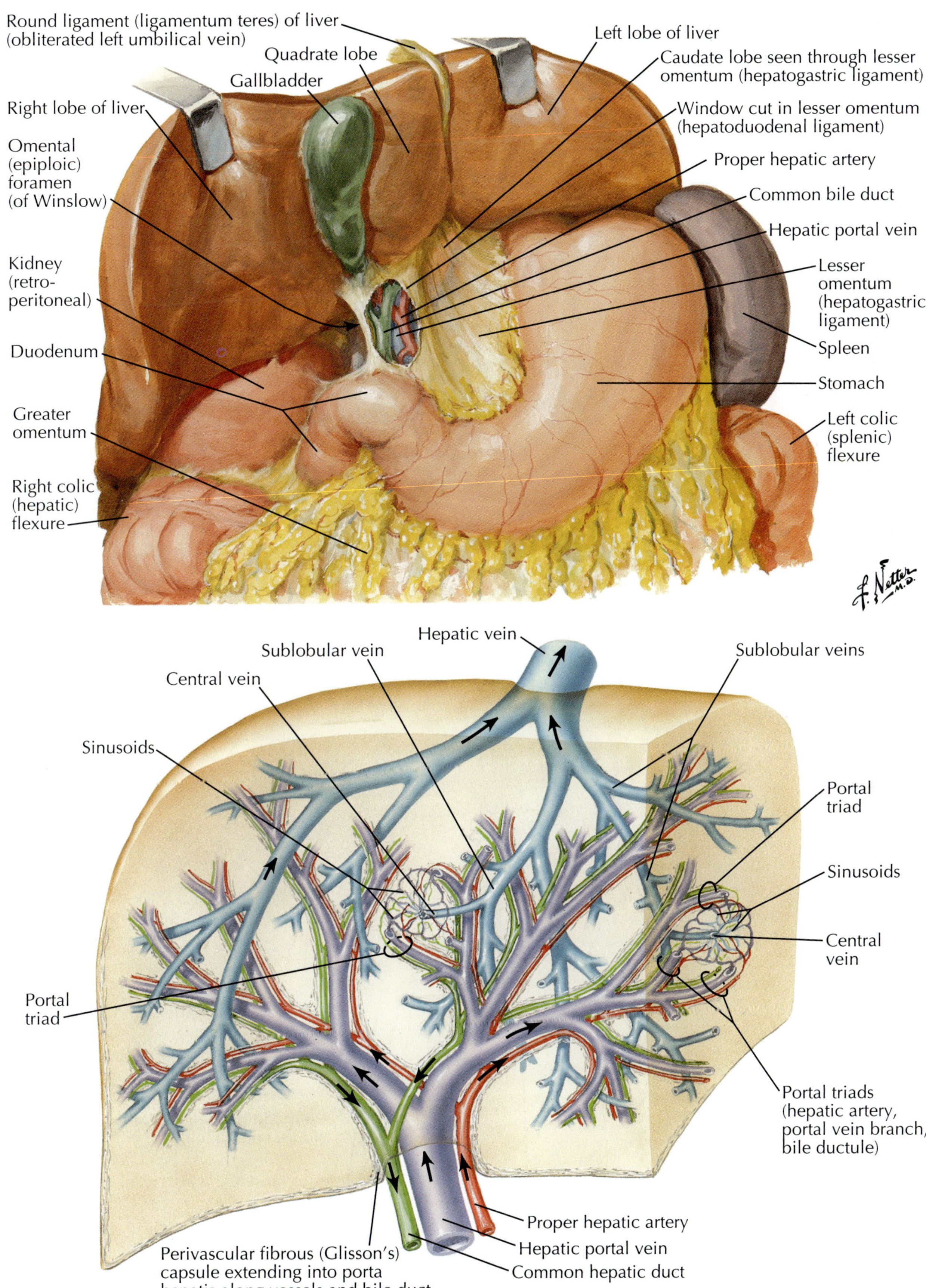

Figure 10-6   Liver and its vascular supply. (*Netter illustration from www.netterimages.com. © Elsevier Inc. All rights reserved.*)

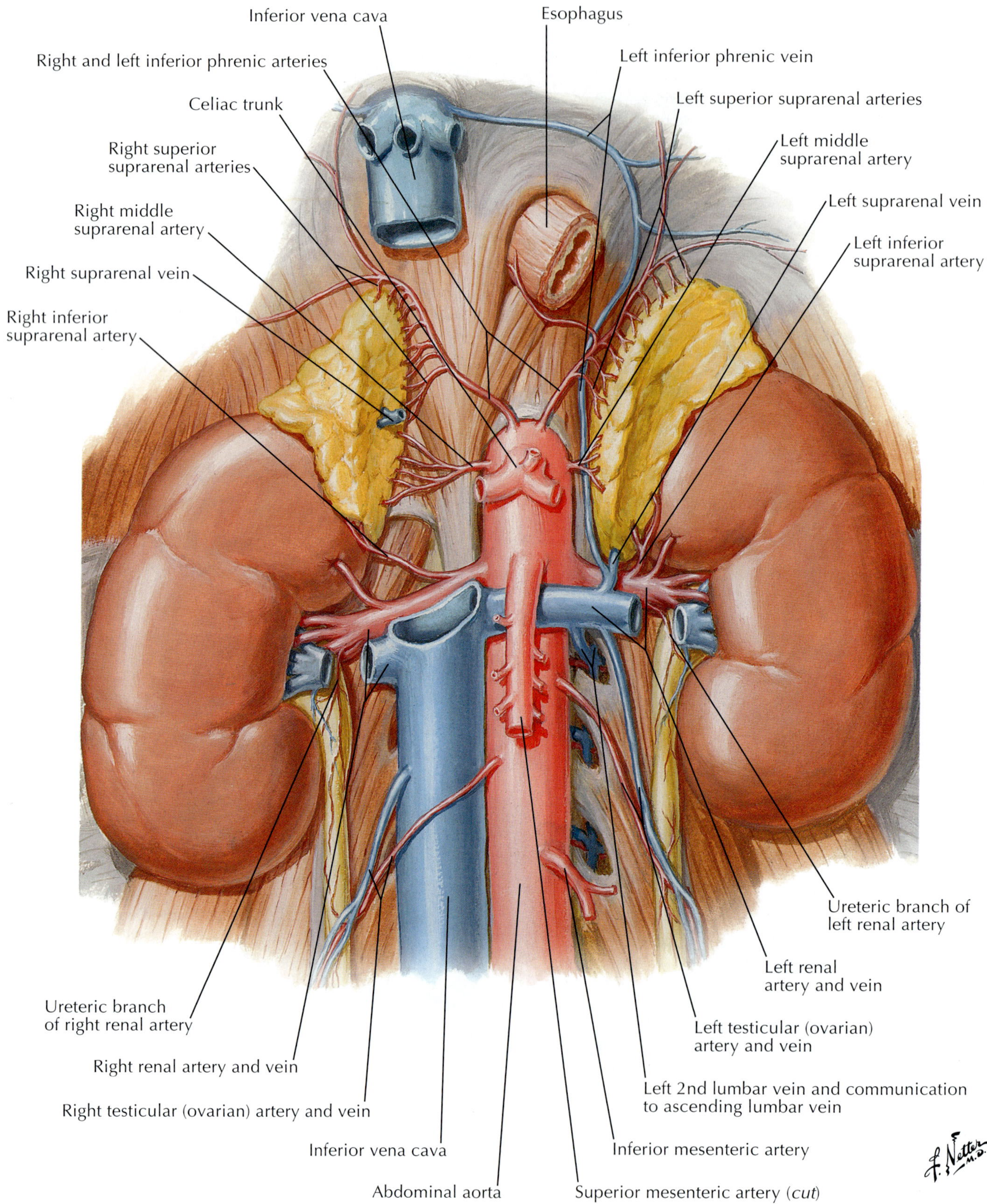

Figure 10-7   Kidneys and their vasculature. (*Netter illustration from www.netterimages.com. © Elsevier Inc. All rights reserved.*)

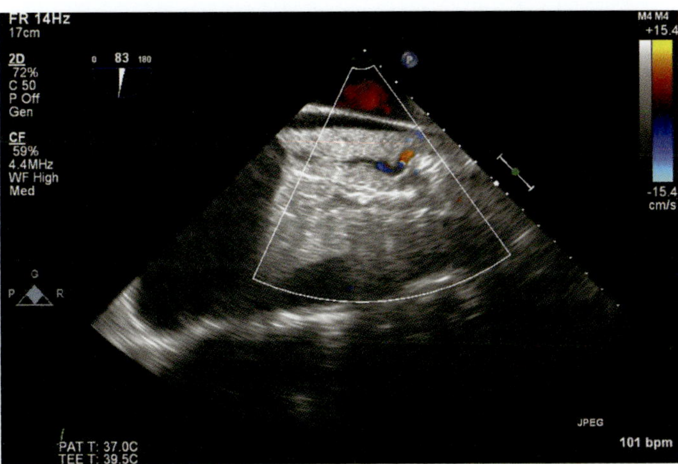

Figure 10-8   Left pleural effusion with collapsed left lung, revealing bronchi and intrapulmonary blood vessels.

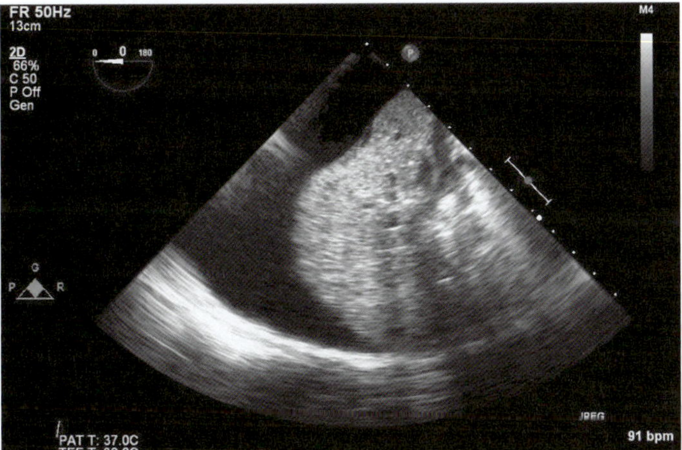

Figure 10-9   Right pleural effusion, atelectatic right lung.

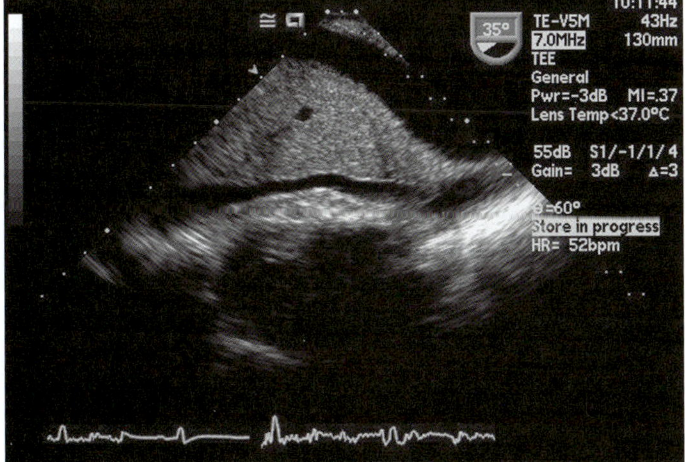

Figure 10-10   Accumulation of intraperitoneal fluid in a patient with constrictive pericarditis.

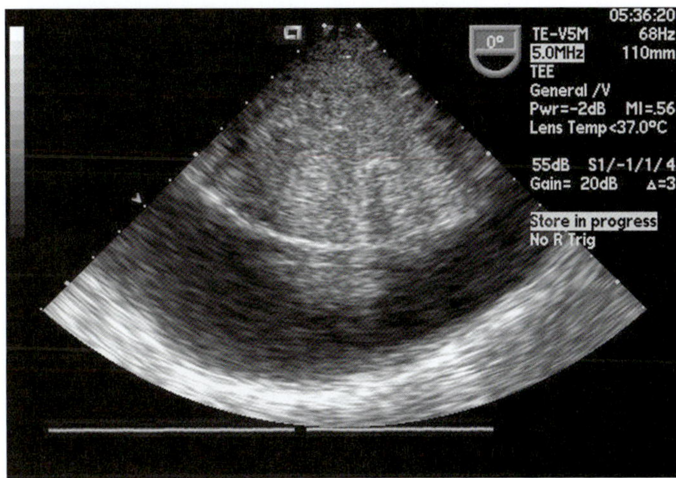

Figure 10-11   Hemoperitoneum in patients with damaged intraabdominal organs (liver, spleen).

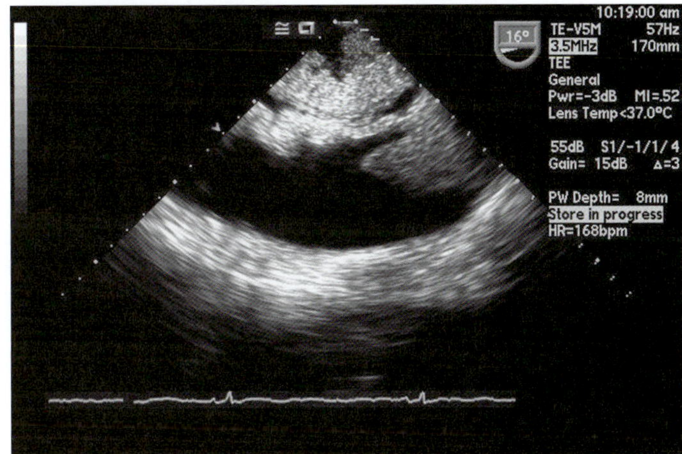

Figure 10-12   Hemoperitoneum in patients with damaged intraabdominal organs (liver, spleen).

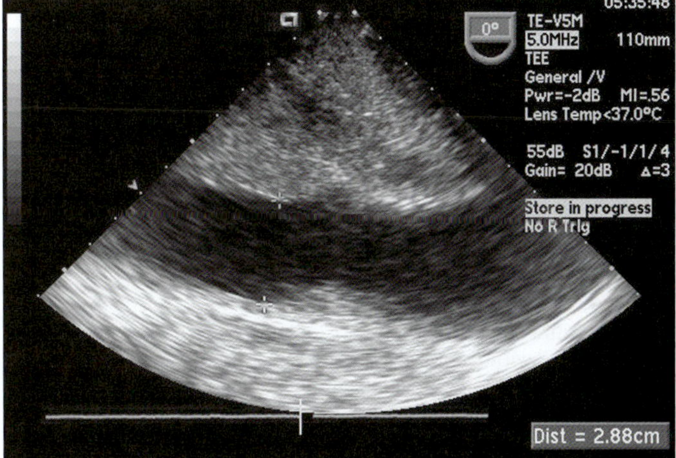

Figure 10-13   Calipers denoting increasing size of intraperitoneal fluid from ongoing bleeding.

(including mobile plaque) is important to obtain and can influence further perioperative management. Intraoperative observation of embolic events, particularly air embolism, is also afforded by TEE. Post-reperfusion intravascular volume and ventricular function can greatly aid the clinician in intraoperative decision making.

Inferior Vena Cava and Hepatic Veins

Hepatic vein engorgement can occur with right heart failure, tamponade, and constrictive or restrictive cardiomyopathies. Estimations of RA pressure have been made with transabdominal ultrasound by assessing

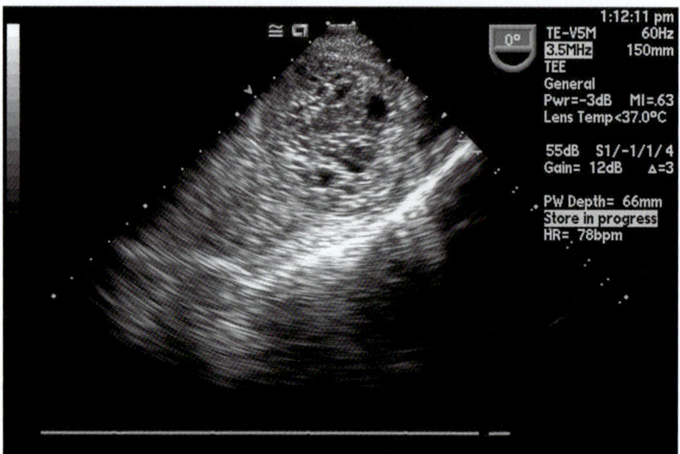

Figure 10-14   Carcinoid tumors in the liver, with cystic or necrotic portions within them.

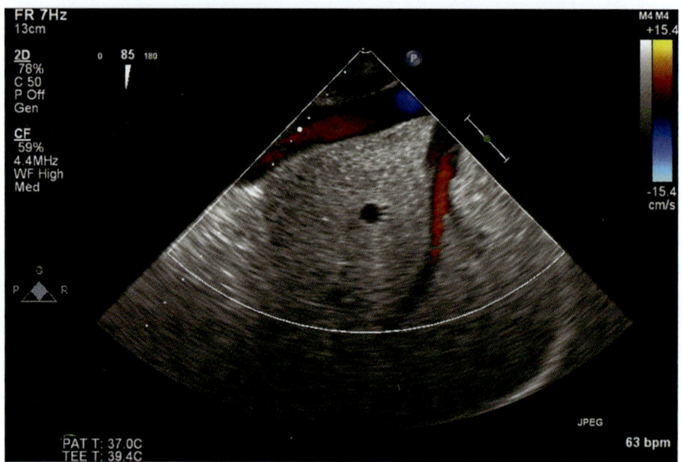

Figure 10-15   Intrahepatic inferior vena cava, right hepatic vein emptying into it, and branch of right portal vein.

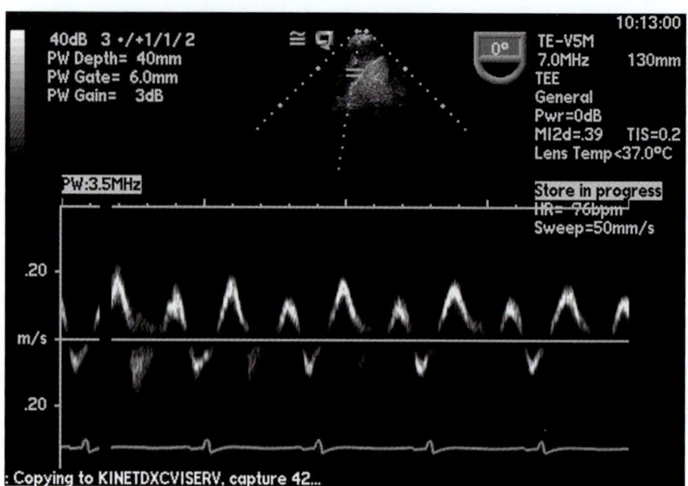

Figure 10-16   Pulsed wave Doppler flow patterns in right hepatic vein, with S, D, V, and AR waves.

changes in IVC end-inspiratory diameter in awake and spontaneously breathing patients.[21] However, in ventilated patients, IVC collapse may not be accurate in predicting RA pressure. IVC diameters obtained by abdominal ultrasound will vary with right heart filling, inspiration, and exhalation, both in spontaneous and positive-pressure ventilation, and with changes in intrathoracic and intraabdominal pressures. Normal IVC diameter with expiration during spontaneous ventilation is about 15 to 17 mm.[22,23] This diameter has been used for assessment of volume loss, fluid replacement, and to support the diagnoses of hypovolemia, tamponade, and (indirectly) pulmonary embolism. A 50% or greater decrease in IVC diameter with spontaneous respiration correlated with an RA pressure of less than 10 mmHg, whereas less than a 50% decrease was associated with RA pressures of 10 mmHg or greater.[23] It is important to note that ventilatory changes in IVC diameter are reversed with positive-pressure ventilation and Valsalva maneuvers.[24] A distended IVC, and one that does not vary in size with respiration, may indicate hypervolemia, cardiac tamponade, pulmonary embolus, or significant tricuspid regurgitation.[25-27] Hypovolemia, on the other hand, may be seen with a small or distally collapsed IVC.

A PWD beam placed parallel to flow in the intrahepatic IVC or right hepatic vein will produce a wave pattern that can be used to assess right ventricular diastolic function.[28,29] It can also be used to quantitate hepatic vein blood flow, which in the case of intraabdominal ultrasound has been used as a marker in evaluating the success of liver transplantation.[30] The actual PWD flow pattern has four phases,

though often it is seen as triphasic, with two forward or positive deflections (S and D waves) and one reversed or negative wave (AR wave). Sometimes a fourth wave is seen as a small negative (reverse) wave (V wave) that follows the S wave (Fig. 10-16).[31-33]

The first forward flow wave is the S wave, which occurs as the RA fills, with the tricuspid annulus moving toward the right ventricular apex as it contracts in systole. The S wave can be timed to occur during the x descent of the RA pressure curve. This passive filling of the RA will depend upon the chamber's compliance and, if present, the degree of tricuspid regurgitation. On occasion, a small reversed or negative wave, the V wave, is seen as the tricuspid annulus returns back toward the base of the heart. The size of this wave is dependent upon the increase in pressure within the atrium, which again is a function of RA compliance.[25]

The second forward or positive deflection, the D wave, occurs as the RA fills during diastolic right ventricular relaxation.[26] This wave is timed to occur with the y descent of the RA pressure curve.

The final inflection seen is the AR wave, which is characterized as a reversed or negative wave pattern. The RA contraction during atrial systole is responsible for the development of this inflection.[33]

In living donor liver transplantation, outflow obstruction is a major determinant in failure of the graft.[34,35] With transabdominal ultrasound in normal individuals, there is a normal hepatic venous triphasic wave pattern and a flow velocity greater than 10 cm/s. Two-dimensional imaging of the intrahepatic IVC may demonstrate narrowing, kinking, or obstruction, and color flow may show a mosaic of color, indicative of flow turbulence.[36]

Loss of pulsatility of the venous wave form is associated with hepatic venous thrombosis. In cardiac cases in which bicaval cannulation has been used, it is imperative that the echocardiographer evaluate the IVC for potential stenosis after cannula removal and tying of the purse string suture.

Color flow mapping can be suggestive of IVC stenosis by displaying a turbulent jet entering the RA. If parallel alignment is possible, spectral Doppler can be used to quantitate the gradient across the stenotic area. If parallel alignment is not feasible, surgeons can measure pressures directly. Normal spectral Doppler of the hepatic artery shows a low resistive index (RI, defined as peak systolic flow − peak end diastolic flow/peak systolic flow) of 0.5 to 0.8, and a high-end diastolic flow.[19]

Changes in hepatic artery Doppler flow patterns obtained with transabdominal ultrasonography can occur with hepatic artery stenosis due to kinking or anastomotic stricture. Lack of color flow would indicate a loss of hepatic artery blood flow, and low intrahepatic arterial flow may produce a spectral Doppler parvus tardus (slow rising and weak pulsation). High peak systolic flows will occur at areas of arterial narrowing.[37-39]

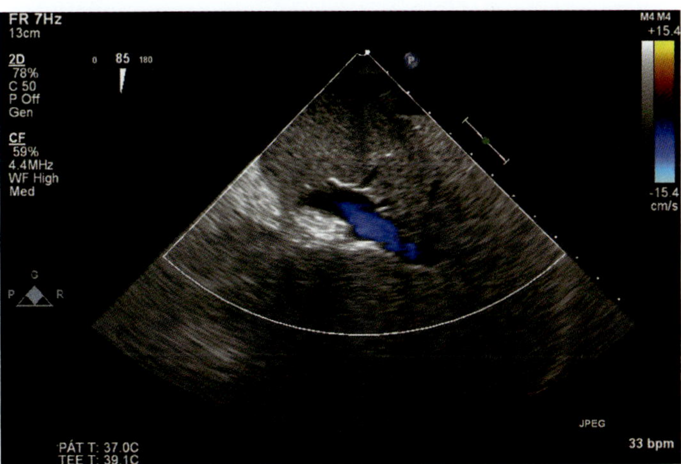

Figure 10-17 Color flow Doppler seen in branch of portal vein.

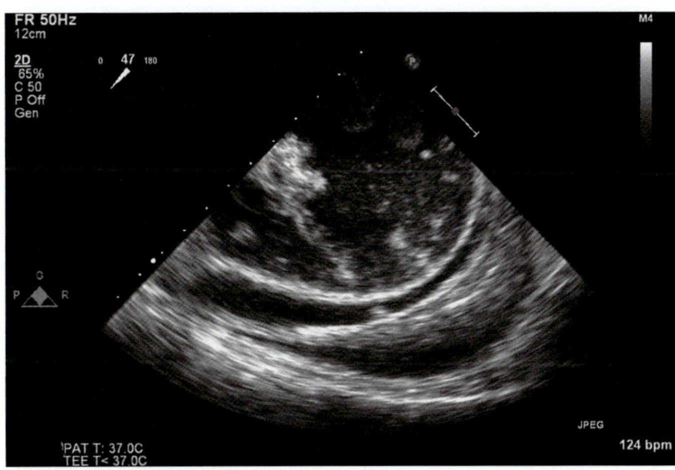

Figure 10-18 Stomach and intragastric fluid.

In practicality, interrogation of the IVC and right hepatic venous flow are the most reliable hepatic vascular assessments obtainable with TEE. There also may be loss of the triphasic flow pattern of hepatic venous flow with Doppler ultrasound when there is parenchymal disease, such as in cirrhosis or graft rejection (Fig. 10-17).

Stomach

In the TG mid–short-axis view, the TEE probe lies inside the cardia or fundus and along the lesser curvature. This enables the echocardiographer to image the stomach as a thick-walled fluid-filled organ situated just below the diaphragm.[40] The stomach is seen on the monitor display just above and to the right of the left ventricle. Because of the thickness of its wall and fluid contents, there are strong specular reflections, and the stomach appears as a brightly echogenic structure with multiple internal convolutions (rugae) with fluid-filled contents (Fig. 10-18). This fluid may be gastric fluid, which appears clear (echolucent), sometimes with multiple air bubbles in suspension or swirls of small bubbles. Over the course of the surgical procedure, there is often an increase in gastric fluid secretion and accumulation, with a subsequent increase in the internal volume of the stomach and more prominence of the rugae of the internal lining of the stomach (Fig. 10-19).

In the setting of esophageal or gastric hemorrhage, the fluid seen in the stomach will have a grayish appearance, a more prominent swirl pattern, and septations as more blood accumulates (see Fig. 10-18). Finally, echogenic clots can be visualized in the lumen.[41,42]

Contractility of the stomach and a decrease in stomach volume may also occasionally be seen, particularly after administration of a prokinetic drug such as metoclopramide. Transabdominal ultrasound has been used in the real-time assessment of gastric motility.[43]

Spleen

The spleen lies in the left upper quadrant of the abdominal cavity. It receives its blood supply from the splenic artery, a branch of the celiac artery. The short gastric arteries arise from the splenic artery and supply a portion of the stomach along the greater curvature. Venous drainage from the spleen occurs via the splenic vein, which empties into the portal venous system.

TEE scanning of the spleen is accomplished by placing the probe in a deep TG position. The spleen appears as a rather homogenous grainy gray structure under the diaphragm and sometimes the left lobe of the liver, adjacent to the stomach. Color Doppler can image blood flow within the spleen when a lower Nyquist limit is chosen (Fig. 10-20).

The spleen is the most common organ (40%) to be injured after blunt abdominal trauma.[44] Focused assessment by sonography in

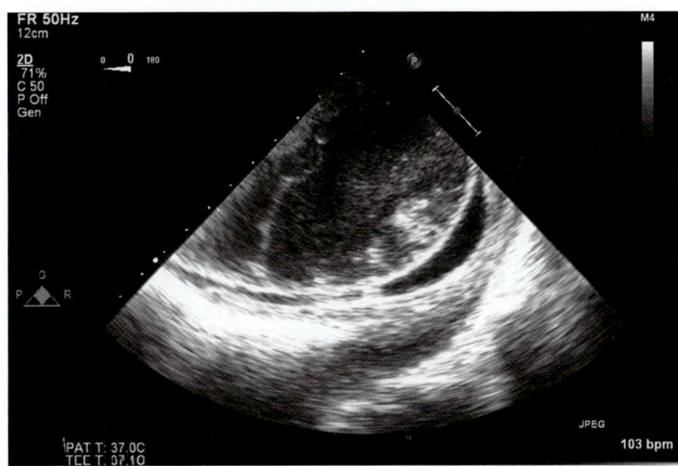

Figure 10-19 Stomach distention.

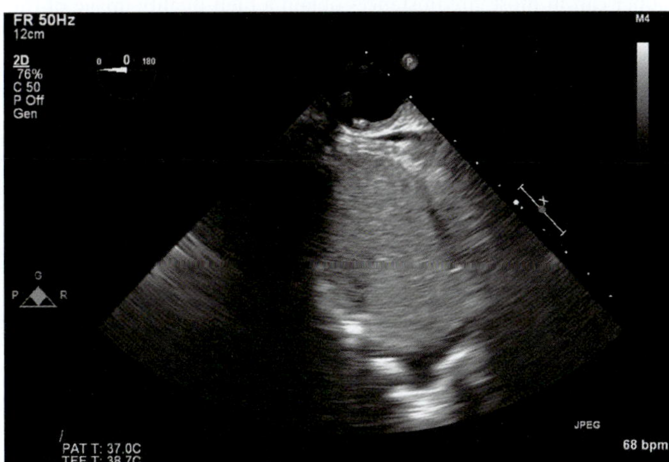

Figure 10-20 Normal spleen and stomach.

trauma (FAST) ultrasonography is used in emergency departments and critical care units to scan the abdomen in patients following blunt trauma.[45] This is accomplished by examining four areas for free fluid. The perihepatic and hepatorenal space (right upper quadrant), the perisplenic area (left upper quadrant), the pelvis (suprapubic view), and the pericardium (subcostal view) are quickly interrogated. Sensitivity is high in multiple prospective and retrospective studies, ranging

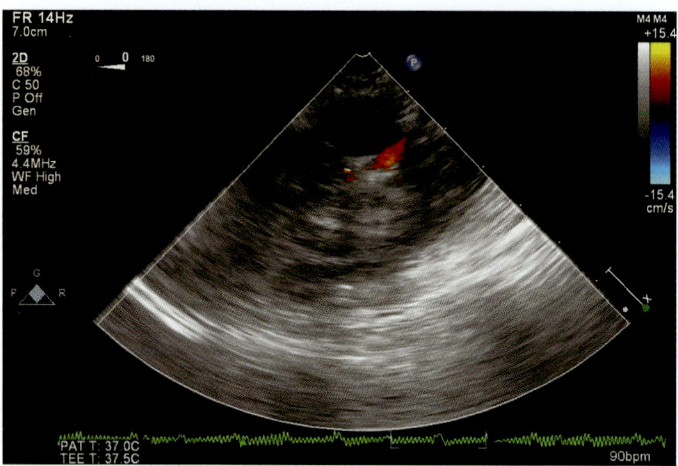

Figure 10-21   Left kidney and intrarenal blood flow.

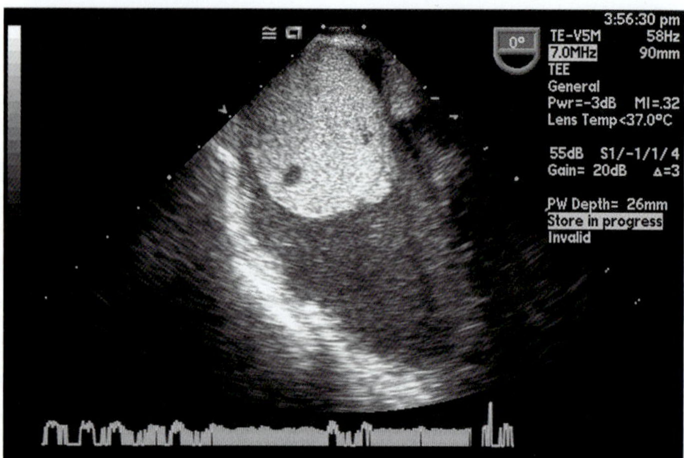

Figure 10-22   Right renal cell carcinoma extending into inferior vena cava and right atrium.

from 86% to 97%, as is a specificity of 90% to 98%.[46,47] Splenic injury can also be seen as a disruption or fragmentation of the spleen, often with an associated lucent area around it and within the peritoneal space, representing a hemoperitoneum (see Fig. 10-12).

There are also case reports of splenic injury following the use of TEE.[48,49] This has been attributed to placing the probe in the cardia of the stomach and anteflexing it, resulting in tension on the splenic hilum by means of the gastrosplenic ligament, and possibly tearing the short gastric blood vessels that lie within it.[49]

Kidney

The kidneys are retroperitoneal organs that may be visualized by TEE in individuals who are not too tall. The probe is placed in a deep TG position to scan them. Under normal anatomic circumstances, the left kidney lies more caudate than the right one. The right kidney is visualized caudally to the liver and is often difficult to see. The left kidney is seen caudally to the spleen. By visualizing the descending aorta from a deep TG position and turning the probe leftwards, the echocardiographer can in most circumstances obtain a high-quality image of this organ. In this view, the kidneys are seen in a cross-sectional plane, and the fibrous outer layer of the kidney capsule appears as an echogenic structure surrounding a rather homogeneous gray parenchyma of both the renal cortex and medulla. The more echogenic calyces are often seen. The renal pelvis where the renal vessels and ureters leave through the renal hilum may occasionally be visualized at 90 degrees (Fig. 10-21).[50]

Tumors of the kidney can be seen, as well as their growth into the IVC, which will sometimes extend all the way into the RA. Use of TEE will allow confirmation of complete tumor removal from the cava and rule out possible embolization of tumor fragments into the right side of the heart and pulmonary arteries during resection (Fig. 10-22). Similarly, renal cysts, which appear as lucent areas within the renal parenchyma, may be seen on occasion as one scans the kidneys. Suprarenal or adrenal neoplasms can be visualized in the region of the cranial pole of the kidneys (Fig. 10-23).

On occasion, a transplanted kidney can be seen by TEE, even though the graft is usually placed within the preperitoneal region of the lower abdomen. Fluid collections around the transplanted kidney may alert the imager to the presence of postoperative hematomas, urinomas or urine leaks, and lymphoceles, which may appear up to a year after the initial procedure.[51,52] Imaging of the graft's parenchyma may reveal changes associated with acute tubular necrosis, acute and chronic rejection, and cyclosporine toxicity. There may be graft enlargement due to edema or loss of parenchymal echogenicity due to swelling, though often there is no specific ultrasound pattern.[53]

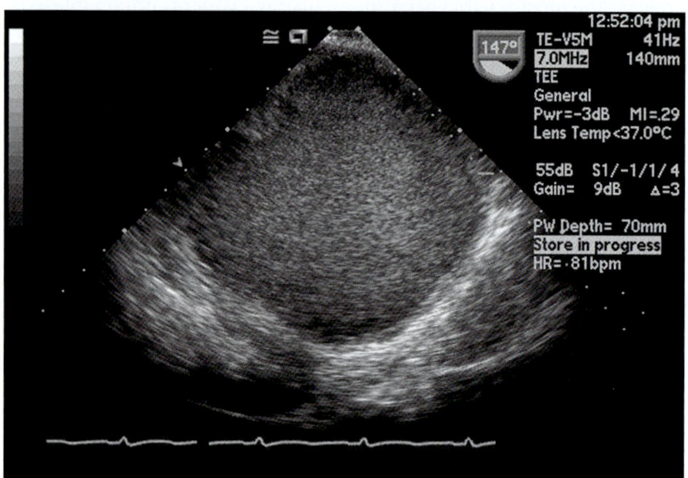

Figure 10-23   Left renal tumor involving adrenal and bowel, proximate to aorta.

Color and spectral Doppler can evaluate renal arterial and venous blood flow patterns and are utilized to assess renal transplant success or failure. Renal vein and arterial thrombosis, though infrequent (1%-2%), can be imaged by color Doppler and will result in graft failure if not treated swiftly.[53]

Renal artery stenosis secondary to neointimal hyperplasia close to the anastomotic site will show turbulent flow, and with spectral Doppler, a higher poststenotic velocity (peak velocity ≥ 2.5 m^2) than the iliac artery to which it is anastomosed, as well as a low RI within the grafted kidney.[54]

Despite the information that can be obtained sonographically, definite diagnosis of renal transplant rejection can only be obtained by performing a biopsy of the transplanted kidney.[55,56]

Spinal Cord

On occasion, by turning the probe further leftwards from the descending aorta, the spinal cord can be visualized. The intervertebral discs allow the imager to view the spinal cord in short axis. As the probe is withdrawn, the echocardiographer intermittently loses the view of the cord because the bony vertebral bodies prohibit continuous visualization. Owing to high variability in obtaining images of high quality, little has been published in regard to the clinical applications of sonographically viewing the spinal cord (Fig. 10-24).

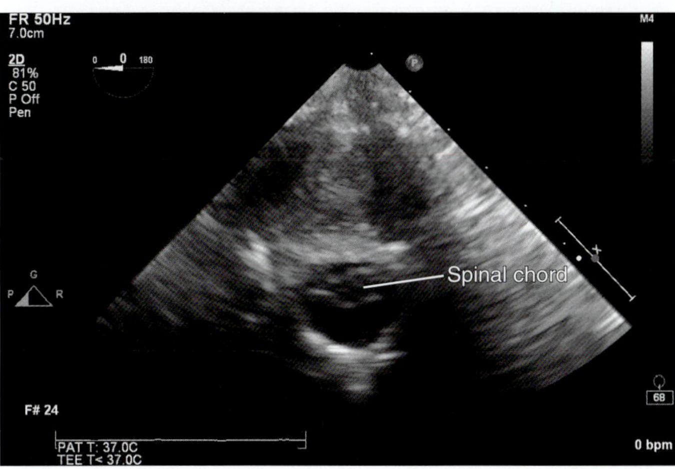

Figure 10-24   Spine with spinal cord.

Summary

TEE can be used to image organs beyond the heart. Careful manipulation and scanning can reveal organ pathology, which will be useful to the anesthesiologist and surgeon in providing more complete patient care.

REFERENCES

1. Hansen JT. *Netter's Clinical Anatomy*. 2nd ed. Philadelphia: Saunders/Elsevier; 2012.
2. Martin K, Ramnarine K. Physics. In: Hoskins PR, Martin K, Thrush A, eds. *Diagnostic Ultrasound, Physics and Equipment*. 2nd ed. Cambridge: Cambridge Univ Press; 2010:4-22.
3. McDicken WN, Anderson T. Basic physics of medical ultrasound. In: Allan PL, Grant MB, Weston MJ, eds. *Clinical Ultrasound*. 3rd ed. London: Churchill Livingstone/Elsevier; 2011:3-15.
4. Beckh S, Bolcskei PL, Lessnau K-D. Real-time chest ultrasonography: a. comprehensive review for the pulmonologist. *Chest*. 2002;122(5):1759-1773.
5. Reuter KL, Bogdan A. Physics of diagnostic ultrasound: creating the image. In: Bollinger CT, Herth FJF, Mayo PH, Miyazawa T, Beamis JF, eds. *Clinical Chest Ultrasound: From the ICU to the Bronchoscopy Suite. Prog Resp Res*. Basel: Karger; 2009:2-10.
6. Soldati G, Testa A, Silva FR, et al. Chest ultrasonography in lung contusion. *Chest*. 2006;130(2):533-538.
7. Koegelenberg CFN, Diacon AH, Bollinger CT. Transthoracic ultrasound for chest wall, pleura, and the peripheral lung. In: Bollinger CT, Herth FJF, Mayo PH, Miyazawa T, Beamis JF, eds. *Clinical Chest Ultrasound: From the ICU to the Bronchoscopy Suite. Prog Resp Res*. Basel: Karger; 2009:22-33.
8. Rahman NM, Gleeson FV. Lung, pleura and chest wall. In: Allan PL, Grant MB, Weston MJ, eds. *Clinical Ultrasound*. 3rd ed. London: Churchill Livingstone/Elsevier; 2011:1005-1021.
9. Henningsen C, Hiett A, Jensen L, et al. *Ultrasound examination of the abdomen and/or retroperitoneum: AUIM practice guidelines*. American Institute for Ultrasound in Medicine. Laurel, MD. April 2012.
10. Goldberg BB, Goodman GA, Clearfield HR. Evaluation of ascites by ultrasound. *Radiology*. 1970;96:15-22.
11. Dinkel E, Lehnart R, Troger J, Peters H, Dittrich M. Sonographic evidence of intraperitoneal fluid. An experimental study and its clinical implications. *Pediatr Radiol*. 1984;14(5):299-303.
12. Goldberg BB. Ultrasonic evaluation of intraperitoneal fluid. *JAMA*. 1976;235(22):2427-2430.
13. Edell SL, Gefter WB. Ultrasonic differentiation of types of ascitic fluid. *AJR Am J Roentgenol*. 1979;133(1):111-114.
14. Chambers JA, Pilbrow WJ. Ultrasound in abdominal trauma: an alternative to peritoneal lavage. *Arch Emerg Med*. 1988;5(1):26-33.
15. Huang MS, Liu M, Wu JK, et al. Ultrasonography for the evaluation of hemoperitoneum during resuscitation: a simple scoring system. *J Trauma*. 1994;36:173-177.
16. McKenney MG, Martin L, Lentz K, et al. 1000 consecutive ultrasounds for blunt trauma. *J Trauma*. 1996;40:607-611.
17. Van Gulik TM, Van Den Esschert JW. James Cantlie's early messages for hepatic surgeons: how the concept of pre-operative portal vein occlusion was defined. *HPB*. 2010;12(2):81-83.
18. Oliveira DA, Feitosa RQ, Correia MM. Segmentation of liver, its vessels and lesions from CT images for surgical planning. *Biomed Eng Online*. 2011;10:30.
19. Smith D, Downey D, Spouge A, et al. Sonographic demonstration of Couinaud's liver segments. *J Ultrasound Med*. 1998;17:375-381.
20. Quinones MA, Otto CM, Stoddard, et al. Recommendations for quantification of Doppler echocardiography: A report from the Doppler quantification task force of the nomenclature and standards committee of the American Society of Echocardiography. *J Am Soc Echocardiogr*. 2002;15(2):167-184.
21. Kircher BL, Himelman RB, Schiller NB. Noninvasive estimation of right atrial pressure from the inspiratory collapse of the inferior vena cava. *Am J Cardiol*. 1990;66:493-496.
22. Lyon M, Blavias M, Brannam L. Sonographic measurement of the inferior vena cava as a marker of blood loss. *Am J Emerg Med*. 2005;23:45-50.
23. Lyon ML, Verma N. Ultrasound guided volume assessment using inferior vena cava diameter. *Open Emerg Med J*. 2010;3:22-24.
24. Natori H, Tamaki S, Kira S. Ultrasonographic evaluation of ventilatory effect on inferior caval configuration. *Am Rev Respir Dis*. 1979;120(2):421-427.
25. Carricart M, Denault AY, Couture P, et al. Incidence and significance of abnormal hepatic venous Doppler flow velocities before cardiac surgery. *J Cardiothorac Vasc Anesth*. 2005;19:751-758.
26. Nomura T, Lebowitz L, Koide Y, et al. Evaluation of hepatic venous flow using transesophageal echocardiography in coronary artery bypass surgery: an index of right ventricular function. *J Cardiothoracic Vasc Anesth*. 1995;9:9-17.
27. Oh JK, Hatle LK, Seward JB, et al. Diagnostic role of Doppler echocardiography in constrictive pericarditis. *J Am Coll Cardiol*. 1994;23:154-162.
28. Reynolds T, Appleton CP. Doppler flow patterns of the superior vena cava, inferior vena cava, hepatic vein, coronary sinus, and atrial septal defect: a guide for the echocardiographer. *J Am Soc Echocardiogr*. 1991;4(5):503-512.
29. Appleton CP, Jensen JL, Hatle LK, Oh JK. Doppler evaluation of left and right diastolic function: a technical guide for obtaining optimal flow velocity. *J Am Soc Echocardiogr*. 1997;10(3):271-292.
30. Huang T-L, Weng HH, Yu PC, et al. the significance of hepatic vein outflow volume in adult-to-adult living donor liver transplantation evaluated by Doppler ultrasound. *Transplant Proc*. 2003;35(1):68-69.
31. Rudski LG, Lai WW, Afilalo J, et al. Guidelines for the echocardiographic assessment of the right heart in adults: a report form the American Society of Echocardiography. *J Am Soc Echocardiogr*. 2010;23:685-713.
32. Dresser TS, Sze DY, Jeffrey RB. Imaging and intervention in the hepatic veins. *AJR Am J Roentgenol*. 2003;180(6):1583-1591.
33. Jequier S, Jequier JC, Hanquinet S, et al. Hepatic vein Doppler studies: variability of flow pattern in normal children. *Pediatr Radiol*. 2002;32(1):49-55.
34. Ryan SM, Sellars MEK, Sidhu PS. Liver transplantation. In: Allan PL, Baxter GM, Weston MJ, eds. *Clinical Ultrasound*. 3rd ed. London: Churchill Livingstone/Elsevier; 2011:199-224.
35. Reid SA, Scoutt LM. Vascular complications of liver transplants: evaluation with duplex Doppler ultrasound. *Ultrasound Clin*. 2011;6(4):513-530.
36. Huang T- L. The role of color Doppler ultrasound in living donor liver transplantation (review). *J Ultrasound Med*. 2008;16(3):177-187.
37. Umphrey HR, Lockhart ME, Robbin ML. Transplant ultrasound of the kidney, liver, and pancreas. *Ultrasound Clin*. 2008;3(1):49-65.
38. Kim KW, Kim TK, Kim MJ, et al. Doppler sonographic abnormalities suggestive of venous congestion in the right lobe graft of living donor liver transplant recipients. *AJR Am J Roentgenol*. 2007;188(3):239-245.
39. Lu O, Wu H, Fan YT, et al. Sonographic evaluation of vessel grafts in living donor liver transplantation recipients of the right lobe. *World J Gastroenterol*. 2009;15(28):3550-3554.
40. Orihashi K, Hong Y, Sisto DA, et al. The anatomic location of the transesophageal echocardiographic transducer during a short-axis view of the left ventricle. *J Cardiothorac Anesth*. 1990;4(6):726-730.
41. Urbanowicz JH, Kernoff RS, Oppenheim G, et al. Transesophageal echocardiography and its potential for esophageal damage. *Anesthesiology*. 1990;72(1):40-43.
42. Gilja OH. Ultrasound of the stomach—the EUROSON lecture 2006. *Ultraschall Med*. 2007;28(1):32-39.
43. Holt S, McDicken WN, Anderson T, et al. Dynamic imaging of the stomach by real-time ultrasound—a method for the study of gastric motility. *Gut*. 1980;21(7):597-601.
44. McGahan JP, Richards J, Gillen M. Focused abdominal ultrasonography for trauma scan–pearls and pitfalls. *J Ultrasound Med*. 2002;21:789-800.
45. Doody O, Lyburn D, Geoghegan T, et al. Blunt trauma to the spleen: ultrasonographic findings *Clin Radiol*. 2005;60(9):968-967.
46. Helling TS, Wilson J, Augustosky K. The utility of focused abdominal ultrasound in blunt trauma abdominal trauma: a reappraisal. *Am J Surg*. 2007;194(6):728-732.
47. Najarian B, Gupta S, Cemaj S, et al. FAST scan: is it worth doing in hemodynamically stable blunt trauma patients? *Surgery*. 2010;148(4):695-700.
48. Chow MS, Taylor MA, Hanson 3rd CW. Splenic laceration associated, with transesophageal echocardiography. *J Cardiothorac Vasc Anesth*. 1998;12(3):314-316.
49. Olenchock Jr SA, Lukaszczyk JJ, Reed 3rd J, et al. Splenic injury after intraoperative transesophageal echocardiography. *Ann Thorac Surg*. 2001;72(6):2141-2143.
50. Allan PL. Kidneys: anatomy and technique. In: Allan PL, Grant MB, Weston MJ, eds. *Clinical Ultrasound*. 3rd ed. London: Churchill Livingstone/Elsevier; 2011.
51. Krumme B. Renal Doppler sonography-update in clinical nephrology. *Nephron Clin Pract*. 2006;103:24-28.
52. Piyasena R, Hamper UM. Doppler ultrasound evaluation of renal transplants. *Appl Radiol*. 2010;39(9):24, 26-27, 30-32.
53. Baxter GM. Renal transplantation. In: Allan PL, Grant MB, Weston MJ, eds. *Clinical Ultrasound*. 3rd ed. London: Churchill Livingstone/Elsevier, 2011.328-349.
54. Tublin ME, Bude RO, Platt JF. The resistive index in renal Doppler sonography: where do we stand? *AJR Am J Roentgenol*. 2003;180(4):885-892.
55. Perrella RR, Duerinckx AJ, Tessler FN, et al. Evaluation of renal transplant dysfunction by duplex Doppler sonography: a prospective study and review of the literature. *Am J Kidney Dis*. 1990;15(6):544-550.
56. Perchik JE, Baumgartner BR, Bernadino ME. Renal transplant rejection. Limited value of duplex Doppler sonography. *Invest Radiol*. 1991;26(5):422-426.

Quantitative and Semiquantitative Echocardiography: Dimensions and Flows

MANISH BANSAL | JAGAT NARULA | PARTHO P. SENGUPTA

Assessing cardiac chamber dimensions and hemodynamics is an integral component of any echocardiographic examination. Estimating chamber size not only helps in evaluating the contractile performance of a particular chamber but also provides valuable information regarding the hemodynamic significance of concomitant lesions such as valve regurgitation and intracardiac shunts. A more detailed assessment of cardiac hemodynamics can be accomplished by directly measuring intracardiac flows and pressures. Altogether, such information has immense diagnostic, prognostic, and therapeutic significance. It allows for judicious administration of medical therapy, especially intravenous fluids, diuretics, vasopressors, and vasodilators. In addition, detailed assessment of cardiac hemodynamics forms the framework required for making crucial decisions such as whether surgical intervention is required for specific cardiac lesions and is also helpful for evaluating the hemodynamic significance of the residual lesions following intervention.

Since its advent in the 1970s, transesophageal echocardiography (TEE) has rapidly evolved into a useful diagnostic modality for assessing cardiac structures and hemodynamics.[1-3] The close proximity of the ultrasound probe to the heart allows better visualization of cardiac structures and permits the use of higher ultrasound frequencies, which significantly improves spatial resolution. More importantly, its relatively noninvasive nature, safety, easy applicability, portability, ability to image the heart in virtually all patients, instant results, and lack of interference with the operating field render TEE the ideal diagnostic tool for cardiac evaluation during the perioperative period.[4-11]

Basic Principles

Although the basic principles of assessing cardiac chamber size and intracardiac flows using TEE are the same as those for transthoracic echocardiography (TTE), there are certain notable differences. Most of the experience regarding quantitative echocardiography has been obtained via transthoracic imaging, so the optimal views for quantifying cardiac chamber dimensions have been standardized only for TTE.[12] It is often quite challenging to reproduce the same standard views during TEE. Similarly, aligning the Doppler beam with the direction of blood flow to obtain velocity measurements across certain cardiac chambers such as the right ventricular outflow tract (RVOT) may also prove to be difficult in TEE. Finally, general anesthesia often produces marked alterations in intracardiac pressures, volumes, and chambers sizes that have to be accounted for while interpreting the information derived from TEE performed in the perioperative setting.

Table 11-1 summarizes the recommended views for performing various dimension and flow measurements during TEE.

Measurement of Cardiac Chamber Dimensions

Qualitative assessment of cardiac chamber dimensions begins the moment the first grayscale image appears on the display screen of the echocardiography machine. The visual impression formed from these initial images permits recognition of the "target" structures and guides the subsequent analysis to conduct a meaningful echocardiographic study. However, the formal quantification of cardiac chamber dimensions is invariably required to yield a correct diagnosis and ensure accurate decision making.

Left Ventricle

Left ventricular systolic function is a key determinant of clinical outcomes in almost every illness affecting the heart. Consequently, assessing left ventricular size and thereby its systolic function is one of the most important goals of any echocardiographic examination. No echocardiogram can be considered complete without an assessment of left ventricular size and systolic function.[12]

Several measurements can be obtained during echocardiography to provide an estimate of left ventricular size and geometry. The most commonly performed measurements include the linear dimensions (minor axis dimension [or internal diameter] and major axis dimension [or length]), left ventricular wall thickness (usually interventricular septum and inferolateral wall), relative wall thickness, left ventricular end-diastolic and end-systolic volumes, and left ventricular mass.

Left Ventricular Linear Dimensions

Measuring the internal dimensions forms the basis of left ventricular size quantification. During TTE, these measurements can be obtained from the M-mode recordings or the two-dimensional (2D) images. M-mode offers better temporal resolution owing to its much higher frame rate but is often limited by the inability to orient the M-mode cursor along the desired imaging plane. This problem is particularly common with TEE, which itself is constrained by the limited imaging planes. Therefore, most of the dimensions in TEE are measured using 2D imaging.

The left ventricular minor axis dimension is the internal diameter of the left ventricular cavity measured at the level of the mitral leaflet tips perpendicular to the long axis of the left ventricular cavity. Because the oblique orientation of the measurement plane will lead to an overestimation of cavity size, great care must be taken to ensure that the measurement plane is perpendicular to the left ventricular long axis.

Earlier guidelines recommended that the measurements be performed using the leading edge–to–leading edge technique.[13] This technique was required because the spatial resolution of the grayscale images at that time was insufficient for accurate delineation of the tissue/blood interfaces. Improvements in echocardiographic instrumentation have now made it possible to accurately identify actual tissue/blood interfaces, so most dimension measurements are currently performed using the inner edge–to–inner edge technique, which allows for measurements of the true cavity size.[12]

During TEE, the left ventricular minor axis dimension can be obtained either from the midesophageal (ME) two-chamber view or from the transgastric (TG) two-chamber view (Figs. 11-1 and 11-2, Videos 11-1 and 11-2). To obtain the ME two-chamber view, a proper ME four-chamber view (0 degrees) first needs to be obtained. From this position, advancement of the omniplane angle forward to 80 to 100 degrees while keeping the probe tip still and the mitral valve in the center will result in the ME two-chamber view. A slight retroflexion of

the tip may be required to direct the imaging plane through the long axis of the left ventricle (LV) (see Video 11-1). The left ventricular diameter is then measured as the distance between the inferior and anterior walls at the level of the mitral leaflet tips.

The TG two-chamber view can be obtained from the TG mid–short-axis view (0 degrees) by advancing the omniplane angle forward to 80 to 90 degrees. A slight anteflexion of the transducer tip may be required to make the LV horizontal (see Video 11-2). The measurement is then performed in the same manner as described previously.

The left ventricular length or major axis dimension is the distance between the midpoint on the mitral annular plane and the left ventricular apex. During TTE, this dimension is usually obtained from the apical four-chamber view. However, its analogous view during TEE—the ME four-chamber view—often results in foreshortening of the LV, so the ME two-chamber view is preferred for measuring left ventricular length during TEE (see Fig. 11-1).[12] It is usually not possible to obtain the same measurement from the TG two-chamber view, because the left ventricular apex is almost invariably excluded from the image sector.

All such measurements should be obtained at ventricular end-diastole and end-systole. An electrocardiogram (ECG) should *not* be used to time these events, since ECG events do not necessarily coincide with the true left ventricular end-diastole and end-systole because of the inherent electromechanical delay during contraction and relaxation. This is particularly problematic in patients with intraventricular conduction defects. Therefore, in echocardiography, end-diastole and end-systole should preferably be identified by direct visualization of the 2D images. The frame showing the maximum left ventricular cavity size, which is usually the frame just preceding the closing of the mitral valve, should be regarded as representative of end-diastole. Similarly, the frame with the smallest cavity size should be taken to represent end-systole. This usually corresponds to the frame immediately prior to the opening of the mitral valve leaflets.

Reference ranges and partition values for left ventricular linear dimensions are presented in Table 11-2. For the reasons mentioned, these values have been derived only from transthoracic imaging; therefore, no such data exist for TEE. However, previous studies have shown that, when carefully performed, measurements obtained by TEE closely match those obtained from TTE.[14,15] Thus, the American Society of Echocardiography recommends using the same reference ranges for left ventricular dimensions in TEE as well.[12]

The major advantage of linear measurements is that they are simple, easy to perform, provide a quick estimate of the left ventricular size and, most importantly, have the least interobserver variability.[16-18] However, because they are performed only in one dimension, linear measurements do not provide a true assessment of left ventricular size in the case of distorted ventricles, which are commonly observed in patients with coronary artery disease. Nevertheless, linear measurements have been shown to be reliable and have proven useful in clinical decision making regarding diseases affecting left ventricular symmetry, such as valvular heart disease, hypertension, and cardiomyopathies.[19]

TABLE 11-1	Recommended Views for Cardiac Chamber Dimension Measurements in Transesophageal Echocardiography	
Chamber	**View**	**Measurement**
Left ventricle	Midesophageal (ME) two-chamber view	• Length • Minor axis diameter • Volume measurement using biplane Simpson's method
	ME four-chamber view	• Volume measurement using biplane Simpson's method
	Transgastric (TG) two-chamber view	• Minor axis diameter
	TG mid–short-axis view	• Short-axis cavity area for volume and mass calculations • Wall thickness
Right ventricle	Right ventricle (RV)–focused ME four-chamber view	• Length • Basal and mid-diameters • Area for fractional area change
	ME right ventricular inflow-outflow view	• Right ventricular outflow tract diameters (proximal and distal)
Left atrium	ME aortic valve short-axis view	• Anteroposterior diameter
	ME aortic valve long-axis view	• Anteroposterior diameter
	ME four-chamber view	• Area • Volume using biplane area-length and Simpson's methods
	ME two-chamber view	• Volume using biplane area-length and Simpson's methods
Right atrium	RV-focused ME four-chamber view	• Length • Diameter • Area
Aorta	ME aortic valve long- and short-axis views	• Aortic annulus (left ventricular outflow tract diameter)
	ME ascending aorta long- and short-axis views	• Aortic root diameters • Ascending aortic diameters
	ME descending aorta short- and long-axis views	• Descending aortic diameters
Pulmonary artery	Upper esophageal aortic arch short-axis view	• Main pulmonary artery size • Right (sometimes left also) pulmonary artery size

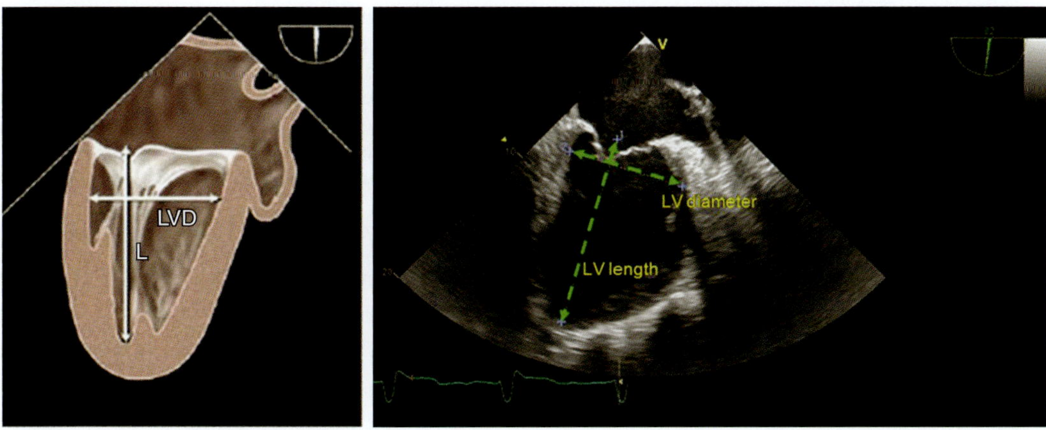

Figure 11-1 Measurement of left ventricular (*LV*) length and minor axis diameter from midesophageal two-chamber view. *L,* Length; *LVD,* left ventricular diameter. (*Modified with permission from Lang RM, Bierig M, Devereux RB, et al. Recommendations for chamber quantification: a report from the American Society of Echocardiography's Guidelines and Standards Committee and the Chamber Quantification Writing Group, developed in conjunction with the European Association of Echocardiography, a branch of the European Society of Cardiology. J Am Soc Echocardiogr. 2005;18:1440-1463.*)

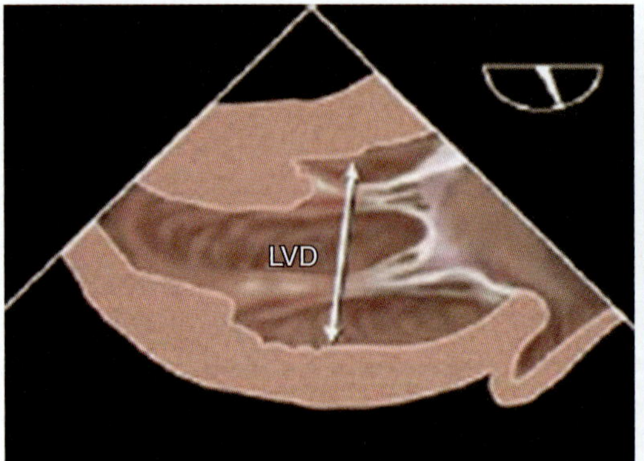

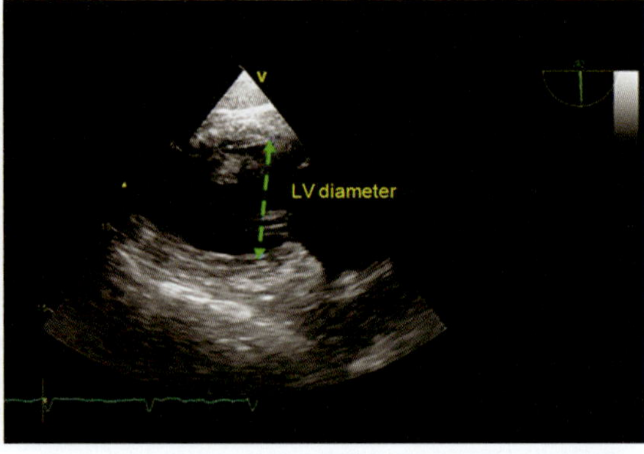

Figure 11-2   Measurement of left ventricular minor axis diameter from transgastric two-chamber view. *LVD,* Left ventricular diameter. *(Modified with permission from Lang RM, Bierig M, Devereux RB, et al. Recommendations for chamber quantification: a report from the American Society of Echocardiography's Guidelines and Standards Committee and the Chamber Quantification Writing Group, developed in conjunction with the European Association of Echocardiography, a branch of the European Society of Cardiology. J Am Soc Echocardiogr. 2005;18:1440-1463.)*

TABLE 11-2   Reference Ranges and Partition Values for Left Ventricle Size

	Men				Women			
	Reference Range	*Mildly Abnormal*	*Moderately Abnormal*	*Severely Abnormal*	*Reference Range*	*Mildly Abnormal*	*Moderately Abnormal*	*Severely Abnormal*
LVIDd (cm)	4.2-5.9	6.0-6.3	6.4-6.8	≥6.9	3.9-5.3	5.4-5.7	5.8-6.1	≥6.2
LVIDd/BSA (cm/m^2)	2.2-3.1	3.2-3.4	3.5-3.6	≥3.7	2.4-3.2	3.3-3.4	3.5-3.7	≥3.8
LVIDd/height (cm/m)	2.4-3.3	3.4-3.5	3.6-3.7	≥3.8	2.5-3.2	3.3-3.4	3.5-3.6	≥3.7
LVEDV (mL)	67-155	156-178	179-201	≥201	56-104	105-117	118-130	≥131
LVEDV/BSA (mL/m^2)	35-75	76-86	87-96	≥97	35-75	76-86	87-96	≥97

BSA, Body surface area; *LVEDV,* left ventricular end-diastolic volume; *LVIDd,* left ventricular internal dimension (diastolic).
Data from Lang RM, Bierig M, Devereux RB, et al. Recommendations for chamber quantification: a report from the American Society of Echocardiography's Guidelines and Standards Committee and the Chamber Quantification Writing Group, developed in conjunction with the European Association of Echocardiography, a branch of the European Society of Cardiology. *J Am Soc Echocardiogr.* 2005;18:1440-1463.

Left Ventricular Wall Thickness and Relative Wall Thickness

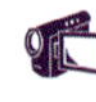

Left ventricular wall thickness is the end-diastolic thickness of the inferolateral wall and the interventricular septum. The recommended view for performing these measurements in TEE is the TG mid–short-axis view (Fig. 11-3, Video 11-3). To obtain this view, the probe should be inserted into the stomach with the omniplane angle kept at 0 degrees. The probe should then be anteflexed and rotated to the right or left to develop the short-axis view of the LV and bring the LV to the center of the image. A slight advancement or withdrawal of the probe may be required to orient the imaging plane through the midportion of the ventricle, which can be recognized by the presence of papillary muscles. The grayscale image gain may have to be adjusted to optimize endocardial definition. From this view, the thicknesses of the inferolateral wall and septum are measured as shown in Figure 11-3.

Relative wall thickness is a measure of myocardial thickness relative to the left ventricular cavity size and is a useful parameter for describing left ventricular geometry. It is calculated using the following equation:

$$\text{Relative wall thickness} = 2ILWIDd/LVIDd$$

where *ILWIDd* is the end-diastolic thickness of the inferolateral wall of the LV, and *LVIDd* is the diameter of the left ventricular cavity at end-diastole.

In patients with left ventricular hypertrophy (defined based on increased left ventricular mass as described later), an increased relative wall thickness (≥0.42) signifies concentric hypertrophy, whereas a normal relative wall thickness (<0.42) indicates the presence of eccentric hypertrophy.[20,21] Concentric left ventricular hypertrophy is observed in conditions causing a pressure overload of the LV, such as hypertension, aortic stenosis, and coarctation of the aorta. In contrast, eccentric hypertrophy is common in diseases causing volume overload, such as aortic and mitral regurgitation. Eccentric hypertrophy is also observed during the late degenerative stages of diseases otherwise characterized by concentric hypertrophy, such as hypertrophic cardiomyopathy and aortic stenosis. Sometimes relative wall thickness is increased without a concomitant increase in left ventricular mass. This is known as *concentric remodeling* and generally occurs in response to pressure overload. The presence of concentric remodeling has been shown to be an adverse prognostic marker in certain disease conditions.[22,23]

The normal ranges and partition values for left ventricular wall thickness are presented in Table 11-3.

Left Ventricular Volume

Measuring left ventricular volume not only provides more accurate information regarding overall left ventricular size compared with linear dimension measurements, but it is also essential for estimating left ventricular ejection fraction (LVEF), which is the most validated and most widely employed measure of left ventricular systolic function. There are several methods for estimating left ventricular volume, and those most commonly used in clinical practice are outlined here.

Linear Method or Cubed Method

The cubed method is the simplest method for estimating left ventricular volume. The volume of the LV is calculated by simply taking the cube of the internal dimension of the LV:

$$\text{Left ventricular volume} = LVID^3$$

where *LVID* is the left ventricular internal dimension.

Based on estimations of left ventricular volumes at end-diastole and end-systole, the LVEF can be derived using the following equation:

$$LVEF = (LVEDV - LVESV)/LVEDV$$

where *LVEDV* is the left ventricular end-diastolic volume, and *LVESV* is the left ventricular end-systolic volume.

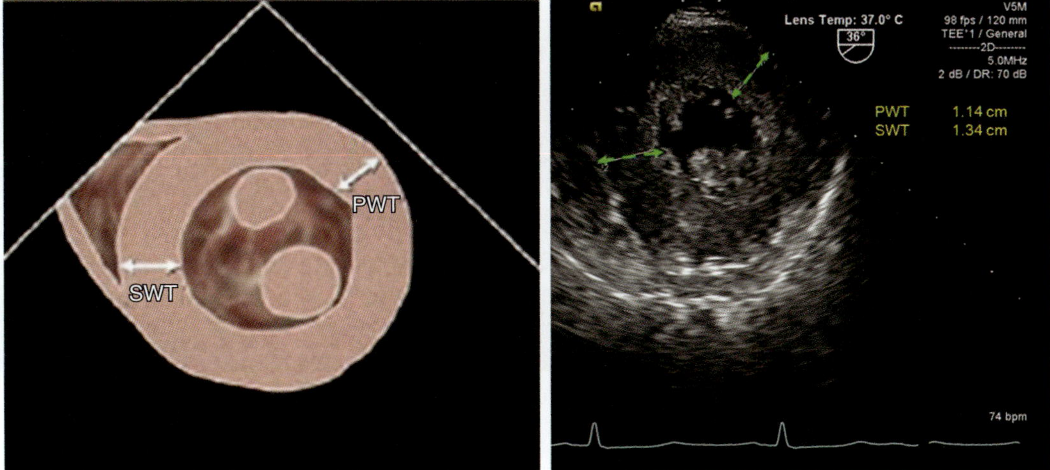

Figure 11-3 Measurement of left ventricular posterior wall and septal thickness from transgastric mid–short-axis view. *PWT, Posterior wall thickness; SWT, septal wall thickness. (Modified with permission from Lang RM, Bierig M, Devereux RB, et al. Recommendations for chamber quantification: a report from the American Society of Echocardiography's Guidelines and Standards Committee and the Chamber Quantification Writing Group, developed in conjunction with the European Association of Echocardiography, a branch of the European Society of Cardiology. J Am Soc Echocardiogr. 2005;18:1440-1463.)*

TABLE 11-3 Reference Ranges and Partition Values for Left Ventricular Wall Thickness and Mass

	Men				Women			
	Reference Range	Mildly Abnormal	Moderately Abnormal	Severely Abnormal	Reference Range	Mildly Abnormal	Moderately Abnormal	Severely Abnormal
Linear Method								
IVSd (cm)	0.6-1.0	1.1-1.3	1.4-1.6	≥1.7	0.6-0.9	1.0-1.2	1.3-1.5	≥1.6
PWd (cm)	0.6-1.0	1.1-1.3	1.4-1.6	≥1.7	0.6-0.9	1.0-1.2	1.3-1.5	≥1.6
Relative wall thickness	0.24-0.42	0.43-0.46	0.47-0.51	≥0.52	0.22-0.42	0.43-0.47	0.48-0.52	≥0.53
LV mass (g)	88-224	225-258	259-292	≥293	67-162	163-186	187-210	≥211
LV mass/BSA (g/m²)	49-115	116-131	132-148	≥149	43-95	96-108	109-121	≥122
Two-Dimensional Method								
LV mass (g)	96-200	201-227	228-254	≥255	66-150	151-171	172-192	≥193
LV mass/BSA (g/m²)	50-102	103-116	117-130	≥131	44-88	89-100	101-112	≥113

BSA, Body surface area; *IVSd*, interventricular septal thickness (diastolic); *LV*, left ventricle; *PWd*, posterior wall thickness (diastolic).
Data from Lang RM, Bierig M, Devereux RB, et al. Recommendations for chamber quantification: a report from the American Society of Echocardiography's Guidelines and Standards Committee and the Chamber Quantification Writing Group, developed in conjunction with the European Association of Echocardiography, a branch of the European Society of Cardiology. *J Am Soc Echocardiogr.* 2005;18:1440-1463.

Given that the cubed method assumes the LV to be spherical, which clearly is not true, it inevitably introduces errors into the estimation of left ventricular volume. Several modifications of this method have been proposed to correct for this error, such as the Teichholz and Quinones methods.[24,25] The Teichholz method is given as[25]

$$\text{Left ventricular volume} = (LVID)^3 \times [7/(LVID + 2.4)]$$

(Please note that for this equation, the LVID must be measured in centimeters.)

The greatest advantage of the cubed method is that it is simple, easy to apply, and provides a quick estimate of left ventricular size. However, the method has several potential limitations. First, as with the method employing linear dimensions, the cubed method is applicable only to ventricles with uniform geometry. In patients with distorted ventricles, the cubed method will over- or underestimate left ventricular volume and ejection fraction depending on the location of the regional wall motion abnormalities (WMAs). If the site of measurement includes the region of WMAs, the ejection fraction will be underestimated. Conversely, when the linear measurement site is away from the infracted territory, the ejection fraction will be overestimated. The latter scenario is encountered more commonly because WMAs usually involve the left ventricular apex, whereas the measurement is performed at the base of the LV. Second, because a single measurement is cubed to obtain the volume, any error in measuring the linear dimension is greatly magnified once the volume is calculated. Finally, as mentioned earlier, the method requires geometrical assumptions whereby the LV is inappropriately assumed to be spherical, which results in systematic inaccuracies.

Two-Dimensional Methods

As mentioned, the cubed method, which is based on a single linear measurement of the LV, has significant limitations and cannot be applied in patients with regional WMAs. By incorporating left ventricular dimensions from more than one plane, 2D methods allow for more accurate estimation of left ventricular volume. There are two different 2D methods that can be used for this purpose: the area-length method and the biplane Simpson's method.[12]

The area-length method assumes the LV to be bullet-shaped (Fig. 11-4). The volume is calculated using the following equation:

$$\text{Volume} = 5/6 \times \text{area} \times \text{length}$$

where *area* is the cross-sectional area of the left ventricular cavity measured at the mid-ventricle level, and *length* is the left ventricular long-axis length as described previously.

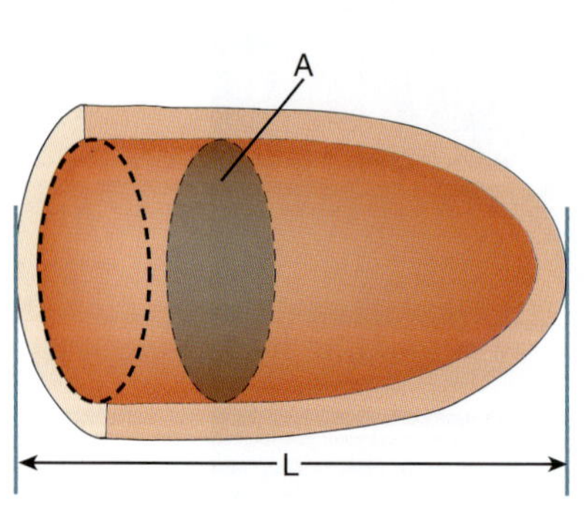

$$V = (A + 2 \times A/3) \times L/2, \text{ or}$$
$$V = 5\,AL/6$$

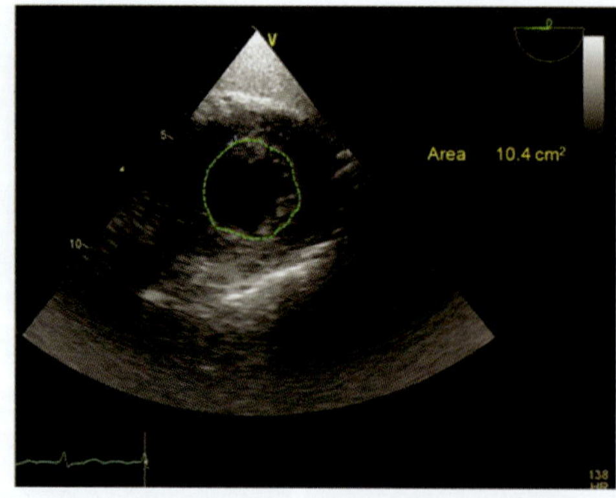

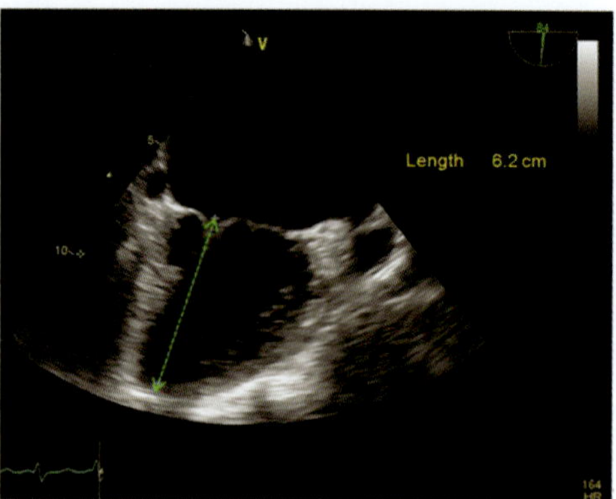

Left ventricular volume (area–length method) = 5/6 × area × length
$$= 5/6 \times 10.4 \times 6.2$$
$$= 53.7 \text{ cm}^3 \text{ or ml}$$

Figure 11-4   **A and B,** Measurement of left ventricular volume using area-length method. Left ventricular cavity cross-sectional area (A) is measured from transgastric mid–short-axis view, and length (L) is measured from midesophageal two-chamber view. Note that papillary muscles are considered to be part of left ventricular cavity. Volume in example will be 53.7 mL (⅚ × 10.4 × 6.2).

The left ventricular cavity cross-sectional area is measured by tracing the endocardial border of the left ventricular cavity in the short-axis view at the papillary muscle level. This can be best accomplished in the TG mid–short-axis view. While tracing the endocardial border, the papillary muscles should be included in the ventricular cavity, and the endocardial border should be traced outside the papillary muscles. Because an optimal endocardial definition is fundamental to obtaining an accurate cross-sectional area, the grayscale image should be optimized by appropriately using gain, contrast, and dynamic range settings. However, despite maximum image optimization, it may not be possible to adequately delineate the endocardial border in the lateral wall and septum in many patients owing to the parallel orientation of the tissue/blood interfaces in these segments to the ultrasound beam.

Although the area-length method provides a more accurate estimation of left ventricular volume than the cubed method, it too does not take into consideration the overall shape of the LV and is therefore not accurate in the presence of significant regional WMAs.

The biplane Simpson's method overcomes many of the geometric assumptions associated with the aforementioned methods. This method divides the entire left ventricular cavity into a stack of elliptical discs (usually 20), and the volume of the left ventricular cavity is calculated by summation of the volumes of each of these discs (Fig. 11-5). The volume of each disc is calculated as the cross-sectional area of the disc multiplied by its height. The cross-sectional area is computed from the two orthogonal diameters obtained from the four-chamber and two-chamber views, and the height is derived from the length of the LV. All of these calculations are performed automatically using built-in software available in all modern echocardiographic equipment.

To obtain left ventricular volume using the biplane Simpson's method, the left ventricular endocardial border must be traced in the ME four-chamber and two-chamber views. The endocardial border is traced manually, starting from one end of the mitral annulus, coursing along the entire left ventricular cavity, and finishing at the other end of the mitral annulus. The base of the ventricle is formed by a straight line joining the mitral valve insertion points at the two ends. The long axis of the ventricular cavity is automatically recognized by the software but can be manually adjusted if it does not appear to conform to the true long axis. The software then computes the left ventricular volume.

While performing these measurements, great caution must be exercised to ensure that the left ventricular cavity is not foreshortened. Slight retroflexion of the tip of the transducer to bring the true left ventricular apex into view may help avoid foreshortening (Video 11-4), but it may still be difficult to obtain a non-foreshortened view of the LV in the ME four-chamber view.

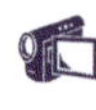

The biplane Simpson's method is currently the most accurate (and the recommended) 2D echocardiographic method for estimating left ventricular volume because it employs the fewest mathematical assumptions regarding the left ventricular cavity shape and also corrects for distortion of left ventricular geometry.[12] However, the accuracy of this method is highly dependent on adequate endocardial border delineation. As already described, the echocardiography machine settings should be adjusted to obtain the best possible endocardial delineation. If, despite these adjustments, the endocardial border cannot be visualized adequately in one of the two requisite views, the single-plane Simpson's method can be used to obtain left ventricular volumes. However, this method will not be accurate enough in the presence of significant regional WMAs. When the endocardial border cannot be adequately visualized in either of the two views, the Simpson's method should be abandoned and the area-length method used to estimate left ventricular volume.

Table 11-2 describes the normal ranges and partition values of left ventricular volumes derived from 2D methods.

Three-Dimensional Methods

The recent advent of three-dimensional (3D) echocardiography has significantly improved our ability to accurately estimate left ventricular volumes by eliminating the need for mathematical assumptions regarding the shape of the LV. The left ventricular cavity can be directly imaged in a 3D space, and its volume can be accurately calculated. Comparative studies using magnetic resonance imaging (MRI) as the gold standard have shown excellent agreement between the two techniques and have demonstrated 3D echocardiography to be superior to 2D echocardiography for estimating left ventricular volumes.[26-30] The availability of live 3D TEE has further improved image quality, and the application of quantitative techniques to these images has the potential to provide an even more accurate estimation of left ventricular volumes than ever before. However, a detailed description of these techniques, including their advantages and potential pitfalls, is beyond the scope of this chapter.

Left Ventricular Mass

Left ventricular hypertrophy is an important prognosis determinant in a number of clinical conditions such as hypertension, aortic stenosis, aortic regurgitation, and cardiomyopathies.[21,31-36] Accordingly, the presence and extent of left ventricular hypertrophy forms the basis of many of the key therapeutic decisions in these disease states. Echocardiography, by allowing for estimation of left ventricular mass, is the most clinically relevant tool for detection and characterization of left

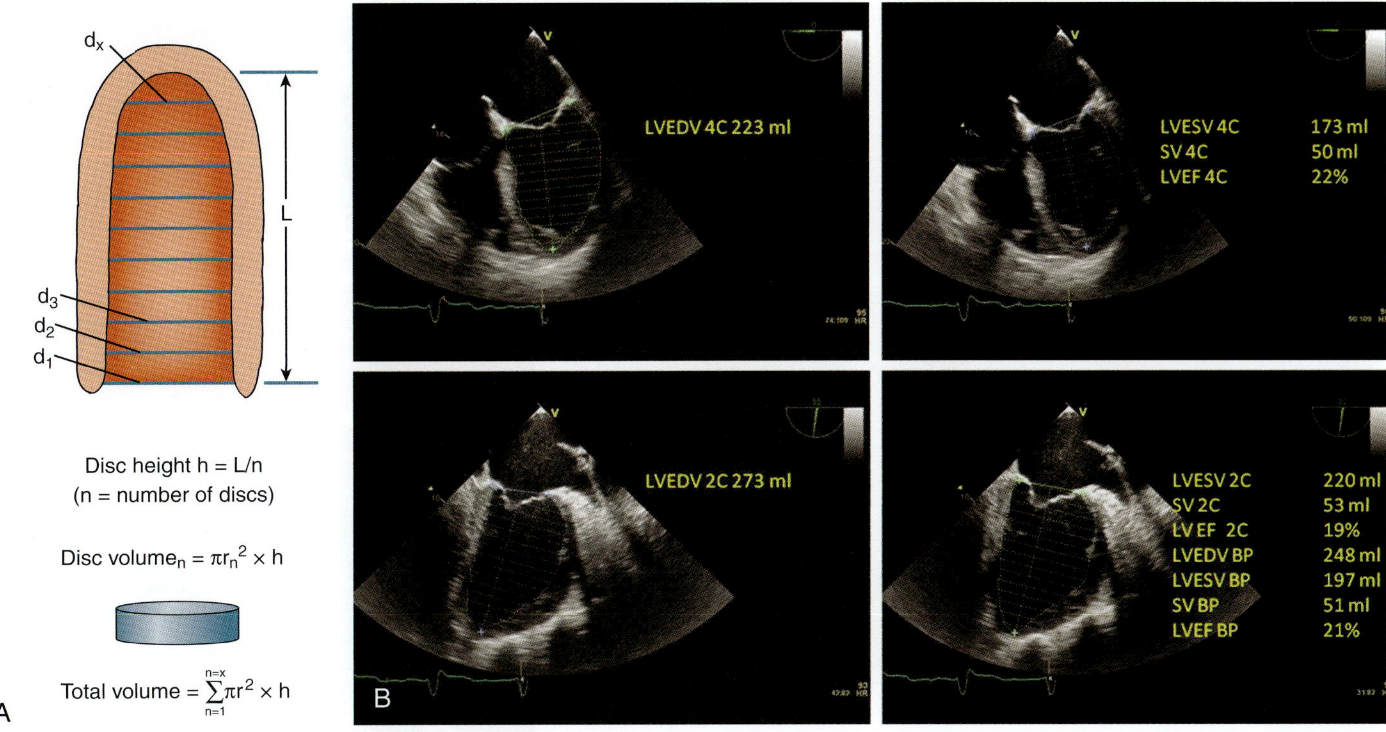

Figure 11-5 **A and B,** Measurement of left ventricular volume using biplane Simpson's method. Endocardial border is traced in midesophageal four-chamber and two-chamber views at end-diastole and end-systole. *2C,* Two-chamber; *4C,* four-chamber; *BP,* biplane; *EDV,* end-diastolic volume; *EF,* ejection fraction; *ESV,* end-systolic volume; *LV,* left ventricular; *SV,* stroke volume. *(Modified with permission from Feigenbaum H, Armstrong W, Ryan T, eds. Feigenbaum's Echocardiography. 6th ed. Philadelphia: Lippincott Williams & Wilkins; 2005.)*

ventricular hypertrophy.[36-38] Assessing left ventricular mass via echocardiography has been extensively used in clinical and research settings for prognostication, guiding treatment, and following the effects of various pharmacologic and nonpharmacologic measures aimed at bringing about regression of left ventricular hypertrophy.[31,36-39]

Although there are several echocardiographic methods for estimating left ventricular mass, the basic principle is the same. First, the left ventricular myocardial volume is calculated, and the volume is then converted to a mass by multiplying it by the specific density of the myocardium. The left ventricular myocardial volume itself is obtained by subtracting the left ventricular cavity volume from the total left ventricular volume, which includes both the left ventricular cavity and the surrounding myocardial shell. All the methods used to estimate left ventricular volume can be used to estimate left ventricular mass as well. Measuring left ventricular mass is performed at end-diastole.

Linear Method

Although the linear method is generally not the preferred method for estimating left ventricular volumes, its simplicity and superior reproducibility have made it the most commonly employed method for estimating left ventricular mass. Using this method, the left ventricular cavity volume is estimated as the $LVIDd^3$, and total left ventricular volume is defined as $(LVIDd + IVSd + ILWd)^3$. From these values, left ventricular mass can then be calculated as:

$$\text{Left ventricular mass (grams)} = 1.04 \times [(LVIDd + IVSd + ILWd)^3 - LVIDd^3] \times 0.8 + 0.6$$

where *1.04* is the myocardial density, and *0.8* is the correction factor. *LVIDd, IVSd,* and *ILWd* represent the end-diastolic left ventricular internal diameter, interventricular septal thickness, and inferolateral wall thickness, respectively.

Two-Dimensional Methods

Using 2D echocardiography, left ventricular mass can be calculated using either the area-length method, the truncated ellipsoid method, or Simpson's method.

For the **area-length method** (Fig. 11-6), the TG mid–short-axis view is obtained at the papillary muscle level, and the left ventricular epicardial and endocardial cross-sectional areas (A_1 and A_2) are measured by tracing the epicardium and endocardium, respectively. When tracing the endocardium, the papillary muscles are included in the cavity, not in the myocardium. Left ventricular length (L) is then measured in the ME two-chamber view as previously described. Left ventricular mass is then calculated using the following equation:

$$\text{Left ventricular mass} = 1.05 \times (\text{total left ventricular volume} - \text{left ventricular cavity volume})$$
$$= 1.05 \times [A_1 (L + t) - A_2 L]$$

where *t* is the mean wall thickness derived by subtracting the left ventricular cavity radius from the left ventricular radius as described in the equation:

$$t = \sqrt{(A_1/\pi)} - \sqrt{(A_2/\pi)}$$

In the example shown in Figure 11-6, *B*, *t* would be 1.16 cm $[\sqrt{(27.8/3.14)} - \sqrt{(10.4/3.14)}]$. Inserting all the values into the equation will yield a left ventricular mass of 122.6 g.

An alternate method for estimating left ventricular mass is based on the **truncated ellipsoid method** (see Fig. 11-6, *A*) and can be calculated with the following equation:

$$\text{Left ventricular mass} = 1.05 \times \{(b + t)^2 [\tfrac{2}{3}(a + t) + d - d^3/3(a + t)^2] - b^2 [\tfrac{2}{3}a + d - d^3/3a^2]\}$$

where *b* is the left ventricular cavity radius, which is back-calculated from the area as $\sqrt{(A_2/\pi)}$, and *a* and *d* are the two segments of the left

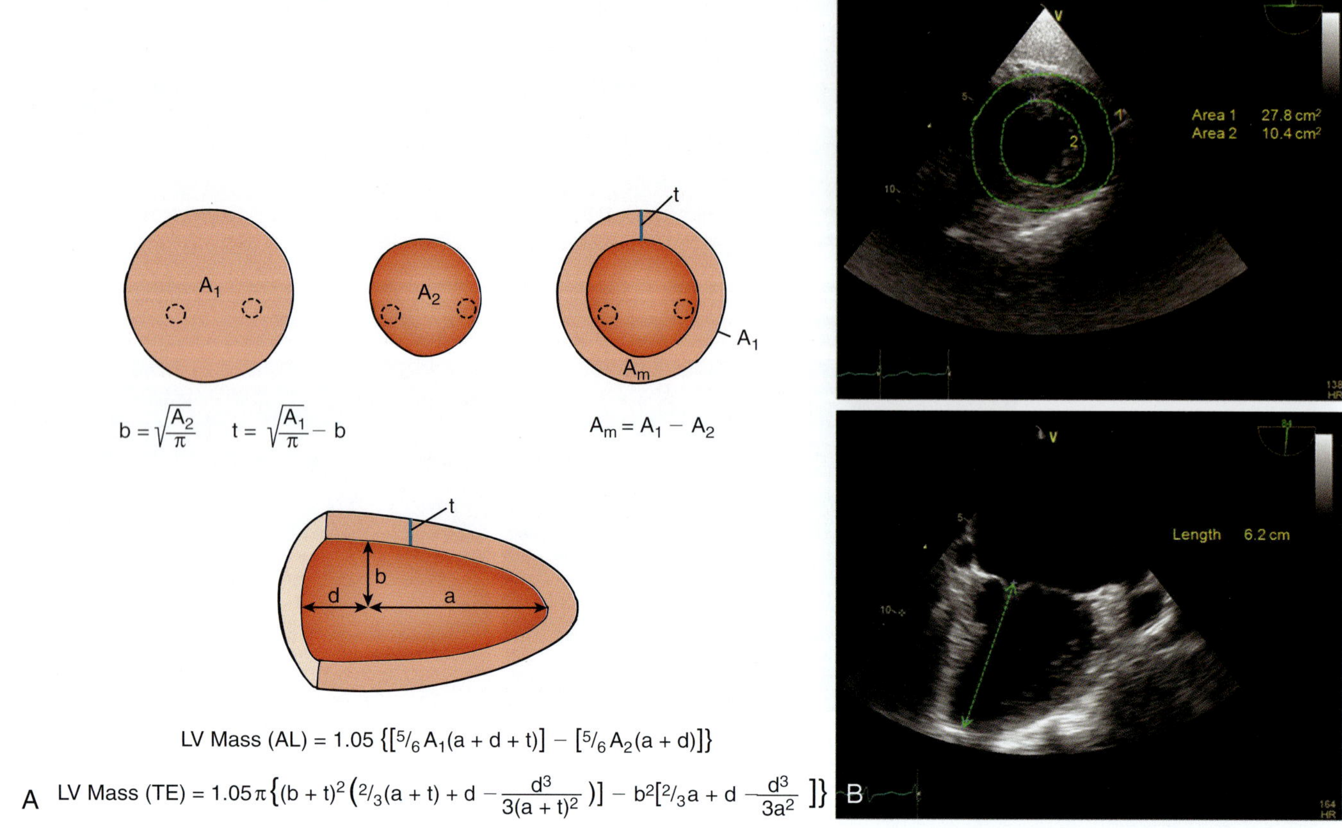

LV Mass (AL) = 1.05 {[⁵⁄₆ A₁(a + d + t)] − [⁵⁄₆ A₂(a + d)]}

$$\text{LV Mass (AL)} = 1.05\left\{\left[\tfrac{5}{6}A_1(a+d+t)\right]-\left[\tfrac{5}{6}A_2(a+d)\right]\right\}$$

$$\textbf{A}\quad\text{LV Mass (TE)} = 1.05\pi\left\{(b+t)^2\left(\tfrac{2}{3}(a+t)+d-\tfrac{d^3}{3(a+t)^2}\right)\right]-b^2\left[\tfrac{2}{3}a+d-\tfrac{d^3}{3a^2}\right]\right\}\quad\textbf{B}$$

Figure 11-6   **A and B,** Estimation of left ventricular *(LV)* mass using area-length *(AL)* formula and truncated-ellipsoid *(TE)* formula. See text for details. A_1, Total LV area; A_2, LV cavity area; *Am*, myocardial area; *a*, length of LV from widest minor axis radius to apex; *b*, short-axis radius of LV cavity (back-calculated from short-axis cavity area); *d*, length of LV from widest minor axis radius to mitral annulus plane; *t*, mean wall thickness. *(Modified with permission from Schiller NB, Shah PM, Crawford M, et al. Recommendations for quantitation of the left ventricle by two-dimensional echocardiography. American Society of Echocardiography Committee on Standards, Subcommittee on Quantitation of Two-Dimensional Echocardiograms. J Am Soc Echocardiogr. 1989;2:358-367.)*

ventricular length measured from the widest minor axis radius to the apex and mitral annulus, respectively.

As emphasized for volume measurements, all given methods for left ventricular mass estimation are applicable only when the LV is not grossly distorted. In the presence of distorted ventricles, the biplane Simpson's method is the most accurate. Using **Simpson's method**, left ventricular volume is calculated at the level of the epicardium and endocardium as described previously, and the built-in software then automatically calculates left ventricular mass from these measurements.

Normal ranges and partition values for left ventricular mass using the linear and 2D methods are summarized in Table 11-3. Although these values are derived from TTE, as mentioned earlier, previous studies using TEE have reported agreement with these values.[14,15] However, inferolateral wall thickness is slightly overestimated using TEE, so the linear method results in overestimation of left ventricular mass by approximately 6 g/m².[14]

Left Atrium

The left atrium is in direct communication with the LV during diastole and is therefore directly exposed to the hemodynamic perturbations taking place within the LV during this phase of the cardiac cycle. As a result, with the development of left ventricular diastolic dysfunction, there is a progressive increase in the mean left atrial pressure paralleling the rise in left ventricular filling pressure. The increase in the mean left atrial pressure eventually leads to an increase in left atrial size.[40,41] Consequently, left atrial size becomes a useful measure of the severity and chronicity of left ventricular diastolic dysfunction and is aptly

regarded as the "HbA1C" of left ventricular diastolic function.[42] A large body of evidence now demonstrates that left atrial size is an independent predictor for recurrence of atrial fibrillation, risk of stroke, heart failure–related hospitalization, and risk of overall mortality in a wide variety of clinical conditions characterized by elevated left ventricular filling pressures.[42-54]

Apart from being an important marker of left ventricular diastolic dysfunction, left atrial size is an important measure of the hemodynamic severity of mitral valve pathologies (mitral stenosis or regurgitation), which are also independent of left ventricular systolic or diastolic function. In addition, left atrial enlargement may also occur secondarily to atrial fibrillation, in which case it serves as an important determinant of immediate success and long-term outcomes of interventions aimed at restoring sinus rhythm.

TEE is the imaging modality of choice for assessing structural abnormalities of the left atrium and left atrial appendage, but measuring left atrial size using TEE is the most challenging. The left atrium is situated in close proximity to the esophagus and therefore falls in the near-field of the TEE transducer where the ultrasound beams have not diverged enough. As a result, the left atrium often cannot be completely included in the image sector, precluding an accurate measurement of its size, and information derived from multiple imaging views must be combined to obtain an overall estimate of left atrial size.[12] However, in some cases, particularly when the left atrium is significantly enlarged, it may be almost impossible to accurately measure left atrial size in any of the available views. In such cases, many investigators have measured left atrial size up to the edge of the image sector, excluding the portion of the left atrium not covered in the imaging sector.[55-57]

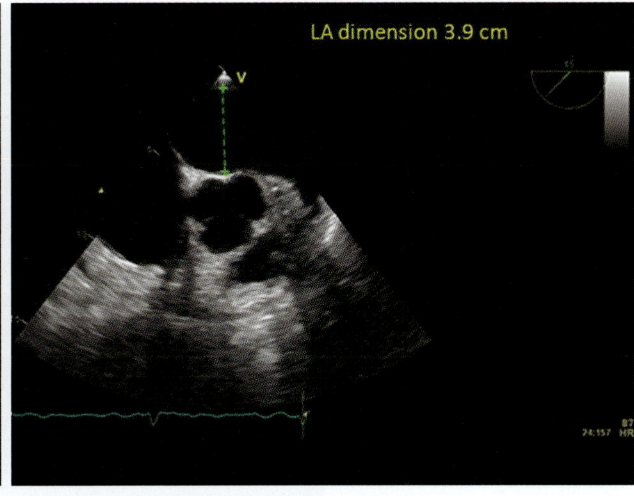

Figure 11-7 Measurement of left atrial *(LA)* anteroposterior diameter from midesophageal aortic valve long-axis and short-axis views.

Left atrial size can be assessed by measuring its anteroposterior diameter, area, or volume. Although left atrial diameter and area are technically simple to measure and provide a quick estimate of left atrial size, they may not be truly representative of left atrial size in disease states, because the left atrium often enlarges non-uniformly.[58,59] Therefore, measuring the volume is considered to be the most accurate method for estimating left atrial size. This is supported by epidemiologic studies showing the strongest association between left atrial volume and adverse cardiovascular outcomes, compared with other measures of left atrial size.[53,60] The American Society of Echocardiography recommends using left atrial volume as the preferred measure of left atrial size.[12] It is important to note that all left atrial size measurements are performed at the end of ventricular systole when left atrial size is at its maximum.

In TTE, the **left atrial anteroposterior diameter** is measured preferably in the parasternal long-axis view. The measurement is performed from the posterior wall of the aorta to the posterior left atrial wall, perpendicular to the long axis of the left atrium. A similar measurement can be obtained from the parasternal short-axis view. In TEE, analogous views, namely the ME aortic valve long-axis view (120 degrees) or the ME aortic valve short-axis view (30-60 degrees), are used to measure left atrial diameter. In the ME aortic valve long-axis view (120 degrees) (Video 11-5), the measurement is performed along a straight line passing perpendicular to the aortic valve and crossing through the posterior wall of the left atrium (Fig. 11-7). In the ME aortic valve short-axis view (30-60 degrees), left atrial diameter is measured as the vertical distance between the aortic root and the posterior wall of the left atrium (see Fig. 11-7). Measurements obtained from both these methods have been shown to have a modest correlation with the measurements obtained from TTE, and it remains debatable which is more accurate.[55-57]

The left atrial area is measured using TTE by performing planimetry of the left atrium in the apical four-chamber view. The endocardial border of the left atrium is traced starting from the insertion of the anterior mitral leaflet at the medial aspect of the mitral annulus and extending up to the insertion point of the posterior mitral leaflet at the other end of the mitral annulus. The tracing should not extend along the mitral valve leaflets. Instead, a straight line joining the two end points, which corresponds to the mitral annular plane, forms the inferior margin of the left atrium. While doing planimetry, it is important to ensure that the pulmonary veins and left atrial appendage are not included in the measurement. One must also be careful to avoid foreshortening the left atrium. This can be ensured by aligning the imaging plane such that the maximum obtainable size of the left atrium is visualized. In TEE, the left atrial area can be measured in a similar manner in the ME four-chamber view (0 degrees) (Fig. 11-8). However, as discussed earlier, inability to include the entire left atrium in the image sector is often a major challenge.

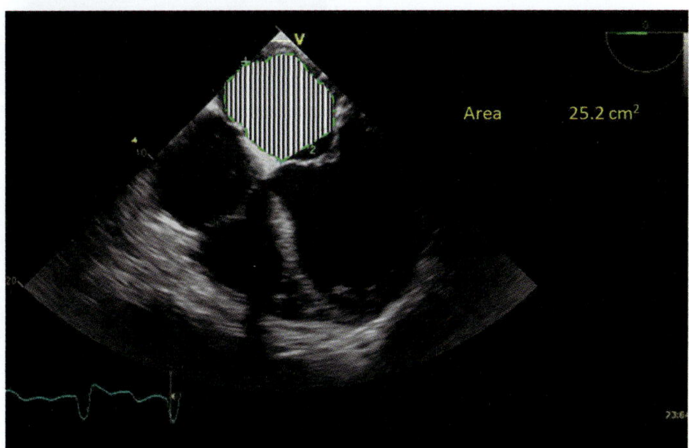

Figure 11-8 Measurement of left atrial area by planimetry from midesophageal four-chamber view. Note that mitral annulus forms inferior margin of left atrium, and endocardial tracing is not extended along mitral valve leaflets.

As already emphasized, measuring **left atrial volume** is the current gold standard for estimating left atrial size, and either the biplane area-length method (based on the ellipsoid model) or Simpson's method can be used for calculation. Given that most existing data were derived from the biplane area-length method, it is the recommended method for this purpose (Figs. 11-9 and 11-10). Left atrial volume can be calculated as.

$$\text{Left atrial volume} = 8/3\pi\,(A_1 \times A_2/L)$$

where A_1 is the planimetered left atrial area in the four-chamber view, and A_2 is the planimetered left atrial area in the two-chamber view. L is the length of the left atrium, measured as the perpendicular distance from the midpoint of the mitral annular plane to the superior aspect of the left atrium. The length is measured in both the four-chamber and two-chamber views, and the shorter of the two is used in the equation. The same method is used to measure left atrial volume during TEE (see Fig. 11-10).

Left atrial volume can also be measured using the Simpson's multiple-disks method. The principle and technique are the same as those described for left ventricular volume estimation.

Table 11-4 describes normal ranges for left atrial size derived from TTE. The same values are used to evaluate left atrial size using TEE, but it must be noted that left atrial size is usually underestimated in TEE.[55-57]

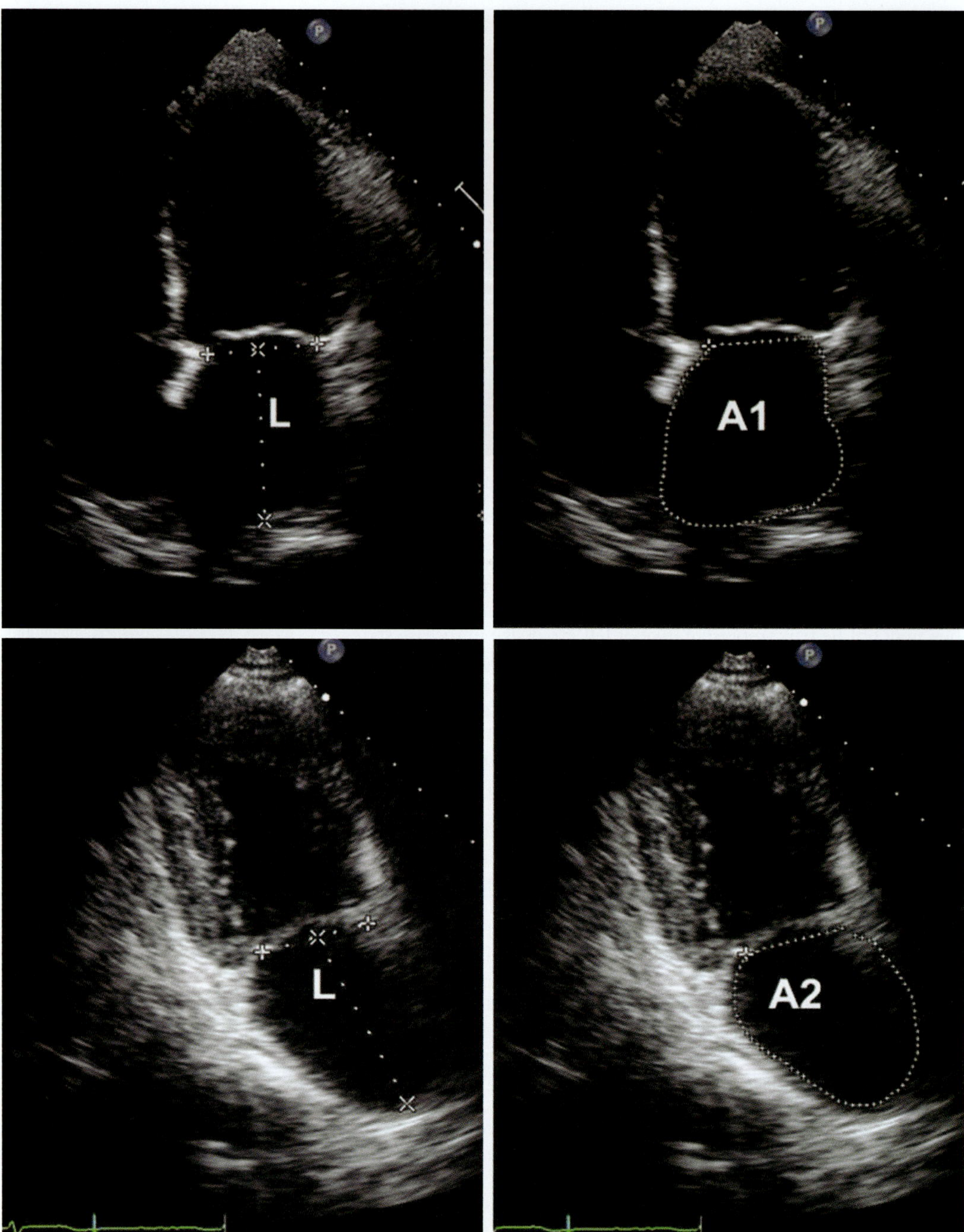

Figure 11-9 Estimation of left atrial volume by biplane area-length method during transthoracic echocardiography. See text for details. *A1 and A2,* Left atrial areas obtained by planimetry from apical four-chamber and two-chamber views; *L,* left atrial length measured from both apical four-chamber and two-chamber views.

Right Ventricle, Right Ventricular Outflow Tract, and Pulmonary Arteries

The right ventricle (RV) plays an important role in maintaining normal cardiac function and contributes significantly to morbidity and mortality in a myriad of clinical conditions, including those affecting the left heart structures, pulmonary vasculature, lungs, and RV.[61-74] Despite its importance, for decades the RV has been regularly ignored during routine echocardiographic studies. Many reasons for this neglect are possible, but the complex shape of the RV, rendering it difficult to image and measure using echocardiography, is the most likely.

As mentioned, the RV has a complex 3D anatomy. It is wrapped around the LV in a crescent shape and has three distinct segments: the body, the inflow portion, and the outflow segment. Because of its complex shape, the entire right ventricular cavity cannot be visualized in any single echocardiographic view. To overcome this limitation, the RV must be imaged from multiple views focusing on its different segments. The information obtained from all views must be integrated to derive comprehensive information regarding the RV's overall size and function.[12,75]

Until recently, assessment of the RV has been largely subjective. Under normal circumstances, in the four-chamber view, the LV appears larger than the RV and forms the cardiac apex. However, as the RV enlarges, it tends to overtake the LV in size and also displaces the LV to become the "apex-forming" ventricle. When right ventricular cavity size visually appears larger than left ventricular size in the four-chamber view, this is an indication that the RV has already become significantly enlarged.

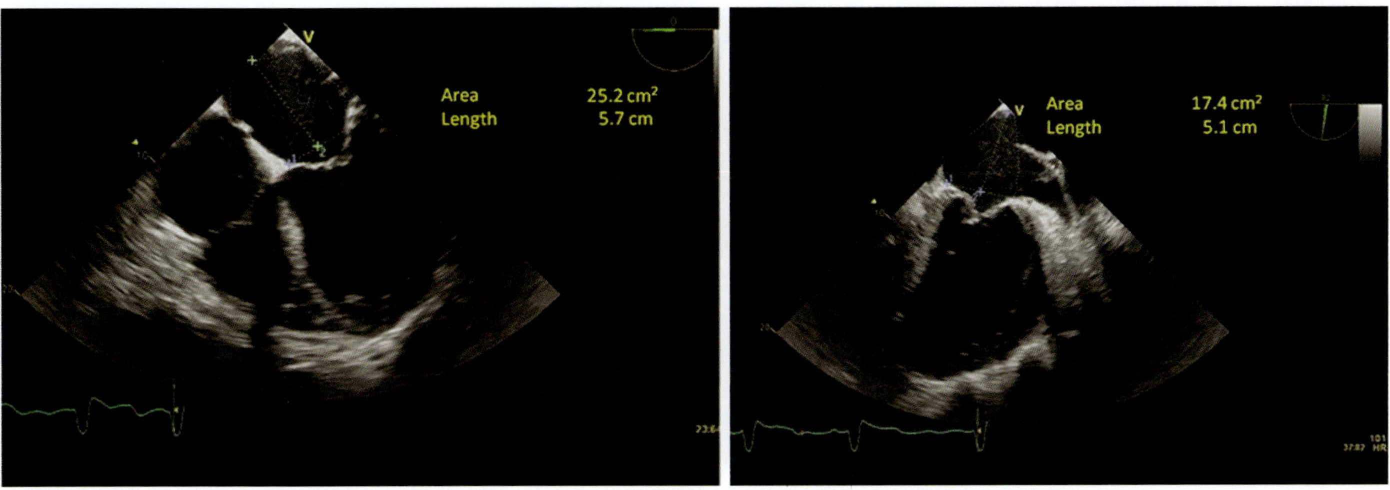

Figure 11-10 Estimation of left atrial volume by biplane area-length method during transesophageal echocardiography. See text for details.

TABLE 11-4	Reference Ranges and Partition Values for Left Atrial Size							
	Men				Women			
	Reference Range	*Mildly Abnormal*	*Moderately Abnormal*	*Severely Abnormal*	*Reference Range*	*Mildly Abnormal*	*Moderately Abnormal*	*Severely Abnormal*
LA diameter (cm)	3.0-4.0	4.1-4.6	4.7-5.2	≥5.2	2.7-3.8	3.9-4.2	4.3-4.6	≥4.7
LA diameter/BSA (cm/m²)	1.5-2.3	2.4-2.6	2.7-2.9	≥3.0	1.5-2.3	2.4-2.6	2.7-2.9	≥3.0
LA area (cm²)	≤20	20-30	30-40	>40	≤20	20-30	30-40	>40
LV volume (mL)	18-58	59-68	69-78	≥79	22-52	53-62	63-72	≥73
LA volume/BSA (mL/m²)	22 ± 6	29-33	34-39	≥40	22 ± 6	29-33	34-39	≥40

BSA, Body surface area; *LA*, left atrium.
Data from Lang RM, Bierig M, Devereux RB, et al. Recommendations for chamber quantification: a report from the American Society of Echocardiography's Guidelines and Standards Committee and the Chamber Quantification Writing Group, developed in conjunction with the European Association of Echocardiography, a branch of the European Society of Cardiology. *J Am Soc Echocardiogr.* 2005;18:1440-1463.

TABLE 11-5	Reference Values for Right Ventricle, Right Atrium, and Pulmonary Artery Sizes	
		Abnormal
Right Ventricle		
Diameter at base (cm)		>4.2
Diameter at midlevel (cm)		>3.5
Length from base to apex (cm)		>8.6
Fractional area change (%)		<35
Right Ventricular Outflow Tract		
Proximal diameter (cm)		>3.3
Distal diameter (cm)		>2.7
Pulmonary artery		
Just distal to pulmonary valve (cm)		>2.1
Right Atrium		
Diameter or minor dimension (cm)		>4.4
Length or major dimension (cm)		>5.3
Area (cm²)		>18

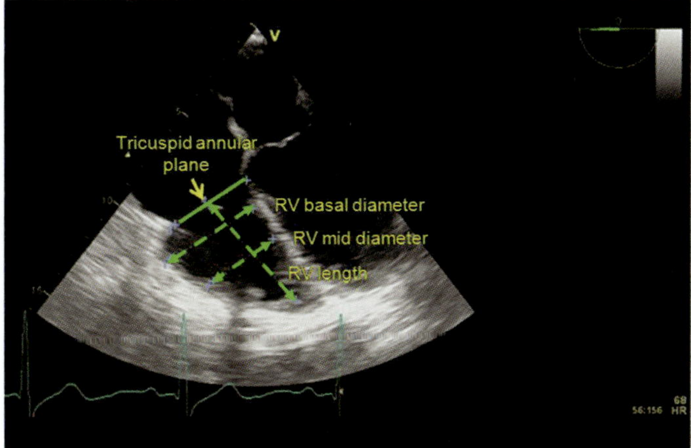

Figure 11-11 Measurement of right ventricular *(RV)* dimensions from RV-focused midesophageal four-chamber view.

Quantitative assessment of right ventricular size and function during echocardiography has been recently standardized.[12,75] Table 11-5 lists the recommended measurements for estimating right ventricular size, along with normal values.

Right ventricular basal and mid-diameters and its length are best obtained from the ME four-chamber view (Fig. 11-11). The basal diameter is the maximal short-axis dimension in the basal one third of the RV, and the mid-cavity diameter is the short-axis dimension measured in the middle third of the RV at the level of the left ventricular papillary muscles. The longitudinal dimension is the linear distance from the plane of the tricuspid annulus to the right ventricular apex. When performing these measurements, it is important to ensure that right ventricular size is not underestimated and that the maximum obtained size of the RV is measured. To achieve this, the image plane has to be adjusted to obtain the "RV-focused" view (Video 11-6). This view can be developed from the standard ME four-chamber view (0 degrees) by increasing the omniplane angle to 10 to 20 degrees to maximize the tricuspid annulus diameter. At the same time, overestimating right ventricular size should be avoided by continuously

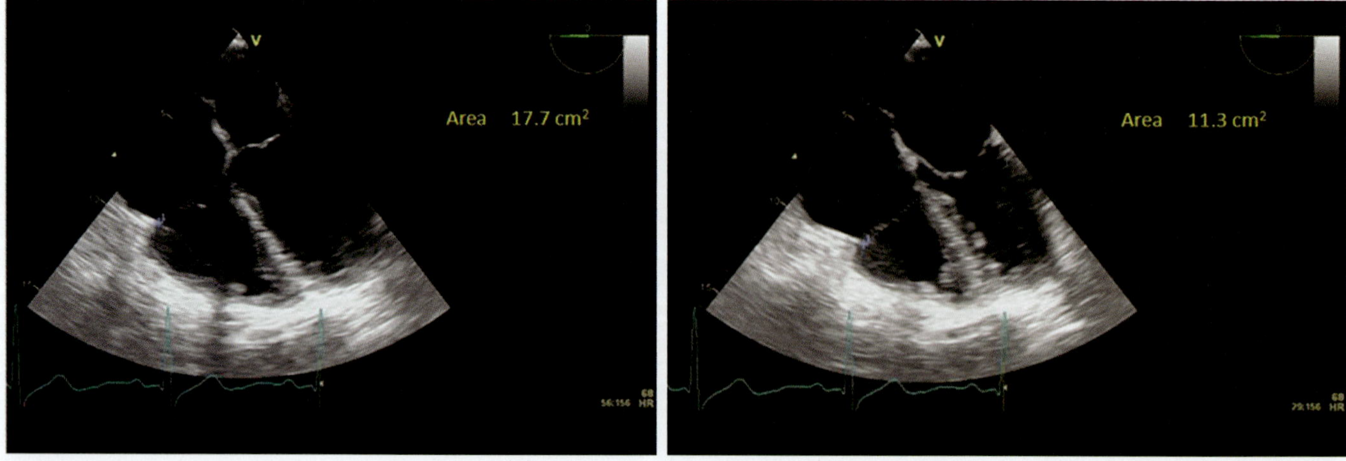

Figure 11-12   Measurement of right ventricular *(RV)* area from RV-focused midesophageal four-chamber view. Area is measured in both end-diastolic and end-systolic frames, and fractional area change is calculated as percentage reduction in RV area during systole.

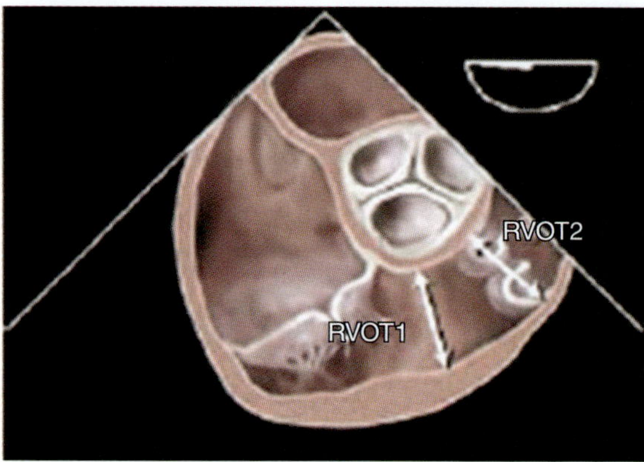
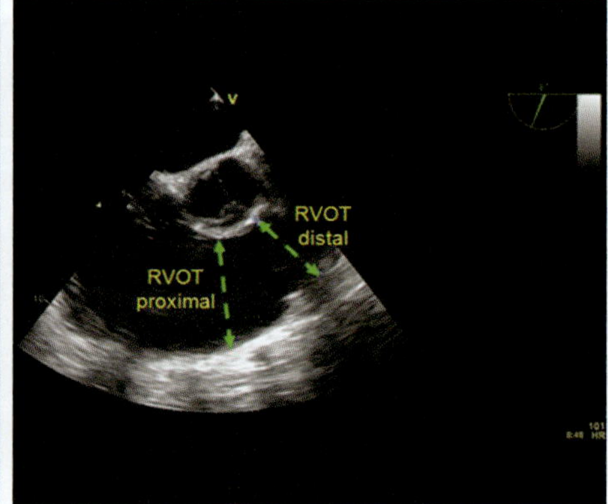

Figure 11-13   Measurement of right ventricular outflow tract *(RVOT)* dimensions from midesophageal RV inflow-outflow view. *RVOT1,* Proximal RVOT diameter; *RVOT2,* distal RVOT diameter.

ensuring that the image plane passes through the cardiac apex. This same view is also used for measuring the right ventricular cavity area and the fractional area change. The latter serves as a measure of right ventricular systolic function (Fig. 11-12).

The RVOT can be best measured in the ME right ventricular inflow-outflow view (Fig. 11-13, Video 11-7). First, the ME aortic valve short-axis view should be obtained (30-60 degrees), and the omniplane angle should then be advanced forward to 60 to 75 degrees to bring the RVOT into view. Further adjustments to the omniplane angle and rotation of the transducer to the right may be required to optimize the view of the tricuspid valve leaflets for the purpose of opening up the RVOT and bringing the pulmonary valve into view. The proximal and distal dimensions of the RVOT diameter can be measured from this view. The proximal dimension is measured at the level of the right ventricular infundibulum by measuring the linear distance between the anterior aortic wall and the anterior wall of the RV. The distal dimension is measured just below the level of the pulmonary valve annulus. Although the diameter of the main pulmonary artery can also be measured from this view, this view generally does not allow for adequate visualization of the pulmonary arteries. An alternate view can be developed from the upper esophageal position and provides good visualization of the main pulmonary artery, its bifurcation, and the proximal segments of the branch pulmonary arteries (usually right) (Fig. 11-14, Video 11-8). For this view, the probe should be inserted into the midesophagus, and the ME descending aorta short-axis view (0 degrees) can then be obtained by rotating the probe to the left. From this position, the probe should be withdrawn to obtain the upper esophageal aortic arch long-axis (0 degrees) view. At this point, the omniplane angle should be advanced forward to 60 to 90 degrees to bring the pulmonary valve and pulmonary artery into

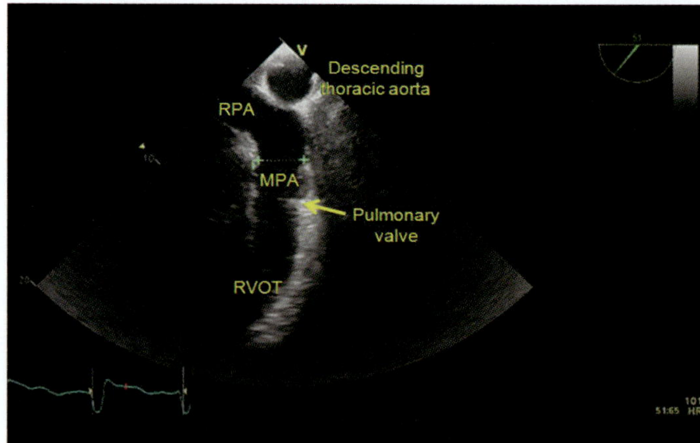

Figure 11-14   Measurement of right ventricular outflow tract *(RVOT)* and pulmonary artery dimensions from upper esophageal pulmonary artery view. *MPA,* Main pulmonary artery; *RPA,* right pulmonary artery.

view. This view not only provides reliable measurements of the main pulmonary artery size, but because it allows for optimal alignment of the ultrasound beam with the direction of blood flow, it is also the best view for measuring blood flow across the pulmonary valve.

Measurement of right ventricular free wall thickness is required for the diagnosis of right ventricular hypertrophy. In TTE, this measurement is best obtained from the subcostal window, but there is no particularly recommended view for this measurement during TEE. Right ventricular wall thickness can be measured from either the ME aortic valve long-axis view (120 degrees) or ME four-chamber view (0 degrees). Care must be taken to avoid including the external epicardial fat, right ventricular trabeculations, and internal papillary muscles in the measurement.

Right Atrium

The best view for assessing right atrial size is the ME four-chamber view (Fig. 11-15). In this view, right atrial length, diameter, and area can be measured. Right atrial length is measured as the maximal long-axis distance from the center of the tricuspid annulus to the center of the superior right atrial wall, parallel to the interatrial septum. Right atrial diameter is the perpendicular distance between the right atrial free wall and the interatrial septum, measured at the midatrial level. Right atrial area is measured by planimetry in the same manner as the left atrium. The endocardial border of the right atrium is traced, beginning at the lateral aspect of the tricuspid annulus and extending up to the septal aspect. The right atrial appendage and vena cava are excluded from the measurement. All measurements are performed at right ventricular end-systole.[12,75]

There are currently no standardized echocardiographic protocols for estimating right atrial volume, so this volume is usually not measured during clinical practice.

Table 11-5 describes the reference ranges for various right atrial dimensions.

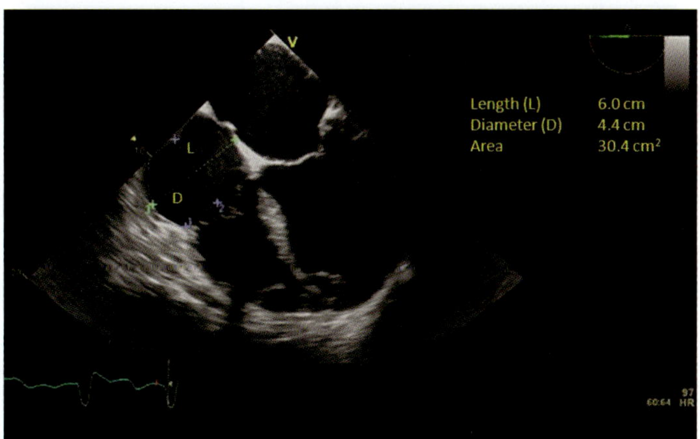

Figure 11-15 Measurement of right atrial dimensions and area from right ventricle–focused midesophageal four-chamber view.

Aorta

A number of methods are used to measure the aortic annulus and ascending aorta, the most common of which involves estimating cardiac output. In addition, assessing aortic size is also required for calculating the aortic valve area by the continuity equation, determining the size of an aortic valve prosthesis to be implanted, and deciding whether surgical repair is required for a dilated aortic root and ascending aorta.

The primary measurements performed to assess aortic size include the left ventricular outflow tract (LVOT) diameter or aortic annulus, the diameter of the aortic root at the level of the sinuses of Valsalva, and the diameter of the sinotubular junction (Fig. 11-16). Additionally, in specific situations, the diameters of the ascending aorta, arch, and descending thoracic aorta may also have to be measured.

For the aortic root and ascending aorta, the ME aortic valve long- and short-axis views and the ME ascending aorta long- and short-axis views provide the best visualization. The ME aortic valve long-axis view can be obtained by rotating the omniplane angle forward to 120 to 150 degrees from the ME four-chamber view (0 degrees) (see Video 11-5). Further adjustments of the probe position and rotation may be required to optimize the view of the aortic annulus and make the sinuses of Valsalva symmetric. The ME ascending aorta long-axis view can be developed from this position by withdrawing the probe to bring the right pulmonary artery into view and then decreasing the omniplane angle slightly by 10 to 20 degrees to make the aortic wall symmetric. To obtain the ME aortic valve short-axis view, the ME four-chamber view (0 degrees) should first be obtained, the probe should be withdrawn to obtain the ME five-chamber view (0 degrees), and the omniplane angle should be advanced forward to 30 to 45 degrees. The aortic valve should be centered and the three aortic valve cusps made symmetric. Further withdrawal of the probe and a decrease in the omniplane angle backward to 0 degrees develops the ME ascending aorta short-axis view.

From the described views, the dimensions of the aortic annulus, aortic root, and ascending aorta can easily be obtained. Imaging planes showing the maximum diameter of the vessel should be used for the measurements, and the measurements should be performed perpendicular to the long axis of the vessel. The aortic annulus is measured as the distance between the hinge points of the two aortic leaflets. The aortic root is measured as the maximum obtainable diameter either at the sinuses of Valsalva or sinotubular junction. The *sinotubular junction* refers to the transition between the sinuses of Valsalva and the tubular portion of the ascending aorta (see Fig. 11-16).[12] Nomograms for the reference values of the aortic root diameter based on age and body surface area have been previously published (Fig. 11-17). These can be used to determine whether the aortic root is dilated in a particular patient.[76]

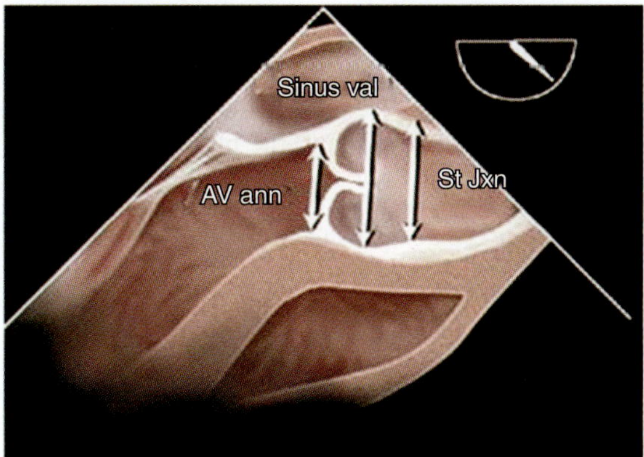

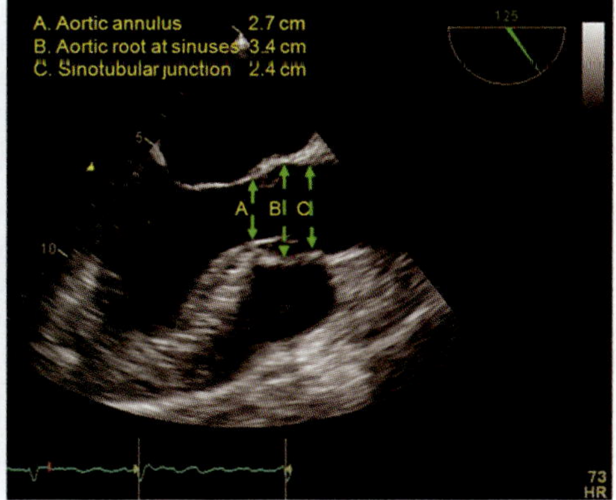

Figure 11-16 Measurement of aortic root dimensions from midesophageal aortic valve long-axis view. *AV ann,* Aortic valve annulus; *Sinus val,* sinus of Valsalva; *St Jxn,* sinotubular junction. *(Modified with permission from Lang RM, Bierig M, Devereux RB, et al. Recommendations for chamber quantification: a report from the American Society of Echocardiography's Guidelines and Standards Committee and the Chamber Quantification Writing Group, developed in conjunction with the European Association of Echocardiography, a branch of the European Society of Cardiology. J Am Soc Echocardiogr. 2005;18:1440-1463.)*

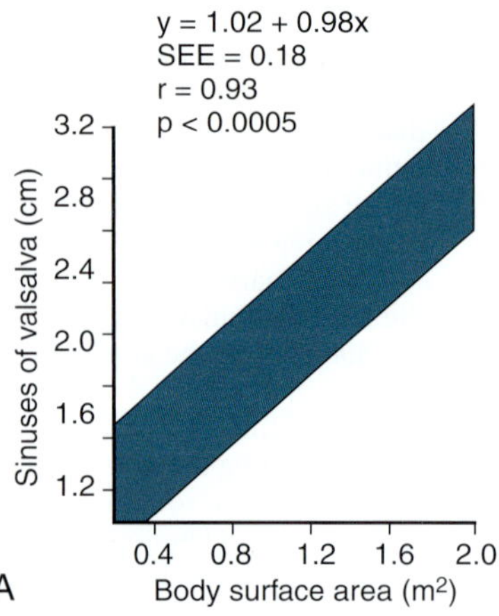
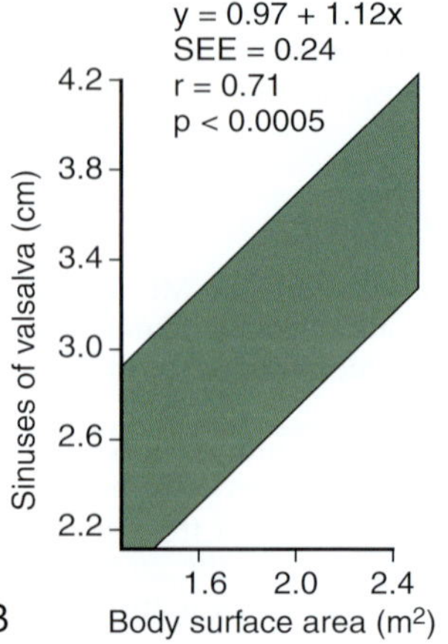
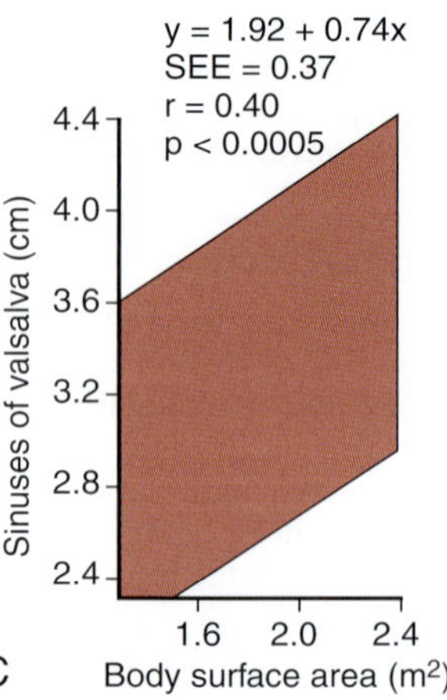

Figure 11-17 The 95% confidence intervals for aortic root diameter at sinuses of Valsalva based on body surface area in three different age groups: **(A)** children and adolescents, **(B)** adults aged 20 to 39 years, and **(C)** and adults aged 40 years or older. *(Modified with permission from Roman MJ, Devereux RB, Kramer-Fox R, O'Loughlin J. Two-dimensional echocardiographic aortic root dimensions in normal children and adults. Am J Cardiol. 1989;64:507-512.)*

As discussed, the leading edge–to–leading edge technique was used to measure cardiac chamber dimensions, including aortic size. However, with refinements in ultrasound technology, the actual cavity size can now be measured with the inner edge–to–inner edge technique. Such an approach permits direct comparisons with analogous measurements obtained from other imaging modalities such as MRI and computed tomography (CT). However, it is important to note that the normal reference values for aortic dimensions in echocardiography were derived using the leading edge–to–leading edge technique.

Descending thoracic aorta dimensions can be obtained from the ME descending thoracic aorta short-axis (0 degrees) and long-axis (90 degrees) views. Withdrawing the transducer from this position and turning it to follow the aortic arch curve also allows for visualization of the distal segment of the arch. However, traversal of the trachea between the esophagus and aorta at this level obstructs the view of the proximal segment of the arch and the distal segment of the ascending aorta with TEE.

Measurement of Intracardiac Flows

Applying the Doppler principle to ultrasound has completely revolutionized the practice of echocardiography. With this addition, echocardiography can now not only provide minute details of cardiac anatomy but has also transformed into an eminently useful modality for comprehensive assessment of intracardiac hemodynamics. Estimating intracardiac flows, assessing ventricular diastolic function, measuring pulmonary arterial pressure, assessing the severity of valve lesions and congenital defects, and evaluating prosthetic heart valve function are just some of its applications currently being used in day-to-day practice.

Measuring cardiac output is a key element of hemodynamic monitoring during the perioperative period and plays a vital role in guiding therapeutic decision making in this setting. In addition, measuring cardiac output (or a modification of it) is also central to assessing valve lesions, intracardiac shunts, and fistulae. Traditionally, invasive monitoring with central venous or pulmonary arterial catheters has been employed to achieve this goal. However, an appreciable risk of complications associated with invasive monitoring has fueled controversy regarding the use of pulmonary artery catheters and has persuaded experts to call for scrutinizing the indications for their use.[77-79] Because it is noninvasive, echocardiography has rapidly evolved into a simple, reliable, and safer alternative for this purpose. Although TEE itself is really not noninvasive, it is often used in the perioperative setting for other reasons (e.g., evaluating cardiac structure and function), and the ability to measure cardiac output simultaneously offers a great advantage.

Measurement of Blood Flow: Basic Principles[13,80]

To understand the basic principle involved in estimating blood flow using the Doppler technique, consider as an example a blood vessel

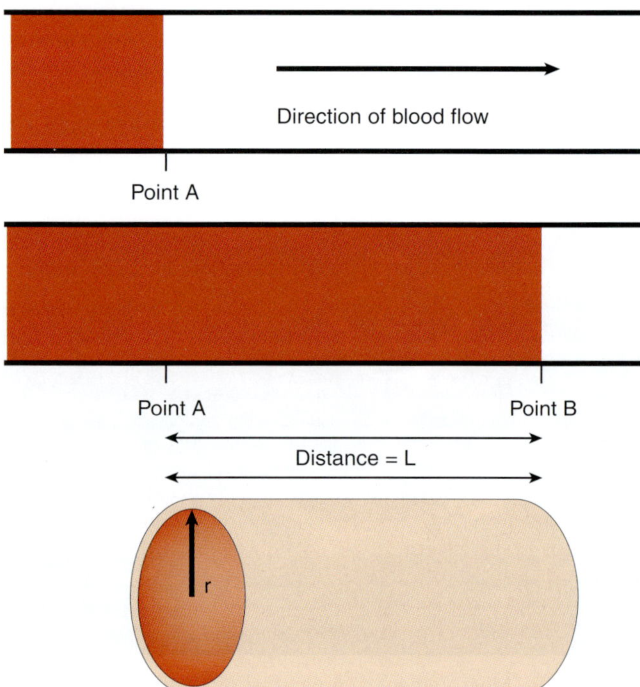

Figure 11-18 Underlying principle of Doppler estimation of blood flow through cardiovascular system. See text for details.

through which blood is flowing (Fig. 11-18). The blood column front is at *Point A* at the beginning of the flow and travels a distance *(L)* during a given time period to move to *Point B*. Thus, the volume of blood that has passed through the blood vessel during this period will be equal to the volume of the blood present in the vessel between points A and B. Given that this column of blood is cylindrical in shape, its volume can be calculated using the following equation:

$$\text{Volume} = \text{cross-sectional area of the cylinder} \times \text{length} = \pi r^2 \times L$$

where *r* is the radius of the cylinder.

The same principle is applied to estimate blood flow through the cardiac structures. The cross-sectional area can be easily derived from the radius measured with the help of M-mode or 2D imaging. However, measuring the distance L is challenging. If blood flow is laminar (i.e., most red blood cells are moving at almost the same velocity) and flow velocity remains constant, the distance L will be equal to the product of the blood velocity and the time during which flow took place:

$$L = \text{velocity} \times \text{time}$$

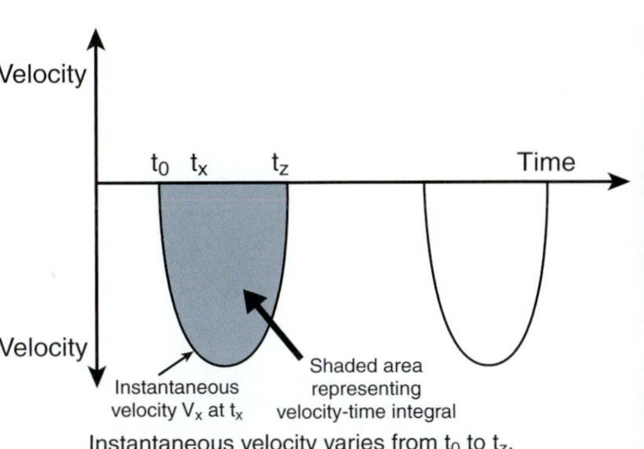

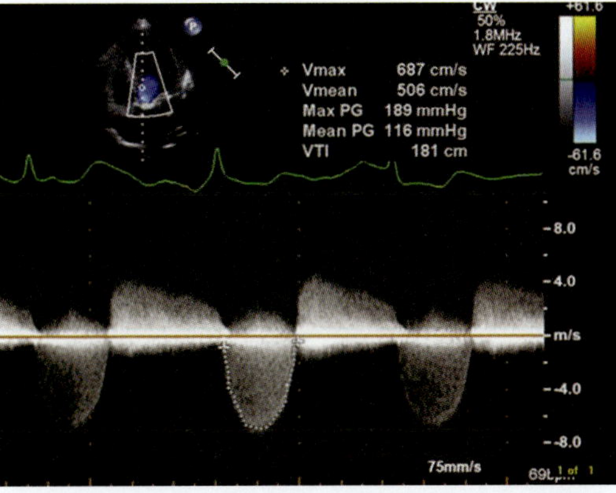

Figure 11-19 Concept of the velocity-time integral (VTI) used to estimate blood flow using the Doppler technique. See text for details. (*Modified with permission from Feigenbaum H, Armstrong W, Ryan T, eds. Feigenbaum's Echocardiography. 6th ed. Philadelphia: Lippincott Williams & Wilkins, 2005.*)

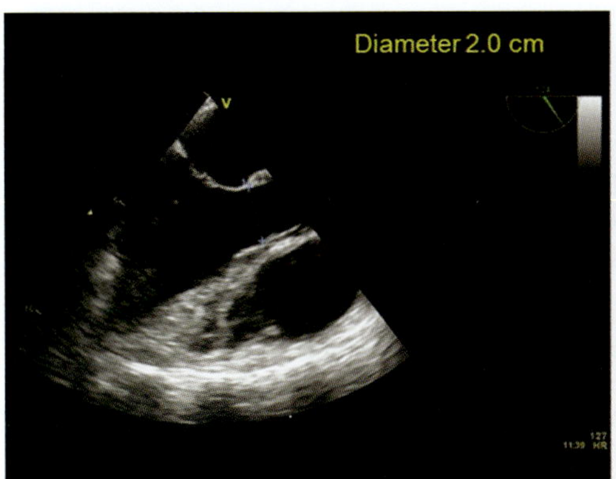

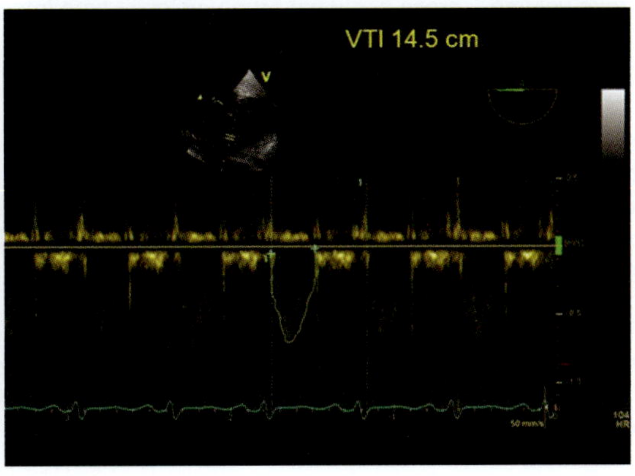

Stroke volume = cross-sectional area × velocity-time integral
$$= (3.14 \times 1 \times 1) \times 14.5$$
$$= 45.5 \text{ cm}^3 \text{ or } 45.5 \text{ ml}$$

Figure 11-20 Estimation of stroke volume at left ventricular outflow tract (LVOT) during transesophageal echocardiography. LVOT diameter is measured from midesophageal aortic valve long-axis view, and LVOT velocity-time integral (*VTI*) is obtained from deep transgastric long-axis view.

Since blood flow in the cardiovascular system is pulsatile, the velocity of the blood is not constant. At every point within the heart, blood flow occurs only during a particular phase of the cardiac cycle. During this phase, blood flow velocity initially increases progressively and then decreases as flow ceases. To measure blood flow in such a situation, the mean velocity within the period during which flow occurred must be calculated. Using echocardiographic equipment, this is accomplished by tracing the spectral Doppler signal of the flow. The built-in software calculates the area under the curve, which is in fact the integral of instantaneous velocities over time and is therefore known as the *velocity-time integral* (VTI) (Fig. 11-19). The VTI is equivalent to the product of the mean velocity and the duration of flow and conveys the same information as L in the equation above. It must be noted that the unit of measurement for the VTI is centimeters because it is the cross-product of velocity (cm/s) and time (seconds).

Flow can then be easily calculated by multiplying the derived "L" by the cross-sectional area of the structure.

Measurement of Cardiac Output

Estimating cardiac output can be performed by measuring blood flow through any cardiac valve that lends itself to an accurate estimation of the size and the blood velocity at that level. In clinical practice, the LVOT is the most commonly used site for cardiac output measurement because it provides the easiest and most accurate estimate of cardiac output, provided there is no significant aortic regurgitation. Cardiac output can also be measured at the mitral valve and RVOT. Although a similar measurement can also be obtained at the tricuspid valve, it is not used in clinical practice because the tricuspid valve often has significant regurgitation, which will lead to an overestimation of blood flow.

Cardiac Output Measurement at Left Ventricular Outflow Tract

As described earlier, estimating blood flow through any cardiac structure requires measuring the cross-sectional area of that structure and the VTI through that structure. In TEE, the LVOT diameter is usually measured in the ME aortic valve long-axis view (120 degrees), which allows the best visualization of the LVOT (Fig. 11-20). In this view, the LVOT is perpendicular to the ultrasound beam, rendering recognition of tissue/blood interfaces easily and diameter measurements accurately. The LVOT diameter is measured as the distance between the insertion points or hinge points of the two aortic valve leaflets. The measurement is performed during early systole when the valve leaflets are fully open. It is extremely critical to obtain an accurate measurement of the LVOT diameter, because any error will become magnified when the cross-sectional area is calculated. Magnifying the image helps minimize any measurement error. The measurement is performed three to five times, and the largest of these measurements is used in the equation.

The LVOT VTI must be measured at the same site used for the diameter measurement. However, this cannot be accomplished in the same views as those used to measure the diameter, because the ultrasound beam direction is almost perpendicular to the direction of blood flow. In TG or deep TG long-axis views, the LVOT is oriented parallel to the ultrasound beam, which makes these views ideal for measuring blood flow velocity (Video 11-9). The pulsed-wave sample volume is placed in the LVOT at a location roughly 5 mm proximal to the aortic valve. Correct placement can be confirmed by the presence of the aortic valve closing click and the absence of the opening click on the spectral Doppler display. In addition, spectral broadening of the signal is minimal at this level, which also helps in confirming correct positioning of the sample volume. After the spectral Doppler signal is obtained, the VTI

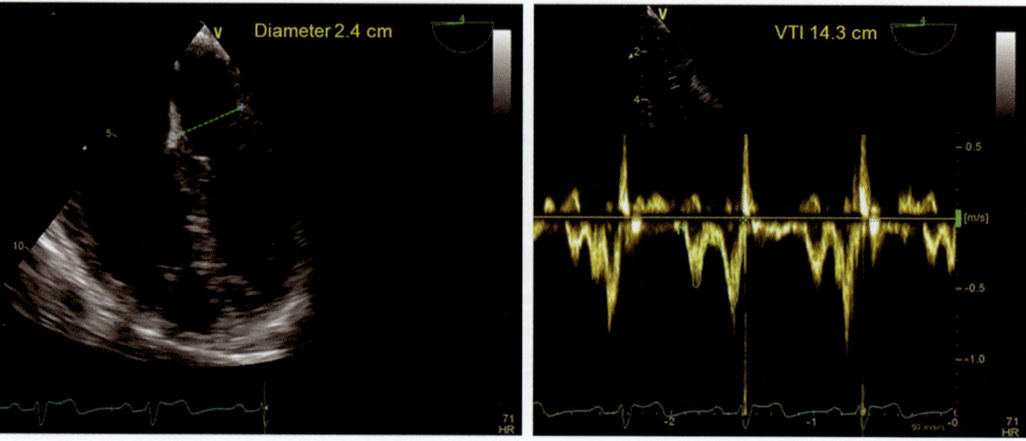

Figure 11-21 Estimation of stroke volume at mitral valve. Mitral annular diameter and velocity-time integral *(VTI)* are both measured from midesophageal four-chamber view.

Stroke volume = cross-sectional area × velocity-time integral
= (3.14 × 1.2 × 1.2) × 14.3
= 64.7 cm³ or 64.7 ml

is derived by tracing the outer border of the signal. The outer edge of the densest portion of the signal should be traced, and the dispersion outside this dense signal (greatest at peak velocity) should be ignored. This is required to ensure that the modal velocity (i.e., velocity of most red blood cells in the jet) is measured. After the described measurements are obtained, stroke volume can be calculated with the equation mentioned earlier. Cardiac output is then calculated by multiplying stroke volume by heart rate.

All Doppler measurements should be obtained at a sweep speed of 50 to 100 mm/s, and the filter settings should be kept at low values. This is required to detect velocities at the beginning and end of the flow and obtain accurate timing of the event. The measurements should be averaged over 3 to 5 cardiac cycles during sinus rhythm and over 5 to 10 cardiac cycles during atrial fibrillation. When the measurements are performed on the right side of the heart, they should be averaged over the entire respiratory cycle because the right-side flow is significantly influenced by respiration.

There are several advantages to performing cardiac output measurement at the LVOT. For example, the LVOT is easily visualized during echocardiography; its shape is presumed to be circular, and its size remains almost constant during the cardiac cycle. In addition, blood flow through the LVOT is mostly laminar, which minimizes the chances of inadvertently sampling velocities that are not truly representative of the actual blood flow at that point. All of these factors contribute to an accurate estimation of the cross-sectional area.

Nevertheless, despite the aforementioned advantages, there are circumstances in which cardiac output cannot be measured accurately at the LVOT. In the presence of significant aortic regurgitation, blood flow through the LVOT is increased and is not representative of true systemic cardiac output. If significant LVOT obstruction is present, flow at the LVOT is turbulent and velocity is increased, thereby precluding an accurate measurement of the VTI at this level. Finally, at times during TEE, it may be challenging to obtain a measurable Doppler signal at the LVOT owing to a suboptimal acoustic window. In such situations, cardiac output must be measured at alternative sites such as the mitral valve or RVOT.

Cardiac Output Measurement at Mitral Valve

Measuring cardiac output at the mitral valve is based on the same principle as described for measurement at the LVOT. The mitral valve cross-sectional area is calculated from the mitral annular diameter (d) obtained from the ME four-chamber view (0 degrees). The diameter measurement should be performed during early to mid-diastole, one frame after the leaflets begin to open following the early rapid filling phase (Fig. 11-21). The transmitral VTI is measured in the same view by placing the pulsed-wave sample volume at the mitral annulus and

tracing the spectral Doppler signal during diastole. Care should be taken to ensure that the sample volume remains at the annulus during diastole.

The mitral annular cross-sectional area is calculated as $\pi d^2/4$, assuming it is circular in shape. However, this is an incorrect assumption because the mitral annular orifice is actually elliptical. An alternative method has been proposed in an attempt to rectify this error. This requires measuring the two diameters from the two orthogonal views: the four-chamber view and the two-chamber view. The mitral orifice area is then calculated as $\pi d_1 d_2/4$. Although this may be geometrically more accurate, obtaining the correct diameter measurements from multiple views is often difficult and is itself a potential source of error. As a result, the former method has been found to have almost similar or even better accuracy than the latter and, given its simplicity, remains the preferred method for measuring cardiac output at the mitral valve.[81,82]

Cardiac output estimation at the mitral valve will not be accurate if there is significant mitral regurgitation or if there is a shunt at the ventricular level.

Cardiac Output Measurement at Right Ventricular Outflow Tract

In the absence of any intracardiac shunt, cardiac output on the right side of the heart is the same as that on the left. Consequently, the RVOT offers another site for cardiac output measurement. However, measuring cardiac output at the RVOT is usually challenging owing to difficulties in aligning the Doppler beam with the blood flow direction (Fig. 11-22). Accurate measurement of RVOT diameter may also be difficult at times.

RVOT diameter is measured from the ME right ventricular inflow-outflow view as described previously. To obtain the flow measurement, the best view for aligning the Doppler beam with the blood flow direction is the upper esophageal pulmonary artery view (see Video 11-8). In this view, the blood flow direction is parallel to the ultrasound beam, thereby providing the most accurate measurement of blood flow velocity at this site. Alternately, blood flow measurement through the RVOT can also be performed in the deep TG long-axis view, in which turning the probe to the right brings the RVOT into view and orients it with the ultrasound beam.

Measuring cardiac output at the RVOT is helpful when this measurement cannot be performed at the LVOT or mitral valve because of significant aortic and mitral regurgitation, respectively. In addition, this measurement is also required for estimating the magnitude of an intracardiac shunt.

Two-Dimensional Method for Estimating Cardiac Output

Although Doppler measurement of cardiac output at the LVOT remains the most commonly employed method for this purpose,

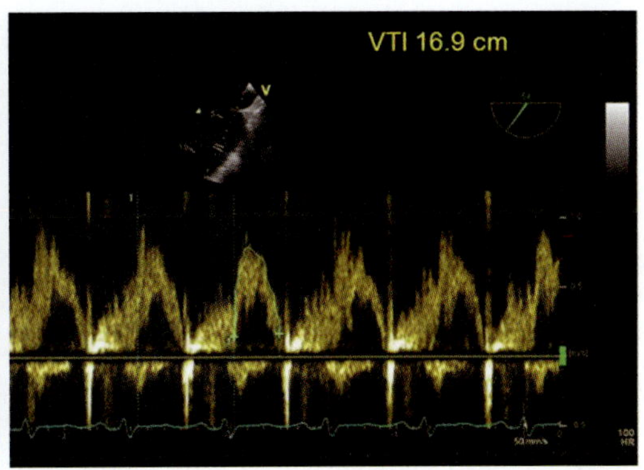

Stroke volume = cross-sectional area × velocity-time integral
= (3.14 × 1.45 × 1.45) × 16.9
= 111.6 cm^3 or 111.6 ml

Figure 11-22 Estimation of stroke volume at right ventricular outflow tract (RVOT). RVOT diameter is measured from midesophageal right ventricular inflow-outflow view, and RVOT velocity-time integral (*VTI*) is obtained from mid- or upper esophageal pulmonary artery view.

cardiac output can also be calculated from 2D images. Left ventricular end-diastolic and end-systolic volumes are measured using one of the volume measurement methods described earlier. The difference between the two volumes is equal to the stroke volume, and multiplying it by the heart rate provides the cardiac output.

Although this method is less commonly used because of technical difficulties involved in obtaining accurate volume measurements, it offers a means to countercheck results obtained using the Doppler method.

Shunts[13]

Estimating the hemodynamic significance of an intracardiac shunt is essential in determining the need to perform a surgical intervention, particularly in the case of left-to-right shunts. In echocardiography, this is usually accomplished by measuring the cardiac chamber dimensions, directly visualizing the jet direction and size, and measuring the pressure gradient across the defect. However, a formal assessment of the shunt magnitude is often required, especially in borderline situations.

Left-to-Right Shunt at Atrial Level

In the presence of a left-to-right shunt at the atrial level, blood flow through the tricuspid and pulmonary valves is increased relative to the flow though the left side of the heart. The difference between the two equals the amount of blood shunted from the left atrium to the right atrium. Cardiac output measured at the RVOT (pulmonary blood flow or Qp) thus represents a combination of systemic blood flow (Qs) and shunt flow. The Qp is measured in the same manner as described earlier (see Fig. 11-22). The Qs can be measured either at the LVOT or mitral valve (see Figs. 11-20 and 11-21). However, for reasons already mentioned, the LVOT is the preferred site for this measurement, provided there is no significant aortic regurgitation. The ratio of Qp to Qs serves as a measure of shunt size, with a value of 2 or greater considered to indicate a hemodynamically significant left-to-right shunt.

Video 11-10, A, shows the ME four-chamber view in a patient with a large ostium secundum atrial septal defect with a visibly significant left-to-right shunt. The ME right ventricular inflow-outflow view in the same patient shows a dilated RV and RVOT (Video 11-10, B). Estimations of Qs and Qp in this patient are depicted in Figures 11-20 and 11-22, respectively. As shown in the figures, the values of Qs and Qp were 45.5 and 111.6 ml, respectively, with a Qp:Qs ratio of 2.45, which indicates a large shunt.

Left-to-Right Shunt at Ventricular Level

In the presence of an interventricular shunt, shunt size is estimated in a manner analogous to that used to estimate the size of an interatrial shunt. However, when the defect is situated very close to the pulmonary valve, as in an outlet ventricular septal defect, the turbulence and streaming produced by the shunt jet precludes an accurate measurement of Qp. In such situations, the cardiac output at the mitral valve can be used as a measure of Qp, provided there is no additional interatrial shunt or significant mitral regurgitation.

Left-to-Right Shunt at Level of Great Arteries

When the shunt exists at the great arterial level (e.g., patent ductus arteriosus or aortopulmonary window), blood flow through the left side of the heart is increased because the entire pulmonary venous return passes through the mitral and aortic valves and into the ascending aorta. At the same time, blood flow through the right side of the heart (tricuspid and pulmonary valves) is not affected. In such situations, cardiac output is measured either at the LVOT or mitral valve, which will actually provide an estimate of pulmonary blood flow or Qp, whereas a similar measurement at the RVOT will reflect true systemic blood flow or Qs. The ratio of the two will allow shunt magnitude to be assessed.

Right-to-Left Intracardiac Shunt

Although the principles described can also theoretically be used to estimate shunt size in right-to-left shunts, it is very difficult and usually not feasible in clinical practice. Right-to-left shunts are most often due to severe right ventricular outflow obstructions or part of complex congenital heart disease pathologies. The former pathology precludes measuring pulmonary blood flow, and the latter makes it difficult to distinguish the relative contributions of left-to-right and right-to-left shunts.

Fistulae

An arteriovenous fistula (AVF) is a channel that allows direct communication between the arterial and venous systems, bypassing the capillaries and precapillary sphincters. Given that the precapillary sphincters are the main site of vascular resistance, a fistula effectively reduces vascular resistance, resulting in increased blood flow through that segment of the vasculature and ultimately leading to volume overload of the heart. The more proximal the fistula, the greater the extent of the bypassed vascular bed and the greater the volume overload produced. An AVF can occur as a congenital malformation (e.g., coronary AVF), as a consequence of another congenital anomaly (e.g., bronchopulmonary collaterals in patients with tetralogy of Fallot), as a consequence of another systemic disease (e.g., pulmonary AVFs observed in patients with chronic liver disease), secondary to trauma (may even be iatrogenic), or by surgical intervention (e.g., AVF created for facilitating hemodialysis).

Because most of the fistulae are situated far from the heart and produce uniform volume overload of the heart, direct echocardiographic assessment of their functional size is usually not feasible. Even in a coronary AVF, blood flow through the fistula cannot be estimated because blood flow is increased across all cardiac chambers and valves. Nevertheless, if an AVF can be temporarily occluded and cardiac output then measured just before and after occlusion, the difference between the two measurements can be used to derive an estimate of fistula size.

Conclusions

TEE remains the diagnostic modality of choice for deriving information instantaneously in perioperative settings. We have reviewed the key principles involved in measuring cardiac dimensions and flow. While recognizing the unique aspects and growing applications of TEE in surgical settings, the necessary skills required for developing requisite imaging views remain critical to ensure optimum utilization of this modality. As miniaturized probes, novel technologies, and new multidimensional approaches emerge, the applications of TEE for chamber quantification and hemodynamic evaluation will likely expand.

REFERENCES

1. Side CD, Gosling RG. Non-surgical assessment of cardiac function. *Nature*. 1971;232:335-336.
2. Frazin L, Talano JV, Stephanides L, Loeb HS, Kopel L, Gunnar RM. Esophageal echocardiography. *Circulation*. 1976;54:102-108.
3. Matsumoto M, Oka Y, Strom J, et al. Application of transesophageal echocardiography to continuous intraoperative monitoring of left ventricular performance. *Am J Cardiol*. 1980;46:95-105.
4. Shanewise JS, Cheung AT, Aronson S, et al. ASE/SCA guidelines for performing a comprehensive intraoperative multiplane transesophageal echocardiography examination: recommendations of the American Society of Echocardiography Council for Intraoperative Echocardiography and the Society of Cardiovascular Anesthesiologists Task Force for Certification in Perioperative Transesophageal Echocardiography. *J Am Soc Echocardiogr*. 1999;12:884-900.
5. Shapira Y, Vaturi M, Weisenberg D, Sagie A. Intraoperative transesophageal echocardiography during valve replacement surgery. A review. *Minerva Cardioangiol*. 2007;55:229-237.
6. Kihara C, Murata K, Wada Y, et al. Impact of intraoperative transesophageal echocardiography in cardiac and thoracic aortic surgery: experience in 1011 cases. *J Cardiol*. 2009;54:282-288.
7. Catena E, Mele D. Role of intraoperative transesophageal echocardiography in patients undergoing noncardiac surgery. *J Cardiovasc Med (Hagerstown)*. 2008;9:993-1003.
8. Rosenhek R, Binder T, Maurer G. Intraoperative transesophageal echocardiography in valve replacement surgery. *Echocardiography*. 2002;19:701-707.
9. Junior CG, Botelho ES, Diego LA. Intraoperative monitoring with transesophageal echocardiography in cardiac surgery. *Rev Bras Anestesiol*. 2011;61:495-512.
10. Gillam LD. Intraoperative transesophageal echocardiography. *Cardiol Rev*. 2000;8:269-278.
11. Sengupta PP, Khandheria BK. Transoesophageal echocardiography. *Heart*. 2005;91:541-547.
12. Lang RM, Bierig M, Devereux RB, et al. Recommendations for chamber quantification: a report from the American Society of Echocardiography's Guidelines and Standards Committee and the Chamber Quantification Writing Group, developed in conjunction with the European Association of Echocardiography, a branch of the European Society of Cardiology. *J Am Soc Echocardiogr*. 2005;18:1440-1463.
13. Feigenbaum H, Armstrong W, Ryan T, eds. *Feigenbaum's Echocardiography*. 6th ed. Philadelphia: Lippincott, Williams and Wilkins; 2005.
14. Colombo PC, Municino A, Brofferio A, et al. Cross-sectional multiplane transesophageal echocardiographic measurements: comparison with standard transthoracic values obtained in the same setting. *Echocardiography*. 2002;19:383-390.
15. Hozumi T, Shakudo M, Shah PM. Quantitation of left ventricular volumes and ejection fraction by biplane transesophageal echocardiography. *Am J Cardiol*. 1993;72:356-359.
16. Ilercil A, O'Grady MJ, Roman MJ, et al. Reference values for echocardiographic measurements in urban and rural populations of differing ethnicity: the Strong Heart Study. *J Am Soc Echocardiogr*. 2001;14:601-611.
17. Palmieri V, Dahlof B, DeQuattro V, et al. Reliability of echocardiographic assessment of left ventricular structure and function: the PRESERVE study. Prospective Randomized Study Evaluating Regression of Ventricular Enlargement. *J Am Coll Cardiol*. 1999;34:1625-1632.
18. Pearlman JD, Triulzi MO, King ME, Newell J, Weyman AE. Limits of normal left ventricular dimensions in growth and development: analysis of dimensions and variance in the two-dimensional echocardiograms of 268 normal healthy subjects. *J Am Coll Cardiol*. 1988;12:1432-1441.
19. Bonow RO, Carabello BA, Chatterjee K, et al. 2008 focused update incorporated into the ACC/AHA 2006 guidelines for the management of patients with valvular heart disease: a report of the American College of Cardiology/American Heart Association Task Force on Practice Guidelines (Writing Committee to revise the 1998 guidelines for the management of patients with valvular heart disease). Endorsed by the Society of Cardiovascular Anesthesiologists, Society for Cardiovascular Angiography and Interventions, and Society of Thoracic Surgeons. *J Am Coll Cardiol*. 2008;52:e1-142.
20. Ganau A, Devereux RB, Roman MJ, et al. Patterns of left ventricular hypertrophy and geometric remodeling in essential hypertension. *J Am Coll Cardiol*. 1992;19:1550-1558.
21. Gaasch WH, Zile MR. Left ventricular structural remodeling in health and disease: with special emphasis on volume, mass, and geometry. *J Am Coll Cardiol*. 2011;58:1733-1740.
22. Berger J, Ren X, Na B, Whooley MA, Schiller NB. Relation of concentric remodeling to adverse outcomes in patients with stable coronary artery disease (from the Heart and Soul Study). *Am J Cardiol*;107:1579-84.
23. Verdecchia P, Schillaci G, Borgioni C, et al. Adverse prognostic significance of concentric remodeling of the left ventricle in hypertensive patients with normal left ventricular mass. *J Am Coll Cardiol*. 1995;25:871-878.
24. Quinones MA, Waggoner AD, Reduto LA, et al. A new, simplified and accurate method for determining ejection fraction with two-dimensional echocardiography. *Circulation*. 1981;64:744-753.
25. Teichholz LE, Kreulen T, Herman MV, Gorlin R. Problems in echocardiographic volume determinations: echocardiographic-angiographic correlations in the presence of absence of asynergy. *Am J Cardiol*. 1976;37:7-11.
26. Mor-Avi V, Sugeng L, Lang RM. Real-time 3-dimensional echocardiography: an integral component of the routine echocardiographic examination in adult patients? *Circulation*. 2009;119:314-329.
27. Tighe DA, Rosetti M, Vinch CS, et al. Influence of image quality on the accuracy of real time three-dimensional echocardiography to measure left ventricular volumes in unselected patients: a comparison with gated-SPECT imaging. *Echocardiography*. 2007;24:1073-1080.
28. Nikitin NP, Constantin C, Loh PH, et al. New generation 3-dimensional echocardiography for left ventricular volumetric and functional measurements: comparison with cardiac magnetic resonance. *Eur J Echocardiogr*. 2006;7:365-372.
29. Jenkins C, Bricknell K, Hanekom L, Marwick TH. Reproducibility and accuracy of echocardiographic measurements of left ventricular parameters using real-time three-dimensional echocardiography. *J Am Coll Cardiol*. 2004;44:878-886.
30. Arai K, Hozumi T, Matsumura Y, et al. Accuracy of measurement of left ventricular volume and ejection fraction by new real-time three-dimensional echocardiography in patients with wall motion abnormalities secondary to myocardial infarction. *Am J Cardiol*. 2004;94:552-558.
31. Devereux RB, Wachtell K, Gerdts E, et al. Prognostic significance of left ventricular mass change during treatment of hypertension. *Jama*. 2004;292:2350-2356.
32. Yasunari K, Maeda K, Nakamura M, Watanabe T, Yoshikawa J, Hirohashi K. Left ventricular hypertrophy and angiotensin II receptor blocking agents. *Curr Med Chem Cardiovasc Hematol Agents*. 2005;3:61-67.
33. Gosse P. Left ventricular hypertrophy as a predictor of cardiovascular risk. *J Hypertens Suppl*. 2005;23:S27-S33.
34. Artham SM, Lavie CJ, Milani RV, Patel DA, Verma A, Ventura HO. Clinical impact of left ventricular hypertrophy and implications for regression. *Prog Cardiovasc Dis*. 2009;52:153-167.
35. Milan A, Caserta MA, Avenatti E, Abram S, Veglio F. Anti-hypertensive drugs and left ventricular hypertrophy: a clinical update. *Intern Emerg Med*. 2010;5:469-479.
36. Mancia G, De Backer G, Dominiczak A, et al. 2007 Guidelines for the management of arterial hypertension: The Task Force for the Management of Arterial Hypertension of the European Society of Hypertension (ESH) and of the European Society of Cardiology (ESC). *Eur Heart J*. 2007;28:1462-1536.
37. Alfakih K, Reid S, Hall A, Sivananthan MU. The assessment of left ventricular hypertrophy in hypertension. *J Hypertens*. 2006;24:1223-1230.
38. Agabiti-Rosei E, Muiesan ML, Salvetti M. Evaluation of subclinical target organ damage for risk assessment and treatment in the hypertensive patients: left ventricular hypertrophy. *J Am Soc Nephrol*. 2006;17:S104-S108.
39. Gottdiener JS, Bednarz J, Devereux R, et al. American Society of Echocardiography recommendations for use of echocardiography in clinical trials. *J Am Soc Echocardiogr*. 2004;17:1086-1119.
40. Tsang TS, Barnes ME, Gersh BJ, Bailey KR, Seward JB. Left atrial volume as a morphophysiologic expression of left ventricular diastolic dysfunction and relation to cardiovascular risk burden. *Am J Cardiol*. 2002;90:1284-1289.
41. Simek CL, Feldman MD, Haber HL, Wu CC, Jayaweera AR, Kaul S. Relationship between left ventricular wall thickness and left atrial size: comparison with other measures of diastolic function. *J Am Soc Echocardiogr*. 1995;8:37-47.
42. Abhayaratna WP, Seward JB, Appleton CP, et al. Left atrial size: physiologic determinants and clinical applications. *J Am Coll Cardiol*. 2006;47:2357-2363.
43. Benjamin EJ, D'Agostino RB, Belanger AJ, Wolf PA, Levy D. Left atrial size and the risk of stroke and death. The Framingham Heart Study. *Circulation*. 1995;92:835-841.
44. Bouzas-Mosquera A, Broullon FJ, Alvarez-Garcia N, et al. Left atrial size and risk for all-cause mortality and ischemic stroke. *CMAJ*. 2011;183:E657-E664.
45. Di Tullio MR, Sacco RL, Sciacca RR, Homma S. Left atrial size and the risk of ischemic stroke in an ethnically mixed population. *Stroke*. 1999;30:2019-2024.
46. Dini FL, Cortigiani L, Baldini U, et al. Prognostic value of left atrial enlargement in patients with idiopathic dilated cardiomyopathy and ischemic cardiomyopathy. *Am J Cardiol*. 2002;89:518-523.
47. Modena MG, Muia N, Sgura FA, Molinari R, Castella A, Rossi R. Left atrial size is the major predictor of cardiac death and overall clinical outcome in patients with dilated cardiomyopathy: a long-term follow-up study. *Clin Cardiol*. 1997;20:553-560.
48. Moller JE, Hillis GS, Oh JK, et al. Left atrial volume: a powerful predictor of survival after acute myocardial infarction. *Circulation*. 2003;107:2207-2212.
49. Nagarajarao HS, Penman AD, Taylor HA, et al. The predictive value of left atrial size for incident ischemic stroke and all-cause mortality in African Americans: the Atherosclerosis Risk in Communities (ARIC) Study. *Stroke*. 2008;39:2701-2706.
50. Ristow B, Ali S, Whooley MA, Schiller NB. Usefulness of left atrial volume index to predict heart failure hospitalization and mortality in ambulatory patients with coronary heart disease and comparison to left ventricular ejection fraction (from the Heart and Soul Study). *Am J Cardiol*. 2008;102:70-76.
51. Sabharwal N, Cemin R, Rajan K, Hickman M, Lahiri A, Senior R. Usefulness of left atrial volume as a predictor of mortality in patients with ischemic cardiomyopathy. *Am J Cardiol*. 2004;94:760-763.
52. Takemoto Y, Barnes ME, Seward JB, et al. Usefulness of left atrial volume in predicting first congestive heart failure in patients > or = 65 years of age with well-preserved left ventricular systolic function. *Am J Cardiol*. 2005;96:832-836.
53. Tsang TS, Barnes ME, Bailey KR, et al. Left atrial volume: important risk marker of incident atrial fibrillation in 1655 older men and women. *Mayo Clin Proc*. 2001;76:467-475.
54. Tsang TS, Barnes ME, Gersh BJ, Bailey KR, Seward JB. Risks for atrial fibrillation and congestive heart failure in patients >/=65 years of age with abnormal left ventricular diastolic relaxation. *Am J Cardiol*. 2004;93:54-58.
55. Block M, Hourigan L, Bellows WH, et al. Comparison of left atrial dimensions by transesophageal and transthoracic echocardiography. *J Am Soc Echocardiogr*. 2002;15:143-149.
56. Singh H, Jain AC, Bhumbla DK, Failinger C. Comparison of left atrial dimensions by transesophageal and transthoracic echocardiography. *Echocardiography*. 2005;22:789-796.
57. Eshoo S, Ross DL, Thomas L. Evaluation of left atrial size on transoesophageal echocardiography: what is the best measure? *Heart Lung Circ*. 2008;17:100-106.
58. Lester SJ, Ryan EW, Schiller NB, Foster E. Best method in clinical practice and in research studies to determine left atrial size. *Am J Cardiol*. 1999;84:829-832.
59. Loperfido F, Pennestri F, Digaetano A, et al. Assessment of left atrial dimensions by cross sectional echocardiography in patients with mitral valve disease. *Br Heart J*. 1983;50:570-578.
60. Pritchett AM, Jacobsen SJ, Mahoney DW, Rodeheffer RJ, Bailey KR, Redfield MM. Left atrial volume as an index of left atrial size: a population-based study. *J Am Coll Cardiol*. 2003;41:1036-1043.
61. Haddad F, Doyle R, Murphy DJ, Hunt SA. Right ventricular function in cardiovascular disease, part II: pathophysiology, clinical importance, and management of right ventricular failure. *Circulation*. 2008;117:1717-1731.
62. Haddad F, Hunt SA, Rosenthal DN, Murphy DJ. Right ventricular function in cardiovascular disease, part I: Anatomy, physiology, aging, and functional assessment of the right ventricle. *Circulation*. 2008;117:1436-1448.
63. de Groote P, Millaire A, Foucher-Hossein C, et al. Right ventricular ejection fraction is an independent predictor of survival in patients with moderate heart failure. *J Am Coll Cardiol*. 1998;32:948-954.
64. Meluzin J, Spinarova L, Hude P, et al. Combined right ventricular systolic and diastolic dysfunction represents a strong determinant of poor prognosis in patients with symptomatic heart failure. *Int J Cardiol*. 2005;105:164-173.
65. Meluzin J, Spinarova L, Hude P, et al. Prognostic importance of various echocardiographic right ventricular functional parameters in patients with symptomatic heart failure. *J Am Soc Echocardiogr*. 2005;18:435-444.
66. O'Rourke RA, Dell'Italia LJ. Diagnosis and management of right ventricular myocardial infarction. *Curr Probl Cardiol*. 2004;29:6-47.
67. Spinarova L, Meluzin J, Toman J, Hude P, Krejci J, Vitovec J. Right ventricular dysfunction in chronic heart failure patients. *Eur J Heart Fail*. 2005;7:485-489.
68. Wroblewski E, James F, Spann JF, Bove AA. Right ventricular performance in mitral stenosis. *Am J Cardiol*. 1981;47:51-55.
69. Wencker D, Borer JS, Hochreiter C, et al. Preoperative predictors of late postoperative outcome among patients with nonischemic mitral regurgitation with 'high risk' descriptors and comparison with unoperated patients. *Cardiology*. 2000;93:37-42.

70. Boldt J, Zickmann B, Ballesteros M, Dapper F, Hempelmann G. Right ventricular function in patients with aortic stenosis undergoing aortic valve replacement. *J Cardiothorac Vasc Anesth.* 1992;6:287-291.

71. Davlouros PA, Niwa K, Webb G, Gatzoulis MA. The right ventricle in congenital heart disease. *Heart.* 2006;92(suppl 1):i27-i38.

72. Chin KM, Kim NH, Rubin LJ. The right ventricle in pulmonary hypertension. *Coron Artery Dis.* 2005;16:13-18.

73. Marcus FI, McKenna WJ, Sherrill D, et al. Diagnosis of arrhythmogenic right ventricular cardiomyopathy/dysplasia: proposed modification of the task force criteria. *Circulation.* 2010;121:1533-1541.

74. MacNee W, Skwarski KM. Right-heat failure and cor pulmonale. In: Crawford MH, DiMarco JP, Paulus WJ, eds. *Cardiology.* 2nd ed. St Louis, Mo: Mosby; 2004:1017.

75. Rudski LG, Lai WW, Afilalo J, et al. Guidelines for the echocardiographic assessment of the right heart in adults: a report from the American Society of Echocardiography endorsed by the European Association of Echocardiography, a registered branch of the European Society of Cardiology, and the Canadian Society of Echocardiography*J Am Soc Echocardiogr.* 2010;23:685-713:quiz 786-8.

76. Roman MJ, Devereux RB, Kramer-Fox R, O'Loughlin J. Two-dimensional echocardiographic aortic root dimensions in normal children and adults. *Am J Cardiol.* 1989;64:507-512.

77. Shah MR, Hasselblad V, Stevenson LW, et al. Impact of the Pulmonary artery catheter in critically ill patients: meta-analysis of randomized clinical trials. *JAMA.* 2005;294:1664-1670.

78. Wheeler AP, Bernard GR, Thompson BT, et al. Pulmonary-artery versus central venous catheter to guide treatment of acute lung injury. *N Engl J Med.* 2006;354:2213-2224.

79. Shure D. Pulmonary-artery catheters–peace at last? *N Engl J Med.* 2006;354:2273-2274.

80. Quinones MA, Otto CM, Stoddard M, Waggoner A, Zoghbi WA. Recommendations for quantification of Doppler echocardiography: a report from the Doppler Quantification Task Force of the Nomenclature and Standards Committee of the American Society of Echocardiography. *J Am Soc Echocardiogr.* 2002;15:167-184.

81. Lewis JF, Kuo LC, Nelson JG, Limacher MC, Quinones MA. Pulsed Doppler echocardiographic determination of stroke volume and cardiac output: clinical validation of two new methods using the apical window. *Circulation.* 1984;70:425-431.

82. Enriquez-Sarano M, Bailey KR, Seward JB, Tajik AJ, Krohn MJ, Mays JM. Quantitative Doppler assessment of valvular regurgitation. *Circulation.* 1993;87:841-848.

Quantitative and Semiquantitative Echocardiography: Ventricular and Valvular Physiology

RENATA G. FERREIRA | MARY W. BRANDON | STEPHEN A. ESPER | MADHAV SWAMINATHAN

Introduction

After a slow start following its introduction in the 1970s,[1] transesophageal echocardiography (TEE) gradually joined mainstream echocardiography and became a staple in cardiac surgical operating rooms from the early 1990s onward.[2,3] With rapid developments in TEE over the last decade, it has become an indispensable intraoperative imaging tool. Its anatomic proximity to the heart and high-frequency transducer enable high-quality images and make TEE ideal for assessment of cardiac function. With the chest usually unavailable for scanning in the surgical setting, TEE becomes the imaging modality of choice. Both ventricles are well visualized in multiple views in the midesophageal (ME) and transgastric (TG) positions, allowing for a comprehensive assessment of structure and function in a quantitative and qualitative manner.

Quantitative echocardiography principally uses Doppler imaging modes to assess velocities. Pulsed wave Doppler (PWD) is ideal for laminar low-velocity flows at specific locations, and continuous wave Doppler (CWD) is used for measurement of high velocities that usually accompany turbulent flows involving valvular lesions. Ventricular pathophysiology can also be assessed by measurement of transvalvular diastolic flows that reflect filling pressures. Color flow Doppler (CFD) is primarily used to evaluate valvular lesions. In conjunction with two-dimensional (2D) echocardiography, Doppler modalities can enable a comprehensive assessment of ventricular and valvular physiology. Real-time three-dimensional (RT-3D) TEE has introduced another method of quantification of ventricular and valvular function that can potentially improve our current techniques.

Ventricular Function in Systole and Diastole

Background

Optimal myocardial performance includes the capacity of the ventricle to appropriately contract in systole and relax during diastole. At the molecular level, ventricular systolic contraction is initiated by an increase in the cytosolic levels of calcium and enhanced interaction between calcium ions and the contractile proteins actin and myosin.[4] During the diastolic period, levels of cytosolic calcium must fall, leading to the relaxation phase. A schematic view of the cardiac cycle is shown in Figure 12-1.

Numerous factors determine left ventricular (LV) myocardial performance. These include loading conditions, the contractile state, and the heart rate. *Preload* reflects the venous filling pressure that fills the left atrium (LA) and subsequently the LV. In response to an increase in the preload, the LV volume increases, stretching the ventricular myocardium, which leads to an increase in the force of contraction (Frank-Starling mechanism) with a resultant increase in stroke volume.[5] An increase in atrial volume stimulates the atrial mechanoreceptors, causing an increase in heart rate and cardiac output.

Interdependence of the LV and right ventricle (RV) is an important phenomenon that also influences myocardial function during the cardiac cycle.[6] Distention of one ventricle owing to increased filling pressures can directly limit diastolic filling of the other ventricle, partly because of pericardial restraint. This eventually results in impaired relaxation of the other ventricle.

Left Ventricular Systolic Function

Contraction Patterns and Pressure-Volume Relationships

Evaluation of systolic function is one of the most frequently performed indications for echocardiography. It is an important component of information gathered by the echocardiographer during the initial TEE examination in the perioperative period. Therefore, an understanding of the physiology of the cardiac cycle, especially pressure-volume relationships, is crucial when utilizing the different methods of assessing global ventricular function. The relationship between LA and LV pressure during each phase of the cardiac cycle is shown in Figure 12-2.

By convention, the mechanical cycle begins at the end of diastole. For the purposes of this discussion, systole can be considered in two phases: (1) isovolumetric contraction and (2) ejection. Diastole can be separated into four distinct phases: (1) isovolumetric relaxation, (2) early diastolic filling, (3) diastasis, and (4) atrial filling.

The period between mitral valve closure and aortic valve opening is defined as the *isovolumetric contraction time* (IVCT). It begins with activation of the actin-myosin complex, which results in a gradual increase in LV pressure triggered by the increased concentration of calcium ions in the cytosol and its interaction with the contractile proteins. Shortly thereafter, the intraventricular pressure exceeds the LA pressure, resulting in mitral valve closure. As the cardiac cycle progresses, an increasing number of myofibers contract and the LV pressure continues to increase. At a critical point, the LV pressure surpasses that in the ascending aorta, leading to opening of the aortic valve followed by the ejection phase.

During LV ejection, the intraventricular pressure rises to a peak and then starts to decline. This decline is a result of the decrease in the cytosolic calcium ion concentration due to uptake of calcium into the sarcoplasmic reticulum.[4] Therefore, an increasing number of myofibers enter a state of relaxation, with a consequent decrease in the rate of ejection of blood from the LV. At the end of LV ejection, the LV pressure falls below the aortic pressure, leading to aortic valve closure and the start of diastole.

The subsequent period, termed the *isovolumetric relaxation time* (IVRT), corresponds to the period in the cardiac cycle between aortic valve closure and mitral valve opening. At this time, LV pressure falls without a change in volume. The IVRT ends when LV pressure falls below LA pressure, leading to opening of the mitral valve. Conditions that delay relaxation of the LV will result in a prolonged IVRT, whereas conditions that increase LA pressure shorten the IVRT.

The subsequent phases correspond to mitral valve opening and early LV filling. As pressure in the atrium and ventricle equilibrates, LV filling ceases. Further filling of the LV is provided by contraction of the LA. At the end of atrial systole, mechanical events outlined previously lead to an increase in LV pressure that result in mitral valve closure and subsequent IVCT.

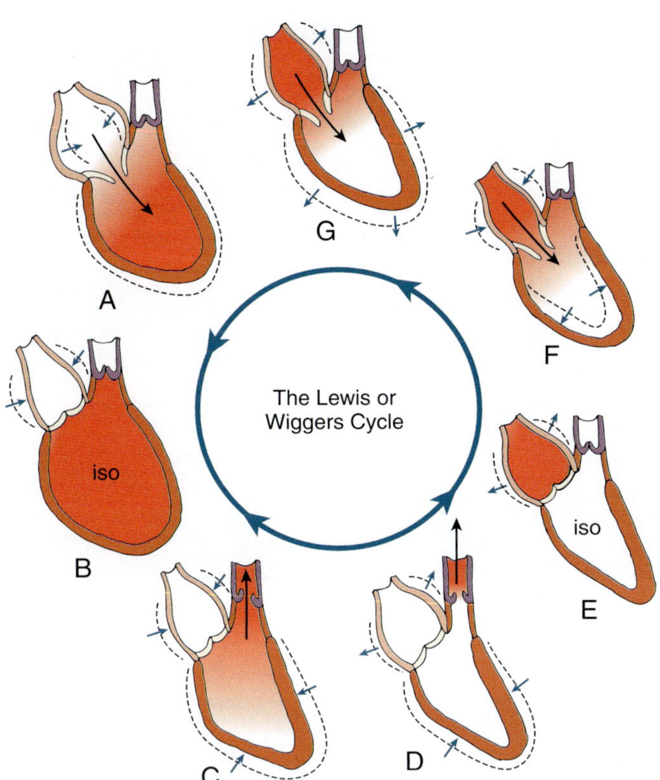

Figure 12-1   Visual phases of cardiac cycle. *iso*, Isovolumic. *(Adapted from Shepherd JT, Vanhoutte PM. The Human Cardiovascular System. New York: Raven Press; 1979:68.)*

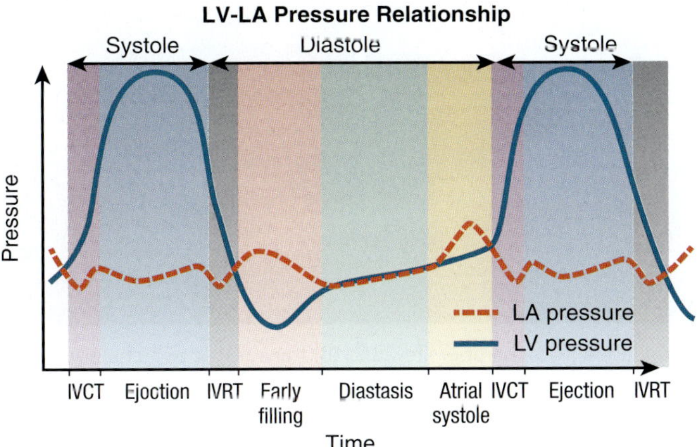

Figure 12-2   Relationship between left atrium and left ventricle throughout various phases of cardiac cycle. *IVCT,* Isovolumic contraction time; *IVRT,* isovolumic relaxation time; *LA,* left atrium; *LV,* left ventricle.

The pressure changes in the LA and LV profoundly affect the amount of volume the LV can accept in diastole and then eject in systole. Impairment of diastolic function can lead to a requirement of higher filling pressures to maintain a given volume of ejection. Similarly, impairment in systolic function directly affects the resulting stroke volume. The pressure-volume relationship of the LV is shown in Figure 12-3.

Chamber Dimensions

Initial quantification of myocardial performance includes measurements of LV dimensions and can be easily accomplished with 2D echocardiography. Gross examination of the LV with 2D echocardiography

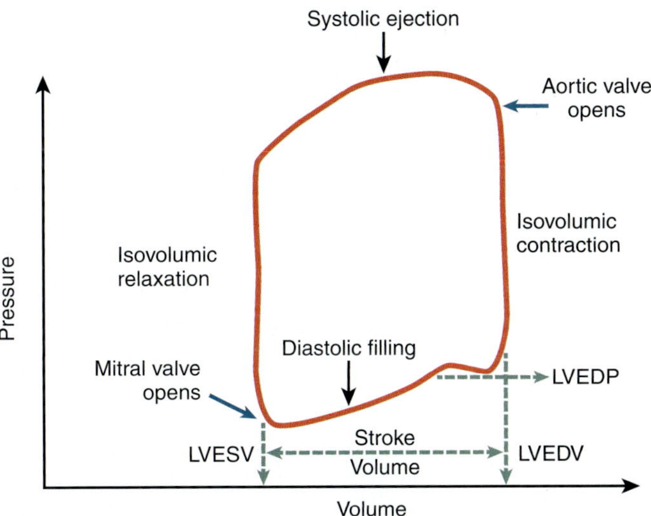

Figure 12-3   The left ventricular pressure-volume loop. *LVEDP,* Left ventricular end-diastolic pressure; *LVEDV,* left ventricular end-diastolic volume; *LVESV,* left ventricular end systolic volume.

will often provide clues to the underlying pathology. Wall thickness, septal hypertrophy, and a dilated or underfilled cavity are often seen with most TEE views of the LV. Measurements for LV chamber dimensions include wall thickness, internal (cavity) dimensions, and mass.

LV wall thickness can be quantified by obtaining linear measurements of the septal wall thickness (SWT) and posterior wall thickness (PWT) at end-diastole.[7] With TEE, these measurements may be made using M-mode or 2D imaging. The advantage of M-mode is its high temporal resolution, which helps distinctly identify end-diastole, whereas 2D imaging with its lower frame rate may miss the exact end-diastolic time point. However, this "inaccuracy" may be clinically insignificant. Conversely, accuracy in M-mode imaging can be limited by a tendency for the cursor to be misaligned with the correct axis of the ventricle, whereas 2D imaging overcomes the angle limitation. By convention, SWT and PWT are measured using the parasternal long-axis view in transthoracic imaging, which is suitable for both M-mode and 2D linear measurements (Fig. 12-4, *A*). With TEE, however, the TG mid–short-axis view enables SWT measurement at the midseptum and PWT at the inferolateral segment.[7] Neither positions in TEE imaging allow M-mode imaging to be used for accurate measurement (Fig. 12-4, *B*). It is important to exclude the papillary muscle in this view when measuring wall thickness.

Internal dimensions of the LV can be obtained from ME two-chamber and TG two-chamber views (Fig. 12-5). The internal LV diameter is measured from the anterior wall to the inferior wall at the junction of the basal and middle thirds of the long axis of the LV. Care must be taken to ensure that foreshortening of the LV is avoided in these views and the maximum obtainable diameter is measured.

Estimation of LV mass is less commonly used in clinical practice and more commonly with transthoracic echocardiography (TTE) in population studies that examine trends and cardiovascular responses to antihypertensive therapies. The formula for estimating LV mass is based on the prolate ellipsoid model and is the method recommended by the American Society of Echocardiography (ASE):[7]

$$\text{LV mass (grams)} = 0.8\{1.04[(\text{LVID} + \text{PWT} + \text{IVST})^3) - \text{LVID}^3]\} + 0.6$$

where *1.04* is the specific density of the myocardium, *LVID* is left ventricular internal diameter, *PWT* is posterior wall thickness, and *IVST* is interventricular septal thickness. The numbers *0.8* and *0.6* are correction factors.

As can be seen in this formula, errors in measurement have profound effects on the calculated LV mass, since critical measured values are cubed.

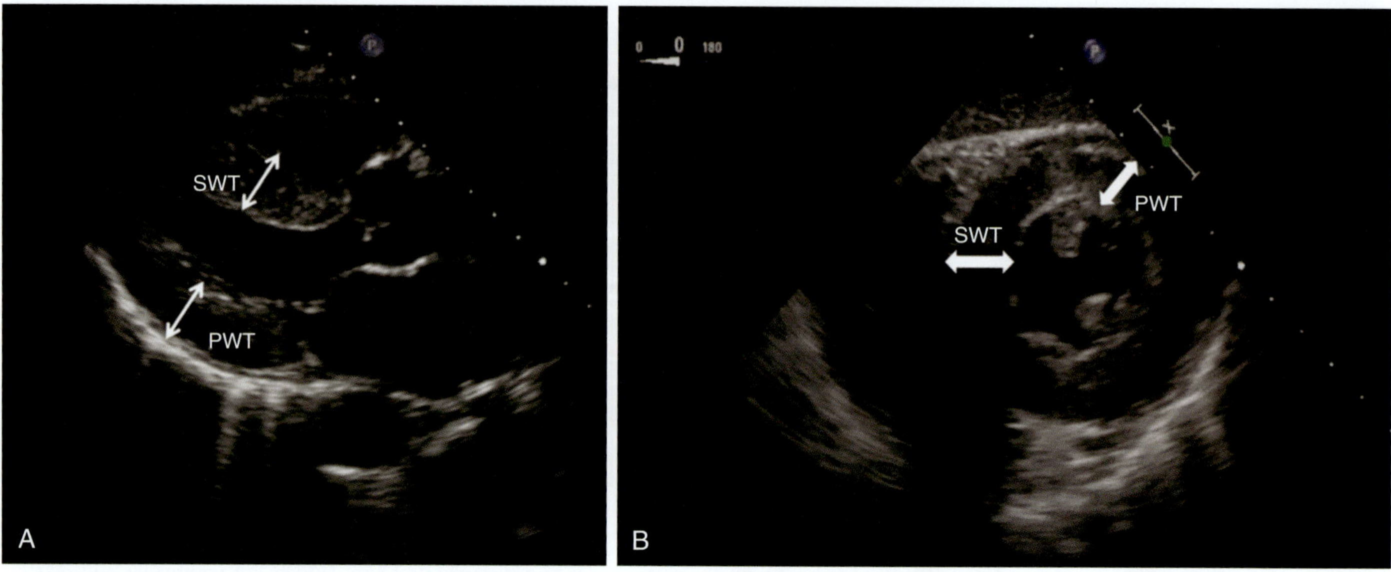

Figure 12-4 Measurement of left ventricular wall thickness with transthoracic **(A)** and transesophageal **(B)** echocardiography. See text for details. *PWT,* Posterior wall thickness; *SWT,* septal wall thickness.

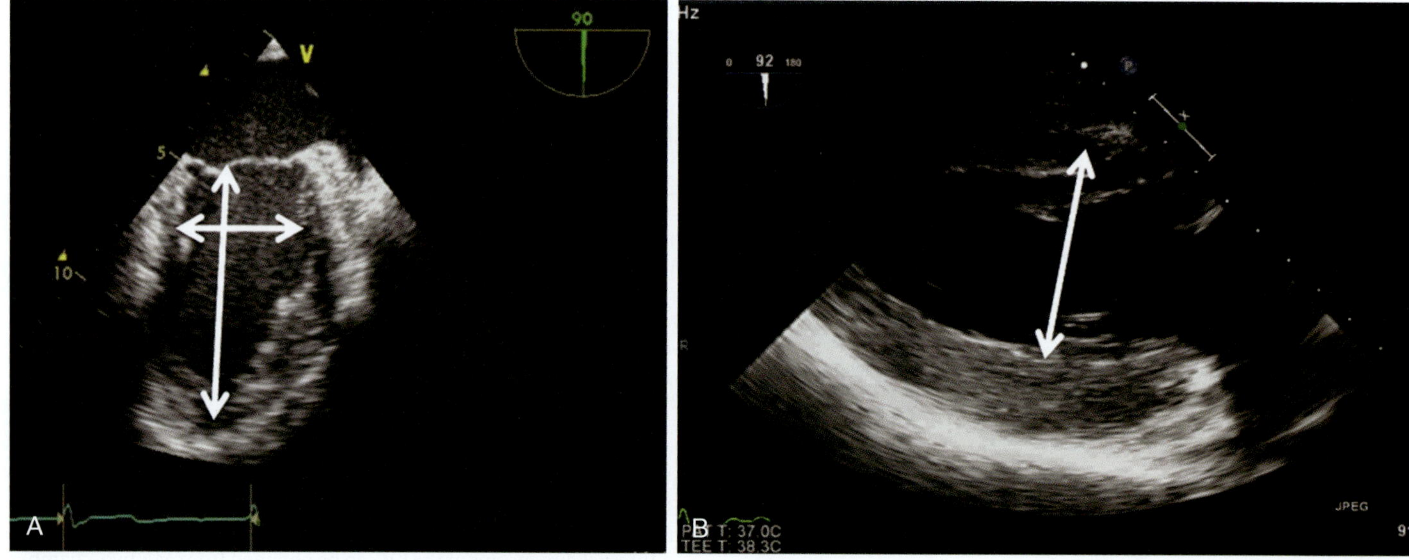

Figure 12-5 Measurement of left ventricular internal dimensions in **(A)** midesophageal two-chamber view and **(B)** transgastric two-chamber view.

Volumetric Parameters

Estimation of LV volumes is common in both clinical practice and research. Echocardiography provides quantitative and qualitative measurement of systolic function by estimating global and regional ventricular function and measuring ventricular volumes and ejection fraction. The ventricular volume measurement can be considered one of the most important components of assessing cardiac function.

Precise evaluation of LV global systolic function can be challenging in the perioperative setting, owing to fluctuations in intracavitary volume due to changes in sympathetic tone, preload, and afterload. The echocardiographer may need to use multiple methods of LV volume estimation to ensure accuracy in measurement. Since its introduction, TEE has undergone continual improvement in imaging quality. Consequently, there are numerous techniques that may be used to assess LV volumes, from M-mode to 3D imaging.

To obtain volumetric measurements, the most important views for 2D quantitation are the midpapillary short-axis view and the apical four- and two-chamber views. Volumetric measurements require manual tracing of the endocardial border. Accurate measurements require optimal visualization of the endocardial border to minimize the need for extrapolation. It is recommended that the basal border of the LV cavity area be delineated by a straight line connecting the mitral valve insertions at the lateral and septal borders of the annulus on the four-chamber view and the anterior and inferior annular borders on the two-chamber view.[7]

The Simpson and area-length methods are the most common quantification techniques using 2D imaging, whereas 3D echocardiography relies on proprietary software for semiautomated volumetric calculations.

Simpson Method

One of the most commonly used methods for LV volume estimation is the biplane method of disks that follows the modified Simpson rule. While it makes some geometric assumptions about the shape of the LV, it remains the method of choice recommended by the ASE.[7]

The Simpson rule states that volume can be calculated by dividing a 3D object into slices of known thickness and surface area. The volume of the object is equal to the sum of the volumes of each slice. It divides

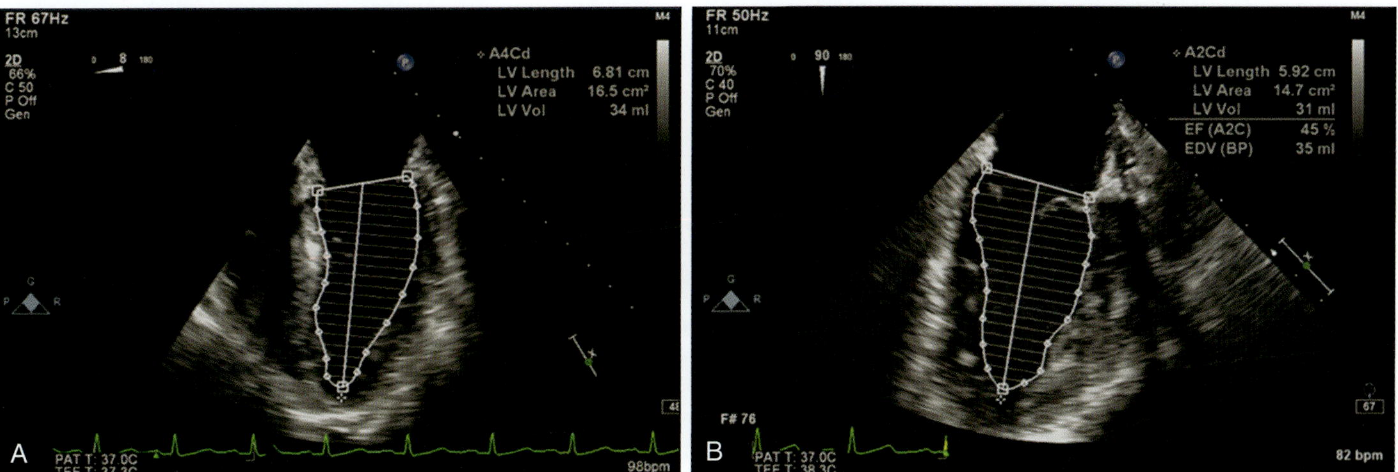

Figure 12-6 Assessment of left ventricular (LV) volume using the Simpson method of disks. **A,** LV endocardium traced in end-diastole in mid-esophageal (ME) four-chamber view. LV area, length, and volume are automated calculations. **B,** Similar tracing in ME two-chamber view. These measurements are repeated in each view in end-systolic frames (not shown). End-diastolic and end-systolic volumes are averaged from both views and ejection fraction automatically calculated.

the ventricular cavity into multiple cylindrical slices (disks) of known volume, with the sum representing LV volume. The height of each disk is calculated as a fraction (usually 1/20) of the LV long axis based on the longer of the two lengths from the two- and four-chamber views. The cross-sectional area of the disk is based on the two diameters obtained from the two- and four-chamber views:

$$V = (\pi \times D_1/2 \times D_2/2)\ H$$

where D_1 and D_2 are orthogonal diameters of the cylinder and H is the longer of the two lengths from the two- and four-chamber views. The volume of the cylinders are calculated and summed to estimate ventricular volume. Most new models of echocardiography machines calculate the end-diastolic and end-systolic volumes and ejection fraction automatically after the echocardiographer traces the endocardium in specified views (Fig. 12-6, Video 12-1).

For practicality, papillary muscles should be excluded from the endocardial border tracings. Accurate measurements require optimal visualization of the endocardial border to minimize the need for extrapolation. It is recommended that the basal border of the LV cavity area be delineated by a straight line connecting the mitral valve insertions at the lateral and septal borders of the annulus in the four-chamber view and the anterior and inferior annular borders on the two-chamber view.

Although quite accurate in ventricular volume estimations, this method of volume analysis is limited by the degree of foreshortening of the ventricular cavity in the four-chamber view, which is common with TEE, leading to underestimation of LV volume. The presence of echo dropout can also compromise accuracy.

Area-Length Method

An alternative method to calculate LV volumes when the lack of endocardial definition precludes accurate tracing is the area-length method, where the LV is assumed to be "bullet" shaped. The area-length method uses the short-axis area of the LV (from the TG mid–short-axis view) and the length of the LV long axis (from the ME four-chamber view) to calculate volume. This method assumes an elliptical shape of the LV, with uniform contraction from base to apex. The measurements are repeated at end-diastole and end-systole, and the volume is computed according to the formula:

$$V = [5\ (\text{area})\ (\text{length})]/6$$

where V is the volume and *area* and *length* are as defined in the text.

As in the Simpson method of disks, papillary muscles should be excluded in the linear measurements. While reasonably accurate, there

are certain limitations. The method assumes that the LV is elliptical in shape. Therefore, it should not be the method of choice in conditions where the shape of the LV is distorted, such as asymmetric septal hypertrophy, LV aneurysm, and dilated cardiomyopathy.[7]

Three-Dimensional Assessment

Although the concept of 3D echocardiography was first introduced in the early 1970s, its utility in the perioperative environment has only recently acquired appropriate recognition. With the availability of RT-3D TEE, volumetric assessment of the LV can be done relatively quickly, with accuracy comparable to the best quantification techniques available.[8]

Optimization of the 2D images before acquiring the full-volume dataset with 3D imaging is crucial. Endocardial borders should be well visualized with 2D echo. Following acquisition of the 3D (raw) data, calculation of LV volumes and mass requires identification of endocardial borders using manual or semiautomated algorithms. These borders are then processed to calculate the cavity or myocardial volume by summation of disks.

The ability to track the endocardium in three dimensions rather than two (as in the Simpson method of disks) makes 3D more suitable when geometric assumptions of LV shape cannot be met, as in LV aneurysms, regional infarction, and dilated cardiomyopathies. The rotate and crop features of 3D imaging without any directional restriction enables an infinite number of viewing perspectives of cardiac infrastructure and is a significant advantage over 2D imaging (Fig. 12-7).[8]

There is considerable enthusiasm pertaining to the utility of 3D TEE technology, but it is important to emphasize that currently, full ventricular volumes are too large to be captured in truly real-time display with the appropriate frame rate or temporal resolution.[8] It requires some degree of reconstruction from sequentially acquired smaller "live" datasets. This technology still relies on stable cardiac rhythms and respiratory and electrocardiographic gating to avoid "stitch" artifacts (Fig. 12-8, Video 12-2). Additionally, the time and expertise required for full-volume acquisition, reconstruction, and "editing" may be challenging in the perioperative setting.[9]

Ejection Phase Parameters

Evaluation of LV systolic function is, in general, dependent on the echocardiographer's ability and trained capacity to interpret data. Visual estimates of ejection fraction are immediately available but less reliable than quantitative methods and insensitive to subtle changes in function.

Initial attempts to assess LV systolic function involved only linear measurements, such as the LV internal dimension in diastole and

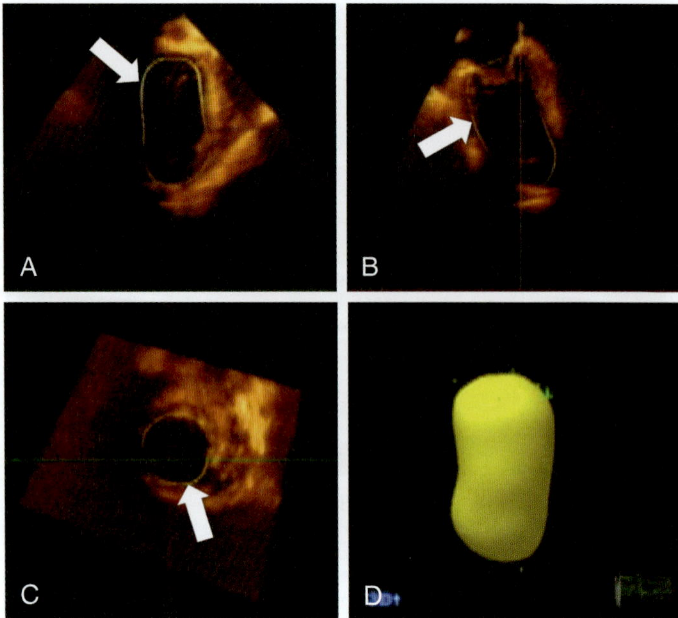

Figure 12-7 Assessment of left ventricular volumes using three-dimensional echocardiography. Following acquisition of full-volume dataset, specific endocardial points are marked on end-systolic and end-diastolic frames, and software automatically tracks endocardial borders on each frame through one cardiac cycle. Borders can be manually adjusted and can be verified in each orthogonal plane *(arrows in A, B, and C)*. Developed volumetric model is shown in **D**.

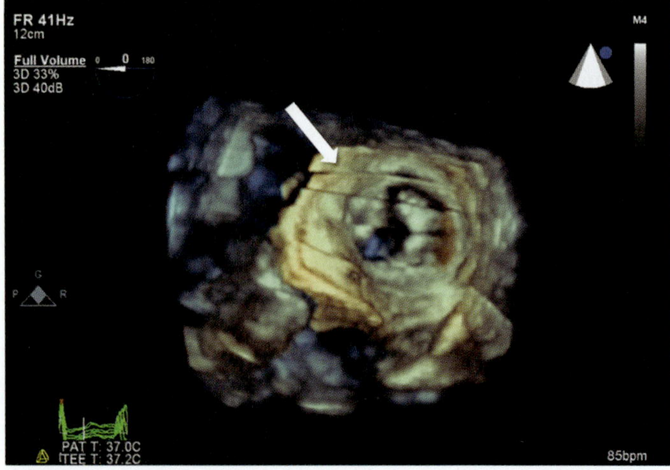

Figure 12-8 "Stitch" artifact *(arrow)* in full-volume dataset created due to unstable cardiac rhythm, translational motion (e.g., due to respiration), or both, leading to inaccurate synchronization of smaller sequential volume datasets.

systole, from which parameters such as fractional shortening and velocity of circumferential shortening could be derived. In the presence of normal ventricular geometry and symmetric function, linear measurements from M-mode and 2D images provide reasonable assessment of ventricular function. They have also proven to be fairly reproducible, with low intraobserver and interobserver variability.[10-12] However, linear measurements have the disadvantage of being able to determine ventricular function only along a single interrogation line.

With the advent of 2D echocardiography, area and volume calculations replaced linear measurements for assessment of LV function. In addition, Doppler echocardiography provides information on systolic flow, which supplements 2D-based measurements, while tissue Doppler and speckle tracking techniques allow a more detailed analysis of myocardial performance.

Fractional Shortening

Although linear measures of LV function are considered inaccurate in the presence of regional abnormalities, patients with uncomplicated hypertension, obesity, or valvular diseases, rarely show regional variation in the absence of clinically recognized infarction. Therefore, fractional shortening (FS) and its relationship to end-systolic stress often provides useful information in the clinical setting. The lower limit of normal is 25% in men and 27% in women.[7]

The formula for fractional shortening is based on M-mode measurements:

$$\mathrm{FS}\,(\%) = [(\mathrm{LVID_d} - \mathrm{LVID_s})/\mathrm{LVID_d}] \times 100$$

where $LVID_d$ is left ventricular internal dimension in diastole and $LVID_s$ is left ventricular internal dimension in systole.

Velocity of Circumferential Fiber Shortening

This is a variant of fractional shortening that takes the ejection time into consideration. Ejection time is measured using M-mode of the aortic valve opening in the ME aortic valve long-axis view or with spectral Doppler of transaortic valve flow in the deep TG long-axis view. Similar to fractional shortening, it is also sensitive to preload and is rarely used in the clinical setting. The lower limit of normal is 1.1 circumferences per second.

The formula for velocity of circumferential fiber shortening (VCFS) is:

$$\mathrm{VCFS} = \text{Fractional shortening} \times \text{Ejection time}$$

Fractional Area Change

Fractional area change (FAC) is frequently used as a surrogate for LV ejection fraction. It measures the percentage of change in area of the ventricular dimension as an estimate of LV contractile performance. The FAC is usually obtained in the TG midpapillary view. Several studies have shown good correlation of FAC and other methods of quantifying ejection fraction, such as angiography and scintigraphy.[13,14] However, it is also limited in accuracy in the presence of regional wall motion abnormalities and is more sensitive to changes in afterload than preload.

The formula for fractional area change (FAC) is:

$$\mathrm{FAC}\,(\%) = [(\mathrm{LV_{EDA}} - \mathrm{LV_{ESA}})/\mathrm{LV_{EDA}}] \times 100$$

where LV_{EDA} is left ventricular area at end-diastole and LV_{ESA} is left ventricular area at end-systole.

Ejection Fraction

Ventricular function is most commonly characterized using ejection fraction. Assessment of ejection fraction can be made with a simple visual estimate or with detailed volumetric measurements using 2D and 3D echocardiography. In TEE, TG images are used to determine ventricular volumes in diastole and systole, from which stroke volume and ejection fraction values are calculated. Several geometric assumptions and formulae have been used to estimate ventricular volumes. The advantage of geometric assumption techniques is that they require only limited visualization for calculation of volume. However, a limitation is that these formulae work only in a symmetrically contracting ventricle and have been supplanted by more direct calculation of ventricular volumes. A simplified method for calculation of ejection fraction involves determining the minor axis dimension in diastole and systole at the base, mid-, and distal LV. These values are combined with a qualitative assessment of apical function (−5% to +15%) to derive the ejection fraction. This methodology has correlated well with standard methods for determination of the ejection fraction.

The formula for ejection fraction (EF) is:

$$\mathrm{EF}\% = [(\mathrm{LV_{EDV}} - \mathrm{LV_{ESV}})/\mathrm{LV_{EDV}}] \times 100$$

where LV_{EDV} is left ventricular volume at end-diastole and LV_{SDV} is left ventricular volume at end-systole.

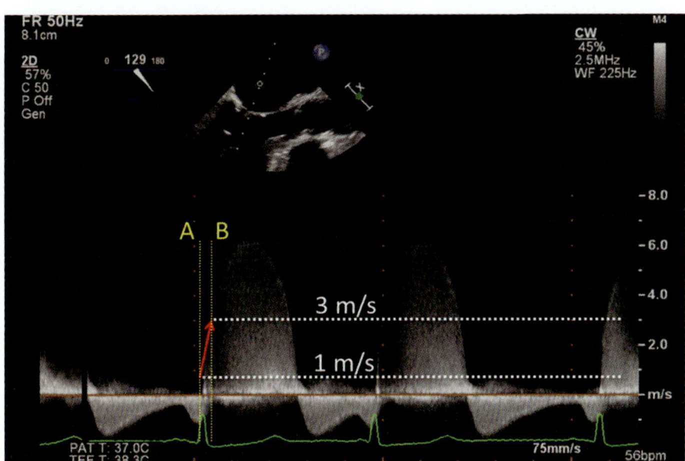

Figure 12-9 Continuous wave spectral Doppler recording of mitral regurgitation jet. Time taken for velocity to rise from *A* (1 m/s) to *B* (3 m/s) is measured to reflect dP/dt. (See text for details.)

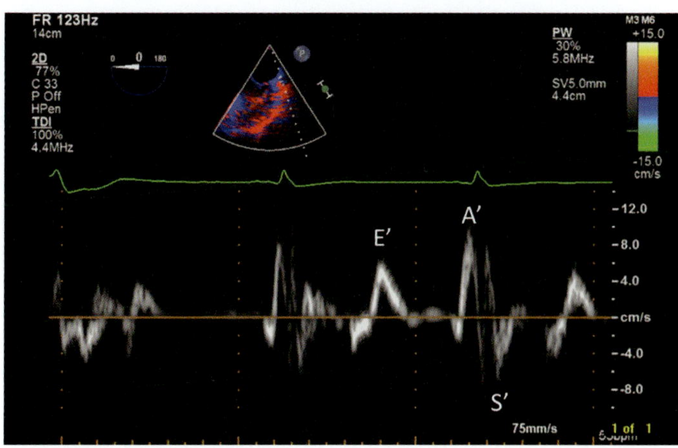

Figure 12-10 Tissue velocities at lateral mitral annulus measured using tissue Doppler imaging. E′ wave indicates tissue motion in early diastole; A′ wave corresponds to atrial contraction; S′ indicates systolic descent of annulus.

Three-dimensional echocardiography is now also widely used for volumetric assessment of the LV. As mentioned previously, acquisition of a full-volume dataset allows the system to use semiautomated methods to track the endocardial border throughout a single cardiac cycle and calculate dynamic volume changes in systole and diastole. This technique does not require geometric assumptions and is sensitive to regional abnormalities in wall motion or asymmetric contraction. However, acquisition of a satisfactory full-volume dataset is also dependent on a stable heart rhythm and absence of translational motion over a sequence of several cardiac cycles (see Video 12-3).[8]

Assessment of Contractility
Isovolumetric Indicators
The rate of rise in ventricular pressure during systole that begins in the isovolumetric contraction phase is a more load-independent indicator of LV systolic function. This parameter is better known as *dP/dt*, and Doppler-derived measurements correlate well with catheter-based invasive measurements. With echocardiography, the measurement of dP/dt is dependent on a mitral regurgitation (MR) jet. The contour of the MR jet reflects the rate of rise of LV systolic pressure until its eventual peak velocity. The time the jet velocity takes to rise from 1 m/s to 3 m/s is considered to indicate the dP/dt (Fig. 12-9). Since it is dependent on an MR jet and the stroke volume, this parameter is also preload sensitive. The corresponding pressure gradient at 1 and 3 m/s is 4 mmHg and 36 mmHg, calculated by the simplified Bernoulli equation [pressure gradient = 4 × (peak velocity)^2]. Therefore, the time taken for the pressure gradient to rise by 32 mmHg reflects the dP/dt according to the formula:

$$dP/dt = 32 \ (mmHg) \times 1000/dT \ (milliseconds)$$

Normal values for this parameter are 1610 ± 290 mmHg/s.[15]

Wall Stress
Ventricular wall stress is another parameter used to assess LV function. Unlike other clinical parameters, such as stroke volume and ejection fraction, wall stress is an index of LV performance that is considered afterload independent, since it accounts for both wall thickness and pressure generation. Wall stress can be calculated either regionally or globally using one of three methods: meridional (longitudinal), circumferential, or radial. In the perioperative period, calculation of stress, either regional or global, has had little utility and acceptance. Calculation of stress indexed to ventricular volume has been used as an index of ventricular performance in valvular heart disease and cardiomyopathy.[16]

Tissue Characterization
For several years, 2D imaging and spectral Doppler analysis were the only methods available for quantification of LV function. More recently, advances in ultrasound technology have enabled more objective and accurate quantification of global and regional ventricular function. Improvements in temporal and spatial resolution allow examination of myocardial structure almost at the level of individual fibers and have provided new insights into the organization and function of the ventricle.[17] While these techniques have been developed and more extensively studied in TTE, increasing use of these tools in TEE is being reported.[18,19]

The following text will discuss the methods of tissue characterization that examine Doppler and 2D signals from the myocardium, allowing the measurement of tissue velocity, strain, twist, and synchrony.

Tissue Velocity
Tissue velocity information can provide early clues to alterations in regional and global LV contractility.[20] Unlike conventional Doppler flow signals that are characterized by high velocity and low amplitude, myocardial motion signals are described as relatively low velocity and high amplitude. Tissue Doppler imaging (TDI) is now available on most ultrasound systems and can be used with TEE imaging as well (see Video 12-3). Current systems that feature TDI have built-in settings for the proper velocity scale and Doppler settings to selectively display the tissue velocities and filter flow signals.

Typically, pulsed Doppler sampling is performed in the lateral and septal wall region of the LV adjacent to the mitral annulus. As with any Doppler modality, the angle of insonation is critical, and minimal angulation (<20 degrees) should be present between the ultrasound beam and the plane of cardiac motion for more precise velocity values. It is important to optimize the frame rate using an image sector as narrow as possible.

According to the Doppler principle, tissue velocities moving toward the transducer are positive, whereas velocities moving away from the transducer are negative (Fig. 12-10). Three distinct velocity signals can be appreciated: peak systolic (S′), peak early diastolic (E′), and late diastolic (A′). The S′ velocity is a quick and reasonable means of estimating LV ejection fraction, and several studies have closely related S′ and LV ejection fraction. However, there are limited data in patients undergoing general anesthesia. Another modality of tissue Doppler is color TDI, where red encodes wall motion toward the transducer (positive velocities), and blue encodes wall motion away from the transducer (negative velocities). On either side of the scale, the brightest shades correspond to the highest velocities (Fig. 12-11).

Ventricular Strain

Ventricular strain refers to the degree of deformation of a segment of myocardium as a result of its pattern of contraction. It is a dimensionless index and is measured according to a formula that accounts for the distance between two specified points in the myocardium and the change in their relative distance from each other through a single cardiac cycle (Fig. 12-12).[21] Ventricular strain is defined by the formula:

$$Strain = (L_0 - L_1)/L_0$$

where L_0 is initial length (distance) and L_1 is final length (distance). Therefore, *lengthening* is defined as a negative strain, whereas *shortening* is defined as a positive strain. The rate of change in strain is the strain rate, or:

$$Strain\ rate\ (SR) = Strain/dT$$

$$dT = duration\ of\ strain\ (seconds)$$

Although 2D echo can provide spatial and temporal information for the myocardium, measurement of the distance between two points in real time is extremely difficult. With Doppler, however, velocities can be measured between two points in real time, and distance information can be extrapolated to reveal strain. This technique is known as *Doppler strain* and is limited by the usual constraints of Doppler imaging such as angle of interrogation.

Another technique for strain measurements that overcomes the angle limitations of Doppler strain is 2D strain. Points in the myocardium are identified by their unique signatures as ultrasound reflectors. The received signal is assigned a property by which the point (or speckle) can be tracked throughout the cardiac cycle until its return to baseline position (or coordinates). Tracking these speckles in real time can simultaneously reveal distance and velocity information along several points in the myocardium. It overcomes Doppler limitations and is the preferred technique for strain measurements (Fig. 12-13, Video 12-5).[21]

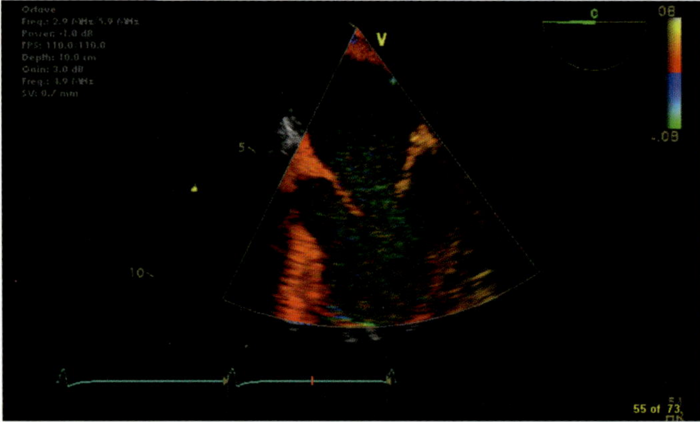

Figure 12-11   Tissue Doppler imaging using color Doppler information. Tissue velocities are color coded according to displayed scale.

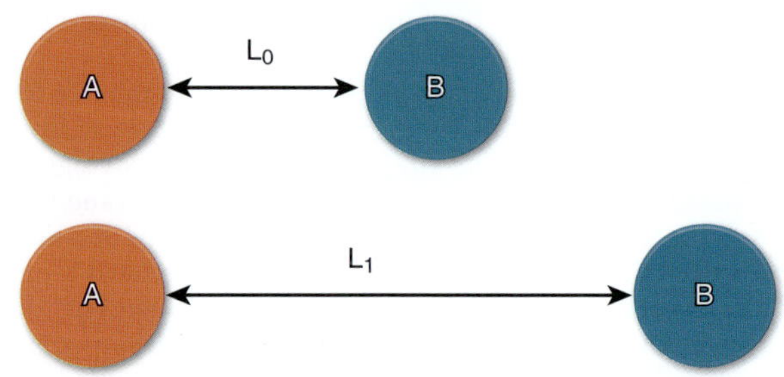

Figure 12-12   Ventricular strain. Points *A* and *B* are shown with relative distances between them before (at rest) and at peak systole. *L₀,* Initial distance; *L₁,* final distance.

Twist

One of the advantages of measuring tissue motion in real time is the ability to quantify circumferential rotation of the ventricle along its longitudinal axis. This rotation occurs in opposing directions at the base and apex, with the middle regions offering little rotation if any. The difference between the base-to-apex rotation can also be quantified as twist or torsion and is relatively independent of loading conditions.[22] It appears to be affected early in the course of ischemia and is also valuable in patients with valve disease, where preload is variable.

Synchrony

Optimal LV function depends on synchronous contraction of the entire ventricle. Premature activation results in areas of early and late contraction that lead to ineffective work. The net result will be an increase in end-systolic volume and a decrease in stroke volume and LV performance. Doppler and 2D techniques can both be used to determine regional differences in time to peak systolic indices. However, Doppler imaging is limited by alignment of angle of interrogation, and 2D imaging may not simultaneously image segments in which dyssynchrony is suspected—limitations that are overcome with 3D synchrony imaging.

Analysis of synchrony can be done by measuring peak systolic velocities and relating the timing of peak velocity to electrical activation of the ventricle (QRS complex). Significantly different time to peak velocity between segments will provide information on electromechanical coupling and intraventricular dyssynchrony.[23]

Left Ventricular Diastolic Function

The importance of diastolic function to LV performance has been known for a long time.[24] The assessment of diastolic function, however, has been limited to surrogate measures of LV filling pressures with both catheter- and Doppler-based techniques. With the recognition that impaired diastolic function may be responsible for a large fraction of heart failure with preserved ejection fraction, identification of diastolic dysfunction has received renewed attention.[25]

Pattern of Relaxation and Phases of Diastole

Diastole is a complex sequence of interrelated events. The two major determinants of LV filling are ventricular relaxation and chamber compliance. Ventricular relaxation is a complex energy-requiring process during which the contractile elements are deactivated and the

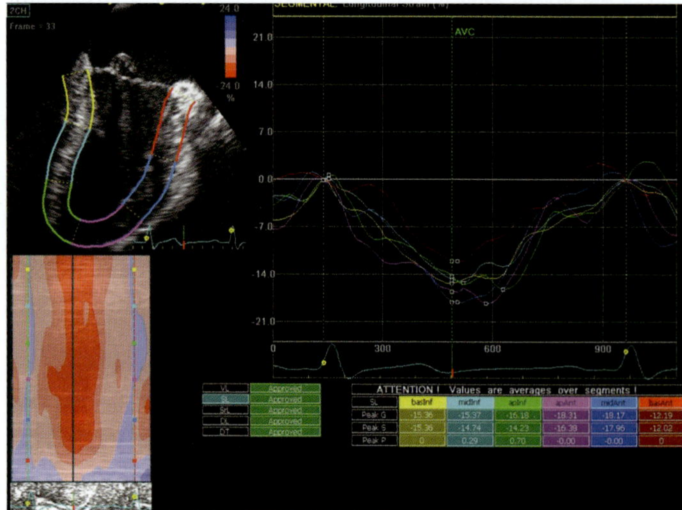

Figure 12-13   Ventricular strain measured using two-dimensional strain. Once myocardium is identified, automated algorithm tracks motion of myocardial reflectors throughout cardiac cycle and calculates strain in various dimensions. Calculation of longitudinal strain is shown here in midesophageal two-chamber view.

myofibrils return to their original (precontraction) length. In a normal heart, ventricular relaxation begins during midsystole and continues throughout the first third of diastolic filling.

There are numerous descriptions of phases of diastole, but they essentially divide diastole into the isovolumetric and filling phases (see Fig. 12-2). The *isovolumetric phase* is characterized by a rapid decline in intraventricular pressure following closure of the aortic valve and results from the decoupling of contractile elements within the myocardium. This phase best represents the ability of the ventricle to relax efficiently, since it receives no volume from any other chamber under normal conditions. The *filling phase* is further divided into *early rapid filling, diastasis,* and *atrial contraction.* The early filling phase begins with the opening of the mitral valve when LV pressure falls below LA pressure. Following rapid filling, the ventricle is quiescent for a period, when there is no flow (diastasis). This is followed by a sudden increase in LA pressure from atrial systole that allows a terminal increase in LV filling in late diastole. Since the LV is already partially full by this time, further filling by atrial contraction will depend on structural compliance of the LV or any external restraint to filling.

Each phase has factors that determine how the ventricle fills during this time. The isovolumetric phase depends on continuity with systole, energy available for initiating relaxation, and LA pressure. Early filling reflects LA-to-LV pressure gradient, LA volume, and elastic recoil. The period of diastasis is most affected by heart rate and rhythm. Tachycardia decreases diastolic time and principally affects diastasis, whereas a prolonged PR interval also shortens diastasis. Atrial compliance, LV compliance/stiffness, and pericardial constraint are the principal determinants of how the LV will fill in late diastole.

Pressure-Volume Relationships in Diastole

The pressure-volume relationships of the LV during the cardiac cycle were described earlier (also see Fig. 12-3). The amount of volume the LV can accept in diastole depends on LA pressure and LV compliance. LA pressure will drive the volume into the LV, but LV compliance will determine the pressure at which the volume may be accepted. As LV compliance decreases and stiffness increases, the chamber pressure for a given amount of volume also increases (see Fig. 12-3), leading to an increase in left ventricular end-diastolic pressure (LVEDP). Therefore, progressive diastolic dysfunction is characterized by LV stiffness and an increase in LA pressure and LVEDP. It should be noted that *any* pericardial constraint will result in the same effects on LVEDP.

Two-Dimensional Assessment of Diastolic Function

Diastolic dysfunction principally remains an echocardiographic diagnosis, but 2D echo can provide important clues to diastolic performance. LV wall thickness, pericardial restraint, and LA size are all indicators of diastolic function.

Although not uncommon in patients with normal LV wall thickness, hypertrophy is an important determinant of diastolic function and is a common finding.[26] The widespread prevalence of hypertension, especially in the elderly, leads to LV hypertrophy and hypertensive heart disease as a common feature of diastolic heart failure.[27] A simple visual assessment of LV relaxation with 2D imaging can provide clues as to whether the ventricle is hypertrophied, stiff, or restrained. LV wall thickness may also be measured using conventional 2D or M-mode techniques.

Diastolic filling of the LV is also dependent on external constraint. Pericardial pathology will significantly influence the capacity of the LV to achieve complete relaxation and accommodate diastolic volume. Pericardial thickening, tamponade, effusions, and inflammation may all interfere with diastolic filling. Pericarditis itself may be difficult to assess with 2D echo, but thickening, effusions, and tamponade are simpler to diagnose.

LA size and function may be the most important indicators of long-term diastolic dysfunction in the presence of a normally functioning mitral valve.[25,28] Any impairment in diastolic function leads to elevation of LA pressures as an adaptation to increased pressure requirements to fill the LV. A chronic increase in LA pressure leads to LA enlargement,

and the presence of an enlarged LA in the absence of mitral valve disease should immediately alert the echocardiographer to suspect significantly impaired diastolic function.

Doppler Assessment

Although 2D echo can provide clues to underlying diastolic function, Doppler imaging provides definitive evidence of dysfunction and helps classify its severity. The principal Doppler-based techniques are PWD of transmitral and pulmonary venous flow and TDI of the lateral mitral annulus. Other techniques such as flow propagation velocity may also be used to quantify diastolic function.[28]

Transmitral Flow

Primary measurements of transmitral inflow include the peak early filling (E wave) and late diastolic filling (A wave) velocities, the E/A ratio, and deceleration time (DT) of the E wave (Fig. 12-14). Secondary measurements include mitral A-wave duration and isovolumetric relaxation time (IVRT), derived using CWD of the left ventricular outflow tract (LVOT) to measure the interval between the end of aortic ejection and the onset of mitral inflow.

The E wave reflects the LA pressure in early diastole and occurs immediately following the IVRT and mitral valve opening. The DT of the E wave is affected by the rate of rise in LV diastolic pressure as a result of early filling. In settings of restrictive diastolic dysfunction, athlete's heart, and pericardial constraint, the early filling shows rapid cessation of flow due either to rapidly rising pressure in the LV or rapid emptying of the LA into a highly compliant LV. The A-wave velocity is affected by LA pressure and LV compliance at the end of diastole. In stiff ventricles, the A wave is smaller and also of shorter duration.

Age is a primary consideration when defining normal values of mitral inflow velocities and time intervals.[28] With increasing age, the mitral E velocity and E/A ratio decrease, whereas DT and A velocity increase. A number of variables other than LV diastolic function and filling pressures affect mitral inflow, including heart rate and rhythm, PR interval, cardiac output, mitral annular size, and LA function. Age-related changes in diastolic function parameters may represent a slowing of myocardial relaxation, which predisposes older individuals to the development of diastolic heart failure.[25]

Transmitral flow patterns have a U-shaped relation with LV diastolic function, with similar values seen in healthy normal subjects and patients with cardiac disease.[29] Sinus tachycardia and first-degree atrioventricular (AV) block can result in partial or complete fusion of the mitral E and A waves. Atrial fibrillation represents a challenge because of variability in LA volume filling the LV. Mechanical ventilation also

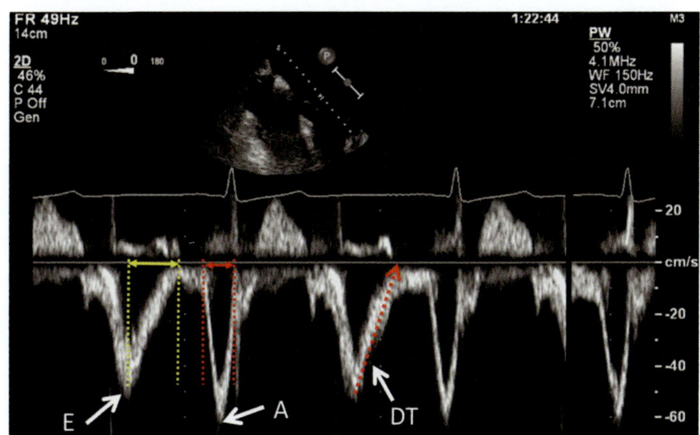

Figure 12-14 Pulsed wave Doppler of transmitral flow. Velocity tracing shows typical diastolic flow pattern. Early filling is measured by peak E-wave velocity (*E*); atrial contribution in late systole is measured by peak A-wave velocity (*A*); E wave deceleration time is shown by yellow double-headed arrow; A wave duration is indicated by red double-headed arrow. Deceleration time (*DT*) is also indicated on adjacent cardiac cycle.

alters loading conditions and can affect flow patterns. Even in healthy subjects, clinical scenarios very common in the perioperative setting (e.g., hypovolemia or a subtle increase in afterload) can mimic pathologic patterns of mitral inflow. Mitral valve diseases will interfere with the analysis in different ways; MR results in an E-dominant trace, but mitral stenosis will reflect flow across the stenosis rather than any intrinsic diastolic function.[28]

Pulmonary Venous Flow

Pulmonary vein flow, when added to the mitral inflow velocity, is very helpful in the assessment of diastolic function. There are two systolic velocities (S_1 and S_2) and two diastolic velocities (D in early diastole and atrial reversal flow [Ar] in late diastole), the latter being a result of atrial contraction. The systolic part often has a biphasic pattern, but the distinction might not be evident in some patients (Fig. 12-15).

The systolic components of pulmonary vein flow are as follows: S_1 (early systole) is a result of atrial relaxation and the subsequent fall in LA pressure. The decreased pressure in the atrial chamber will lead to forward flow from the pulmonary vein into the LA. The S_2 wave is a result of a further decrease in LA pressure, this time caused by the descent of the base of the LV during contraction.

The diastolic components of pulmonary vein flow are as follows: peak diastolic velocity represents the pulmonary vein forward flow during diastole and therefore occurs after mitral valve opening. Atrial reversal flow velocity is dependent on LA contraction as well as compliance of the pulmonary venous bed, LA, and LV.

In addition to the S_1, S_2, D, and Ar velocities, the S/D ratio, the duration of the Ar wave, and the difference between the Ar and mitral A-wave duration (Ar − A) are other measurements that can be used to study the diastolic function of the LV.

On occasion, pulmonary vein flow can be difficult to obtain and interpret, especially when there is translational motion that creates tissue motion artifacts during atrial contraction. Sinus tachycardia and AV block can also complicate measurement of the Ar wave.

Tissue Doppler Imaging

Spectral PWD patterns of transmitral and pulmonary venous flow are influenced by loading conditions that can be quite variable during the surgery and might not always represent actual diastolic properties of the LV. TDI of the lateral annular velocities track ventricular motion through diastole and can be very helpful in diagnosing diastolic dysfunction in the perioperative setting.[30,31]

The basic concept of TDI was described earlier (see Figs. 12-10 and 12-11). In diastole, tissue velocity rarely exceeds 15 cm/s. A typical display of the lateral mitral annular velocity shows one negative systolic velocity (S′) and two positive peak velocities (E′ and A′). While

E′ represents movement of the mitral annulus during early diastole, A′ represents atrial contraction. The E′ wave is related to diastolic properties of the LV (e.g., elastic recoil, relaxation) and is largely independent of filling pressures or systolic function. The A′ wave represents passive myocardial distention caused by atrial contraction, due either to retraction of the annular ring or subsequent late ventricular filling.

Once the TDI settings on the system have been activated, the sample volume of the pulsed wave cursor is placed on the lateral mitral annulus to obtain spectral recordings. This is generally done in the ME four-chamber view. Prostheses in the mitral position (valves, rings) and calcification can render this technique inaccurate because velocities will not appropriately reflect ventricular diastolic motion. As with all spectral Doppler recordings, a sweep speed of 50 to 100 mm/s should be chosen, and a minimum of three cardiac cycles should be recorded and measurements averaged. An E′ value less than 8 cm/s is consistent with diastolic dysfunction.[28] Some studies have suggested that the threshold values of E′ used to identify diastolic dysfunction should be approximately 12.5 cm/s in young adults and 8.5 cm/s for older individuals. In those with normal diastolic function, the E′/A′ ratio is usually greater than 1.

Flow Propagation Velocity

The principal disadvantage of PWD is that it only detects flow at a single location determined by the sample volume. Color M-mode combines the superior temporal and spatial resolution of M-mode imaging with superimposed color-coded velocity data. The result is a color-coded display of velocities along a linear path extending from the LA to the LV apex across the mitral valve (Fig. 12-16). Flow propagation velocity can identify relaxation abnormalities with reasonable certainty and is also useful in the perioperative setting.[32,33]

The ME four-chamber view is the preferred view for this modality. A color Doppler window is selected, with a narrow sector extending along the length of the image (from the tip of the LA to the tip of the LV apex) across the mitral valve. The M-mode modality is then selected to obtain the color M-mode display. The color scale baseline is reduced to about 20 cm/s to enable visualization of the first aliasing velocity. The slope of this first aliasing velocity column from the tips of the mitral leaflets to the LV apex is the propagation velocity of early diastolic filling (Vp). Highest velocities are seen at or just below the level of the mitral leaflets.

This parameter is also less affected by preload, compared with transmitral flow and pulmonary venous flow. In younger patients with normal LV function, the early diastolic suction effect may result in higher velocities near the LV apex rather than the mitral leaflets.[28] In patients with diastolic dysfunction and cardiomyopathies, the same column of blood moves at a slower pace toward the LV apex, resulting in a more

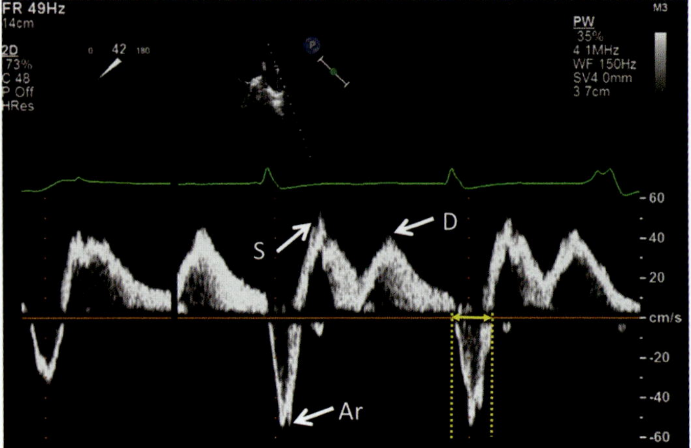

Figure 12-15 Pulsed wave Doppler of pulmonary vein flow. Three distinct waves are seen: S wave in systole, D wave in early diastole, and Ar wave in late diastole. Measurement of Ar duration is also shown.

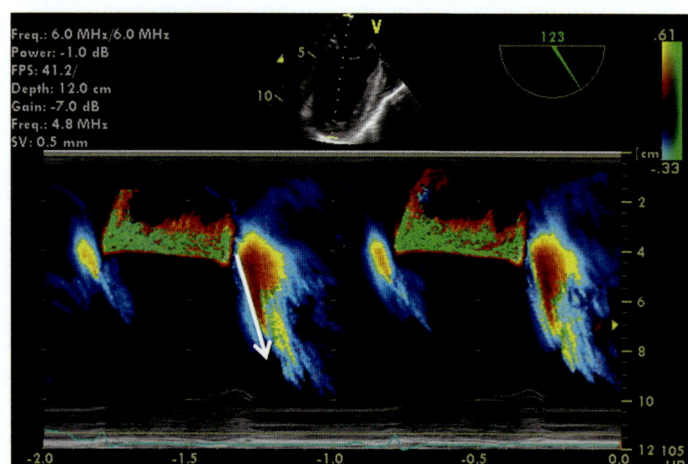

Figure 12-16 Flow propagation velocity measured using color M-mode. White arrow indicates the slope of flow propagation.

obtuse slope and a Vp that is typically less than 45 cm/s. However, the eccentric direction of flow within the LV in advanced LV dysfunction may preclude accurate detection of a slope using this modality. Since determination of Vp depends on blood flow in line with the M-mode cursor, eccentrically directed flows result in loss of slope definition.

Twist and Untwist

Measurements of LV twist and untwisting rate[34] are not currently recommended for routine clinical use but may become an important part of diastolic function evaluation in the future. Untwisting starts in late systole but mostly occurs during the IVRT and is largely complete at the time of mitral valve opening. Diastolic untwist represents elastic recoil due to the release of restoring forces that have been generated during the preceding systole.[34] The rate of untwisting is also known as the *recoil rate*. Diastolic untwisting contributes to LV filling through suction generation. It has been assumed that the reduction in LV untwisting with attenuation or loss of diastolic suction contributes to diastolic dysfunction in diseased hearts.[35] Interestingly, diastolic dysfunction associated with normal aging, however, does not appear to be due to a reduction in diastolic untwist.

Grading of Diastolic Dysfunction

The concept of grading diastolic dysfunction is important. Classification of diastolic dysfunction according to severity allows stratification of risk and tailoring of therapy. It also allows for longitudinal follow-up and identification of trends in progression of diastolic dysfunction. Diastolic dysfunction has been conventionally graded according to progression of disease from normal function through impaired relaxation and reduced compliance.[28,29,36,37] Since early attempts to assign grade were based on transmitral flow patterns, the grading nomenclature has reflected these patterns: normal, impaired relaxation, pseudonormal, and restrictive (Fig. 12-17).

Each progressive stage of diastolic dysfunction leads to increasing LA pressure as an adaptation to increasing LV filling pressure requirements. Transmitral pulmonary venous flow patterns represent these changes in LA pressure relative to LV filling pressure. Tissue Doppler profiles reflect decreasing early motion and excursion of the lateral mitral annulus as LV compliance keeps declining. Grading diastolic dysfunction therefore requires measuring a number of parameters that reflect these changes.

ASE guidelines for evaluating diastolic function reviewed several measurement modalities and identified an approach to grading diastolic dysfunction based on alignment of several 2D and Doppler parameters.[28] These guidelines also recognized the differences in estimation of filling pressures in patients with depressed versus normal systolic function. A significant drawback in the proposed guidelines is assessment of LA volume, for which there are acknowledged limitations using TEE. They also acknowledged that the proposed algorithm was complex and suggested that a simpler approach would be desirable in the clinical setting.

We examined and evaluated the utility and validity of a simplified algorithm in the operative setting, using TEE in a large cohort of coronary artery bypass graft surgery patients.[30] The simple algorithm consisted only of peak transmitral E velocity and TDI-derived E′ velocity, both of which are easier to obtain in the operating room than other parameters, indicating improved utility of the algorithm (Fig. 12-18). Most patients were assigned a grade, and those with worse grades of diastolic dysfunction were at increased risk of long-term adverse outcomes, suggesting validity of the algorithm.

Right Ventricular Systolic and Diastolic Function

Right Ventricular Structure and Function

Evaluation of the RV continues to evolve as we recognize the importance of RV function and interventricular dependence. Both the structure and function of the RV are significantly different from the LV. Its non-geometric shape, pattern of contraction, and lack of equivalent contractile mass make quantitative and qualitative assessment of the RV an echocardiographic challenge.

The RV is elliptical, typically extending two-thirds the length of the LV as assessed in the ME four-chamber view. Both anatomic and embryologic divisions of the RV can be assessed from the RV

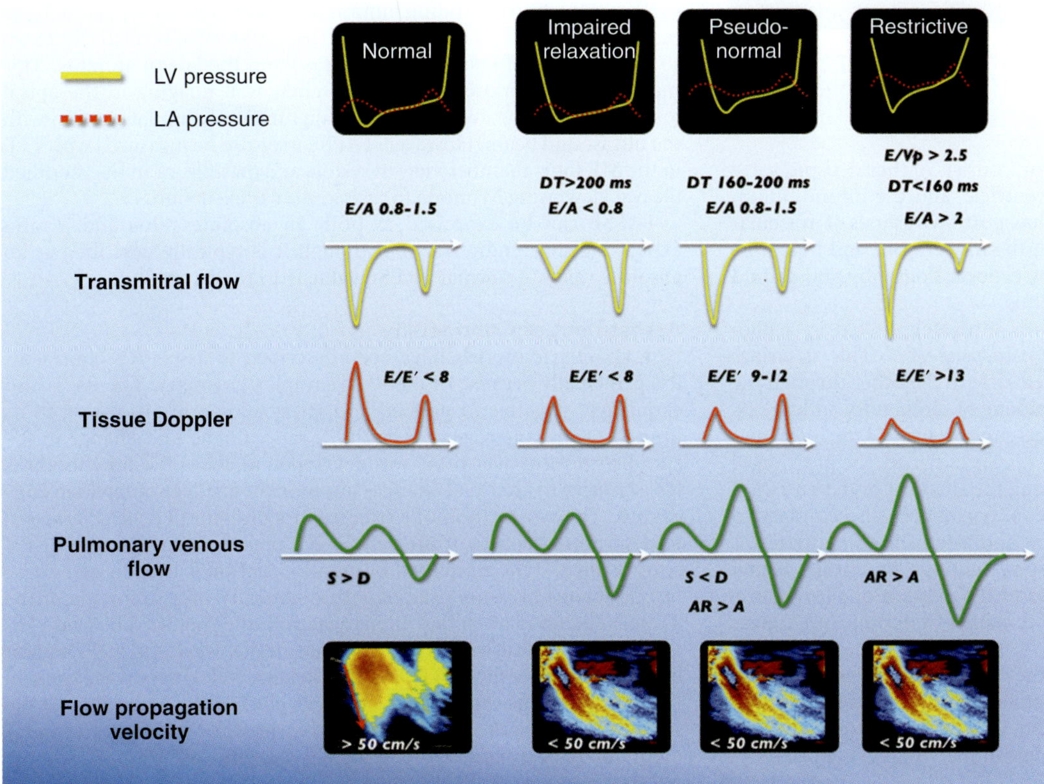

Figure 12-17 Grading of left ventricular *(LV)* diastolic dysfunction. *A,* Transmitral A velocity; *AR,* pulmonary venous diastolic atrial reversal velocity; *D,* pulmonary venous diastolic D velocity; *DT,* deceleration time of E wave; *E,* transmitral E velocity; *E′,* tissue Doppler early velocity; *LA,* left atrium; *S,* pulmonary venous systolic velocity; *Vp,* propagation velocity.

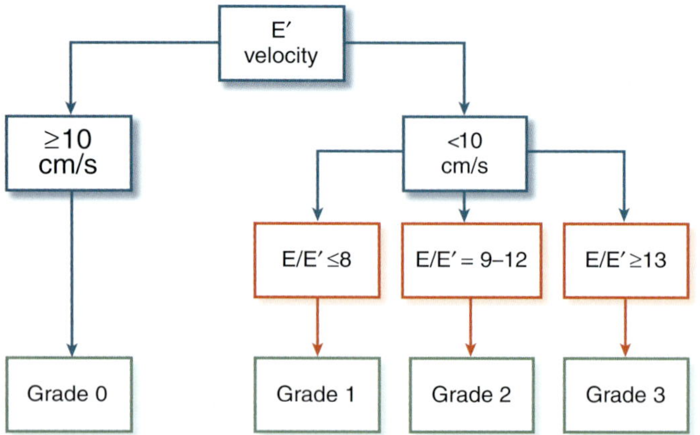

Figure 12-18 Simplified algorithm for grading diastolic dysfunction. Tissue Doppler velocity of lateral mitral annulus (*E'*) and transmitral pulsed Doppler of peak early velocity (*E*) are the only two variables used in this algorithm. Grades: 0 = normal; 1 = impaired relaxation; 2 = pseudonormal; 3 = restrictive.

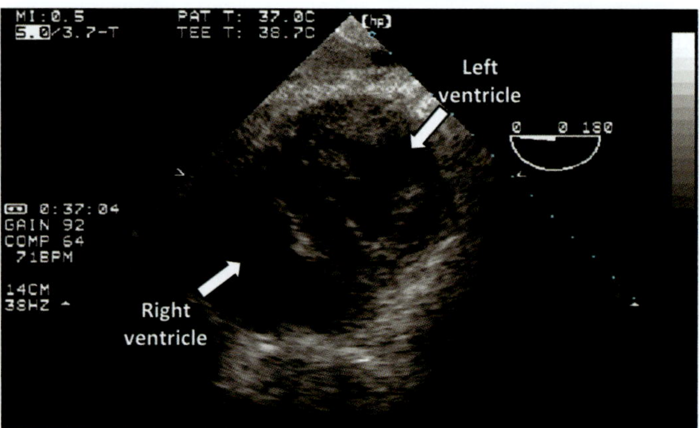

Figure 12-19 Transgastric mid–short-axis view of both ventricles, demonstrating a D-shaped ventricle due to right ventricular dysfunction.

inflow-outflow view. The inflow portion consists of the tricuspid valve and the trabeculated portion of the ventricle, and the infundibulum and pulmonic valve comprise the outflow portion. A series of muscular bands separate the two divisions, with the moderator band being the most prominent. This is often seen by echocardiography and should not be confused with a mass or thrombus.

The functioning of both ventricles is intricately linked in a phenomenon aptly termed *ventricular interdependence*.[6] This describes the transmission of forces from one ventricle to the other through the myocardium or pericardium, independent of circulatory influences. Normally, the interventricular septum is concave toward the LV. However, under conditions of pressure or volume overload, the position of the septum can change, thereby affecting the shape of both ventricles. Septal flattening may occur if the RV is hypertrophied secondary to pressure overload, changing the shape and size of both ventricles.[38] This commonly results in the D-shaped ventricle in systole. Septal motion may also be abnormal in cases of RV dilation due to volume overload, and the septum may appear to flatten in diastole but appear normal at end-systole (Fig. 12-19).

Echocardiographic assessment of the RV is challenging, given its unique shape and function. Intraoperative echocardiographers should use all modalities at their disposal for quantitative and qualitative assessment, including methods for determining volume, contractility, and transvalvular flow.

Volumetric Methods

Volumetric assessment of the RV can be performed using both 2D and 3D TEE. With 2D echocardiography, the assessment of volume—a 3D entity—involves several geometric assumptions to derive a volume measurement from a series of 2D measurements. Although 2D methods like the Simpson method of disks and 3D methods of direct volume assessment have been largely validated for the LV, extrapolation to the RV cannot be assumed, owing to differences in shape and function. Planimetry by tracing the endocardial border can be challenging because of trabeculations within the RV.

Determination of RV ejection fraction (i.e., fractional area change [FAC]) is similar to fractional shortening and can be calculated as follows:

$$FAC = [(\text{End-diastolic area} - \text{End-systolic area})/\text{End-diastolic area}] \times 100$$

This measurement is made using planimetry in either ME four-chamber or TG short-axis views. The degree of FAC suggests the degree of RV dysfunction, with a normal FAC being 32% to 60%.

Volumetric assessment using 3D TEE continues to evolve and currently includes ejection fraction calculation from the summation of geometric volumes.[39] This is similar to the Simpson method but has not been validated for the RV. More recent technology offers 3D modeling of the RV that makes no geometric assumptions and closely correlates with magnetic resonance imaging (MRI) findings.

Internal Dimensions

Global assessment of RV size and function is dependent on several of the ASE/Society of Cardiovascular Anesthesiologists (SCA) views. The ME four-chamber view allows for measurement of the long and short axis for evaluation of RV enlargement. The short axis is measured at the mid-cavitary level, with a normal value of 2.7 to 3.3, and the long axis has a normal value of 7.1 to 7.9. Shortening fraction, a unidimensional index of the shortening of either the long or short axis, can provide a measure of global RV systolic function.

Tricuspid annular plane systolic excursion (TAPSE) is a variant of the shortening fraction in the long axis. TAPSE has been shown to better correlate with RV ejection fraction, because the major contribution to RV contraction is a sliding motion of the longitudinal smaller muscle mass.[40] The septal attachment of the tricuspid valve is relatively fixed, so the majority of systolic excursion is from the lateral annulus. This measurement is more feasible with chest wall imaging in the apical four-chamber view, owing to better alignment of annular motion with the ultrasound beam. However, TAPSE may also be measured with TEE in the ME four-chamber view in systole and diastole, or in the modified bicaval view using M-mode to assess annular excursion.

TAPSE can be expressed as both an absolute value and a ratio expressing shortening fraction, though it is typically described as an absolute value. A normal TAPSE value is 15 to 25 mm.[41]

Assessment of Contractility

Non-geometric models have been described to assess RV contractility, principally because of the RV's complex geometry. The RV is also exquisitely sensitive to preload and afterload conditions owing to its limited contractile reserve. The dP/dt ratio, or the unit change in RV systolic pressure over time, was developed to assess RV function; it is less sensitive to afterload changes but more dependent on preload conditions. The acceleration of a tricuspid regurgitant (TR) jet is assessed to determine the rate of increase in RV pressure as a measure of RV contractility.[42] The simplified Bernoulli equation is used to determine instantaneous pressure gradients from velocity measurements of the TR jet. The jet is often best interrogated in the modified bicaval view after identification with CFD. The continuous wave spectral Doppler beam is aligned with the TR jet. First, the flow velocities on the spectral Doppler envelope are marked at 1 m/s and 2 m/s. According to the simplified Bernoulli equation (ΔP $4V^2$, where ΔP is the pressure gradient and V is instantaneous velocity), the pressure gradient at these points are 4 mmHg and 16 mmHg, respectively. The time interval

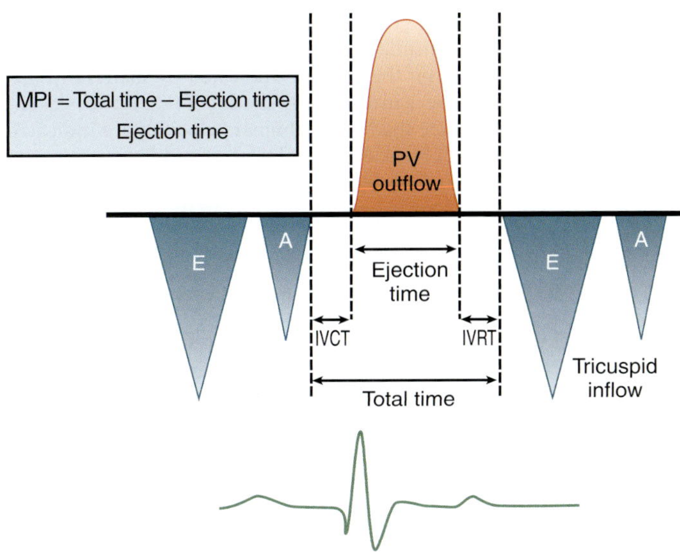

Figure 12-20 Right ventricular myocardial performance index (MPI). *A,* late diastolic flow; *E,* early diastolic flow; *IVCT,* Isovolumetric contraction time; *IVRT,* isovolumetric relaxation time; *PV,* pulmonic valve.

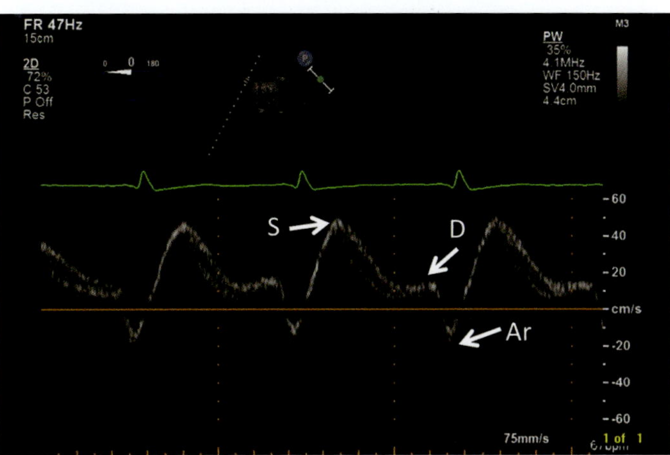

Figure 12-21 Hepatic venous flow pattern. There is usually a single systolic *(S)* wave and two diastolic waves: an early D wave and a late Ar wave from atrial contraction.

between the two is measured, and the time taken by the RV to generate a change in pressure from 4 to 16 mmHg (i.e., a change of 12 mmHg) is measured and the result expressed as mmHg/s. A normal value for dP/dt is greater than 1000 mmHg/s. There is also some evidence that dP/dt/P(max) may be superior to dP/dt alone for assessment of RV systolic function.[43]

An additional quantitative assessment, the myocardial performance index (MPI), is also free of geometric limitations.[44] A significant advantage of MPI is that it is minimally affected by heart rate, preload, and afterload. It is defined as the sum of isovolumic contraction and relaxation divided by ejection time. Ejection time is obtained from pulmonary artery flow and total time including ejection time, and the isovolumic time is measured as the interval between the end of the A wave and the start of the E wave (Fig. 12-20). The isovolumic period is total time minus ejection time. Normal values are 0.3 to 0.4.

Right Ventricular Diastolic Function

Diastolic function and RV filling can be evaluated by obtaining tricuspid inflow velocities and patterns. This is analogous to mitral inflow patterns to assess LV diastolic function. Maximal velocities across the tricuspid valve are lower than across the mitral valve, because the tricuspid annulus is larger and the inflow time longer.[41] Normal inflow, as seen with PWD with the sample volume located just beneath the leaflet tips, reveals an early diastolic (E) wave and late diastolic (A) wave. Impaired relaxation of the RV results in a decrease in E-wave peak velocity, with an increase in A-wave velocity (E/A <1). A restrictive RV inflow pattern is characterized by a tall E wave and a small A wave (E/A >1.5).[45]

Tissue Doppler may be used to assess tricuspid annular motion as a measure of diastolic function. With TEE, a normal tracing shows one negative systolic wave (away from the probe, below the baseline) and positive diastolic E′ and A′ waves, analogous to the trans-tricuspid E and A waves. Impaired relaxation is indicated by a decreased E′ and E′/A′ of less than 1, along with an increased deceleration time. Restrictive RV diastolic function reveals E′/A′ less than 1, which will continue to decline as function worsens.[41,45]

Hepatic vein flow is another way to assess filling and RV function (Fig. 12-21).[40] The initial positive deflection or forward flow is related to the decline in atrial pressure from relaxation, as well as apical movement of the tricuspid valve during ventricular systole. Diastolic flow is evidenced by a positive deflection resulting from a fall in right atrial (RA) pressure during passive RV filling in early diastole. Atrial systole is evidenced by a negative deflection, indicating reverse flow. Blunting of the systolic peak and augmentation of the diastolic peak suggest RV dysfunction, whereas severe TR can result in systolic flow reversal.

Measuring Stenosis

Physiologic Effect of a Stenosed Valve

The function and purpose of the intracardiac valves is to permit forward unidirectional flow of blood and prevent backward flow. A dysfunctional valve may either restrict forward flow (stenosis) or allow backward flow (regurgitation). In either situation, the total amount of forward flow is compromised, with serious physiologic ramifications. The following describes the physiologic effect of valve stenosis.

When the valve area of an AV valve is reduced, a higher pressure gradient across the valve from the atrium to the ventricle is required to maintain adequate forward flow. Atrial enlargement or dilation often results, along with bowing of the interatrial septum away from the side of enlargement. Dilation can also cause stasis of flow seen by spontaneous echo contrast, or "smoke." This stagnant flow can lead to thrombus formation within regions that have very little flow, such as in the atrial appendage. A thrombus formed in the RA may become dislodged and flow into the pulmonary circulation, resulting in pulmonary embolism, and LA thrombi may lead to stroke if dislodged. There is also a possibility of an RA clot traversing a patent foramen ovale to result in a left-sided lesion. Arrhythmias due to a distended atrium, especially atrial fibrillation, are also common. Elevated LA pressures translate to elevated pulmonary pressures and increased afterload for the RV. Both right and left ventricular dysfunction may result. The ventricular chamber of a stenosed AV valve is typically underfilled owing to chronically reduced forward flow.

Increased afterload created by a stenosed ventriculo-arterial valve leads to concentric hypertrophy of the respective ventricle and consequent diastolic dysfunction. As this condition progresses, atrial pressures become elevated, leading to atrial enlargement and atrial fibrillation. Late in the disease process, ventricular dilation occurs. Regurgitation of the respective AV valve can result. Poststenotic dilation of the aorta or pulmonary artery can also be seen.

Fundamental Difference Between a Stenosed Atrioventricular Valve and a Ventriculo-Arterial Valve

AV valves, namely the mitral and tricuspid valves, are affected in diastole by stenosis. In contrast, ventriculo-arterial (aortic and pulmonic valves) are affected in systole.

Normally functioning AV valves open during diastole, allowing low-pressure forward flow of blood from the atrium to the respective ventricle. Stenosis of the valve causes an increase in back pressure, resulting in the described physiologic changes. Each one of those changes (i.e., increased atrial size, stasis of blow flood, arrhythmias, elevated filling pressures) can be attributed to the stenotic valve in question. Additionally, there is often underfilling of the ventricles.

Ventriculo-arterial valve stenosis also reduces forward flow but results in a different set of adaptations. Valve stenosis results in a low cardiac output state, which in turn requires the ventricle to generate a higher systolic pressure to maintain pressure and flow downstream of the valve. The need for higher ventricular systolic pressure to overcome the increase in afterload from a stenosed valve results in an increase in contractile mass. This initial ventricular adaptation takes the form of ventricular hypertrophy, more impressively seen in the LV than the RV. Ventricular hypertrophy can overcome the flow limitations posed by a stenosed valve, but chronic progression of the disease can lead to ventricular fatigue with eventual dilation and failure. The onset of failure is more rapid with the RV, owing to its limited contractile reserve compared to the LV.

Echo Assessment: Two-Dimensional Methods

Views

Echo assessment of any valve begins with the standard ASE/SCA views[46] that will be described for each valve in detail in the next chapter. Once the appropriate view is obtained, attention is initially focused on the appearance of the valve. The diagnosis of a stenotic valve is suggested by thickening and calcification of the leaflets in addition to restricted motion. Excessive thickening or calcification can also lead to acoustic shadow artifacts in the far field. Attention can then be turned to the subvalvular apparatus in the case of AV valves, which too can be thickened, calcified, or shortened. Annular calcification may also be present. From the same views, the size of the atria should also be assessed. Atrial adaptation to valve stenoses can be seen as dilation and spontaneous echo contrast due to sluggish flow. Ventricular adaptations should also be assessed with 2D imaging, with hypertrophy suggesting ventriculo-arterial valve stenosis or a small ventricular cavity in AV valve stenosis. Other standard views may reveal poststenotic dilation of the aorta or pulmonary artery. Most of these changes can be seen without using CFD. The authors suggest an initial comprehensive assessment with 2D echo prior to CFD; it is easy to overlook key features of valve stenosis if only the valve is evaluated rather than the subvalvular apparatus and chambers connected by the valve.

Planimetry

Planimetry is another method of assessing effective valve opening area as one of the quantitative measures used to assess valvular stenosis. Planimetry is performed by tracing the area of a valve at its point of maximal opening. The advantage of planimetry is that it is fast and simple and can theoretically be performed on any of the four valves, though it is less reliable than some of the other methods described in greater detail in the next chapter. While it seems like an ideal method to quantify valve area, there are significant limitations. First, there is substantial interobserver variability because there is a subjective component to the measurement owing to the difficulty in defining the border of the leaflets secondary to heavy calcification and acoustic shadowing. Second, valve area can be under- or overestimated depending on the character of the leaflets and the point at which the ultrasound beam intersects them. Finally, it must be recognized that planimetry is the estimation of a 3D structure using a single 2D image plane.

Echo Assessment: Doppler Techniques

Color Flow Doppler

CFD provides information about blood flow through a region and is extremely useful in assessing valve stenosis. Whereas pulsed wave spectral Doppler displays the peak velocity at a single location within a defined sample volume, CFD displays mean velocities that are color coded according to magnitude of velocity and direction of flow. By convention, flow away from the probe is indicated by shades of blue, and flow toward the probe is indicated by shades of red. Lower velocities are indicated by darker shades, and higher velocities are indicated by lighter shades. Areas of black on the color spectrum indicate an area where no Doppler shift is detected. The actual color displayed is indicated by the color map. Variance in the color map indicates regions of turbulent blood flow (Fig. 12-22).

Following initial inspection of the valve on 2D echo, CFD provides basic information on the direction of flow and mean velocity in a specific area. It is yet another tool in assessing stenosis, which is indicated by high velocities and turbulent flow. Associated valvular regurgitation in the presence of a stenotic valve may also be easily detected by CFD. Because it is based on PWD, CFD is also subject to the same limitations. Aliasing is one major pitfall; if the sampling velocity exceeds one half the pulse repetition frequency (Nyquist limit), aliasing of color occurs (see Fig. 12-22). In the presence of a variance map, a mosaic color or velocities exceeding the Nyquist limit can suggest turbulent flow. Another major limitation of CFD is the relatively lower temporal and spatial resolution compared to 2D echo. The low temporal resolution is important when measurements such as vena contracta are made. With low frame rates, the point of maximum jet width may be missed, leading to potentially inaccurate measurements. As with most other echo imaging modalities, CFD is also subject to artifacts including ghosting or reverberation. Ghosting may occur from strong reflectors such as calcified leaflets of a valve.

Spectral Doppler
Velocity and Gradient

Spectral Doppler is the gold standard for quantification of stenosis. Both CWD and PWD can be applied to assess a valve. The high velocities seen with a stenotic valve require CWD for more accurate measurement of peak velocities. The phenomenon of aliasing makes PWD inappropriate for measurement of high-velocity jets (Fig. 12-23). The Doppler beam is aligned with the direction of flow across the valve, and a velocity and gradient can be determined. Both peak and mean gradients can be determined by tracing the Doppler envelope.

Beyond the stenosis, there is a drop in downstream pressure. Definitions for valve-specific mild, moderate, and severe stenosis will be addressed in subsequent sections. From these Doppler envelopes, a velocity-time integral (VTI) can be calculated, and the continuity equation can be employed to determine valve area, assuming no other lesions exist that would affect this calculation. The VTI can also be used as part of the dimensionless index (DI, defined as LVOT VTI/aortic valve VTI), which specifically describes aortic stenosis. The density and contour of the Doppler envelope can also provide important clues about the severity of the stenosis. Increased density of the envelope suggests a higher velocity and a higher number of cells passing through the orifice. The contour of the jet can suggest where the stenosis actually exists. One shape of the envelope may suggest that obstruction to flow is occurring at the valvular apparatus, where another shape may suggest subvalvular obstruction. Jet contour can also suggest a fixed or dynamic obstructive lesion.[47]

Pressure Half-Time

Pressure half-time (PHT) is another method used to assess the severity of stenosis and valve area, though it has only been validated for a few specific valvular lesions.[47] The principle of PHT is equilibration of pressures between two chambers during diastole. The PHT is the amount of time it takes the pressure gradient to fall to half the peak value. This time is prolonged in stenotic AV valve lesions because there is a smaller orifice, forcing equilibration of pressure to occur over a longer period of time. The PHT is particularly valuable for estimating the valve area in mitral stenosis. Since PHT is dependent on the peak pressure gradient, any factor that affects the peak velocity across the valve will affect the time taken to reach half the peak gradient. Similarly, factors that affect chamber pressure equalization (e.g., associated

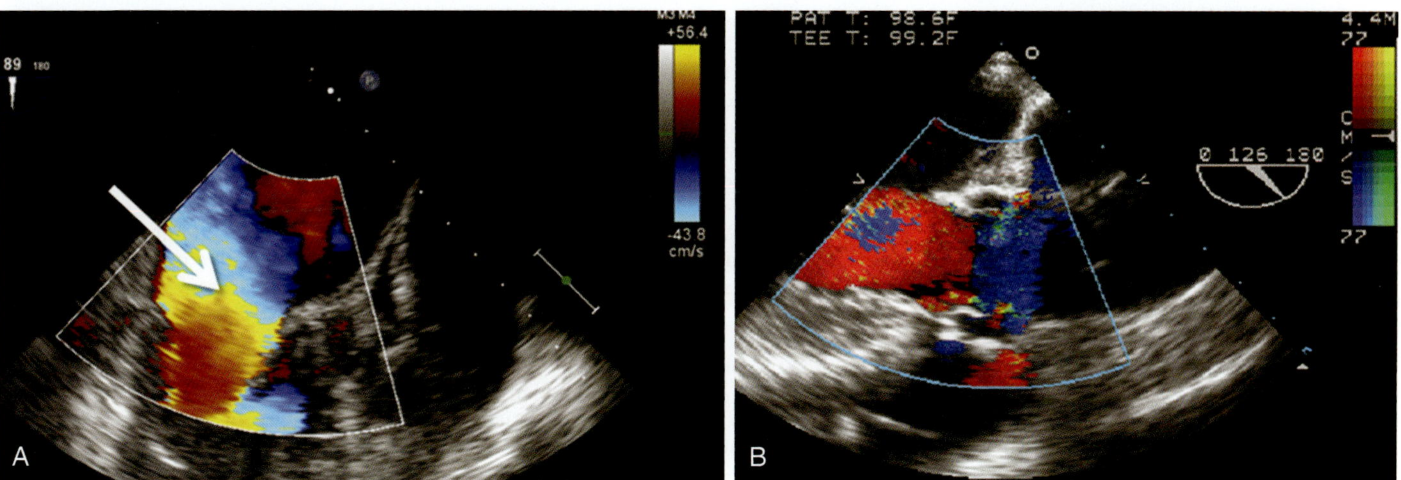

Figure 12-22 Color flow Doppler. **A,** Velocity map with flow through mitral valve. **B,** Variance map with flow across aortic valve. Arrow indicates point at which aliasing occurs. (See text for details.)

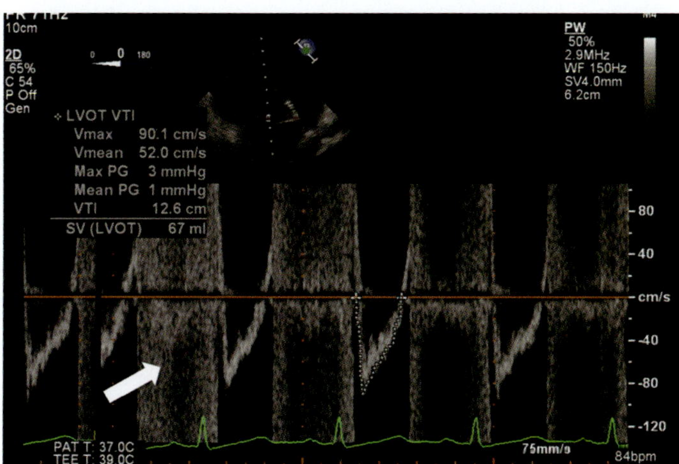

Figure 12-23 Pulsed wave Doppler of left ventricular outflow tract *(LVOT)*. Arrow indicates aliasing from aortic regurgitation jet. Actual jet is directed above baseline, but high velocity exceeds Nyquist limit and aliasing occurs.

observations with 2D and CFD. In PISA calculations, small changes in the radius can cause large variations in the calculated area of the orifice. These calculations are also time consuming and plagued by interobserver variability. Moreover, PISA assumes a hemispherical convergence, which may not be true.

Three-Dimensional Assessment

RT-3D TEE is changing the way we assess both ventricular and valvular function; 3D imaging of valves allows for more accurate planimetry measurements as well as better visualization of the subvalvular apparatus.[8] More accurate quantification of valvular size and other measurements (e.g., LVOT diameter) are attainable with RT-3D TEE, and abnormalities are often identified that may have been missed with traditional 2D imaging; 3D imaging is particularly helpful with volumetric measurements such as ventricular volumes, ejection fraction, and mass. RT-3D TEE relies less upon geometric modeling and image plane position, resulting in more accurate quantification.[23] Recent studies have confirmed a pre- and post-valvuloplasty role for RT-3D TEE in patients with mitral stenosis.[48,49] This technology is not new but still in its infancy; as it advances and improves our imaging capabilities, novel applications for 3D imaging will also continue to evolve.

Measuring Regurgitation

Physiologic Effect of a Regurgitant Valve

A valve rendered incompetent by a pathologic process can have profound effects, depending on its location and the chambers it separates. In each case, there are "upstream" and "downstream" effects. Upstream effects relate to development of abnormal pressures in the transmitting chamber, and downstream effects relate to decreased forward flow. All four cardiac valves can be subject to processes that destroy the natural one-way mechanism and cause regurgitation. Valvular incompetence usually results from malcoaptation of the leaflets caused by conditions that affect the structural integrity of the valve leaflets or their support structures.

Fundamental Difference Between a Regurgitant Atrioventricular Valve and a Ventriculo-Arterial Valve

The fundamental difference between the cuspid valves (mitral and tricuspid) and the semilunar valves (aortic and pulmonic) is that whereas the chordae tendineae prevent the cuspid valves from prolapsing into the atria during ventricular systole, the semilunar valves are designed

valve lesions, diastolic stiffness) will also affect the slope of the jet and thus the PHT.

Flow Convergence

Flow convergence is a phenomenon that can be used for stenosis assessment in the form of proximal isovelocity surface area (PISA).[47] As flow moves toward a small area, such as a stenotic orifice, the flow velocity increases over an area which assumes a hemispherical shape. Flow rate at the surface of this hemisphere equals flow across the orifice (conservation of flow). Across the surface area of the hemisphere, the velocities are the same. Using CFD, the velocities on the color map are adjusted in the direction of flow, so the aliasing will occur earlier (at a lower velocity) in a semicircular pattern. The stenotic orifice area is calculated using the PISA formula based on the conservation of flow (orifice area = PISA × aliasing velocity/peak velocity across stenotic valve) (see Chapter 4).

Often, several diagnostic tools are used to assess any one valvular lesion, because there are intrinsic errors within the system that make no one of these calculations perfect or the gold standard. Many of these calculations require CWD, which has the inherent issue with range ambiguity. Multiple velocities are sampled on a single line, but the exact location of the highest velocity cannot be determined. One can suspect where the highest velocity is located based on other to close during diastole and prevent backflow from the great arteries into the ventricles.

As retrograde flow through a valve progressively worsens, the heart musculature remodels to deal with this phenomenon. For AV valve regurgitation, the atria will enlarge to accommodate the increased amount of blood volume. Initially, the ventricles may enlarge to deal with the volume overload from the regurgitant flow. Late in disease progression, the ventricular cavity dilates, its capacity to achieve adequate forward flow is compromised, and ejection fraction declines. A vicious cycle ensues, and as the ventricle becomes dilated, the valvular annulus also dilates, leading to further malcoaptation of the leaflets and a greater regurgitant fraction.

Stretching of the atria can lead to increased pressure that is transmitted back through the circulation, resulting in pulmonary or hepatic venous congestion. In the case of MR, this can be characterized by pulmonary edema, and in TR, ascites, peripheral edema, and elevated jugular venous pulse can occur. Owing to distortion of the electrical system, this stretch can also lead to conduction abnormalities and arrhythmias, especially atrial fibrillation. Late in the progression of chronic MR, pulmonary vascular resistance due to chronic overload of the pulmonary circulation can occur and result in RV failure.

The ventriculo-arterial (aortic and pulmonary) valves share some similarities in that the heart will also remodel when these valves are incompetent, sometimes to the same degree. The same symptoms may be seen, although for different reasons. In the case of aortic regurgitation, the LVEDP increases secondary to diastolic volume overload. Chronic volume overload then leads to ventricular dilation and congestive heart failure. The LA then has to generate a higher pressure during atrial systole to propel blood across the mitral valve into an LV with a high LVEDP. As LA pressure increases, the back pressure through the pulmonary circulation can result in pulmonary edema, increases in pulmonary vascular resistance, and right heart failure. The same pathophysiology exists for pulmonary valve regurgitation, except the RV fails first, cardiac output decreases, and pedal edema, jugular venous distention, and hepatic congestion ensue.

The underlying concept in all valvular regurgitant lesions is that forward flow is compromised and cardiac output is reduced when adaptive mechanisms eventually fail.

Echo Assessment

Echocardiography is an ideal imaging modality for assessment of regurgitant valve lesions. In patients presenting for cardiac surgery, intraoperative TEE is invaluable for assessment of the severity of regurgitant lesions.[50] Echo assessment of a regurgitant valve can confirm known preoperative findings or quantify previously unknown lesions that could impact immediate surgical management. Several modalities are available to the echocardiographer to help assess the nature of the valve lesion in question.

Two-Dimensional Methods

When characterizing a regurgitant lesion, the structure and integrity of the valve must first be examined. All four valves are located in the same plane within the fibrous skeleton of the heart, so most valve lesions can be appreciated in ME views. However, to align a Doppler beam for assessment of transvalvular velocity, other views may have to be used (e.g., deep TG view for aortic valve lesions). It is also important to realize that regurgitation can often be diagnosed without Doppler examination, based on the effects of the regurgitant valve on associated cardiac structures.

Annulus

The annulus is a ring of non-conductive tissue that provides support for the valve leaflets. When the annulus becomes dilated, the leaflets are pulled apart from the coaptation point, with resulting regurgitation. Annular dilation can usually be assessed in ME views.

Leaflet Prolapse

Excessive retrograde movement of the valve leaflet beyond the coaptation point can occur into the upstream chamber. Prolapse does not necessarily lead to regurgitation unless leaflet coaptation is affected.

Flail

A valve leaflet is termed *flail* when part of its subvalvular support mechanism fails and the leaflet is rendered incapable of coaptation. The flail mechanism is seen most commonly with mitral valves, owing to the high systolic pressure gradients the valve must tolerate and a subvalvular apparatus that relies on LV integrity.

Chamber Size

Chronic regurgitation is generally associated with a size increase for the right and left ventricular cavities for all regurgitant lesions. It can also result in atrial enlargement. As the regurgitant lesion progresses in severity, the regurgitant volume rises and increases the volume burden on the ventricle. For aortic regurgitation, chamber size may appear normal because the ventricle has not yet adapted to the volume overload. However, with chronic regurgitation, progressive chamber dilation usually results.

Leaflet Excursion

How the leaflet moves during forward flow can be just as important as how the leaflet moves during regurgitant flow. For example, in the case of aortic stenosis, calcification of the valve can restrict leaflet movement during forward flow. This may also lead to the valve's inability to coapt appropriately, and regurgitation follows. A regurgitant jet may also affect the excursion of other leaflets. A moderate or severe aortic regurgitant jet directed anteriorly can cause fluttering of the anterior leaflet of the mitral valve in diastole.

Color Doppler Assessment

CFD is commonly used to assess the orientation, origin, and severity of regurgitant jets. According to the ASE guidelines for assessment of regurgitant lesions, knowledge of instrument settings such as gain, output power, Nyquist limit, size and depth of the image sector, and transducer frequency is necessary for optimal image acquisition and accuracy of interpretation.[50] CFD allows the operator to visualize the origin of the regurgitation, direction of the jet and spatial orientation within the receiving chamber, and flow convergence through the regurgitant orifice. Each of these is an important consideration for quantification of regurgitation.

Jet Area

A regurgitant lesion can be characterized by the area of the jet relative to the receiving chamber. Generally, a larger proportional area indicates a larger defect and breech of valvular integrity. However, since preload, driving pressure, and size of the receiving chamber can all affect the jet area, it should not be used as the sole determinant of the severity of the regurgitant lesion.

Jet Direction and Dimension

The direction of the jet is an extremely important feature of a regurgitant lesion. In the mitral valve, for example, jet direction can help determine the etiology of the lesion. A central jet may suggest annular dilation from ischemia, whereas an eccentric wall-hugging jet implies a prolapsed or flail leaflet. Starting with a larger color box allows the echocardiographer to search for the regurgitant lesion. Once the site of the lesion is established, the CFD box should be narrowed to that specific area to allow a high frame rate to create a smooth and accurate picture. Lesions may sometimes be complex, so scanning through all views to visualize the jet direction may characterize the origin of the lesion.

Vena Contracta

Characterized by a high speed yet laminar flow, this is the narrowest portion of the jet close to the regurgitant orifice. Although the vena

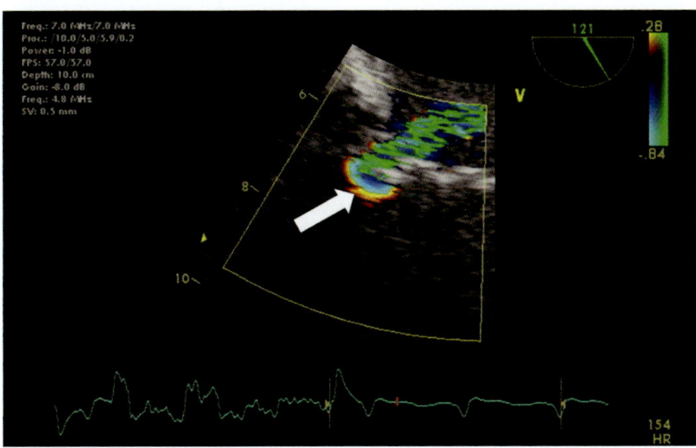

Figure 12-24   Color flow Doppler across mitral valve, indicating regurgitation. Flow convergence is shown with proximal isovelocity surface area (PISA) formed *(arrow)* at the point of aliasing velocity.

contracta is somewhat smaller than the anatomic orifice area, it represents a measure of the effective regurgitant orifice area and is considered to be independent of flow or pressure of the regurgitant jet. While generally true for centrally directed jets, the vena contracta may be difficult to accurately define with eccentric regurgitant jets.

Proximal Isovelocity Surface Area

As blood flow approaches a regurgitant orifice, its velocity increases, forming concentric roughly hemispheric shells of increasing velocity and decreasing surface area (Fig. 12-24). Calculating the PISA provides instantaneous peak flow rate and can be used to calculate the regurgitant orifice area. The PISA method also has its limitations. When compared with central jets, eccentric jets are less likely to be accurately characterized by PISA. Additionally, a circular regurgitant orifice is assumed, which may not always be true.

Spectral Doppler Quantification

Spectral Doppler, when combined with 2D measurements discussed earlier, can help further quantify regurgitation. While using spectral Doppler, it is important to consider the differences in regurgitant lesions originating from an AV valve versus a ventriculo-arterial valve. The severity of mitral and tricuspid valve regurgitation is defined by the contour and density of the jet on CWD, and by the effect of the regurgitation on pulmonary and hepatic venous flow on PWD. For the aortic and pulmonic valves, regurgitation is primarily characterized by the rate of deceleration of the regurgitant jet.

Jet Contour

The shape of the jet can give insight into the severity of regurgitation and is a useful qualitative feature of the lesion. The shape of the waveform can be parabolic, which may indicate a milder form of regurgitation, or triangular/early peaking in more severe forms.

Jet Density

The density of the regurgitant jet waveform with CWD is directly proportional to the regurgitant blood volume and is a qualitative index of regurgitation severity.

Pressure Half-Time

Used to characterize aortic and pulmonic valve insufficiency (see earlier discussion), PHT is the time taken for the peak pressure to decline to half its peak value. It reflects the rate of equilibration of diastolic arterial and ventricular pressures. With severe regurgitation, pressures tend to equalize rapidly, leading to a steep decline in velocity of flow and consequently a shorter PHT. With milder lesions, flow velocity is sustained, since pressures take longer to equilibrate, resulting in longer PHTs. This phenomenon is based on sound principles of flow dynamics,

but it should be interpreted with caution. The pressure equilibration is critically dependent on the arterial (transmitting chamber) pressure distal to the valve and on the diastolic ventricular (receiving chamber) pressure.

Pulmonary and Hepatic Venous Flow

Flow through the pulmonary and hepatic veins depends on the pressure in the receiving atrial chamber. Regurgitation of the mitral and tricuspid valves results in an increase in systolic pressure within the receiving atrium. This in turn results in a decrease in systolic flow velocity (systolic blunting) in the veins that empty into the atria. With severe regurgitation, systolic flow reversal may be seen.

Three-Dimensional Assessment

The mitral valve remains one of the most complex cardiac structures to evaluate comprehensively using 2D echocardiography, but 3D echo is useful for evaluating the spatial relationships between cardiac structures and particularly suited for assessing the mitral valve. There are three principal advantages of 3D over 2D echo. First, the etiology of MR can be established more accurately by determining the precise location of leaflet abnormality, such as flail or prolapse. Second, the need for geometric assumptions is eliminated, since color 3D can permit direct measurement of effective regurgitant orifice area without the need for mathematical equations. It also allows for direct assessment of the vena contracta. Finally, the location of regurgitant jets can be precisely determined using color 3D TEE. Importantly, in the assessment of prosthetic valve dysfunction in the mitral position, the location of a paravalvular jet can be very useful when the surgical team is planning a percutaneous closure. Color 3D TEE, however, is limited by the necessity of processing a large quantity of data in a short time span, resulting in lower temporal resolution compared to non-color 3D modes.[8]

Summary

Intraoperative TEE has evolved tremendously in the last decade, with better imaging technology and more user-friendly systems leading to widespread use in surgical settings. Quantification of ventricular function and assessment of valvular dysfunction is now simpler than ever to perform. Additionally, with 3D TEE, complex geometric assumptions may no longer be necessary, making echo even easier to adopt into routine clinical practice.

REFERENCES

1. Frazin L, Talano JV, Stephanides L, Loeb HS, Kopel L, Gunnar RM. Esophageal echocardiography. *Circulation.* Jul 1976;54(1):102-108.
2. Ungerleider RM, Greeley WJ, Sheikh KH, Kern FH, Kisslo JA, Sabiston Jr DC. The use of intraoperative echo with Doppler color flow imaging to predict outcome after repair of congenital cardiac defects. *Ann Surg.* Oct 1989;210(4):526-533.
3. Ungerleider RM, Greeley WJ, Sheikh KH, et al. Routine use of intraoperative epicardial echocardiography and Doppler color flow imaging to guide and evaluate repair of congenital heart lesions. A prospective study. *J Thorac Cardiovasc Surg.* Aug 1990;100(2):297-309.
4. Bers DM. Cardiac excitation-contraction coupling. *Nature.* Jan 10 2002;415(6868):198-205.
5. Allen DG, Kentish JC. The cellular basis of the length-tension relation in cardiac muscle. *J Mol Cell Cardiol.* Sep 1985;17(9):821-840.
6. Bove AA, Santamore WP. Ventricular interdependence. *Prog Cardiovasc Dis.* 1981;23(5):365-388.
7. Lang RM, Bierig M, Devereux RB, et al. Recommendations for chamber quantification: a report from the American Society of Echocardiography's Guidelines and Standards Committee and the Chamber Quantification Writing Group, developed in conjunction with the European Association of Echocardiography, a branch of the European Society of Cardiology. *J Am Soc Echocardiogr.* Dec 2005;18(12):1440-1463.
8. Lang RM, Badano LP, Tsang W, et al. EAE/ASE recommendations for image acquisition and display using three-dimensional echocardiography. *J Am Soc Echocardiogr.* Jan 2012;25(1):3-46.
9. Jungwirth B, Mackensen GB. Real-time 3-dimensional echocardiography in the operating room. *Semin Cardiothorac Vasc Anesth.* Dec 2008;12(4):248-264.
10. Pearlman JD, Triulzi MO, King ME, Newell J, Weyman AE. Limits of normal left ventricular dimensions in growth and development: analysis of dimensions and variance in the two-dimensional echocardiograms of 268 normal healthy subjects. *J Am Coll Cardiol.* Dec 1988;12(6):1432-1441.
11. Nidorf SM, Picard MH, Triulzi MO, et al. New perspectives in the assessment of cardiac chamber dimensions during development and adulthood. *J Am Coll Cardiol.* Apr 1992;19(5):983-988.
12. Ilercil A, O'Grady MJ, Roman MJ, et al. Reference values for echocardiographic measurements in urban and rural populations of differing ethnicity: the Strong Heart Study. *J Am Soc Echocardiogr.* Jun 2001;14(6):601-611.
13. Clements FM, Harpole DH, Quill T, Jones RH, McCann RL. Estimation of left ventricular volume and ejection fraction by two-dimensional transesophageal echocardiography: comparison of short axis imaging and simultaneous radionuclide angiography. *Br J Anaesth.* Mar 1990;64(3):331-336.

14. Urbanowicz JH, Shaaban MJ, Cohen NH, et al. Comparison of transesophageal echocardiographic and scintigraphic estimates of left ventricular end-diastolic volume index and ejection fraction in patients following coronary artery bypass grafting. *Anesthesiology.* Apr 1990;72(4):607-612.

15. Loutfi H, Nishimura RA. Quantitative evaluation of left ventricular systolic function by Doppler echocardiographic techniques. *Echocardiography.* May 1994;11(3):305-314.

16. Douglas PS, Reichek N, Plappert T, Muhammad A. St John Sutton MG. Comparison of echocardiographic methods for assessment of left ventricular shortening and wall stress. *J Am Coll Cardiol.* Apr 1987;9(4):945-951.

17. Marcucci C, Lauer R, Mahajan A. New echocardiographic techniques for evaluating left ventricular myocardial function. *Semin Cardiothorac Vasc Anesth.* Dec 2008;12(4):228-247.

18. Marcucci CE, Samad Z, Rivera J, et al. A comparative evaluation of transesophageal and transthoracic echocardiography for measurement of left ventricular systolic strain using speckle tracking. *J Cardiothorac Vasc Anesth.* Feb 2012;26(1):17-25.

19. Tousignant C, Desmet M, Bowry R, Harrington AM, Cruz JD, Mazer CD. Speckle tracking for the intraoperative assessment of right ventricular function: a feasibility study. *J Cardiothorac Vasc Anesth.* Apr 2010;24(2):275-279.

20. Gorcsan 3rd J, Strum DP, Mandarino WA, Gulati VK, Pinsky MR. Quantitative assessment of alterations in regional left ventricular contractility with color-coded tissue Doppler echocardiography. Comparison with sonomicrometry and pressure-volume relations. *Circulation.* May 20 1997;95(10):2423-2433.

21. Yip G, Abraham T, Belohlavek M, Khandheria BK. Clinical applications of strain rate imaging. *J Am Soc Echocardiogr.* Dec 2003;16(12):1334-1342.

22. Buckberg G, Hoffman JI, Mahajan A, Saleh S, Coghlan C. Cardiac mechanics revisited: the relationship of cardiac architecture to ventricular function. *Circulation.* Dec 9 2008;118(24):2571-2587.

23. Gorcsan 3rd J, Abraham T, Agler DA, et al. Echocardiography for cardiac resynchronization therapy: recommendations for performance and reporting–a report from the American Society of Echocardiography Dyssynchrony Writing Group endorsed by the Heart Rhythm Society. *J Am Soc Echocardiogr.* Mar 2008;21(3):191-213.

24. Ross Jr J, Covell JW, Sonnenblick EH. The mechanics of left ventricular contraction in acute experimental cardiac failure. *J Clin Invest.* Mar 1967;46(3):299-312.

25. Aurigemma GP, Gaasch WH. Clinical practice. Diastolic heart failure. *N Engl J Med.* Sep 9 2004;351(11):1097-1105.

26. Bonow RO, Udelson JE. Left ventricular diastolic dysfunction as a cause of congestive heart failure. Mechanisms and management. *Ann Intern Med.* 1992;117(6):502-510.

27. Sanderson JE. Heart failure with a normal ejection fraction. *Heart.* Feb 2007;93(2):155-158.

28. Nagueh SF, Appleton CP, Gillebert TC, et al. Recommendations for the evaluation of left ventricular diastolic function by echocardiography. *J Am Soc Echocardiogr.* Feb 2009;22(2):107-133.

29. Khouri SJ, Maly GT, Suh DD, Walsh TE. A practical approach to the echocardiographic evaluation of diastolic function. *J Am Soc Echocardiogr.* Mar 2004;17(3):290-297.

30. Swaminathan M, Nicoara A, Phillips-Bute BG, et al. Utility of a simple algorithm to grade diastolic dysfunction and predict outcome after coronary artery bypass graft surgery. *Ann Thorac Surg.* Jun 2011;91(6):1844-1850.

31. Groban L, Dolinski SY. Transesophageal echocardiographic evaluation of diastolic function. *Chest.* Nov 2005;128(5):3652-3663.

32. Matyal R, Hess PE, Subramaniam B, et al. Perioperative diastolic dysfunction during vascular surgery and its association with postoperative outcome. *J Vasc Surg.* Jul 2009;50(1):70-76.

33. Djaiani GN, McCreath BJ, Ti LK, et al. Mitral flow propagation velocity identifies patients with abnormal diastolic function during coronary artery bypass graft surgery. *Anesth Analg.* Sep 2002;95(3):524-530.

34. Buckberg G, Hoffman JI, Nanda NC, Coghlan C, Saleh S, Athanasuleas C. Ventricular torsion and untwisting: further insights into mechanics and timing interdependence: a viewpoint. *Echocardiography.* Aug 2011;28(7):782-804.

35. Takeuchi M, Borden WB, Nakai H, et al. Reduced and delayed untwisting of the left ventricle in patients with hypertension and left ventricular hypertrophy: a study using two-dimensional speckle tracking imaging. *Eur Heart J.* Oct 19 2007.

36. Paulus WJ, Tschope C, Sanderson JE. How to diagnose diastolic heart failure: a consensus statement on the diagnosis of heart failure with normal left ventricular ejection fraction by the Heart Failure and Echocardiography Associations of the European Society of Cardiology. *Eur Heart J.* Oct 2007;28(20):2539-2550.

37. Rakowski H, Appleton C, Chan KL, et al. Canadian consensus recommendations for the measurement and reporting of diastolic dysfunction by echocardiography: from the Investigators of Consensus on Diastolic Dysfunction by Echocardiography. *J Am Soc Echocardiogr.* Sep-Oct 1996;9(5):736-760.

38. Kaul S. The interventricular septum in health and disease. *Am Heart J.* Sep 1986;112(3):568-581.

39. Karhausen J, Dudaryk R, Phillips-Bute B, et al. Three-dimensional transesophageal echocardiography for perioperative right ventricular assessment. *Ann Thorac Surg.* 2012;94:468-474.

40. Mishra M, Swaminathan M, Malhotra R, Mishra A, Trehan N. Evaluation of right ventricular function during CABG: transesophageal echocardiographic assessment of hepatic venous flow versus conventional right ventricular performance indices. *Echocardiography.* Jan 1998;15(1):51-58.

41. Rudski LG, Lai WW, Afilalo J, et al. Guidelines for the echocardiographic assessment of the right heart in adults: a report from the American Society of Echocardiography endorsed by the European Association of Echocardiography, a registered branch of the European Society of Cardiology, and the Canadian Society of Echocardiography. *J Am Soc Echocardiogr.* Jul 2010;23(7):685-713.

42. Pai RG, Bansal RC, Shah PM. Determinants of the rate of right ventricular pressure rise by Doppler echocardiography: potential value in the assessment of right ventricular function. *J Heart Valve Dis.* Mar 1994;3(2):179-184.

43. Kanzaki H, Nakatani S, Kawada T, Yamagishi M, Sunagawa K, Miyatake K. Right ventricular dP/dt/P(max), not dP/dt(max), noninvasively derived from tricuspid regurgitation velocity is a useful index of right ventricular contractility. *J Am Soc Echocardiogr.* Feb 2002;15(2):136-142.

44. Tei C, Dujardin KS, Hodge DO, et al. Doppler echocardiographic index for assessment of global right ventricular function. *J Am Soc Echocardiogr.* Nov-Dec 1996;9(6):838-847.

45. Schroeder RA, Bar-Yosef S, Mark JB. Evaluation of right heart function. In: Mathew JP, Swaminathan M, Ayoub CM, eds. *Clinical Manual and Review of Transesophageal Echocardiography.* New York: McGraw Hill; 2010:298-315.

46. Shanewise JS, Cheung AT, Aronson S, et al. ASE/SCA guidelines for performing a comprehensive intraoperative multiplane transesophageal echocardiography examination: recommendations of the American Society of Echocardiography Council for Intraoperative Echocardiography and the Society of Cardiovascular Anesthesiologists Task Force for Certification in Perioperative Transesophageal Echocardiography. *Anesth Analg.* 1999;89(4):870-884.

47. Baumgartner H, Hung J, Bermejo J, et al. Echocardiographic assessment of valve stenosis: EAE/ASE recommendations for clinical practice. *J Am Soc Echocardiogr.* Jan 2009;22(1):1-23.

48. Soliman OI, Anwar AM, Metawei AK, McGhie JS, Geleijnse ML, Ten Cate FJ. New scores for the assessment of mitral stenosis using real-time three-dimensional echocardiography. *Curr Cardiovasc Imaging Rep.* Oct 2011;4(5):370-377.

49. Anwar AM, Attia WM, Nosir YF, et al. Validation of a new score for the assessment of mitral stenosis using real-time three-dimensional echocardiography. *J Am Soc Echocardiogr.* Jan 2010;23(1):13-22.

50. Zoghbi WA, Enriquez-Sarano M, Foster E, et al. Recommendations for evaluation of the severity of native valvular regurgitation with two-dimensional and Doppler echocardiography. *J Am Soc Echocardiogr.* Jul 2003;16(7):777-802.

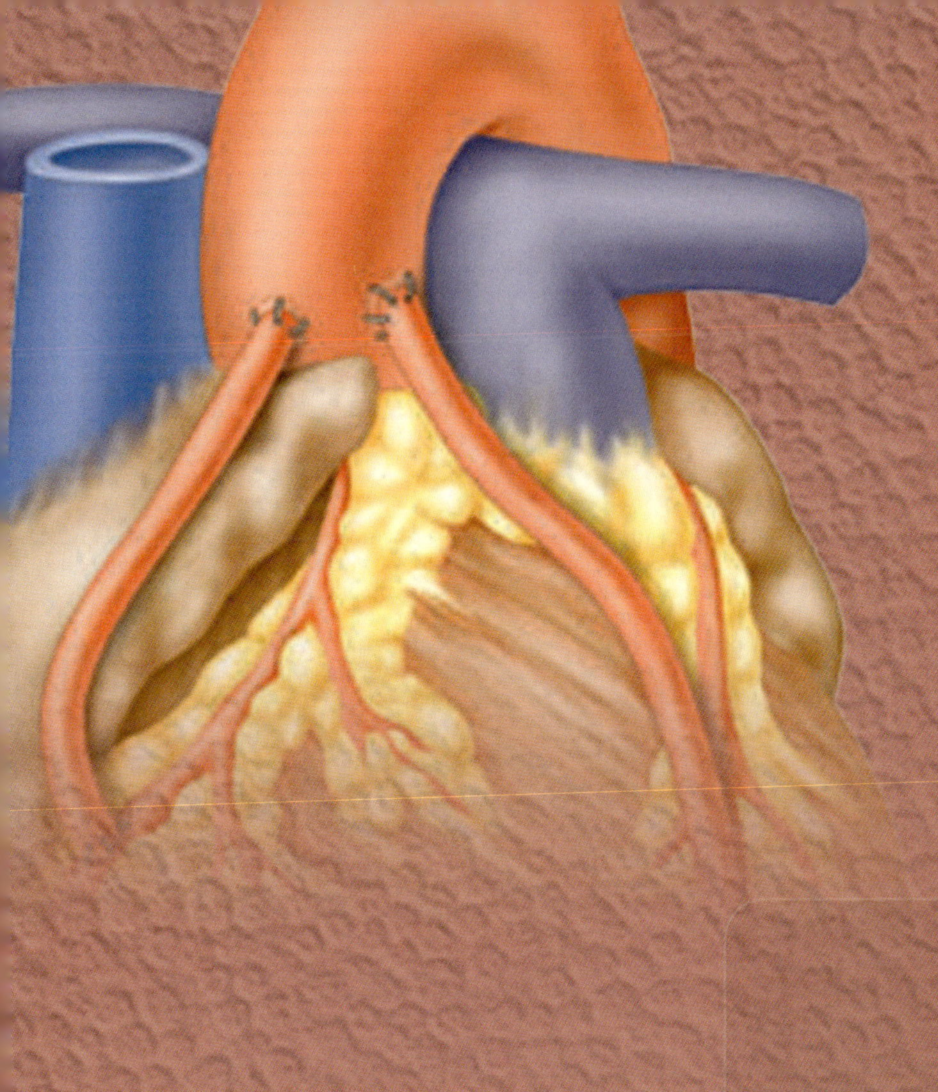

Understanding How Transesophageal Echocardiography Demonstrates Cardiovascular Pathology

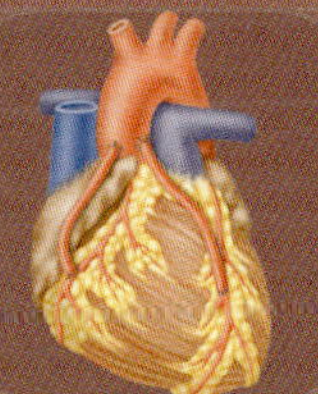

Myocardial Ischemia and Aortic Atherosclerosis

ANTOINE G. ROCHON | PIERRE COUTURE | ALAIN DESCHAMPS | ANDRÉ Y. DENAULT

Transesophageal echocardiography (TEE) has become a powerful diagnostic tool in the perioperative period. A recent updated report of practice guidelines for perioperative TEE by the American Society of Anesthesiologists (ASA) and the Society of Cardiovascular Anesthesiologists (SCA) recommends its use in all open heart surgeries and thoracic aortic procedures, and that its use be considered in coronary artery bypass grafting (CABG) surgeries.[1] This chapter will focus on TEE's uses in the evaluation of perioperative myocardial ischemia, complications of coronary artery disease, and assessment of aortic atherosclerosis.

Coronary Anatomy and Myocardial Function

The coronary arteries provide blood flow to the myocardium. They originate from the sinuses of Valsalva. The left main coronary artery gives rise to the left anterior descending coronary artery (LAD) and to the circumflex coronary artery from the left sinus of Valsalva. The LAD descends to the left ventricular (LV) apex in the anterior ventricular groove and gives diagonal and septal branches. The circumflex coronary artery courses laterally in the left atrioventricular groove, dividing into obtuse marginal branches. The right coronary artery (RCA) originates in the right sinus of Valsalva and descends medially in the right atrioventricular groove. The left main coronary and the right coronary arteries can sometimes be visualized at their origin in the sinuses of Valsalva in the midesophageal long-axis view and in the midesophageal short-axis view of the aortic valve (Fig. 13-1).

Studies correlating coronary angiography and echocardiography have described the specific coronary perfusion of each LV segment.[2] The LAD supplies blood to the anterior segments of the interventricular septum (IVS), to the anterior LV free wall, and to the septal and anterior segments of the apex. The circumflex artery provides blood to the inferolateral and anterolateral LV segments as well as to the lateral apex. The RCA provides blood to the right ventricle, the LV inferior free wall, the inferior half of the septum, and the inferior apex. Given the coronary distribution, ischemic lesions will translate into regional wall motion abnormalities (WMAs) that can identify the coronary culprit (Fig. 13-2).

Myocardial Segments

The American Heart Association (AHA) recommends the use of the 17-segment model,[2] whereas the American Society of Echocardiography (ASE) recommends the use of the 16-segment model (Fig. 13-3).[3] In both models, the LV is divided from its base to the apex into different levels or imaging planes: basal, midpapillary, apical and, in the AHA model, an apical cap that corresponds to the 17th segment. The levels correspond to the proximal, middle, and apical territories of the coronary arteries. The basal and midpapillary levels each have six segments (anteroseptal, anterior, anterolateral, inferoseptal, inferior, and inferolateral), whereas there are four apical segments (septal, anterior, lateral, and inferior). Confusion can arise with the segment numbering adopted by the AHA and the ASE. In the AHA 17-segment model,

starting with the basal anterior segment, each segment is numbered in a clockwise fashion (see Fig. 13-3, *A*), whereas in the ASE 16-segment model, starting with the basal anteroseptal segment, each segment is numbered in a counterclockwise fashion (see Fig. 13-3, *B*). Most TEE views allow identification of some of the LV segments, and WMAs can be correlated with the coronary artery perfusion territory, helping identify the stenotic/problematic vessel.

Normal Segmental Function

As the LV contracts, its endocardial border moves toward the center of the ventricular cavity (endocardial excursion or radial shortening), resulting in LV myocardium thickening and reduced LV cavity area. Normal LV radial shortening and myocardial thickening is greater than 30%.[4] The regional wall motion scoring index provides a subjective yet effective means to assess LV function and detect and quantify acute myocardial ischemia (Table 13-1). However, heterogeneity of normal segmental wall motion, left bundle branch block, right ventricular volume overload, constrictive pericarditis, pacemaker rhythm, and post–cardiac surgery period must all be taken into account, since these elements can alter interventricular septal wall motion.

Evaluation of WMA has many limitations, including important regional differences in normal myocardial contractility.[5] In fact, a reduced myocardial thickening is more specific than WMA for identifying ischemia.[6] Furthermore, movements of the ventricular segments are affected by the rotation and translation of the heart, so a floating frame should be used (Fig. 13-4). These movements can also be subject to tethering of the adjacent myocardium. This can result in overestimation of the ischemic area. The transgastric (TG) midpapillary short-axis view is often used to detect ischemia. However, in this view, only 6 segments (7, 8, 9, 10, 11, and 12) are evaluated. One study[7] found that the midpapillary short-axis view allowed detection of only 17% of new WMAs, whereas an additional 48% of WMAs were detected by the concomitant evaluation of other short-axis planes and an additional 35% of new WMAs in the long-axis views alone. This emphasizes the importance of carrying out the analysis of WMA in more than one plane and, ideally, in all 17 segments. Finally, intraoperative regional WMAs are diagnosed on real-time TEE (on-line), and some ischemic episodes may be missed.[8]

The distinction between stunned or hibernating myocardium and infarcted or ischemic myocardium is another limitation of the evaluation of WMAs. A stunned myocardium suffers from prolonged post-ischemic contractile dysfunction and has been clinically observed in stress-induced angina, unstable angina, post-thrombolysis, post-percutaneous transluminal angioplasty (PTCA), and post-CABG surgery. It may take several weeks for the stunned myocardium to recover normal function.

Segmental Wall Motion Analysis

Segmental WMAs take place in the myocardium seconds after myocardial blood flow to the affected segment is interrupted, long before electrocardiographic (ECG) changes and angina occur. WMAs are classified as *hypokinetic* when ventricular contraction is reduced in magnitude, *akinetic* when it is absent, and *dyskinetic* in the presence of

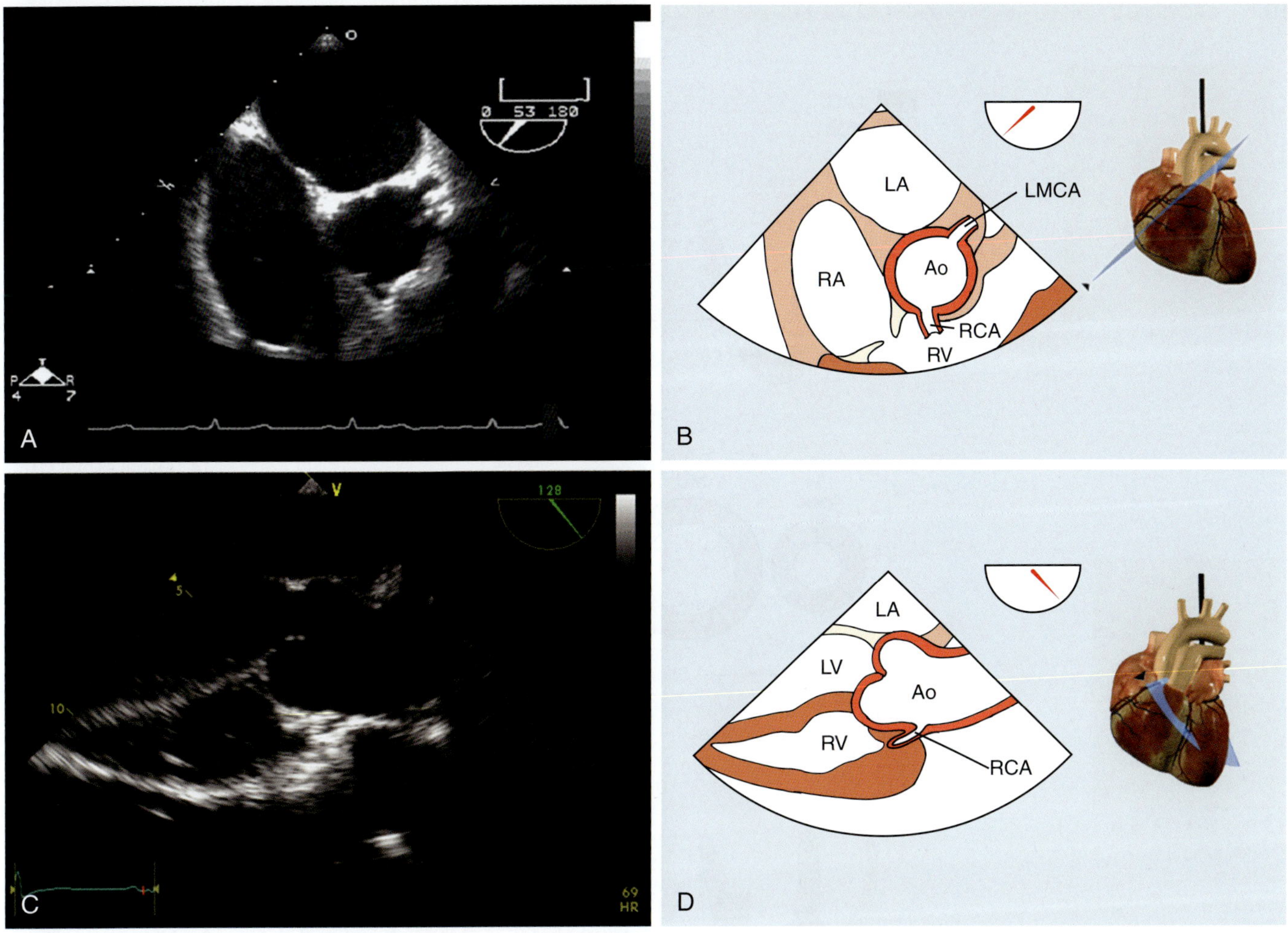

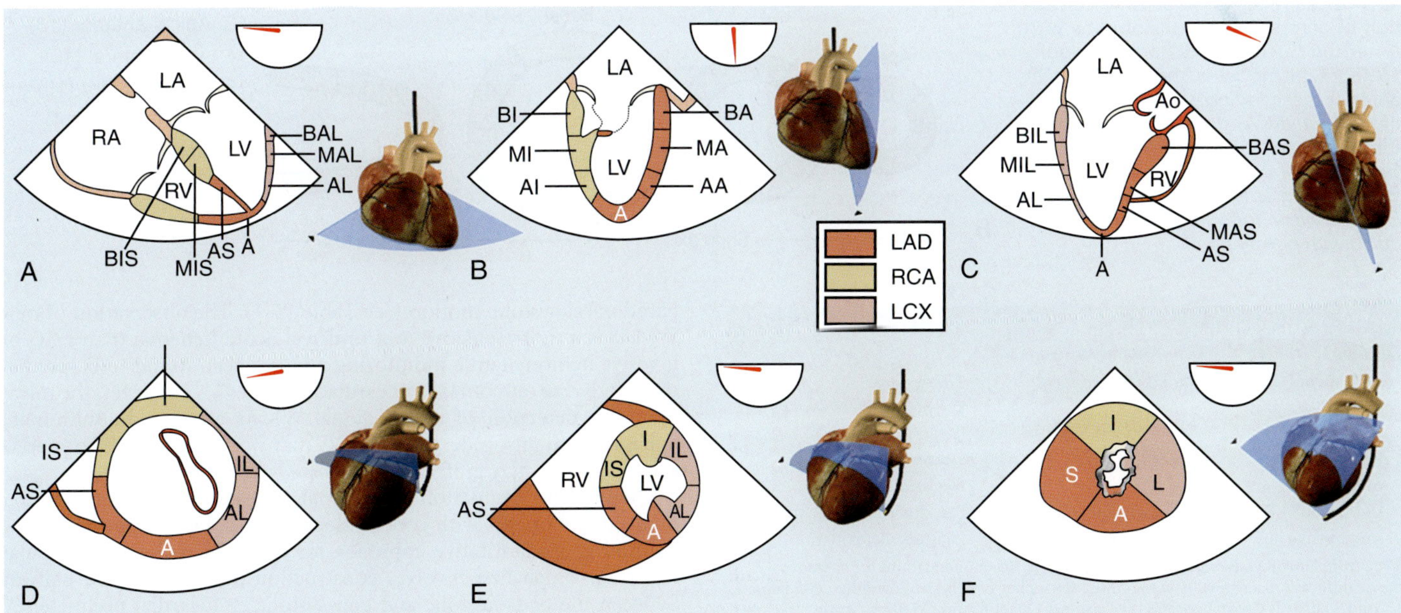

Figure 13-1 Coronary ostia. **A** and **B,** Midesophageal short-axis view of ascending aorta, with both coronary ostia visualized above aortic valve. **C** and **D,** Midesophageal long-axis view with proximal ascending aorta showing right coronary artery ostium. *Ao,* Aorta; *LA,* left atrium; *LMCA,* left main coronary artery; *LV,* left ventricle; *RA,* right atrium; *RCA,* right coronary artery; *RV,* right ventricle. *(From Denault AY, Couture P, Vegas A, Buithieu J, Tardif J-C. Transesophageal Echocardiography Multimedia Manual. 2nd ed. New York: Informa Healthcare; 2011, with permission.)*

Figure 13-2 Left ventricular *(LV)* function. **A, B,** and **C,** Midesophageal views to evaluate right ventricular and LV function: four-chamber, two-chamber, and long-axis views. *A,* Apex; *AA,* apical anterior; *AI,* apical inferior; *AL,* apical lateral; *Ao,* aorta; *AS,* apical septal; *BA,* basal anterior; *BAL,* basal anterolateral; *BAS,* basal anteroseptal; *BI,* basal inferior; *BIL,* basal inferolateral; *BIS,* basal inferoseptal; *LA,* left atrium; *LAD,* left anterior descending; *LCX,* left circumflex artery; *LV,* left ventricle; *MA,* mid-anterior; *MAL,* mid-anterolateral; *MAS,* mid-anteroseptal; *MI,* mid-inferior; *MIL,* mid-inferolateral; *MIS,* mid-inferoseptal; *RA,* right atrium; *RCA,* right coronary artery; *RV,* right ventricle. **D, E,** and **F,** Basal, mid-, and apical transgastric short-axis views. *A,* Anterior; *AL,* anterolateral; *AS,* anteroseptal; *I,* inferior; *IL,* inferolateral; *IS,* inferoseptal; *L,* lateral; *LAD,* left anterior descending; *LCX,* left circumflex artery; *LV,* left ventricle; *RCA,* right coronary artery; *RV,* right ventricle; *S,* septal. *(Adapted from Denault AY, Couture P, Vegas A, Buithieu J, Tardif J-C. Transesophageal Echocardiography Multimedia Manual. 2nd ed. New York: Informa Healthcare; 2011, with permission.)*

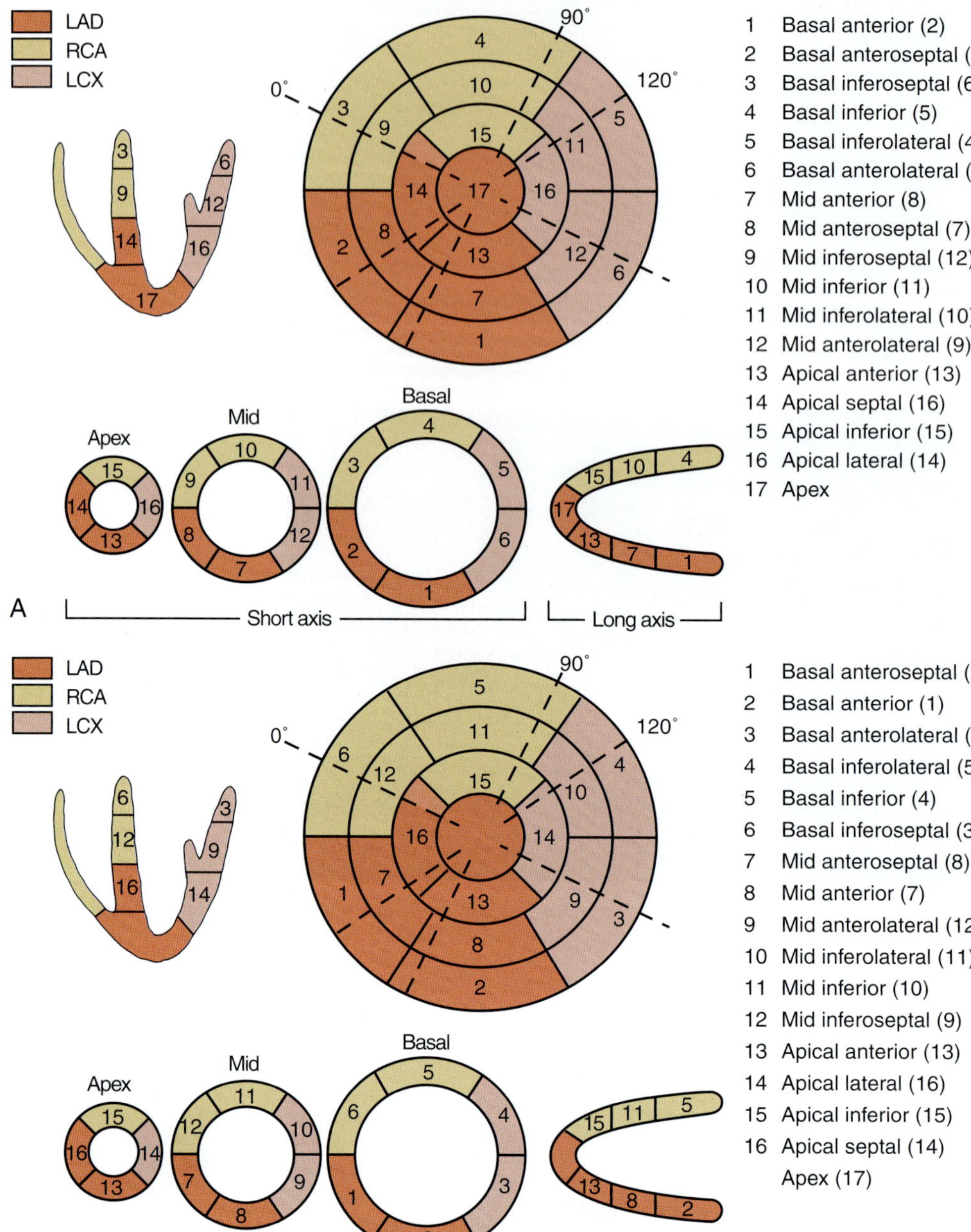

Figure 13-3 **A,** Segmental model of left ventricle. Transesophageal echocardiographic correlation of coronary artery distribution with American Heart Association 17-segment model is shown. **B,** Segmental model of left ventricle. Transesophageal echocardiographic correlation of coronary artery distribution with American Society of Echocardiography 16-segment model is shown. *LAD,* Left anterior descending; *LCX,* left circumflex artery; *RCA,* right coronary artery. *(From Denault AY, Couture P, Vegas A, Buithieu J, Tardif J-C. Transesophageal Echocardiography Multimedia Manual. 2nd ed. New York: Informa Healthcare; 2011, with permission.)*

TABLE 13-1	Wall Motion Scoring Index		
Movement	*Radial Displacement*	*Thickening*	
Normal or hyperkinesis = 1	>30%	Normal	
Hypokinesis = 2	0-30%	Decreased	
Akinesis = 3	0%	Negligible	
Dyskinesis = 4	Systolic lengthening	Paradoxical systolic motion	
Aneurysmal = 5	Paradoxical displacement	Diastolic deformation	

Data from Lang RM, Bierig M, Devereux RB, et al. Recommendations for chamber quantification: a report from the American Society of Echocardiography's Guidelines and Standards Committee and the Chamber Quantification Writing Group, developed in conjunction with the European Association of Echocardiography, a branch of the European Society of Cardiology. *J Am Soc Echocardiogr.* 2005;18:1440-1463.

paradoxical systolic motion (see Table 13-1). The observation of new WMAs is a more sensitive tool to detect acute ischemia than ECG or invasive hemodynamic monitoring and has been found to be predictive of adverse outcomes after cardiac surgery.[4,9,10] However, the intraoperative detection of new regional WMAs after cardiopulmonary bypass in patients undergoing CABG may not be as reliable to predict acute postoperative graft failure.[11]

Quantitative evaluation of regional LV systolic function requires high-quality images with good endocardial resolution. The centerline method is a quantitative approach for assessing regional ventricular function, which first involves construction of a line located halfway between the end-diastolic and end-systolic endocardial perimeters.[12] The endocardial excursion is determined along 100 equally spaced chords perpendicular to the centerline. Motion is then normalized for heart size by dividing it by the length of the end-diastolic perimeter. The normalized length of each line is then converted into units of standard deviation (SD) from the mean excursion along a given chord. This method allows the regional heterogeneity of ventricular contraction to be taken into account (Fig. 13-5). By convention, negative and positive values indicate hypokinetic and hyperkinetic chords, respectively. The extent of abnormal wall motion is calculated as the number of hypokinetic chords equal to or more severe than two SDs. The severity of WMAs is calculated as the area under the curve below the zero SD line.

Wall Motion Score Index

The Wall Motion Score Index (WMSI) is a semiquantitative assessment of regional LV contraction. Each of the 17 segments is given a score on a scale of 1 to 5. A score of 1 is given to normally contracting or hyperkinetic segments (>30% thickening), 2 for hypokinetic segments (10%-30% thickening), 3 for akinetic segments (<10% thickening), 4 for dyskinetic segments (paradoxical systolic motion), and 5 for aneurysmal (diastolic deformation) segments (see Table 13-1).[13] The WMSI is equal to the sum of the regional scores divided by the number of evaluable segments. It ranges from 1.0 in the normal heart to 3.9 in severe systolic dysfunction. The WMSI has been shown to have prognostic value in clinical studies. Berning et al.[14] found that patients in acute myocardial infarction with a higher (i.e., worse) WMSI had a higher cardiovascular mortality at 1 year (51%) than patients with a lower (i.e., better) WMSI (cardiovascular death at 1 year of 8%). Kan et al.[15] observed similar results and found a mortality rate of 61% in patients with a higher WMSI by comparison to 3% in patients with a lower WMSI.

Tissue Doppler Imaging

Tissue Doppler imaging (TDI) filters out the high-velocity signals from blood to isolate the low-velocity, high-amplitude signals of movement of the myocardium. Combined with pulsed wave (PW) Doppler, it allows for the analysis of direction and velocity of individual segments of myocardium to quantify regional wall motion (Fig. 13-6).[16] Mean values of 5.5 cm/s and maximum velocities below 7.5 cm/s are indicative of myocardial failure. Decreases in regional myocardial velocities during ischemia have been observed in clinical studies.[17-19] However, the simultaneous analysis of multiple segments is only possible offline, even though this can be done intraoperatively. Furthermore, because they are based on the Doppler equation, measured velocities will be inaccurate if the Doppler beam is not parallel to the movement of the interrogated segment. Finally, akinetic segments tethered by the adjacent contracting myocardium will have near-normal velocities, and because of poor spatial resolution, the differentiation between subendocardium and subepicardium is not possible.

Color Tissue Doppler Imaging

Color TDI superimposes color-coded tissue velocity onto a real-time live two-dimensional (2D) image. Color TDI evaluates mean velocities from each pixel so that the velocity is lower than that of PW spectral TDI, which measures peak velocities at the sample volume. Compared to pulsed TDI, color TDI has superior spatial resolution, which enables simultaneous evaluation of multiple segments. It can be displayed in different formats as velocity against time for each segment or as a curved M-mode (see Fig. 13-6).

Strain and Strain Rate

In systole, the myocardium shortens its length, while it elongates during diastole. *Strain* is used to measure this deformation during the cardiac

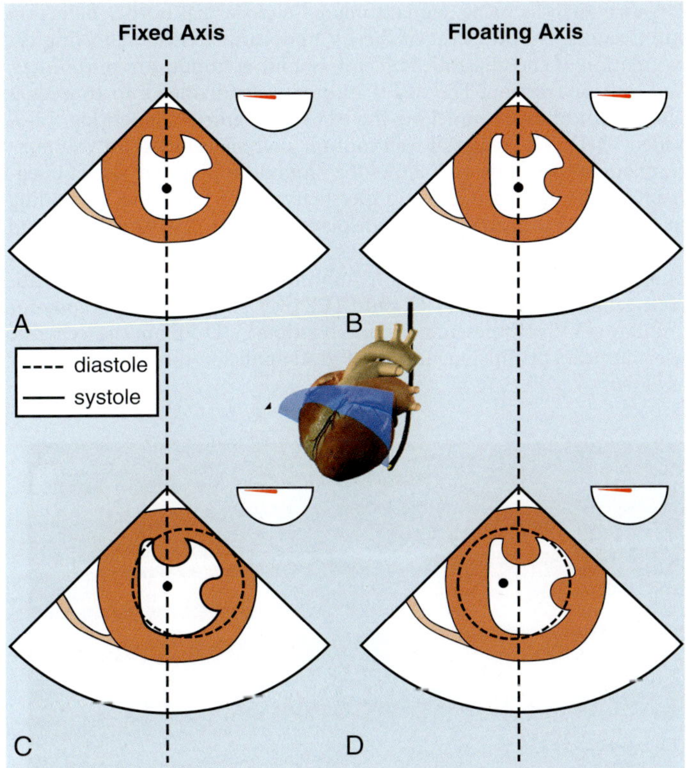

Figure 13-4 Abnormal septal motion. Transgastric mid–short-axis view using a fixed axis (**A, C**) or a floating axis (**B, D**). In a patient with left bundle branch block, with a fixed axis, abnormal septal motion is identified without rotational artifact. With a floating axis, center of image is displaced to the left, but normal segment appears hypokinetic. (*Adapted from Denault AY, Couture P, Vegas A, Buithieu J, Tardif J-C. Transesophageal Echocardiography Multimedia Manual.* 2nd ed. *New York: Informa Healthcare; 2011, with permission.*)

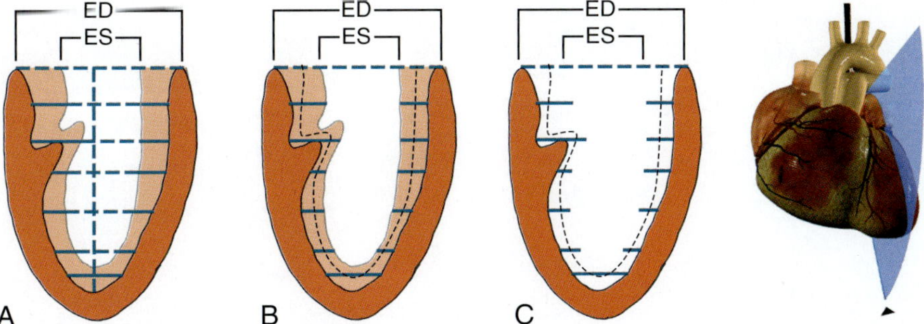

Figure 13-5 Centroid reference systems. **A,** Parallel chords drawn from centroid (long axis) trace endocardial border during end-systole (*ES*) and end-diastole (*ED*) in this midesophageal two-chamber view. **B** and **C,** Centerline method traces ED and ES endocardial borders, and computer draws a centerline midway between these endocardial borders. Note slightly greater systolic thickening in anterior wall. (*Adapted from Denault AY, Couture P, Vegas A, Buithieu J, Tardif J-C. Transesophageal Echocardiography Multimedia Manual.* 2nd ed. *New York: Informa Healthcare; 2011, with permission.*)

cycle. It is defined as the change in myocardial length in relation to myocardial initial length divided by the initial length. The rate of myocardial deformation is called *strain rate* (SR) (Fig. 13-7). Myocardial ischemia translates into a decreased deformation and causes reductions in systolic strain and SR. By convention, myocardial shortening has a negative SR, while myocardial lengthening has a positive strain. Radial strain is measured in the TG midpapillary short-axis (SAX) view and will be positive during systole (Fig. 13-8). Longitudinal strain is measured in midesophageal views and is positive during diastole.

Strain is an off-line measure obtained from saved TDI loops or using 2D speckle tracking technology. It corresponds to the integration of SR over time. Strain and SR can be displayed as a function of time or as curved anatomic M-mode images. Radial and segmental strain and SR will have different values depending on the interrogated myocardial segment (Table 13-2).[20] Strain will be reduced in the ischemic myocardium and absent in the infarcted heart muscle. The ratio of systolic strain to the sum of postsystolic strain and systolic strain relates to the level of ischemia.[21]

Limitations of strain and SR include their high sensitivity to noise and their dependence on the Doppler equation, the accuracy of which depends on the proper alignment of the ultrasound beam to the direction of tissue motion.

Speckle Tracking

Speckle tracking is a technique based on the tracking of interference patterns and natural acoustic reflections created by B-mode imaging.[22] These reflections are described as "speckles" and will have unique patterns for each myocardial segment. With this technique, the myocardial velocities are not dependent on the Doppler angle, thus permitting simultaneous 2D radial and longitudinal assessments (see Fig. 13-8).

Three-Dimensional TEE

Three-dimensional (3D) TEE is a promising new analytic modality that has been shown to correlate well with cardiac computed tomography (CT) and magnetic resonance imaging (MRI) analysis of LV morphology and function.[23] However, poor 2D TEE images will result in a poor-quality full-volume 3D dataset, emphasizing the importance of acquiring high-quality 2D images. Full-volume acquisition and off-line software analysis using semiautomated endocardial border detection will create a dynamic cast of the LV endocardial cavity, allowing for calculation of end-diastolic and end-systolic volumes, stroke volumes, and ejection fraction. The cast is automatically divided into 16 wedges plus an apical cap, mimicking the AHA 17-segment model (Fig. 13-9, Video 13-1). The regional wall motion analysis is based on volumetric changes over time and allows for rapid detection of dyskinetic segments with high sensitivity and specificity.[24] ASE guidelines pertaining to the acquisition, analysis, and display of cardiac structures in 3D and including a description of current and potential clinical applications of 3D echocardiography recently published recommend 3D transthoracic echocardiography (TTE) and TEE over 2D echocardiography for evaluating LV volumes and ejection fraction.[25] 3D TEE in the ischemic heart appears promising, and its clinical application has to be further assessed.

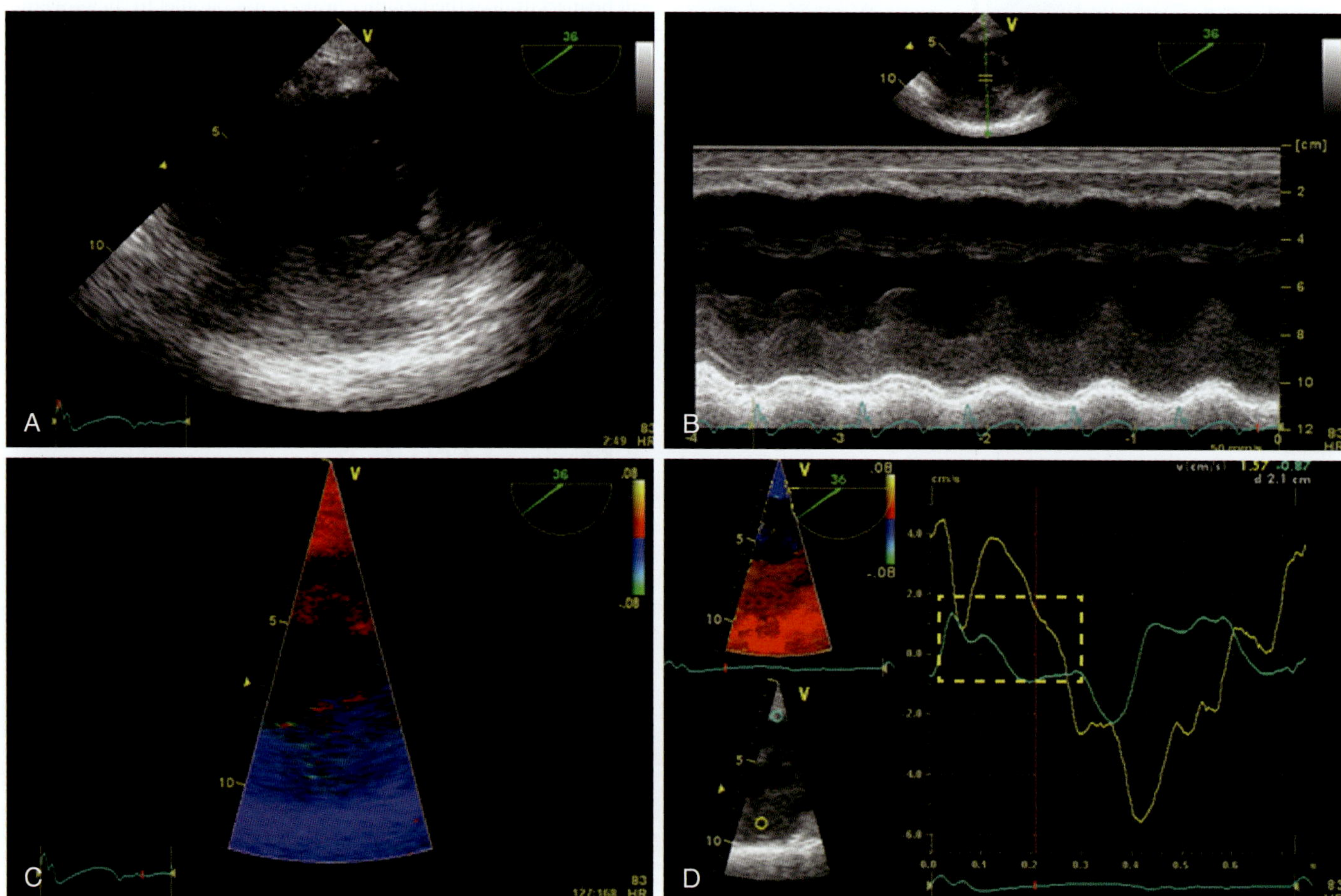

Figure 13-6 Tissue Doppler imaging (TDI) with inferior hypokinesis. **A,** Midpapillary transgastric view of a 77-year-old man with a previous inferior wall myocardial infarction. Corresponding M-mode is shown. Note reduced excursion of inferior wall **(B)**. **C,** TDI on same region. TD velocities are obtained on anterior wall *(yellow)* and inferior wall *(blue)*. Note abnormal systolic excursion of inferior wall **(D)** indicated in dotted red square. TD velocities are characteristic of regional dyskinesia.

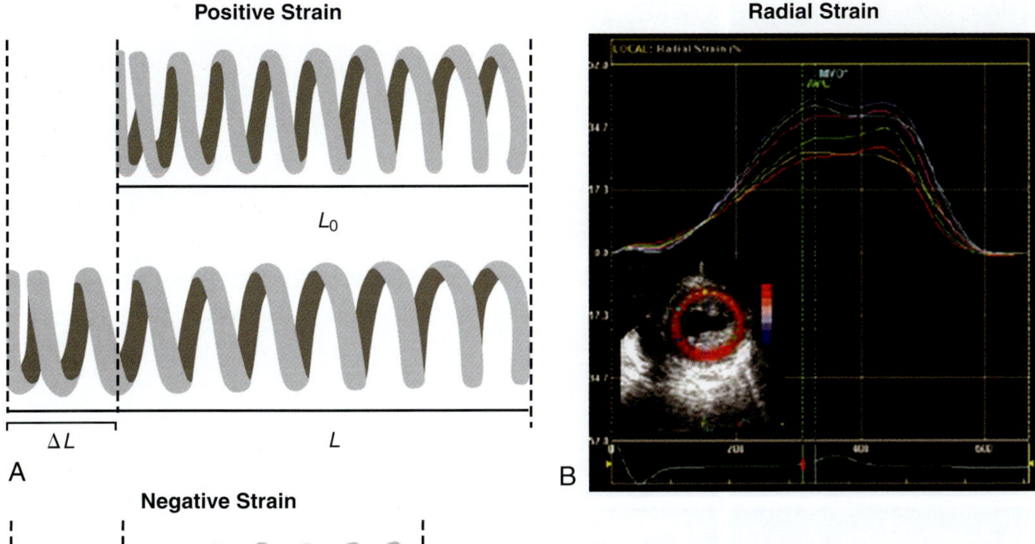

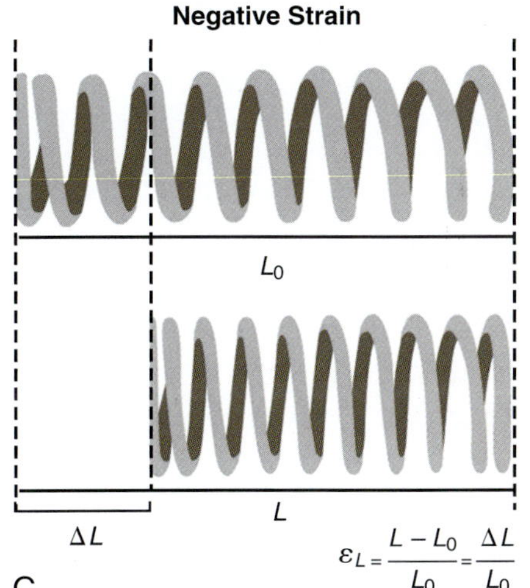

$$\varepsilon_L = \frac{L - L_0}{L_0} = \frac{\Delta L}{L_0}$$

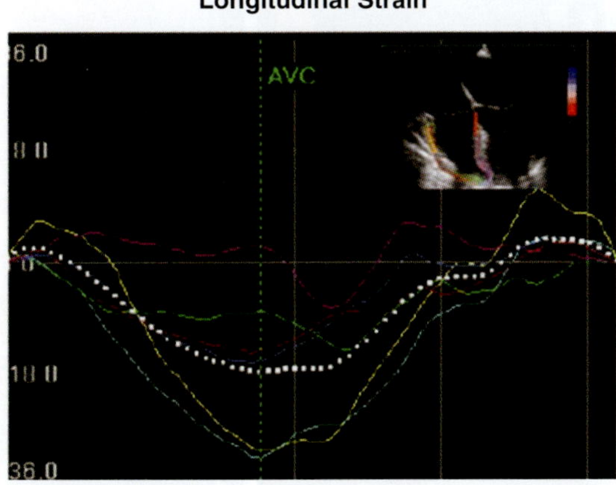

Figure 13-7 Strain (ε), or deformation concept. **A** and **B,** When strain is positive, initial length value (L_0) is smaller than the final one (L). For instance, in transgastric mid–short-axis view, myocardial thickness increases during radial shortening. The radial strain obtained from this view will be positive (thickening). **C** and **D,** The opposite applies for a negative strain. Typically the longitudinal contraction of left ventricle obtained from a midesophageal four-chamber view has a negative systolic strain. *(From Denault AY, Couture P, Vegas A, Buithieu J, Tardif J-C.* Transesophageal Echocardiography Multimedia Manual. *2nd ed. New York: Informa Healthcare; 2011, with permission.)*

Dobutamine Stress Echocardiography

New segmental WMAs may be the consequence of inadequate myocardial revascularization, ongoing ischemia, or stunned myocardium. Dobutamine is a positive inotrope at low doses (5-10 µg/kg/min) and has chronotropic effects at higher doses. The increased contractility observed in a hypokinetic or akinetic segment of a heart subjected to dobutamine suggests that regional systolic function may improve following revascularization in the hibernating myocardium[26] or spontaneously in the stunned heart segment.[27] Dobutamine stress echocardiography is not routinely performed in the intraoperative setting.

Diastolic Function

The onset of ischemia rapidly translates into diastolic dysfunction, often faster than the appearance of systolic dysfunction and regional WMAs. Patterns of diastolic abnormalities can be identified and are associated with impaired myocardial relaxation and/or compliance (Fig. 13-10).

Impaired LV relaxation results in an increased delay between aortic valve closure and mitral valve (MV) opening, as seen by prolonged isovolumic relaxation time (IVRT ≥100 ms), slower decay of the atrioventricular gradient in early diastole (deceleration time ≥270 ms), reduced rapid ventricular filling (reduced E-wave velocity) due to a reduced pressure gradient between the atrium and the ventricle after MV opening, and a greater contribution of left atrium (LA) contraction to ventricular filling (increased A-wave velocity), resulting in an E/A ratio less than 1. Mild diastolic dysfunction (relaxation abnormality) will usually be associated with a prominent systolic component of the pulmonary venous inflow. Moderate diastolic dysfunction (pseudonormal pattern), which is associated with an elevation of the left ventricular end diastolic pressure (LVEDP), is manifested in the pulmonary veins by an increase in the maximal velocity (peak velocity ≥35 cm/s) and duration (at least 30 milliseconds more than the mitral A-wave duration) of the A-reversal wave during atrial contraction. This pattern is characterized by a normal E/A ratio, and the deceleration time is normal because of an increase in the left atrial pressure (LAP).

In severe diastolic dysfunction (restriction to filling secondary to poor compliance), the Doppler pattern is different. The peak E-wave velocity will be increased and accompanied by a short deceleration time as LV and left atrial pressures rapidly equilibrate (Fig. 13-11). There is a markedly shortened or nonexistent diastasis plateau. Because of the elevated LV diastolic pressure, the atrial contraction A-wave is decreased. The E/A ratio is greater than 2, the deceleration time less than 150 milliseconds, and the IVRT less than 70 milliseconds.

A pseudonormal pattern characterized by a normal E/A ratio and normal deceleration time exists between these two opposite abnormalities because of an increase in the left atrial pressure (see Fig. 13-10).

Complications of Myocardial Ischemia and Associated Findings

Left Ventricular Thrombus

With the advent of thrombolytic therapy, LV thrombus formation is now a relatively infrequent complication of acute myocardial

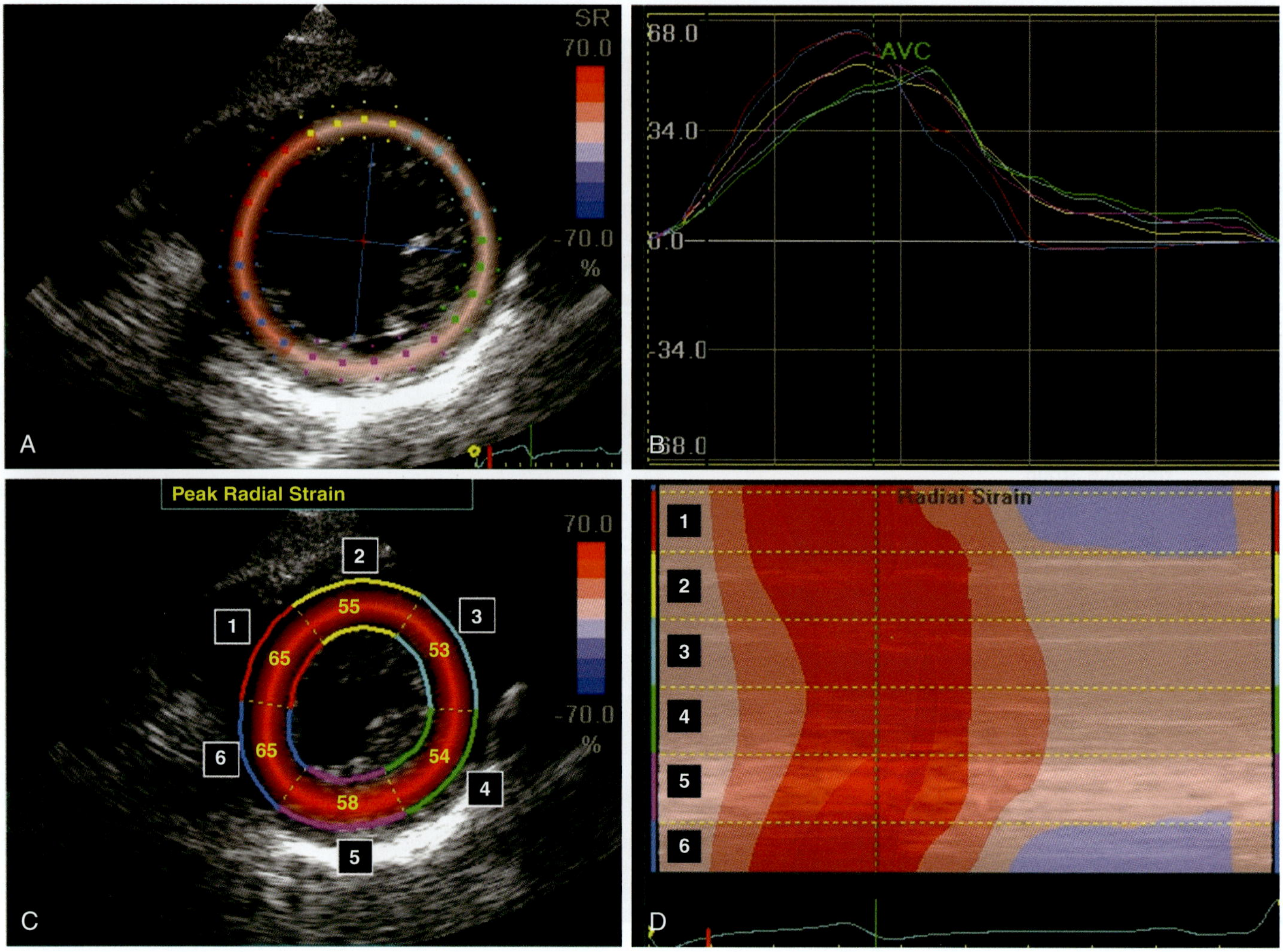

Figure 13-8 Radial strain by two-dimensional speckle tracking in a normal patient. **A** and **C**, Transgastric mid–short-axis view with radial strain overlay. Peak radial strain has a positive value for all left ventricular (LV) segments because of myocardial thickening during systole. **B** and **D**, The change in peak radial strain of each LV segment can be displayed as individual tracings over time (**B**) or as a curved M-mode map over time (**D**). *(From Denault AY, Couture P, Vegas A, Buithieu J, Tardif J-C. Transesophageal Echocardiography Multimedia Manual. 2nd ed. New York: Informa Healthcare; 2011, with permission.)*

TABLE 13-2	Strain Rate of Individual Segments			
	Septum	*Lateral*	*Inferior*	*Anterior*
Peak Systolic Wave (Ssr)				
Basal	0.99 ± 0.49	1.5 ± 0.74	0.88 ± 0.39	1.64 ± 0.9
Mid	1.25 ± 0.73	1.29 ± 0.58	0.95 ± 0.54	0.98 ± 0.68
Apical	1.15 ± 0.5	1.09 ± 0.59	1.38 ± 0.45	1.05 ± 0.63
Early Diastolic Wave (Esr)				
Basal	1.95 ± 0.89	1.92 ± 1.11	1.85 ± 0.89	2.03 ± 0.99
Mid	1.94 ± 0.97	1.71 ± 0.66	1.92 ± 1.2	1.7 ± 0.82
Apical	1.91 ± 0.66	1.81 ± 0.87	2.29 ± 0.88	1.76 ± 0.98
Late Diastolic Wave (Asr)				
Basal	1.54 ± 0.93	0.93 ± 0.59	1.18 ± 0.78	1.49 ± 0.96
Mid	1.29 ± 0.86	1.48 ± 0.77	0.78 ± 0.62	1.04 ± 0.57
Apical	0.95 ± 0.54	1.07 ± 0.68	1.68 ± 0.76	0.68 ± 0.65

Peak systolic (Ssr), early (Esr), and late (Asr) diastolic strain rates shown in 1/s.
Data from Denault AY, Couture P, Vegas A, Buithieu J, Tardif J-C. *Transesophageal Echocardiography Multimedia Manual.* 2nd ed. New York: Informa Healthcare; 2011.

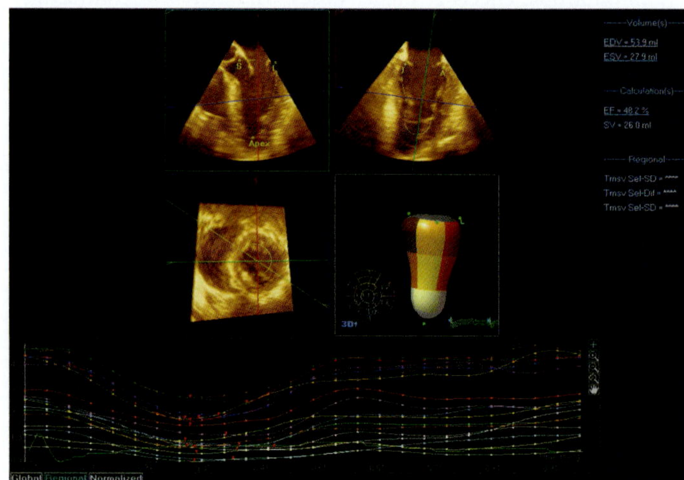
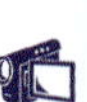

Figure 13-9 Three-dimensional (3D) cast of left ventricle (LV) (see Video 13-1), with ejection fraction calculated using automated border detection. American Heart Association LV segments are represented with color, and change in volume of each of the 17 segments is plotted over time and displayed in lower diagram.

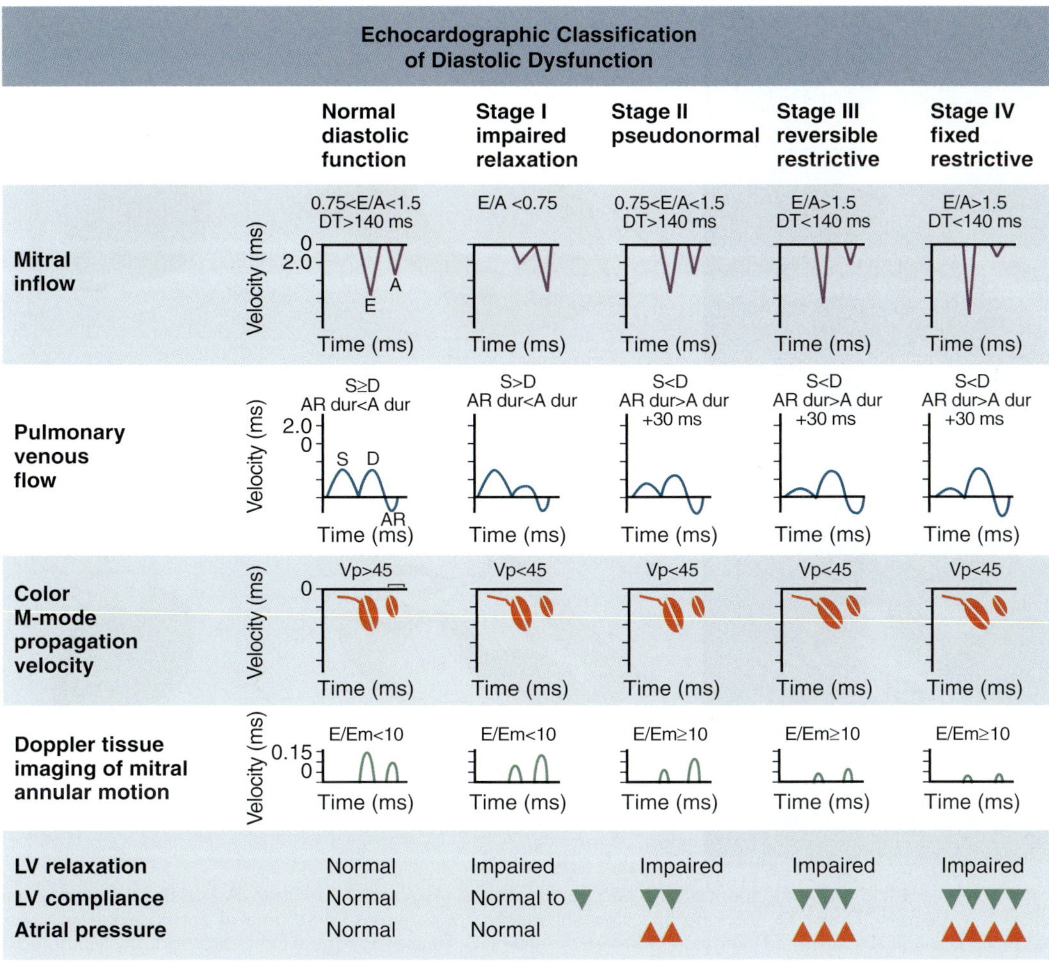

Figure 13-10 Diastolic dysfunction classification. Echocardiographic classification of diastolic dysfunction adapted for transesophageal echocardiography is shown. *A*, Peak late diastolic transmitral flow velocity; *A dur*, duration of mitral inflow A-wave; *AR dur*, peak pulmonary venous atrial reversal flow velocity duration; *D*, peak diastolic pulmonary venous flow velocity; *DT*, deceleration time; *E*, peak early diastolic transmitral flow velocity; *Em*, peak early diastolic myocardial velocity; *LV*, left ventricle; *S*, peak systolic pulmonary venous flow velocity; *Vp*, flow propagation velocity. (*Adapted from Denault AY, Couture P, Vegas A, Buithieu J, Tardif J-C. Transesophageal Echocardiography Multimedia Manual. 2nd ed. New York: Informa Healthcare; 2011, with permission.*)

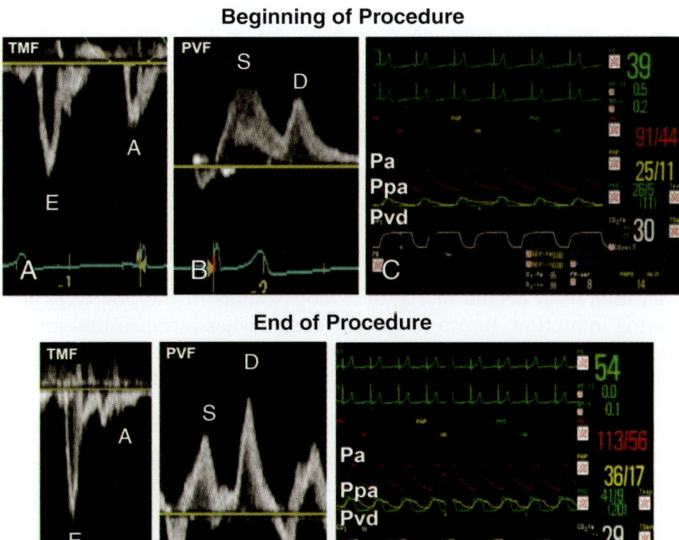

Figure 13-11 Diastolic function. Transmitral flow *(TMF)* **(A)** and pulmonary venous flow *(PVF)* **(B)** with corresponding hemodynamic waveforms **(C)** before and after coronary revascularization **(D, E,** and **F)** in a 65-year-old man. Note change from a normal to a restrictive left ventricular diastolic pattern with associated increase in filling pressure. *A*, Atrial TMF velocity; *D*, diastolic PVF velocity; *E*, early TMF velocity; *Pa*, arterial pressure; *Ppa*, pulmonary artery pressure; *Pvd*, right ventricular pressure; *S*, systolic PVF velocity.

infarction. Large anterior wall infarction puts the patient particularly at risk of thrombus formation (Fig. 13-12), especially in the presence of a ventricular aneurysm. TEE may not be as efficient as TTE for detecting LV thrombi, compared to LA thrombi, because of the difficulty in visualizing the apex from the esophagus. In a study[28] comparing TTE to TEE, LV thrombi were identified with certainty in only 53% of patients with TEE compared to TTE, advocating for the complementarity of the two ultrasound modalities. The deep TG or TG two-chamber views are the most useful for their detection.

The risk of LV thrombus embolization during intraoperative heart manipulation warrants LV cavity exploration if an LV thrombus is suspected or possible.

Ischemic Mitral Regurgitation

Although rare (<1% of myocardial infarction), acute mitral regurgitation (MR) caused by partial or complete rupture of a papillary muscle, leading to severe mitral regurgitation and heart failure, requires emergent surgical intervention. Ischemic MR is more common, less severe, and results from segmental WMA. The posteromedial papillary muscle is particularly at risk in inferior wall infarction because of its single blood supply from the RCA, contrary to the anterolateral papillary muscle which receives blood from both the diagonal branches of the LAD and the circumflex coronary arteries.

Papillary muscle rupture is obvious when the head of the papillary muscle prolapses into the LA during systole. A flail mitral leaflet pointing toward the LA in systole may be observed. The regurgitant orifice will be large and the regurgitant flow less turbulent than in non-ischemic MR. Systolic reversal of the PW Doppler of the pulmonary

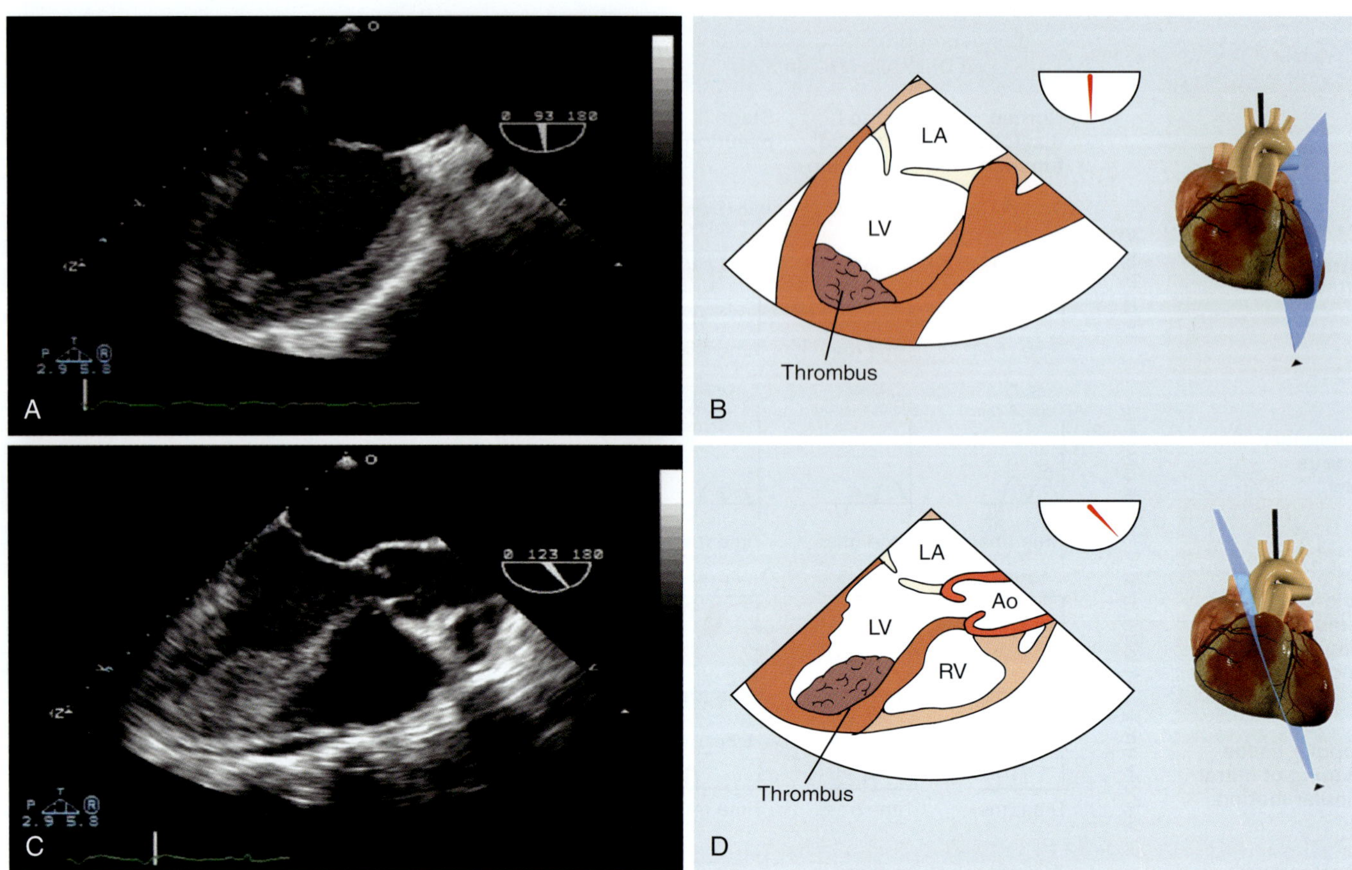

Figure 13-12   Thrombus and hematoma in left ventricle *(LV)* in a patient after a large anteroseptal myocardial infarction. **A** and **B**, Midesophageal (ME) two-chamber view with thrombus seen at LV apex. **C** and **D**, ME long-axis view showing a concomitant hematoma of anteroseptal wall. *Ao,* Aorta; *LA,* left atrium; *RV,* right ventricle. *(From Denault AY, Couture P, Vegas A, Buithieu J, Tardif J-C. Transesophageal Echocardiography Multimedia Manual. 2nd ed. New York: Informa Healthcare; 2011, with permission.)*

venous flow is important in evaluating the severity of MR in this setting because color Doppler techniques are often unreliable. Systolic reversal of pulmonary venous flow indicates severe MR.

Ventricular Dilation and Aneurysm

Within 48 hours of myocardial infarction, the infarcted zone may undergo stretching and thinning, leading to an increase in LV end-diastolic volume, which in turn leads to LV dilation, aneurysm formation, and myocardial wall rupture. Characteristics of LV dilation include an abrupt angulation of the contour of the proximal anteroseptal wall in the long-axis (LAX) view and a segmental dilation in the TG midpapillary short-axis (SAX) view. In the acute setting of transmural infarction, ventricular dilation will most likely involve the infarcted segment. However, complete remodeling of the entire LV cavity involving nonischemic segments may be observed later.

LV aneurysm is a common complication among survivors of non-reperfused transmural myocardial infarctions. Aneurysms occur four times more often at the apex and at the anterior wall than at the inferobasal wall (Fig. 13-13, Video 13-2). True aneurysms result from expansion of the infarcted area and thinning of the myocardium. All three layers of the ventricular wall are preserved. The aneurysm may cause angina, heart failure, or ventricular arrhythmias. On TEE, the aneurysmal segments are dyskinetic or akinetic, distorting the LV shape, and consist of an outpouching of ventricular myocardium with well-defined borders and a wide neck persisting in diastole.

In LV pseudoaneurysm, there is a rupture of the ventricular free wall, with a localized hemopericardium contained by the parietal pericardium (Fig. 13-14, Video 13-3). By contrast, in a true aneurysm, there is no myocardial rupture with outside blood loss (Fig. 13-15). LV

pseudoaneurysm is a rare complication of myocardial infarction. It can also be caused by trauma, laceration, or abscess. On TEE, it will appear as an outpouching connected to the LV cavity by a narrow neck, with an abrupt rupture of the myocardial wall. Bidirectional blood flow will be evidenced to and from the pseudoaneurysmal sac, which may contain thrombus material. In systole, expansion of the LV pseudoaneurysm contrasts with the LV cavity getting smaller.

Ventricular Septal Defect

A ventricular septal defect (VSD) complicating an anterior or inferior wall infarction occurs in 1% to 2% of patients in the first week following infarction. Rupture typically occurs when a transmural infarction is in a territory supplied by a single vessel without collaterals, thus increasing the shear stress between the necrotic myocardium and the intact heart muscle.

On TEE, VSD often presents as a single perforation (Figs. 13-16 and 13-17; Videos 13-4 and 13-5), but it can be irregular in shape and serpiginous. A VSD resulting from an anterior wall infarction is usually located near the apex and associated with anterior akinesis. A VSD resulting from an inferior wall infarction usually spares the apex and is located in the basal septum, with extensive inferior wall dyskinesis. PW Doppler and color flow Doppler can identify the defective site, with a mosaic pattern secondary to the turbulent flow. Thorough assessment of RV function is crucial because it is a major predictor of outcome.

Myocardial Rupture

Rupture of the LV free wall is usually a sudden event that accounts for 8% to 17% of all in-hospital deaths in the postinfarction period. It

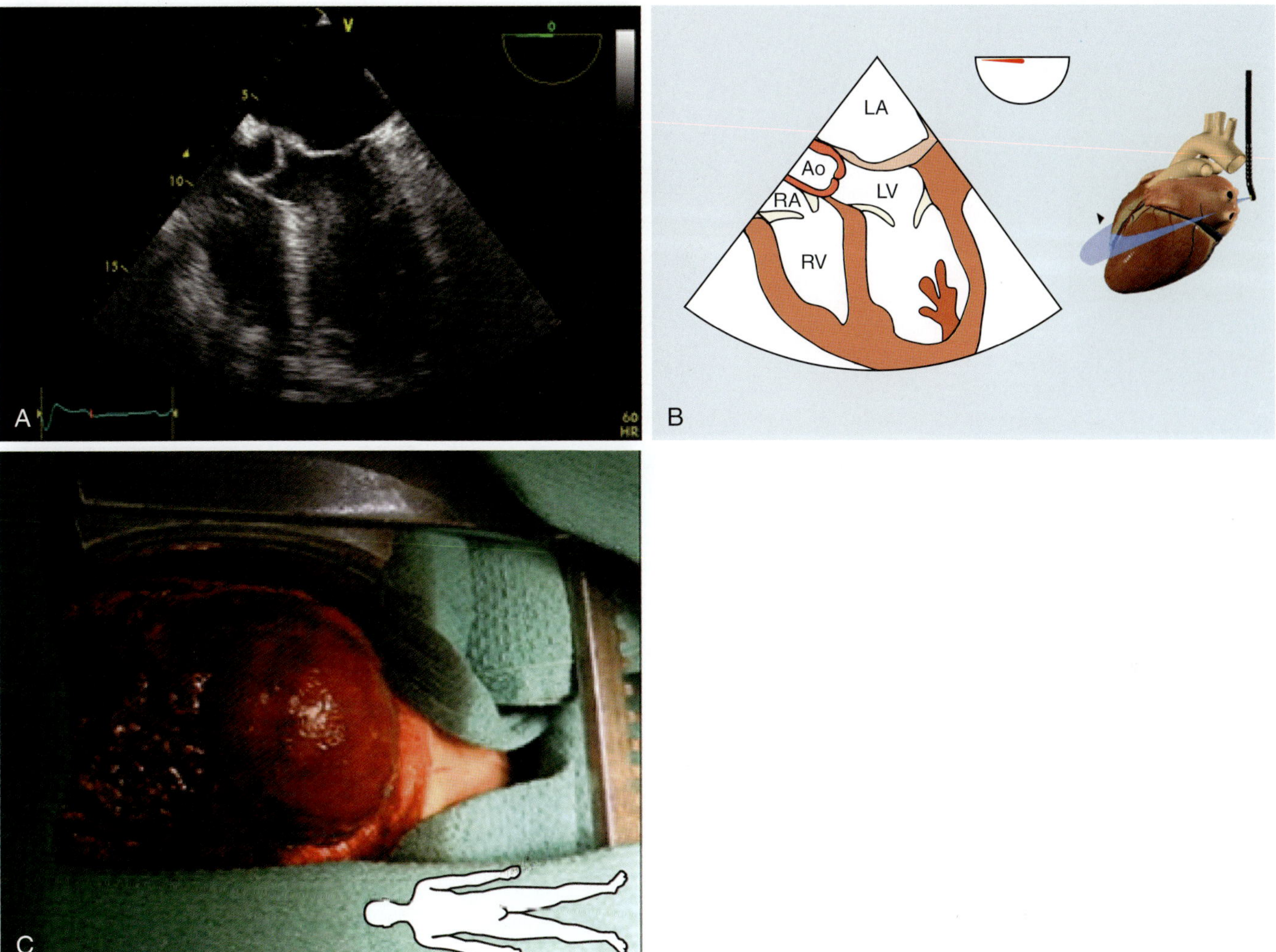

Figure 13-13   Left ventricular (*LV*) aneurysm (see Video 13-2). Midesophageal view from a 61-year-old man with ischemic cardiomyopathy and apical akinesis. LV spontaneous contrast is present (**A** and **B**). **C,** Intraoperative aspect of LV aneurysm. *Ao,* Aorta; *LA,* left atrium; *RA,* right atrium; *RV,* right ventricle.

equally affects the anterior, inferior, and lateral walls. It is an acute and devastating complication with massive hemopericardium, fast hemodynamic deterioration leading to electromechanical dissociation, and death within minutes. TEE will demonstrate a pericardial effusion and pericardial thrombus. The association of cardiac tamponade (Fig. 13-18, Video 13-6), pericardial effusion greater than 5 mm, and pericardial thrombus has a diagnostic sensitivity of 70% and a specificity of 90% for the diagnosis of myocardial rupture.[29]

Right Ventricular Infarction

Inferior myocardial infarction may extend into the RV free wall and compromise RV function. TEE findings will include RV regional wall motion hypokinesis, akinesis, or global RV dysfunction.[30] The LV inferior wall is usually also affected. The TG SAX view has been shown to have the highest sensitivity (82%), with a specificity ranging from 62% to 93% for hemodynamically significant RV infarction.[31] Other signs of RV infarction include RV dilation, abnormal interventricular septal motion, tricuspid regurgitation, reduced systolic excursion of the tricuspid annulus, and dilation of the inferior vena cava (Figs. 13-19 and 13-20; Videos 13-7 and 13-8). Bowing of the interatrial septum toward the LA is a negative marker associated with a high incidence of hypotension, heart block, and mortality.[32]

Aortic Atherosclerosis

Aortic atherosclerosis is present in up to 58% of patients undergoing cardiac surgery.[33-35] Atherosclerotic plaques have a non-uniform distribution throughout the aorta,[36] which may impact on the surgical management and outcome of a patient undergoing cardiac operations, particularly during routine aortic manipulations such as aortic cannulation and aortic cross-clamping.

A stroke is a devastating complication of cardiac surgery, and the risk of stroke has been associated with the presence and severity of aortic atherosclerosis.[33-35] Grading systems of aortic atherosclerosis have been proposed.[37-44] A widely used grading system is the one devised by Katz (Fig. 13-21).[37] However, none of these grading systems have been proven superior one over another in predicting the risk of stroke. Consistent risk factors between studies appear to be (1) plaque height greater than 3 mm, (2) any mobile components, and (3) location in the ascending aorta.[36] Cardiac surgeons usually place the aortic cannula in the distal anterior segment of the ascending aorta, which is the area most commonly affected by atherosclerosis and often not well visualized with TEE.[36] In one study,[36] van der Linden found that atherosclerotic disease in the mid-lateral segment was a significant independent risk factor for postoperative stroke (incidence of 26%). What is certain is that the more severe the aortic disease, the higher the risk of stroke.

Text continued on p. 16

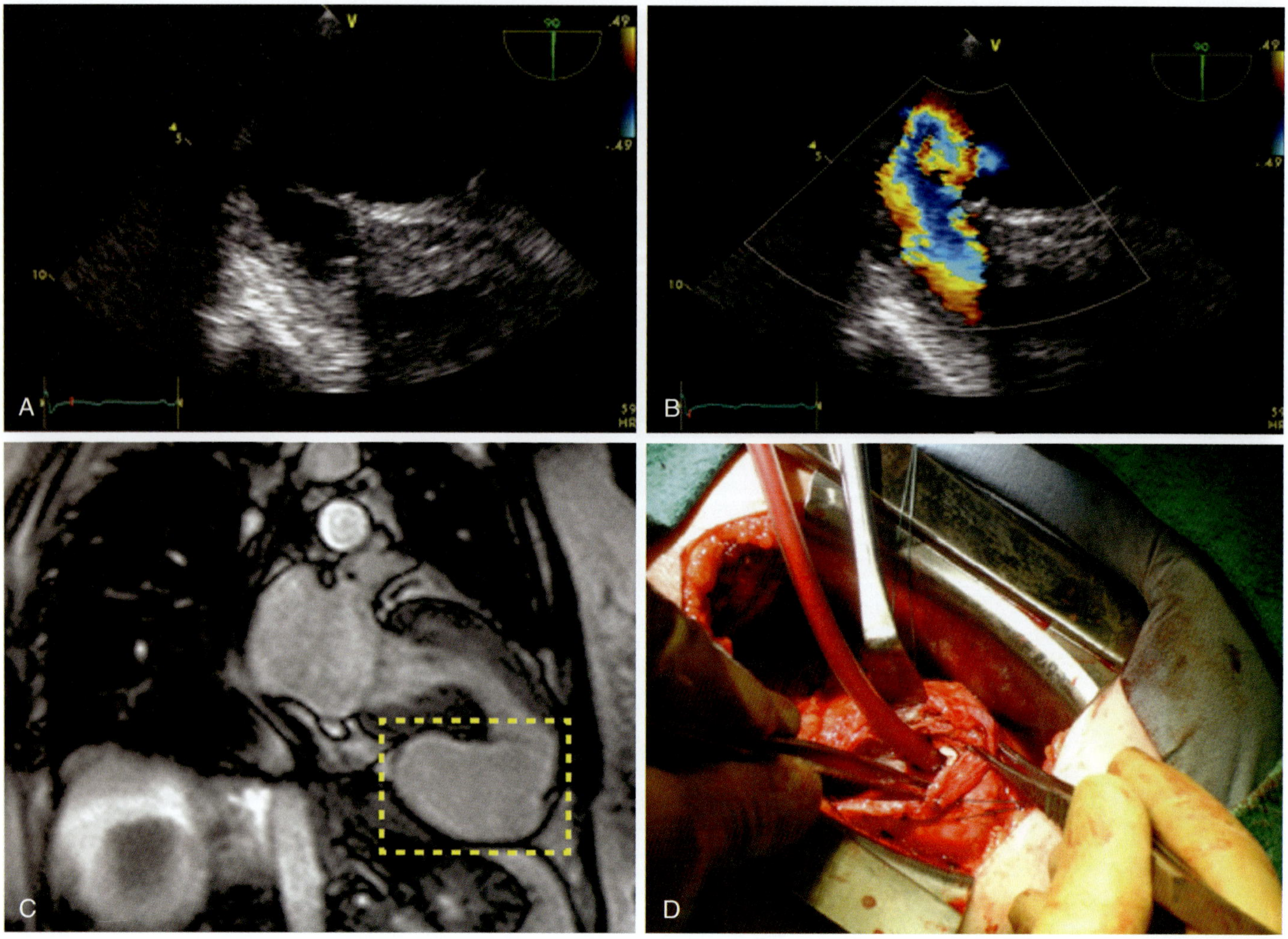

Figure 13-14   Left ventricular (LV) pseudoaneurysm (see Video 13-3) in a 60-year-old woman. The 90-degree transgastric view illustrates communication between LV into pseudoaneurysm (**A**), which is confirmed by color Doppler imaging (**B**). Magnetic resonance imaging (*dotted square*) (**C**) and intraoperative view (**D**) are shown. (*D courtesy Dr. Denis Bouchard.*)

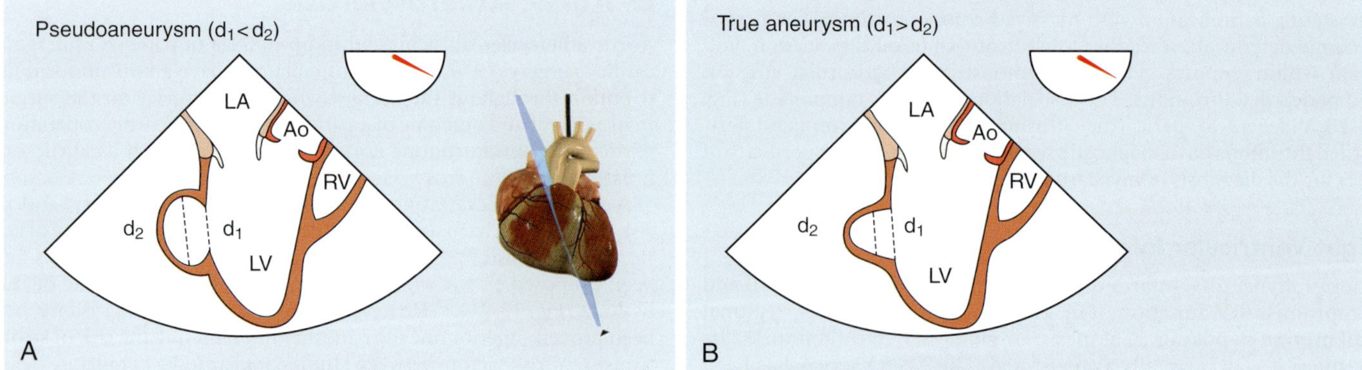

Figure 13-15   Pseudoaneurysm and true aneurysm. Differences between a pseudo- and true aneurysm are illustrated. **A,** In a pseudoaneurysm, diameter of orifice (d_1) is smaller than diameter of aneurysm (d_2). **B,** The opposite is found in a true aneurysm. *Ao,* Aorta; *LA,* left atrium; *LV,* left ventricle; *RV,* right ventricle. (*From Denault AY, Couture P, Vegas A, Buithieu J, Tardif J-C. Transesophageal Echocardiography Multimedia Manual. 2nd ed. New York: Informa Healthcare; 2011, with permission.*)

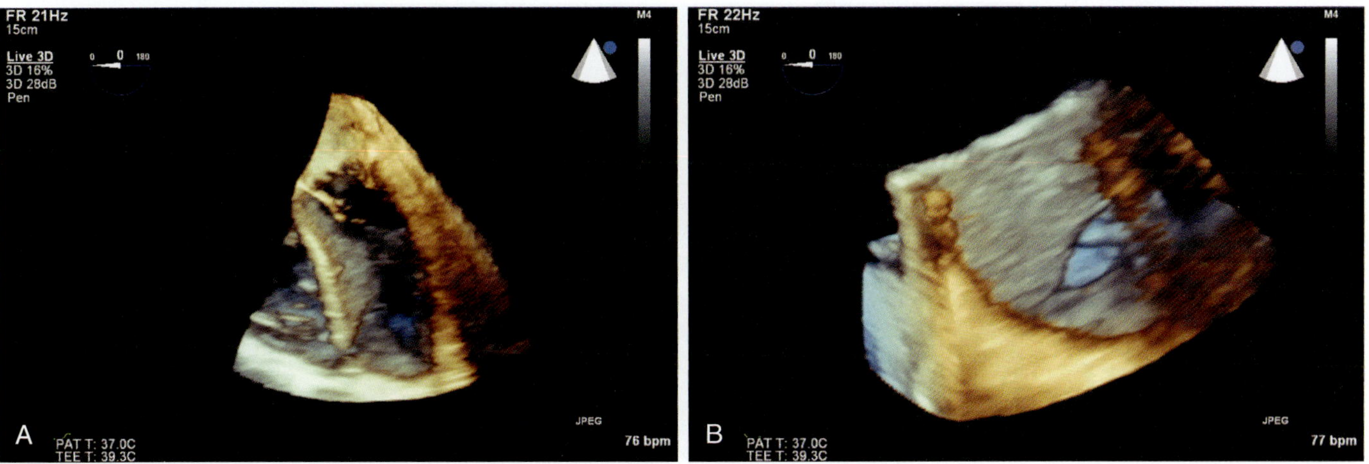

Figure 13-16   Ventricular septal defect (VSD; see Video 13-4). **A** and **B,** VSD in a 65-year-old man 10 days following myocardial infarction resulting from a left anterior descending coronary artery occlusion. VSD is located in apical septal region.

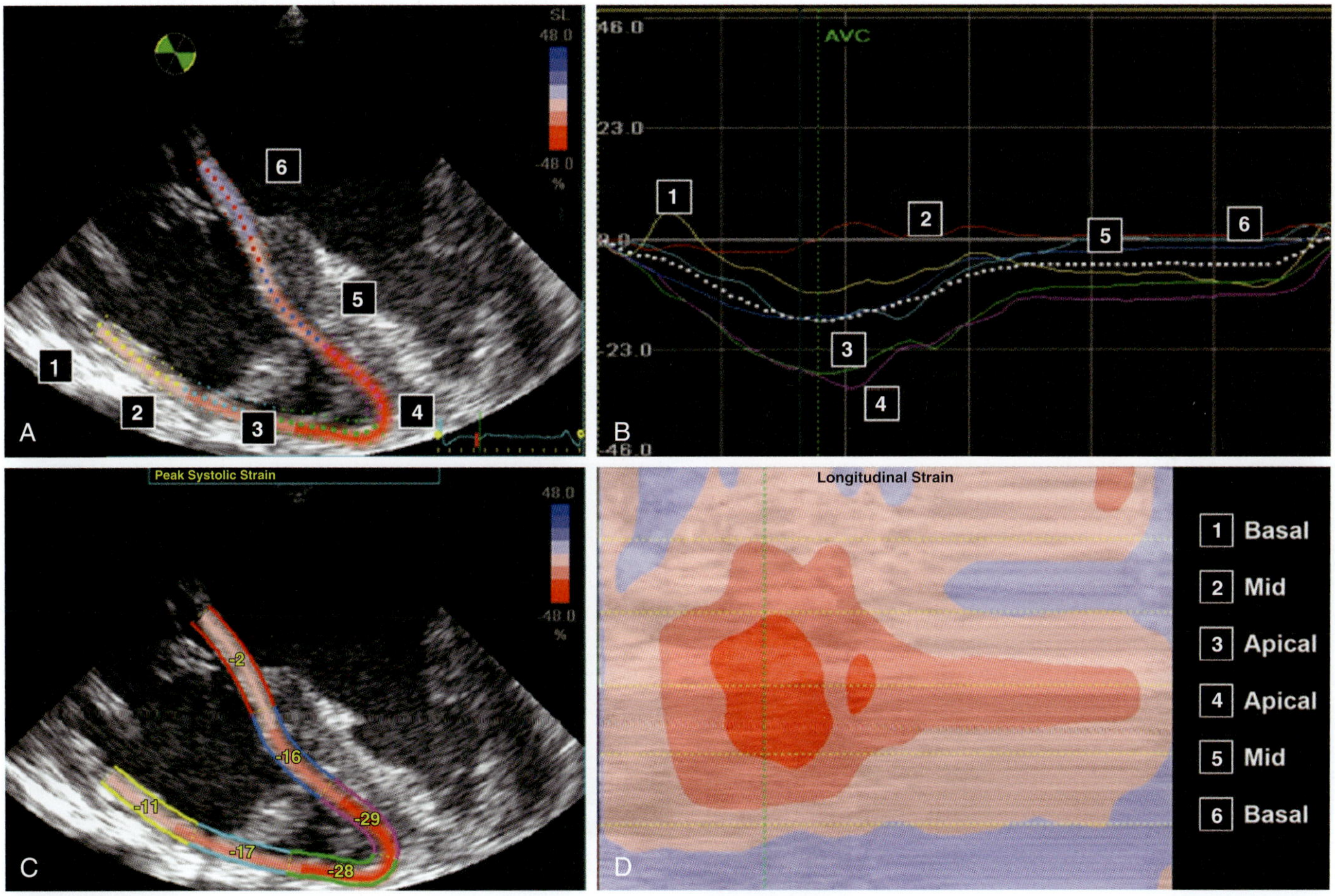

Figure 13-17   Ventricular septal defect and strain (see Video 13-5). Longitudinal strain by two-dimensional speckle tracking from a patient with an intraventricular septal defect. Midesophageal four-chamber view with global longitudinal strain overlay (**A**). Individual sampling curves (**B**), regional peak (**C**), and curved M-mode mapping (**D**) show that basal regions *(1,6)* have a lower strain value than apical regions *(3,4)*. *AVC,* Aortic valve closure; *FR,* frame rate.

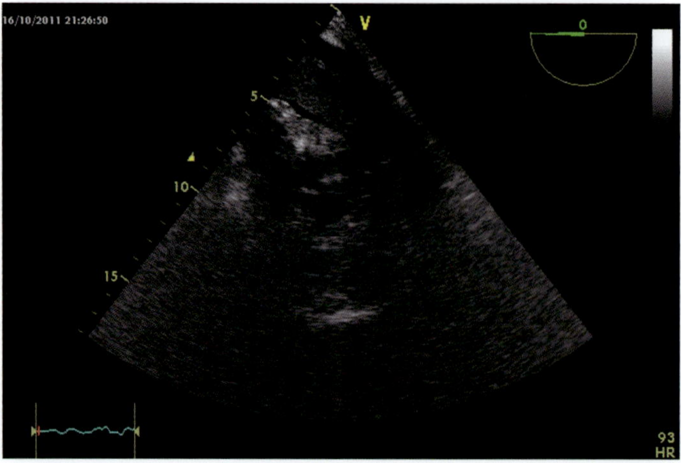

Figure 13-18   Myocardial rupture (also see Video 13-6) in a 56-year-old man after inferior wall myocardial infarction. Note significant pericardial effusion (>5 mm) and large pericardial thrombus.

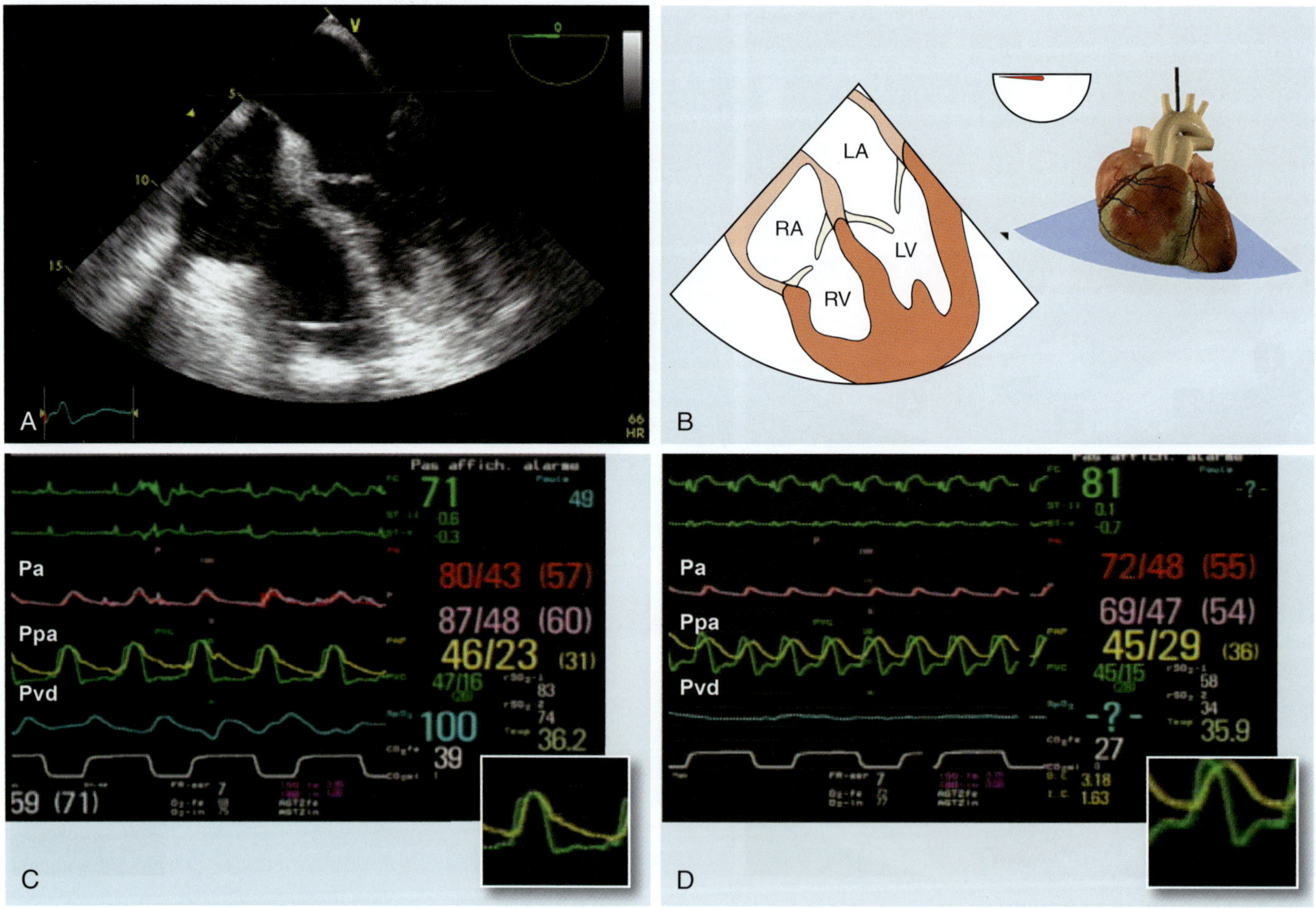

Figure 13-19   Right ventricular failure (see Video 13-7). Midesophageal four-chamber view in a 67-year-old man with severe right ventricular failure after cardiac surgery (**A** and **B**). Hemodynamic waveforms before and after cardiopulmonary bypass. Note change in the aspect of right ventricular pressure waveform (Pvd) from horizontal diastolic slope (**C**) to a square root pattern (**D**). Also note reduction in end-tidal carbon dioxide from 39 to 27 mmHg; lower peripheral (83% to 58%) and brain saturation (74% to 34%) are consistent with reduced cardiac performance resulting from right ventricular dysfunction. *IAS,* Interatrial septum; *LA,* left atrium; *LV,* left ventricle; *Pa,* arterial pressure; *Ppa,* pulmonary artery pressure; *Prv,* right ventricular pressure; *RA,* right atrium; *RV,* right ventricle.

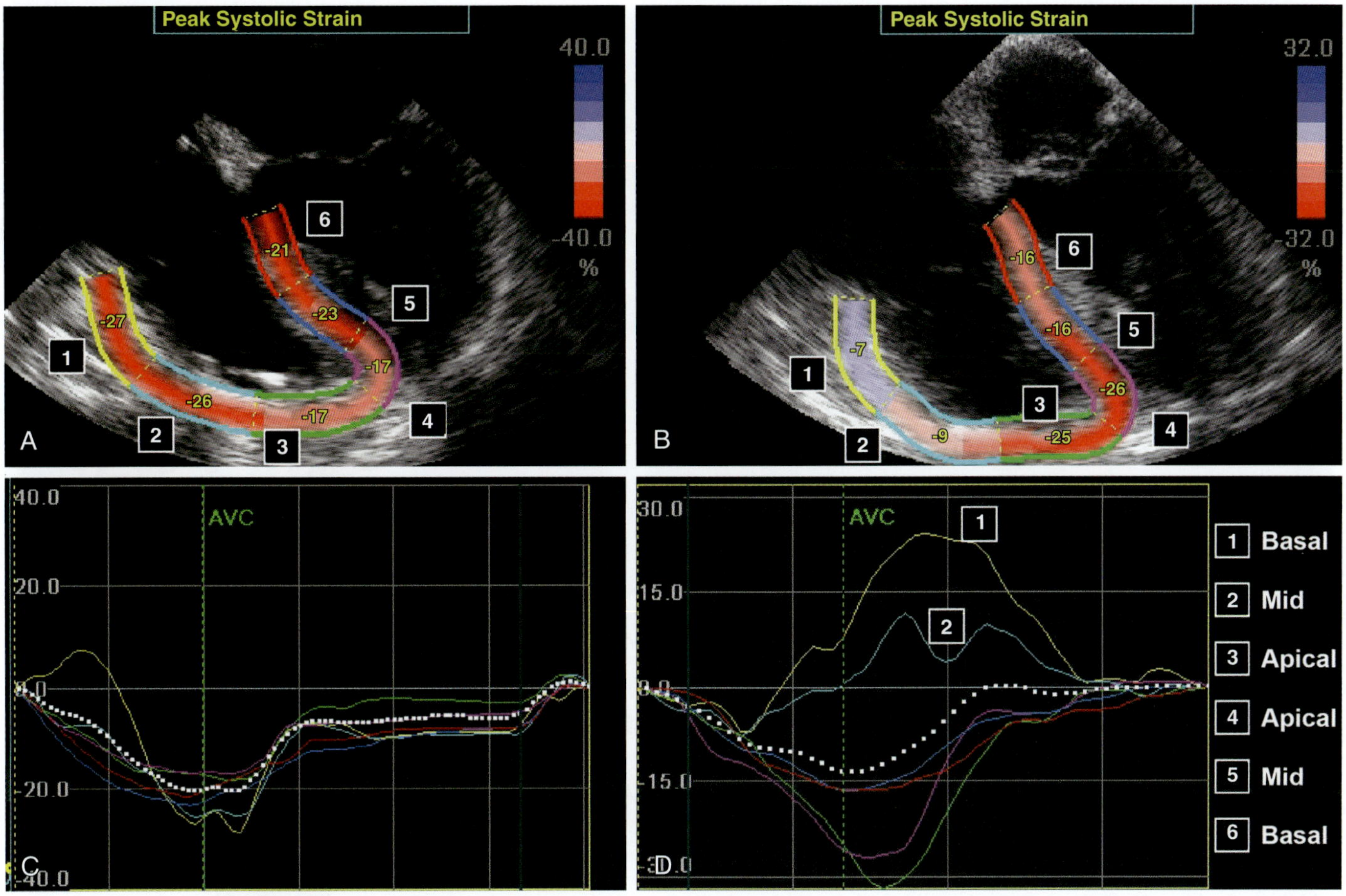

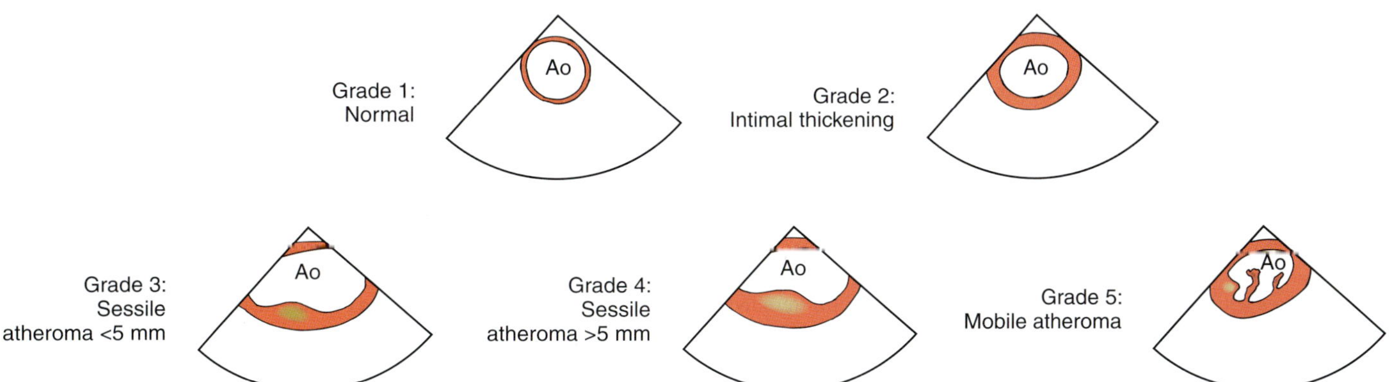

Figure 13-20 Right ventricular failure and strain (see Video 13-8). Longitudinal strain using two-dimensional speckle tracking in a 72-year-old woman undergoing coronary revascularization. Right ventricular regional peak systolic strain obtained before revascularization (**A**) was reduced after cardiopulmonary bypass (**B**), particularly in basal (*1*) and midlateral (*2*) region. Global strain went from −20.7% to −13.5%. Individual sampling curves are shown before (**C**) and after (**D**) surgery.

Figure 13-21 Classification of atheromatosis of the aorta. Grades of atheromatous disease of aorta are represented. *Ao*, Aorta. (*Adapted from Denault AY, Couture P, Vegas A, Buithieu J, Tardif J-C. Transesophageal Echocardiography Multimedia Manual. 2nd ed. New York: Informa Healthcare; 2011, with permission.*)

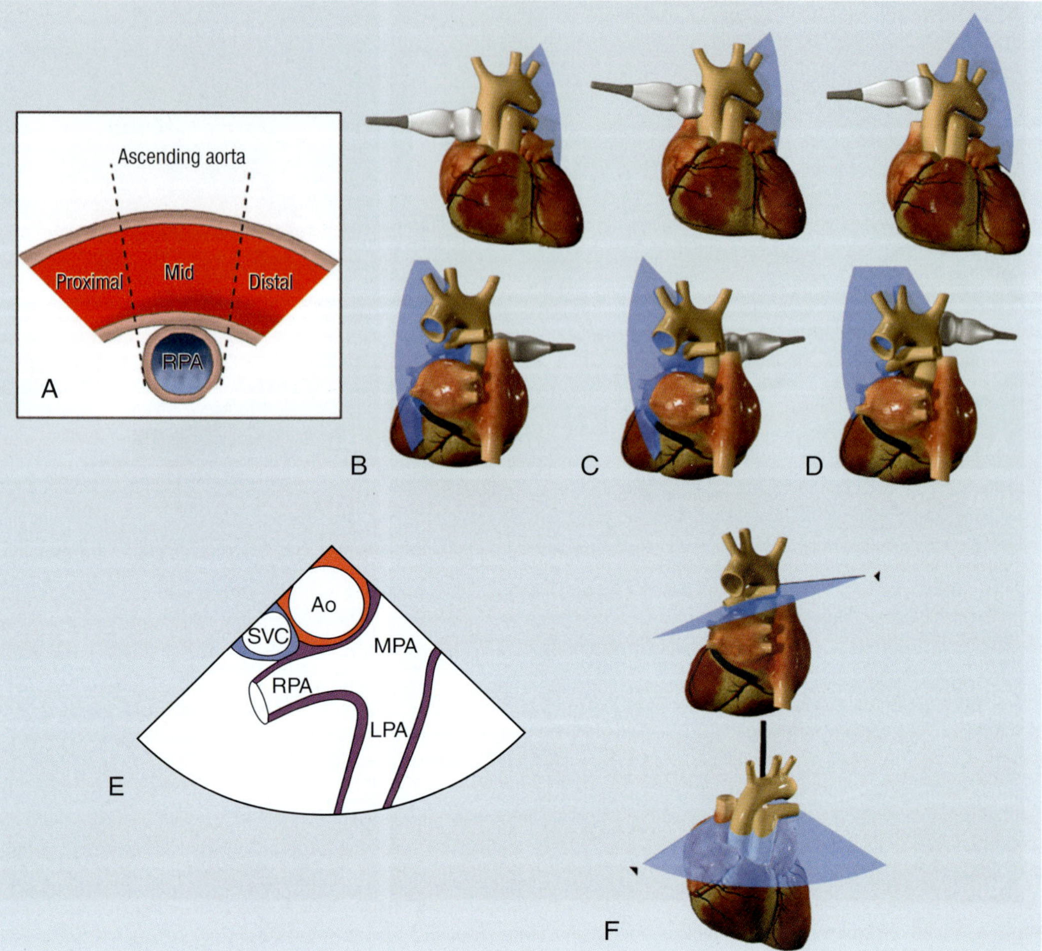

Figure 13-22 Epiaortic ultrasound (EAU) long- and short-axis views. EAU scanning is performed with a high-resolution (>7 MHz) ultrasound transducer inserted in a sterile sheath. Longitudinal ascending aorta *(Ao)* is divided into proximal, mid-, and distal regions **(A)**. EAU scan of ascending aorta in short-axis view also shows bifurcation of main pulmonary artery *(MPA)* into right pulmonary artery *(RPA)* and left pulmonary artery *(LPA)* **(E)**. **B, C, D,** and **F,** Anterior and posterior positions of probe during EAU scanning are shown. *SVC,* Superior vena cava. *(Adapted from Denault AY, Couture P, Vegas A, Buithieu J, Tardif J-C. Transesophageal Echocardiography Multimedia Manual. 2nd ed. New York: Informa Healthcare; 2011, with permission.)*

Epiaortic ultrasound (EAU) imaging is the gold standard modality for evaluation of aortic atherosclerosis,[45] and guidelines for its performance have been published.[46] However, EAU is not widely used. TEE presents many advantages with regard to examination of the aorta. Indeed, the close proximity of the esophagus to the thoracic aorta and the use of high-frequency transducers convey images of great resolution. By comparison to CT and MRI scanning, TEE is low cost as well as readily performed at the bedside and intraoperatively. Using short and long-axis views, most of the ascending aorta can be visualized, with the exception of its distal segment and the initial segment of the aortic arch, which are often hidden to ultrasound by the interposition of the right mainstem bronchus and/or trachea but can be visualized by EAU (Fig. 13-22).

Cardiac surgeons often evaluate aortic cannulation and cross-clamping sites with digital palpation alone. Digital palpation to detect aortic atherosclerotic plaque has reported sensitivities ranging from 4% to 55%.[39,45,47,48] By comparison, TEE sensitivity to detect aortic atherosclerosis is only slightly better, with ranges from 30% to 58%.[39,48,49]

EAU remains the best method for detecting atherosclerotic plaques, as illustrated in a study[49] where TEE detected 179 lesions in 60 patients, and EAU detected 362 lesions in the same 60 patients (Fig. 13-23).

Given the advantages of each evaluation technique, a combined approach using palpation, TEE, and EAU should be recommended. An algorithm for management of the surgical patient with aortic atherosclerosis has been proposed (Fig. 13-24),[50] although this approach has not yet been evaluated in clinical studies.

Conclusion

TEE is a powerful perioperative diagnostic tool for the clinician to detect, identify, follow, and quantify segmental myocardial ischemia. It is an essential tool to evaluate many mechanical complications caused by myocardial ischemia. Its use in a systematic multimodal evaluation of aortic atherosclerosis may have a dramatic impact on postoperative outcome if stroke can be avoided.

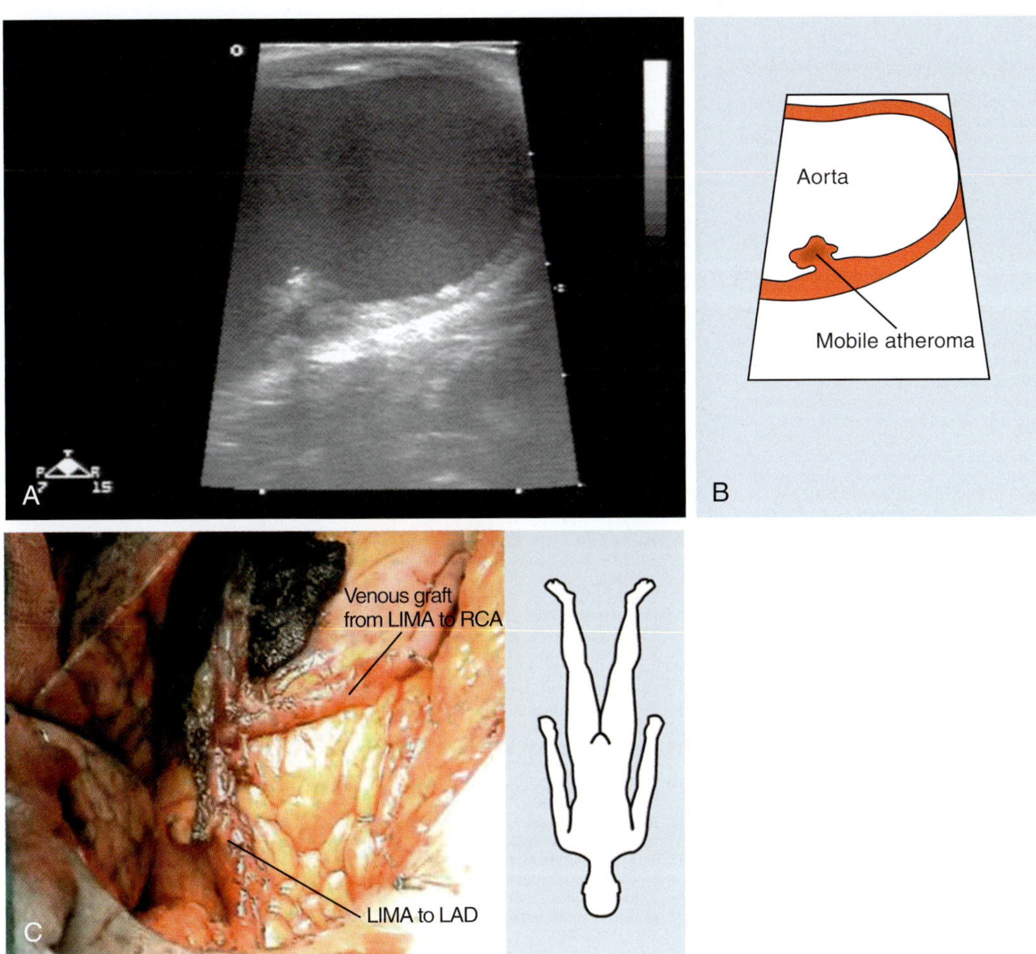

Figure 13-23 Epiaortic scanning. **A** and **B,** Epiaortic images of aortic arch reveal a mobile atheroma (Grade 5) in a 74-year-old woman before cardiopulmonary bypass. **C,** To avoid aortic clamping during off-pump coronary artery bypass grafting, saphenous vein graft to right coronary artery *(RCA)* was anastomosed to left internal mammary artery *(LIMA)* graft rather than on the aorta as is usually the case. *LAD,* Left anterior descending coronary artery. *(Adapted from Denault AY, Couture P, Vegas A, Buithieu J, Tardif J-C. Transesophageal Echocardiography Multimedia Manual. 2nd ed. New York: Informa Healthcare; 2011, with permission. C courtesy Dr. Louis P. Perrault.)*

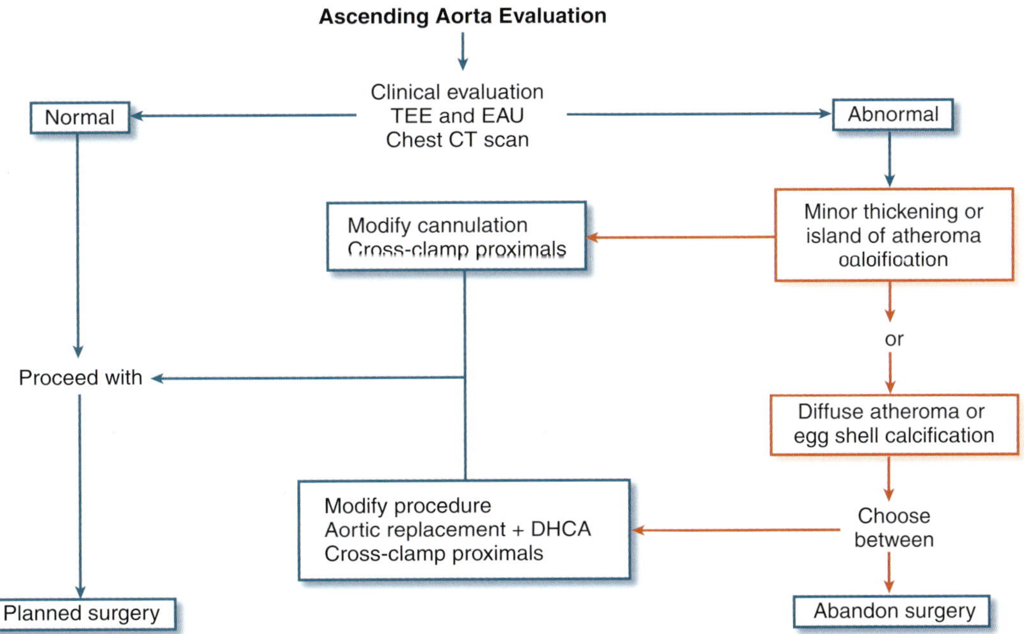

Figure 13-24 Aortic disease. Algorithm for management of ascending aorta during cardiac surgery is shown. *CT,* Computed tomography; *DHCA,* deep hypothermic cardiac arrest; *EAU,* epiaortic ultrasound; *TEE,* transesophageal echocardiography. *(Adapted from Denault AY, Couture P, Vegas A, Buithieu J, Tardif J-C. Transesophageal Echocardiography Multimedia Manual. 2nd ed. New York: Informa Healthcare; 2011, with permission.)*

REFERENCES

1. Thys DM, Abel MD, Brooker RF, et al. Practice guidelines for perioperative transesophageal echocardiography. *Anesthesiology*. 2010;112(5):1084-1096.
2. Cerqueira MD, Weissman NJ, Dilsizian V, et al. Standardized myocardial segmentation and nomenclature for tomographic imaging of the heart. *Circulation*. 2002;105(4):539-542.
3. Schiller NB, Shah PM, Crawford M, et al. Recommendations for quantitation of the left ventricle by two-dimensional echocardiography. American Society of Echocardiography Committee on Standards, Subcommittee on Quantitation of Two-Dimensional Echocardiograms. *J Am Soc Echocardiogr*. 1989;2(5):358-367.
4. Smith JS, Cahalan MK, Benefiel DJ, et al. Intraoperative detection of myocardial ischemia in high-risk patients: electrocardiography versus two-dimensional transesophageal echocardiography. *Circulation*. 1985;72(5):1015-1021.
5. Shapiro E, Marier DL, St John Sutton MG, et al. Regional non-uniformity of wall dynamics in normal left ventricle. *Br Heart J*. 1981;45(3):264-270.
6. Gallagher KP, Kumada T, Koziol JA, et al. Significance of regional wall thickening abnormalities relative to transmural myocardial perfusion in anesthetized dogs. *Circulation*. 1980;62(6):1266-1274.
7. Rouine-Rapp K, Ionescu P, Balea M, et al. Detection of intraoperative segmental wall-motion abnormalities by transesophageal echocardiography: the incremental value of additional cross sections in the transverse and longitudinal planes. *Anesth Analg*. 1996;83(6):1141-1148.
8. Couture P, Bolduc L, De Mey N, et al. Real-time compared to off-line evaluation of segmental wall motion abnormalities with transesophageal echocardiography using dobutamine stress testing. *J Cardiothorac Vasc Anesth*. 2011:(in press).
9. van Daele ME, Sutherland GR, Mitchell MM, et al. Do changes in pulmonary capillary wedge pressure adequately reflect myocardial ischemia during anesthesia? A correlative preoperative hemodynamic, electrocardiographic, and transesophageal echocardiographic study. *Circulation*. 1990;81(3):865-871.
10. Leung JM, O'Kelly B, Browner WS, et al. Prognostic importance of postbypass regional wall-motion abnormalities in patients undergoing coronary artery bypass graft surgery. *Anesthesiology*. 1989;71(1):16-25.
11. De Mey N, Couture P, Laflamme M, et al. Intraoperative changes in regional wall motion: Can we predict postoperative coronary artery bypass graft failure? *J Cardiothorac Vasc Anesth*. 2012:(in press).
12. Sheehan FH, Bolson EL, Dodge HT, et al. Advantages and applications of the centerline method for characterizing regional ventricular function. *Circulation*. 1986;74(2):293-305.
13. Lang RM, Bierig M, Devereux RB, et al. Recommendations for chamber quantification: a report from the American Society of Echocardiography's Guidelines and Standards Committee and the Chamber Quantification Writing Group, Developed in Conjunction with the European Association of Echocardiography, a branch of the European Society of Cardiology. *J Am Soc Echocardiogr*. 2005;18(12):1440-1463.
14. Berning J, Steensgaard-Hansen F. Early estimation of risk by echocardiographic determination of wall motion index in an unselected population with acute myocardial infarction. *Am J Cardiol*. 1990;65(9):567-576.
15. Kan G, Visser CA, Koolen JJ, et al. Short- and long-term predictive value of admission wall motion score in acute myocardial infarction. A cross-sectional echocardiographic study of 345 patients. *Br Heart J*. 1986;56(5):422-427.
16. MacLaren G, Kluger R, Prior D, et al. Tissue doppler, strain, and strain rate echocardiography: principles and potential perioperative applications. *J Cardiothorac Vasc Anesth*. 2006;20(4):583-593.
17. Bach DS, Armstrong WF, Donovan CL, et al. Quantitative Doppler tissue imaging for assessment of regional myocardial velocities during transient ischemia and reperfusion. *Am Heart J*. 1996;132(4):721-725.
18. Derumeaux G, Ovize M, Loufoua J, et al. Doppler tissue imaging quantitates regional wall motion during myocardial ischemia and reperfusion. *Circulation*. 1998;97(19):1970-1977.
19. Edvardsen T, Aakhus S, Endresen K, et al. Acute regional myocardial ischemia identified by 2-dimensional multiregion tissue Doppler imaging technique. *J Am Soc Echocardiogr*. 2000;13(11):986-994.
20. Sun JP, Popović ZB, Greenberg NL, et al. Noninvasive quantification of regional myocardial function using Doppler-derived velocity, displacement, strain rate, and strain in healthy volunteers: effects of aging. *J Am Soc Echocardiogr*. 2004;17(2):132-138.
21. Skulstad H, Urheim S, Edvardsen T, et al. Grading of myocardial dysfunction by tissue Doppler echocardiography: a comparison between velocity, displacement, and strain imaging in acute ischemia. *J Am Coll Cardiol*. 2006;47(8):1672-1682.
22. Amundsen BH, Helle-Valle T, Edvardsen T, et al. Noninvasive myocardial strain measurement by speckle tracking echocardiography: validation against sonomicrometry and tagged magnetic resonance imaging. *J Am Coll Cardiol*. 2006;47(4):789-793.
23. Jenkins C, Bricknell K, Chan J, et al. Comparison of two- and three-dimensional echocardiography with sequential magnetic resonance imaging for evaluating left ventricular volume and ejection fraction over time in patients with healed myocardial infarction. *Am J Cardiol*. 2007;99(3):300-306.
24. Corsi C, Coon P, Goonewardena S, et al. Quantification of regional left ventricular wall motion from real-time 3-dimensional echocardiography in patients with poor acoustic windows: effects of contrast enhancement tested against cardiac magnetic resonance. *J Am Soc Echocardiogr*. 2006;19(7):886-893.
25. Lang RM, Badano LP, Tsang W, et al. EAE/ASE recommendations for image acquisition and display using three-dimensional echocardiography. *J Am Soc Echocardiogr*. 2012;25(1):3-46.
26. Cigarroa CG, deFilippi CR, Brickner ME, et al. Dobutamine stress echocardiography identifies hibernating myocardium and predicts recovery of left ventricular function after coronary revascularization. *Circulation*. 1993;88(2):430-436.
27. Smart SC, Sawada S, Ryan T, et al. Low-dose dobutamine echocardiography detects reversible dysfunction after thrombolytic therapy of acute myocardial infarction. *Circulation*. 1993;88(2):405-415.
28. Chen C, Koschyk D, Hamm C, et al. Usefulness of transesophageal echocardiography in identifying small left ventricular apical thrombus. *J Am Coll Cardiol*. 1993;21(1):208-215.
29. López-Sendón J, González A, López de Sá E, et al. Diagnosis of subacute ventricular wall rupture after acute myocardial infarction: sensitivity and specificity of clinical, hemodynamic and echocardiographic criteria. *J Am Coll Cardiol*. 1992;19(6):1145-1153.
30. Haddad F, Couture P, Tousignant C, et al. The right ventricle in cardiac surgery, a perioperative perspective: i. anatomy, physiology, and assessment. *Anesth Analg*. 2009;108(2):407-421.
31. Lopez-Sendon J, Garcia-Fernandez MA, Coma-Canella I, et al. Segmental right ventricular function after acute myocardial infarction: Two-dimensional echocardiographic study in 63 patients. *Am J Cardiol*. 1983;51(3):390-396.
32. López-Sendón J, López de Sá E, Roldán I, et al. Inversion of the normal interatrial septum convexity in acute myocardial infarction: incidence, clinical relevance and prognostic significance. *J Am Coll Cardiol*. 1990;15(4):801-805.
33. Dávila-Román VG, Barzilai B, Wareing TH, et al. Atherosclerosis of the ascending aorta. Prevalence and role as an independent predictor of cerebrovascular events in cardiac patients. *Stroke*. 1994;25(10):2010-2016.
34. Hogue Jr CW, Murphy SF, Schechtman KB, et al. Risk factors for early or delayed stroke after cardiac surgery. *Circulation*. 1999;100(6):642-647.
35. van der Linden J, Bergman P, Hadjinikolaou L. The topography of aortic atherosclerosis enhances its precision as a predictor of stroke. *Ann Thorac Surg*. 2007;83(6):2087-2092.
36. van der Linden J, Hadjinikolaou L, Bergman P, Lindblom D. Postoperative stroke in cardiac surgery is related to the location and extent of atherosclerotic disease in the ascending aorta. *J Am Coll Cardiol*. 2001;38(1):131-135.
37. Katz ES, Tunick PA, Rusinek H, Ribakove G, Spencer FC, Kronzon I. Protruding aortic atheromas predict stroke in elderly patients undergoing cardiopulmonary bypass: experience with intraoperative transesophageal echocardiography. *J Am Coll Cardiol*. 1992;20(1):70-77.
38. Amarenco P, Cohen A, Tzourio C, et al. Atherosclerotic disease of the aortic arch and the risk of ischemic stroke. *N Engl J Med*. 1994;331(22):1474-1479.
39. Dávila-Román VG, Phillips KJ, Daily BB, et al. Intraoperative transesophageal echocardiography and epiaortic ultrasound for assessment of atherosclerosis of the thoracic aorta. *J Am Coll Cardiol*. 1996;28(4):942-947.
40. Acaturk E, Demir M, Kanadas M. Aortic atherosclerosis is a marker for significant coronary artery disease. *Jpn Heart J*. 1999;40:775-781.
41. Ferrari E, Vidal R, Chevallier T, et al. Atherosclerosis of the thoracic aorta and aortic debris as a marker of poor prognosis: benefit of oral anticoagulants. *J Am Coll Cardiol*. 1999;33(5):1317-1322.
42. Blackshear JL, Pearce LA, Hart RG, et al. Aortic plaque in atrial fibrillation: prevalence, predictors, and thromboembolic implications. *Stroke*. 1999;30(4):834-840.
43. Trehan N, Mishra M, Kasliwal RR, et al. Reduced neurological injury during CABG in patients with mobile aortic atheromas: a five-year follow-up study. *Ann Thorac Surg*. 2000;70(5):1558-1564.
44. Nohara H, Shida T, Mukohara N, Obo H, Higami T. Ultrasonic plaque density of aortic atheroma and stroke in patients undergoing on-pump coronary artery bypass surgery. *Ann Thorac Cardiovasc Surg*. 2004;10:235-240.
45. Marshall Jr WG, Barzilai B, Kouchoukos NT, et al. Intraoperative ultrasonic imaging of the ascending aorta. *Ann Thorac Surg*. 1989;48(3):339-344.
46. Glas KE, Swaminathan M, Reeves ST, et al. Guidelines for the performance of a comprehensive intraoperative epiaortic ultrasonographic examination: recommendations of the American Society of Echocardiography and the Society of Cardiovascular Anesthesiologists; endorsed by the Society of Thoracic Surgeons. *Anesth Analg*. 2008;106(5):1376-1384.
47. Bolotin G, Domany Y, de Perini L, et al. Use of Intraoperative Epiaortic ultrasonography to delineate aortic atheroma*. *Chest*. 2005;127(1):60-65.
48. Suvarna S, Smith A, Stygall J, et al. An intraoperative assessment of the ascending aorta: a comparison of digital palpation, transesophageal echocardiography, and epiaortic ultrasonography. *J Cardiothorac Vasc Anesth*. 2007;21(6):805-809.
49. Ibrahim KS, Vitale N, Tromsdal A, et al. Enhanced intra-operative grading of ascending aorta atheroma by epiaortic ultrasound vs echocardiography. *Int J Cardiol*. 2008;128(2):218-223.
50. Bainbridge D, Murkin J, Calaritis C, et al. Aortic dissection in a patient with a previous ascending aortic dissection and repair: the role of new monitoring devices in the high-risk patient. *Semin Cardiothoracic Vascular Anesth*. 2004;8(1):3-7.

14

Aortic Valve Anatomy and Embryology

JONATHAN K. FROGEL | WILLIAM J. VERNICK | JACOB T. GUTSCHE |
JOSEPH S. SAVINO

The aortic valve (AV), located at the base of the aorta, comprises three semilunar cusps and functions to allow unidirectional blood flow from the left ventricle into the systemic circulation. AV closure prevents blood from flowing backward into the left ventricular outflow tract (LVOT) and left ventricle. The AV's three cusps are named for their relationships to the coronary ostia (right, left, and noncoronary cusps) and have three corresponding sinuses of Valsalva (right, left, and noncoronary sinuses). The AV ascends at the level of the commissures between the cusps and descends toward (but not into) the LVOT at the base or nadir of the cusps.[1-3] The sinuses of Valsalva become continuous with the left ventricle at the lower margin of the aortic root and meet the ascending aorta at the upper margin.[4] The upper margin of the sinuses (where they meet the tubular portion of the aorta) is the sinotubular junction. The aortic wall and LVOT have both muscular and fibrous components. The LVOT consists of a muscular membranous septal component and a fibrous posterior quadrant that is continuous with the fibrous skeleton of the heart. The base of the anterior leaflet of the mitral valve has a fibrous connection to the left and noncoronary cusps and constitutes the aortomitral continuity. The AV lacks a discrete annulus. The attachments of the AV cusps to the aorta and left ventricle are curvilinear. The three cusps meet centrally during diastole at the nodule of Arantius.[3]

The AV and its supporting sinuses develop within a turret of cardiac muscle.[5,6] The initial muscular walls of the intrapericardial trunks become transformed to arterial structures with separation of the adjacent aorta and pulmonary trunks. The sinus walls of the roots are also formed of arterial tissues.[7] The aortic and pulmonary valves are quite similar histologically in the fetus. Histologic differences develop after birth between the aortic and pulmonary valves related to molecular stability and cross-linking of collagen. After birth, the neonatal AV collagen becomes more unstable owing to the increase in transvalvular pressure compared to the low transvalvular gradients exerted on the pulmonic valve. Changes in the molecular stability and cross-linking of collagen of the AV during the transition from fetal to neonatal circulation appear to be due to increased transvascular pressure gradients.[8] In the adult, the AV cusps become thicker and are composed of denser collagen fibers with compartmentalization of vascular interstitial cells, compaction, and stratification of the extracellular matrix into a trilaminar structure.[8-10] The pulmonic valve remains thin with less collagen compared to the AV.[8] These differences in the semilunar valves can be seen with both visual inspection and transesophageal echocardiography (TEE). The applicability of these insights become useful in both achieving a better understanding of the anatomy and embryology of the AV and in production and tissue engineering of prosthetic heart valve replacements for both the pulmonic and aortic positions.[9] The other application of these structural differences in the semilunar valves is in the surgical explant and transfer of the pulmonary valve to the aortic position during the Ross procedure.[11] The central position of the AV relative to the atria, pulmonary trunk, and ventricles render these adjacent structures susceptible to involvement (e.g., fistula) in the setting of endocarditis and abscess.[12]

In a small percentage of individuals, excessive fusion between cushions or ridges of the aortic cusp can produce a septum in the developing outflow tract.[7] Bicuspid AVs develop when excessive fusion of ridges results in conjoined leaflets. This most often occurs between the

leaflets arising from the sinuses of the right and left coronary cusps. A less common mechanism in the formation of a bicuspid AV is a relative paucity of endothelial nitric oxide synthase, which may result in a phenotype in which the conjoined leaflets represent fusion of the noncoronary and right coronary cusps.[12,13] In either case, the presence of a bicuspid AV predisposes to both aortic insufficiency and early calcification and stenosis; this is one of the most common etiologies of aortic pathology in patients presenting for AV surgery.

Transesophageal Echocardiographic Views for Aortic Valve Assessment

TEE imaging of the AV uses four standard imaging planes, each providing a distinct advantage to addressing specific functional and anatomic data.

Midesophageal Aortic Valve Short-Axis View

The midesophageal (ME) AV short-axis (SAX) view (Fig. 14-1 and Video 14-1) is generated with the tip of the TEE probe in the esophagus and the ultrasound transducer rotated to approximately 35 to 50 degrees. The images generate an en face view of the AV akin to the view of the surgeon when peering through an aortotomy incision. The valve is inspected by echocardiography in diastole (closed) and systole (open). In normal valves, the cusps are thin and freely mobile. The systolic orifice area can be measured by planimetry (or calculated via the continuity equation using other views). "Normal" individuals may have a tiny jet of trace aortic regurgitation (AR), often located in the center of the AV. In the presence of AR, the SAX view is particularly useful in defining the locus of the regurgitant orifice. Ostia of the left main and right coronary arteries are easily detected emanating from the corresponding coronary sinuses. Slight withdrawal of the TEE probe demonstrates the proximal ascending aorta. Advancement of the probe depicts the LVOT.

Midesophageal Aortic Valve Long-Axis View

The ME-AV long-axis (LAX) view (Fig. 14-2 and Video 14-2) is produced by rotating the transducer to approximately 120 to 150 degrees. Blood flow is mostly perpendicular to the ultrasound beam. The LVOT, valve cusps, sinuses, sinotubular junction, and ascending aorta are seen in a single image. The mobile cusps of the AV produce a zone of coaptation and effacement during diastole that spans several millimeters. The cusps separate widely during systole in normal patients (where the AV area is $\approx 2.6\text{-}3.5\ cm^2$). The sinuses of Valsalva are seen as symmetric outpouchings that form an aortic root bulb that joins the ascending aorta at the sinotubular junction. The AV LAX view is suitable for assessing the grade of AR with color Doppler. Application of color Doppler in the normal AV demonstrates no transvalvular flow during diastole but laminar flow during systole.

Deep Transgastric Long-Axis View of Aortic Valve

The deep transgastric (TG) LAX view of the AV (Fig. 14-3 and Video 14-3) is obtained by insertion and anteflexion of the probe from the TG SAX imaging plane and can be difficult to attain without significant flexion

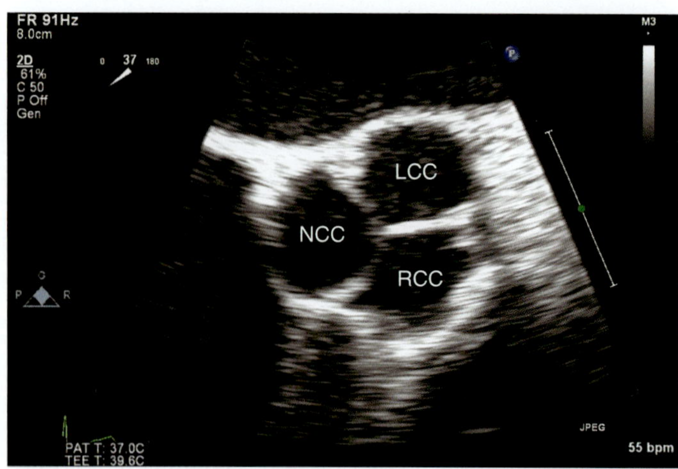

Figure 14-1 Midesophageal aortic valve short-axis view in diastole demonstrating left (*LCC*), right (*RCC*) and noncoronary (*NCC*) cusps.

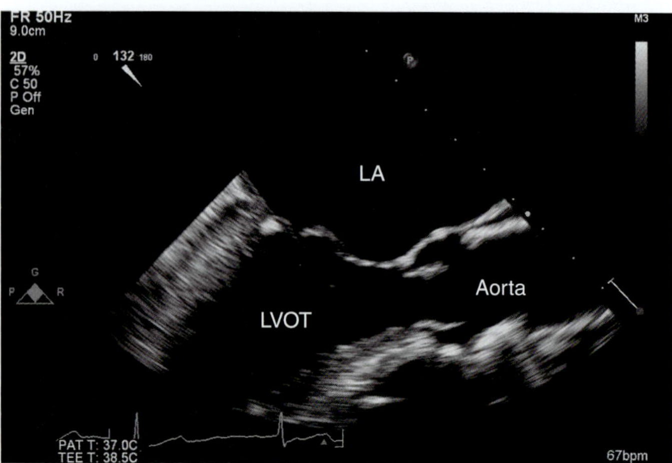

Figure 14-2 Midesophageal aortic valve long-axis view in systole. Aortic valve leaflets are seen in open position. *LA*, Left atrium; *LVOT*, left ventricular outflow tract.

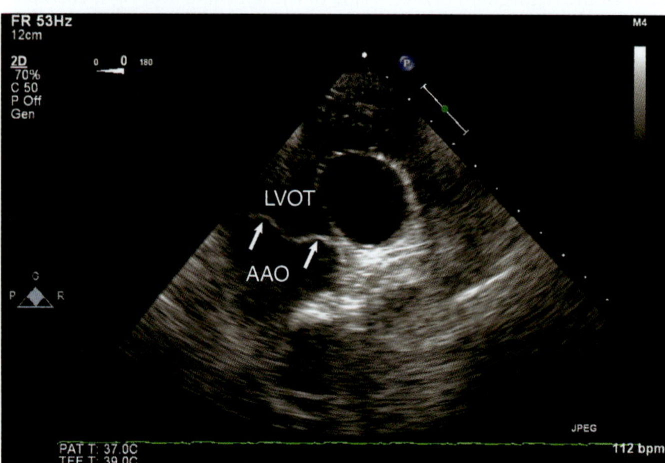

Figure 14-3 Deep transgastric long-axis view in diastole. Arrows point to aortic valve. *AAO*, Ascending aorta; *LVOT*, left ventricular outflow tract.

of the probe in the stomach. However, the TG view can often align the transvalvular flow parallel to the ultrasound beam, rendering TEE reliable in detecting and quantifying transvalvular blood flow velocities. It is the preferred view for spectral Doppler measurements of flow velocities to generate estimates of AV gradients and spectral displays of regurgitant jets.

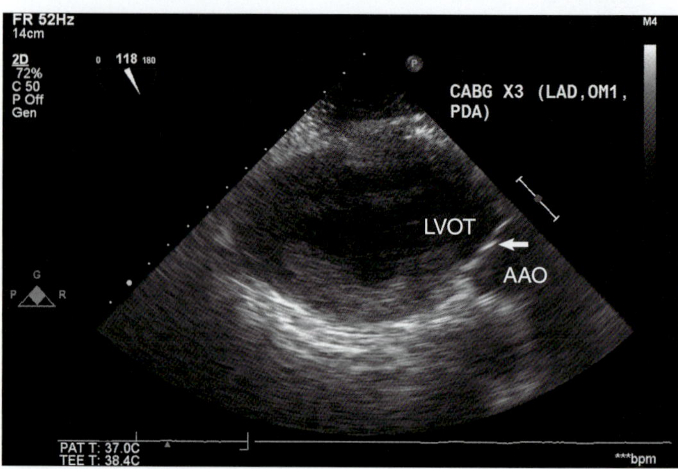

Figure 14-4 Transgastric long-axis view in diastole. Arrow points to aortic valve. *AAO*, Ascending aorta; *LVOT*, left ventricular outflow tract.

Transgastric Long-Axis View of Aortic Valve

The TG LAX view of the AV (Fig. 14-4) is obtained at an angle of 110 to 135 degrees from the TG SAX view of the left ventricle. Like the deep TG view, it allows for parallel alignment of the ultrasound beam with transaortic flow, making it an excellent choice for spectral Doppler interrogation of the AV. In addition, ME views of the AV may be obscured by echo shadowing in patients with significant mitral annular calcification or in patients with prosthetic mitral valves and mitral annuloplasty rings. In these scenarios, both deep TG and TG LAX views often allow imaging of the AV without overlying shadowing.

Aortic Stenosis

The intraoperative echocardiographer encounters aortic stenosis in several scenarios. Patients presenting for AV replacement commonly have symptomatic and well-delineated aortic stenosis. The echocardiographer's role in these cases is to confirm the diagnosis and rule out the presence of additional pathology or anatomic variants that may alter the surgical plan. A second, not uncommon, scenario is the patient who presents for cardiac surgery with an abnormal-appearing AV but without adequate preoperative recognition or quantification of the degree of stenosis. It is critically important for intraoperative echocardiographers to have the ability to accurately identify aortic stenosis and interpret the significance of the lesion.

Anatomic Imaging in Aortic Stenosis

A thorough two-dimensional (2D) echocardiographic examination of the AV usually yields the first evidence of stenosis. Increased valve echogenicity secondary to calcifications is typically present in patients with aortic stenosis (see Video 14-4). Although increased echogenicity can be due solely to leaflet sclerosis, the calcifications seen in true aortic stenosis are associated with leaflet thickening and a reduction in valve opening. The pattern of calcification can also provide insight into the underlying etiology of the valve stenosis (Fig. 14-5). In senile calcific degeneration of tricuspid AVs, the bodies of the leaflets are most affected. In rheumatic stenosis, commissural fusion may be the most outstanding feature. With advanced rheumatic or bicuspid aortic stenosis, the degree of calcification may be so great that echocardiographic distinction between entities is impossible. A full anatomic evaluation should also include an assessment of both the subvalvular (Fig. 14-6) and supravalvular areas to rule out nonvalvular stenosis.[14]

In addition to qualitative evaluation, 2D imaging can be used to quantify the severity of the stenosis. The simplest technique for quantification is to measure leaflet separation in long axis. This is best accomplished in the ME-AV LAX view (Fig. 14-7), although the deep

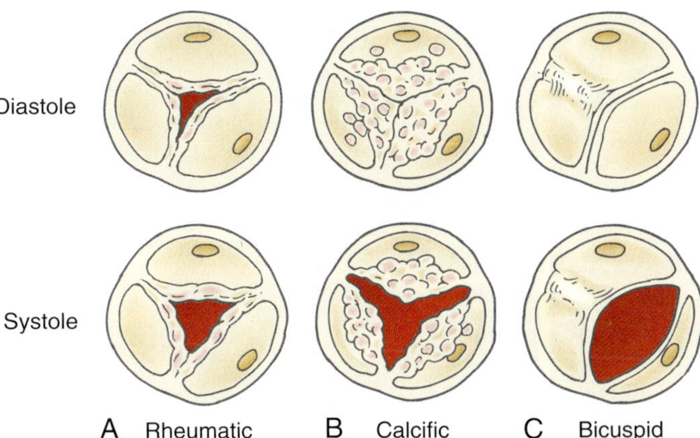

Figure 14-5 Morphology of valve calcification and etiology of stenosis. **A,** Rheumatic disease with commissural fusion. **B,** Senile calcific degeneration of leaflet bodies. **C,** Bicuspid valve with fused raphe. *(Adapted from Baumgartner H, Hung J, Bermejo J, et al. Echocardiographic assessment of valve stenosis: EAE/ASE recommendations for clinical practice. J Am Soc Echocardiogr. 2009;22:1-23.)*

TG LAX view can yield acceptable results as well. When the separation is greater than 15 mm, significant obstruction can be reliably excluded.[15] When using this quantification technique, it is important to align the 2D image in the center of the valve; a sector cut closer to a commissure may lead to overestimation of the degree of stenosis. In the ME-AV LAX view, a 2D-guided M-mode measurement of leaflet separation can also be used. Given the more complex leaflet orientation seen in congenital valve stenosis, use of leaflet separation to estimate the severity of stenosis may be less accurate.[15]

Direct valve orifice area measurements can be obtained using valve planimetry in the ME-AV SAX view. Planimetry is performed by tracing the area of the valve orifice using echocardiographic software packages (Fig. 14-8). To increase accuracy, it is important to trace the valve orifice at the level of the leaflet tips, because measurements obtained near the base of the leaflets may overestimate valve area and underestimate the severity of stenosis. Planimetry is usually straightforward in patients without significant leaflet calcification (Fig. 14-9), but in those with significant calcification, the ability to clearly visualize and define the true valve orifice may be impeded. This limitation will also apply if the valve has a complex 3D orientation leading to a nonplanar orifice (Fig. 14-10) and may be even more relevant in congenital lesions (Fig. 14-11).[3]

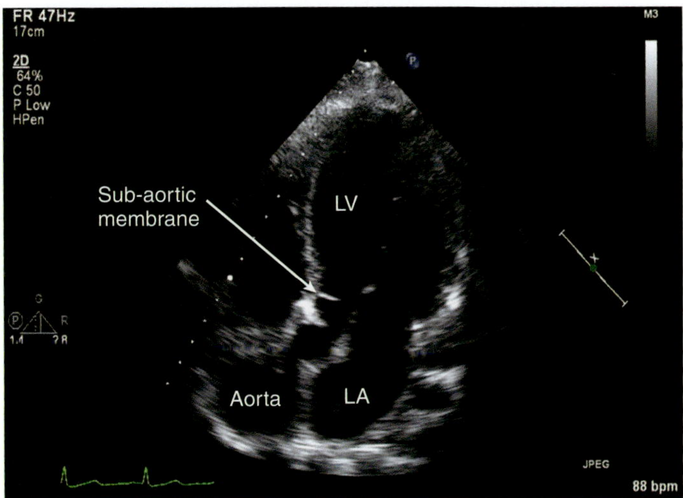

Figure 14-6 Subaortic membrane. In this deep transgastric long-axis image, membrane is seen within left ventricular outflow tract, creating stenosis proximal to aortic valve. *LA,* Left atrium; *LV,* left ventricle.

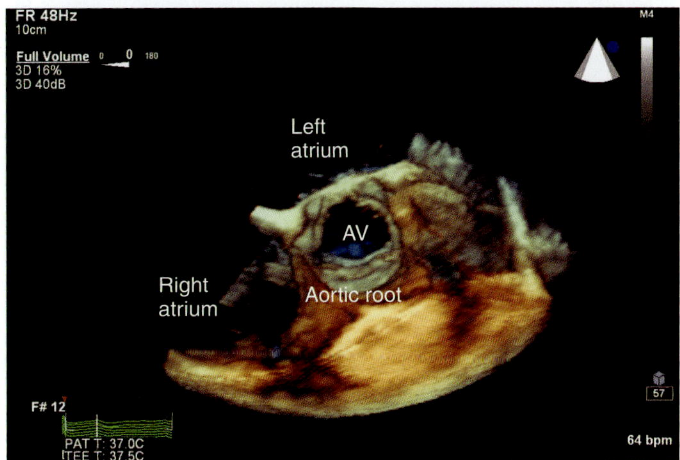

Figure 14-8 Full-volume three-dimensional image focused on aortic root with normal trileaflet aortic valve *(AV)* seen in center of image. Note cylindrical nature of this normal valve orifice, which facilitates ability to measure leaflet separation or valve area planimetry.

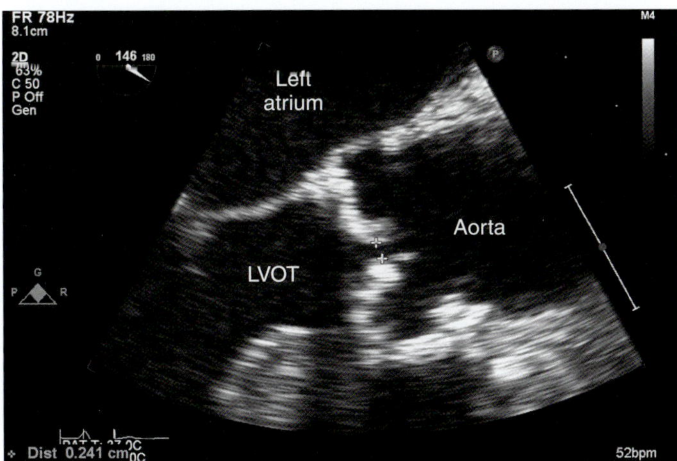

Figure 14-7 Measurement of leaflet separation in trileaflet valve. Transesophageal echocardiographic image obtained from zoomed midesophageal aortic valve long axis. Effort is made to image through center of aortic valve. NOTE: leaflet edges are parallel to each other and within aortic root. *LVOT,* Left ventricular outflow tract.

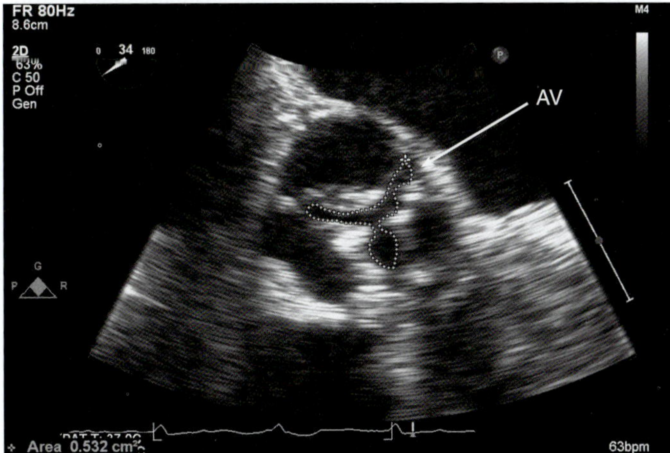

Figure 14-9 Planimetry of aortic valve (AV): zoomed midesophageal AV short-axis view. AV is seen in its short axis in center of image, with its area traced. To optimize accuracy, multiple measurements should be made to ensure smallest planar area is measured.

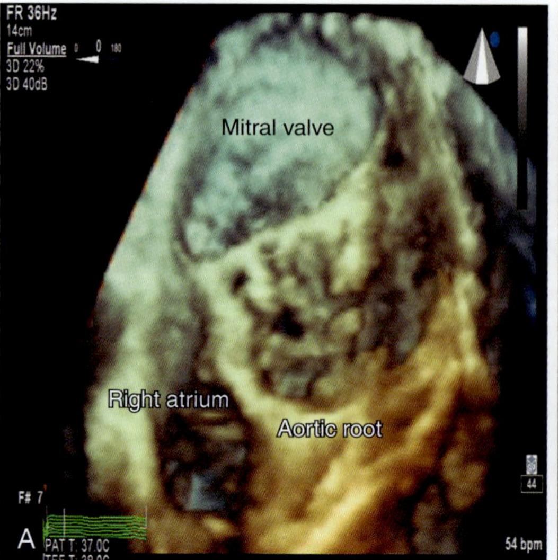

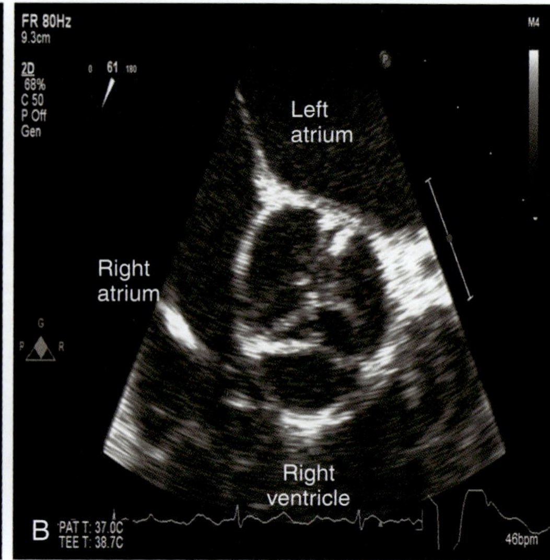

Figure 14-10 In comparison to Figure 14-8, note the complex three-dimensional (3D) height of this severely stenotic aortic valve in **A**. This complexity is not readily apparent in corresponding two-dimensional (2D) image in **B**. This inability to appreciate 3D orientation limits accuracy when performing planimetry of 2D images.

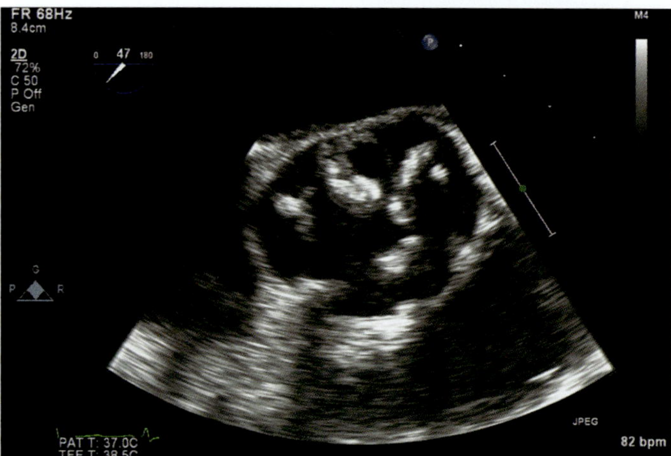

Figure 14-11 Planimetry of bicuspid aortic valve: midesophageal aortic valve short-axis view zoomed. Given the complex nature of this bicuspid valve with dense calcifications, the ability to reliably measure planimetry at the valve orifice is severely limited.

Doppler-Derived Quantification of Aortic Stenosis

While 2D valve analysis provides invaluable qualitative information regarding valve function and orientation as well as important (although somewhat limited) quantitative data, Doppler-derived measurements have emerged as the cornerstone of aortic stenosis quantification.

To properly interpret Doppler-derived measurements, an understanding of the nature of fluid dynamics through a stenotic orifice is important. Acceleration of blood flow during ventricular systole into a naturally occurring tapered ventricular outflow tract (LVOT) creates a uniform velocity flow profile throughout the entire outflow tract. As blood from the LVOT approaches a stenotic AV, flow accelerates and converges just proximal to the stenosis (Figs. 14-12 and 14-13 and Video 14-5). This acceleration continues as the jet crosses the stenosis. The jet reaches its narrowest width and highest velocity just downstream from the stenotic valve. This point is called the *vena contracta* (Fig. 14-14; also see Fig 14-13).

Distal to the vena contracta, flow expands and the jet velocity begins to fall. The pressure in the aorta distal to the vena contracta rises as blood flow velocity decreases, eventually reaching a level corresponding to the overall "pressure drop" across the stenosis. The distance the high-velocity jet travels into the ascending aorta will also be dependent on the angle of blood flow.[16,17] Blood flow adjacent to the high-velocity jet is typically disturbed and characterized by disorganized movement

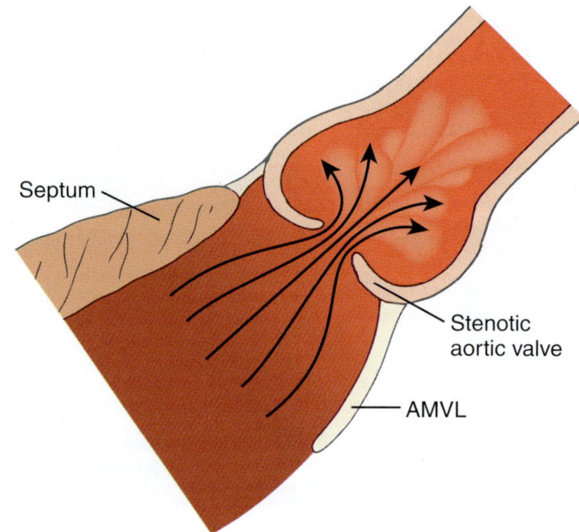

Figure 14-12 Flow through a stenotic orifice. *AMVL,* Anterior mitral valve leaflet. *(From Otto CM, ed.* Textbook of Clinical Echocardiography. *Philadelphia: WB Saunders; 2000.)*

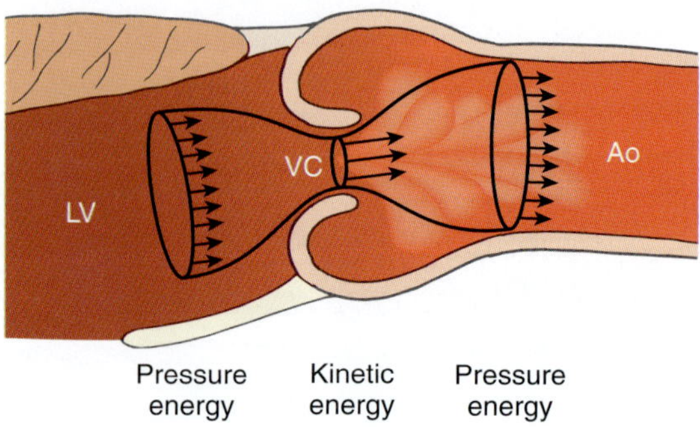

Figure 14-13 Recovery of pressure distal to a stenosis. Distal to the vena contracta *(VC),* the flow stream expands and kinetic energy is converted back to pressure energy in the aorta *(Ao)* minus any irrecoverable energy losses due to frictional and heat losses. *LV,* Left ventricle. *(Adapted from Bach DS. Echo/Doppler evaluation of hemodynamics after aortic valve replacement: principles of interrogation and evaluation of high gradients. JACC Cardiovasc Imaging. 2010;3:296-304.)*

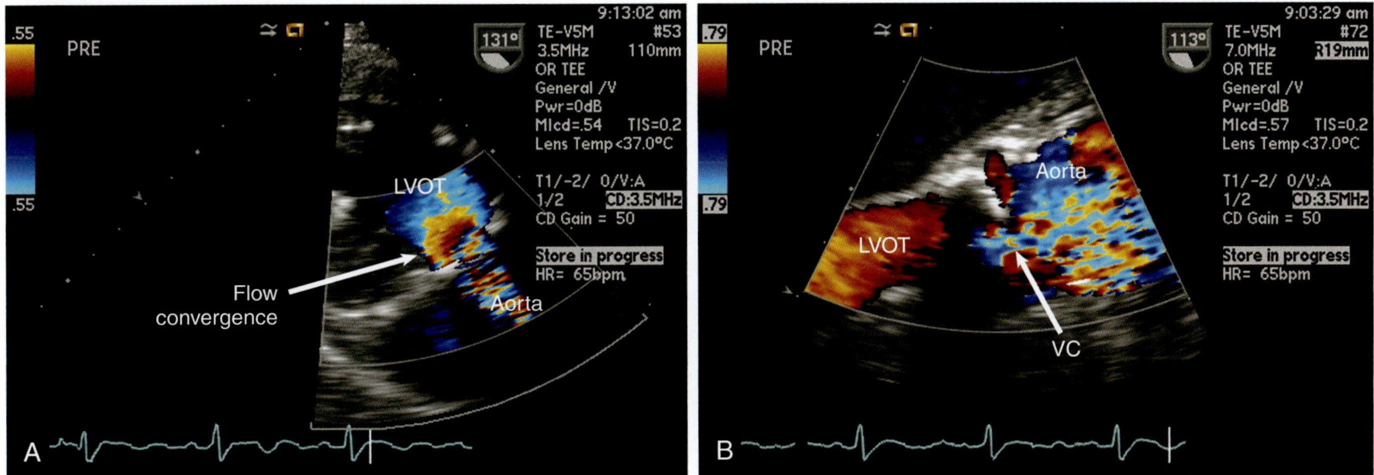

Figure 14-14   **A,** Deep transgastric long-axis (LAX) view with color flow Doppler (CFD) demonstrating prestenotic flow convergence in patient with aortic stenosis. **B,** Zoomed midesophageal aortic valve LAX view with CFD demonstrating vena contracta *(VC)* at level of stenotic valve. *LVOT,* Left ventricular outflow tract.

with varying velocities (see Fig. 14-12).[15] The degree of flow disturbance is most related to the severity of the stenosis but will also be affected by the geometry of both the valve and ascending aorta.[18]

Use of the Bernoulli Equation

Because the pressure gradient across a stenotic valve is directly related to the degree of valve narrowing, calculation of peak and mean gradients are frequently used to quantify the degree of aortic stenosis. Although pressure gradients cannot be measured directly via echocardiography, they can be derived from flow velocities obtainable using spectral Doppler. As described in Chapter 4, pressure gradients are related to jet velocity through the use of the modified Bernoulli equation:

$$\Delta Pmax = 4Vmax^2$$

Thus, by simply measuring the maximum velocity across the valve, the peak pressure gradient can be easily and reliably calculated.[19,20] The mean gradient can be determined by tracing the obtained velocity curve and using the instrument software package to average the instantaneous velocities over the entire ejection period (Fig. 14-15).

The velocity profile in aortic stenosis is best obtained from TG imaging planes that allow for parallel alignment of the Doppler beam with transaortic flow. Because the velocity of blood flow in clinically significant aortic stenosis is usually elevated, continuous wave Doppler (CWD) should be used to avoid pulsed wave Doppler (PWD) aliasing. Use of the simplified Bernoulli equation has been well validated, but there are some potential pitfalls. Most critically, the Doppler beam must be aligned parallel to the transaortic flow, because angles of intercept greater than 30 degrees can produce significant error and underestimation of the severity of stenosis.[14] To this end, it is helpful to utilize color flow Doppler (CFD) to visualize the jet crossing the valve (see Fig. 14-14, *A*) to help align the spectral Doppler beam. However, it is important to remember that even if the jet and Doppler beam appear well aligned in the visualized tomographic plane, the eccentric nature of many jets makes it impossible to know with certainty whether the alignment is optimized in the elevational plane.

For the most accurate results, multiple recordings should be made and ideally in more than one echocardiographic view, searching for the largest velocity obtainable. The recorded Doppler envelope with the highest velocity and a well-defined smooth velocity curve should then be used to derive gradients. In patients with significant stenosis, the ejection period is longer, creating a more rounded curve rather than more triangular. Patients with irregular rhythms will require additional effort to select representative tracings while avoiding use of post-PVC (premature ventricular contraction) beats.[14]

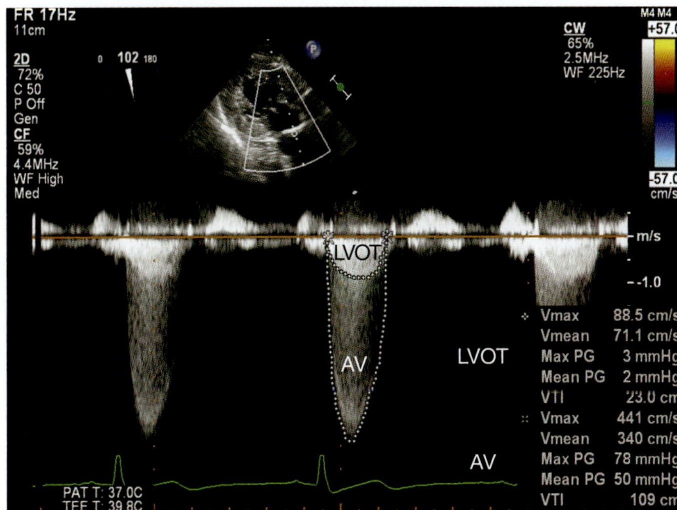

Figure 14-15   Double envelope technique; image obtained in deep transgastric long-axis view with continuous wave cursor placed crossing aortic valve *(AV)*. Once obtained, the lower-velocity but denser left ventricular outflow tract *(LVOT)* curve is traced, as is the larger-velocity transvalvular curve, producing peak and mean gradients and velocity-time integrals (VTIs) for both velocity curves.

It is also important to understand that factors other than valve area can impact transvalvular velocity and gradient. Chief among these factors is variation in the stroke volume (i.e., flow rate across the valve). For example, pressure gradients increase with exercise and/or stress secondary to increased stroke volume. The presence of significant concomitant AR will also increase volume flow rate across the AV and may cause overestimation of the severity of stenosis. Underestimation of the severity of stenosis in patients with low-volume flow rate may also occur. For example, patients with depressed left ventricular function or other low cardiac output states may present with low transvalvular gradients despite severe aortic stenosis.

When trying to explain these discrepancies, it is important to remember that the simplified Bernoulli equation eliminates LVOT velocity from the pressure gradient calculation. In patients with elevated LVOT velocities (>1.5 m/s), including those with AR, the proximal velocity term in the simplified Bernoulli equation cannot be ignored. Similarly, when the maximum transaortic velocity is less than 3 m/s, the LVOT velocity should also be reintroduced to provide for more accurate results.[14]

Continuity Equation

Because of the major influence trans-AV flow exerts on pressure gradients, use of the continuity equation to calculate AV area has become an important tool for quantification of stenosis severity. As described in Chapter 4, the continuity equation is based on the concept of the continuity of flow or mass. In the case of the AV, stroke volume through the LVOT should remain equal to that of stroke volume through the AV.

$$\text{Stroke volume (LVOT)} = \text{Stroke volume (AV)}$$

Measurement of LVOT diameter is best obtained in the ME-AV LAX view and should be measured leading edge to leading edge, just proximal to the AV and as parallel to the valve plane as possible (Fig. 14-16). Because the diameter is squared in calculating LVOT area, small variations in its measurement can lead to substantial error. To minimize this effect, effort should be made to optimize imaging, and multiple measurements should be made and averaged.

Stroke volume through the LVOT is obtained by placing the PWD sample volume within the LVOT and tracing the resultant velocity curve. This is best accomplished in the deep TG LAX or TG LAX views where LVOT flow is most parallel to the Doppler ultrasound beam. The software package will generate the velocity-time integral (VTI) (Fig. 14-17). The sample volume should be placed just proximal to the valve. If a smooth velocity curve cannot be obtained because of significant flow convergence at the annulus level, the sample volume should be relocated 0.5 to 1 cm proximal to the valve. The diameter of the LVOT should than be remeasured at this corresponding point. However, it must be considered that the LVOT in this more proximal position may be more elliptical in shape.[21]

The VTI through the AV can be obtained using CWD to interrogate trans-AV flow in the deep TG LAX or TG LAX views (identical to obtaining a peak or mean gradient) and using the echocardiographic software package to trace the velocity curve. If a well-defined second lower velocity envelope is seen within the CW envelope used for the AV interrogation, this second velocity profile can then be used as the LVOT velocity envelope. The "double envelope" technique has the advantage of using a single cardiac ejection and minimizing the effects of beat-to-beat variability (see Fig. 14-15). The obtained velocity will represent the highest LVOT velocity, which owing to flow convergence should correspond to a site immediately proximal to the valve.

After obtaining all three measures, the cross-sectional area of the AV in cm² can be solved for:

$$CSA_{\text{aortic valve}} = CSA_{\text{LVOT}} \times \frac{VTI_{\text{LVOT}}}{VTI_{\text{aortic valve}}}$$

The continuity equation can also be simplified by substituting the VTI of the LVOT and AV with their respective peak velocities. Finally, the velocity or VTI ratio is a dimensionless measure comparing the peak velocity in the LVOT to that of the valve itself. A lower ratio signifies more severe stenosis.[22] The advantage of this technique is avoiding errors associated with incorrect LVOT diameter measurement:

$$\text{Velocity or VTI ratio} = \frac{\text{Velocity or VTI}_{\text{LVOT}}}{\text{Velocity or VTI}_{\text{aortic valve}}}$$

Interpreting Results

Obtaining data regarding the severity of aortic stenosis is only part of the echocardiographic evaluation of aortic stenosis. Proper interpretation is a critical component of the examination as well. Because patients may present with widely varying body habitus, any calculated valve area should be indexed to patient size. This is particularly important for equivocal cases. Classification of valve stenosis based on indexed effective orifice area has been previously published (Table 14-1). The ability to properly index valve area in patients with obesity remains a challenge.

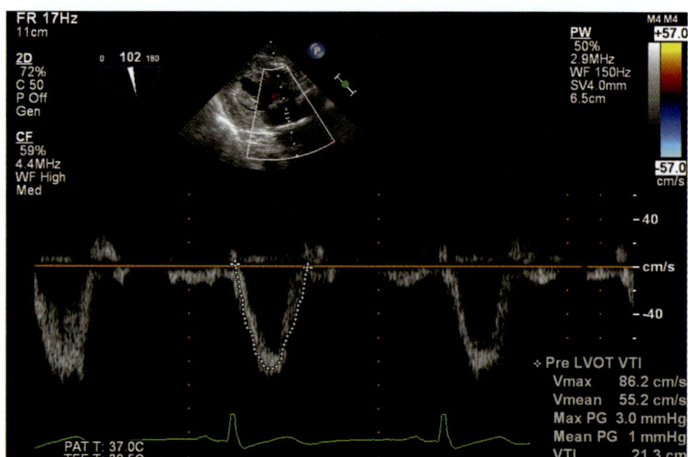

Figure 14-17 Obtaining left ventricular outflow tract (LVOT) velocity-time integral (VTI). Image obtained in deep transgastric long-axis view with pulsed wave cursor placed just proximal to aortic valve. Once obtained, velocity curve is traced, producing a peak and mean gradients and VTI within LVOT.

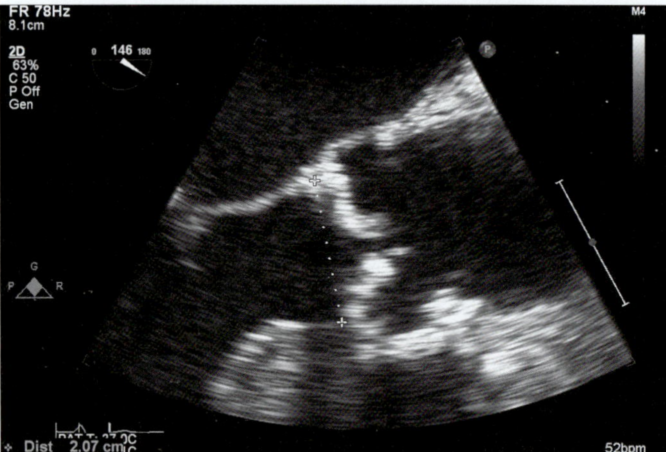

Figure 14-16 Left ventricular outflow tract (LVOT) diameter measurement; transesophageal echocardiographic image obtained from zoomed midesophageal aortic valve long-axis view. Effort is made to achieve parallel alignment of leaflets and rest of aortic root to achieve accurate measurement of true diameter. LVOT diameter is best obtained at aortic valve annular level, the most circular location. Because many patients with aortic stenosis have annular as well as leaflet calcification, estimation may be required to distinguish between LVOT and annulus.

TABLE 14-1	Quantification of Aortic Stenosis Severity			
	Aortic Sclerosis	Mild	Moderate	Severe
Aortic jet velocity (m/s)	<2.5 m/s	2.6-2.9	3.0-4.0	>4.0
Mean gradient (mmHg)	—	<20 (<30*)	20-40† (30-50*)	>40† (>50*)
AVA (cm²)	—	>1.5	1.0-1.5	<1.0
Indexed AVA (cm²/m²)		>0.85	0.60-0.85	<0.6
Velocity ratio		>0.50	0.25-0.50	<0.25

*ESC guidelines.
†AHA/ACC guidelines.
AVA, Aortic valve area.
From Baumgartner H, Hung J, Bermejo J, et al. Echocardiographic assessment of valve stenosis: EAE/ASE recommendations for clinical practice. *J Am Soc Echocardiogr.* 2009;22:1-23.

Even with proper valve interrogation and area indexing, the clinical picture may remain equivocal in some cases. There are several reasons why this occurs. An important yet often overlooked factor is the effect of the "pressure recovery" phenomenon. The nature of fluid dynamics through a stenotic valve (discussed earlier) causes recovery of pressure distal to a stenosis to always occur. However, the degree of this recovery can vary considerably depending on several factors. Because Doppler techniques only measure the largest difference in velocity (and thus pressure) that occurs between the LVOT and vena contracta, any significant recovery of pressure distal to the valve is not appreciated. In contrast, because of the obligatory displacement of the catheter tip away from the vena contracta, the gradient measured by cardiac catheterization is a fundamentally different quantity than the Doppler-derived gradient.[23] The presence of elevated Doppler-derived gradients compared to catheter gradients—which cannot be explained simply by differences in peak-to-peak versus instantaneous measurements—have been demonstrated in some subsets of patients.[24,25]

Based mostly on in vitro models, factors that have been shown to promote the occurrence of significant "pressure recovery" are the size of the ascending aorta and the degree of stenosis. The degree of pressure recovery is related to the extent of irreversible energy loss distal to the stenosis. In patients with severe stenosis, the increased amount of surrounding disturbed and chaotic blood flow will increase energy losses. Interaction of the stenotic jet and stagnant blood within the sinuses of Valsalva and along the aortic wall in patients with enlarged aortas will also increase energy loss and limit recovery. Consequently, "pressure recovery" only becomes relevant in patients with mild to moderate aortic stenosis who have normal to small-sized ascending aortas.

A formula to adjust for the effect of pressure recovery and provide a "corrected" AV effective orifice area, or so-called energy loss coefficient, is:

$$\text{Energy loss coefficient} = \left(\frac{\text{EOA}_{\text{continuity}} \times \text{CSA}_{\text{aorta}}}{\text{EOA}_{\text{continuity}} - \text{CSA}_{\text{aorta}}} \right)$$

where *EOA* is the effective orifice area and *CSA* is the cross-sectional area.

However, this formula has not been well validated. One of the biggest issues is that it does not account for several factors that affect the degree of pressure recovery. For example, the degree of jet flow angulation is believed to be an important variable.[17] In addition, in patients with no or mild stenosis, viscous forces likely predominate over the effects of pressure recovery, making the formula inapplicable in these patients.[26] Although the ability to accurately account for pressure recovery effects may be limited, it is important to consider its presence when making clinical decisions in patients with borderline surgical indications.

When evaluating the clinical significance of aortic stenosis, it is important to consider how the disease process affects the left ventricle and vice versa. The adaptation of the left ventricle to chronic pressure overload is increased ventricular mass due to chamber hypertrophy. The degree of hypertrophy and presence of diastolic dysfunction should be noted. Ventricular systolic dysfunction can develop later in the course of the disease. In patients with ventricular dysfunction and concomitant aortic stenosis, it is important to exclude the presence of pseudosevere aortic stenosis, which may occur secondarily to contractile dysfunction, leading to a reduced force of valve opening. With the semirigid leaflets seen in moderate (but not necessarily severe) stenosis, this reduced force may lead to valve area calculations consistent with severe stenosis even though the actual valve disease is not truly severe. This distinction may be significant, since pseudosevere aortic stenosis likely portends a worse prognosis. An inotropic challenge may help differentiate pseudosevere stenosis from severe stenosis,[27] but questions regarding individual variability in flow improvement exist.[28]

It is also necessary to consider the interaction of the valve and the aorta. Poststenotic aortic dilation is not an uncommon finding (Fig. 14-18). In addition, the association of bicuspid AV with ascending aortic aneurysm is well known.[29] The resulting "pressure drop" or energy loss across an AV stenosis may be exacerbated in patients with ascending aortic aneurysm. Consequently, these patients may develop symptomatic aortic stenosis despite relatively large AV orifice areas.

Patients with senile degenerative aortic stenosis often have concomitant decreased arterial compliance, since both disease processes share histologic features consistent with atherosclerotic disease.[28] Patients who have reduced arterial compliance with aortic stenosis experience even greater left ventricular afterload elevations and will typically develop worsening compensatory hypertrophy.[30] The resultant smaller chamber size and afterload elevation may limit stroke volume, which might lead to lower peak and mean velocities than would be expected for a given degree of stenosis.

TEE for Transcatheter Aortic Valve Replacement

Transcatheter aortic valve replacement (TAVR) is an exciting new technique currently under investigation in North America and Europe for the treatment of aortic stenosis. The superiority of TAVR over medical management in patients who are not candidates for conventional surgery has been demonstrated.[31] In addition, data comparing conventional AV replacement to TAVR in high-risk patients demonstrates comparable outcomes at 1-year follow-up.[32]

TEE plays multiple crucial roles in TAVR. Prior to implantation, TEE may be used for patient selection and prosthesis sizing. During implantation, TEE can help ensure proper placement and deployment of the valve. Finally, following implantation, TEE can be used to assess valve function, detect paravalvular leaks, and rule out injury to adjacent structures. As the indications for TAVR expand and availability increases, a working knowledge of the echocardiographic considerations for TAVR will become essential for perioperative echocardiographers.

There are currently two transcatheter valve systems approved for use in the United States—the Edwards SAPIEN (Fig. 14-19) and the Medtronic CoreValve systems (Fig. 14-20).[33] Access for SAPIEN implantation is achieved with a retrograde transfemoral approach or, when the femoral-iliac tree is not suitable, with an antegrade trans–left ventricular apical approach. Access for CoreValve implantation is achieved with the transfemoral approach or via the subclavian artery when the transfemoral route is contraindicated. Transthoracic approaches to the ascending aorta via a small-incision thoracotomy may also be used. Whereas many echocardiographic considerations for the two systems are similar, there are important differences that will be highlighted throughout this section.

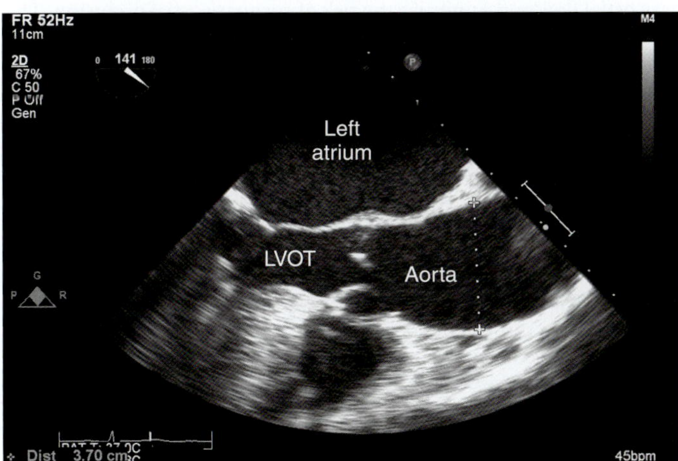

Figure 14-18 Poststenotic aortic dilation; transesophageal echocardiographic image obtained from midesophageal aortic valve long-axis view, showing patient with aortic stenosis and dilation (diameter 3.7 cm) of ascending aorta. *LVOT*, Left ventricular outflow tract.

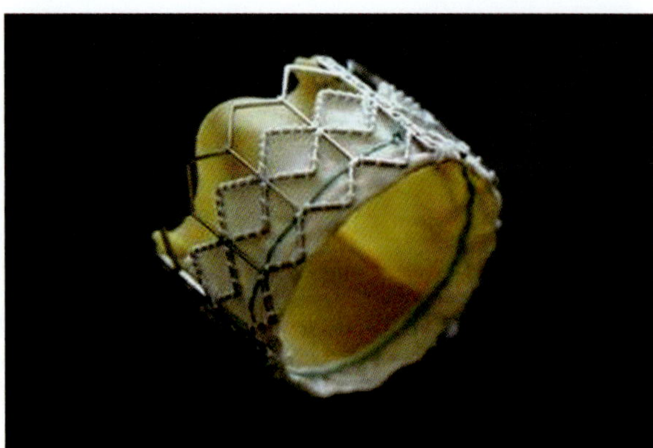

Figure 14-19 Edwards SAPIEN valve consisting of a tissue valve mounted on a balloon-expandable metallic frame. When deployed, frame traverses native aortic annulus, and valve sits in a slightly supra-annular position.

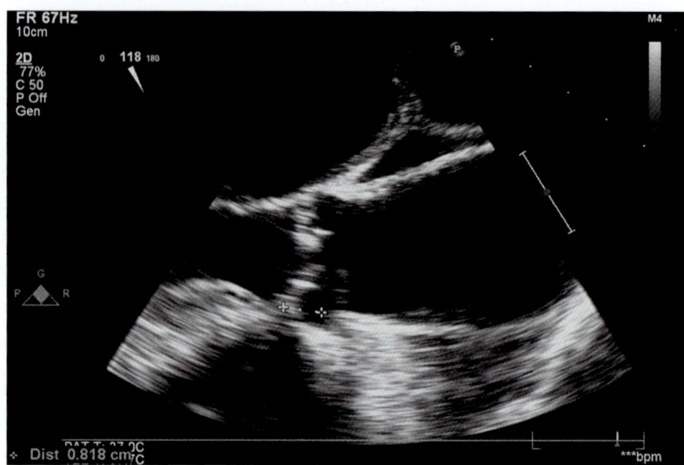

Figure 14-21   Zoomed midesophageal aortic valve long-axis view demonstrating aortic valve annulus–to–right coronary ostia measurement.

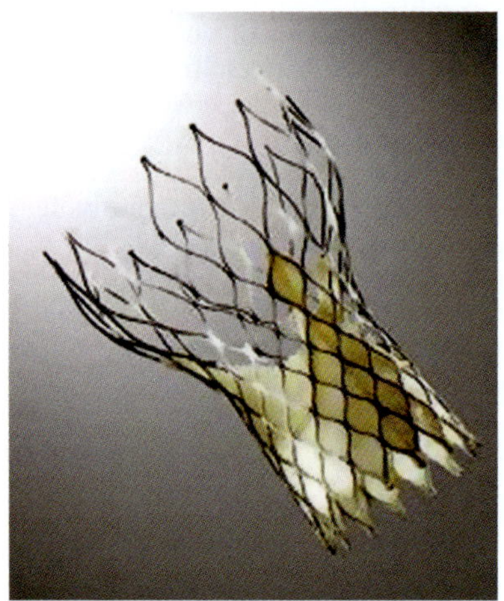

Figure 14-20   Medtronic CoreValve system for transcatheter aortic valve replacement (TAVR) consists of biological valve on self-expanding metal frame. When deployed, proximal edge of frame sits in distal left ventricular outflow tract, and distal end sits in proximal ascending aorta. Valve rests in a supra-annular position. Concavity of central portion of cylinder prevents coronary ostial occlusion.

Predeployment Evaluation

Patient selection and echocardiographic evaluation of suitability for TAVR are typically determined well in advance of the procedure. Nonetheless, intraoperative TEE should be performed when feasible.

Prior to deployment, subvalvular stenosis should be ruled out. Obvious asymmetric septal hypertrophy, particularly of the upper septum adjacent to the LVOT, may make implantation challenging even in the absence of frank subaortic stenosis. Significant hypertrophy may also lead to prosthesis dislodgement after deployment.[34] The presence of focal calcification of the aortic annulus and aortic root, best appreciated in the ME-AV LAX view, should be noted. Focal annular calcification will predispose to postimplantation paravalvular leak, and focal root calcification may be a risk factor for root perforation or rupture during valve deployment. In addition, a small root diameter with a relatively flat sinus segment is believed to be a risk factor for root rupture.[33]

Left ventricular thrombus is considered a contraindication to TAVR because of the risk of thrombus dislodgement and embolization during valve deployment. Similarly, high-grade aortic atheroma of the descending thoracic aorta and aortic arch is considered a relative contraindication to transfemoral implantation and should prompt consideration of alternate access routes when encountered. Finally, because

both the CoreValve and SAPIEN systems require balloon valvuloplasty of the native AV prior to deployment, patients with excessively long leaflets or those who have a relatively short distance from the aortic annulus to the coronary ostia are at risk for postdeployment coronary occlusion. When possible, the annular-ostial distance and relative leaflet heights should be assessed to identify patients at high risk. The annular-to–right coronary ostia distance can usually be ascertained in the ME-AV LAX view (Fig. 14-21), but the annular-to–left coronary ostia distance measurement requires three-dimensional (3D) imaging.[35]

Preimplantation Aortic Annular and Root Sizing

Measurements of the AV annulus and aortic root are required to determine patient suitability for TAVR and for prosthetic valve sizing. Proper sizing is critical because undersized valves are associated with a high risk of postprocedural paravalvular aortic insufficiency,[36] and oversized valves have been associated with increased risks of aortic root rupture and postoperative rhythm disturbances.[37]

The CoreValve revalving system consists of a tissue trileaflet valve mounted on a self-expanding stent. The system is designed such that the stent is anchored just proximal to the AV annulus and in the proximal ascending aorta. The intervening length of the stent (which traverses the aortic root) is slightly concave to allow for adequate coronary ostial flow and minimize the risk of coronary ostial occlusion. The biological valve sits in a slightly supra-annular position when the prosthesis is properly deployed. Because of this design, careful measurement of the AV annulus, aortic root, and proximal ascending aortic diameters are necessary for sizing. In addition, the height of the sinuses of Valsalva must be measured to ensure appropriate stent selection. Knowledge of selection and sizing criteria for the CoreValve is required when applying these measurements in clinical practice (Table 14-2). All measurements are best obtained in systole in the ME-AV LAX view zoomed on the AV annulus, root, and proximal ascending aorta (Fig. 14-22). The measurement of the AV annulus should be taken at the leaflet insertion or hinge points. Because of the significant leaflet calcification seen in most patients with aortic stenosis, care should be taken to exclude areas of calcification when measuring.

The SAPIEN valve consists of a bovine pericardial valve with a fabric cuff mounted on a balloon-expandable stainless steel frame. This prosthesis is affixed 2 to 4 mm below (on the ventricular side) the AV annulus. Like the CoreValve system, accurate measurements of the native valve annulus are critical for appropriate prosthesis sizing. In addition, because of the presence of the fabric cuff (designed to minimize postdeployment paravalvular leaks), the height of the sinuses of Valsalva must be sufficient to minimize the risk of coronary occlusion.[33] Once again,

TABLE 14-2	Measurement Guidelines for CoreValve Prosthesis	
Structure	**Measurement**	
Aortic valve area	<1 cm^2	
Aortic annulus diameter	20-23 mm for a 26-mm valve 24-27 mm for a 29-mm valve	
Sinus of Valsalva		
Width	≥27 mm for a 28-mm valve ≥29 mm for a 29-mm valve	
Height	≥15 mm for a 28-mm valve ≥15 mm for a 29-mm valve	
Left ventricular outflow tract	Septal thickness < 17 mm No obstruction due to membranes or protuberant calcium	
Ascending aorta diameter	≤40 mm for a 28-mm valve ≤43 mm for a 29-mm valve	

From Patel PA, Fassl J, Thompson A, Augoustides JGT. Transcatheter aortic valve replacement—part 3: the central role of perioperative transesophageal echocardiography. *J Cardiothorac Vasc Anesth.* 2012;26:698-710.

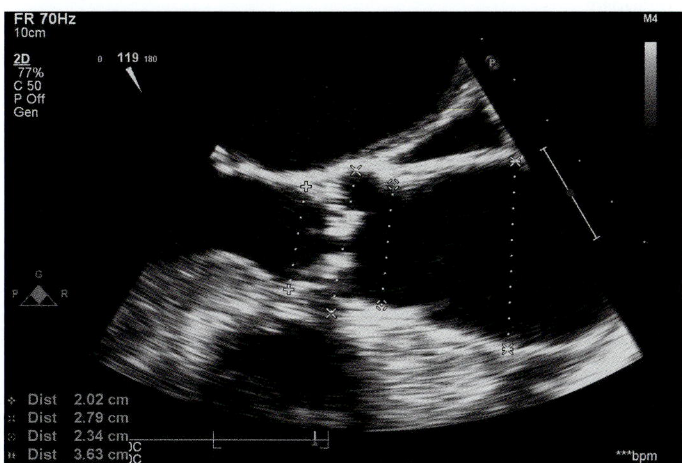

Figure 14-22 Zoomed midesophageal aortic valve long-axis view with measurements of aortic annular, sinus of Valsalva, sinotubular junction, and proximal ascending aorta diameters.

TABLE 14-3	Measurement Guidelines for Edwards SAPIEN Prosthesis	
Structure	**Measurement**	
Aortic valve area	<0.8 cm^2	
Aortic annulus diameter	18-21 mm for a 23-mm valve 22-24.5 mm for a 25-mm valve	
Sinus of Valsalva		
Width	Not applicable	
Height	≥10 mm for a 23-mm valve ≥11 mm for a 25-mm valve	
Ascending aorta diameter	Not applicable	

From Patel PA, Fassl J, Thompson A, Augoustides JGT. Transcatheter aortic valve replacement—part 3: the central role of perioperative transesophageal echocardiography. *J Cardiothorac Vasc Anesth.* 2012;26:698-710.

a working knowledge of the SAPIEN valve selection and sizing criteria is necessary for clinical application of these measurements (Table 14-3).

Valve Deployment

TEE plays a vital role during valve deployment in both assisting proper positioning of the prosthesis and identifying complications during the procedure. The first phase of valve deployment is placement of a guidewire across the AV (retrograde when the femoral or subclavian routes are used, or antegrade during transapical procedures). Transvalvular placement of the guidewire is best confirmed in the ME-AV LAX view (Fig. 14-23).

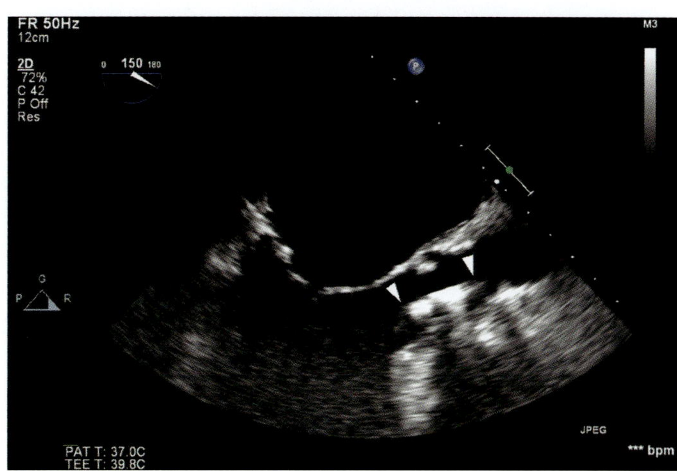

Figure 14-23 Midesophageal aortic valve long-axis view demonstrating proper positioning of valvuloplasty balloon across aortic valve prior to inflation (borders of balloon marked with arrowheads).

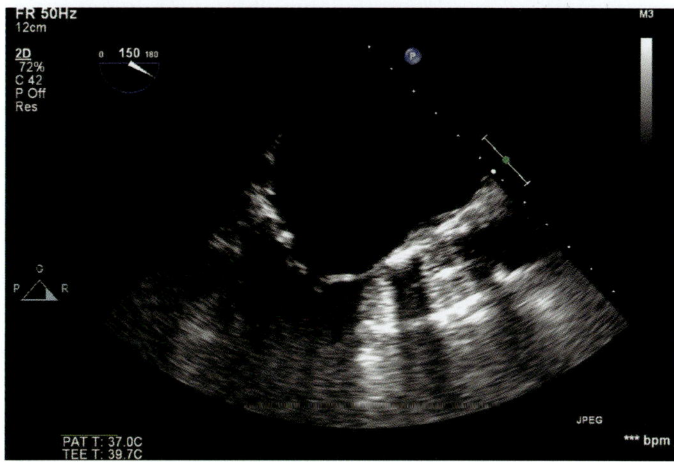

Figure 14-24 Midesophageal aortic valve long-axis view during balloon valvuloplasty.

The rare but catastrophic complications of guidewire placement should be excluded. Ventricular perforation can be diagnosed by identification of a new-onset pericardial effusion. Iatrogenic injury of the mitral subvalvular apparatus can be diagnosed with 2D imaging of the mitral valve and CFD identification of new-onset eccentric mitral regurgitation. In addition, iatrogenic aortic dissection should be ruled out, particularly when difficulty is encountered during guidewire passage.[38]

Once the guidewire has been successfully placed, balloon valvuloplasty of the native valve is performed. The ME-AV LAX view is once again ideal for confirming proper balloon placement and inflation (Fig. 14-24 and Video 14-6).  Following balloon valvuloplasty, the degree of aortic insufficiency should be assessed. In addition, annular rupture and iatrogenic ventricular septal defect and/or ventricular outflow tract tear can be ruled out in the ME-AV LAX view.

After balloon valvuloplasty, TEE can assist in confirming proper prosthesis positioning prior to valve deployment. For the CoreValve, the ventricular border of the device should sit approximately 5 to 10 mm below the aortic annulus. The ventricular edge of the SAPIEN valve should be 2 to 4 mm below the annulus. Excessive ventricular placement can impinge on proper anterior mitral leaflet function, particularly with the CoreValve prosthesis. Conversely, aortic malpositioning can lead to coronary ostial occlusion and increases the likelihood of paravalvular regurgitation. Positioning can usually be confirmed in the ME-AV LAX view, although in cases with significant shadowing secondary to calcification, 3D imaging may be useful.[37]

After proper prosthesis positioning has been confirmed, TEE can be used to visualize valve deployment. For the SAPIEN valve, this involves reinflation of the valvuloplasty balloon to expand the metal stent. For the CoreValve this, involves withdrawal of its encasing sheath followed by self-expansion. As with balloon valvuloplasty, valve expansion and deployment can result in annular rupture, aortic rupture, outflow tract tears, and iatrogenic ventricular septal defects. Valve embolization is a rare complication of this stage that can be readily identified with TEE.[39]

Postdeployment Examination

Following deployment, TEE is invaluable for confirming proper prosthetic valve function and positioning. As mentioned, the ideally positioned SAPIEN valve sits with the ventricular edge 2 to 4 mm proximal to the native aortic annulus (Fig. 14-25), whereas the ventricular edge of the CoreValve system sits 5 to 10 mm proximal to the native annulus (Fig. 14-26). Proper positioning is best confirmed in the ME-AV LAX view.

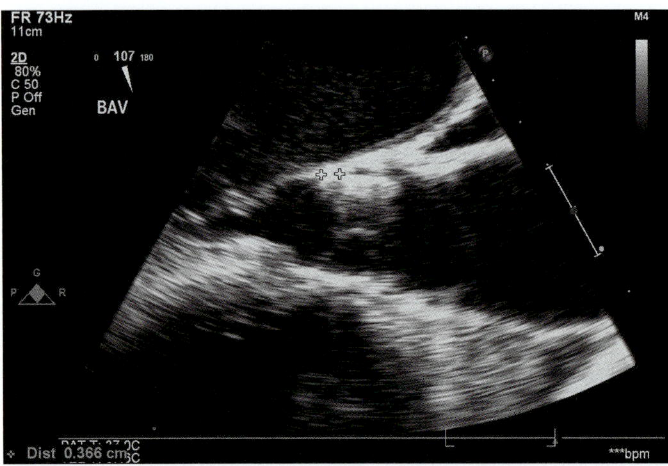

Figure 14-25 Midesophageal aortic valve long-axis view of properly deployed SAPIEN valve. Ventricular edge of prosthesis sits approximately 3.5 mm proximal to native aortic valve annulus.

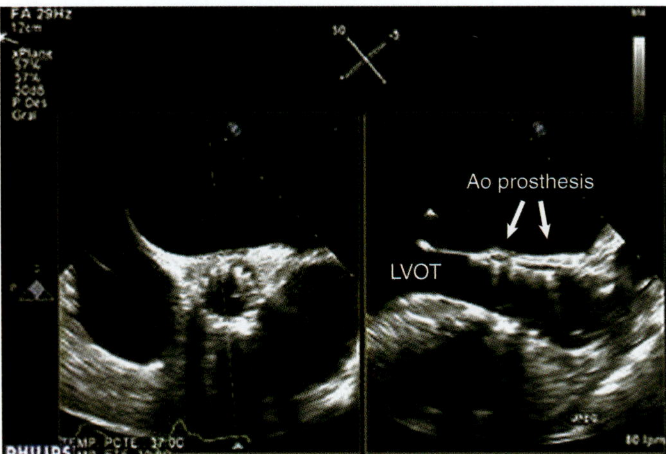

Figure 14-26 Biplane image (midesophageal [ME] aortic valve [AV] short axis on right, ME-AV long axis on left) of properly deployed Core-Valve. Note ventricular edge of prosthesis in left ventricular outflow tract (*LVOT*) and distal end in proximal ascending aorta (*Ao*). (*From Zamorano JL, Badano LP, Bruce C, et al. EAE/ASE recommendations for the use of echocardiography in new transcatheter interventions for valvular heart disease. J Am Soc Echocardiogr. 2011;24:937-965.*)

Hemodynamically insignificant postdeployment paravalvular regurgitation is present in the majority of patients after TAVR.[38] Nonetheless, careful examination of the prosthesis for significant paravalvular regurgitation is mandatory. The ME-AV LAX view with CFD is usually sufficient for this purpose (Fig. 14-27 and Video 14-7). Unfortunately, this view can be obscured by calcification and echo shadowing. When this occurs, both the deep TG LAX and TG LAX views offer windows that are typically free of shadowing. The ME-AV SAX view may be useful in identifying specific origins of paravalvular regurgitation.[35]

Significant intravalvular regurgitation is less commonly encountered after TAVR. In the immediate postdeployment period, some intravalvular regurgitation may be present as long as the guidewire or delivery system is across the valve and may persist for several minutes after wire removal.[35]

The ME-AV SAX view is useful to confirm normal mobility of the prosthetic valve leaflets. This can be confirmed in the ME-AV LAX, TG LAX, and deep TG LAX views as well. The transvalvular gradient should be obtained in either the TG LAX or deep TG LAX view. The valve area can be calculated with the continuity equation as described previously.

Finally, mechanical complications related to the newly deployed valve should be ruled out. The presence of new-onset wall motion abnormalities should raise the suspicion of coronary ostial occlusion. The mitral valve and subvalvular apparatus should be examined to rule out iatrogenic injury and associated regurgitation.

Aortic Regurgitation

Echocardiographic Evaluation of Aortic Regurgitation

AR is best described as retrograde flow across the AV and into the left ventricle during diastole.[40] AR can be caused by a variety of pathologies from congenital valvular malformations to acutely acquired processes such as leaflet destruction secondary to endocarditis. In the United States, AR is most commonly caused by progressive valve degeneration due to leaflet calcification or thickening or annular dilation and aortic root distortion. In developing countries, rheumatic disease is still the leading cause of chronic AR.[41] In patients with prosthetic valvular AR, intravalvular and paravalvular mechanisms may both play a role in the genesis of regurgitation.

AR of some degree is present in 10% of the population of the United States. Approximately 10% of these individuals (or 1% of the general population) suffer from moderate or severe disease.[40] Given this prevalence, the perioperative echocardiographer can expect to encounter AR during clinical practice on a regular basis. In some cases, the patient

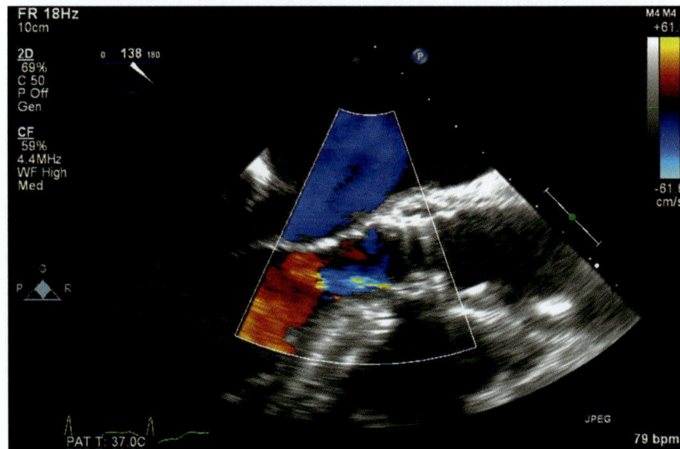

Figure 14-27 Midesophageal aortic valve long-axis view with color flow Doppler demonstrating anterior paravalvular leak following Edwards SAPIEN prosthetic valve deployment.

may be presenting with known surgical AR. The role of the echocardiographer is then to both confirm the diagnosis and evaluate the etiology of the disease to assist in surgical decision making. In other cases, the echocardiographer may discover concomitant AR during the perioperative exam in patients presenting with other surgical indications. Clearly, in these scenarios, it is critical to be able to accurately identify AR that requires surgical intervention. In addition, even when the AR itself is considered "nonsurgical," it may have significant implications for the conduct of the procedure. For example, moderate preoperative AR may prevent effective antegrade cardioplegia and may prompt consideration of coronary sinus cannulation and administration of retrograde cardioplegia. Likewise, in patients presenting for ventricular assist device (VAD) placement or those requiring intraaortic balloon pump (IABP) placement, AR that initially appears mild or moderate may prove to have significant hemodynamic consequences after insertion and should be carefully considered.

Accurate identification, quantification, and evaluation of aortic insufficiency require the application of multiple echocardiographic modalities. A summary of the most commonly used methods to grade severity of AR can be found in Table 14-4.

Two-Dimensional Examination

Although 2D imaging cannot on its own identify the presence of AR, it provides important information regarding possible mechanisms of any identified regurgitation. Careful examination of the leaflet anatomy and aortic root architecture will often yield the first evidence of pathology. Several TEE windows are particularly useful for this evaluation. The ME-AV SAX view allows careful examination of the valve leaflets. The presence of obvious leaflet abnormalities that may predispose to AR should be noted, including leaflet thickening, calcification, fenestration, vegetations, and destruction. In addition, congenital anomalies that may cause AR (e.g., bicuspid or quadricuspid valve) should be appreciated in this window. The ME-AV LAX view allows for good visualization of leaflet prolapse or restriction when those problems are present.

The ME-AV LAX view also offers the ideal window for examination of aortic root architecture and dimensions. Aortic annular or root dilation, with the accompanying increased tension on valve leaflets that can lead to abnormal coaptation and/or leaflet fenestration, are important causes of AR.[42] Therefore, routine measurement of annular, sinus segment, sinotubular junction, and proximal ascending aortic diameters in patients with aortic insufficiency is indicated (see Fig. 14-22). Many echocardiographers report these measurements using the inner edge–to–inner edge technique, which accurately matches radiographic methods. It is important to note, however, that the normative values were obtained using the leading edge–to–leading edge technique.[42]

Two additional TG imaging planes may be useful in the 2D examination of patients with AR. While the deep TG LAX and TG LAX views do not offer the resolution of the ME windows, TG views offer an excellent alternative when severe anterior mitral annular calcification or in situ prosthetic mitral valves obscure ME imaging of the AV.

In addition, there are several associated 2D echocardiographic findings that may provide insight into the severity of the disease process. In patients with chronic significant AR, a decline in left ventricular function and an increase in left ventricular end-diastolic dimensions typically is evident.[43] However, it should be noted that in patients with acute AR, compensatory left ventricular dilation may not occur. Left ventricular ejection fraction is usually preserved in these patients unless wall stress increases sufficiently to prevent diastolic coronary perfusion.

Early mitral valve closure in diastole secondary to premature increases in left ventricular diastolic pressures may occur with significant AR. In addition, fluttering of the anterior leaflet of the mitral valve may be evident, particularly in patients with eccentric jets directed at the underside of the mitral leaflet.

Doppler Evaluation

Doppler-derived interrogation of the AV forms the cornerstone of echocardiographic assessment of AR severity. Doppler is a powerful tool, but it is important for the echocardiographer to understand the limitations inherent in each of the Doppler modalities. To compensate for these limitations, the echocardiographer's ability to utilize multiple techniques when evaluating the severity of AR is critical.

Color Flow Doppler: Jet Dimensions

When assessing AR, the simplest technique uses CFD to visualize the turbulent jet emanating from the AV during diastole. This jet is typically best visualized using the ME-AV LAX view with the color sector applied to the AV and LVOT (see Video 14-8 and 14-9). In addition to demonstrating the regurgitant jet(s), for a rapid evaluation of severity, jet direction may provide information regarding the mechanism. Central jets are often caused by aortic annulus or root dilation, whereas eccentric jets often indicate leaflet pathology, although there is certainly crossover. 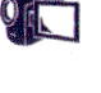

Several semiquantitative methods for assessing AR with CFD in this view have been developed. The ratio of jet width to LVOT diameter in central regurgitant jets can estimate the severity of AR. To properly obtain the ratio, measurements of the jet width and LVOT diameter just below the AV should be obtained (Fig. 14-28). A ratio less than 0.25 is considered mild; a ratio greater than 0.65 is considered severe.[44] Measurements of the area of the color flow jet or the depth of the color flow jet into the left ventricle have not been well correlated with the severity of AR.[44]

The vena contracta is the narrowest central flow region at or just downstream from the regurgitant orifice. Measurement of vena contracta diameter has been validated as a useful tool for quantifying the severity of AR.[45] In the ME-AV LAX view, measurement of the vena contracta is obtained using CFD interrogation of the AV. The CFD jet should consist of three regions: (1) proximal flow acceleration on the aortic side of the valve as blood velocity increases as it approaches the regurgitant orifice, (2) the vena contracta at or just above the level of

TABLE 14-4	Quantitative and Semiquantitative Techniques for Grading Severity of Aortic Insufficiency			
Parameter	**Mild**		**Moderate**	**Severe**
Continuous wave Doppler pressure half-time (m/s)	>500		500-200	<200
Vena contracta width (cm)	<0.3		0.3-0.6	>0.6
Aortic flow reversal	—		—	Holodiastolic flow in abdominal aorta
	Mild	**Mild-Moderate**	**Moderate-Severe**	**Severe**
Jet width/LVOT width (%)	<25	25-45	46-64	≥65
Jet CSA/LVOT CSA (%)	<5	5-20	21-59	≥60
EROA (cm²)	<0.10	0.10-0.19	0.20-0.29	≥0.30
Regurgitant volume (mL)	<30	30-44	45-59	≥60
Regurgitant fraction (%)	<30	30-39	40-49	≥50

CSA, Cross-sectional area; *EROA,* effective regurgitant orifice area; *LVOT,* left ventricular outflow tract.

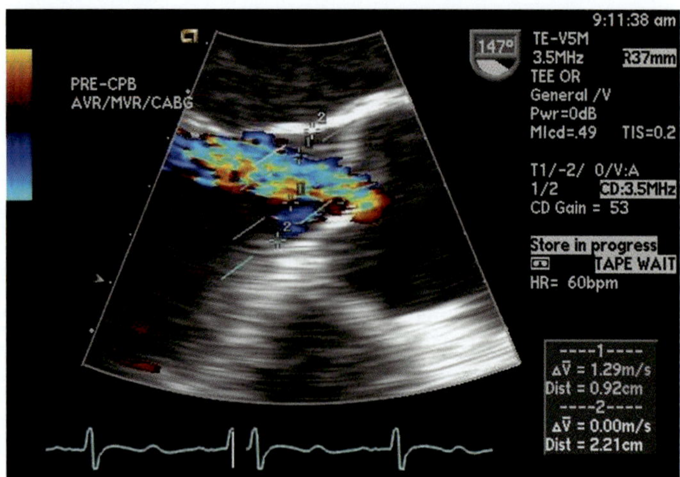

Figure 14-28   Midesophageal aortic valve long-axis view with color flow Doppler demonstrating central aortic insufficiency jet with a jet width. Left ventricular outflow tract diameter of 0.41 corresponds to moderate aortic insufficiency.

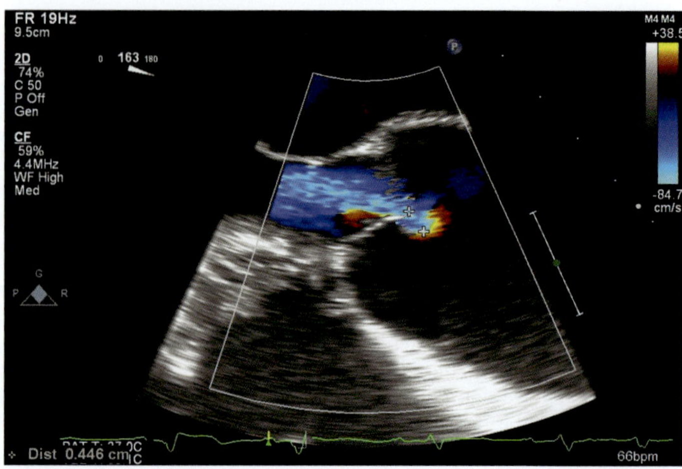

Figure 14-30   Midesophageal aortic valve long-axis view with measurement of proximal isovelocity surface area (PISA). Note that PISA radius is measured from leaflet tips to aliasing zone of proximal flow acceleration portion of regurgitant jet.

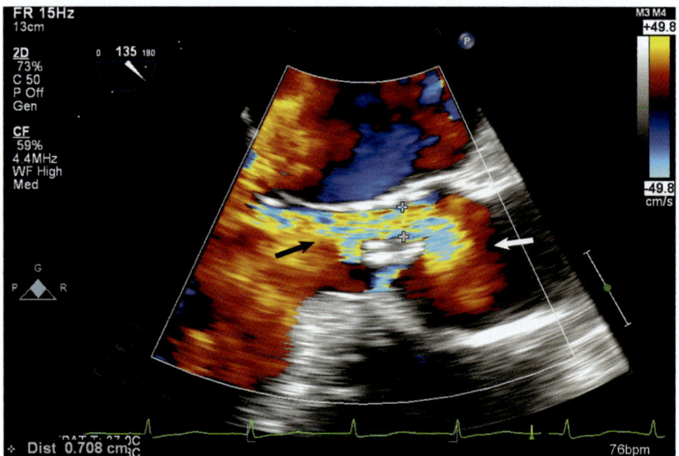

Figure 14-29   Midesophageal aortic valve long-axis view with color flow Doppler demonstrating vena contracta (VC) measurement for aortic insufficiency quantification. VC measurement of 0.71 corresponds to severe insufficiency. White arrow indicates proximal acceleration; black arrow, distal blooming.

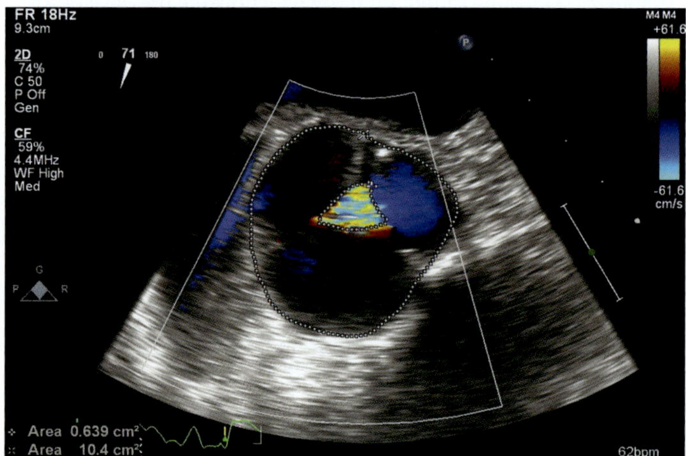

Figure 14-31   Modified midesophageal aortic valve short axis (ME-AV SAX) with color flow Doppler (CFD) and jet area: left ventricular outflow tract (LVOT) area. To obtain this image, a standard ME-AV SAX view with CFD is obtained, then probe is advanced slightly to obtain LVOT SAX view. Cross-sectional area ratio of 0.639:10.4 = 6.1% indicates mild to moderate aortic regurgitation.

the valve, and (3) distal blooming of the jet in the LVOT.[46] When all three components of the jet are present, the vena contracta is measured at the narrowest portion of the jet at or just above the regurgitant orifice (Fig. 14-29). A vena contracta width of 6 mm or greater reliably correlates with severe AR.[47,48]

Measurement of the proximal isovelocity surface area (PISA) can be used to calculate effective regurgitant orifice area (EROA) and thereby quantify the severity of AR.[49] To use the PISA method, an area of flow convergence must be visualized on the aortic side of the regurgitant orifice under CFD examination.[49] The flow convergence area represents concentric hemispheres of blood of increasing velocity as flow converges on the regurgitant orifice. The velocity of blood where the color map transitions from red to blue occurs at the aliasing velocity and is equal to the color flow Nyquist limit. As described in Chapter 4, the distance from the center of the regurgitant orifice to the edge of this hemisphere demonstrating aliasing velocity is the radius of the hemisphere (Fig. 14-30).[50] Next, the peak velocity (V_{max}) of the regurgitant jet must be obtained using CWD (best acquired in the deep TG apical or TG LAX view to optimize alignment of the spectral Doppler axis with regurgitant jet flow).

Once this has been obtained, we can derive the AR EROA using the continuity equation:

$$A_1 \times V_1 = A_2 \times V_2$$
$$EROA \times V_{max} = A_{hemisphere} \times Nyquist\ limit$$
$$EROA = 2\pi r^2 \times Nyquist\ limit/V_{max}$$

An EROA of 0.3 cm^2 or greater is considered severe AR.[51]

CFD can also be used in a modified ME-AV SAX view to assess AR severity. After obtaining the ME-AV SAX view with CFD over the AV, the probe is inserted slightly until the proximal LVOT is visualized in short axis along with a SAX view of the regurgitant jet. Measurement of the jet and LVOT cross-sectional areas in this view and the resulting ratio of jet CSA to LVOT CSA correlate with AR severity (Fig. 14-31). A ratio less than 5% is considered mild, and a ratio greater than 60% is considered severe.[51]

Spectral Doppler: Jet Deceleration Rate

CWD may be used in the TG LAX and deep TG LAX views to quantify the severity of AR. By measuring the deceleration slope of the

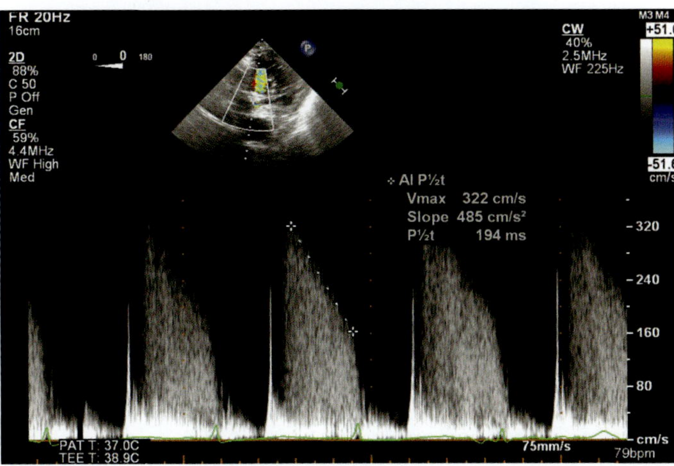

Figure 14-32 Continuous wave Doppler interrogation of aortic insufficiency jet with measured pressure half-time of 194 ms, corresponding to severe aortic insufficiency.

regurgitant jet, a semiquantitative estimation of the severity of AR can be derived (Fig. 14-32).[50] This is based on the principle that the velocity of the AR directly correlates with the difference in pressure between the aorta and left ventricle during diastole. This pressure difference will quickly approach zero in severely regurgitant lesions, and the descending slope of the CWD regurgitant jet envelope will be steeper. The accuracy of this method is dependent on interrogating the center of the regurgitant jet, which may be impossible in patients with eccentric AR. Other limitations with this method include the presence of physiology that would alter the pressure relationship between the aorta and ventricle, such as changes in systemic vascular resistance or left ventricular compliance. A hypertrophic noncompliant left ventricle would cause rapid equalization in pressure between the aorta and ventricle even in the setting of non-severe AR. Conversely, the presence of significant mitral regurgitation may result in a lengthening of the pressure half-time and underestimation of the severity of AR.

Flow Quantitation

Regurgitant volume and regurgitant fraction utilizing flow calculations are still considered reasonable diagnostic tools to assess the severity of AR.[51] The regurgitant volume is calculated by subtracting the right ventricle stroke volume from the left ventricle stroke volume measured at the level of the LVOT. To derive the right ventricular stroke volume, the area of the pulmonary artery is calculated by first measuring the diameter of the pulmonary artery in the ME ascending aortic SAX view and then using the formula: $\pi(d/2)^2$. PWD of pulmonary arterial flow in the same view proximal to the bifurcation of the pulmonary artery will yield the VTI, which when multiplied by the pulmonary artery area yields right ventricle stroke volume. Measurements for the left ventricle can be obtained just proximal to the AV in the LVOT.[52] These measurements are then entered into the equation:

$$\text{Regurgitant volume} = \text{Left ventricle stroke volume} - \text{Right ventricle stroke volume}$$

$$\text{Regurgitant volume} = (\text{LVOT area} \times \text{LVOT VTI}) - (\text{Pulmonary artery area} \times \text{pulmonary artery VTI})$$

The use of regurgitant fraction has been validated as a method to quantitate the severity of AR using the formula:

$$\text{Regurgitant fraction} = \text{Regurgitant volume} / \text{Left ventricle stroke volume}$$

A regurgitant fraction of 50% or greater is considered severe AR.

TABLE 14-5

TABLE 14-5	El Khoury Functional Classification of Aortic Insufficiency
Type of Aortic Regurgitation	**Mechanism of Aortic Regurgitation**
IA	Dilated sinotubular junction (normal cusp mobility)
IB	Dilated sinuses of Valsalva (normal cusp mobility)
IC	Dilated ventriculoaortic junction (normal cusp mobility)
ID	Aortic cusp perforation (normal cusp mobility)
II	Aortic cusp prolapse (excessive cusp mobility)
III	Restricted cusp mobility (thickening, fibrosis, calcification)

From Augoustides JG, Andritsos M. Innovations in aortic disease: the ascending aorta and aortic arch. *J Cardiothorac Vasc Anesth.* 2010;24:198-207.

Aortic Flow Reversal

PWD may be used to reveal retrograde flow in the aorta during ventricular diastole.[53] Absence of retrograde flow in the descending thoracic and abdominal aorta rules out the presence of severe AR, but the presence of flow reversal in the descending thoracic aorta does not necessarily indicate severe AR.[54] Holodiastolic retrograde flow in the abdominal aorta is considered sufficient to distinguish severe AR from mild AR.[53]

TEE for Aortic Valve Repair

The traditional approach to surgical management of AR has been AV replacement. More recently with advances in surgical technique, AV repair/resuspension has become a viable option for many patients presenting with AR. This approach was initially reserved for patients with AR secondary to aortic root pathology,[55] but its application has been expanded to include patients with AR and normal root architecture.[56] AV repair avoids some of the disadvantages of AV replacement, including the need for anticoagulation following mechanical valve replacement and limited valve durability following bioprosthetic valve implantation. Unlike echocardiography for AV replacement, where the surgical decision to replace the valve hinges chiefly on AR severity, echocardiography for AV repair is crucial for deciding whether the valve is reparable and directing the surgical approach. As described earlier, there are a wide variety of AR etiologies. An early functional classification of AR mechanism proposed three main categories of pathology: aortic annular dilation (type I), excessive leaflet tissue/prolapse (type II), and leaflet restriction (type III).[57] More recently, El Khoury introduced a modification of this classification system that further divides type I lesions into four subcategories (Table 14-5).[43] In the El Khoury system, the aortic root and its components, the aortic annulus (or ventriculoaortic junction), sinuses of Valsalva, and sinotubular junction are treated as a functional unit. While dilation of any single component of the root can result in AR, this refined classification is useful in guiding the surgical approach to valve repair.

Pre-Repair Evaluation

The literature suggests that perioperative TEE accurately predicts feasibility of repair in 90% of cases.[58] The cornerstone of the pre-repair evaluation is close inspection of the AV cusps to determine the mechanism of AR and identify specific leaflet pathology. The ME-AV LAX view with CFD can be used to distinguish central jets that may arise because of annular or root dilation (Fig. 14-33) from eccentric jets that imply leaflet pathology. In type II lesions, where leaflet prolapse is present, the jet will be directed away from the diseased cusp. When prolapse is encountered, the offending cusp should be identified. Right coronary cusp prolapse is usually easily diagnosed in the ME-AV LAX view, with the eccentric jet directed toward the anterior leaflet of the mitral valve and the anterior prolapsing cusp visualized with 2D imaging (Fig. 14-34 and Video 14-10). When left or noncoronary cusp prolapse is present, the ME-AV LAX view alone cannot reliably distinguish between the two posterior leaflets. In these cases, the ME-AV SAX view may be helpful in delineating the cusp in need of repair; 3D imaging modalities may 

also be of use in distinguishing between the left and noncoronary cusps. Isolated cusp prolapse can often be corrected with excision of excessive cusp tissue, cusp plication, and/or patch repair. These repairs are usually reinforced with subcommissural annuloplasty sutures.[59]

Type III lesions (leaflet restriction) are the least amenable to repair.[60] In these cases, leaflet calcification, thickening, and/or fibrosis may be present, resulting in limited cusp mobility and suboptimal coaptation. The ME-AV LAX view with CFD will usually demonstrate a central jet with or without additional regurgitant orifices near the leaflet commissures.

As implied by the El Khoury classification system, aortic root pathology can have a profound impact on AV function. Consequently, a detailed examination of the aortic root anatomy is a central component of the pre-repair examination. The ME-AV LAX view allows excellent visualization of all the components of the aortic root as well as the proximal ascending aorta (see Fig. 14-22). Measurements of the aortic annular, sinuses of Valsalva, sinotubular junction, and proximal ascending aortic diameters should be obtained. The specific site of root aneurysm can have major implications for the planned surgical repair. Patients with type Ia aneurysms and normal valve cusps (limited to the sinotubular junction and proximal ascending aorta) will often see improvement or complete resolution of AR with placement of a properly sized ascending aortic graft. Type Ib lesions (sinus of Valsalva aneurysm) with normal leaflet mobility are often amenable

to AV resuspension/reimplantation and root replacement. Type Ic lesions (annular dilation) are often reparable with subcommissural annuloplasty.[59]

Type Id lesions (leaflet perforation) may occur secondary to endocarditis. In patients who receive adequate preoperative antibiotics, patch repair and subcommissural annuloplasty may be considered. Leaflet fenestrations are also encountered with high frequency (30%) in patients with sinus of Valsalva aneurysms.[61] These fenestrations are often not visible on 2D examination of the valve; 3D imaging may, on occasion, reveal fenestrations (Fig. 14-35), although inappropriate gain settings can give the leaflets a fenestrated appearance even in the absence of pathology. The coexistence of type Ib and Id lesions demonstrates that multiple mechanisms and pathologies may be at play in a single patient.[62]

Postrepair Evaluation

The immediate postrepair period should be used to confirm adequate results of the surgical intervention. CFD interrogation of the repaired valve in the ME-AV LAX view should rule out significant residual regurgitation. When this window is obscured by acoustic shadowing or postsurgical changes, TG imaging planes should allow adequate visualization. Residual regurgitation is a strong predictor of late repair failure and may prompt surgical revision of the repair.[63] The nature of the regurgitation can, on occasion, help direct the revision. For example, a central jet following repair of a type Ia lesion may indicate that the ascending aortic graft has to be downsized to allow for adequate AV cusp coaptation. The deep TG LAX and TG LAX views should also be used for spectral Doppler examination of the valve to rule out the presence of iatrogenic stenosis.

In addition to assessment of the functional adequacy of the repair, its structural integrity should be confirmed as well. Cusp coaptation below the level of the AV annulus is an independent risk factor of AR recurrence and the need for repeat AV surgery even in the absence of residual AR.[64] The presence of subannular coaptation is best appreciated in the ME-AV LAX view and may indicate the need for immediate surgical revision of the repair. In addition, the coaptation length or zone of cusp apposition can be predictive of risk of recurrent AR. Residual AR coupled with a coaptation zone less than 4 mm has been associated with elevated risk of both AR recurrence and the need for reoperation.[63] The coaptation zone can be measured in the ME-AV LAX view at end-diastole (Fig. 14-36). The presence of a short coaptation zone with residual AR may suggest the need for repair revision.

Since the coronary ostia arise from the sinuses of Valsalva, there is a risk of iatrogenic coronary injury. Careful examination of the left and right ventricles to rule out new-onset regional wall motion

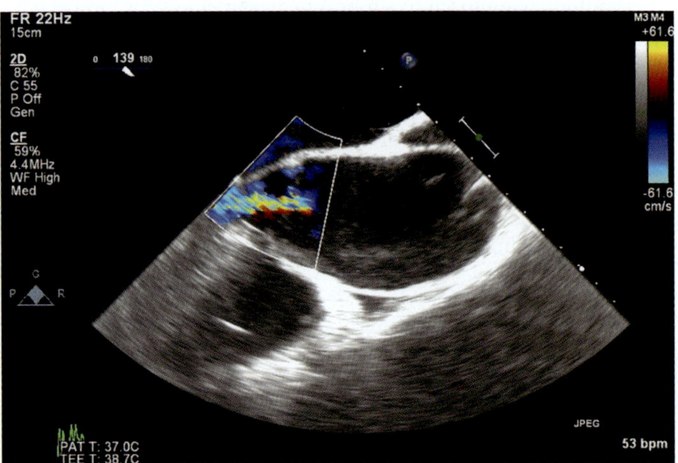

Figure 14-33 Midesophageal aortic valve long-axis view with color flow Doppler demonstrating central aortic insufficiency secondary to sinus of Valsalva dilation.

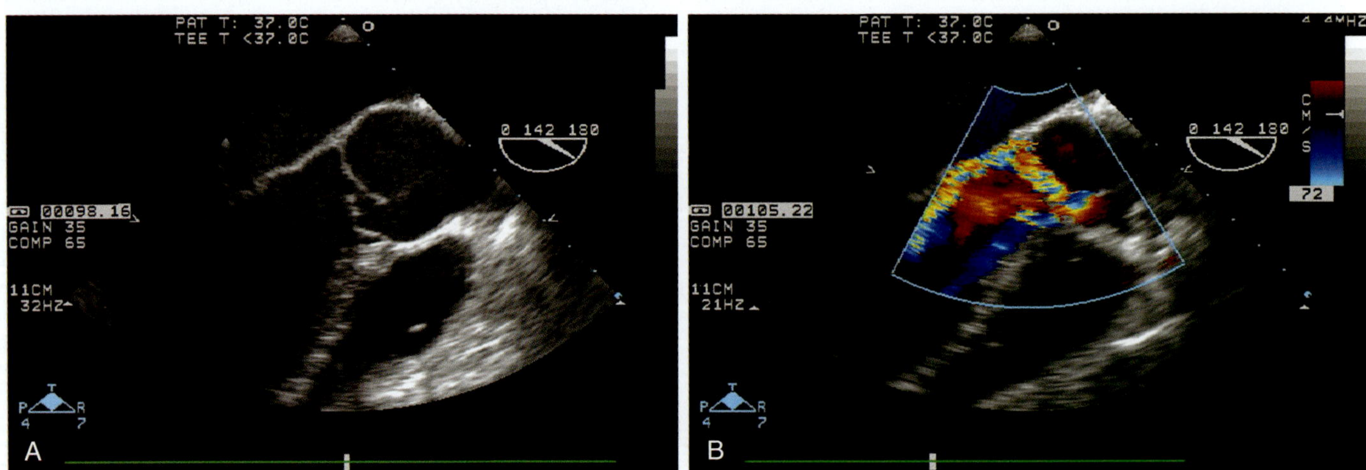

Figure 14-34 **A,** Midesophageal aortic valve long-axis view demonstrating prolapse of right coronary cusp. **B,** Resulting eccentric jet directed toward anterior leaflet of mitral valve.

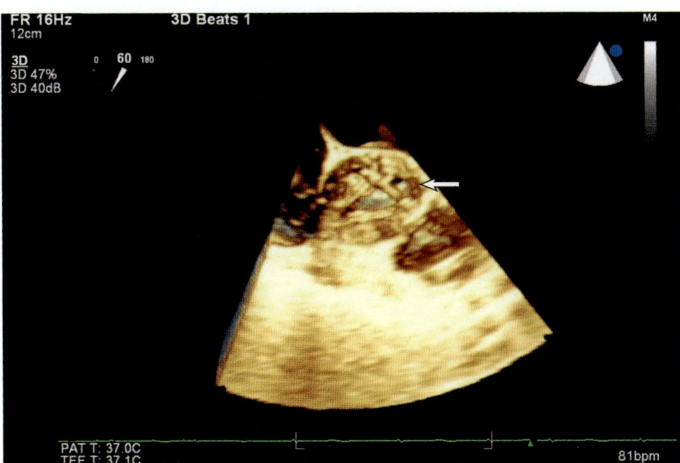

Figure 14-35 Full-volume three-dimensional image of aortic valve with color flow Doppler, demonstrating fenestrations of all three leaflets *(arrow)* in patient with ascending aortic aneurysm and associated aortic insufficiency.

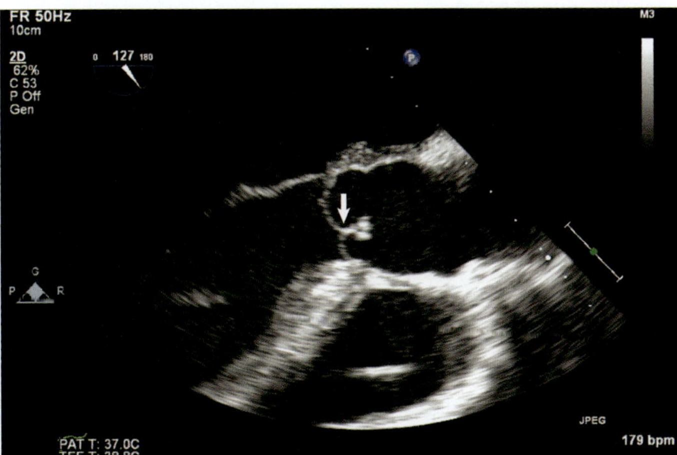

Figure 14-36 Midesophageal aortic valve long-axis view demonstrating resuspended aortic valve in diastole following repair. Note coaptation zone, measuring 9 mm.

abnormalities is warranted. The likelihood of iatrogenic ischemia may be highest following AV resuspension with sinus of Valsalva aneurysm repair, since this procedure necessitates coronary reimplantation.

Echocardiographic Evaluation of Prosthetic Valves

The perioperative echocardiographer may encounter prosthetic AVs immediately following implantation or in patients with in situ valves returning for surgery. Evaluating prosthetic AVs in many ways mimics evaluation of native valves, particularly regarding the quantification principles of stenosis and regurgitation. However, there are important aspects of the prosthetic valve evaluation that are unique, and there are significant differences in the respective evaluations of bioprosthetic and mechanical valves. It is important for the echocardiographer to appreciate these differences when assessing prosthetic valve function.

Two-Dimensional Examination

The 2D evaluation of prosthetic valves begins with identification of the valve type. Several different models of mechanical valves have been used in clinical practice over the past 5 decades, but by far the most commonly encountered mechanical prosthetic valve today is the bileaflet mechanical valve.[65] Most bioprosthetic valve models consist of bovine or porcine trileaflet valves mounted on a stented sewing ring (Fig. 14-37*A* and *B*). Stentless valves may offer potentially better flow dynamics but are technically more complicated to place.

When assessing valve function, it is important to use multiple acoustic windows; acoustic shadowing from the valve housing may obscure visualization of the leaflets, particularly in ME views (Fig. 14-38). Both deep TG LAX and TG LAX views should be used in this scenario to obtain unobstructed images of the leaflets (Fig. 14-39). All leaflets should be visualized moving freely without evidence of obstruction or restriction. In addition, excessive movement or rocking of the valve relative to the aortic root or annulus is often a sign of valve dehiscence and should prompt further careful inspection of the valve.

In patients presenting with in situ valves, an examination for signs of valve degeneration is warranted. Bioprosthetic valves may exhibit signs of leaflet fibrosis or calcification affecting either systolic or diastolic function (or both) (Fig. 14-40 and Video 14-11). Alternatively, leaflet breakdown or prolapse may occur with 2D evidence of malcoaptation. Mechanical valves should be inspected for the presence of adherent 

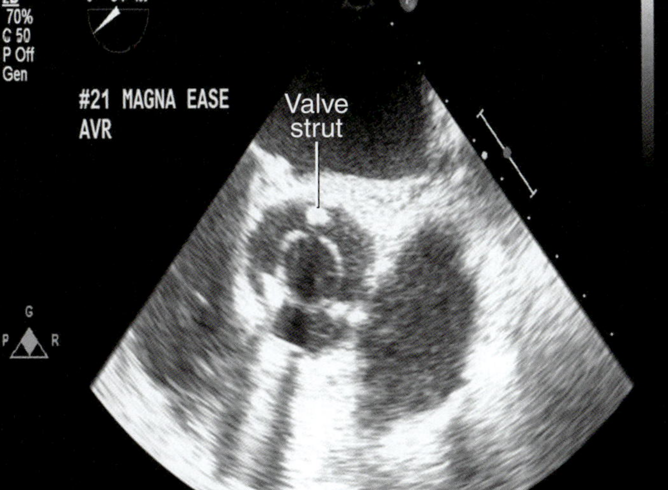

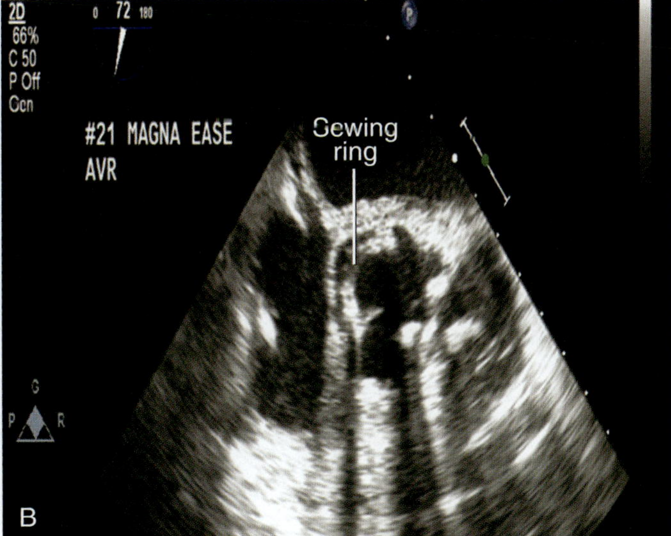

Figure 14-37 Two midesophageal short-axis images of bioprosthetic aortic valve. In **A**, all three struts of stent can be visualized. In **B**, sector is altered to visualize part of sewing ring.

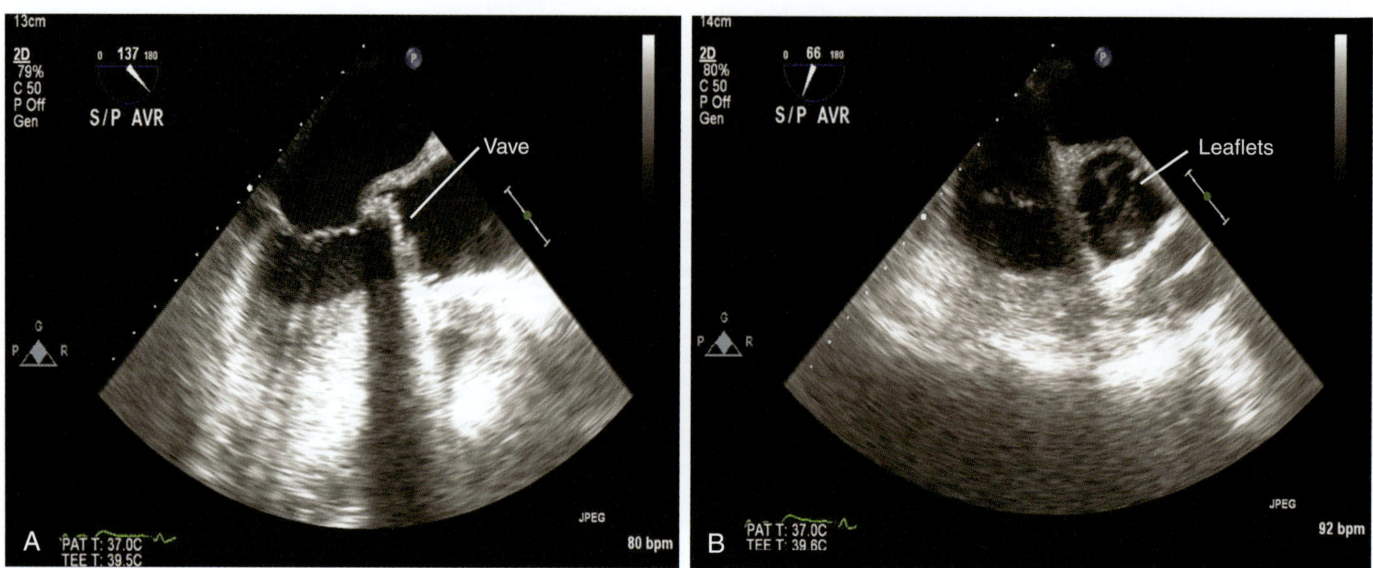

Figure 14-38 *A* and *B*, Long- and short-axis views of freshly implanted bileaflet mechanical aortic valve replacement *(AVR)*. Note acoustic shadowing in long-axis image that limits visualization. In short-axis image, the two leaflets are seen opening.

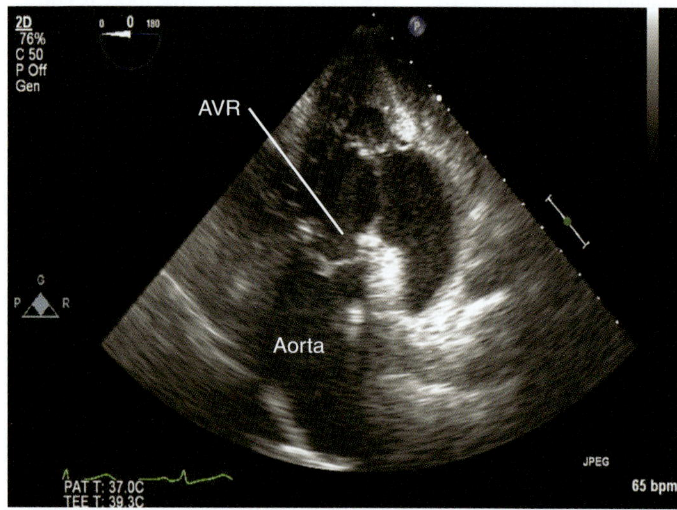

Figure 14-39 Deep transgastric image of a freshly implanted bioprosthetic aortic valve replacement *(AVR)*. Sewing ring does not obscure prosthetic valve leaflets in this imaging plane.

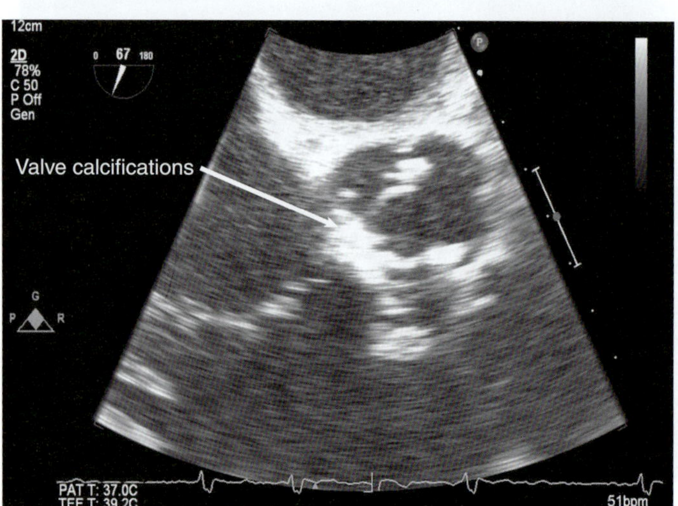

Figure 14-40 Midesophageal aortic valve short-axis image of in situ bioprosthetic valve with calcifications that limit overall leaflet mobility.

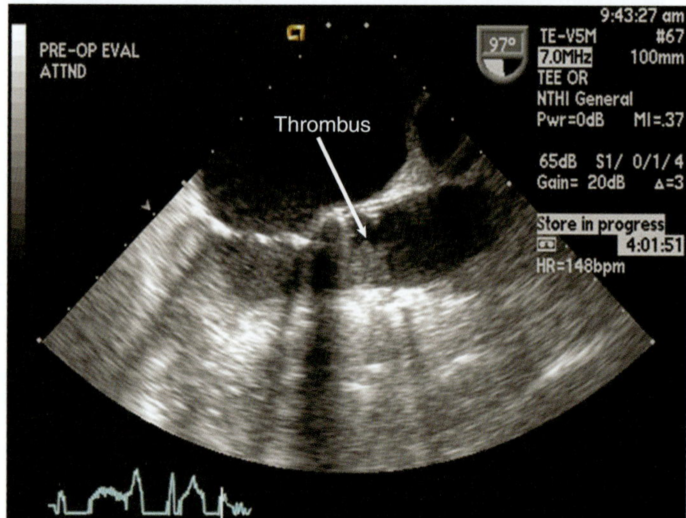

Figure 14-41 Midesophageal long-axis image of thrombus obstructing mechanical aortic valve.

thrombus (Fig. 14-41). Thrombus formation can cause intermittent or complete leaflet fixation. Hemodynamically, fixation can result in stenosis when the leaflet is stuck in the closed position, insufficiency when the leaflet is stuck in the open position, or both when the leaflet is stuck in an intermediate position. Pannus formation within the valve housing may also limit mechanical valve leaflet function (Fig. 14-42).

Newly implanted valve leaflet motion is typically normal, but full excursion should be confirmed with TEE because manufacturer defects and technical difficulties with implantation can lead to restricted leaflet motion. Because of the close proximity of the AV to the coronary ostia, a high index of suspicion for coronary ostial occlusion is appropriate (Fig. 14-43). This is particularly true after aggressive valve oversizing in the supra-annular position or in patients with aberrant coronary anatomy. Careful postimplantation inspection of regional wall motion is mandatory to rule out this potentially devastating complication.

Prosthetic Valve Stenosis

The diagnosis of prosthetic AV stenosis can be challenging. In addition to the aforementioned potential issues surrounding 2D imaging, there are also several important limitations with Doppler quantification of stenosis after TAVR. In the immediate postoperative period, patients often exhibit a hyperdynamic state that can lead to elevated transvalvular gradients even in the absence of significant stenosis. Theoretically, calculation of valve area using the continuity equation should resolve this dilemma. However, postoperative changes and acoustic shadowing complicate LVOT diameter measurement, a critical component of the continuity equation. Some authors have advocated using the known dimensions of the implanted valve to define the LVOT diameter.[66] However, variations in the position of valve implantation (intra-annular vs. supra-annular) as well as variations in aortic root architecture may undermine the accuracy of the calculation with this approach. In fact, significant differences in continuity-derived valve areas have been demonstrated when known prosthetic dimensions are substituted for directly measured LVOT diameter in the equation.[67] Use of the Doppler Velocity Index (DVI) ratio to estimate the severity of stenosis may be useful in situations where direct measurement of the LVOT is particularly limited.

When presented with elevated gradients and either a calculated valve area or a DVI ratio suggesting stenosis in a prosthetic valve with normal or equivocal-appearing leaflet opening on 2D examination, it is useful to know the expected effective orifice area (EOA) of the implanted valve. This is necessary because residual stenosis may occur with a properly functioning valve owing to the phenomenon of patient-prosthesis mismatch (PPM).[68] With PPM, the EOA of an implanted valve may be too small for the recipient patient despite normal valve function, resulting in residual stenosis. To account for patient size variability, PPM is generally defined as an indexed effective orifice area (iEOA). The clinical significance of PPM is a subject that is currently being debated in the literature, with some studies suggesting that PPM significantly increases both short- and long-term mortality following valve replacement.[69,70] Other data suggest that the effects of PPM are much more modest.[71,72]

In addition to PPM, pressure recovery phenomena may lead to detection of elevated Doppler transvalvular gradients in normal-appearing valves. In vitro[25] and in vivo[24] studies have shown discrepancies between simultaneously measured prosthetic AV Doppler and catheter gradients. As discussed earlier, this potential overestimation of the true physiologic gradient is most likely to occur in patients with small ascending aortic dimensions and milder degrees of aortic stenosis. Angled and high-velocity flow can also increase the degree of "pressure recovery,"[73] and thus, overestimation may be a more prominent concern in the immediate postoperative hypertrophic patient.[74] In summary, when elevated gradients are encountered in prosthetic valves, careful 2D inspection to rule out leaflet dysfunction is mandatory. In valves that appear to be functioning normally on 2D examination, the possibilities of PPM and pressure recovery should be considered before concluding that prosthetic dysfunction is the etiology of the elevated gradient.

Prosthetic Valve Insufficiency

The echocardiographer must also evaluate prosthetic valves for the presence of AR. Mechanical bileaflet valves are designed to produce small intravalvular jets known as *leakage backflow*.[65] In bileaflet mechanical valves, these jets can be seen emanating from the four hinge points of the valve leaflets. Physiologic intravalvular jets found with bioprosthetic valves may be central and emanate from leaflet coaptation zones or eccentric due to leakage from the fabric covering of the valve struts. These mild physiologic jets seen early after implantation often resolve over time. More significant intravalvular AR is most often associated with in situ valves with degeneration or other processes such as endocarditis, thrombus, or pannus formation.

In the immediate postoperative period, it is important to distinguish between intravalvular and paravalvular AR jets; this distinction may dictate the need for surgical intervention (see Video 14-12). Intravalvular 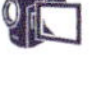

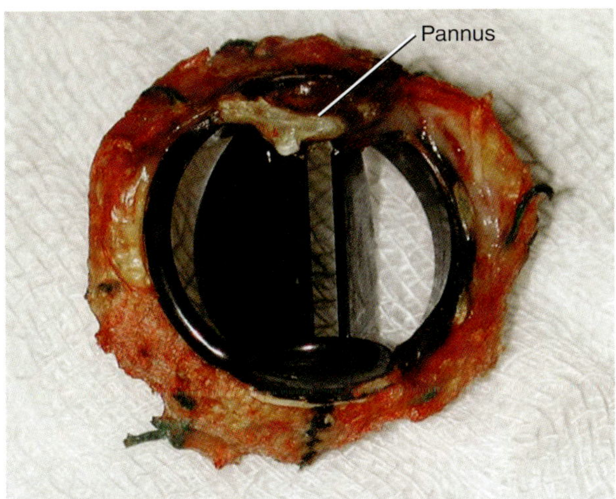

Figure 14-42 Excised bileaflet mechanical valve with pannus formation seen within valve housing, leading to limited leaflet motion.

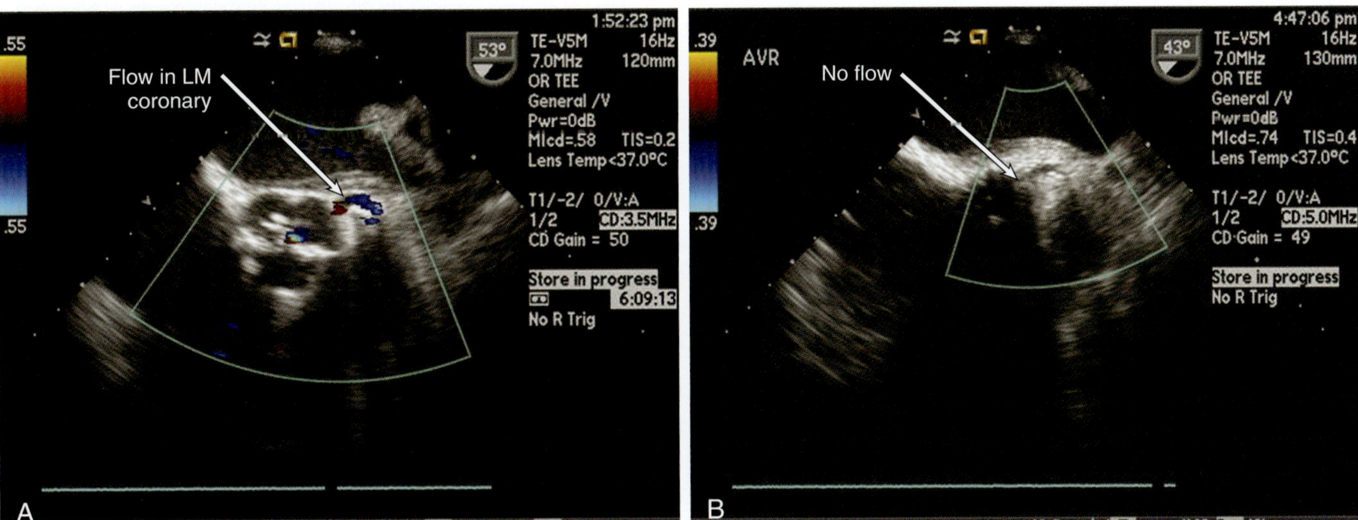

Figure 14-43 Two midesophageal aortic valve short-axis images. **A,** Pre–aortic valve replacement (*AVR*), with flow seen in left main (*LM*) coronary during diastole. **B,** After implantation of bioprosthetic AVR with no flow detected in LM.

leaks arise from within the sewing ring and in the vast majority of cases do not require surgical intervention. Paravalvular leaks are caused by incomplete fixation of the sewing ring to the native annulus, resulting in jets that arise from outside the sewing ring and may require surgical revision.[67] Although this distinction sounds obvious, demonstrating conclusive echocardiographic evidence can be extremely challenging because of acoustic shadowing and postoperative changes. Careful examination with both ME and TG windows is often necessary to confirm the diagnosis. Furthermore, because paravalvular jets are by nature highly eccentric, accurate quantification of severity can be difficult. If surgical intervention is necessary, identification of the jet origin can facilitate surgical correction of the lesion.

REFERENCES

1. Hicks GH. *Cardiopulmonary Anatomy and Physiology*. Philadelphia, PA: W.B. Saunders Company; 2000;40:42.
2. Des Jardins T. *Cardiopulmonary Anatomy & Physiology*. 4th ed. Albany, NY: Delmar Thomson Learning; 2002;182:183.
3. Mill MR, Anderson RH, Cohn LH. *Surgical Anatomy of the Heart in Cardiac Surgery in the Adult*. 4th ed. New York: McGraw Hill; 2012:21-41.
4. Thubrikar Mano. *The aortic valve*. Boca Raton, FL: CRC Press, Inc; 1990:2-3.
5. Anderson RH, Webb S, Brown NA, Lamers W, Moorman A. Development of the heart: (3) formation of the ventricular outflow tracts, arterial valves, and intra pericardial arterial trunks. *Heart*. 2005;89:1110-1118.
6. Ya J, Van Den Hoff MJB, De Boer PAJ, et al. The normal development of the outflow tract in the rat. *Circ Res*. 1998;82:464-472.
7. Anderson RH, Thompson RP, Kern CB. Development of aortic valves with 2 and 3 leaflets. *J Am Coll Cardiol*. 2009;54:2319-2320.
8. Aldous IG, Lee MJ, Well SM. Differential changes in the molecular stability of collagen from the pulmonary and aortic valves during the fetal-neonatal transition. *Ann Biomed Eng*. 2010;38:3000-3009.
9. Aikawa E, Whittaker P, Farber M, et al. Human semilunar cardiac valve remodeling by active cells from fetus to adult: implications for postnasal adaption, pathology, and tissue engineering. *Circulation*. 2006;113:1344-1352.
10. Hinton Jr RB, Lincoln J, Deutsch GH, et al. Extracellular matrix remodeling and organization in developing and disease aortic valves. *Circ. Res*. 2006;98:1431-1438:Circulation Research 2006.
11. Ross D. Pulmonary valve autotransplantation (the Ross operation). *J. Card Surg*. 1988;3:313-319.
12. Lee TC, Zhao YD, Courtman DW, Stewart DJ. Abnormal aortic valve development in mice lacking endothelial nitric oxide synthase. *Circulation*. 2000;101:2345-2348.
13. Angelini A, Ho SY, Anderson RH, et al. The morphology of the normal aortic valve as compared with the aortic having two leaflets. *J Thorac Cardiovasc Surg*. 1989;98:362-.
14. Baumgartner H, Hung J, Bermejo J, et al. Echocardiographic assessment of valve stenosis: EAE/ASE recommendations for clinical practice. *J Am Soc Echocardiogr*. 2009;22:1-23:quiz 101-102.
15. Otto CM. *Clinical Echocardiography*. Philadelphia: WB Saunders Company; 2000:229-264.
16. Donal E, Novaro GM, Deserrano D, et al. Planimetric assessment of anatomic valve area overestimates effective orifice area in bicuspid aortic stenosis. *J Am Soc Echocardiogr*. 2005;18(12):1392-1398.
17. VanAuker MD, et al. Jet eccentricity: a misleading source of agreement between Doppler/catheter pressure gradients in aortic stenosis. *J Am Soc Echocardiogr*. 2001;14(9):853-862.
18. Niederberger J, et al. Importance of pressure recovery for the assessment of aortic stenosis by Doppler ultrasound. Role of aortic size, aortic valve area, and direction of the stenotic jet in vitro. *Circulation*. 1996;94(8):1934-1940.
19. Currie PJ, et al. Continuous-wave Doppler echocardiographic assessment of severity of calcific aortic stenosis: a simultaneous Doppler-catheter correlative study in 100 adult patients. *Circulation*. 1985;71(6):1162-1169.
20. Simpson IA, et al. Clinical value of Doppler echocardiography in the assessment of adults with aortic stenosis. *Br Heart J*. 1985;53(6):636-639.
21. Baumgartner H, et al. Determination of aortic valve area by Doppler echocardiography using the continuity equation: a critical evaluation. *Cardiology*. 1990;77(2):101-111.
22. Oh JK, et al. Prediction of the severity of aortic stenosis by Doppler aortic valve area determination: prospective Doppler-catheterization correlation in 100 patients. *J Am Coll Cardiol*. 1988;11(6):1227-1234.
23. Garcia D, et al. Discrepancies between catheter and Doppler estimates of valve effective orifice area can be predicted from the pressure recovery phenomenon: practical implications with regard to quantification of aortic stenosis severity. *J Am Coll Cardiol*. 2003;41(3):435-442.
24. Aljassim O, et al. Doppler-catheter discrepancies in patients with bileaflet mechanical prostheses or bioprostheses in the aortic valve position. *Am J Cardiol*. 2008;102(10):1383-1389.
25. Baumgartner H, et al. "Overestimation" of catheter gradients by Doppler ultrasound in patients with aortic stenosis: a predictable manifestation of pressure recovery. *J Am Coll Cardiol*. 1999;33(6):1655-1661.
26. Cape EG, et al. Turbulent/viscous interactions control Doppler/catheter pressure discrepancies in aortic stenosis. The role of the Reynolds number. *Circulation*. 1996;94(11):2975-2981.
27. Clavel MA, et al. Validation of conventional and simplified methods to calculate projected valve area at normal flow rate in patients with low flow, low gradient aortic stenosis: the multicenter TOPAS (True or Pseudo Severe Aortic Stenosis) study. *J Am Soc Echocardiogr*. 2010;23(4):380-386.
28. Dumesnil JG, Pibarot P, Akins C. New approaches to quantifying aortic stenosis severity. *Curr Cardiol Rep*. 2008;10(2):91-97.
29. Keane MG, et al. Bicuspid aortic valves are associated with aortic dilatation out of proportion to coexistent valvular lesions. *Circulation*. 2000;102(19 Suppl 3):III35-III39.
30. Briand M, et al. Reduced systemic arterial compliance impacts significantly on left ventricular afterload and function in aortic stenosis: implications for diagnosis and treatment. *J Am Coll Cardiol*. 2005;46(2):291-298.
31. Leon MB, Smith CR, Mack M, et al. Transcatheter aortic-valve implantation for aortic stenosis in patients who cannot undergo surgery. *N Engl J Med*. 2010;363(17):1597-1607.
32. Smith CR, Leon MB, Mack MJ, et al. Transcatheter versus surgical aortic valve replacement in high risk patients. *N Engl J Med*. 2011;364:2187-2198.
33. Jayasuriya C, Moss RR, Munt B. Transcatheter aortic valve implantation in aortic stenosis: the role of echocardiography. *J Am Soc Echocardiogr*. 2011;24(1):15-27.
34. Piazza N, De Jaegere P, Schultz C, et al. Anatomy of the aortic valvular complex and its implications for transcatheter implantation of the aortic valve. *Circ Cardiovasc Interv*. 2008;1:9-15.
35. Zamorano JI, Badano LP, Bruce C, et al. EAE/ASE recommendations for the use of echocardiography in new transcatheter interventions for valvular heart disease. *Eur Heart J*. 2011;32:2189-2214.
36. Detaint D, Lepage L, Himbert D, et al. Determinants of significant paravalvular regurgitation after transcatheter aortic valve implantation. *J Am Coll Cardiol Interv*. 2009;2:821-827.
37. Bleiziffer S, Ruge H, Horer J, et al. Predictors of new onset complete heart block after transcatheter aortic valve implantation. *J Am Coll Cardiol Interv*. 2010;3:524-530.
38. Patel PA, Fassl J, Thompson A, Augoustides JG. Transcatheter aortic valve replacement—part 3: the central role of perioperative transesophageal echocardiography. *J Cardiothorac Vasc Anesth*. 2012:in press.
39. Masson JB, Kovac J, Schuler G, et al. Transcatheter aortic valve implantation: review of the nature, management and avoidance of complications. *JACC Cardiovasc Interv*. 2009;2:811-820.
40. Singh JP, Evans JC, Levy D, et al. Prevalence and clinical determinants of mitral, tricuspid, and aortic regurgitation (the Framingham Heart Study). *Am J Cardiol*. Mar 15 1999;83(6):897-902.
41. Stout KK, Verrier ED. Acute valvular regurgitation. *Circulation*. 2009;119:3232-3241.
42. Enriquez-Sarano M, Tajik AJ. Clinical practice. Aortic regurgitation. *N Engl J Med*. 2004;351:1539-1546.
43. El Khoury G, Glineur D, Rubay J, et al. Functional classification of aortic root/valve abnormalities and their correlation with etiologies and surgical procedures. *Curr Opin Cardiol*. 2005;20:115-121.
44. Bonow RO, Carabello BA, Chatterjee K, et al. 2008 Focused update incorporated into the ACC/AHA 2006 guidelines for the management of patients with valvular heart disease: a report of the American College of Cardiology/American Heart Association Task Force on Practice Guidelines (Writing Committee to Revise the 1998 Guidelines for the Management of Patients With Valvular Heart Disease): endorsed by the Society of Cardiovascular Anesthesiologists, Society for Cardiovascular Angiography and Interventions, and Society of Thoracic Surgeons. *Circulation*. 2008;118:e523-e661.
45. Lang RM, Bierig M, Devereux RB, et al. Recommendations for chamber quantification: a report from the American Society of Echocardiography's Guidelines and Standards Committee and the Chamber Quantification Writing Group, developed in conjunction with the European Association of Echocardiography, a branch of the European Society of Cardiology. *J Am Soc Echocardiogr*. 2005;18:1440-1463.
46. Perry GJ, Helmcke F, Nanda NC, et al. Evaluation of aortic insufficiency by Doppler color flow mapping. *J Am Coll Cardiol*. 1987;9:952-959.
47. Willett DL, Hall SA, Jessen ME, et al. Assessment of aortic regurgitation by transesophageal color Doppler imaging of the vena contracta: validation against an intraoperative aortic flow probe. *J Am Coll Cardiol*. 2001;37:1450-1455.
48. Tribouilloy CM, Enriquez-Sarano M, Bailey KR, et al. Assessment of severity of aortic regurgitation using the width of the vena contracta: A clinical color Doppler imaging study. *Circulation*. 2000;102:558-564.
49. Tribouilloy CM, Enriquez-Sarano M, Fett SL, et al. Application of the proximal flow convergence method to calculate the effective regurgitant orifice area in aortic regurgitation. *J Am Coll Cardiol*. 1998;32:1032-1039.
50. Grayburn PA, Handshoe R, Smith MD, et al. Quantitative assessment of the hemodynamic consequences of aortic regurgitation by means of continuous wave Doppler recordings. *J Am Coll Cardiol*. 1987;10:135-141.
51. Zoghbi WA, Enriquez-Sarano M, Foster E, et al. Recommendations for evaluation of the severity of native valvular regurgitation with two-dimensional and Doppler echocardiography. *J Am Soc Echocardiogr*. 2003;16:777-802.
52. Lewis JF, Kuo LC, Nelson JG, et al. Pulsed Doppler echocardiographic determination of stroke volume and cardiac output: clinical validation of two new methods using the apical window. *Circulation*. 1984;70:425-431.
53. Takenaka K, Sakamoto T, Dabestani A, et al. [Pulsed Doppler echocardiographic detection of regurgitant blood flow in the ascending, descending and abdominal aorta of patients with aortic regurgitation]. *J Cardiol*. 1987;17:301-309.
54. Sutton DC, Kluger R, Ahmed SU, et al. Flow reversal in the descending aorta: a guide to intraoperative assessment of aortic regurgitation with transesophageal echocardiography. *J Thorac Cardiovasc Surg*. 1994;108:576-582.
55. David TE, Feindel CM. An aortic valve-sparing operation for patients with aortic incompetence and aneurysm of the ascending aorta. *J Thorac Cardiovasc Surg*. 1992;103:617-621.
56. Lausberg HF, Aicher D, Kissinger A, Langer F, Fries R, Schafers HJ. Valve repair in aortic regurgitation without root dilatation–aortic valve repair. *Thorac Cardiovasc Surg*. 2006;54:15-20.
57. Haydar HS, He GW, Hovaguimian H, et al. Valve repair for aortic insufficiency: surgical classification and techniques. *Eur J Cardiothorac Surg*. 1997;11:258-265.
58. De Vinuesa PGG, Castro A, Barquero JM, et al. Functional anatomy of aortic regurgitation. Role of transesophageal echocardiography in aortic valve-sparing surgery. *Rev Esp Cardiol*. 2010;63:536-543.
59. Van Dyck MJ, Watremez C, Boodhwani M, et al. Transesophageal echocardiographic evaluation during aortic valve repair surgery. *Anesth Analg*. 2010;111:59-70.
60. De Waroux JBLP, Pouleur AC, Goffinet C, et al. Functional anatomy of aortic regurgitation: accuracy, prediction of surgical reparability and outcome implications of transesophageal echocardiography. *Circulation*. 2007;116:1264-1269.
61. Boodhwani M, de Kerchove L, Glineur D, et al. Repair oriented classification of aortic insufficiency: impact on surgical techniques and clinical outcomes. *J Thorac Cardiovasc Surg*. 2009;137:286-294.
62. Augoustides JGT, Szeto WY, Bavaria JE. Advances in aortic valve repair: focus on functional approach, clinical outcomes and central role of echocardiography. *J Cardiothorac Vasc Anesth*. 2010;24:1016-1020.
63. De Waroux JBLP, Pouleur AC, Robert A, et al. Mechanisms of recurrent aortic regurgitation after aortic valve repair: predictive value of intraoperative transesophageal echocardiography. *JACC Cardiovasc Imaging*. 2009;2:931-939.
64. Pethig K, Milz A, Hagl C, et al. Aortic valve reimplantation in ascending aortic aneurysm: risk factors for early valve failure. *Ann Thorac Surg*. 2002;73:29-33.
65. Zoghbi WA, et al. Recommendations for evaluation of prosthetic valves with echocardiography and doppler ultrasound: a report from the American Society of Echocardiography's Guidelines and Standards Committee and the Task Force on Prosthetic Valves, developed in conjunction with the American College of Cardiology Cardiovascular Imaging Committee, Cardiac Imaging Committee of the American Heart Association, the European Association of Echocardiography, a registered branch of the European Society of Cardiology, the Japanese Society of Echocardiography and the Canadian Society of Echocardiography, endorsed by the American College of Cardiology Foundation, American Heart Association, European Association of Echocardiography, a registered branch of the European Society of Cardiology, the Japanese Society of Echocardiography, and Canadian Society of Echocardiography. *J Am Soc Echocardiogr*. 2009;22(9):975-1014:quiz 1082-4.
66. Mohty D, et al. Impact of prosthesis-patient mismatch on long-term survival in patients with small St Jude Medical mechanical prostheses in the aortic position. *Circulation*. 2006;113(3):420-426.
67. Chafizadeh ER, Zoghbi WA. Doppler echocardiographic assessment of the St. Jude Medical prosthetic valve in the aortic position using the continuity equation. *Circulation*. 1991;83(1):213-223.
68. Dumesnil JG, Pibarot P, Akins C. New approaches to quantifying aortic stenosis severity. *Curr Cardiol Rep*. 2008;10(2):91-97.

69. Pibarot P, et al. Impact of prosthesis-patient mismatch on hemodynamic and symptomatic status, morbidity and mortality after aortic valve replacement with a bioprosthetic heart valve. *J Heart Valve Dis.* 1998;7(2):211-218.
70. Mohty D, et al. Impact of prosthesis-patient mismatch on long-term survival after aortic valve replacement: influence of age, obesity, and left ventricular dysfunction. *J Am Coll Cardiol.* 2009;53(1):39-47.
71. Cotoni DA, et al. Defining patient-prosthesis mismatch and its effect on survival in patients with impaired ejection fraction. *Ann Thorac Surg.* 2011;91(3):692-699.
72. Garatti A, et al. Aortic valve replacement with 17-mm mechanical prostheses: is patient-prosthesis mismatch a relevant phenomenon? *Ann Thorac Surg.* 2011;91(1):71-77.
73. VanAuker MD, et al. Jet eccentricity: a misleading source of agreement between Doppler/catheter pressure gradients in aortic stenosis. *J Am Soc Echocardiogr.* 2001;14(9):853-862.
74. Kwon DH, et al. Steep left ventricle to aortic root angle and hypertrophic obstructive cardiomyopathy: study of a novel association using three-dimensional multimodality imaging. *Heart.* 2009;95(21):1784-1791.

Mitral Valvular Disease

GREGORY W. FISCHER | **PAULA TRIGO**

Introduction

Transesophageal echocardiography (TEE) has evolved dramatically over the last 3 decades and is now considered an indispensable tool for the practice of cardiac anesthesia. There is arguably no other aspect of cardiac surgery in which perioperative echocardiography plays a more profound role in surgical decision making as in surgery for mitral valve disease. Additionally, surgical philosophy in treating mitral valve disease is constantly changing, making it imperative that the echocardiographer adapt to this very dynamic subspecialty.

Mitral valve disease is now as common as aortic valve disease in the developed world, especially in the aging population,[1] and mitral valve regurgitation is the primary mechanism of valve disease. In the developing world, however, mitral stenosis (MS) continues to play an important role.[2] While contemporary surgical practice recommends mitral valve repair as the standard of care for many regurgitant lesions,[3-5] leading valve surgeons are also advocating repair techniques in the setting of mitral valve stenosis.

The information acquired during a perioperative TEE exam for mitral valve disease has a different focus than that obtained by cardiologists during the preoperative evaluation. Determining the severity of regurgitation or stenosis is no longer the sole focus of the exam. Instead, precise valve analysis in determining mechanisms of dysfunction plays a more important role in planning the correct surgical procedure. Which segments are prolapsing or restricted and whether or not the commissures are calcified in the setting of rheumatic MS are commonly asked questions that must be addressed to determine repair feasibility. Intraoperative TEE provides a roadmap for a successful procedure and controls the quality of the reconstruction.

Although these new demands placed upon the perioperative echocardiographer increase both responsibility and liability, they also solidify the role of the perioperative echocardiographer as an integral member of the surgical team.

Functional Anatomy of the Mitral Valve

The foundation to understanding pathologies of the mitral valve apparatus lies in the echocardiographer's knowledge of normal valvular anatomy from the surgeon's perspective. While the surgeon will always examine the mitral valve apparatus once on cardiopulmonary bypass (CPB), many subtle pathologies could be missed. Many nuances of mitral valve disease can only be diagnosed by imaging the moving heart and evaluating the topographic relationship among different aspects of the valve.

Normal Mitral Valve Anatomy

Two-dimensional (2D) echocardiography has become the standard of care in imaging the mitral valve apparatus. However, the mitral valve is a complex three-dimensional (3D) structure. It lies in the left atrioventricular groove, ensuring unidirectional flow of blood from the left atrium (LA) into the left ventricle (LV). From a clinical perspective, five distinct anatomic features are relevant.

Leaflets

The mitral valve is the only cardiac valve to have, under normal circumstances, two leaflets instead of three. Carpentier et al. described a useful nomenclature for segmental anatomy of the mitral valve.[6] Other classifications are described in the literature, but the Carpentier classification has been adopted by the American Society of Echocardiography (ASE). It may not matter which classification is used, so long as the echocardiographer and surgeon share a common classification for segmental differentiation of the leaflets.

The posterior leaflet of the mitral valve is quadrangular in shape and is attached to three fifths of the annular circumference in the region of the parietal atrioventricular grove. The posterior leaflet typically has two well-defined indentations that divide the leaflet into three individual scallops. These indentations are believed to aid leaflet opening during diastole. By definition, P1 designates the anterior or lateral scallop, P2 the middle scallop, and P3 the posterior or medial scallop. The three opposing segments of the anterior leaflet are continuous without indentations and designated as A1 (anterior segment), A2 (middle segment), and A3 (posterior segment) (Fig. 15-1, Video 15-1). The anterior (or aortic mitral) leaflet has a semicircular shape and attaches to approximately two fifths of the annular circumference in the region of the fibrous trigone. A fibrous continuity exists between the anterior leaflet and the aortic valve in the area of the left and noncoronary cusp. This region is referred to as the *aortic-mitral curtain*. The motion of the anterior leaflet defines an important boundary between the inflow (during diastole) and outflow (during systole) tracts of the LV. The height of the normal posterior leaflet is less than half of the anterior leaflet; however, both leaflets have similar surface areas because of the difference in their circumferences.

A rough zone or coaptation zone (CZ) can be found on the atrial side of the leaflets at the free edge. This rough zone represents the coaptation surface of the valve. The coaptation zone of the valve must provide an adequate surface to maintain valve competency during systole.[7] The non-coapting portions of the valve leaflets are relatively smooth and referred to as the *smooth zone* (Fig. 15-2).

Commissures

The commissures define a distinct area where the leaflets adjoin and function in a manner similar to the corner of the human mouth where the upper and lower lips meet. Dysfunction in this region often leads to severe degrees of regurgitation. The amount of commissural tissue varies greatly, and occasionally commissures may exist as distinct leaflet segments. More commonly, the commissure represents several millimeters of valve leaflet tissue that provides continuity between the anterior and posterior leaflets at their insertion into the annulus. Commissural chordae have a distinct configuration, providing support to the commissure as well as the adjacent anterior and posterior segments. The commissure where A1 and P1 abut is referred to as the *anterior* or *anterolateral commissure* (AC), and the commissure at A3/P3 is the *posterior* or *posteromedial commissure* (PC) (see Fig. 15-1).

Chordae

The chordae tendineae make up the leaflet suspension system that ultimately determine and maintain the position and tension on the valve

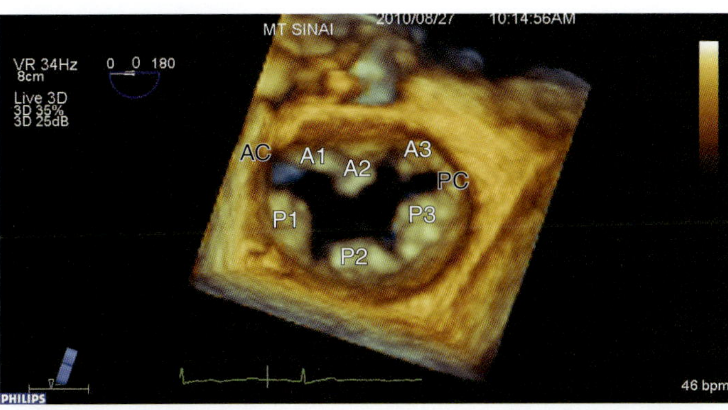

Figure15-1   Surgeon's view of mitral valve apparatus with segmental division. *AC,* Anterior commissure; *PC,* posterior commissure.

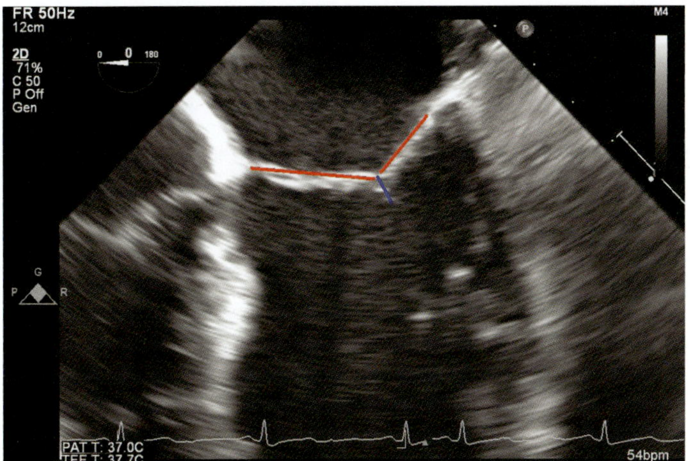

Figure15-2   Importance of zone of coaptation to ensure optimal valvular competence during systole. Red line indicates "smooth zone," blue line marks actual coaptation between leaflets ("rough zone").

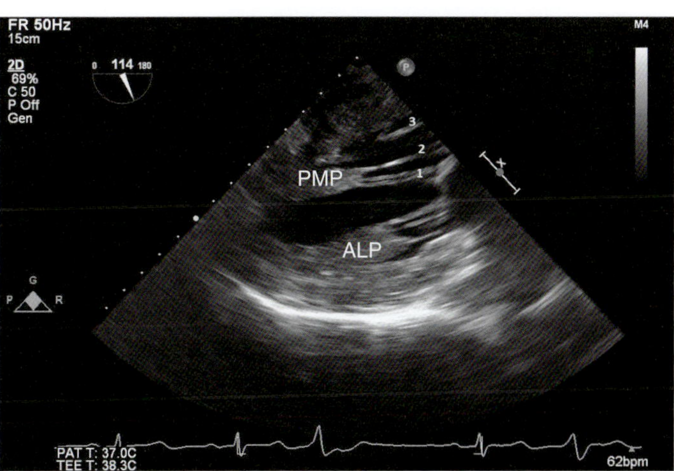

Figure15-3   Primary chords attach to leaflet margins, secondary chords to leaflet body, and tertiary chords (only found in posterior leaflet) to leaflet base. *ALP,* Anterolateral papillary muscle; *PMP,* posteromedial papillary muscle.

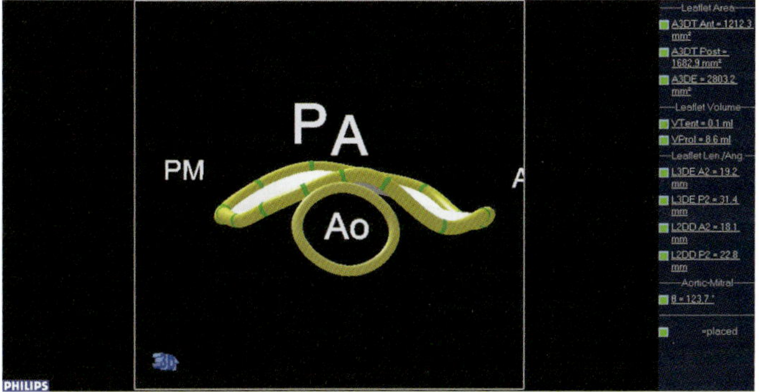

Figure15-4   Three-dimensional (3D) reconstruction of mitral valve annulus with integrated software. Note 3D structure and saddle shape of annulus. *P,* posterior; *A,* posterior; *Ao,* aorta; *PM,* posteriomedial.

leaflets at end of systole. The chordae originate from the fibrous heads of the papillary muscles and may be classified according to their site of insertion on the leaflet. Marginal or "primary" chordae insert on the free margin of the leaflets and prevent marginal leaflet prolapse in addition to aligning the rough zones and ensuring coaptation. Intermediate or "secondary chordae" insert on the ventricular surface of the body of the leaflets at the junction of the rough and clear zones and primarily prevent billowing and reduce and distribute tension across leaflet tissue. They may also play a role in dynamic ventricular shape and function, owing to their contribution to ventricular-valve continuity. Basal or "tertiary chordae" connect the posterior leaflet base and mitral annulus to the papillary muscles and help maintain ventricular-valve continuity (Fig. 15-3 and Video 15-2).

Annulus

The mitral annulus represents an anatomic junction between the LV and LA and serves as an insertion site for the two leaflets. It can be divided segmentally according to the site of leaflet insertion (anterior or posterior annulus). The anterior portion of the mitral annulus is contiguous with the fibrous trigones. The right fibrous trigone represents a fibrous area between the mitral valve, tricuspid valve, noncoronary cusp of the aortic annulus, and the membranous septum. The left fibrous trigone is an area made up of the left fibrous borders of the aortic mitral curtain. The posterior mitral annulus is only rudimentarily developed, explaining why this portion of the annulus is prone to dilation. The mitral annulus has a 3D saddle shape, with the highest point being the mid-aspect of the anterior leaflet; this saddle is exaggerated during systole as the annulus contracts

and commissural areas move apically while the aortic root bulges, thus narrowing the circumference during systole.[8] The annulus relaxes during diastole, increasing the annular area by 20% to 40% compared to systole. A loss of such annular relaxation may predispose to functional mitral valve stenosis after rigid ring annuloplasty (Fig. 15-4).

Papillary Muscles and Left Ventricle

There are typically two papillary muscles arising from the area between the apical and middle thirds of the LV free wall. The anterolateral papillary muscle is often composed of one body or head, whereas the posteromedial papillary muscle may have two or more heads. Each papillary muscle provides chordae to both leaflets, and the axial relationship of the chordae prevents chordal abrasion or dyssynchrony. The attachment of the papillary muscles to the lateral wall of the LV indicates that the ventricle is also an important part of the mitral valve complex. Any change in ventricular geometry that affects papillary muscle position can change the axial relationship of the chordae and leaflets, resulting in valve dysfunction (see Fig. 15-3 and Video 15-2).

Mitral Valve Dysfunction and Etiology of Disease

The foundation to understanding the types of valvular dysfunction that comprise mitral valve disease was set forth in Carpentier's landmark

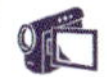

TABLE 15-1	Types of Mitral Valve Dysfunction	
Dysfunction	*Leaflet Motion in Regard to Annular Plane*	*Surgical Approach to Repair*
Type I	Normal leaflet motion	Annuloplasty ring, closure of clefts or endocarditis lesions
Type II	Excessive leaflet motion	Complex reconstruction
Type IIIa	Restricted leaflet motion in systole and diastole	Complex reconstruction, leaflet augmentation with pericardial patch
Type IIIb	Restricted leaflet motion in systole	Annuloplasty ring, possible chordal release

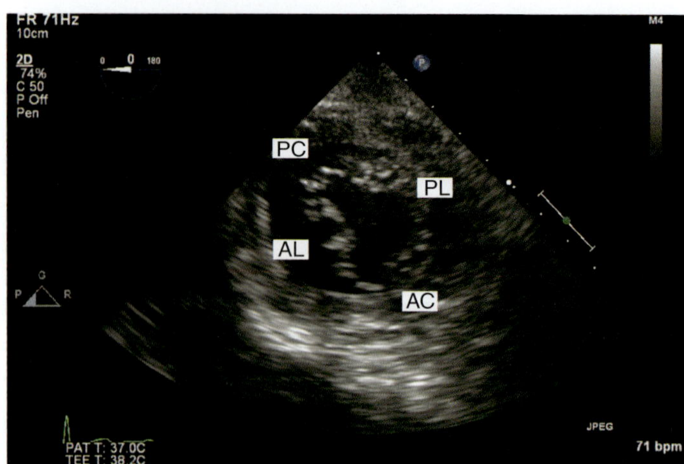

Figure 15-5 Transgastric basal short axis view, also known as "fish mouth" view. *AC,* Anterior commissure; *AL,* anterior leaflet; *PC,* posterior commissure; *PL,* posterior leaflet.

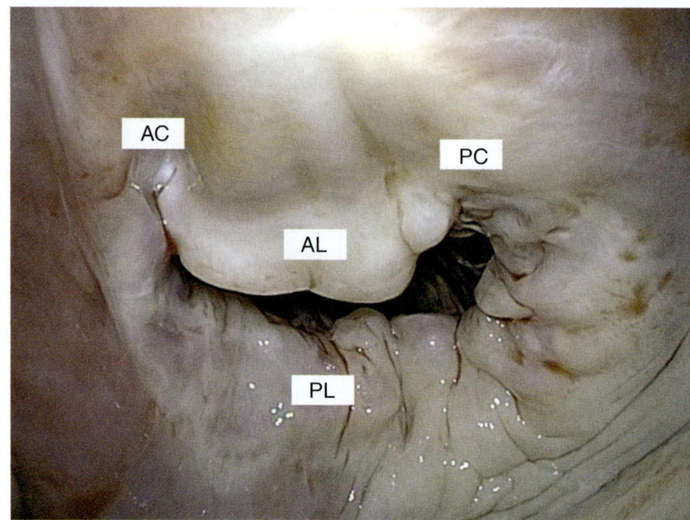

Figure 15-6 Similar to corner of mouth ("fish mouth" view), commissures provide a transitional zone from anterior to posterior leaflet while maintaining valve competency. *AC,* Anterior commissure; *AL,* anterior leaflet; *PC,* posterior commissure; *PL,* posterior leaflet.

paper "The French Correction," in which the different segments of the mitral valve were defined.[6] In addition to defining this segmental approach, Carpentier also proposed a pathophysiologic triad that is a useful adjunct to clearly differentiating the particular causes of mitral regurgitation (MR). The triad consists of: (1) the *etiology* (underlying disease causing MR [e.g., Barlow disease, ischemic cardiomyopathy]), (2) the *lesions* (pathologic changes in the valve that result from the disease process [e.g., chordal rupture, chordal elongation, leaflet tethering, annular dilation, calcification]), and (3) the *dysfunctions.*

It is highly recommended that the echocardiographer take a similar organized approach when evaluating the mitral valve. Frequently, however, the imager will first start by identifying the dysfunction (e.g., presence of leaflet prolapse or restriction). Once a dysfunction has been identified, the cause should be determined. In other words, the imager needs to search for the lesion responsible for the dysfunction (e.g., chordal elongation or rupture, leaflet perforation). Finally, in certain cases, it is possible to propose likely etiologies (e.g., thickened calcified leaflets in type IIIa dysfunction are frequently associated with rheumatic mitral valve disease) (Table 15-1).

Preprocedural Valve Analysis by TEE

In 1996, the ASE/Society of Cardiovascular Anesthesiologists (SCA) published guidelines for performing a comprehensive intraoperative multiplane TEE examination.[9] In this landmark paper, 20 standard TEE views were defined (see Chapter 1). Once acquired, many of these views can be correctly interpreted even by the non-echocardiographer (e.g., transgastric short-axis view for LV function), but assessment of a complex structure like the mitral valve apparatus requires thorough understanding of both the anatomy and the spatial relationship of the 2D interrogating plane to the valvular apparatus.

Once on CPB, the surgeon views the valve in its entirety in a flaccid state from the LA looking downward toward the LV. In this view, the patient's left and right side correspond to the surgeon's left and right side, while the anterior and posterior mitral valve leaflets appear in the appropriate positions. The lateral and medial aspects of the mitral valve are to the left and right, respectively. This is in contrast to the echocardiographer's view, who sees the images at angles that are by definition 180 degrees reversed from the surgical view. In other words, the left and right sides of the image on the monitor are reversed relative to the surgeon's perspective (Figs. 15-5 and 15-6).

Seven standard views are used to evaluate the mitral valve apparatus. Four views are transesophageal (TE); three are transgastric (TG). The order in which these seven views are obtained is a matter of individual preference so long as the comprehensive exam acquires all of the pertinent information.

Two-dimensional echocardiography provides the examiner with an overview of the anatomy of the mitral valve apparatus and should always be performed prior to additional Doppler-based diagnostic studies (e.g., color flow Doppler [CFD], spectral analysis). Although 2D TEE cannot directly assess the severity of valve regurgitation, its strength lies in its contribution to understanding the mechanisms underlying the regurgitant lesion. Most questions posed by Carpentier's pathophysiologic triad (etiology, lesion, and dysfunction) can

be answered by a comprehensive 2D exam. The following is an overview of the seven views frequently used to examine the mitral valve apparatus.

Four-Chamber View

According to the ASE/SCA guidelines, the two scallops being interrogated with this view are A3 and P1.[9] Reiterating Carpentier's classification of the mitral valve complex, it is apparent that the *zone of coaptation* cannot be unambiguously defined with this view, since A3 and P1 by definition do not share a common coaptation surface (Fig. 15-7 and Video 15-3). The inability to properly define which scallop is currently in view at the zone of coaptation is due to this view's oblique cross-section of the mitral valve. Analysis of the zone of coaptation, rather than the smooth zone of the leaflet, is pivotal to understanding the mechanism(s) of MR. In this view, the anterior leaflet is interrogated posteromedially from the base of A3 to a more anterolateral aspect at its free edge (A2). If the imaging plane is directed more anterolaterally, the left ventricular outflow tract (LVOT) and aortic valve are imaged,

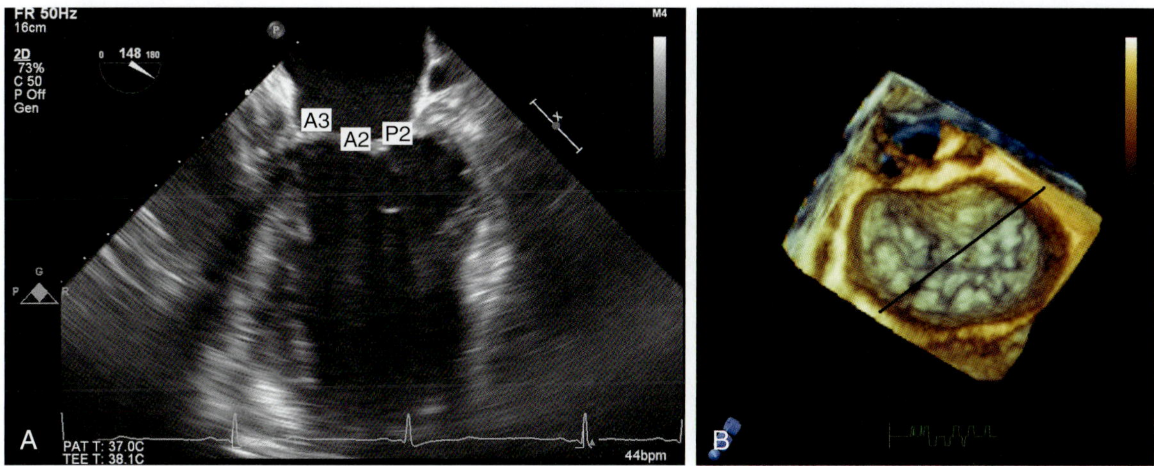

Figure 15-7 **A,** Midesophageal four-chamber view; A3, A2, and P2 segments. **B,** En face three-dimensional view of mitral valve. Black line represents interrogation plane for two-dimensional four-chamber view.

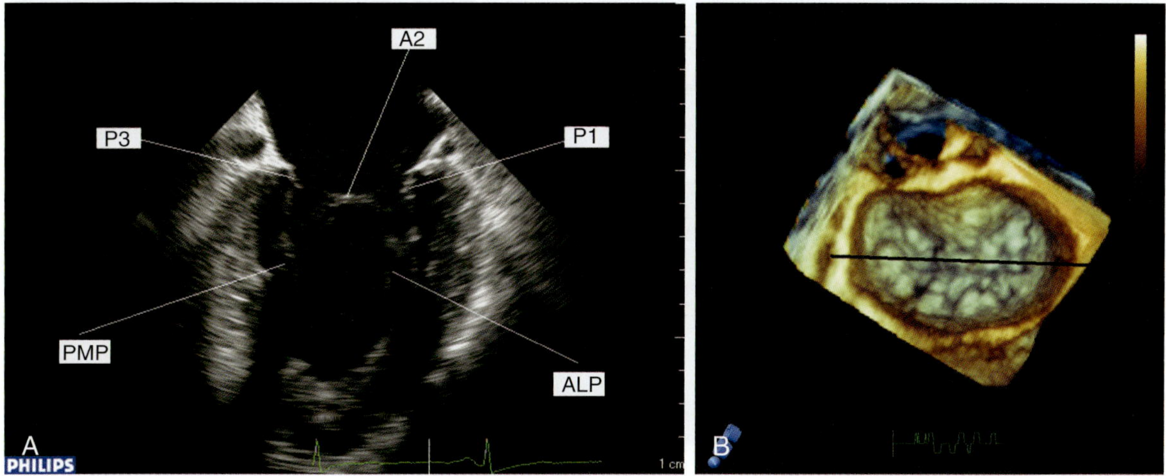

Figure 15-8 **A,** Commissural view during diastole. **B,** En face three-dimensional view of mitral valve. Black line represents interrogating plane for two-dimensional commissural view. *A2,* A2 segment of anterior leaflet; *ALP,* anterolateral papillary muscle; *P1,* P1 segment of posterior leaflet; *P3,* P3 segment of posterior leaflet; *PMP,* posteromedial papillary muscle.

and the portion of the coaptation zone imaged would represent A1/P1. Obtaining the more anterolateral view is often facilitated by either by anteflexing the probe or rotating the multiplane transducer to approximately 20 degrees.

In the standard four-chamber view, the posterior leaflet is imaged at the region of the P1/P2 indentation. Because of this leaflet's short height, the angle of the interrogating plane will determine whether P1 (more anterior angle) or P2 (less anterior angle) will be imaged at the zone of coaptation.

Anteflexing and retroflexing the probe across the valve represents a "sweeping" maneuver that enables the echocardiographer to visualize all eight anatomic components of the mitral valve using only this one view. Defining the anterolateral commissure (AC) as the starting point, which can be obtained by maximally anteflexing the probe until the mitral valve apparatus can no longer be visualized, the echocardiographer gradually retroflexes the probe. At first, the AC will be interrogated, and then the A1/P1 segments can be examined. Upon further retroflexion, the A2/P2 region will be imaged. Finally, the A3/P3 region and the posteromedial commissure (PC) will be imaged. If the more posterior regions of the valve cannot be visualized under maximal retroflexion, the probe can be advanced slightly further into the esophagus. This will result in identification of the PC (see Video 15-3).

Commissural View

The commissural view is obtained by rotating the multiplane transducer to approximately 60 degrees. In this view, the interrogating plane bisects the oblique coaptation surface, providing the echocardiographer with the ability to examine the P1/P3 scallops, the A2 region of the anterior leaflet, and both commissural regions of the valve (Fig. 15-8 and Video 15-4). Proper acquisition of this view results in a "seagull-like" picture during diastole. With standard orientation, the P3 scallop is seen to the left and the P1 scallop will be on the right on the monitor. The middle segment is A2. Once this image is optimized, rotation of the probe counterclockwise brings the P2 scallop into view, thus completing visualization of the entire posterior leaflet. Clockwise rotation of the probe will enable visualization of the anterior leaflet in its entirety.

Two-Chamber View

The two-chamber view is imaged by further rotating the multiplane probe to approximately 90 degrees. The plane of interrogation is now perpendicular to that of the four-chamber view. As described for the four-chamber view, a similar ambiguity exists with respect

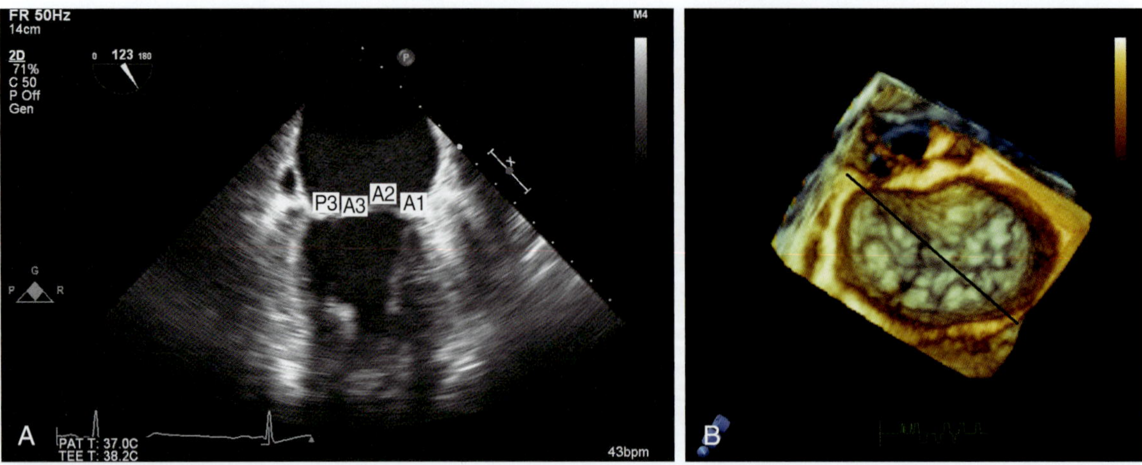

Figure 15-9   **A,** Midesophageal two-chamber view; A1, A2, A3, and P3 segments. **B,** En face three-dimensional view of mitral valve. Black line represents interrogation plane for two-dimensional two-chamber view.

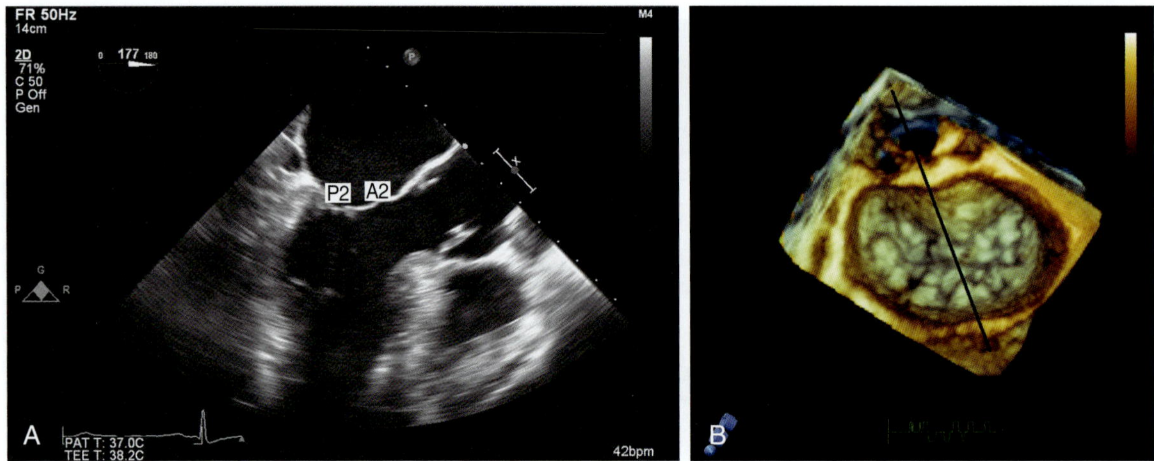

Figure 15-10   **A,** Midesophageal long-axis view, A2 and P2 segments. **B,** En face three-dimensional view of mitral valve. Black line represents interrogation plane for two-dimensional long-axis view.

to determining which segments comprise the zone of coaptation. The posterior leaflet is now seen on the left side of the screen. The interrogating plane transects the posterior leaflet at the region of the P2/P3 indentation (Fig. 15-9 and Video 15-5). As previously described for the four-chamber view, the more posteriorly the interrogation plane is directed, the higher the likelihood that the P3 scallop and PM commissure will be imaged. The anterior leaflet is on the right side of the screen, with the base of the leaflet representing the A1 segment. Toward the zone of coaptation, the A2 segment is encountered.

Long-Axis View

The long-axis view is obtained by rotating the multiplane transducer to approximately 120 degrees. The interrogating plane now transects the mitral valve apparatus through the midportion of both the mitral and aortic valves (Fig. 15-10 and Video 15-6). In this view, neither papillary muscle should be visualized. The strength of this view lies in the ability to unambiguously determine the two segments (A2, P2) that comprise the zone of coaptation. By rotating the TEE probe counterclockwise, the examiner sweeps from the midportion of the valve toward the anterior commissure. Clockwise rotation allows the posteromedial aspect of the valve, including the posterior commissure, to be examined.

The long-axis view can also be used to provide a rough estimate of the annuloplasty ring size that should be used for valve repair. Assuming the valve is imaged correctly, the length (or "height") of the anterior leaflet equals the ring size.

Transgastric Basal Short-Axis View

Commonly referred to as the "fish mouth" view, all eight segments of the mitral valve are potentially imaged. As noted earlier, the images acquired in this view are rotated 180 degrees from the "surgeon's view" once the LA is opened. To aid in orientation, the echocardiographer can imagine that the valve complex is being viewed from the LV looking upward into the LA. The PC will be found on the left side of the screen, and the AC will be on the right. The anterior leaflet is in the far field, and the posterior leaflet lies closest to the probe.

This view is difficult to obtain consistently. After acquiring the TG midpapillary short-axis view, the probe is further anteflexed. Minor changes (≈20 degrees) in the interrogating angle are sometimes required to optimize the image.

Especially in the setting of rheumatic disease with commissural fusion, this view can be used to assess the degree of fusion and calcification of the commissures, which in return will determine reparability (Fig. 15-11 and Video 15-7).

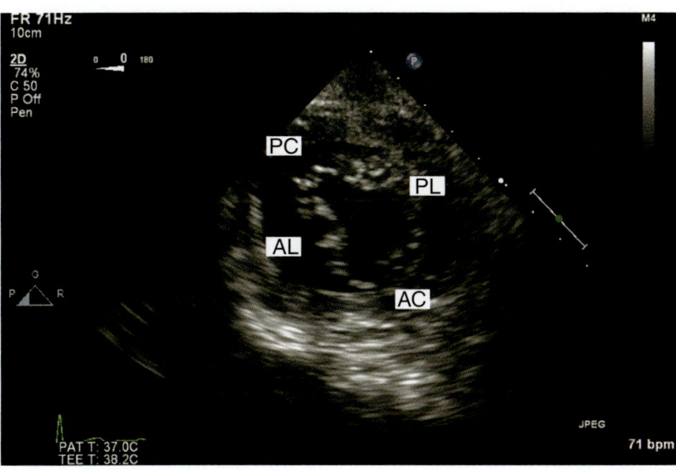

Figure 15-11 Transgastric basal short-axis view ("fish mouth"). *AC*, Anterior commissure; *AL*, anterior leaflet; *PC*, posterior commissure; *PL*, posterior leaflet.

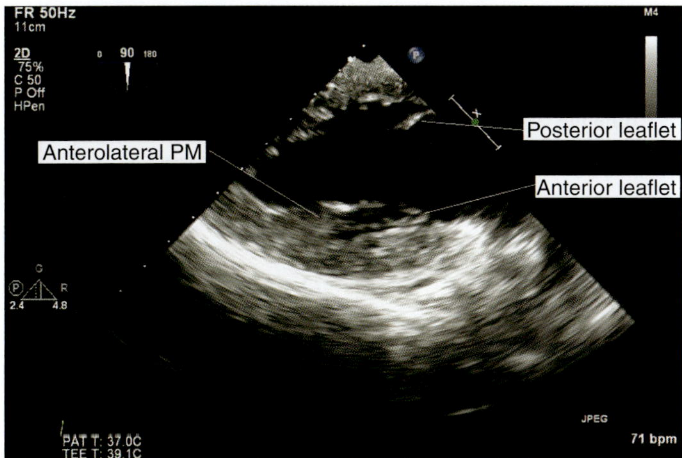

Figure 15-12 Transgastric two-chamber view. Inferior wall of left ventricle and posterior mitral valve leaflet are seen in near field; anterior wall anterior leaflet and anterolateral papillary muscle *(PM)* are seen in far field.

Transgastric Two-Chamber View

By first acquiring the TG midpapillary short-axis view and then rotating the probe to 90 degrees, the echocardiographer can easily obtain this view. The inferior wall of the LV and the posteromedial papillary muscle are seen in the near field. From the head of the papillary muscle, multiple chordae can be identified stretching from the head of the papillary muscle and inserting at different zones of the posterior leaflet. The anterior leaflet, anterolateral papillary muscle, and anterior wall of the LV make up the far field (Fig. 15-12 and Video 15-8).

Deep Transgastric Long-Axis View

This view is not classically associated with imaging of the mitral valve apparatus and is more commonly used for the purpose of aligning the Doppler cursor to estimate pressure gradients across the LVOT and aortic valve. It is particularly useful, however, in patients with annuloplasty rings (especially in the postrepair period) to analyze the coaptation zone of the leaflets. Because of the probe's position near the apex of the heart, and with maximal anteflexion, a clear and unobstructed view of the subvalvular apparatus can frequently be obtained. The posterior leaflet, which is difficult to visualize post repair in the classic views (as described earlier) because of excessive

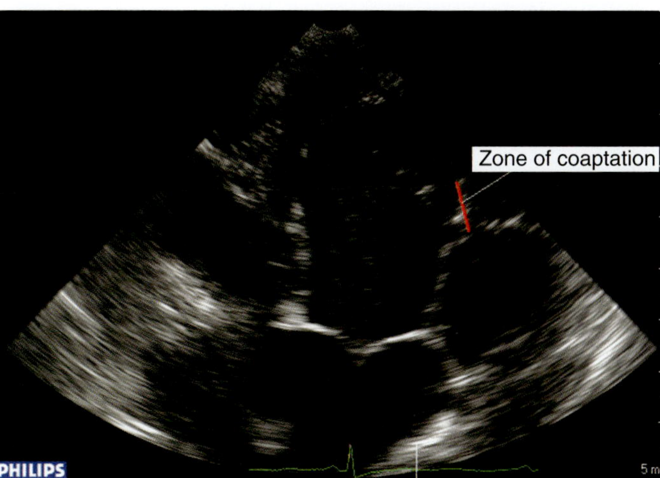

Figure15-13 Deep transgastric long-axis view during systole. This imaging plane permits evaluation of zone of coaptation. Mitral annuloplasty rings do not cause acoustic shadowing of zone of coaptation in this view.

shadowing caused by the annuloplasty ring, can easily be seen from this approach. The zone of coaptation can be measured, which represents one of the important parameters for judging the success of mitral valve reconstruction (Fig. 15-13 and Video 15-9). 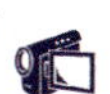

Assessing Degree of Mitral Regurgitation

The method of choice for determining the mechanism(s) of mitral valve disease is 2D echocardiography, but to quantitate the severity of the dysfunction (stenosis, regurgitation), Doppler imaging modalities must be used. Most patients presenting to the operating room for mitral valve surgery have already undergone an extensive preoperative workup. The patient's cardiologist and cardiac surgeon have preoperatively determined the degree of MR or stenosis as well as the indication for surgery. Consequently, the early intraoperative TEE exam is generally not indicated to quantify the degree of MR/MS, but to give the surgeon important information regarding etiology, lesions, and dysfunction of the mitral valve apparatus that will influence the strategy for successfully reconstructing the valve. Important to note is that general anesthesia influences loading conditions of the cardiovascular system and may result in a downgrading of severity, especially in functional MR, as can be seen in type I and type IIIb dysfunction (see below).[10]

Occasionally, a patient will present to the operating room with an incidental finding of MR or MS that will require quantification (e.g., CABG with concurrent MR). Additionally, any residual regurgitation after separation from CPB will require thorough evaluation and quantification. Consequently, the cardiac anesthesiologist must have a thorough understanding of methods of quantifying the degree of MR.

Assessing the severity of MR is based primarily on CFD visualization of the regurgitant jet (length, height, area, and direction) and the width of the vena contracta. In conjunction with spectral Doppler–based modalities, the effective regurgitant orifice area (ERO) and pulmonary vein flow velocity characteristics can be analyzed.[11-14]

Mitral Valve Dysfunction and Reconstructive Valve Techniques

The information given to the surgeon by the echocardiographer is instrumental in guiding the surgical strategy. While in many cases the surgeon can perform a good repair just based on direct inspection of

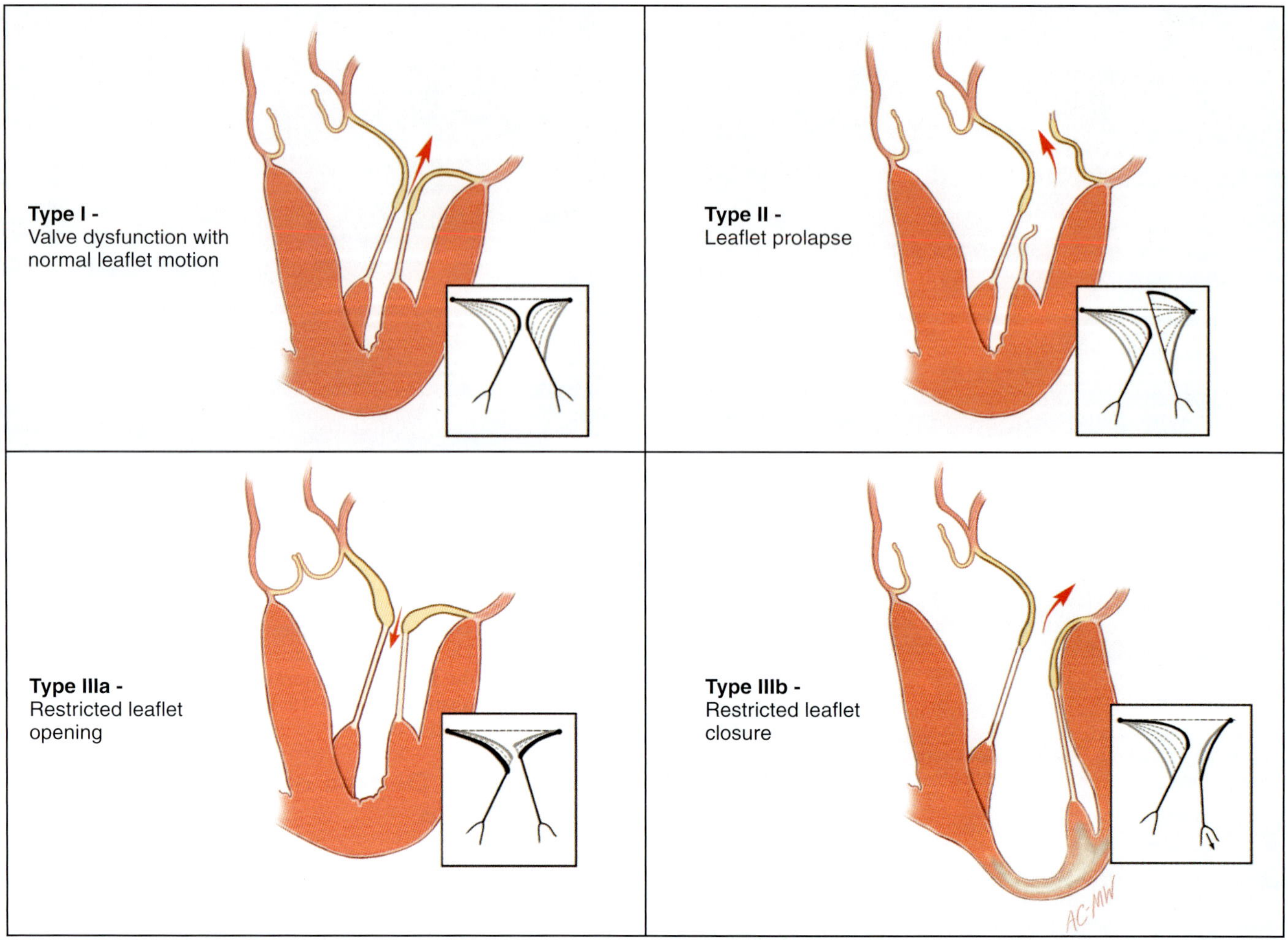

Figure 15-14   Carpentier's functional classification. *Type I*, Normal leaflet motion. *Type II*, Increased leaflet motion (leaflet prolapse). *Type IIIa*, Restricted leaflet motion during diastole and systole. *Type IIIb*, Restricted leaflet motion, predominantly during systole. *(From Carpentier A, Adams DH, Filsoufi F. Carpentier's Reconstructive Valve Surgery: From Valve Analysis to Valve Reconstruction. Philadelphia: Saunders; 2010.)*

the valve, a surgeon cannot achieve a high repair rate in all cases without accurate interpretation of the echocardiogram. A wrong echocardiographic diagnosis can result in the wrong surgical treatment, hence the importance of complete evaluation and reporting of findings by segment and according to the pathophysiologic triad (Fig. 15-14).

Type I Dysfunction

If the echocardiographer tells the surgeon the patient has type I dysfunction due to annular dilation, the implication is that the only technique the surgeon should use is an annuloplasty ring. An annuloplasty ring reduces the dimensions of the posterior mitral annulus to restore coaptation of the leaflets. It is important to note that annular dilation also occurs in the majority of regurgitant valves, so a diagnosis of type I dysfunction should not be made solely on this basis, but only when all eight segments of the valve have been examined and found to be neither prolapsing nor restricted. In the circumstance where the leaflets are neither prolapsing nor restricted and seem to coapt well, the cause of the type I dysfunction would be a leaflet perforation or cleft. The treatment would usually involve pericardial patch repair of a leaflet, so it is important to communicate this to the surgeon early so autologous pericardium can be procured and a patch prepared before CPB is instituted (Video 15-10).

Type II Dysfunction

Type II dysfunction refers to leaflet prolapse. Attempts should be made to use echocardiography to differentiate the disease causing the prolapse.[15] The echocardiographer needs to determine whether there is excess leaflet tissue in all valve segments (Barlow disease) (Video 15-11), whether there is a relatively normal-sized valve with prolapse secondary to a ruptured chord (fibroelastic deficiency) (Video 15-12), or whether the valve has characteristics of both etiologies (e.g., advanced fibroelastic deficiency or a forme fruste of Barlow disease) (Video 15-13). The amount of leaflet tissue will guide the surgeon in the techniques to use during the repair. The commissural view is very useful for determining the height of the posterior leaflet segments. If the P1 and/or P3 segments are 2 cm or greater, this would imply Barlow disease, and the surgical therapy would usually require some form of resection or imbrication to reduce the height of this leaflet. Otherwise, a residual tall leaflet would predispose to systolic anterior motion (SAM) post repair. The standard technique for reducing the height of a tall posterior leaflet is the sliding leaflet-plasty (Fig. 15-15). If only the P2 segment is tall and prolapsing and the adjacent P1 and P2 are of normal height, excision of this prolapsing segment (quadrangular or triangular resection) would provide an effective repair. If all posterior leaflet segments are thin and short (1 to 1.5 cm), the echocardiographer must caution the surgeon because resection of tissue in this

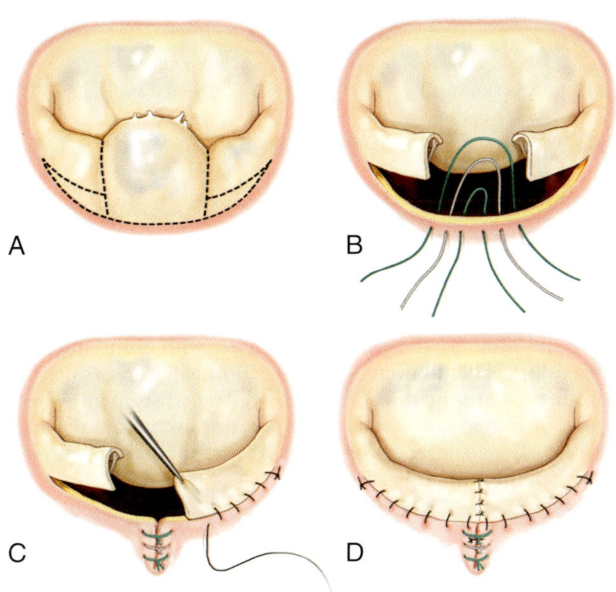

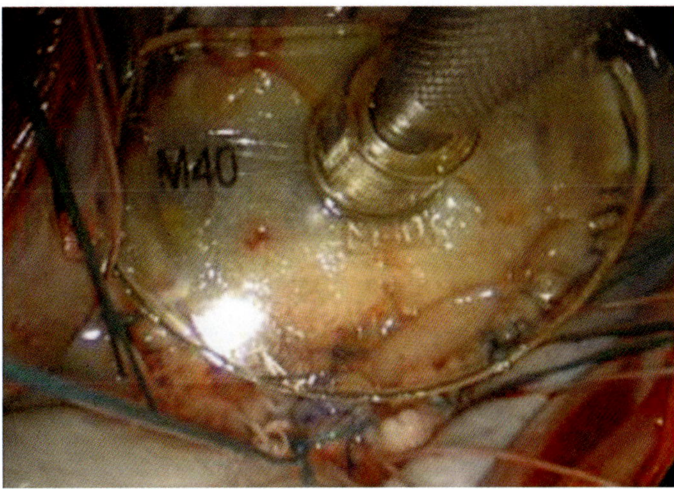

Figure 15-16 Correct annuloplasty ring size is determined by measuring height of anterior leaflet.

Figure 15-15 Posterior leaflet quadrangular resection and sliding plasty. **A,** Quadrangular resection including detachment of P1 and P3 to shorten their height. **B,** Vertical plication of posterior annulus. **C,** Reattachment of leaflet segments to annulus. **D,** Leaflet edges are re-approximated prior to a remodeling annuloplasty. *(From Carpentier A, Adams DH, Filsoufi F. Carpentier's Reconstructive Valve Surgery: From Valve Analysis to Valve Reconstruction. Philadelphia: Saunders; 2010.)*

circumstance could leave insufficient posterior leaflet tissue to reconstruct the gap after resection. In such a case, chordal replacement by implanting artificial chords to the prolapsing segment or transferring intact secondary chords from another part of the valve would be the technique of choice.

Anterior leaflet prolapse is treated by limited triangular resection, chordal transfer, and/or artificial chordoplasty. Prolapse of the commissures is treated by any of these techniques but can also be treated by closing the commissure at its angle to improve coaptation (commissuroplasty). Where the posterior leaflet has been resected or a sliding plasty has been undertaken, most surgeons will perform an annular plication to take tension off the leaflet repair. Prominent clefts in either leaflet are closed, and a ring annuloplasty is generally performed. Sizing of the ring must reflect the height of the anterior leaflet, otherwise there will be a risk of SAM (Fig. 15-16).

Type IIIa Dysfunction

Type IIIa dysfunction must be differentiated from all others because it has the lowest rate and durability of repair. The echocardiographer can easily distinguish this from other dysfunctions, because the leaflet body and margins do not rise to the annular plane and the leaflet margins have only limited movement in diastole (Video 15-14). Some patients may also have a diastolic gradient across the valve. The echocardiographer may note specific lesions, including leaflet thickening, leaflet retraction, minimal height of the posterior leaflet, leaflet calcification, annular calcification, and chordal calcification. Special attention should be paid to the anterior leaflet, since this is the key determinant of reparability of the valve. If the anterior leaflet is very mobile, repair is usually feasible, but if the anterior leaflet is very thickened, calcified, or limited in movement, the chances of a successful repair are low. The degree of commissural fusion and calcification should also be evaluated by the imager. Commissural calcification is usually an indication to abort valve repair and perform valve replacement.

Repairs for type IIIa dysfunction involve techniques that improve leaflet mobility and typically involve division or fenestration of restricting chords and pericardial patch augmentation of retracted leaflets.

The most common etiology for type IIIa dysfunction is rheumatic mitral valve disease. Other rare causes, such as radiation therapy or carcinoid heart disease in the setting of a patent foramen ovale, can lead to a similar picture. When there is significant MS, spontaneous echo contrast can be seen in the LA. In this setting, a frequent finding is LA thrombus, particularly in the LA appendage. If a thrombus is detected, it should be removed during surgery and the LA appendage closed.

Percutaneous mitral balloon valvuloplasty (MBV) is a safe nonsurgical procedure for the treatment of severe rheumatic MS. This modality generally renders favorable immediate results and is widely used.

Some patients affected with rheumatic MS are not candidates to undergo balloon valvuloplasty. For example, subvalvular calcification or the presence of substantial mitral or tricuspid regurgitation may make the valve morphology unsuitable. These patients must undergo open heart surgery—either valve repair or replacement. The procedure can involve commissurotomy, chordal splitting, and decalcification of the annulus or the valve leaflets.

After surgical repair, it is important to assess the degree of residual stenosis or regurgitation. Although mitral valve replacement poses a lesser surgical challenge than valve repair, it is essential for the echocardiographer to evaluate the function of the prosthesis. Both biological and metal valves should be assessed for proper function. If a "stuck" prosthetic leaflet or paravalvular leak are identified, these findings have to be discussed with the surgeon *prior to* decannulation and reversal of heparin (Video 15-15). 

Type IIIb Dysfunction

The echocardiographer must differentiate restriction of the posterior leaflet from prolapse of the anterior leaflet; treatments for these are very different (Fig. 15-17 and Video 15-16). Typically in IIIb dysfunction,  tethering of the posterior leaflet (sometimes also anterior) causes this leaflet to have restricted closure, though the opening is preserved. The standard therapy for this is a downsized annuloplasty. The echocardiographer must seek markers of advanced stages of IIIb dysfunction and, if present, should alert the surgeon. In particular, if the LV end-diastolic diameter is greater than 65 mm[16] or the tenting height is greater than 15 mm, the effect of the annuloplasty may be limited, and the surgeon may want to consider adjunctive measures such as chordal cutting, papillary muscle repositioning, or even mitral valve replacement.

Postrepair Valve Analysis by TEE

After separation from CPB and prior to removal of cannulae, the quality of the surgical procedure should be analyzed in the seven views described earlier. Initially, the valve is inspected with 2D

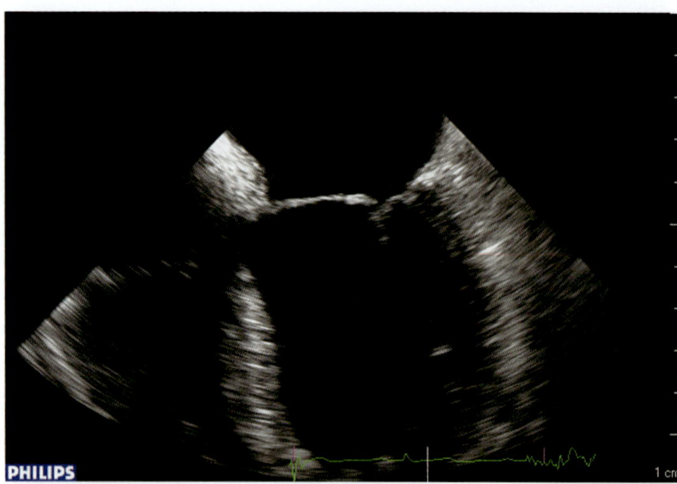

Figure 15-17 Midesophageal four-chamber view. Pseudoprolapse. Note restriction of posterior leaflet. Anterior leaflet overrides posterior but does not come above annular plane.

echocardiography to evaluate leaflet structure and motion. For mitral valve repair procedures, a CFD map is added to the 2D picture to exclude the presence of a residual leak. Leaks can occur at the coaptation surface, within the body of the leaflet (e.g., residual cleft, perforation during suturing of annuloplasty ring), or outside the annuloplasty ring (paravalvular leak). If a leak is found, an attempt must be made to again define it according to Carpentier's triad, since this information is crucial in directing the surgeon to the problem's solution. Most importantly, the dysfunction should be identified. Type I would imply either the ring size is too big, a residual cleft, or an iatrogenic perforation. Type II would imply residual or new prolapse that (if localized) should be easily correctable. Type III would imply insufficient correction of restriction, over-restriction resulting from leaflet-plasty, malpositioning of the annuloplasty ring, or excessive tissue resection.

Using segmental analysis, an attempt should be made to localize the site of the residual dysfunction. The lesion causing the residual leak should also be sought. For example, excessive tissue height of P1 could result in SAM. The surgeon can then reinstitute CPB and directly remedy the culprit lesion and dysfunction, or promptly proceed to valve replacement if the identified lesions are deemed irreparable. Without segmental analysis of the lesion and identification of the dysfunction causing the residual leak, the surgeon will likely have difficulty understanding the mechanism of the residual leakage, even with direct reinspection of the valve. This information can be critical in deciding how to manage a residual leak. The surgeon may opt for a short second CPB run to fix a mild leak due to a perforation at the base of a leaflet, but less inclined to go back on CPB if the echocardiographer cannot find a clear mechanism for the leak or if the mechanism is such that a complex or protracted solution is required.

For prosthetic valves, the function of the valve is inspected. The echocardiographer looks specifically at the opening and closing mechanism to be certain all leaflets are coapting well. It is not uncommon to find a small central jet in a normally functioning bioprosthesis. Normal-functioning mechanical valves show multiple tiny "washing" jets. These findings represent normal valve function (Video 15-17).

As after repair with an annuloplasty ring, prosthetic valves can also have paravalvular leaks. The echocardiographer should grade the severity, note the location, and communicate the findings with the surgical team.

Assessment of a Mitral Regurgitation Jet

If a regurgitant jet is detected, its direction, size, and duration during systole must be analyzed. The severity of the jet can be assessed both qualitatively and quantitatively.

TABLE 15-2	Vena Contracta
Vena Contracta Diameter	**Severity of Mitral Regurgitation**
<3 mm	Mild
4-6 mm	Moderate
>7 mm	Severe

Qualitative Assessment

Jet Direction
An eccentric jet will be seen in the presence of segmental restriction or prolapse and provides the echocardiographer with useful information with regard to leaflet dysfunction. Restriction will lead to an eccentric jet pointing toward the direction of the restricted segment, whereas a jet caused by prolapse will lead to a jet pointing away from the diseased segment. A concentric jet is seen in the presence of malcoaptation (e.g., oversizing of the annuloplasty ring).

Jet Duration
The duration of the jet during systole is important to recognize and quantify. Early systolic jets (closing jet) are generally considered harmless. They result from tiny clefts, indentations, or irregularities along the coaptation surface that require closing pressure to create firm coaptation. Pansystolic jets, however, represent structural defects and have to be discussed with the surgical team.

Jet Area
The area of the LA occupied by the regurgitant jet can also be used as a qualitative measurement of the severity of MR. Jets occupying less than 20% of the LA are associated with mild MR, while jets that fill out more than 40% are consistent with severe MR.[17] Although frequently utilized in daily practice, this method is very dependent upon loading conditions of the ventricle and proper use of Doppler settings by the echocardiographer. Generally, a Nyquist limit of 0.55 to 0.65 m/s is recommended for interrogating MR.[17] Lower settings of the Nyquist limit will result in overestimation; higher settings will result in underestimation of the severity of the lesion. Eccentric jets that are directed against (or "hug") the atrial wall are generally underestimated, and central jets are overestimated in their severity by less experienced echocardiographers.

Vena Contracta
The vena contracta is reported to be mostly independent of loading conditions and represents a good method of assessing the severity of MR during the perioperative period (Table 15-2).[5]

Proximal Isovelocity Surface Area
Flow convergence will only be seen in situations where significant regurgitation is present, so the presence of a proximal isovelocity surface area (PISA) "shell" should always alert the echocardiographer to the likelihood of significant MR and prompt further investigation. It must be emphasized that all CFD examinations be performed with a standardized Nyquist limit (Fig. 15-18 and Video 15-18).

Quantitative Assessment

If uncertainty persists with qualitative assessments, quantitative Doppler-based measurements must be obtained. These include determining the estimated regurgitant orifice (ERO), and calculating the regurgitant volume (RV) and regurgitant fraction (RF).

Estimated Regurgitant Orifice
ERO measurement best correlates with the severity of the lesion.[18] Based on the continuity equation, the ERO can be calculated using the following equation:

$$ERO = 2\pi r^2 \times V_{nl}/V_{max}$$

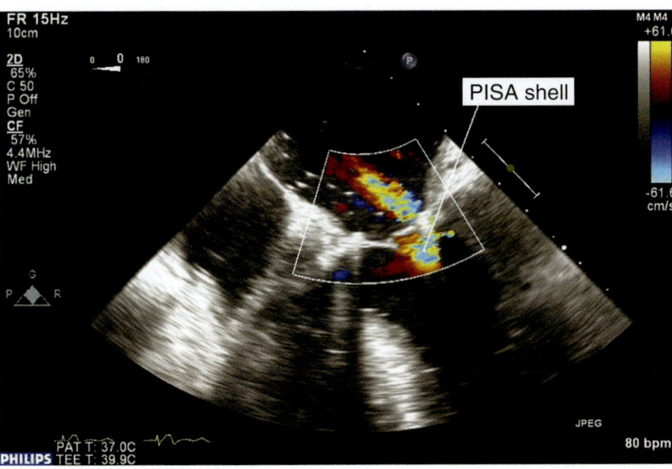

Figure 15-18 Presence of a proximal isovelocity surface area (PISA) shell should alert echocardiographer to likelihood of severe residual leak after mitral valve repair.

TABLE 15-4	Grading of Mitral Stenosis		
	Mild	*Moderate*	*Severe*
Mean gradient (mm Hg)	<5	5-10	>10
PA systolic pressure (mm Hg)	<30	30-50	>50
Valve area (cm^2)	>1.5	1.0-1.5	<1

PA, Pulmonary artery.
Data from 2008 focused update incorporated into the ACC/AHA 2006 guidelines for the management of patients with valvular heart disease. *Circulation.* 2008;118:e523-661.

can potentially lead to under- or overestimation of the severity of MR. To properly diagnose the degree of MR, a comprehensive assessment must be performed so that diagnostic conclusions are based upon multiple parameters.

Quantification of residual MR is important because this determines whether further action is required by the surgeon. Moderate or severe regurgitation is an unacceptable postsurgical result and associated with inferior early and midterm outcomes. This implies that if the anesthesiologist reports residual MR as either moderate or severe, it is a direct communication to the surgeon that CPB must be reinstituted (providing the general condition of the patient is acceptable) and further repair or replacement employed. If the regurgitation is reported as trivial, that is a direct communication to the surgeon that a second period of CPB is *not* required. Where residual MR is reported as mild, then depending on the identified mechanism of MR and the clinical condition of the patient, the surgeon may or may not elect for a return to CPB.

Grading Mitral Stenosis

The most common etiology for MS remains rheumatic heart disease. Rarer causes include stenosis as a complication after mitral valve repair, severe annular calcification, pulmonary vein obstruction, LA myxoma, and cor triatriatum.

After valve repair, especially in the setting of ischemic regurgitation with the use of a downsized annuloplasty ring, it is imperative to measure the mitral transvalvular gradient to ensure the patient is not left with functional MS. The same principles applied for evaluation of a primary stenotic valve can be used. On the basis of the mitral valve area and the transvalvular pressure gradients, severity of MS is classified as mild, moderate, and severe (Table 15-4).

Miscellaneous Aspects of Mitral Stenosis
TEE Imaging

Among the nonvalvular features of MS, the LA is dilated, often with marked left-to-right bulging of the atrial septum. Severe MS is usually associated with signs of right ventricular failure, such as tricuspid regurgitation, right atrial enlargement, and pulmonary hypertension. With prolonged diastolic filling of the LV, septal displacement, and ventricular interdependence, LV diastolic compliance is reduced and the LV can be underfilled.

Transmitral Pressure Gradient
The pressure across a stenotic valve can be calculated using the simplified Bernoulli equation (see Chapter 4):

$$\text{Pressure gradient (mm Hg)} = 4v^2$$

where *v* is instantaneous velocity.

The CWD waveform of the transmitral inflow allows estimation of pressure gradients across the valve. Doppler interrogation of the inflow velocities is performed using the midesophageal four-chamber, two-chamber, or long-axis view.

Once the manual tracing of the diastolic spectral profile is made, the echocardiographic machine software displays a mean gradient measured in millimeters of mercury (Fig. 15-19). The peak transmitral pressure gradient can be obtained using the caliper function.

TABLE 15-3	Quantifying Mitral Regurgitation	
ERO	*Degree of MR*	
0.1 cm^2	Trace	+
0.2 cm^2	Mild	++
0.3 cm^2	Moderate	+++
0.4 cm^2	Severe	++++

ERO, Effective regurgitant orifice area; *MR,* mitral regurgitation.

where *ERO* is the estimated regurgitant orifice, *r* is the radius of the PISA shell, V_{nl} is the Nyquist limit flow velocity, and V_{max} is the maximal systolic transmitral flow velocity (see Chapter 4).

During the perioperative period, a simplified method can be used to assess severity of regurgitation. Under the assumption that V_{max} is roughly 5 m/s in most individuals, the Nyquist limit can be set by the echocardiographer to 0.4 m/s; this in turn leads to the following simplified equation:

$$\text{ERO} = 1/2 \, r^2$$

Mitral regurgitation can be quantified using the system shown in Table 15-3.[5]

Regurgitant Volume
RV is an absolute measure of volume overload and may be calculated in two ways. Utilizing pulsed wave Doppler (PWD) technology, the forward stroke volume across the LVOT and mitral valve, respectively, can be determined. RV is calculated by subtracting the inflow volume across the mitral valve during diastole from the LVOT stroke volume during systole. Alternatively, the velocity-time integral of the mitral regurgitant jet is determined using continuous wave Doppler (CWD), and this is multiplied by the ERO (see Chapter 4).

In degenerative valve disease, an RV greater than 60 mL is consistent with severe MR, whereas amounts less than 30 mL are generally considered mild. If the etiology is ischemic MR, an RV greater than 40 mL is considered severe.

Regurgitant Fraction
This method represents a relative measure of volume overload. RF is the ratio of RV to the sum of RV and forward (or LVOT) stroke volume. Values greater than 50% are considered severe, and values less than 30% are associated with mild MR.

While in theory these methods to quantify the severity of MR sound appealing, the echocardiographer must realize that many of these calculations are based on geometrical assumptions (e.g., hemispheric shape of the PISA shell, ellipsoid form of the mitral annulus and LVOT) that

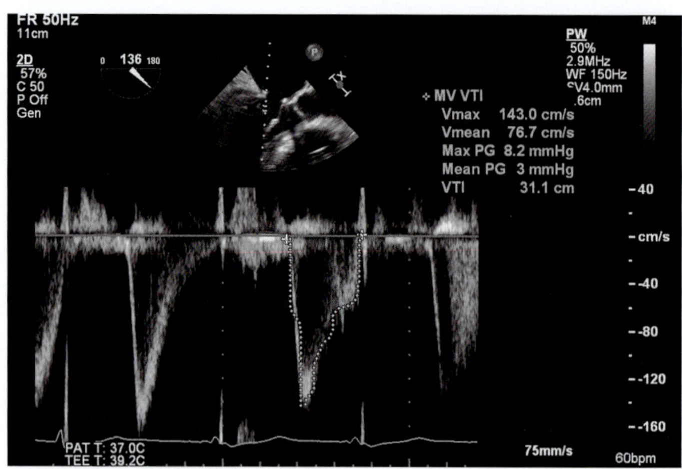

Figure 15-19   After mitral valve repair, diastolic spectral profile was traced, and mean pressure gradient was calculated to be 3 mm Hg.

The echocardiographer must be aware that pressure gradients vary according to flow, such as with elevated or diminished cardiac output states. For instance, in cases of concomitant MR, the transmitral gradient is higher, resulting in overestimation of the severity of MS.

Another problem results when the angle between the sampling beam and the flow vector is greater than 20 degrees, which can lead to pressure gradient underestimation. To avoid this problem, it is important to align the Doppler beam with the mitral inflow. A mean transmitral pressure gradient of greater than 10 mmHg indicates severe MS.

Continuity Equation

Applying the continuity principle that assumes forward stroke volume in one part of the heart equals forward flow in another, flow across the MV in diastole is assumed to be equivalent to flow across the LVOT in systole:

$$\text{VTI MV} \times \text{CSA MV} = \text{VTI LVOT} \times \text{CSA LVOT}$$

The mitral valve area (MVA) can be calculated by rearranging the equation:

$$\text{MVA} = \text{VTI LVOT} \times \text{CSA LVOT/VTI MV}$$

This assumption would be incorrect in patients with MR or aortic insufficiency.

Pressure Half-Time and Deceleration Time

The pressure half-time (PHT) measures the rate at which the pressure difference between the LA and LV diminishes. The PHT constitutes a quick estimation of the valve area in patients with MS, and its value is directly related to the severity of stenosis. The PHT can be obtained from the transmitral inflow velocity profile. In MS, during the early passive filling of the LV, the pressure gradient is maintained longer in diastole, and the transmitral CWD shows a prolonged E-wave deceleration time and a decrease in the E-wave slope. Therefore, the more severe the MS, the slower the rate of pressure decline between the LA and LV and the longer the PHT.

To calculate the PHT, the CWD beam is aligned with the mitral inflow, the flow velocity is acquired, and the time it takes to decrease by a factor of the square root of 2 is traced and measured. The echocardiography machine software displays the PHT calculated in milliseconds, which can be used to calculate the MVA in square centimeters:

$$\text{MVA} = 220/\text{PHT}$$

This formula is not accurate in cases of moderate or severe aortic regurgitation, following mitral valve repair, or immediately after mitral balloon valvuloplasty.

In a normal mitral valve, the PHT is usually less than 60 milliseconds. In cases of mild MS, the PHT is 100 milliseconds; in moderate MS, it is approximately 200 milliseconds, and more than 300 milliseconds in cases of severe MS.

Another useful measurement to estimate MVA and the severity of MS is the deceleration time (DT), defined as the time from the peak velocity to the time at which the velocity reaches baseline. The formula to calculate the MVA based on the DT measured is:

$$\text{MVA} = 759/\text{DT}$$

One of the caveats encountered with these parameters is that both PHT and DT are influenced by hemodynamic conditions and other valve pathologies. For instance, states of high cardiac output, MR, mild aortic insufficiency, and restrictive diastolic pattern are situations that can overestimate MVA.

Underestimation of MVA, and therefore overestimation of MS severity, can occur with bradycardia and impaired LV relaxation.

Planimetry Valve Area

Images of the mitral valve opening can be obtained from the TG basal short-axis view, acquiring the area by tracing the minimal orifice seen. This method is limited by virtue of the difficulty of positioning the 2D TEE plane to "cut" the mitral valve at the correct angle, making planimetric evaluation of the MVA an inaccurate technique.

Other errors have been shown to interfere with the results, such us the gain settings. If the gain is set too low, "echo dropout" will occur and the valve area will be overestimated. Likewise, when the gain is set too high or the annulus and leaflets are heavily calcified, acoustic shadowing limits the accuracy of this method, and the area measured by the tracing will be falsely low.

Proximal Flow Convergence and PISA Analysis

The PISA method is based on the continuity principle, where color aliasing and PISA formation on the LA side of the mitral valve is obtained using CFD mapping during diastole.

Unlike the ERO estimation obtained using the PISA method in cases of MR, an angle correction is necessary when calculating the MVA for mitral valve stenosis. Therefore, the formula for MVA is:

$$\frac{2\pi r^2 \times \dfrac{\alpha}{180} \times NL}{Ve}$$

where α is the angle between the mitral leaflets in diastole, *NL* is the Nyquist limit, and *Ve* is the maximum aliasing velocity across the MV in diastole. This method remains accurate in the presence of mitral or aortic regurgitation.

Potential Problems Seen After Mitral Valve Repair

Systolic Anterior Motion

Leaflet motion should be smooth, with both the anterior and posterior leaflets rising to the annular plane and their marginal edges forming a coaptation zone of at least 5 mm in length during systole. Especially after repair of degenerative disease, the echocardiographer must be certain to examine for the presence of SAM, in which the anterior leaflet is dynamically entrained into the LVOT during systole (Video 15-19). This in turn leads to dynamic obstruction, impeding the LV's ejection into the ascending aorta. Depending upon the degree of obstruction, a severe reduction in cardiac output can occur, leading to hemodynamic instability. Displacement of the anterior leaflet into the LVOT also results in loss of coaptation and integrity of the mitral valve apparatus. This results in MR, increased end-diastolic filling pressures, and pulmonary vascular congestion. The underlying cause of SAM is usually that one of the leaflets has been left "too tall" after repair relative to the size of the annuloplasty ring. A tall posterior leaflet will displace the anterior leaflet into the outflow tract, whereas a tall anterior leaflet will not be accommodated within the annuloplasty ring, such that the excess tissue remains in the LV. Treatment consists of increasing afterload, decreasing contractility, and correcting hypovolemia. Correct medical management is usually successful, and return to CPB for resistant SAM is rare (Video 15-20).[19] 

Zone of Coaptation

One of the primary goals of current mitral valve repair techniques is to create a large zone of coaptation between the anterior and posterior leaflets. The deep TG short-axis view is valuable for assessing the zone of coaptation, because the annuloplasty ring does not create acoustic shadowing of the coaptation zone from this view. After surgical mitral valve repair, it has been recommended that the zone of coaptation be at least 8 mm in length.[20] A coaptation zone less than 5 mm is inadequate, and although the valve may be competent in the operating room, these patients are likely to experience recurrent MR postoperatively (see Fig. 15-13).[20]

Future Directions

Over the course of the previous 50 years, echocardiography has evolved from a one-dimensional (A-mode, M-mode) to a 2D imaging modality. It is only logical that the technology would advance so as to image the heart in 3D (see Chapter 9). This would certainly result in a better understanding of anatomic relationships between cardiac structures. Although 3D echocardiography has been available since the 1970s, its use in the operating room environment has been limited by the prolonged acquisition times necessary to reconstruct images obtained through electrocardiographic and respiratory gating methods. With the introduction of matrix-based technology that has enabled real-time 3D image acquisition, another evolutionary step in echocardiography has taken place. Advances in imaging will result in a better understanding of pathophysiology and may guide refinement of surgical techniques. Minimally invasive approaches to mitral valve treatment are becoming increasingly popular, and these require echocardiographic guidance for placement of CPB and cardioplegia cannulae. Interventional cardiologists and surgeons are addressing mitral valve disease with innovational ideas (e.g., endovascular valve prosthesis delivery and coronary sinus devices), and these techniques are performed under echocardiographic guidance. Whether these new techniques will bring an improvement in outcome will require future investigation.

One aspect of mitral valve repair is clear. The field is dynamic and continually evolving. It is important that cardiac anesthesiologists keep pace with these developments for the good of our profession and the health of our patients.

REFERENCES

1. Nkomo VT, Gardin JM, Skelton TN, Gottdiener JS, Scott CG, Enriquez-Sarano M. Burden of valvular heart diseases: a population-based study. *Lancet*. 2006 Sep 16;368(9540):1005-1011.
2. Rose AG. Etiology of valvular heart disease. *Curr Opin Cardiol*. 1996 Mar;11(2):98-113.
3. Sand ME, Naftel DC, Blackstone EH, et al. A comparison of repair and replacement for mitral valve incompetence. *J Thorac Cardiovasc Surg*. 1987;94:208-219.
4. Goldman ME, Mora F, Guarino T, et al. Mitral valvuloplasty is superior to valve replacement for preservation of left ventricular function an intraoperative two-dimensional echocardiographic study. *J Am Coll Cardiol10*. 1987:568-575.
5. Bonow RO, Carabello BA, Chatterjee K, et al. 2006 Writing Committee Members; American College of Cardiology/American Heart Association Task Force. 2008 Focused update incorporated into the ACC/AHA 2006 guidelines for the management of patients with valvular heart disease: a report of the American College of Cardiology/American Heart Association Task Force on Practice Guidelines (Writing Committee to Revise the 1998 Guidelines for the Management of Patients With Valvular Heart Disease): endorsed by the Society of Cardiovascular Anesthesiologists, Society for Cardiovascular Angiography and Interventions, and Society of Thoracic Surgeons. *Circulation*. 2008 Oct 7;118(15):e523-e661.
6. Carpentier A. Cardiac valve surgery–the "French correction." *J Thorac Cardiovasc Surg*. 1983;86:323-337.
7. Anyanwu AC, Adams DH. The intraoperative "ink test": a novel assessment tool in mitral valve repair. *J Thorac Cardiovasc Surg*. 2007;133:1635-1636.
8. Salgo IS, Gorman 3rd JH, Gorman RC, et al. Effect of annular shape on leaflet curvature in reducing mitral leaflet stress. *Circulation*. 2002;106:711-717.
9. Shanewise JS, Cheung AT, Aronson S, et al. ASE/SCA guidelines for performing a comprehensive intraoperative multiplane transesophageal echocardiography examination: recommendations of the American Society of Echocardiography Council for Intraoperative Echocardiography and the Society of Cardiovascular Anesthesiologists Task Force for Certification in Perioperative Transesophageal Echocardiography. *Anesth Analg*. 1999;89:870-884.
10. Aklog L, Filsoufi F, Flores KQ, et al. Does coronary artery bypass grafting alone correct moderate ischemic mitral regurgitation? *Circulation*. 2001;18:104:I68-75.
11. Smith MD. Evaluation of valvular regurgitation by Doppler echocardiography. *Cardiol Clin*. 1991;9:193-228.
12. Grayburn PA, Fehske W, Omran H, et al. Multiplane transesophageal echocardiographic assessment of mitral regurgitation by Doppler color flow mapping of the vena contracta. *Am J Cardiol*. 1994;74:912-917.
13. Enriquez-Sarano M, Seward JB, Bailey KR, et al. Effective regurgitant orifice area: a noninvasive Doppler development of an old hemodynamic concept. *J Am Coll Cardiol*. 1994;23:443-451.
14. Klein AL, Obarski TP, Stewart WJ, et al. Transesophageal Doppler echocardiography of pulmonary venous flow: a new marker of mitral regurgitation severity. *J Am Coll Cardiol*. 1991;18:518-526.
15. Adams DH, Anyanwu AC, Sugeng L, et al. Degenerative mitral valve regurgitation: surgical echocardiography. *Curr Cardiol Rep*. 2008;10:226-232.
16. Braun J, van de Veire NR, Klautz RJ, et al. Restrictive mitral annuloplasty cures ischemic mitral regurgitation and heart failure. *Ann Thorac Surg*. 2008;85:430-436.
17. Zoghbi WA, Enriquez-Sarano M, Foster E, et al. American Society of Echocardiography. Recommendations for evaluation of the severity of native valvular regurgitation with two-dimensional and Doppler echocardiography. *J Am Soc Echocardiogr*. 2003;16:777-802.
18. O'Gara P, Sugeng L, Lang R, et al. The role of imaging in chronic degenerative mitral regurgitation. *J Am Coll Cardiol Imaging*. 2008;1:221-237.
19. Brown ML, Abel MD, Click RL, et al. Systolic anterior motion after mitral valve repair: is surgical intervention necessary? *J Thorac Cardiovasc Surg*. 2007;133:136-143.
20. Yamauchi T, Taniguchi K, Kuki S, et al. Evaluation of the mitral valve leaflet morphology after mitral valve reconstruction with a concept. *coaptation length index*." *J Card Surg*. 2005;20:432-435.

Tricuspid Valvular Disease

JOANNA CHIKWE

Overview

The distinction between *organic tricuspid regurgitation*—where pathology (most commonly rheumatic valve disease, endocarditis, carcinoid valve disease, and trauma) results in structural leaflet damage—and *secondary* or *functional tricuspid regurgitation*—where the leaflets appear macroscopically normal—was made in the 1950s.[1] By far the most common reason for tricuspid valve surgery is functional tricuspid regurgitation (TR) in a patient whose primary indication for surgery is mitral valve disease. Functional TR may be due to any combination of right heart dysfunction or dilation, pulmonary hypertension, or left heart dysfunction, and it occurs in the setting of an otherwise normal tricuspid valve. It is commonly seen in patients presenting for mitral, aortic, and coronary bypass surgery, where the indications for concomitant tricuspid repair remain somewhat controversial, and accurate evaluation is complicated by the highly dynamic nature of the dysfunction. Organic tricuspid disease such as endocarditis, carcinoid, and rheumatic valve disease is relatively uncommon in cardiac surgical patients.

Irrespective of the underlying etiology, patients undergoing tricuspid repair as a concomitant procedure represent a very different cohort of patients than those undergoing isolated tricuspid surgery. In the latter, severe right ventricular (RV) dysfunction, pulmonary hypertension, hepatic dysfunction, and previously operated left-sided valvular heart disease often present significant additional perioperative challenges and much greater operative mortality and major morbidity.

Functional Tricuspid Regurgitation

Functional TR occurs in the absence of pathology affecting the tricuspid valve leaflets. It results from poor leaflet coaptation due to annular dilation and chordal tethering associated with right ventricular dilation and/or left ventricular (LV) dysfunction (Video 16-1): the most common underlying pathophysiology is congestive heart failure, followed by pulmonary hypertension and aortic or mitral valve dysfunction. It is a common finding in severe ischemic and dilated cardiomyopathy. Significant functional TR is found in up to a third or more of patients presenting for mitral surgery.[2] Although severe TR is a widely accepted indication for surgical intervention, moderate TR is highly dynamic, and its impact on prognosis and functional capacity is not well defined. Indications and optimal strategy for treatment of moderate functional TR at the time of concomitant cardiac surgery remain controversial.

Functional Anatomy

The tricuspid valve maintains its competence through the integrity of its three valve leaflets, the subvalvular apparatus (which consists of thin chordae arising from the RV papillary muscles attaching to the margins and body of the leaflet), and the saddle-shaped valve annulus.[3] Distortion in the three-dimensional geometry of any of these components results in regurgitation. This can be described using Carpentier's pathophysiologic triad and classification of regurgitation (Table 16-1).[4] This terminology is most commonly used in reference to the mitral valve but was applied to the tricuspid valve in his original manuscript on the subject and remains a useful nomenclature. Functional TR is due to RV and annular dilation (which cause type I leaflet dysfunction) and/or papillary muscle displacement and leaflet tethering (which cause type IIIb leaflet dysfunction). Both of these mechanisms, which frequently coexist, result in loss of leaflet coaptation and have been described as occurring in three phases:[5]

1. An initial phase in which RV and annular dilation are present, with or without TR
2. Significant TR due to progressive annular and RV dilation
3. Papillary muscle displacement as a result of right and/or LV dysfunction causes leaflet tethering and more severe TR.

Annular dilation is an early consequence of RV dilation or dysfunction due to lack of an anatomic fibrous annulus and may increase the annular circumference from around 100 mm to 170 mm. Annular dilation does not occur symmetrically; the posterior and anterior annulus—which are relatively unsupported—dilate more rapidly than the septal annulus (Fig. 16-1). Structures in close proximity to the tricuspid annulus, and that may be compromised by disease processes or tricuspid valve surgery, include the atrioventricular conduction tissue that lies at the apex of the triangle of Koch (formed by the coronary sinus, septal annulus, and tendon of Todaro), the midportion of the right coronary artery, and the noncoronary cusp of the aortic valve (Fig. 16-2).

Pathophysiology

The primary mechanism causing regurgitation is transmission of pressure overload to the valve in the form of pulmonary hypertension; this assumption underpins medical and surgical management. In the absence of pulmonary hypertension, the primary mechanisms underlying TR are annular dilation and leaflet tethering.

Pulmonary Hypertension

Severe left-sided cardiomyopathy and valvular heart disease are usually characterized by elevated left atrial filling pressures that are directly transmitted to the pulmonary vasculature. Pulmonary hypertension is due to a combination of the resultant increased afterload and compensatory pulmonary vasoconstriction and chronic vascular remodeling, resulting in RV pressure overload, which may directly result in TR. Pulmonary hypertension appears to determine the degree of secondary TR to a limited extent, but the relationship is not a direct one.[6] The finding that functional TR may also develop in the absence of demonstrable pulmonary hypertension suggests additional underlying mechanisms.

Annular Dilation

Annular dilation results in loss of leaflet coaptation, causing type I regurgitation, and has been shown to be a strong independent predictor of functional TR.[6] It has more recently become apparent that in addition to dilation, several other annular abnormalities characterize functional TR. Three-dimensional (3D) echocardiography has been used to show how valves with functional TR lose their normal saddle-shaped annular geometry, becoming flattened and circular as they dilate, with an associated asymmetric loss of annular contraction.[6]

TABLE 16-1	**Carpentier's Classification of Regurgitation, Listing Lesions Commonly Associated with Each Leaflet Dysfunction**
Valve Dysfunctions	*Lesions*
Type I: Valve dysfunction with normal leaflet motion	Annular dilation and deformation Leaflet perforation
Type II: Leaflet prolapse	Chordae rupture Chordae elongation Papillary muscle rupture Papillary muscle elongation
Type III: Restricted leaflet motion	
IIIa: Diastolic	Leaflet thickening and retraction Commissure fusion Chordae thickening Chordae fusion Calcification
IIIb: Systolic	Ventricular aneurysm Ventricular fibrous plaque Ventricular dilation Leaflet entrapment

From Carpentier A, Adams DH, Filsoufi F. *Carpentier's Reconstructive Valve Surgery: From Valve Analysis to Valve Reconstruction.* Philadelphia: Saunders; 2010:188.

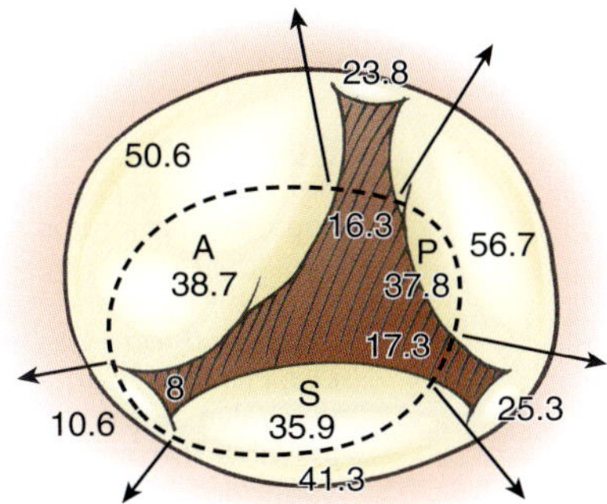

Figure 16-1 Segmental dimensions in millimeters are reported for normal *(dotted line)* and pathologic conditions. Note greater tendency of anterior *(A)* and posterior *(P)* annulus to dilate compared to septal *(S)* annulus. *(Adapted from Deloche A, Guerinon J, Fabiani JN. Etude anatomique des valvulopathies rhumatismales tricuspidiennes: application à l'étude des différentes valvuloplasties. Ann Chir Thorac Cardiovasc. 1973;12:343-349.)*

Leaflet Tethering

Leaflet tethering that results in Carpentier type IIIb regurgitation may be the result of chordal or papillary muscle shortening or papillary muscle displacement, most commonly due to ventricular dilation. Functional TR due to septal leaflet tethering may be observed in the context of normal RV function, dimensions, and pulmonary pressure. This really leaves only LV pathology as a potential explanation for functional TR in this setting. The right and left ventricles are interdependent at the septum, where the papillary muscles giving rise to the chordae of the tricuspid valve's septal leaflet take origin. Where LV pathology results in a dysfunctional or displaced interventricular septum, tethering of the septal tricuspid leaflet may result, even if the RV appears echocardiographically normal.[7,8] This may be why LV dysfunction is associated with functional TR. In an analysis of 75 patients with dilated RVs, *eccentricity* of the RV and tricuspid valve tethering area were most strongly predictive of the severity of functional TR, whereas RV function, dimension, and pulmonary artery pressures were insignificant determinants.[9]

Organic Tricuspid Disease

Organic tricuspid disease requiring surgery is uncommon (Table 16-2). Right-sided infective endocarditis is suggestive of intravenous drug use but is also seen in patients with indwelling catheters for dialysis or chemotherapy. Multiple vegetations attached to indwelling catheters and wires

and extending over the atrial and ventricular surfaces of the leaflets, which are frequently thickened, are common; leaflet perforations and annular abscesses less so. Trauma can cause TR, most commonly as a result of iatrogenic mechanisms such as endomyocardial biopsies in heart transplant patients, fibrosis around pacing wires, or extraction of long-term intracardiac lines. Blunt trauma is an unusual cause of TR due to papillary muscle rupture (Video 16-1). 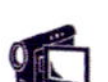 Rheumatic valve disease, rheumatoid arthritis, systemic lupus erythematosus, and antiphospholipid syndrome are all associated with organic leaflet lesions that may result in significant tricuspid valve dysfunction. Rheumatic tricuspid valve disease is often predominantly functional, but it is occasionally characterized by leaflet involvement with thickened, shortened leaflets and commissural fusion. Carcinoid valve disease usually involves the tricuspid and pulmonary valve, causing very pronounced leaflet thickening and mixed stenotic and regurgitant lesions (regurgitation is usually predominant). In these patients, one of the goals of valve surgery is to facilitate subsequent resection of hepatic metastases. Tricuspid valve stenosis, which is predominantly caused by rheumatic valve disease and occasionally a feature of carcinoid valve disease, is an extremely rare entity in developed countries.

Indications for Tricuspid Valve Surgery

Severe symptomatic TR is an American College of Cardiology/American Heart Association (ACC/AHA) and European Society of Cardiology class I indication for surgical intervention (Boxes 16-1 and 16-2).[10,11] It is equally accepted that moderate TR in isolation is *not* an indication for surgery. A large portion of patients fall in a gray area between the two extremes. These are patients who usually present for mitral valve surgery (although occasionally the question arises in patients undergoing aortic valve or coronary bypass surgery) in whom functional TR is an incidental finding. Should these patients undergo tricuspid repair in addition to their primary surgical procedure? The rationale for surgical correction of functional TR in this setting stems from somewhat circumstantial evidence. Over a third of patients undergoing isolated left-sided valve surgery without concomitant tricuspid repair will develop significant TR during long-term follow-up.[12,13] Is this associated with poorer clinical outcomes? In nonsurgical series, moderate TR has been associated with increased early and late mortality[14,15] and decreased functional outcome; this may be applicable to the population of patients undergoing mitral surgery. Most studies comparing the outcomes of concomitant tricuspid annuloplasty for moderate functional TR at the time of mitral repair to isolated mitral repair have been inadequately powered to demonstrate any clear survival benefit. However, there is limited evidence from two nonrandomized studies suggesting that tricuspid annuloplasty in this setting may be associated with an improvement in both functional status and survival.[16,17] This may be due to the beneficial effects of repairing severe (rather than moderate) TR. Although the established consensus is that severe TR should be repaired at the time of concomitant mitral surgery, the indications for repair of lesser degrees of TR are less well defined, and there is wide variation between groups in the prevalence of concomitant tricuspid repair.

Rationale for Concomitant Tricuspid Repair

Moderate Tricuspid Regurgitation

Moderate TR may be identified for the first time on routine intraoperative transesophageal echocardiography (TEE) prior to institution of cardiopulmonary bypass (CPB), and its presence in this setting is highly suggestive of significant valvular dysfunction. Atrioventricular valve regurgitation is usually reduced in severity by at least one grade by the decreased preload, afterload, and RV function that occurs in patients under general anesthesia.[18] Furthermore, quantitative methods may underestimate TR.[19]

Traditional consensus was that correction of mitral and aortic valve disease was sufficient to address moderate TR by improving pulmonary hypertension and allowing RV remodeling, but this view has been

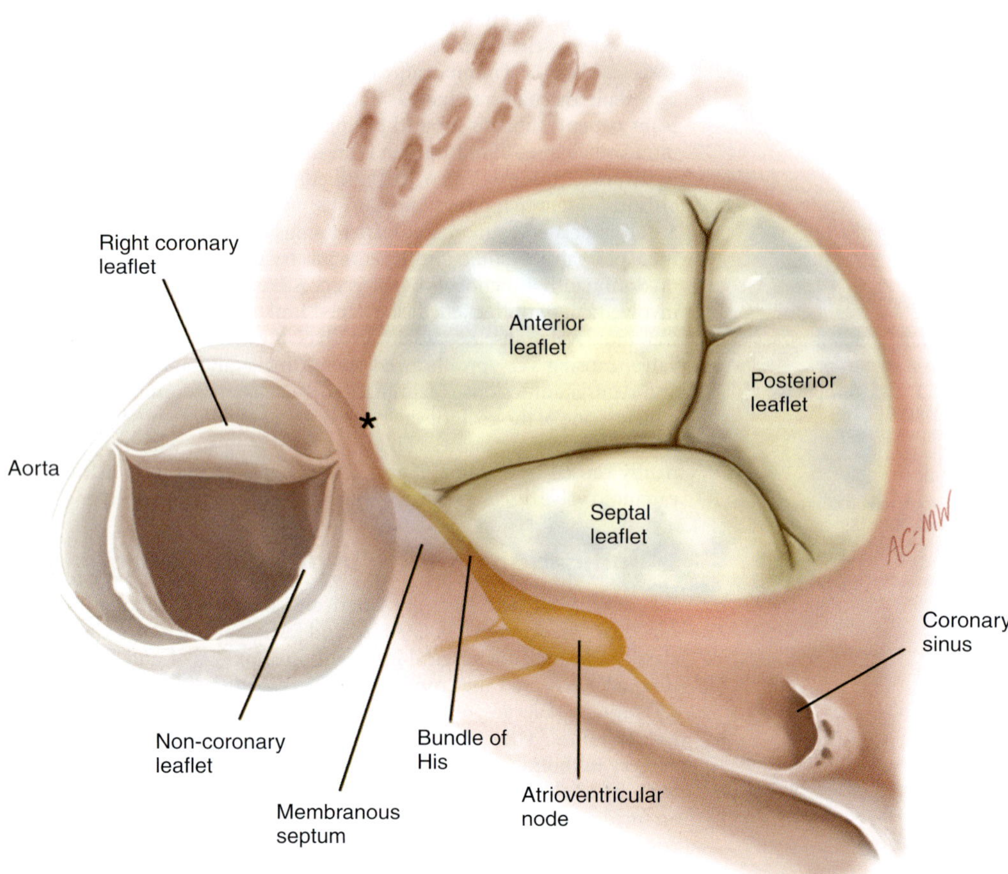

Figure 16-2 Surgeon's view of tricuspid valve and coronary sinus, showing anatomic structures close to tricuspid annulus. Asterisk denotes commissure between right and noncoronary aortic sinuses. *(From Carpentier A, Adams DH, Filsoufi F. Carpentier's Reconstructive Valve Surgery: From Valve Analysis to Valve Reconstruction. Philadelphia: Saunders; 2010:178.)*

TABLE 16-2	Indications for Intervention in Tricuspid Valve Disease	
Indication		*Class*
Severe TR in a patient undergoing left-sided valve surgery		IC
Severe primary TR and symptoms despite medical therapy without severe RV dysfunction		IC
Severe TS (±TR) with symptoms despite medical therapy*		IC
Severe TS (±TR) in a patient undergoing left-sided valve intervention*		IC
Moderate organic TR in a patient undergoing left-sided valve surgery		IIaC
Moderate secondary TR with dilated annulus (>40 mm) in a patient undergoing left-sided valve surgery		IIaC
Severe TR and symptoms after left-sided valve surgery, in the absence of left-sided myocardial, valve, or RV dysfunction and without severe pulmonary hypertension (systolic pulmonary artery pressure >60 mmHg)		IIaC
Severe isolated TR with mild or no symptoms and progressive dilation or deterioration of RV function		IIbC

*Percutaneous technique can be attempted as a first approach if TS is isolated.
RV, Right ventricular; *TR*, tricuspid regurgitation; *TS*, tricuspid stenosis.
From Vahanian A, Baumgartner H, Bax J, et al. Guidelines on the management of valvular heart disease: the Task Force on the Management of Valvular Heart Disease of the European Society of Cardiology. *Eur Heart J.* 2007;28:230-268.

BOX 16-1. ETIOLOGY OF ORGANIC TRICUSPID VALVULAR DISEASE

Primary Valve Diseases
- Congenital malformations
- Inflammatory diseases
  1. Rheumatic
  2. Lupus erythematosus
- Degenerative diseases
  1. Barlow disease
  2. Marfan disease
  3. Fibroelastic deficiency
- Bacterial endocarditis*
- Trauma
- Valvular tumors
- Carcinoid valve
- Radiation therapy

Secondary to Myocardial Diseases
- Ischemic cardiomyopathy
- Dilated cardiomyopathy
- Endomyocardial fibrosis
- Myocardial tumors
- Cardiac transplantation

Other Causes
- Permanent pacemaker or defibrillator lead
- Right ventricular sternal adhesions
- Medication induced

*Bacterial endocarditis may be a primary valve disease or may complicate the course of a preexisting valve disease.
From Carpentier A, Adams DH, Filsoufi F. *Carpentier's Reconstructive Valve Surgery: From Valve Analysis to Valve Reconstruction.* Philadelphia: Saunders; 2010:185.

undermined by available observational data. Tricuspid regurgitation has been reported to either persist or increase in up to two thirds of patients after isolated mitral valve surgery.[12,13] Two thirds of patients who undergo isolated mitral surgery and then need reoperative tricuspid surgery for late development of severe TR had only mild tricuspid insufficiency at the time of their initial operation. (Reoperative tricuspid valve surgery is a particularly high-risk procedure, not because of the intrinsic risk of the surgery but because of the associated severe congestive cardiac failure and pulmonary dysfunction.) This appears

BOX 16-2. MANAGEMENT OF PATIENTS WITH TRICUSPID REGURGITATION

Class I
Tricuspid valve repair is beneficial for severe TR in patients with MV disease requiring MV surgery. (Level of Evidence: B)

Class IIa
1. Tricuspid valve replacement or annuloplasty is reasonable for severe primary TR when symptomatic. (Level of Evidence: C)
2. Tricuspid valve replacement is reasonable for severe TR secondary to diseased/abnormal tricuspid valve leaflets not amenable to annuloplasty or repair. (Level of Evidence: C)

Class IIb
Tricuspid annuloplasty may be considered for less than severe TR in patients undergoing MV surgery when there is pulmonary hypertension or tricuspid annular dilation. (Level of Evidence: C)

Class III
1. Tricuspid valve replacement of annuloplasty is not indicated in asymptomatic patients with TR whose pulmonary artery systolic pressure is less than 60 mmHg in the presence of a normal MV. (Level of Evidence: C)
2. Tricuspid valve replacement or annuloplasty is not indicated in patients with mild primary TR. (Level of Evidence: C)

MV, Mitral valve; *TR*, tricuspid regurgitation.
From Bonow RO, Carabello B, Chatterjee K, et al. ACC/AHA 2006 guidelines for the management of patients with valvular heart disease: a report of the ACC/AHA Task Force on Practice Guidelines. *J Am Coll Cardiol.* 2006;48:e1-148, with permission.

to be less of a problem in patients undergoing early mitral repair for degenerative valve disease.[20] It is difficult to accurately distinguish between patients in whom moderate TR will or will not progress, so it is increasingly the view that moderate functional TR should probably be repaired at the time of concomitant mitral valve surgery.

Annular Dilation

Because annular dilation is a strong predictor of functional regurgitation, and annular diameter is a less dynamic measure than the regurgitant jet, annular size is commonly used to identify patients who would benefit from tricuspid repair. Obtaining accurate and reproducible measurements of tricuspid annular dimensions, however, is challenging. The asymmetric saddle shape of the tricuspid valve means that even small variations in the angle of the ultrasound beam can result in quite large discrepancies. Tricuspid annular dilation may be defined as an intercommissural distance of over 35 mm in any two-dimensional (2D) echocardiographic view, but the echocardiographic threshold for surgical repair has variously been suggested to be greater than 27 mm in either maximal early systolic or minimal late end-systolic diameters,[21] greater than 40 mm maximum end-systolic diameter in the four-chamber view,[22] greater than 51 mm mean diastolic annulus diameter in the four-chamber view and 54 mm in the short-axis view,[22] or greater than 70 mm in the transgastric view (Fig. 16-3).[3] Tricuspid dilation may be more accurately analyzed with 3D echocardiography. Intraoperatively, direct assessment can be used to obtain a definitive answer. In the absence of a history of significant TR, reasonable indications for tricuspid annuloplasty include a maximal intercommissural distance greater than 70 mm in the flaccid heart[17] or annulus circumference significantly larger than combined posterior and anterior leaflet surface area.

Pulmonary Hypertension

In the presence of tricuspid valve dysfunction, pulmonary hypertension is a relative indication for tricuspid valve repair, even in the absence of significant TR, since it frequently persists despite correction of the left-sided valve lesion and predicts residual and progressive

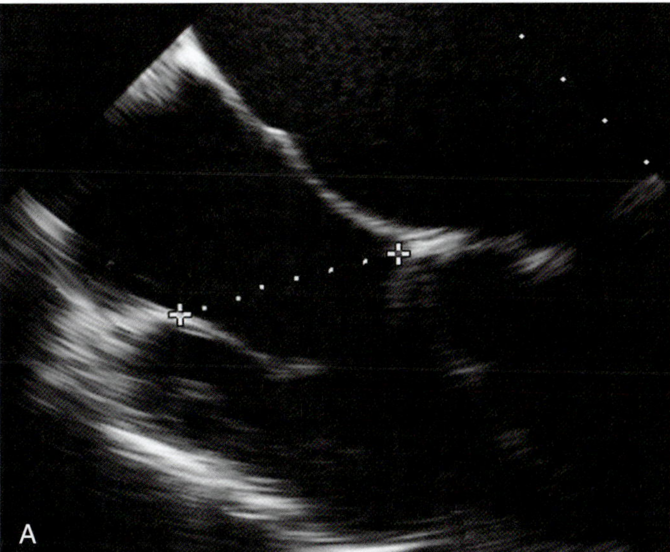

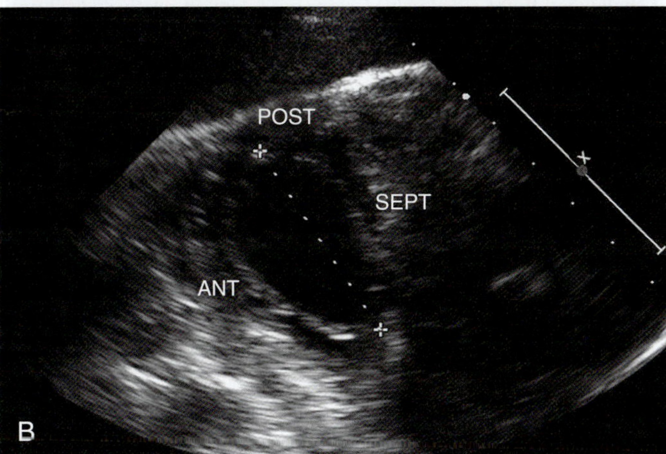

Figure 16-3 Significantly dilated annulus is indicated by a cutoff value of 40 mm in four-chamber view (**A**) and 70 mm in transgastric view (**B**). *ANT*, Anterior; *POST*, posterior; *SEPT*, septal. (*From Carpentier A, Adams DH, Filsoufi F. Carpentier's Reconstructive Valve Surgery: From Valve Analysis to Valve Reconstruction. Philadelphia: Saunders; 2010:185.*)

functional TR as outlined earlier. It is probably reasonable to perform tricuspid annuloplasty for mild functional regurgitation or annular dilation in the presence of moderate pulmonary hypertension.

Systematic Tricuspid Valve Repair

Should tricuspid annuloplasty be routinely performed at the time of mitral surgery? Routine tricuspid annuloplasty is probably *not* indicated in the absence of annular dilation or moderate regurgitation, because the small but present hazard posed by complications (described later) may outweigh any potential benefit in these patients.

Surgical Considerations

The tricuspid valve may be approached via a median sternotomy or right anterolateral thoracotomy, most commonly using an oblique right atriotomy. Bicaval cannulation, which may be direct or indirect (via the right atrial appendage and body of the right atrium, or transjugular or transfemoral in minimally invasive approaches and reoperations), is required together with caval snares and/or vacuum-assisted venous drainage to eliminate airlocks abruptly terminating venous drainage. The additional CPB time required to repair the tricuspid valve is 15 to 20 minutes, which may represent a significant addition to the ischemic time if the repair is performed with the cross-clamp on. There are two alternatives in situations where minimizing ischemic time is a particular priority: (1) performing the tricuspid repair on the beating heart on bypass prior to cross-clamping the aorta (using the opportunity to directly verify placement of the retrograde coronary sinus catheter) or (2) carrying out the tricuspid repair after removal of the cross-clamp during a period of de-airing and reperfusion.

The goals of operative management of TR are to address abnormal anatomy and pathophysiology. This includes annular reduction, correction of significant left-sided pathology, treatment of pulmonary hypertension, and ventricular remodeling. In practice, this is achieved through surgical and pharmacologic modalities. As outlined earlier, elimination of pulmonary hypertension or left-sided valve disease alone cannot be relied upon to eliminate TR in all patients. Similarly, annular reduction without addressing severe leaflet tethering is unlikely to yield a durable repair. Functional TR resulting from ventricular remodeling may also require a ventricular solution or replacement.

Isolated Tricuspid Surgery

Patients undergoing isolated tricuspid valve surgery present a unique set of challenges. Right-sided valve lesions are tolerated relatively well until very late in the disease process when severe RV dysfunction and severe pulmonary hypertension become common. Severe TR makes accurate assessment of RV dysfunction and pulmonary hypertension very challenging. In this context, preoperative right heart catheterization to quantify pulmonary hypertension, pulmonary vascular resistance, and RV stroke work is particularly helpful. Cardiac magnetic resonance imaging (MRI) to identify the etiology of the cardiomyopathy and quantify valvular and ventricular dysfunction is also valuable. Careful attention should be paid to assessing liver function. Moderate degrees of dysfunction due to hepatic congestion often improve after surgery, but advanced cirrhosis (often present despite relatively mild derangements of liver enzymes and bilirubin) is commonly characterized postoperatively by refractory coagulopathy, vasoplegia, and hepato-renal failure. Patients frequently present with isolated severe TR several years after left-sided valve surgery. The problems inherent in mediastinal reentry in the setting of advanced cardiomyopathy and pulmonary and hepatic dysfunction are reflected in the high rate of postoperative vasoplegia, cardiogenic shock, and respiratory failure in these patients, in whom multiorgan dysfunction and sepsis are among the most common modes of death. In carcinoid valve disease, one of the goals of surgery is to facilitate subsequent hepatic resection of metastases, which may be extensive. Management of these patients is complicated by carcinoid syndrome associated with hepatic metastases, which requires infusion of octreotide and avoidance of exogenous catecholamines to reduce the incidence of carcinoid crises, residual effects of prior chemotherapy, and hepatic dysfunction.

Surgical Treatment of Functional Tricuspid Regurgitation

Annular dilation and abnormal geometry are effectively addressed by tricuspid annuloplasty, the most widely used repair technique. The many annuloplasty options can be divided into either suture or ring annuloplasty. Rings may be flexible, semirigid, or rigid, and most are incomplete. Tricuspid valve replacement is not indicated for repair of moderate functional regurgitation, since it introduces the additional risks of thromboembolic and hemorrhagic complications (inherent with mechanical prostheses) or the risk of structural valve degeneration requiring reoperation (associated with bioprostheses).

Tricuspid Annuloplasty

Essentially, there are two surgical approaches to restoring the dilated annulus to its physiologic size and stabilizing an annulus of normal size (Fig. 16-4).[3] *Remodeling annuloplasty* permanently fixes the annulus in a systolic position by suturing in a rigid or semirigid ring and reducing the size of the tricuspid orifice (Video 16-2).[4] The alternative to this method is *reduction annuloplasty*—often using the De Vega suture

annuloplasty technique and its derivatives or a completely flexible band to reduce annulus size by using a continuous suture to "purse string" the annulus, relying on continued integrity of the suture and annular contraction and fibrosis to maintain the new annular dimensions. Both methods stabilize the anterior and posterior annulus, which is most at risk of dilation. Depending on the choice of annuloplasty ring, the septal annulus is kept relatively free of sutures, particularly in the anteroseptal commissural area where the conduction tissue is at risk.

Methods of plicating the posterior annulus or sewing the leaflet edges together have fallen out of favor because long-term results have shown relatively poor freedom from residual and recurrent regurgitation. A remodeling ring may offer the best long-term durability; observational studies suggest that ring repairs are more durable than suture repairs.[23] Data from the surgical literature suggest that over 85% of patients who have a ring annuloplasty will be free from moderate or severe TR 5 to 10 years after surgery.[2,23]

Repair of Organic Tricuspid Disease

In tricuspid endocarditis, the tricuspid valve may be repaired after careful débridement of vegetations, repairing small leaflet perforations primarily and larger ones with autologous pericardium, and stabilizing the annulus with a ring. Tricuspid regurgitation due to long-term pacing wires usually requires resection of the fibrotic mass from the leaflets, which may then require patch repair. Flail leaflets can be resuspended using neochordae or chordal translocation.

Tricuspid Valve Replacement

Unlike left-sided valve prostheses, where the primary consideration is balancing the lifetime risk of embolic and hemorrhagic complications associated with mechanical valves against the risk of structural valve degeneration carried by bioprostheses, the main issue in tricuspid valve selection is usually the inability of most patients requiring replacement to comply with anticoagulation. In the case of patients with carcinoid valve disease requiring liver resection (with significant baseline hepatic dysfunction), the difficulties inherent in anticoagulation must be weighed against the levels of tumoral activity, which are inversely related to the longevity of bioprostheses in that position. High serotonin or 5HIAA levels may be associated with severe structural valve degeneration in as little as 2 years.[24] In patients undergoing tricuspid valve replacement, permanent epicardial pacing wires are often placed, in view of the increased risk of postoperative complete heart block and the contraindication to transvalvular pacing wires.

Technical Pitfalls

The tricuspid valve is in close proximity to the noncoronary and right coronary aortic sinuses, atrioventricular conduction tissue, and middle right coronary artery; exposure of the valve requires specific cannulation techniques outlined earlier. There are several potential complications specific to tricuspid surgery. The sinoatrial node is at risk if direct cannulation of the superior vena cava is performed too proximally or caval snares are incorrectly positioned. The atrioventricular node may be injured by suture placement in the region of the apex of the triangle of Koch. Most annuloplasty techniques are designed to avoid this area to reduce the risk of complete heart block and need for a permanent pacemaker, which has been reported to be around 3% after tricuspid surgery.[25] Acute aortic insufficiency is a recognized complication of excessively deep suture placement in the region of the anteroseptal annulus, distorting the adjacent aortic sinuses or even impinging on the aortic valve leaflets.

Outcomes of Tricuspid Surgery

Isolated Tricuspid Surgery

Tricuspid valve surgery has been associated with operative mortality of up to 25% in historic series.[26] Currently, isolated tricuspid valve surgery has an associated mortality of 10% to 15% in national registries[27,28]—much

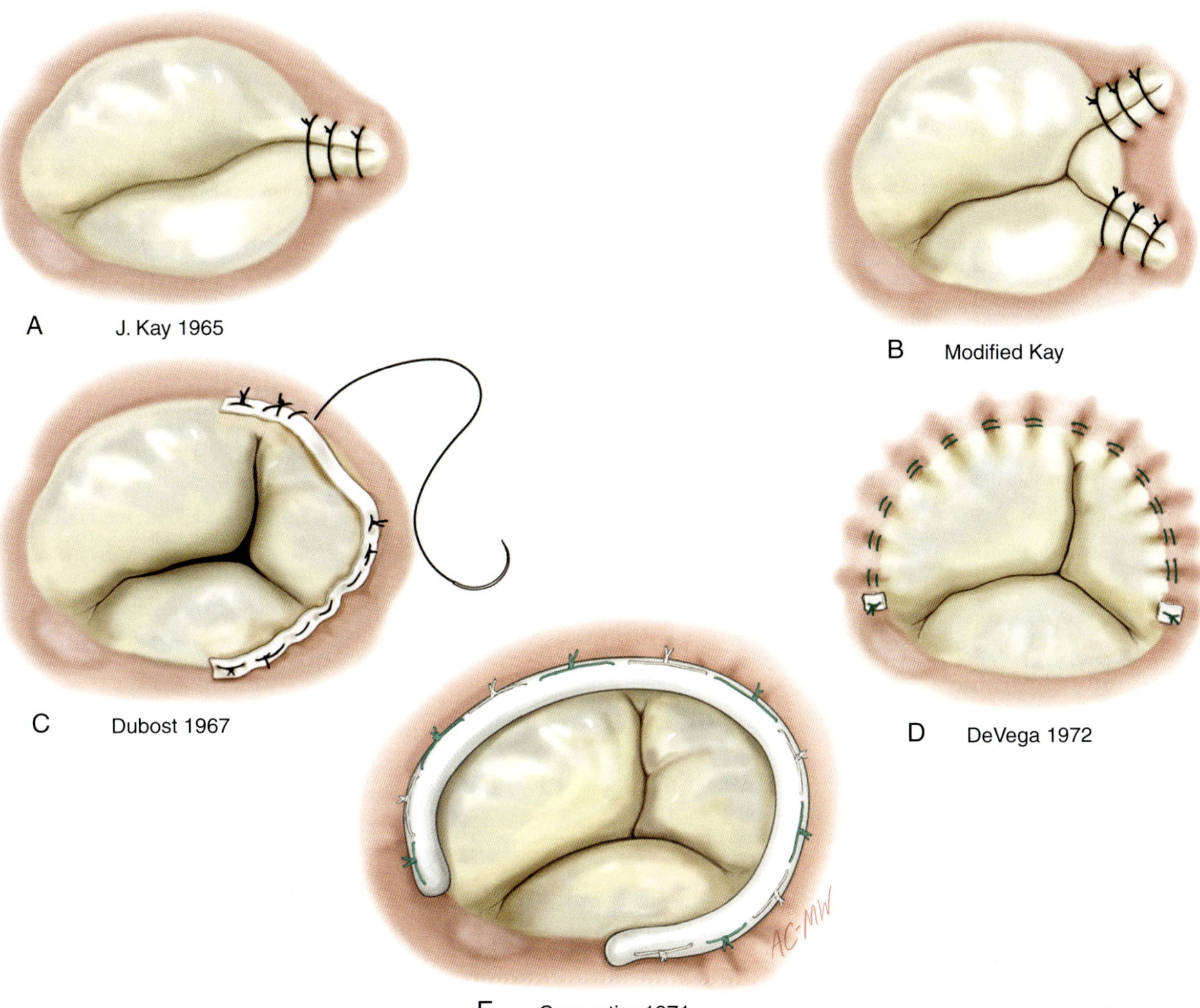

Figure 16-4 Selected techniques of tricuspid annuloplasty. Kay bicuspidalization techniques (**A** and **B**) have shown less long-term durability than suture (**C** and **D**) and ring (**E**) annuloplasty techniques and are consequently much less common. (*From Carpentier A, Adams DH, Filsoufi F. Carpentier's Reconstructive Valve Surgery: From Valve Analysis to Valve Reconstruction. Philadelphia: Saunders; 2010:195.*)

higher than that for isolated surgery of other valves, reflecting the significant burden of comorbidity in these patients. The apparent decrease in mortality compared to historical series has probably been achieved through incremental changes in patient selection and preoperative optimization; refining strategies for mediastinal reentry; more aggressive use of inhaled pulmonary vasodilators (e.g., nitric oxide, epoprostenol, and oral pulmonary inodilators like sildenafil); management of RV dysfunction using inotropes and mechanical support where necessary; and prevention and effective treatment of end-organ dysfunction, coagulopathy, and sepsis in the postoperative period. Prolonged dependence on mechanical ventilation and inotropic support is common. Long-term data on event-free survival are limited. In one recent series, the 10-year survival of patients undergoing isolated tricuspid repair was 69%, compared to 50% for those undergoing tricuspid valve replacement. Ten-year freedom from reoperation for patients with bioprostheses has been reported to be 95% and for those with mechanical valves, 80%.[29,30] The combined challenges of hepatic dysfunction, right heart failure, and carcinoid crises mean that valve replacement for carcinoid disease is associated with a mortality of 10% to 20%.

Concomitant Tricuspid Repair

In contrast to outcomes for isolated tricuspid surgery, the incremental mortality risk posed by concomitant tricuspid annuloplasty at the time of mitral valve surgery in contemporary practice appears to be almost negligible.[17] Tricuspid valve repair takes an additional 15 to 20 minutes but can be performed with the cross-clamp off and the heart perfused and beating, so although the procedure does add significantly to the CPB time, there is no particular need to prolong the ischemic clamp time if this is a concern. The incidence of heart block requiring pacemaker insertion is potentially greater with concomitant tricuspid surgery, but this has not been shown to be the case in most comparative series[17] and is highly dependent on choice of annuloplasty technique. Similarly, the theoretical incremental risk of postoperative bleeding incurred by the addition of a right atriotomy suture line has not been confirmed by studies available to date.[17] Midterm freedom from significant TR appears significantly greater in patients with tricuspid annular dilation or moderate functional TR undergoing concomitant tricuspid annuloplasty, compared to those undergoing isolated mitral surgery, with some evidence of associated improvement in functional status.[17]

REFERENCES

1. Anyanwu AC, Chikwe J, Adams DH. Tricuspid valve repair for treatment and prevention of secondary tricuspid regurgitation in patients undergoing mitral valve surgery. *Curr Cardiol Rep.* 2008;10: 110-117.
2. Chan V, Burwash IG, Lam BK, et al. Clinical and echocardiographic impact of functional tricuspid regurgitation repair at the time of mitral valve replacement. *Ann Thorac Surg.* 2009;88:1209-1215.

3. Carpentier A, Adams DH, Filsoufi F. *Carpentier's Reconstructive Valve Surgery: From Valve Analysis to Valve Reconstruction*. Philadelphia: Saunders; 2010.

4. Carpentier A. Cardiac valve surgery–the "French correction." *J Thorac Cardiovasc Surg*. 1983;86: 323-337.

5. Dreyfus GD, Chan KM. Functional tricuspid regurgitation: a more complex entity than it appears. *Heart*. 2009;95:868-869.

6. Park YH, Song JM, Lee EY, Kim YJ, Kang DH, Song JK. Geometric and hemodynamic determinants of functional tricuspid regurgitation: a real-time three-dimensional echocardiography study. *Int J Cardiol*. 2008;124:160-165.

7. Fukuda S, Saracino G, Matsumura Y, et al. Three-dimensional geometry of the tricuspid annulus in healthy subjects and in patients with functional tricuspid regurgitation: a real-time, 3-dimensional echocardiographic study. *Circulation*. 2006;114:I492-I498.

8. Fukuda S, Gillinov AM, McCarthy PM, et al. Determinants of recurrent or residual functional tricuspid regurgitation after tricuspid annuloplasty. *Circulation*. 2006;114:I582-I587.

9. Kim HK, Kim YJ, Park JS, et al. Determinants of the severity of functional tricuspid regurgitation. *Am J Cardiol*. 2006;98:236-242.

10. Bonow RO, Carabello BA, Kanu C, et al. ACC/AHA 2006 guidelines for the management of patients with valvular heart disease: a report of the American College of Cardiology/American Heart Association Task Force on Practice Guidelines (writing committee to revise the 1998 Guidelines for the Management of Patients With Valvular Heart Disease), developed in collaboration with the Society of Cardiovascular Anesthesiologists, endorsed by the Society for Cardiovascular Angiography and Interventions and the Society of Thoracic Surgeons. *Circulation*. 2006;114:e84-231.

11. Vahanian A, Baumgartner H, Bax J, et al. Guidelines on the management of valvular heart disease: the Task Force on the Management of Valvular Heart Disease of the European Society of Cardiology. *Eur Heart J*. 2007;28:230-268.

12. Porter A, Shapira Y, Wurzel M, et al. Tricuspid regurgitation late after mitral valve replacement: clinical and echocardiographic evaluation. *J Heart Valve Dis*. 1999;8:57-62.

13. Matsunaga A, Duran CM. Progression of tricuspid regurgitation after repaired functional ischemic mitral regurgitation. *Circulation*. 2005;112:I453-I457.

14. Sagie A, Schwammenthal E, Newell JB, et al. Significant tricuspid regurgitation is a marker for adverse outcome in patients undergoing percutaneous balloon mitral valvuloplasty. *J Am Coll Cardiol*. 1994;24:696-702.

15. Nath J, Foster E, Heidenreich PA. Impact of tricuspid regurgitation on long-term survival. *J Am Coll Cardiol*. 2004;43:405-409.

16. Calafiore AM, Gallina S, Iaco AL, et al. Mitral valve surgery for functional mitral regurgitation: should moderate-or-more tricuspid regurgitation be treated? a propensity score analysis. *Ann Thorac Surg*. 2009;87:698-703.

17. Dreyfus GD, Corbi PJ, Chan KM, Bahrami T. Secondary tricuspid regurgitation or dilatation: which should be the criteria for surgical repair? *Ann Thorac Surg*. 2005;79:127-132.

18. Grewal KS, Malkowski MJ, Piracha AR, et al. Effect of general anesthesia on the severity of mitral regurgitation by transesophageal echocardiography. *Am J Cardiol*. 2000;85:199-203.

19. Grossmann G, Stein M, Kochs M, et al. Comparison of the proximal flow convergence method and the jet area method for the assessment of the severity of tricuspid regurgitation. *Eur Heart J*. 1998;19:652-659.

20. Yilmaz O, Suri RM, Dearani JA, et al. Functional tricuspid regurgitation at the time of mitral valve repair for degenerative leaflet prolapse: the case for a selective approach. *J Thorac Cardiovasc Surg*. 2011;142:608-613.

21. Ubago JL, Figueroa A, Ochoteco A, Colman T, Duran RM, Duran CG. Analysis of the amount of tricuspid valve anular dilatation required to produce functional tricuspid regurgitation. *Am J Cardiol*. 1983;52:155-158.

22. Come PC, Riley MF. Tricuspid anular dilatation and failure of tricuspid leaflet coaptation in tricuspid regurgitation. *Am J Cardiol*. 1985;55:599-601.

23. McCarthy PM, Bhudia SK, Rajeswaran J, et al. Tricuspid valve repair: durability and risk factors for failure. *J Thorac Cardiovasc Surg*. 2004;127:674-685.

24. Castillo JG, Filsoufi F, Rahmanian PB, Zacks JS, Warner RR, Adams DH. Early bioprosthetic valve deterioration after carcinoid plaque deposition. *Ann Thorac Surg*. 2009;87:321.

25. Ghoreishi M, Brown JM, Stauffer CE, et al. Undersized tricuspid annuloplasty rings optimally treat functional tricuspid regurgitation. *Ann Thorac Surg*. 2011;92:89-95:discussion 6.

26. King RM, Schaff HV, Danielson GK, et al. Surgery for tricuspid regurgitation late after mitral valve replacement. *Circulation*. 1984;70:I193-I197.

27. Rankin JS, Hammill BG, Ferguson Jr TB, et al. Determinants of operative mortality in valvular heart surgery. *J Thorac Cardiovasc Surg*. 2006;131:547-557.

28. Bridgewater B, Keogh B. The Society for Cardiothoracic Surgery in Great Britain and Ireland Sixth National Adult Cardiac Surgical Database Report 2008: Dendrite Clinical Systems ; 2009.

29. Moraca RJ, Moon MR, Lawton JS, et al. Outcomes of tricuspid valve repair and replacement: a propensity analysis. *Ann Thorac Surg*. 2009;87:83-88:discussion 8–9.

30. Filsoufi F, Anyanwu AC, Salzberg SP, Frankel T, Cohn LH, Adams DH. Long-term outcomes of tricuspid valve replacement in the current era. *Ann Thorac Surg*. 2005;80:845-850.

Pulmonic Valvular Disease

SHUBHIKA SRIVASTAVA | PUNEET BHATLA

Diseases of the pulmonary valve (PV) are most often congenital and only rarely acquired in origin. Disorders of the right ventricular outflow tract (RVOT) encompass conditions that cause obstruction to flow and/or regurgitation across the PV. Pulmonary valve stenosis can be isolated or associated with more complex malformations, such as tetralogy of Fallot (TOF) or transposition of the great arteries. This chapter focuses on preoperative echocardiography of isolated abnormalities of the RVOT. The abnormalities can be divided into PV stenosis, subpulmonary stenosis, main pulmonary artery (MPA) stenosis, and dysplastic PV. When imaging the PV, the subpulmonary infundibulum and MPA must also be imaged.

Pulmonary Valve Stenosis

Pulmonary valve stenosis is defined as obstruction at the level of the PV and is found in 80% to 90% of all patients with RVOT obstruction. It is the fourth most common congenital heart lesion, occurring in approximately 53 (35-83) per 100,000 live births.[1] The recurrence risk of cardiac disease (pulmonary stenosis [PS] or TOF) in siblings of patients with PS has been reported as 2.1%.[2] The second natural history study of congenital heart defects reported an incidence of definite and possible congenital cardiac defects as 1.1% and 2.1%, respectively.[3] The associated genetic abnormalities include Noonan, Williams, and Alagille syndromes. The MPA and left pulmonary artery are often dilated with isolated PV stenosis. Absence of MPA dilation is seen in conjunction with a dysplastic PV or isolated supravalvar stenosis.

Subvalvar Pulmonary Stenosis

Primary fibromuscular narrowing limited to the RVOT is an extremely rare phenomenon that is probably part of the spectrum of illness associated with a double-chambered RV.[4] In comparison, varying degrees of secondary outflow tract narrowing are commonly seen as part of the overall muscular hypertrophy of the RV induced by PS. This secondary obstruction often regresses following valvotomy or valvuloplasty.[5] Supravalvular pulmonic stenosis—isolated or multiple areas of narrowing of the MPA or branches—has been described but is a rare de novo finding in the adult.[6]

Morphology

The most common morphology seen in isolated PS is that of a normal PV that is trileaflet, with a normal annulus dimension and three commissures with varying degrees of fusion.[7] Rarely, bicuspid and unicuspid valves are seen in isolated PS, though these are a more common finding in association with TOF. A small proportion of patients (particularly those with Noonan syndrome) have a markedly dysplastic valve with myxomatous and thickened leaflets, little commissural fusion, and often a hypoplastic annulus and proximal pulmonary artery.[8] These valves are often severely stenotic and usually require repair during childhood. Secondary changes typical of patients with long-standing valvar stenosis include poststenotic dilation of the pulmonary artery, varying degrees of right ventricular hypertrophy, and ultimately, right ventricular dysfunction and dilation.

Transesophageal Echocardiography for Pulmonary Valve Assessment

The PV is the farthest valve from the esophagus; it is anterior and superior in location, and the leaflets are thin. Hence, both its position and morphology make it more difficult to image with transesophageal echocardiography (TEE). The direction of flow across the PV is somewhat anterior to posterior, right to left, and hence, it is difficult to align parallel to the flow using standard midesophageal (ME) views. Thus, reliable spectral Doppler interrogation of the PV may be limited.

Imaging Planes Used to Evaluate Right Ventricular Outflow Tract and Pulmonary Valve

1. **ME RV inflow-outflow view.** In the RV inflow-outflow (RVOT) view (60-75 degrees), the imaging plane is directed through the left atrium to image the RV inflow from the tricuspid valve (displayed on the left) and RV outflow through the PV (displayed on the right) in a single view (Fig. 17-1). Two-dimensional (2D) long-axis imaging of the PV, MPA, and RVOT in a single view is best imaged using this plane. This plane is excellent for assessing additional levels of obstruction involving both the supravalvar and infundibular regions, and in assessment of pulmonary regurgitation (PR).[9]
2. **ME ascending aorta short axis (SAX).** From ME RV inflow-outflow (60 degrees), withdraw probe from the ascending aorta (AAo) SAX, and rotate the omniplane angle back to 0 degrees. 2D imaging of the right pulmonary artery (RPA) and MPA in long axis is performed using this plane (Fig. 17-2). The left pulmonary artery (LPA) arches over the left mainstem bronchus after originating from the MPA and is often difficult to visualize because of the interference of the airway (Videos 17-1 and 17-2).
3. **Upper esophageal (UE) aortic arch SAX.** From the ME AAo SAX (0 degrees), withdraw probe to obtain the UE aortic arch LAX (0 degrees) view, rotate the omniplane angle to 60 to 90 degrees, and turn the probe to the left to bring the PV and MPA into view (Fig. 17-3). Retroflexion of the probe at this level will improve the view of the PV. This is also a good imaging plane to align the continuous wave Doppler parallel to flow through the PV and MPA and is useful in assessment of severity of obstruction at these levels.
4. **Transgastric (TG) LAX.** From the deep TG view, with hard antiflexion, rotate the omniplane angle between 70 and 110 degrees (usually at 90 degrees) with rightward flexion to profile the RVOT (Fig. 17-4). This will provide a good imaging plane and an insonation angle parallel to flow that will allow for accurate and a more reliable spectral Doppler interrogation across the RVOT (Videos 17-3 and 17-4; also see Fig. 17-3).

Usual Indications for Assessment

Indications for perioperative assessment of the pulmonic valve include:
1. Preoperative assessment of congenital heart disease (TOF, double-chambered RV, valvar and supravalvar PS, transposition and PS, anomalous origin of coronary artery from the pulmonary artery, coronary artery fistulae). Prior to the Ross procedure, it is very

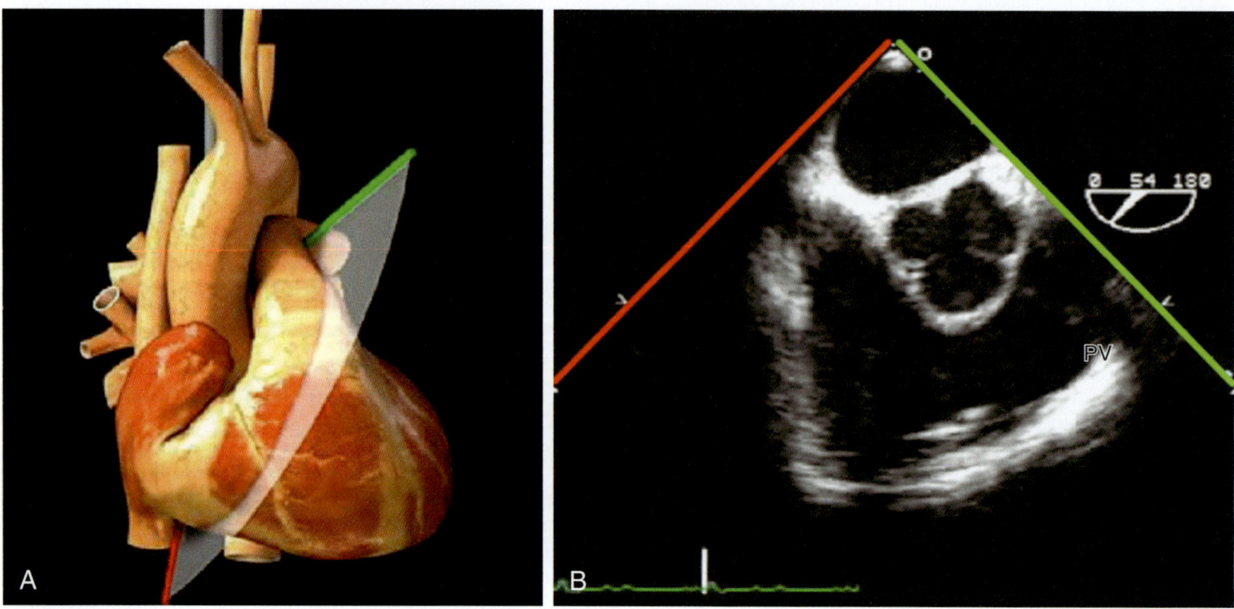

Figure 17-1   **A,** Midesophageal (ME) right ventricular (RV) inflow-outflow view simulation on three-dimensional heart model. **B,** ME RV inflow-outflow view. *PV,* Pulmonary vein.

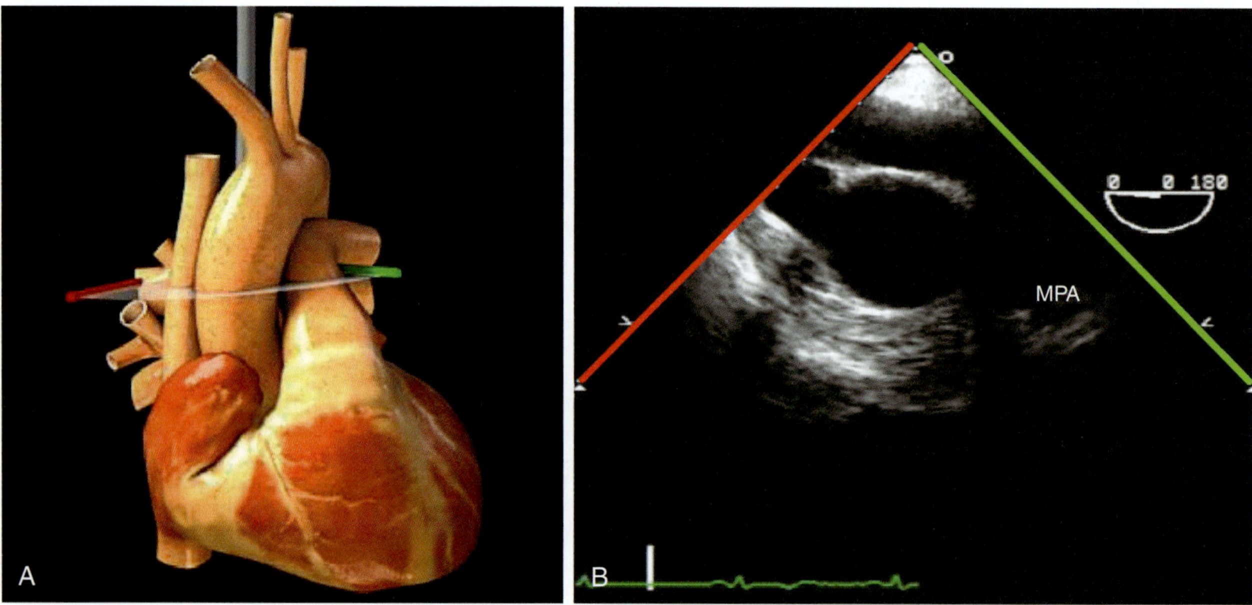

Figure 17-2   **A,** Midesophageal (ME) ascending aorta short-axis (SAX) three-dimensional simulation on heart model. **B,** ME ascending aorta SAX. *MPA,* Main pulmonary artery.

important to define normal PV morphology and function, since a bicuspid PV is a contraindication for a successful Ross procedure. It is also imperative to image the atrial septum and confirm that it is intact prior to PV or conduit replacement surgery in order to avoid air embolism.

2. Intraoperative assessment for these conditions. Following an initial attempt at repairing a lesion of the RVOT, PV, or PA, the indications for returning to cardiopulmonary bypass (CPB) to revise the repair would be significant residual obstruction at any level of the RVOT, including the MPA. It is recommended that Doppler gradients be confirmed by direct intraoperative measurement prior to going back on CPB. Some ventricular septal defects (VSDs), such as doubly committed subarterial or subpulmonary VSDs, are closed

surgically via the PV approach. Hence, imaging for residual PV regurgitation and MPA stenosis should also be part of the routine exam. Supra-annular stenosis should also be examined following PV replacements and conduit revisions.

3. Post–catheter-based interventions to assess for residual lesions and the degree of PR. Residual PV gradients greater than 20 to 30 mm Hg or anything greater than mild regurgitation would be considered suboptimal results.

4. PV tumors (fibroelastoma, fibroma, and Lambl excrescence) and for endocarditis.

5. Carcinoid syndrome.

6. TEE guidance is not currently used for assisting placement of percutaneous transcatheter PVs (e.g., the "Melody" valve).

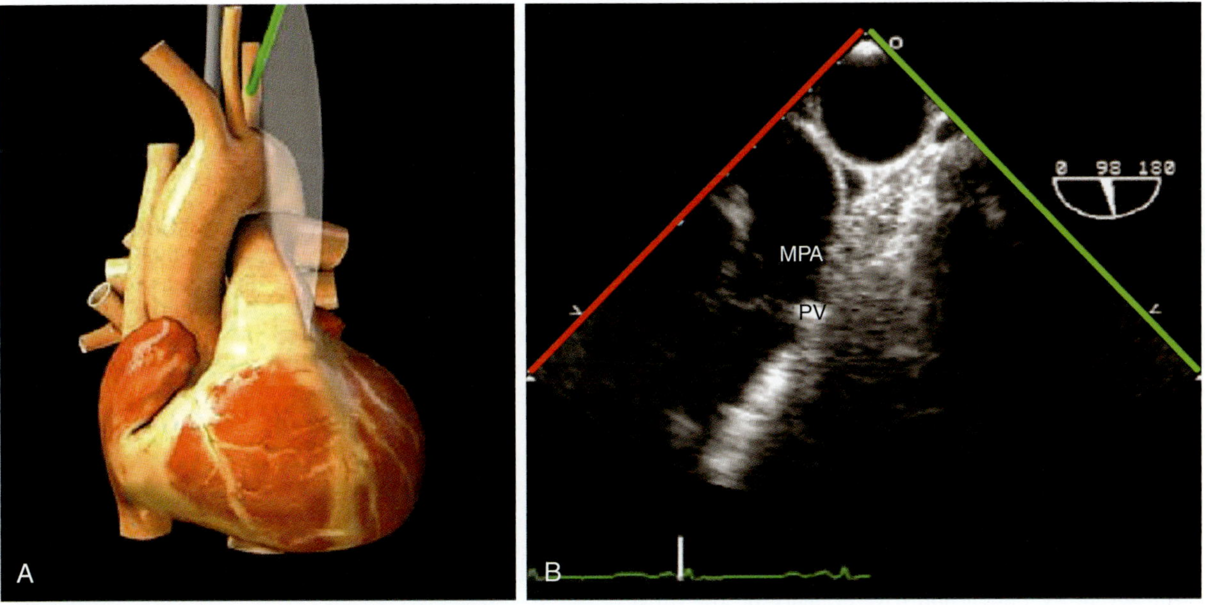

Figure 17-3   **A,** Upper esophageal (UE) aortic arch short-axis (SAX) simulation on three-dimensional heart. **B,** UE aortic arch SAX. *MPA,* Main pulmonary artery; *PV,* pulmonary vein.

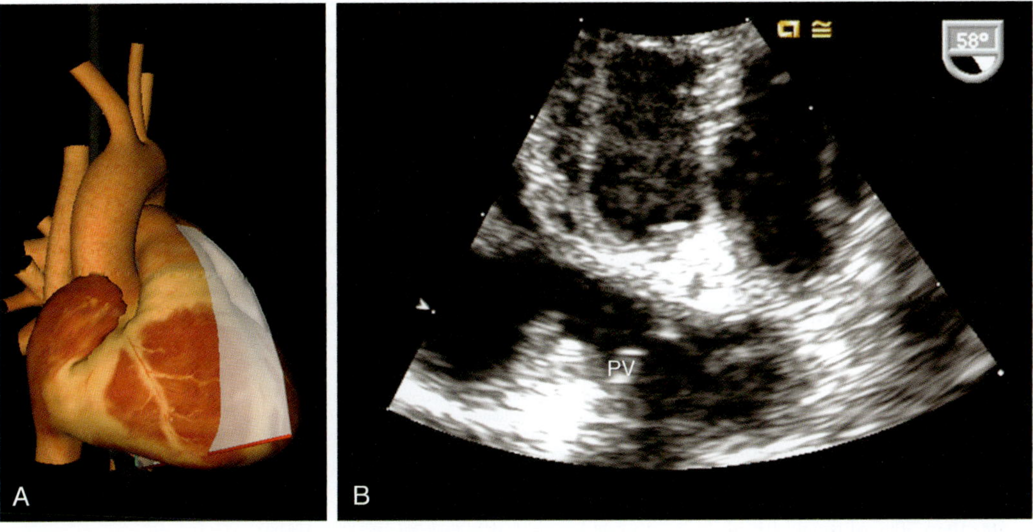

Figure 17-4   **A,** Transgastric (TG) right ventricular outflow tract (RVOT) long-axis (LAX) simulation on three-dimensional heart model. **B,** TG RVOT LAX. *PV,* Pulmonary vein.

Goals for TEE Evaluation of the Pulmonary Valve

The following represent the elements of a comprehensive evaluation of the PV using TEE:

1. Imaging PV leaflet excursion and thickness
2. Measurement of PV annular and supra-annular dimensions
3. Imaging the branch pulmonary arteries in 2D, and using color flow and spectral Doppler
4. Imaging the RVOT to assess whether obstruction is present at the subvalvar level
5. Color flow and spectral Doppler assessment for PS and regurgitation
6. Determining the degree of RV dilation and hypertrophy
7. Assessing RV function
8. Assessing the magnitude of the tricuspid valve regurgitation gradient so as to estimate the systolic RV pressure
9. Evaluating for associated congenital defects, such as tricuspid valve abnormalities, atrial septal defects, patent ductus arteriosus, VSDs, and coronary fistulae
10. Determining whether anomalous origin of the left coronary artery from the pulmonary artery (ALCAPA) or an abnormal coronary

artery course is present. Anomalous origin of a coronary artery from the wrong sinus can course between the aorta and pulmonary artery. Dual left anterior descending or left main origin from the right coronary cusp can course anteriorly across the RV infundibulum or have an intramyocardial course just below or at the level of the PV annulus.

Assessing Severity of Pulmonary Stenosis

The following are criteria for assessing the severity of PS:[10]

1. Mild PS: RV pressures less than half systemic pressures and a peak instantaneous gradient by continuous wave Doppler of less than 35 to 40 mm Hg
2. Moderate PS: RV pressures 50% to 75% of systemic pressures and a peak instantaneous gradient by continuous wave Doppler of 40 to 70 mm Hg
3. Severe PS: RV pressures greater than 75% of systemic pressures and a peak instantaneous gradient by continuous wave Doppler of greater than 70 mm Hg

Pulsed wave Doppler interrogation below, at, and above the PV would differentiate among different levels of stenosis if present. In the absence of accurate or suboptimal angles for interrogation of the RVOT, the tricuspid valve regurgitation (TR) gradient can be used to estimate RV pressures.

Natural History of Pulmonary Stenosis

Patients with mild PS have a benign prognosis, excellent survival, and a normal response to exercise. This mild degree of stenosis does not progress, as observed in the natural history study,[3] so in this subset of patients, recommendations are to follow patients without intervention. One exception noted is in neonates and infants; of the 56 patients younger than 1 month of age with mild obstruction, 16 progressed to moderate stenosis, and 50% of these patients did so in the first 6 months of life.[3]

In patients with moderate obstruction, more controversy surrounds follow-up and treatment. This degree of obstruction is more likely to progress and carries a higher likelihood that intervention will be required. It has also been shown that asymptomatic adults with moderate obstruction have a suboptimal cardiac output response and higher RV end-diastolic pressure when exposed to formal exercise testing. This suggests that these patients have evidence of both systolic and diastolic dysfunction of the RV.

Patients with severe PV obstruction have evidence of low stroke index and higher RV end-diastolic pressure at rest, and this worsens with exercise. The effects have shown to be irreversible when left untreated beyond childhood.

The treatment option for isolated PS is transcatheter balloon dilation in most patients. Surgical treatment is infrequently required. Surgical treatment is required when there are other levels of obstruction, such as in the supra- or subvalvar regions. The 2006 American College of Cardiology/American Heart Association guidelines for management of PS recommend balloon valvotomy in asymptomatic patients with peak-to-peak catheterization gradients greater than 40 mm Hg (Class 1c indication).[11] In symptomatic patients, treatment is recommended for peak-to-peak catheterization gradients greater than 30 mm Hg (Class 1c). Measuring the PV annulus is required to plan for the intervention. Typically a balloon size of 1.1 to 1.3 times the size of the PV annulus is used for dilation. Surgery is still usually required for the dysplastic valves that are often seen in Noonan's syndrome, supravalvar PS, and double-chambered RVs.

Pulmonary Regurgitation

PR is usually an acquired lesion that follows pulmonary valvotomy, transannular patch repairs for TOF, and is often seen with carcinoid syndrome or endocarditis. The echocardiographic criteria that define moderate severity or greater are:

1. The width of the vena contracta is greater than 50% of the width of the PV annulus.
2. There is diastolic flow reversal in the branch pulmonary arteries.
3. The duration of PR exceeds two thirds of the duration of diastole.
4. The pressure half-time is less than 100 milliseconds.[12]

TEE that is performed preoperatively can confirm the degree of PV regurgitation. Imaging and measurement of the PV annulus is important to guide the sizing of prosthetic PV replacements. A poor result is present when greater than mild pulmonary insufficiency is noted by TEE following surgical valve replacement, catheter interventions, or valved conduit placement or revision.

Assessment of Prosthetic and Conduit Pulmonary Valves

There is a paucity of data that address assessment of the prosthetic PV in isolation or as part of a valved conduit. This is largely related to the technical limitations that affect imaging of the PV using either transthoracic echo or TEE. The usual measures of prosthetic valve function, such as effective orifice area, cannot be used because of the invalidity of the continuity equation related to the presence of a "funnel-shaped" infundibulum. The characterization of pulmonary prostheses is limited to pulmonary homograft valved conduits or xenografts in patients needing PV replacements due to congenital heart disease, or to the cryopreserved homografts that are used in the Ross procedure.[13]

Current guidelines recommend that a complete evaluation of prosthetic PV function include:

1. Noting cusp or leaflet thickening or immobility
2. Determining whether there is narrowing of forward flowing color map
3. Assessing whether peak velocity is greater than 2 to 3 m/s through a homograft
4. Monitoring for an increase in the peak velocity on serial studies
5. Assessing RV function and RV systolic pressure

For prosthetic PV regurgitation, there are no definite TEE criteria. The criteria discussed for estimation of PR can be applied for estimation of the degree of prosthetic PV regurgitation.

Three-Dimensional TEE

The utility of three-dimensional (3D) TEE has not yet been defined for imaging of the PV. In present applications of 3D TEE, PV imaging is limited by the thinness of the leaflets and its distance from the esophagus. Its potential utility has yet to be established.

Summary

TEE guidance for PV interventions is challenging, and one needs to use adjunct information from imaging and spectral Doppler interrogation of adjacent structures, including the RV, tricuspid valve, and pulmonary arteries. Since the perioperative use of TEE for PV surgery in congenital heart disease often involves reoperations for PV replacements and conduit revisions, imaging using standard views alone may not suffice. Assistance from echocardiographers experienced in congenital heart disease is recommended.

REFERENCES

1. Hoffman JI, Kaplan S. The incidence of congenital heart disease. *J Am Coll Cardiol.* 2002 Jun 19;39(12):1890-1900.
2. Campbell M. Factors in the aetiology of pulmonary stenosis. *Br Heart J.* 1962;24:625-632.
3. Hayes CJ, Gersony WM, Driscoll DJ, et al. Second natural history study of congenital heart defects. Results of treatment of patients with pulmonary valvar stenosis. *Circulation.* 1993 Feb;87(suppl 2): I28-I37.
4. Cabrera A, Martinez P, Rumoroso JR, et al. Double-chambered right ventricle. *Eur Heart J.* 1995 May;16(5):682-686.
5. Robertson M, Benson LN, Smallhorn JS, et al. The morphology of the right ventricular outflow tract after percutaneous pulmonary valvotomy: long-term follow up. *Br Heart J.* 1987 Sep;58(3):239-244.
6. Kreutzer J, Landzberg MJ, Preminger TJ, et al. Isolated peripheral pulmonary artery stenosis in the adult. *Circulation.* 1996 Apr 1;93(7):1417-1423.
7. Moore GW, Hutchins GM, Brito JC, Kang H. Congenital malformations of the semilunar valves. *Hum Pathol.* 1980 Jul;11(4):367-372.
8. Koretzky ED, Moller JH, Korns ME, Schwartz CJ, Edwards JE. Congenital pulmonary stenosis resulting from dysplasia of valve. *Circulation.* 1969 Jul;40(1):43-53.
9. Shanewise JS, Cheung AT, Aronson S, et al. ASE/SCA guidelines for performing a comprehensive intraoperative multiplane transesophageal echocardiography examination: recommendations of the American Society of Echocardiography Council for Intraoperative Echocardiography and the Society of Cardiovascular Anesthesiologists Task Force for Certification in Perioperative Transesophageal Echocardiography. *J Am Soc Echocardiogr.* 1999 Oct;12(10):884-900.
10. Prieto LR, Latson LA. Pulmonary stenosis. In: Allen HD, Driscoll DJ, Shaddy RE, Feltes TF, eds. *Moss & Adams' Heart Disease in Infants, Children, and Adolescents.* 7th ed. Philadelphia: Lippincott Williams & Wilkins; 2008:835-848.
11. American College of Cardiology/American Heart Association Task Force on Practice Guidelines, Society of Cardiovascular Anesthesiologists, Society for Cardiovascular Angiography and Interventions, Society of Thoracic Surgeons, Bonow RO, Carabello BA, et al. ACC/AHA 2006 guidelines for the management of patients with valvular heart disease: a report of the American College of Cardiology/American Heart Association Task Force on Practice Guidelines (Writing Committee to Revise the 1998 Guidelines for the Management of Patients with Valvular Heart Disease), developed in collaboration with the Society of Cardiovascular Anesthesiologists, endorsed by the Society for Cardiovascular Angiography and Interventions and the Society of Thoracic Surgeons. *Circulation.* 2006 Aug 1;114(5):e84-231.
12. Renella P, Aboulhosn J, Lohan DG, et al. Two-dimensional and Doppler echocardiography reliably predict severe pulmonary regurgitation as quantified by cardiac magnetic resonance. *J Am Soc Echocardiogr.* 2010 Aug;23(8):880-886.
13. Zoghbi WA, Chambers JB, Dumesnil JG, et al. Recommendations for evaluation of prosthetic valves with echocardiography and Doppler ultrasound: a report from the American Society of Echocardiography's Guidelines and Standards Committee and the Task Force on Prosthetic Valves, developed in conjunction with the American College of Cardiology Cardiovascular Imaging Committee, Cardiac Imaging Committee of the American Heart Association, the European Association of Echocardiography, a registered branch of the European Society of Cardiology, the Japanese Society of Echocardiography and the Canadian Society of Echocardiography, endorsed by the American College of Cardiology Foundation, American Heart Association, European Association of Echocardiography, a registered branch of the European Society of Cardiology, the Japanese Society of Echocardiography, and Canadian Society of Echocardiography. *J Am Soc Echocardiogr.* 2009 Sep;22(9):975-1014:quiz 1082-4.

18

Cardiomyopathies

KENT H. REHFELDT | WILLIAM J. MAUERMANN | GREGORY A. NUTTALL |
WILLIAM C. OLIVER, JR.

Cardiomyopathy

Cardiomyopathy is any structural and functional abnormality of the heart muscle unattributable to specific causes or disease processes such as coronary artery disease (CAD), congenital heart disease, or valvular disease. Over the years, classification of this condition has been updated by the rapid advancement of genetic, imaging, and clinical investigation. In 2006 in association with the American Heart Association (AHA), the classification of heart muscle disease was updated with an intention to bridge the gap between rapidly expanding genetic knowledge and existing clinical experience. An expert panel proposed this definition:

Cardiomyopathies are a heterogeneous group of diseases of the myocardium associated with mechanical and/or electrical dysfunction that usually (but not invariably) exhibit inappropriate ventricular hypertrophy or dilatation and are due to a variety of causes that frequently are genetic. Cardiomyopathies either are confined to the heart or are part of generalized systemic disorders, often leading to cardiovascular death or progressive heart failure–related disability.[1]

This new classification divided cardiomyopathies into two major groups—primary and secondary—based on the predominant organ involvement. It retained the common clinical cardiomyopathies synonymous with worsening myocardial performance due to diastolic or systolic dysfunction, but for the first time included diseases with electrical abnormalities that cause life-threatening arrhythmias (differentiated by their specific molecular nature). *Primary cardiomyopathies* include those conditions with only or mostly myocardial involvement (genetic, mixed, acquired) (Fig. 18-1). This places a traditional cardiomyopathy like hypertrophic cardiomyopathy (HCM) with disorders that cause tachyarrhythmias because of genomic changes that encode for ion channel dysfunction.[1] *Secondary cardiomyopathies* are defined as the result of any disease process that includes the heart but is not limited to the heart. These were previously referred to as *specific cardiomyopathies* or *specific heart muscle diseases*. Box 18-1 lists some of the major disease processes that may be associated with cardiomyopathy but are not considered "primary" cardiomyopathies under the new classification. Also excluded are cardiomyopathies due to myocardial conditions such as valvular, congenital heart, and atherosclerotic disease. The common use of "ischemic cardiomyopathy" is excluded.

The importance of echocardiography in cardiomyopathy diagnosis, research, and patient care is evident. Using the AHA classification of cardiomyopathies, this chapter will first provide an overview of primary cardiomyopathy in the adult in association with a range of echocardiographic imaging, including during the perioperative period. This patient population may need a wide range of cardiac surgical procedures (including heart transplantation) that will necessitate perioperative transesophageal echocardiography (TEE). TEE may be especially valuable for optimal care in this patient population during noncardiac surgical procedures, such as cholecystectomy or hip replacement.

Enormous work has been done identifying genetic causes for cardiomyopathies. Genetic testing is advancing rapidly to identify disease-causing mutations in family members at risk but asymptomatic.[2] The primary cardiomyopathies have a very complex genetic profile, with mutations that affect clinical expression of the same disease. The result is heightened clinical surveillance and possibly earlier intervention and prevention of the sequelae of cardiomyopathies. At this time, genetic testing is not 100% sensitive, so it is usually performed once the disease has been diagnosed and confirmed clinically. Genetic screening's greatest use is to identify carriers within a family. This may allow family members that carry the same genetic mutation to be followed, since they may have a reduced penetrance that leads to a lesser form of the disease or even asymptomatic expression.[3]

Most inherited cardiomyopathies demonstrate a mendelian autosomal dominant inheritance. It has been accepted that HCM is largely a genetic defect of the contractile proteins. In contrast, the genetic trail of dilated cardiomyopathy (DCM) is really only solid as it pertains to familial DCM. The more common sporadic DCM has not been found to have a genetic basis. Arrhythmogenic right ventricular cardiomyopathy/dysplasia (ARVC/D) is primarily related to genetic mutations that encode proteins of the desmosome. Desmosomes, cell-cell adhesion organelles, are especially abundant in heart tissue.[4] A genetic basis for restrictive cardiomyopathy (RCM) has not been identified, but a familial form exists and is caused by mutations in the troponin I gene.[5] The genetic basis for left ventricular noncompaction (LVNC) has not been found (and the diagnostic criteria for LVNC continue to be debated),[6] but it is frequently familial, with at least 25% of asymptomatic relatives having a range of echocardiographic abnormalities.[5] More extensive information about the genetics of primary cardiomyopathies is available.[7-10]

Dilated Cardiomyopathy

Formerly referred to as *congestive cardiomyopathy* or *idiopathic cardiomyopathy*, DCM is by far the most common of the four major cardiomyopathies in adults (60%), with a prevalence of 1:2500 individuals.[1] It is the third leading cause of heart failure overall, with nearly 550,000 individuals diagnosed each year. Not surprisingly, it is the most common indication for cardiac transplantation, because survival for adults at 1 and 5 years after diagnosis is 76% and 35%, respectively.[11] Since DCM was classified as a primary cardiomyopathy in 2006, the term *idiopathic* has rarely been applied, because the heart is the main organ involved. The disease process is of mixed etiology; both genetic and acquired cases have been described.[1] It is now appreciated that there is a genetic basis for DCM when all the more common causes have been excluded. More recently, the familial prevalence rate of DCM has been shown to range from 20% to 50%.[8] More than 20 genes have been identified as causes of DCM. Most genetic inheritance is autosomal dominant. The familial form of DCM shows age-dependent penetrance, so that even a normal echocardiogram does not exclude onset later in life.[10] Incomplete penetrance may account for differences in disease severity and progression in familial DCM, despite identical mutations.[12] Interestingly, 30% of patients diagnosed with DCM are asymptomatic.[13] If medical treatment is begun immediately, there is extended quality of life and survival for those individuals. Improved survival supports the vast potential benefits of genetic research in cardiomyopathies.

Numerous causes of acquired DCM exist that include a variety of viral, bacterial, and parasitic infections; autoimmune disorders; neuromuscular diseases (Duchenne muscular dystrophy); exposure to toxic agents, including chemotherapeutic drugs, ethanol, mercury, and lead; as well as certain dietary deficiencies. In North America, myocarditis is the major cause of DCM, usually secondary to a viral illness.[12]

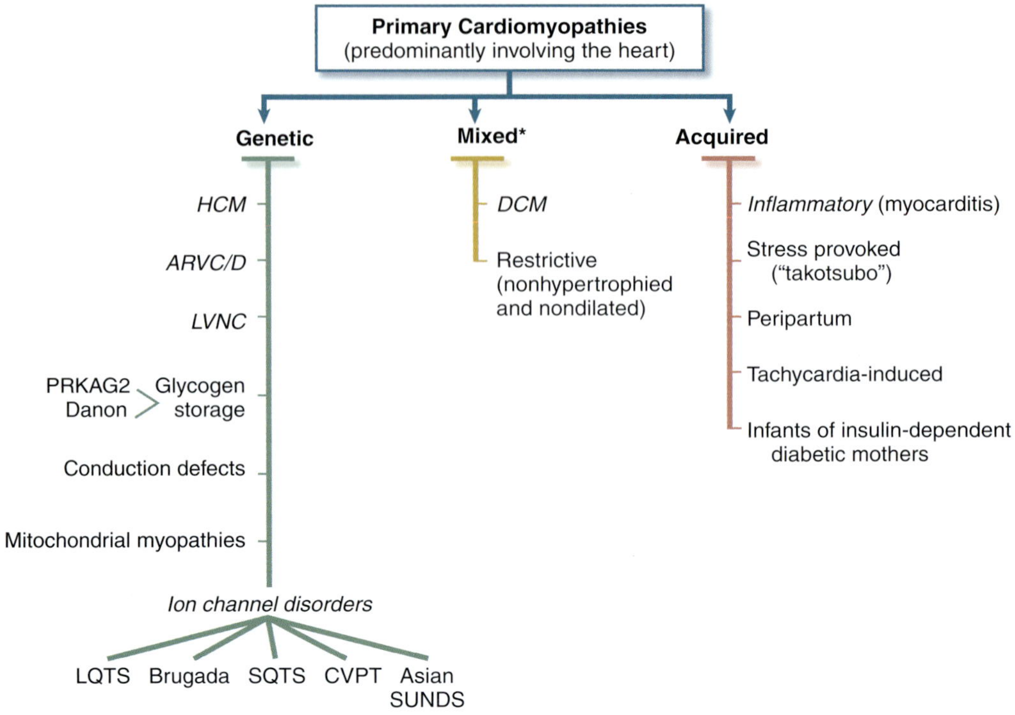

Figure 18-1 Primary cardiomyopathies in which clinically relevant disease processes solely or predominantly involve myocardium. Conditions have been segregated according to their genetic or nongenetic etiologies.* Predominantly nongenetic; familial disease with a genetic origin has been reported in a minority of cases. *(From Maron BJ, Towbin JA, Thiene G, et al. Contemporary definitions and classification of the cardiomyopathies: an American Heart Association scientific statement from the Council on Clinical Cardiology, Heart Failure and Transplantation Committee; Quality of Care and Outcomes Research and Functional Genomics and Translational Biology Interdisciplinary Working Groups; and Council on Epidemiology and Prevention. Circulation. 2006;113:1807-1816.)*

BOX 18-1. SECONDARY CARDIOMYOPATHIES

Infiltrative*
- Amyloidosis (primary forms)
- Gaucher disease[†]

Storage‡
- Hemochromatosis
- Fabry disease[†]

Toxicity
- Drugs, heavy metals, chemical agents

Endomyocardial
- Endomyocardial fibrosis
- Hypereosinophilic syndrome (Loeffler endocarditis)

Inflammatory (granulomatous)
- Sarcoidosis

Endocrine
- Hypothyroidism

Pheochromocytoma

Cardiofacial
- Noonan syndrome[†]

Neuromuscular/neurological
- Friedreich ataxia[†]
- Duchenne-Becker muscular dystrophy[†]

Nutritional deficiencies
- Beriberi (thiamine)

Autoimmune/collagen
- Systemic lupus erythematosus
- Scleroderma

Consequence of cancer therapy
- Anthracyclines: doxorubicin (Adriamycin), daunorubicin
- Cyclophosphamide
- Radiation

*Accumulation of abnormal substances between myocytes (i.e., extracellular).
[†]Genetic (familial) origin.
‡Accumulation of abnormal substances within myocytes (i.e., intracellular).
Adapted from Maron, BJ, Towbin JA, Thiene G, et al. Contemporary definitions and classification of the cardiomyopathies: an American Heart Association Scientific Statement from the Council on Clinical Cardiology, Heart Failure and Transplantation Committee; Quality of Care and Outcomes Research and Functional Genomics and Translational Biology Interdisciplinary Working Groups; and Council on Epidemiology and Prevention. Circulation 2006;113:1807-1816.

DCM is characterized morphologically by right and left ventricular cavity enlargement, with hypertrophied muscle fibers without an appropriate increase in the ventricular septal or free wall thickness, giving an almost spherical shape to the heart. The heart is often two to three times larger than normal.[12] The valve leaflets may be normal, but dilation of the heart may cause a regurgitant lesion secondary to displacement of the papillary muscles and tethering of the chordae tendineae. Histologic changes are nonspecific and not associated with positive immunohistochemical, ultrastructural, or microbiological tests. Microscopically, instead of large losses of myocardium, there is patchy and diffuse loss of tissue, with interstitial fibrosis and scarring uncharacteristic of ischemic myocardium.[12]

With DCM, there is more impairment of systolic function even though diastolic function is affected. As contractile function diminishes, stroke volume is initially maintained by augmentation of end-diastolic volume. Despite a severely decreased ejection fraction (EF), stroke volume may be almost normal. Eventually, increased wall stress due to marked left ventricular (LV) dilation and normal or thin LV wall thickness occurs.[14] The echocardiographic diagnostic criteria for DCM are a dilated LV (Fig. 18-2) together with reduced systolic function and normal or thin walls (Fig. 18-3). However, for greater diagnostic accuracy, the patient should not have abnormal LV loading conditions (e.g., severe valvular heart disease, significant CAD).[15] Some experts have suggested specific diagnostic criteria for measurements of LV size and systolic function that include an LVEF less than 45%, a fractional shortening less than 25%, and an LV end-diastolic diameter greater than 112%.[15] Criteria should be corrected for age, gender, and body surface area (Box 18-2).

Increasing left atrial (LA) size may indicate worsening diastolic dysfunction in these patients contributing to functional mitral regurgitation (MR).[16] Dilation combined with valvular regurgitation compromises the metabolic capabilities of heart muscle and produces overt circulatory failure. Compensatory mechanisms may allow symptoms of myocardial dysfunction to go unnoticed for an extended period of time. However, the onset of MR signals a poor prognosis because ventricular function progressively worsens without intervention. The importance of corresponding neurohumoral influences (e.g., renin-angiotensin system) in this pathologic process has only recently been appreciated as a major factor in the appearance of common signs

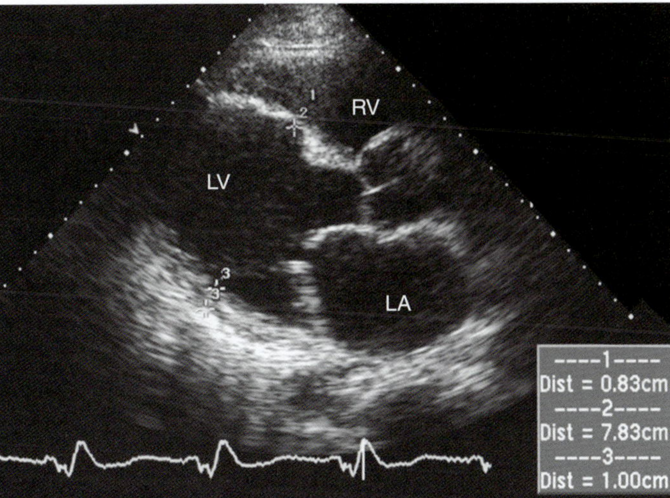

Figure 18-2 Transthoracic parasternal long-axis image of patient with dilated cardiomyopathy. In this diastolic frame, left ventricle is noted to be severely enlarged with normal wall thickness. *LA,* Left atrium; *LV,* left ventricle; *RV,* right ventricle.

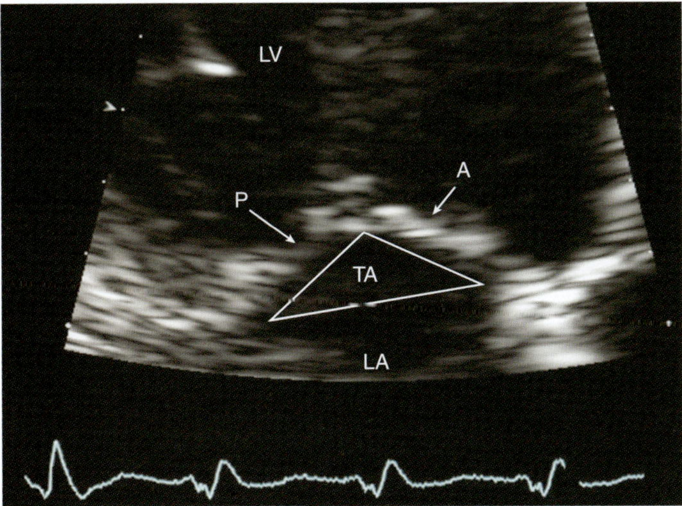

Figure 18-3 Zoomed transthoracic apical long-axis view of mitral valve showing anterior (*A*) and posterior (*P*) leaflets. Note significant valve tenting; tenting area (*TA*) is outlined. *LA,* Left atrium; *LV,* left ventricle.

BOX 18-2. ECHOCARDIOGRAPHIC DIAGNOSTIC CRITERIA FOR DILATED CARDIOMYOPATHY

- Left ventricular enlargement (LV end-diastolic diameter >112% predicted for age, gender, BSA)
- Left ventricular systolic dysfunction
  - LV ejection fraction <45%
  - LV fractional shortening <25%
- Normal or reduced LV wall thickness
- Absence of abnormal loading conditions as the cause of LV dysfunction (e.g., severe valvular heart disease)
- Absence of significant ischemic heart disease

BSA, Body surface area; *LV,* left ventricle.
Adapted from Elliott P. Cardiomyopathy. Diagnosis and management of dilated cardiomyopathy. *Heart.* 2000;84:106-112.

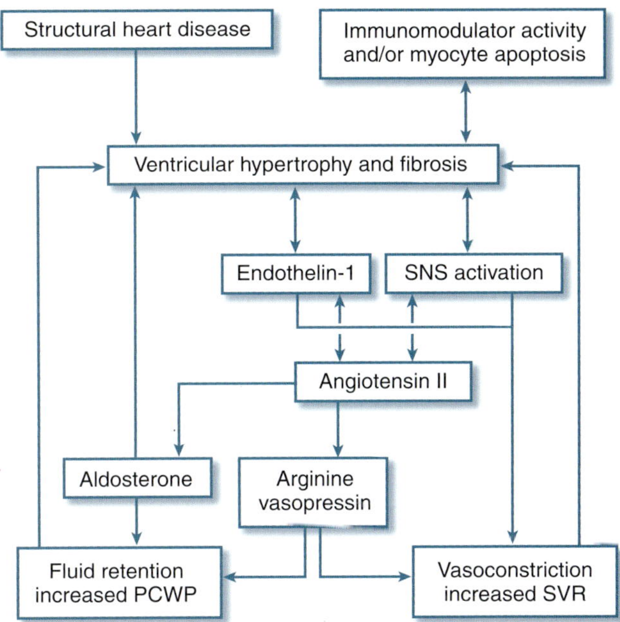

Figure 18-4 Impact of pathophysiologic mediators on hemodynamics in patients with heart failure. *PCWP,* Pulmonary capillary wedge pressure; *SNS,* sympathetic nervous system; *SVR,* systemic vascular resistance. (From McBride BF, White CM. Acute decompensated heart failure: a contemporary approach to pharmacotherapeutic management. Pharmacotherapy. 2003;23:1002.)

and symptoms of congestive heart failure (CHF) and development of therapeutic options (Fig. 18-4).[17,18]

DCM usually presents in the fourth and fifth decades of life.[12] The clinical picture typically includes signs and symptoms of CHF often corresponding to months of fatigue, weakness, and reduced exercise tolerance prior to diagnosis.[15] One third of individuals complain of chest pain.[14] However, the first indication of DCM may be a stroke, arrhythmia, or even sudden death. Increasingly, individuals presenting for routine medical screening are found to have cardiomegaly on a routine chest roentgenogram. Symptoms may appear insidiously over a period of years or evolve rapidly after an unrelated illness. Physical signs of DCM depend on the disease's progression but may include pulsus alternans, jugular venous distention, murmurs of atrioventricular valvular regurgitation, tachycardia, gallop heart sound, rales, cool extremities, and leftward displacement of the apex with palpation of the precordium.

A chest roentgenogram demonstrates variable degrees of cardiomegaly and pulmonary venous congestion (Fig. 18-5, *A*). An electrocardiogram (ECG) may be surprisingly normal or depict low QRS voltage, abnormal axis, nonspecific ST-segment abnormalities,

LV hypertrophy, conduction defects, and evidence of atrial enlargement. Atrial fibrillation is common, and about a fourth of patients have nonsustained ventricular tachycardia (VT).[15] B-type natriuretic peptide (BNP) levels also increase dramatically with ventricular wall stress and are predictive of mortality in acute decompensated CHF.[19] Coronary catheterization would reveal marked LV dilation (Fig. 18-5, *B*) and typically normal coronary vessels, which has therapeutic and prognostic implications. An endomyocardial biopsy is rarely valuable or indicated to identify the etiology of DCM but may be useful to rule out other pathologies with presentations similar to DCM.[12]

Echocardiography is the primary diagnostic modality by which clinicians diagnose DCM. It can be used to exclude findings such as severe primary valvular heart disease as the cause of LV dysfunction and to assess and quantitate associated cardiac conditions such as functional MR. Serial echocardiography studies are used to quantify LV size, shape, and systolic function and to assist physicians in assessing the response to therapy.

The approach to diagnosing DCM with echocardiography begins by demonstrating LV chamber enlargement and systolic dysfunction

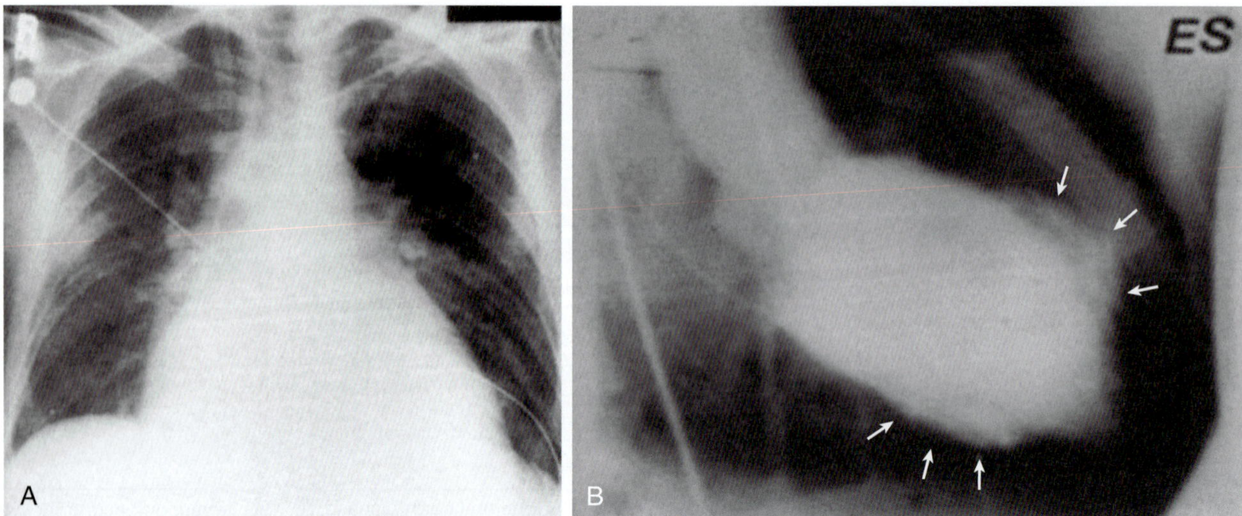

Figure 18-5   **A,** Chest radiography showing marked cardiomegaly in patient with AIDS who developed dilated cardiomyopathy following treatment for *Pneumococcus carinii* pneumonia. **B,** Left ventriculogram of different patient with sarcoidosis and dilated cardiomyopathy at end-systole, demonstrating uneven wall motion abnormalities with discrete dyskinetic or akinetic regions *(arrows)*. There is marked dilation even in end-systole. *ES,* End-systole. (*A* from Corboy JR, Fink L, Miller WT. Congestive cardiomyopathy in association with AIDS. Radiology. 1987;165:139-141. *B* from Yazaki Y, Isobe M, Hiramitsu S, et al. Comparison of clinical features and prognosis of cardiac sarcoidosis and idiopathic dilated cardiomyopathy. Am J Cardiol. 1998;82:537-540.)

in the setting of normal or reduced wall thickness (Videos 18-1 and 18-2). Indeed, all markers of systolic function (EF, fractional shortening, stroke volume, cardiac output [CO]) are uniformly decreased.[20] Specific diagnostic echocardiographic criteria have been noted (see Box 18-2).

With progressive dilation, LV geometry changes and the LV assumes a more spherical rather than ellipsoid shape. Alterations in mitral valve geometry accompany ventricular remodeling. Geometric abnormalities resulting from LV remodeling can be quantitated in patients with DCM. In particular, the sphericity index allows echocardiographers to quantitate the progression of LV shape from ellipsoid to spherical that characterizes DCM. More than one method has been reported for calculating the *sphericity index*, potentially leading to confusion during report interpretation. One method calculates the sphericity index as the calculated LV volume divided by the volume of a sphere whose diameter is the major-axis (long-axis) linear measurement of the LV.[21] Others use simple linear measurements rather than volumes. Matsumoto et al. calculated sphericity index as the ratio of the LV major axis (long axis) to the LV minor axis (short axis) as determined from a four-chamber echocardiography view.[22] These two methods yield different results, with the former producing a value less than 1 and the latter generating a value greater than 1. For instance, Matsumoto used simple linear measurements and noted that the sphericity index in patients with DCM averaged 1.5 ± 0.2 while the index in normal controls averaged 1.9 ± 0.3.[22] Sadeghpour et al.[23] showed that increases in sphericity parallel worsening of functional MR.

Functional MR is a common finding in patients with DCM. Despite structurally normal leaflets, remodeling of the LV leads to changes in the mitral apparatus. The mitral annulus dilates and the coaptation point of the leaflets occurs closer to the apex, leading to the appearance of valve tenting (see Fig. 18-3). Both the tenting area and tenting distance can be measured (Fig. 18-6). The degree of MV tenting correlates well with functional MR severity. Sadeghpour et al.[23] noted that tenting distance correlated more closely with functional MR severity than annular dilation or sphericity index. In particular, these investigators found that in patients with mild functional MR, the tenting distance (distance from the mitral leaflet coaptation point to the plane of the mitral annulus) averaged 1.1 ± 0.25 cm. However, the tenting distance in patients with severe functional MR averaged 1.56 ± 0.25 cm ($P < 0.001$).

A thorough echocardiographic examination in a patient with DCM should include assessment of right ventricular (RV) size and systolic function. Variable RV involvement in the disease process characterizes

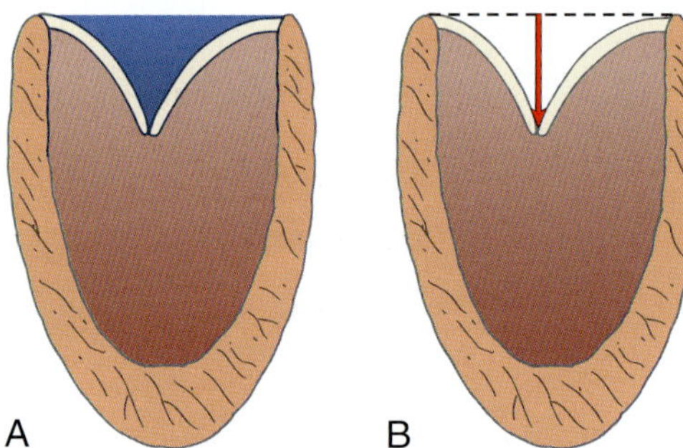

Figure 18-6   **A,** Mitral valve tenting area *blue shaded area.* **B,** Tenting distance, or distance from plane of mitral annulus to leaflet coaptation point *(arrow). (Used with permission of Mayo Foundation for Medical Education and Research. All rights reserved.)*

patients with DCM. RV dysfunction (when present) tends to be associated with worse LV systolic function[15] and is associated with a greater degree of heart failure symptoms and worse clinical outcome.[24] Similarly, assessment of diastolic function may be helpful. Faris et al. noted that patients with DCM who also have a restrictive diastolic filling pattern have a mortality rate three times higher than DCM patients without a restrictive filling pattern.[25] The usual methods of diastolic assessment include Doppler flow patterns of mitral inflow, pulmonary veins, and tissue Doppler interrogation of the mitral annulus (see Chapter 12).

Intracardiac thrombus formation is possible in the setting of reduced LV systolic function due to intracavitary stasis. A comprehensive echocardiographic examination in patients with DCM should include a search for intracardiac thrombus, particularly in the LV apex and LA appendage. However, the risk of thromboembolic complications is relatively low (1%-3%/yr) even with very poor EF and echocardiographic evidence of intracardiac thrombi.[26] The rates are so low that it is difficult to determine a difference in outcome with anticoagulation. Patients with DCM may be on anticoagulation if they have experienced a prior embolic event or paroxysmal or persistent atrial fibrillation,[27] but the benefit remains unclear.

Color Doppler imaging is also useful in assessing the presence or absence of valvular regurgitation. Pulsed wave and continuous wave Doppler (PWD, CWD) are used to quantify CO and evaluate filling pressures and pulmonary artery pressures. Well-compensated patients with DCM may have only mild impairment of diastolic function. As the disease progresses and patients become less well compensated, the LV diastolic filling pattern changes to that of restricted filling. While systolic function may not change in these patients, the increased filling pressures associated with restrictive LV filling will often worsen their CHF symptomatology.

Compared to ischemic CHF, patients with nonischemic DCM show greater improvement in symptoms, LV function, and remodeling with contemporary therapy than in the past.[28] Guidelines are available for clinical care of patients with DCM along the entire spectrum of the disease, presymptomatic to end stage.[26] Treatment revolves around management of symptoms and progression of DCM, while other measures are designed to prevent complications such as pulmonary thromboembolism and arrhythmias. The mainstay of therapy for DCM is an ACE inhibitor or angiotensin II receptor blocker, diuretic, and a β-blocker. Recent trials have supported selective use of spironolactone in DCM owing to its association with improved survival, but renal function must be carefully followed.[26] Afterload-reducing agents such as selective phosphodiesterase-3 inhibitors (e.g., milrinone) may improve quality of life but do not affect mortality so are rarely administered chronically in DCM. Digoxin is not considered a first-line drug for CHF and DCM but may play a role in a few selected patients,[26] since it has been clinically beneficial in two large adult trials.[29]

Use of β-blockers in DCM has not only provided symptomatic improvement but substantial reductions in sudden and progressive death in New York Heart Association (NYHA) class II and III heart failure.[30] This is especially significant because almost 50% of deaths are sudden.[31] Experience with β-blockers suggests that if taken long term, symptoms improve and there is improvement in both clinical status and overall sense of well-being. Like the angiotensin-converting enzyme (ACE) inhibitors, β-blockers reduce risk of death and the combined risk of death and hospitalizations.[26]

High-grade ventricular arrhythmias are common with DCM. Some 12% of all patients with DCM die suddenly,[32] but overall prediction of sudden death in an individual with DCM is poor.[31] Electrophysiologic (EP) testing has a poor negative predictive value that limits its usefulness. The best predictor of sudden death remains the degree of LV dysfunction. Patients who have sustained VT or out-of-hospital ventricular fibrillation are at increased risk for sudden death, but more than 70% of patients with DCM have nonsustained VT during ambulatory monitoring.[33] Prophylactic administration of antiarrhythmic drugs to suppress premature ventricular depolarizations and nonsustained ventricular arrhythmias has not been shown to improve survival.[26] Consequently, antiarrhythmic agents should not be considered part of routine treatment in patients with DCM, even with frequent premature ventricular depolarizations or asymptomatic nonsustained VT. Furthermore, most antiarrhythmic medications have a negative inotropic effect. Amiodarone is the safest agent and most effective when antiarrhythmic therapy is necessary to prevent recurrent atrial fibrillation or symptomatic ventricular arrhythmias.[26]

The role of the implantable cardioverter-defibrillator (ICD) is complex in these patients in terms of balancing the benefits with the risks. There is evidence that with previous cardiac arrest or sustained VT, more benefit was gained from an ICD.[34] More recently, Kadish et al.[35] enrolled 458 patients with nonischemic DCM, LVEF less than 36%, and premature ventricular complexes or nonsustained VT. A total of 229 patients were randomly assigned to receive standard medical therapy, and 229 to receive standard medical therapy plus a single-chamber ICD. There were 17 sudden deaths from arrhythmia: 3 in the ICD group and 14 in the standard therapy group ($P = 0.006$). In this population of patients, the ICD significantly reduced the risk of sudden death, and there was a nonsignificant reduction in risk of death from any cause ($P = 0.08$). Complications associated with ICD insertion (e.g., bleeding, infection) can be serious. The study could not say that ICDs should be routinely placed in all patients with DCM, but should be considered on a case-by-case basis.

Patients who are resistant to pharmacologic therapy for CHF with DCM have received left ventricular assist devices (LVAD), cardiac surgery (mitral valve repair or replacement), and transplantation in recent years. Transplantation is still the most viable surgical approach to end-stage DCM and can substantially prolong lives,[36] but limited organ availability and drug-related morbidity looks to future improvements in assist devices for increased survival. Mechanical devices like LVADs have become implantable, so discharge from the hospital is possible. LVADs are currently used primarily as "bridges" to transplantation, but they have also been considered as "destination" therapy in some patients who are not candidates for transplantation. Completion of a study looking at destination therapy with LVADs compared to medical management in patients with DCM who were ineligible for transplant showed a 2-year survival of 23% with an LVAD, compared to 8% of patients who received only medical therapy.[37] Although efficacy was demonstrated, there are a number of serious complications such as bleeding, stroke, sepsis, and device failure. Occasionally the mechanical device can be removed several months after placement in the patient if the resting ventricle has recovered enough for explantation.

Finally, cardiac surgery is not too dangerous when necessary for patients even with severely depressed EF and DCM. Sometimes if MR develops in an individual with DCM, mitral valve repair or replacement is safe to perform and has been shown to improve NYHA classification and survival.[38]

Hypertrophic Cardiomyopathy

HCM is the most common genetic cardiac disease, with marked heterogeneity in clinical expression, pathophysiology, and prognosis. The overall prevalence for adults in the general population is 0.2%,[39] affecting men and women equally. It is the most common cause of sudden death in athletes, yet most HCM patient have a normal life expectancy without disability or the need for major therapeutic interventions.[40]

HCM is a disease of the cardiac sarcomere. This is a primary myocardial disease with myocyte disarray, diastolic dysfunction, and asymmetric LV hypertrophy (Fig. 18-7, *A*). The extent of sarcomeric disarray distinguishes HCM from other conditions, but this pattern is also seen in pressure-overloaded ventricles.[41] The hypertrophied muscle is composed of cells with bizarre shapes and multiple intercellular connections arranged in a chaotic "whorling" pattern characteristic of HCM (Fig. 18-7, *B*).[39,42] Increased connective tissue combined with markedly disorganized and hypertrophied myocytes contribute to the diastolic abnormalities present in all HCM patients. It manifests as a stiffer ventricular chamber, impaired and prolonged relaxation of the ventricular muscle, severely impaired filling, and an unstable electrophysiologic substrate that causes complex arrhythmias and sudden death.[39] Doppler imaging techniques may be utilized to evaluate diastolic function in patients with HCM, but many of the parameters typically used to grade diastolic function are less reliable in HCM than in other disease states. In particular, E-wave deceleration time and transmitral E/A ratios tend to correlate poorly with LV end-diastolic pressure in HCM.[43] Pulmonary vein velocities also appear less reliable in HCM and in other cardiomyopathies. The E/e' (tissue Doppler imaging–derived e') appears more reliable in estimating left-sided filling pressures,[44] but in one study, 25% of patients with an E/e' ratio above 15 still had LA pressures less than 15 mmHg.[45] It is worth noting that in patients with normal LA size (LA volume index ≤28 cm^3/m^2) LV filling pressures are likely to be normal.[46]

Besides diastolic dysfunction, the other major abnormality and fundamental characteristic of HCM is unexplained LV hypertrophy in a nondilated ventricular chamber in the absence of another cardiac or systemic disease capable of generating this degree of muscle hypertrophy.[1] This nonuniform asymmetric hypertrophy typically occurs in the basal anterior ventricular septum and anterior free wall, with a disproportionate increase in ventricular wall thickness relative to the posterior free wall, as shown in the gross specimen in Figure 18-7, *A*. The extent and pattern of hypertrophy varies greatly. The LV wall thickness is the most extensive of all cardiac conditions,[39] yet heart size may be deceptive in that it may vary from normal to more than 100% enlarged.

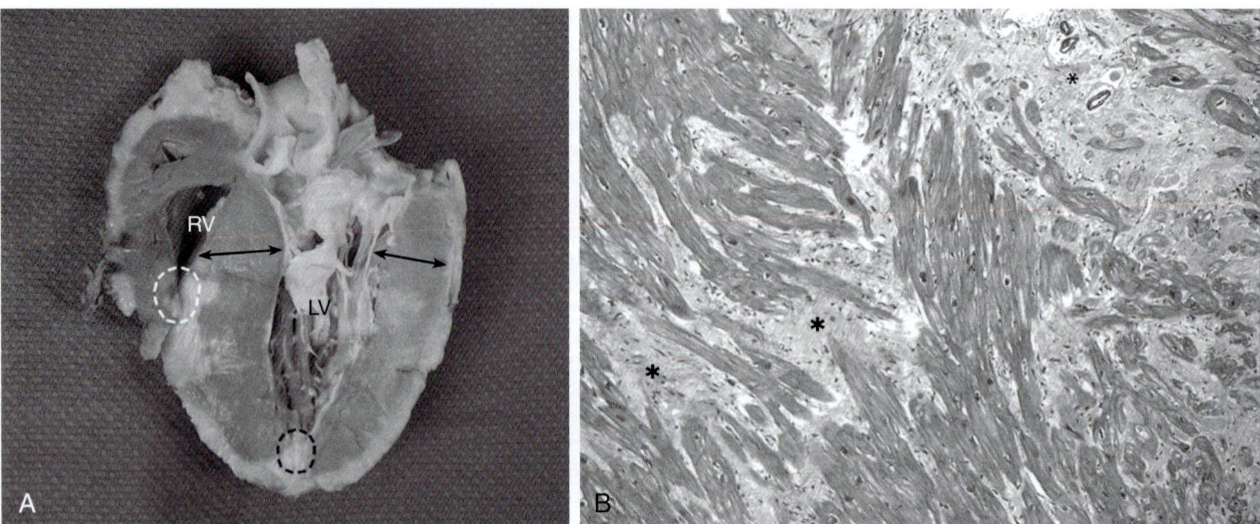

Figure 18-7 **A,** Hypertrophic cardiomyopathy (HCM) from saggital section of explanted native heart. Arrows indicate asymmetric myocardial thickening. Ventricular cavity is small. Thickening is predominately in subaortic region but also occurs in midventricular and apical regions as well as lateral and posterior wall. Apical aneurysms in left *(black dashed circle)* and right *(white dashed circle)* ventricles are observed. Note narrowing of left ventricular outflow tract caused by thickened ventricular septum and anterior leaflet of mitral valve. **B,** Photomicrograph of septal myocardium in HCM. Note pronounced disarray and hypertrophy of individual muscle fibers, resulting in a "whorled" appearance. Normal myocytes run in straight parallel bundles, but these often are identified as running at oblique angles. Interstitial fibrosis is found in many areas. In this figure, with increased magnification, myofibril disarray is evident in many of myocytes. Variation in size of nuclei is also evident. *Areas of significant interstitial myocardial fibrosis. (Movat pentachrome stain ×6400.) *(From Soor GS, Luk A, Ahn E, et al. Hypertrophic cardiomyopathy: current understanding and treatment objectives. Clin Pathol. 2009;62:226-235.)*

Increases in wall thickness, *not* chamber enlargement, are responsible for the increase in ventricular mass.

Two-dimensional (2D) and Doppler echocardiography easily identify LV hypertrophy. Although ventricular hypertrophy is typically asymmetric and most commonly involves the interventricular septum, nearly any myocardial segment can be involved (Fig. 18-8).[47-49] Asymmetric septal hypertrophy is more common than diffuse concentric patterns of LV hypertrophy, and thickening of the basal and mid-anterior septal walls are common.[48,50,51] Typically, patients will present with a maximal wall thickness measuring between 20 and 30 mm, but in some it may reach 35 to 40 mm.[42] Confusion may arise when the LV hypertrophy is concentric, which may arise from other causes like hypertension or aortic stenosis that result in increased afterload.[40] Hypertrophy of the ventricular septum is most easily appreciated from the midesophageal (ME) four-chamber and long-axis (LAX) echocardiographic views (Fig. 18-9). Concentric ventricular hypertrophy is best seen in transgastric (TG) short-axis (SAX) images. Oftentimes there will be near-obliteration of the LV cavity during systole when imaged from the TG window. The 2D echocardiographic criteria used to diagnose HCM include maximal wall thickness greater than 15 mm in any myocardial segment that cannot be explained by other causes (confusion may arise when maximum wall thickness is 13-15 mm[40]), septal/posterior wall thickness ratio greater than 1.3 in non-hypertensive patients, and septal/posterior wall thickness ratio greater than 1.5 in hypertensive patients.[47]

Systolic function of the LV in HCM is usually normal or hyperdynamic, with only a small subset of patients having impaired systolic function. If there is severely depressed systolic function, it is often accompanied by LV dilatation and thinning of the ventricular walls.[47]

HCM is inherited in an autosomal dominant manner.[41] It may be caused by over 1400 mutations in any of 8 genes;[40] however, three genes that encode proteins of the cardiac sarcomere predominate in frequency.[49] The similarity of the genes accounts for the many different expressions of HCM that resemble one disease entity. The causal mutations of the genes encode the changes in sarcomeric function, leading to hypertrophy and fibrosis beginning as early as puberty.[8] There may be any number of abnormalities generated, such as alterations of protein structure that change interactions or sensitivity to regulators (e.g., calcium), resulting in changes in force or velocity of myocyte contraction.[42]

At present, the pathway from gene mutation to clinical expression is still only partially understood. Not all patients who possess a gene for HCM will manifest clinical features of the disease, reflecting incomplete genetic expression.[39] The phenotype appears not only to depend on the mutation but also on other modifier genes and environmental factors.[49,52] Patients without a family history of HCM may have sporadic gene mutations or simply a very mild form of the disease. A preclinical diagnosis in an asymptomatic person is possible with gene testing but is not routine, nor can it be used to establish a treatment strategy.

HCM is unique for its range of clinical presentations from infancy to 90 years of age. While major referral centers described a disease with severe symptomatology, many elderly individuals with mild to asymptomatic disease were unaccounted for in past studies, resulting in an annual mortality rate of 3% to 6% per year; more recent studies show it to be closer to 1% per year.[39] Most HCM patients are asymptomatic or have mild symptoms that progress slowly or not at all.[14] If symptoms appear, it is usually in the second or third decade. However, LV hypertrophy can occur at any age and increase or decrease dynamically throughout the person's life.[39]

Symptoms of HCM are nonspecific and include chest pain, palpitations, dyspnea, and syncope. Dyspnea occurs in 90% of patients secondary to diastolic abnormalities that increase filling pressures, causing pulmonary congestion. Syncope occurs in only 20% of patients, but 50% may have presyncopal symptoms. The ECG is abnormal in most individuals (showing increased QRS voltage, ST-segment and T-wave abnormalities, QRS axis shift, and LV hypertrophy with strain pattern) but may be normal in 5% of patients.[42] There is little correlation between ECG voltages and degree of LV hypertrophy.[39] Normal sinus rhythm predominates, but patients with ambulatory monitoring show supraventricular tachycardia (46%) and nonsustained VT (26%). Atrial fibrillation may occur in 25% to 30% of older patients, with serious consequences.[42] A chest roentgenogram may show LA enlargement or be normal.

The most important clinical decision is to identify whether the patient has a nonobstructive or obstructive form of HCM, because management strategy will be largely centered on the presence or absence of symptoms that ensue. Two thirds of patients will have left ventricular outflow tract (LVOT) obstruction.[40] In a recent prospective

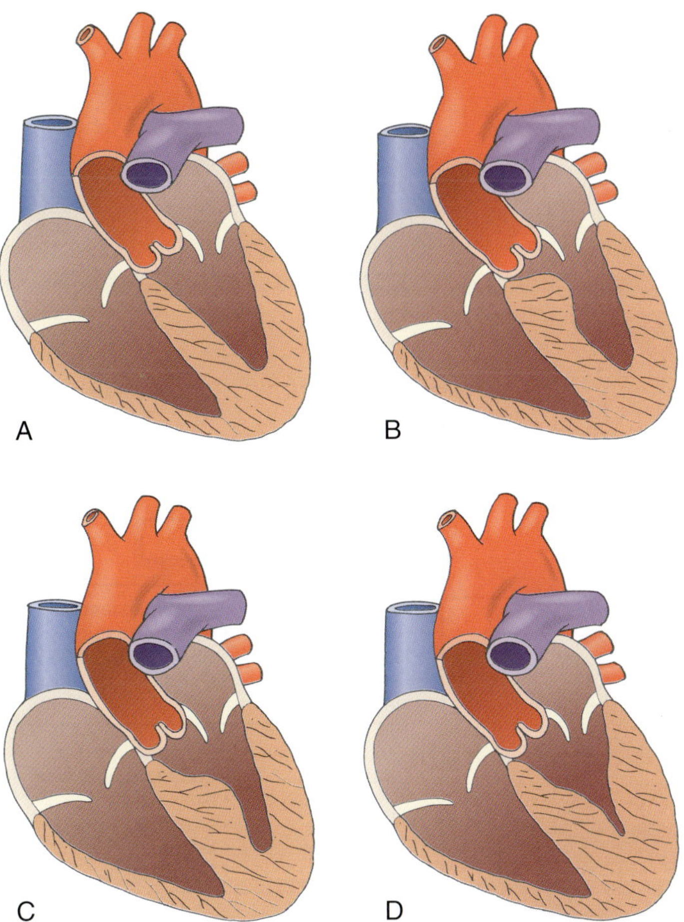

Figure 18-8 Types of hypertrophic obstructive cardiomyopathy. **A,** A normal heart. **B,** Hypertrophic disease isolated to basal portion of interventricular septum. **C,** Hypertrophic disease of midventricular septum resulting in midventricular outflow obstruction. **D,** Apical hypertrophic disease resulting in small left ventricular cavity and small apical pouch. *(Used with permission of Mayo Foundation for Medical Education and Research. All rights reserved.)*

study of 320 patients with HCM and their gradient, 37% had LVOT obstruction at rest and 33% required provocation.[53] This may add to the unreliability of clinical diagnosis of HCM, because classic physical findings associated with LVOT obstruction are not always present.

Septal hypertrophy and anterior displacement of the papillary muscles and mitral leaflets narrows the LVOT. High-velocity blood flow during ventricular systole creates a drag that mobilizes the mitral valve (particularly the anterior leaflet) into the LVOT, further decreasing the functional LVOT orifice, with the anterior mitral leaflet making contact with the ventricular septum in midsystole, causing abrupt cessation of LV emptying and closure of the aortic valve. Elongation of the mitral leaflets results in coaptation of the body of the leaflets instead of the tips. The part of the anterior leaflet distal to the coaptation is subjected to strong Venturi forces that provoke systolic anterior motion (SAM), mitral septal contact, and ultimately LVOT obstruction (Fig. 18-10).[49] SAM of the mitral leaflets occurs in roughly 30% to 60% of patients with HCM. The end result of this dynamic process is early closure of the aortic valve due to obstruction to outflow, decreased stroke volume, and MR if the SAM results in a coaptation defect between the mitral leaflets. SAM can occur prior to the opening of the aortic valve by the generation of maximum Venturi effect due to the position of the mitral leaflets on the LVOT, reflecting its importance in SAM compared to traditional explanations. Longitudinal flow in the ventricle may push the mitral valve into the LVOT.[54] SAM of the anterior leaflet may also cause MR unlike that seen with intrinsic structural abnormalities of the valve. Both SAM and LVOT obstruction can be readily appreciated with 2D echocardiographic imaging, an important method of differentiating obstructive from nonobstructive HCM (see Fig. 18-9).

The onset and duration of mitral leaflet–septal contact determine the magnitude of the gradient and the degree of MR. The pressure gradient between the aorta and LV is worsened by decreased end-diastolic volume, increased contractility, or decreased aortic outflow resistance (Fig. 18-11).[55] The cavity of the LV is often very small in those with severe gradients. Doppler echocardiography is essential to defining the presence, location, and severity of LVOT obstruction when present. CWD is helpful for measuring the absolute magnitude of gradient across the LVOT, whereas PWD can define the anatomic location of the obstruction, whether it be in the midventricle or at the base of the heart.

TEE CWD may be used from deep TG, ME four-chamber, or ME LAX views to measure the maximum instantaneous gradient (Fig. 18-12). The typical CWD appearance of the LVOT signal is that of a high-velocity "dagger-shaped" configuration. Particularly when

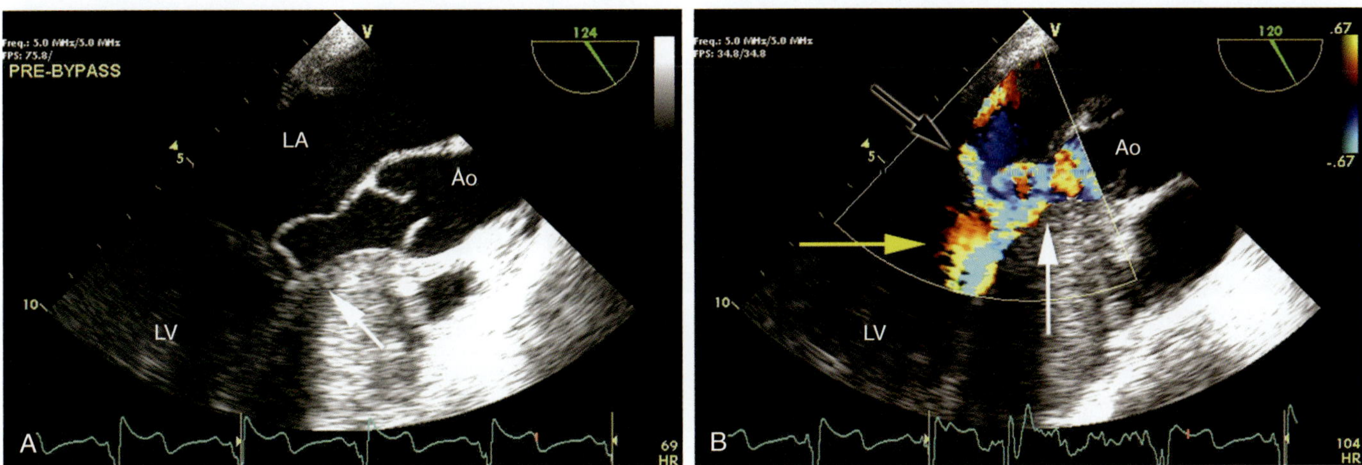

Figure 18-9 **A,** Typical two-dimensional appearance of hypertrophic obstructive cardiomyopathy. Image is a midesophageal view with a probe angle of 124 degrees. Note hypertrophy of the basal septum *(arrow)*. In this image from midsystole, entire mitral apparatus has been drawn into left ventricular outflow tract (LVOT), causing obstruction to left ventricular emptying and a coaptation defect between mitral leaflets. **B,** Similar view with color Doppler imaging added. Note typical posteriorly directed jet of mitral regurgitation *(black arrow)*. Color aliasing indicating obstruction to ventricular emptying begins at base of heart just below site of hypertrophy *(yellow arrow)* and worsens in LVOT, indicating high-velocity turbulent flow *(white arrow)*. These color signals often combine to form the appearance of a Y. *Ao,* Aorta; *LA,* left atrium; *LV,* left ventricle.

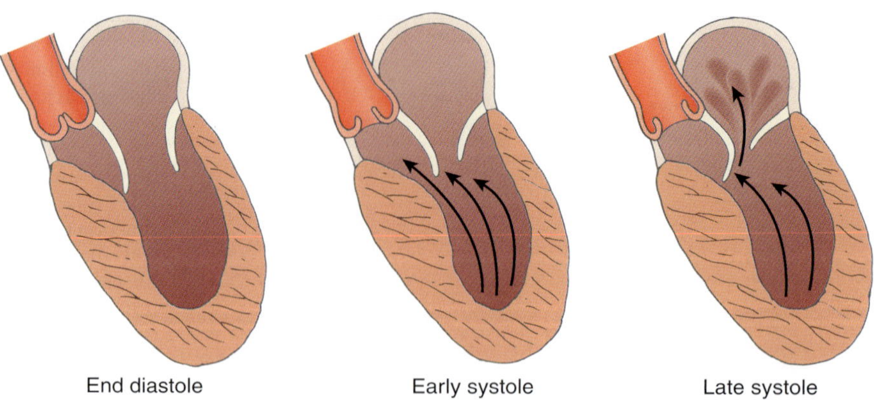

Figure 18-10 Depiction of modern concepts of mechanism of left ventricular outflow tract obstruction in hypertrophic cardiomyopathy. In early systole, abnormal flow around hypertrophied septum pushes mitral valve into outflow tract and results in obstruction and mitral valve regurgitation. *(From Ommen SR, Shah PM, Tajik AJ. Left ventricular outflow tract obstruction in hypertrophic cardiomyopathy: past, present and future. Heart. 2008;94:1276-1281.)*

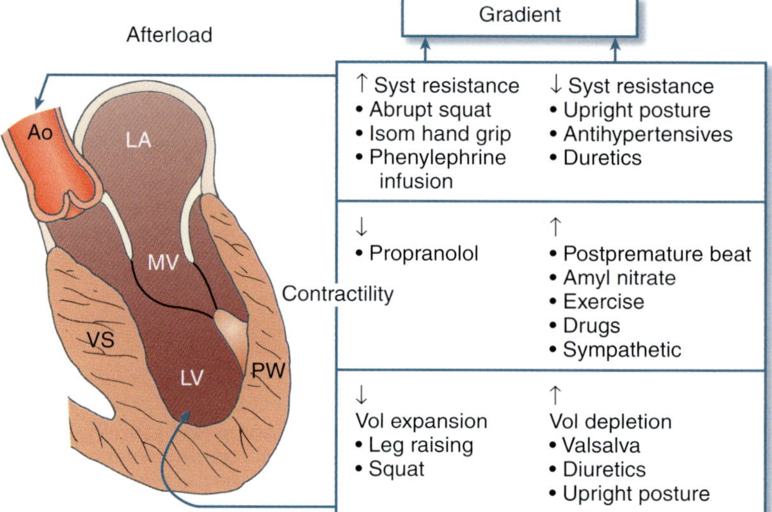

Figure 18-11 Interventions that change outflow gradient in hypertrophic cardiomyopathy (HCM), with resultant change in intensity of systolic murmur in HCM. Outflow gradient is affected by changes in afterload, preload, and contractility. *Ao,* Aorta; *LA,* left atrium; *LV,* left ventricle; *MV,* mitral valve; *PW,* posterior wall; *VS,* ventricular septum. *(From Giuliani ER, Fuster V, Gersh BJ, et al. Cardiology: Fundamentals and Practice. St. Louis: Mosby; 1991.)*

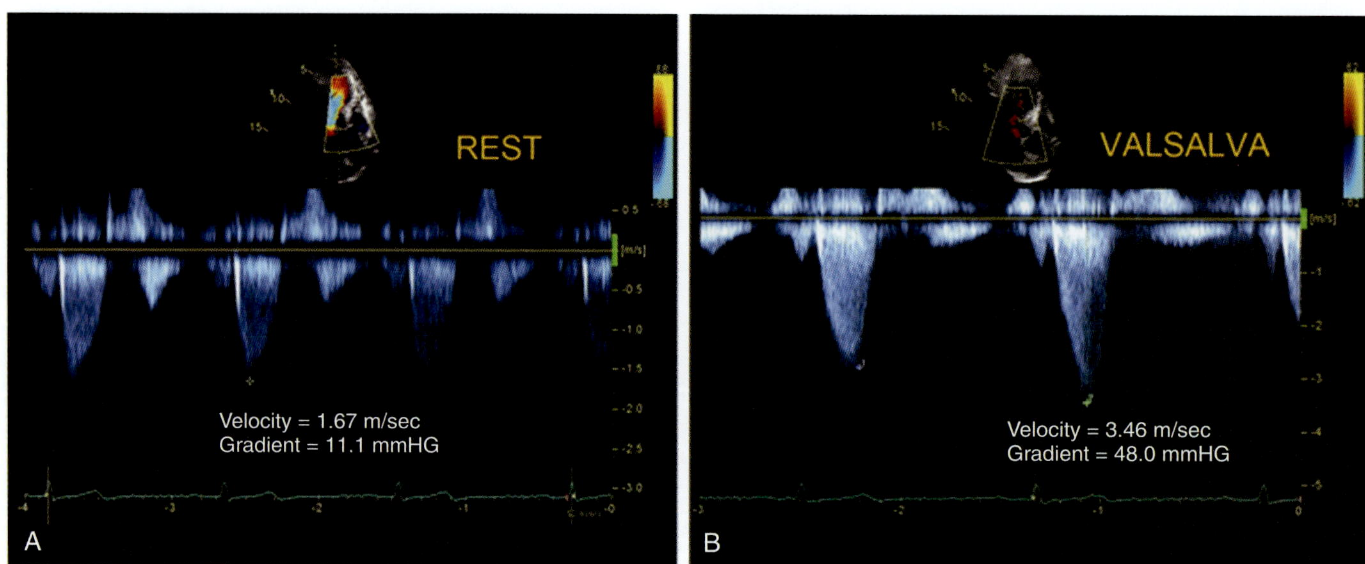

Figure 18-12 Continuous wave Doppler spectra obtained from apex, demonstrating dynamic left ventricular outflow tract obstruction. Note typical late-peaking configuration resembling a dagger or ski slope (**A** and **B**). The baseline (**A**) velocity is 1.67 m/s, corresponding to the peak LV outflow tract of 11.1 mmHg (4 × 1.672). With the Valsalva maneuver (**B**), the velocity increased to 3.46 m/s, corresponding to a gradient of 48 mmHg.

imaging from the esophagus, the LVOT signal is relatively easy to confuse with that of MR. Velocities from both signals may be similar, but the signal due to MR tends to be more symmetric and rounded, lacking the dagger-shaped appearance of the LVOT signal (Fig. 18-13).

To induce a gradient in the awake patient undergoing transthoracic echocardiography (TTE), the strain phase of a Valsalva maneuver, exercise, or administration of amyl nitrate may be effective. In the anesthetized patient, it may be possible to elicit the gradient by applying sustained positive pressure via the ventilatory circuit. It is more common to administer isoproterenol in 2 to 4 µg boluses to obtain tachycardia and decrease systemic vascular resistance.

Although CWD is helpful to determine the maximum gradient, it cannot discern *where* along the pathway the gradient occurs during ventricular emptying. In particular, some patients' primary obstruction to outflow will lie midventricle. Sequential imaging with PWD beginning with the sample volume near the apex of the heart and moving in a stepwise fashion toward the aortic valve allows the examiner to determine where the predominant obstruction occurs. This is relatively easy to perform with TTE from apical views. TEE imaging may be more difficult owing to the foreshortened nature of the deep TG view. However, in patients with adequate imaging windows, sequential PWD imaging may be performed using the ME four-chamber and LAX views.

Color Doppler imaging reveals a multitude of subjective findings in patients with obstructive HCM. Typical findings in patients with obstructive disease include flow acceleration in midventricle or at the base of the LV as blood flow begins to accelerate upon approaching the LVOT. Aliasing is seen in the LVOT as blood flow reaches maximum acceleration due to LVOT obstruction, and the jet of MR is also seen (see Fig. 18-9). Indeed, the classic description of color Doppler imaging in obstructive HCM is that of acceleration → obstruction (to LVOT flow) → leak (MR). Along with PWD findings, the point of flow acceleration seen with color Doppler imaging can give valuable insight as to the point of obstruction to LV emptying. This finding has important implications when planning the surgical approach to septal myectomy.

Dynamic pressure gradients do not necessarily correlate with symptoms of HCM. Significant functional limitation, disability, and sudden death may all occur without a gradient, but gradients exceeding

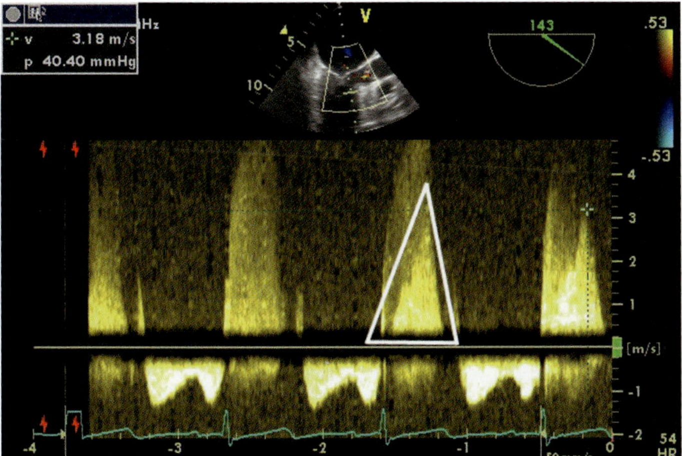

Figure 18-13 The probe is in the midesophagus with an angle of 143 degrees. A continuous wave Doppler signal has been placed through mitral valve and left ventricular outflow tract. Note in the Doppler signal tracing that denser signal from outflow tract is seen within lighter-shaded, higher-velocity signal of mitral regurgitation (outflow tract signal outlined by white triangle). Signal has a steep upslope due to rapidly increasing velocity as obstruction to outflow worsens throughout systole, giving signal the appearance of a "dagger." In the subsequent cardiac cycle, echocardiographer is able to measure the gradient through the outflow tract even though it is confined within mitral regurgitation signal. Velocity of outflow tract signal is 3.18 m/s, yielding a gradient of 40.4 mmHg.

30 mmHg are usually of physiologic and prognostic importance in HCM patients.[49] Two thirds of individuals with LVOT obstruction will become severely symptomatic, and there is 10% mortality within 4 years of diagnosis. LVOT obstruction is an independent predictor of death in HCM.[56]

CAD may be absent angiographically, but these patients are predisposed to myocardial ischemia. Thallium redistribution scans demonstrate that HCM patients may experience myocardial ischemia often associated with atypical chest pain and not relieved with nitrates.[57] Blunted coronary perfusion despite angiographically normal coronary arteries is characteristic of a coronary microvascular dysfunction that increases the risk of ischemia, especially in the subendocardium. More recently, the degree of LVOT obstruction and wall stress was found to exacerbate microvascular dysfunction.[58] This may have implications for treatments that reduce LV mass and wall stress instead of increasing diastolic filling time with medications (e.g., β- and calcium channel blockers) and may partially explain the benefit of myectomy. Thallium abnormalities may represent relatively underperfused myocardium with abnormal intramyocardial coronary arteries that exist in patients with HCM. A mismatch between myocardial oxygen demand resulting from systolic and diastolic abnormalities, increased ventricular mass, and coronary circulation may exacerbate myocardial ischemia. Myocardial death and scarring may then serve as a substrate for VT and fibrillation.[39]

The clinical course and treatment of HCM are complex and have been determined by the American College of Cardiology (ACC) Foundation/AHA Task Force on Practice Guidelines.[40] Medical treatment for asymptomatic HCM patients is not clearly indicated. However, because symptoms are primarily attributed to the diastolic abnormality, symptomatic relief is achieved by improving ventricular relaxation. Medications with negative inotropic effect are generally successful in relieving symptoms of exercise intolerance and dyspnea associated with CHF,[59] but symptoms may return in up to 60% of pharmacologically treated patients.[60] In general, high-dose β-blockers have been a mainstay of therapy for years in adults and are preferred over calcium channel blockers. The combination of β-blockers and calcium channel blockers has not proven beneficial. β-Blockers relieve symptoms of angina and dyspnea and improve exercise tolerance by limiting the gradient associated with exercise. The gradient is not reduced at rest by these medications.[49] Other beneficial effects of β-blockers include heart rate reduction, lower myocardial oxygen demand, and longer diastolic filling times, but diastolic function is not improved nor long-term survival prolonged. Patients with obstructive symptoms may worsen with calcium channel blockers that contain strong vasodilator properties. Disopyramide, a negative inotrope that alters calcium kinetics and produces a vasoconstrictor effect, has been recommended instead of calcium channel blockers in obstructive HCM.[49] Disopyramide is the most effective agent to reduce LVOT obstruction and gradient as well as relieve symptoms.[61] Combined with β-blockers, disopyramide prolongs exercise times more successfully than verapamil.

Surgical correction of HCM is directed primarily at relieving symptoms of LVOT obstruction in the 5% of patients who are refractory to medication.[40,49] In general, these are individuals with subaortic gradients in excess of 50 mmHg, with or without provocation, and frequently associated with severe CHF.[14,39] A myotomy-myectomy through a transaortic approach is the primary method used to relieve the obstruction (Fig. 18-14). The muscle is excised from the proximal septum extending just beyond the mitral valve leaflets that widens the LVOT. Currently, the classic Morrow technique has been replaced by a more extensive resection that is described in greater detail elsewhere.[61,62] This is a technically challenging operation owing to the limited exposure and precise area in which the muscle is excised. It is usually reserved for centers with considerable experience with myectomy.[40]

Diagnosis and ventricular anatomy, including the site of obstruction to ventricular outflow, should be determined before the time of operation, but intraoperative TEE is extremely useful during the surgical procedure. Initially, the diagnosis of obstructive HCM should be confirmed. As noted earlier, 2D imaging of the intraoperative patient typically reveals basal septal hypertrophy (see Fig. 18-9). The point of obstruction may be determined by noting where on the ventricular septum contact with the anterior mitral leaflet is made and measuring the distance from this point to the aortic annulus. The site of obstruction may also be seen with color Doppler imaging. The gradient across the LVOT may be measured from the deep TG view, TG LAX view, or from the ME four-chamber or LAX views using CWD. It is our practice to confirm the gradient by direct pressure simultaneous measurements with needles in the LV and aorta. A post–premature ventricular contraction (PVC) beat will show an increased gradient as the compensatory pause between beats allows for increased preload and subsequent increased contractility of the LV.

Particular attention should be paid to the mitral valve during the preoperative exam (Fig. 18-15). Patients with HCM frequently have structural abnormalities of the mitral apparatus. Elongation of the mitral leaflets along with anterior displacement of the papillary muscles predispose some patients to SAM and LVOT obstruction.[63,64] Other patients may have short chordae tendineae or anomalous insertion of the papillary muscle into the mitral leaflet.[48] Typically, patients with obstructive HCM will present with moderate to severe MR due to the coaptation defect created by SAM. When viewed with color Doppler, the regurgitant jet should be posteriorly directed. If the jet appears directed toward the midline of the LA or anteriorly, the mitral valve has to be further evaluated for other causes of regurgitation such as mitral valve prolapse or ruptured chordae. A subset of patients with

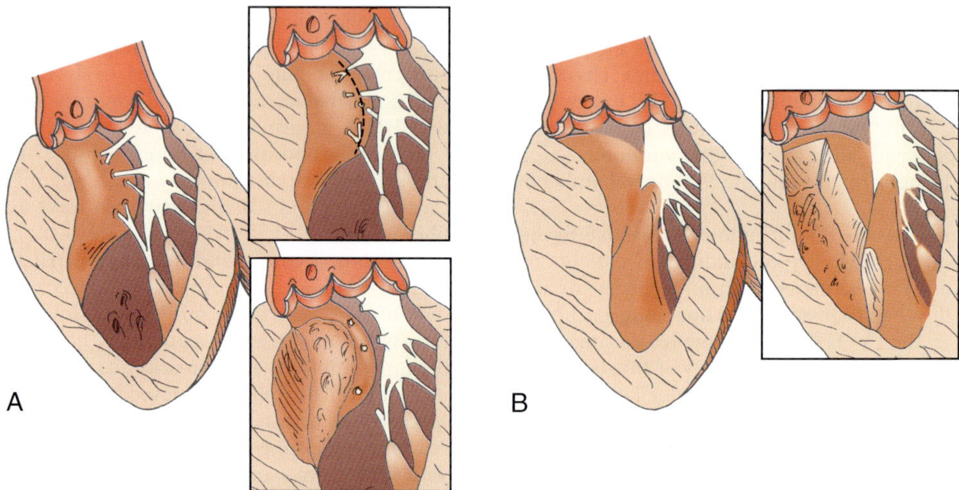

Figure 18-14   Two operative approaches for performing septal myectomy in obstructive hypertrophic cardiomyopathy. **A**, *Right insert*, Typical outflow tract morphology with predominant basal septal hypertrophy and subaortic obstruction caused primarily by systolic anterior motion of mitral valve. Endocardial thickening at line of apposition of anterior mitral leaflet to septum (friction lesion) can be seen (**A**, *left insert*). A standard rectangular myectomy trough (Morrow procedure) is created from 1 cm below aortic valve apically to a point beyond the line of mitral-septal contact and intraventricular obstruction, allowing relief of outflow tract gradient and preservation of sinus rhythm. **B**, In the presence of muscular mid-cavity obstruction caused by anomalous papillary muscles with direct insertion into mitral valve or to extensive diffuse septal hypertrophy extending to bases of the papillary muscles, a much more substantial myectomy is performed by combining the standard operation with an extended midventricular resection. Apical portion of myectomy trough is much wider and includes distal third of right side of septum. (*From Dearani JA, Ommen SR, Gersh BJ, Schaff HV, Danielson GK. Surgery insight: septal myectomy for obstructive hypertrophic cardiomyopathy—the Mayo Clinic experience. Nat Clin Pract Cardiovasc Med. 2007;4:503-512.*)

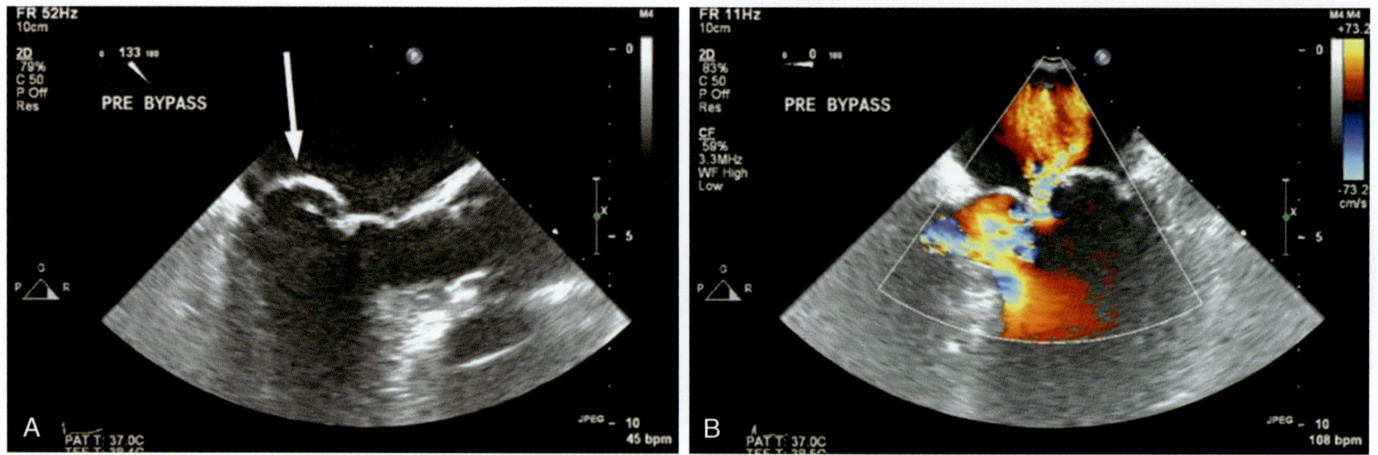

Figure 18-15   Midesophageal long-axis view of left ventricle and mitral and aortic valves. Posterior mitral valve leaflet is prolapsing into left atrium during diastole (**A**, *arrow*). Also note hypertrophy of basal septum in **A**. **B**, Color Doppler is added, revealing a jet of central regurgitation. Less well seen is mild degree of systolic anterior motion of mitral apparatus. If mitral regurgitation (MR) were due solely to prolapse of posterior mitral leaflet, one would expect regurgitant jet to be directed anteriorly. If MR were due to systolic anterior motion of mitral leaflet, jet should be directed posteriorly. In this case, both mechanisms contribute and resultant jet is central in origin. This patient requires both a septal myectomy and mitral valve repair to treat MR.

HCM will present with morphologic abnormalities of the mitral valve that will have to be addressed with mitral valve repair (Fig. 18-16 and Video 18-3).

In the post–cardiopulmonary bypass period, TEE is essential for evaluating adequacy of the operation. The SAM should be nearly completely relieved (Fig. 18-17). Presence of a small amount of residual SAM by 2D imaging may be inconsequential because it will typically resolve with medical therapy by the time of hospital discharge.[65] Gradients through the LVOT should be obtained as evidence of resolution of the obstruction. Evaluation of the mitral valve should reveal

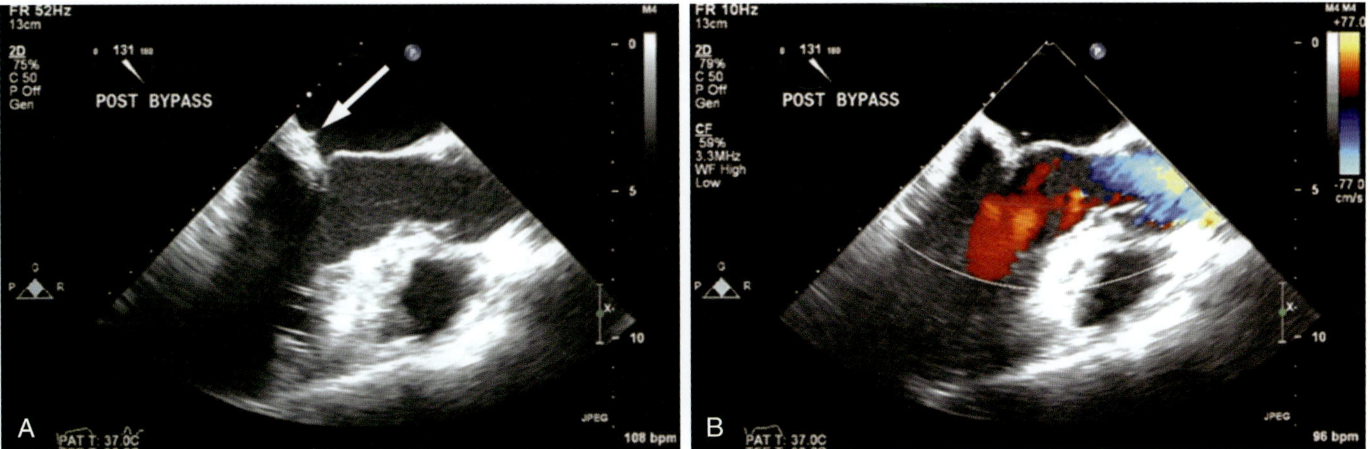

Figure 18-16 Same patient as in Figure 18-15 after undergoing repair of prolapsing posterior mitral leaflet and a septal myectomy. **A,** Note typical shortened, thickened appearance of posterior mitral leaflet *(arrow)* as well as resection of basal septum, with a widely patent left ventricular outflow tract (LVOT). **B,** Color Doppler is shown during systole, with no mitral regurgitation and completely laminar flow in LVOT.

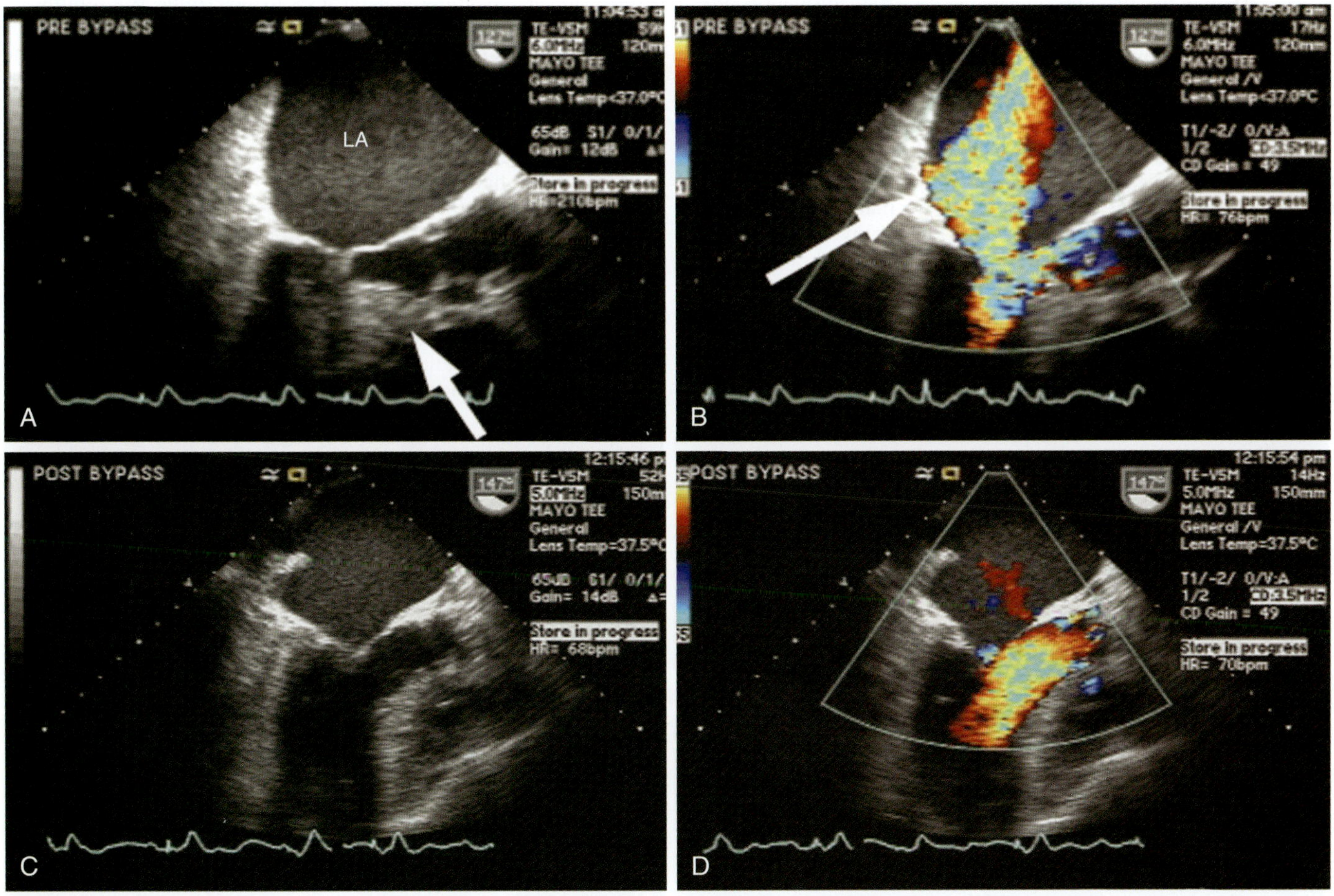

Figure 18-17 Sequential imaging of patient undergoing septal myectomy for hypertrophic obstructive cardiomyopathy. **A,** Two-dimensional (2D) midesophageal long-axis (ME LAX) view showing septal hypertrophy *(arrow)* with systolic anterior motion of mitral leaflets during systole. **B,** Same as **A** with color Doppler imaging added. Note severe posteriorly directed mitral regurgitation (MR) *(arrow)* and aliasing in left ventricular outflow tract (LVOT) due to obstruction to ventricular emptying. **C,** 2D ME LAX view, again in systole. Compared to **A,** there is no systolic anterior motion of mitral leaflets, and hypertrophied ventricular septum has been resected, yielding a wider LVOT. **D,** Color Doppler imaging added. MR seen in **B** has resolved, and color signal in outflow tract shows lower velocity and more laminar flow after relief of obstruction. *LA,* Left atrium.

resolution of MR. The interventricular septum should be carefully evaluated for signs of a ventricular septal defect (VSD). It should be noted that it is not uncommon with color Doppler imaging to see jets of flow into the LV that represent transection of coronary arteries in the septum (Fig. 18-18). These small coronary arterial–cameral fistulae should not be confused with flow from a VSD. When trying to determine the origin of flow into the LV, it is helpful to remember that flow from transected coronary arteries will typically be most prominent during diastole, whereas flow from a VSD will occur predominantly during systole. Lastly, with a surgical approach through the aortic valve, aortic valve integrity must be ensured after completion of the operation.

When myectomy is successful, the LVOT is widened and SAM, MR, and outflow gradient are all much improved. Mitral valve repair or replacement has accompanied myectomy when there is coexistent primary mitral valve structural abnormalities, but mitral valve replacement is not indicated for treating LVOT obstruction alone.[54] If the valve is not repaired during myectomy, incomplete or temporary relief of obstruction may occur. Recently Wan et al.[66] described the use of mitral valve repair in those with LVOT obstruction and degenerative mitral valve disease. Mitral valve repair was effective compared to replacement, with low early mortality and successful treatment of both obstruction and mitral valve regurgitation. Mitral valve replacement is rare.

Surgery provides persistent long-lasting relief from symptoms that exceeds any form of current medical treatment.[59,67] Five years after myectomy, 85% of patients have improved enough to advance one NYHA functional class.[68] The concomitant reduction in LA size may partially account for the lower incidence of atrial fibrillation after myectomy.[49] Septal myectomy results in reduction in LV mass that exceeds the myocardium resected over time, indicating a relief of the pressure overload.[69] Myectomy is also associated with a mortality rate of less than 1% in major institutions.[60] This low mortality rate is even more noteworthy because surgical patients usually have more severe disease than those treated medically. Long-term survival at 1, 5, and 10 years is 98%, 96%, and 83%, respectively. Surgical patients have an overall survival that is equivalent to the age-matched and gender-matched general population.[70] Complications of myectomy such as complete heart block or septal perforation (0%-2%) are rare.[61] Similarly, recurrence of LVOT gradient or SAM requiring repeat myectomy is less than 2%.[54]

Surgery is the most appropriate treatment today in patients with obstructive HCM and no relief of symptoms with medical management.[40] It is not recommended if there is no obstructive component or if the individual is asymptomatic to mildly symptomatic because (1) better survival with surgery versus medical therapy is not established, (2) operative mortality may exceed the risk of HCM in mildly affected patients, (3) LVOT obstruction may be compatible with longevity in selected individuals, and (4) there is no evidence surgery halts the progression of HCM to end stage.[49] End-stage patients with nonobstructive HCM who have severely reduced systolic function are effectively treated with heart transplantation, with 7-year survival of 90%, comparable to those with DCM who require transplantation.[71]

All patients with HCM should undergo a comprehensive assessment for sudden cardiac death.[40] However, only a minority of diagnosed patients is at increased risk for sudden cardiac death, with a rate of about 1% per year. Often these patients are asymptomatic or mildly symptomatic and constitute a very small part of the HCM population. Sudden death is not age restricted but occurs more commonly in younger individuals, frequently in association with physical exertion. HCM is the most common cause of sudden death in otherwise healthy young individuals, reaching up to 6% per year in those 20 to 30 years of age.[72]

Risk stratification for sudden death is useful now that it has been found that VT or ventricular fibrillation are the culprits.[39,73] Multiple risk factors have been identified.[49,72] Two or more risk factors are associated with a risk of sudden death of 4% to 5% per year. The value of EP testing as it relates to prediction of sudden death is mixed.[49,74,75] Extreme LV wall thickness has been associated with greater incidence of spontaneous ventricular arrhythmias and sudden death. In the future, genotyping may reliably define the risk of sudden death, but currently there are no screening genetic tests to determine risk stratification for such clinical characteristics as sudden death.[76] Septal myectomy reduces the risk of sudden death in HCM patients compared to those with LVOT obstruction and no surgery and those with nonobstructive HCM. The mechanism for this improved survival is undetermined.[70]

At present, the only effective modality to prevent sudden death associated with HCM is the ICD. Pharmacologic therapy for prevention of sudden death has recently been shown to reduce symptoms but not risk of sudden death.[77] The decision to place an ICD should include clinical judgment, discussion of the strength of evidence, benefits, and risks (Fig. 18-19).[40] Long-term follow-up of patients receiving ICDs for HCM has shown a worrisome rate of inappropriate (5.3%/yr) versus appropriate (4%/yr) shocks.[78] The overall incidence (36%) of device complications was concerning during a 5-year period. The ICD can save high-risk patients' lives, but its risk of complications should factor into the decision about whether one should be implanted.

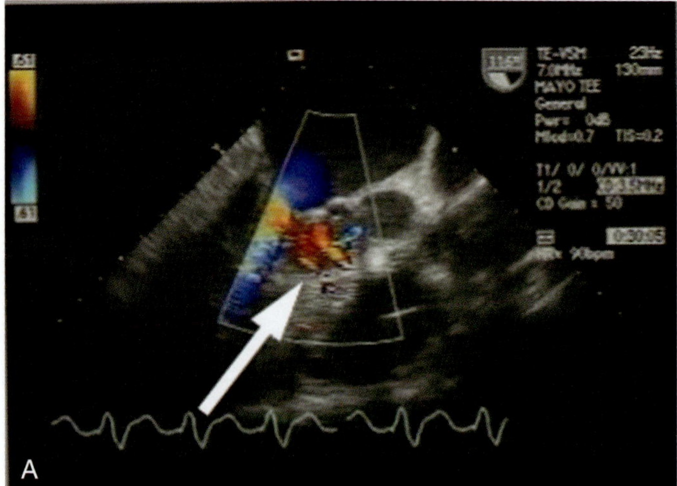
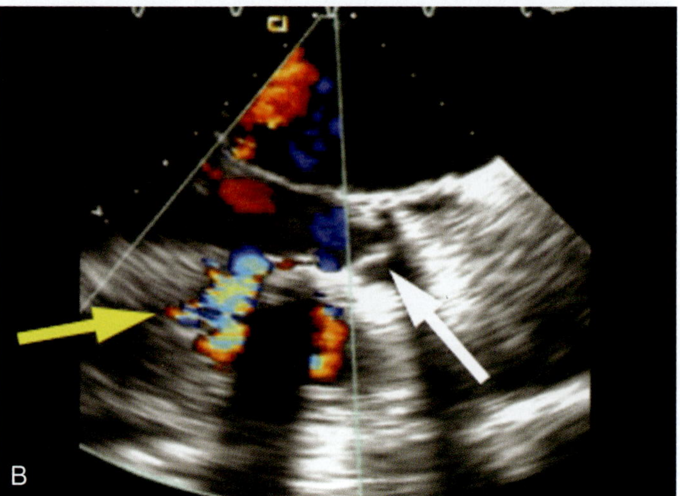

Figure 18-18   **A,** Midesophageal (ME) long-axis view with a color signal in left ventricular outflow tract (LVOT). Note the two red jets of flow into LV at site of myectomy *(arrow).* Jets are due to transection of coronary perforators of septum. Flow from these jets occurs primarily during diastole and essentially results in a left-to-left shunt of no consequence. It is important that they not be confused with flow secondary to an iatrogenic ventricular septal defect (VSD) created by the myectomy. **B,** VSD *(yellow arrow)* seen in ME image taken during systole as aortic valve is opening *(white arrow).* Flow is seen between LVOT and right ventricle and occurs predominantly during systole, resulting in left-to-right shunt.

Possible alternatives to surgery have included dual-chamber pacing and percutaneous alcohol septal ablation. Previously, atrioventricular sequential pacing had been shown to decrease subaortic gradients, possibly by causing abnormal septal motion, so was considered a possible treatment even though the mechanism had not been proven.[59] Pacing has become the most rigorously evaluated treatment of all therapies for HCM. A series of nonrandomized and randomized studies have shown reductions in the LVOT gradient and improvement in symptoms, but others have found no differences in gradient, NYHA class, quality of life score, exercise duration, or maximal oxygen uptake, reflecting a significant placebo effect.[79] Within groups, there appear to be responders but no variables that identified these patients.[54] Consequently, the optimal use of pacing in HCM requires continued reevaluation.[59] When pacing was compared to surgical therapy, LVOT gradient was reduced below 20 mmHg in only 26% of patients compared to over 90% of surgical patients,[54] creating drastically fewer indications for pacing. Furthermore, symptoms were improved in all patients with surgery, compared to only 50% with pacing. The role of pacing has been relegated to one where there are absolute contraindications to other therapies.

Septal ablation with alcohol is a nonsurgical myocardial reduction first attempted in 1994 based on interruption of blood supply to the interventricular septum, causing infarction. This causes reduced septal thickness and LVOT remodeling, with resolution of symptoms. Alcohol septal ablation utilizes technology aimed at management of CAD to treat HCM. Alcohol is administered through an angioplasty balloon to the first major septal perforator of the left anterior descending coronary artery. Myocardial contrast may be injected into the catheter and imaged with either TTE or TEE (Fig. 18-20). TTE imaging is usually adequate and obviates the need for a general anesthetic or deep sedation to tolerate TEE. After contrast is injected, enhancement of the hypertrophic part of the septum—and *only* that part—should be showing. If there is enhancement in areas of the myocardium where injection of ethanol would be undesirable, assessment of the coronary vasculature should be reevaluated in an attempt to find a more suitable point for ethanol administration (see Fig. 18-20). The LVOT gradient may show immediate improvement, likely due to myocardial stunning in the area of alcohol injection. Rebound in the gradient 24 hours later after recovery of the myocardium is common. Ultimately, the gradient slowly declines over the course of 6 to 12 months owing to remodeling of the ventricular septum. Overall LV function is usually minimally affected.[49]

The success rate has been good based on a recent systematic review of ablation incorporating 42 studies and nearly 3000 patients.[80] The study revealed effective gradient reduction and improvement in NYHA class comparable to myectomy 12 months after ablation. However, 20% of patients required a second procedure, and some even required myectomy after alcohol ablation. A retrospective review of 375 patients who underwent alcohol ablation identified 20 patients who underwent subsequent surgical myectomy for recurrent dynamic LVOT obstruction.[81] The surgery was successful in all failed ablation patients, indicating myectomy as rescue therapy for failed alcohol septal ablation. Although myectomy and alcohol ablation both produce hemodynamic and symptomatic benefit, some comparative observational and nonrandomized studies and one recent meta-analysis show that compared to alcohol ablation, surgery can provide the most consistent, complete, and rapid relief of symptoms, especially in those older than 65 years of age.[67]

There is concern about the incidence of complications and mortality accompanying alcohol ablation. Annual mortality with alcohol septal ablation in the best centers in the United States is 2%; Canada reports 4% to 10%.[54] Besides mortality, the incidence of nonfatal complications is a concern compared to surgical myectomy. Recently, Maron et al.[67] also reported from comparative observational and nonrandomized studies that myectomy is associated with lower postintervention gradients and fewer procedural complications and interventions. Heart block necessitating pacemaker placement has been reported in 11% to 38% of patients undergoing septal ablation.[82] The toxic effect of alcohol to both the coronary circulation and the myocardium has the potential to generate morbidity.[59]

Management of HCM continues to evolve as new information is made available. Figure 18-21 displays a treatment algorithm for patients with HCM that is an excellent summary of current practice.

Restrictive Cardiomyopathy

In 2006, an AHA scientific council updated the definition of RCM to "a rare form of heart muscle disease and a cause of heart failure that is characterized by normal or decreased volume of both ventricles associated with biatrial enlargement, normal LV wall thickness and atrioventricular valves, impaired ventricular filling with restrictive physiology, and normal (or near normal) systolic function. Both sporadic and familial forms have been described."[1] However, RCM has always been difficult to define because it occurs among a wide range of pathologies. The exact prevalence is unknown, but it is probably the least common of the cardiomyopathies, with few actual series in adults.[5,83,84] Recent molecular genetic investigations in RCM without any associated systemic disease has revealed that most of it is due to mutations in sarcomeric genes that have been associated with HCM, DCM, and LVNC.[85]

RCM is associated with many conditions (e.g., amyloidosis, carcinoid, sarcoidosis) and can be classified into five major causes (Box 18-3).[86,87] One can also characterize the types of processes involved in producing restrictive physiology: extracellular infiltration, intracellular accumulation of abnormal substances, inflammation, or endocardial disease.[84,85] Restrictive myocardial disorders are characteristically atypical in presentation and may appear in the final stages of other cardiac conditions such as DCM or HCM. With "true" idiopathic RCM, the cause is entirely unknown and lacks any identifiable histopathologic distinctiveness.

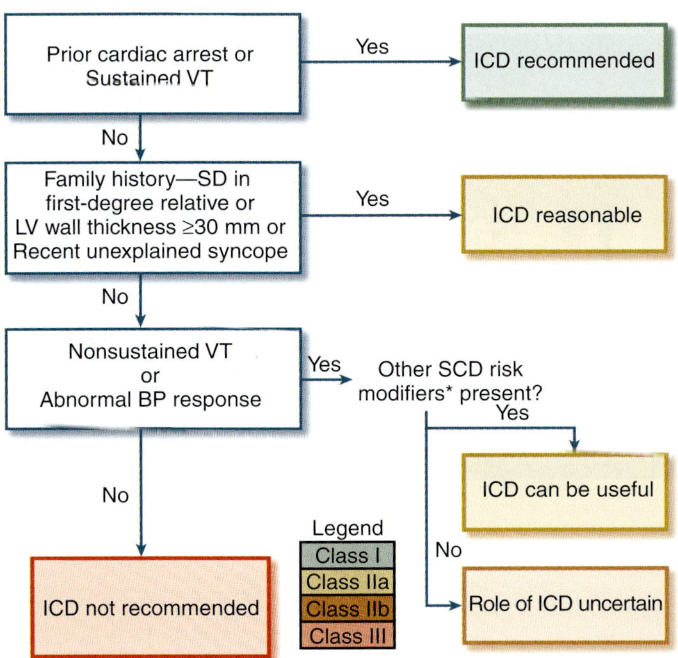

Figure 18-19 Indications for implantable cardioverter-defibrillators *(ICDs)* in hypertrophic cardiomyopathy. *, Sudden cardiac death *(SCD)* risk modifiers include established risk factors and emerging risk modifiers [Section 6.3.1.2]. *BP,* Blood pressure; *LV,* left ventricular; *SD,* sudden death; *VT,* ventricular tachycardia. *(From Gersh BJ, Maron BJ, Bonow RO, et al. 2011 ACCF/AHA guideline for the diagnosis and treatment of hypertrophic cardiomyopathy: a report of the American College of Cardiology Foundation/American Heart Association Task Force on Practice Guidelines Writing Committee Members. Circulation. 2011;124:e783-e831.)*

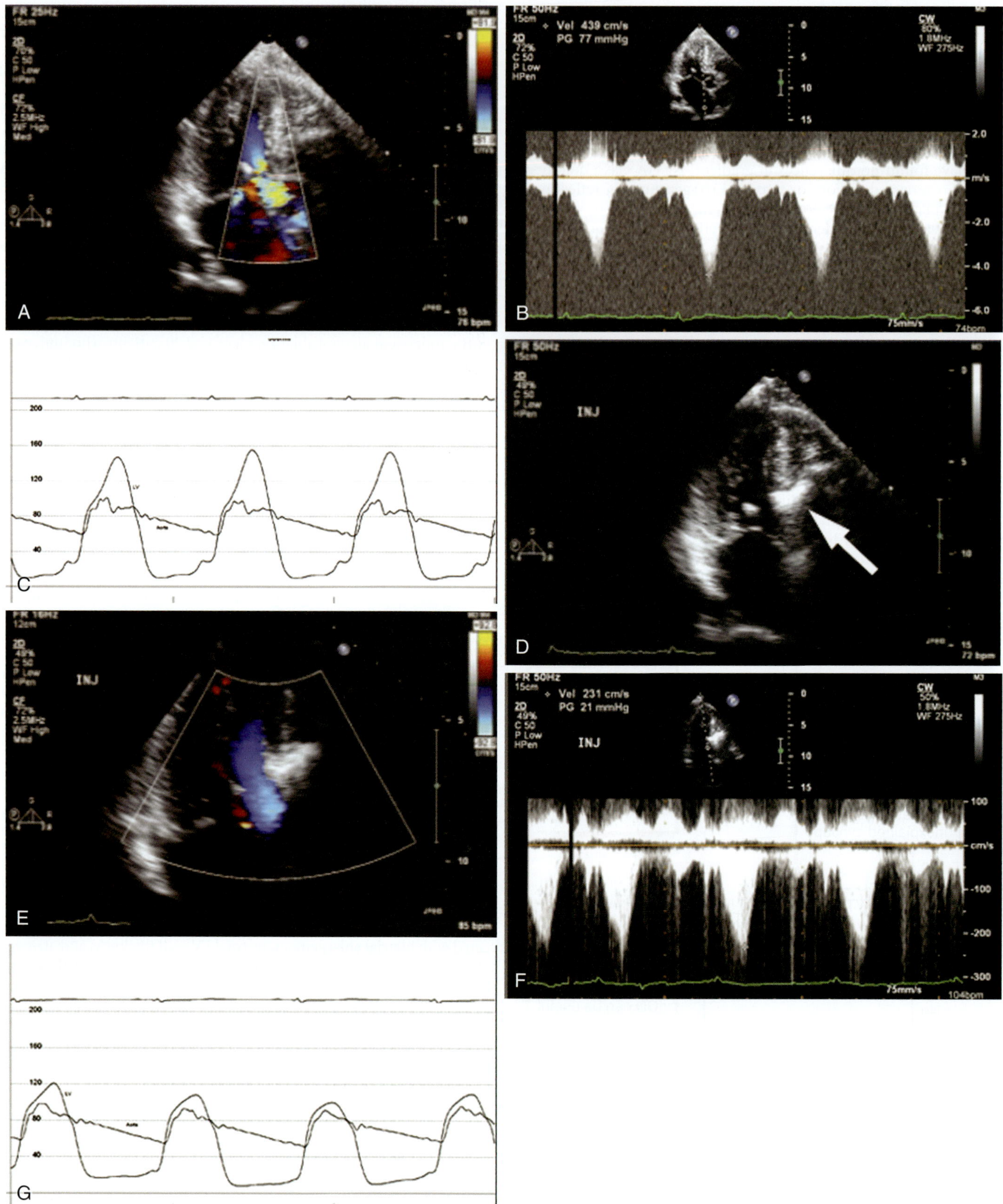

Figure 18-20   Sequential transthoracic imaging and pressure gradients from a patient undergoing alcohol ablation of isolated septal hypertrophy for hypertrophic obstructive cardiomyopathy. **A, B,** and **C,** Transthoracic apical long-axis view with color aliasing in left ventricular outflow tract due to obstruction. Continuous wave Doppler signal through outflow tract yields a gradient of 77 mmHg, and this is confirmed by simultaneous catheter-based pressure measurements in aorta and left ventricle. **D,** Injection of contrast and alcohol into a coronary artery feeding ventricular septum is seen as bright white in septum *(arrow).* **E, F,** and **G,** Resolution of obstruction to outflow. Apical long-axis view **(E)** reveals laminar flow in outflow tract. Gradient by Doppler measurements **(F)** has decreased to 21 mmHg, and catheter-based measurements **(G)** show similar reduction in gradient after injection.

Restrictive physiology is characterized by stiffness in the ventricle that results in a precipitous rise in ventricular pressure after small changes in volume; however, cardiomegaly or ventricular dilation should not be present. Diastolic dysfunction is evident by abnormalities of ventricular relaxation that later lead to poor myocardial compliance. Filling is accentuated early in diastole and impeded during the rest of diastole, owing to reduced ventricular distensibility. This causes the characteristic ventricular diastolic waveform of "dip and plateau" (so-called square root sign). The ventricles appear thick with small cavities. The atria appear dilated despite normal LV volumes. Systolic function has classically been reported to be minimally affected, but this is probably incorrect.[5] Once ventricular filling is restricted, prognosis worsens.

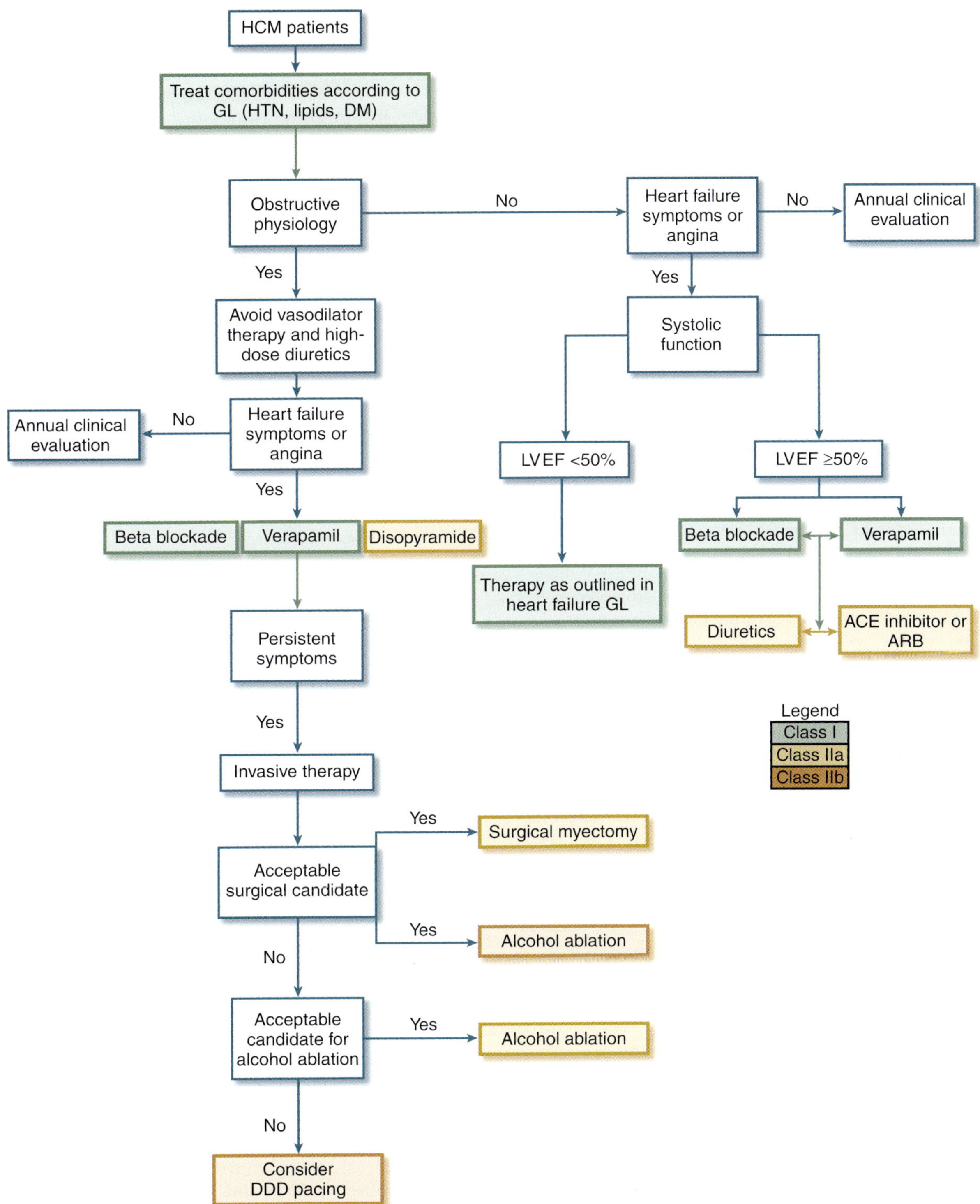

Figure 18-21 Treatment algorithm for HCM. *ACE,* Angiotensin-converting enzyme; *ARB,* angiotensin receptor blocker; *DM,* diabetes mellitus; *GL,* guidelines; *HCM,* hypertrophic cardiomyopathy; *HTN,* hypertension; *LVEF,* left ventricular ejection fraction. *(From Gersh BJ, Maron BJ, Bonow RO, et al. 2011 ACCF/AHA guideline for the diagnosis and treatment of hypertrophic cardiomyopathy: a report of the American College of Cardiology Foundation/American Heart Association Task Force on Practice Guidelines. Circulation. 2011;124:e783-831.)*

BOX 18-3. CAUSES OF RESTRICTIVE CARDIOMYOPATHY

Idiopathic restrictive cardiomyopathy
Radiation-induced cardiomyopathy
Eosinophilic endomyocardial disease
Infiltrative disorders:
- Amyloidosis
- Sarcoidosis
- Gaucher disease
- Hurler disease

Storage diseases:
- Hemochromatosis
- Fabry disease
- Glycogen storage disease

Data from Nihoyannopoulos P, Dawson D. Restrictive cardiomyopathies. *Eur J Echocardiogr.* 2009;10:iii23-33; Kushwaha SS, Fallon JT, Fuster V. Restrictive cardiomyopathy. *N Engl J Med.* 1997;336:267-276.

BOX 18-4. DOPPLER CRITERIA SUPPORTING DIAGNOSIS OF RESTRICTIVE CARDIOMYOPATHY

E-wave deceleration time < 140 ms
Mitral E/A ratio > 2
Mitral E/e′ > 15
Pulmonary and hepatic vein flow systolic velocity < diastolic velocity*
Increased diastolic flow reversal in hepatic vein during inspiration*
Increased atrial flow reversal velocity and duration in pulmonary vein

*Assume spontaneous respirations.

Typically, adult patients present with insidious onset of fatigue and exertional dyspnea. Because the right, left, or both ventricles may be involved, symptoms may present as either right- or left-sided heart failure or a combination of the two. The chest roentgenogram usually shows evidence of pulmonary congestion and a normal or smaller-than-anticipated heart size with dilated atria. ECG evidence of biatrial enlargement may be present.[85] Clinically, it is often challenging to distinguish "restrictive" physiology from "constrictive," especially since this physiology is not solely limited to RCM but occurs in mitral stenosis, tricuspid stenosis, and aortic stenosis. It is important to differentiate RCM from constrictive pericarditis (CP) because of differences in prognosis and treatment. Greater details about the diagnosis of RCM and CP are available elsewhere.[88,89] Advances in echocardiography and other noninvasive methods have been used to try to reliably discriminate between pericardial disease and RCM and remain the mainstay of diagnosis. However, it has been difficult to obtain consensus regarding uniform diagnostic criteria for RCM.[85]

If one excludes other cardiomyopathies that may lead to restrictive-type physiology (i.e., DCM), the echocardiographic findings of patients with RCM tend to be similar regardless of the cause (infiltrative vs. noninfiltrative). In the majority of patients, 2D echocardiographic findings reveal ventricles of normal size and normal to low-normal systolic function.[83] The ventricular walls may be of normal thickness or may appear hypertrophied, depending on the cause of restriction. Biatrial enlargement secondary to chronically elevated ventricular filling pressures is seen. When compliance of the ventricle is decreased, a small increase in ventricular volume causes a large increase in ventricular pressure. The result is a shortened deceleration time (DT) of early rapid filling (E wave) when measuring mitral inflow (DT < 160 milliseconds). Because LA pressure is high, the mitral valve opens at a high pressure and intraventricular relaxation time is decreased. In addition, the elevated atrial pressure leads to high-velocity inflow during early diastole, with an E-wave velocity greater than 1 m/s. As the pressure quickly rises in the noncompliant LV, atrial contraction adds little to ventricular filling, so the velocity of the A wave is low, resulting in an E/A ratio greater than 2.[90]

When LA pressure is high, little atrial filling from the pulmonary veins occurs during systole. Essentially, the LA acts as a conduit such that significant atrial filling occurs only during ventricular diastole. This results in a large D wave and a small S wave when measuring pulmonary venous flow velocities. An additional consequence of high atrial pressure is an increase in atrial flow reversal velocity and duration in the pulmonary veins during atrial contraction. This finding is mimicked on the right side of the heart with prominent atrial reversal flow waves seen in the hepatic veins during atrial contraction. Measuring inferior vena cava and hepatic vein flows may be less reliable in the anesthetized patient undergoing perioperative TEE, however.

Lastly, tissue Doppler imaging reveals the expected pattern of severe relaxation abnormalities. Mitral annular e′ velocity is less than 7 cm/s, and given the high E wave velocity discussed earlier, the resultant E/e′ is typically greater than 15.[91] Tissue Doppler imaging has demonstrated some success in providing differentiation between RCM and CP by measuring E velocity to determine ventricular relaxation, with 89% sensitivity and 100% specificity.[92]

Echocardiographic Doppler criteria do not exist for diagnosing RCM, but Box 18-4 provides a summary of supporting criteria. Doppler findings may indicate the severity of RCM once the diagnosis is certain.

Cardiac catheterization is still performed to differentiate between RCM and CP. During catheterization, increased left and right venous pressures with large A and V waves may be observed in RCM. It is not uncommon to see right atrial (RA) pressures of 15 mmHg to 20 mmHg. The ventricular pressure curve may display the diastolic dip-and-plateau pattern (square root sign) described previously. Recently, more advanced catheterization criteria for RCM and CP differentiation have been devised.[93]

Endomyocardial biopsy may differentiate RCM from CP; the biopsy in RCM is rarely normal, in contrast to CP. A biopsy can identify specific causes of restrictive physiology, such as cardiac sarcoidosis, amyloidosis, and Fabry disease.[84,94] However, more often the biopsy only shows patchy endocardial and interstitial fibrosis with some myofibril hypertrophy.[83,95] If a biopsy is nondiagnostic and tests such as radionuclide angiography, Doppler, or echocardiography are inconclusive, exploratory surgery may be needed because it is the most definitive method of differentiating RCM from CP. There has been some concern about subjecting the patient with RCM to anesthesia,[96] but to determine a proper diagnosis, this is a lesser concern in modern practice.

There is no specific treatment for RCM. A surgical option for RCM is rare, with the exception of endomyocardial fibrosis with eosinophilic cardiomyopathy. The fibrotic endocardium may be excised in combination with mitral or tricuspid valve replacement. Survival with RCM depends largely on the etiology but rarely goes beyond 2 years without transplantation,[85] which is not always an option for adults with RCM, because the processes responsible for the disease would invariably affect the newly transplanted heart.

Although there are many causes of RCM, there are three conditions that merit additional discussion: idiopathic RCM, amyloidosis, and hypereosinophilic syndrome. Idiopathic RCM is the purest form of the disease. Ventricular wall thickness appears normal on 2D imaging, and there is no identifiable cause on histopathology. Idiopathic RCM tends to be a rare diagnosis, with 5-year survival of 64%.[83]

Amyloidosis is the most common cause of RCM. In fact, most of the literature about RCM actually refers to patients with amyloid disease. Amyloidosis is a systemic disorder that results in extracellular deposition of protein subunits. Deposition can occur in a variety of tissue beds, including the heart. There are a variety of types of amyloidosis, and the incidence of cardiac involvement depends on the type of amyloid disease affecting the patient. For example, in primary amyloidosis, up to 50% of patients may show cardiac involvement, whereas with secondary amyloidosis, less than 5% of patients will have cardiac manifestations.[97] Protein deposition in the myocardium ultimately leads to thickening of the myocardium, and on autopsy the myocardium is often described as "rubbery" in texture. Echocardiographic findings may support the diagnosis, but ultimately a myocardial biopsy

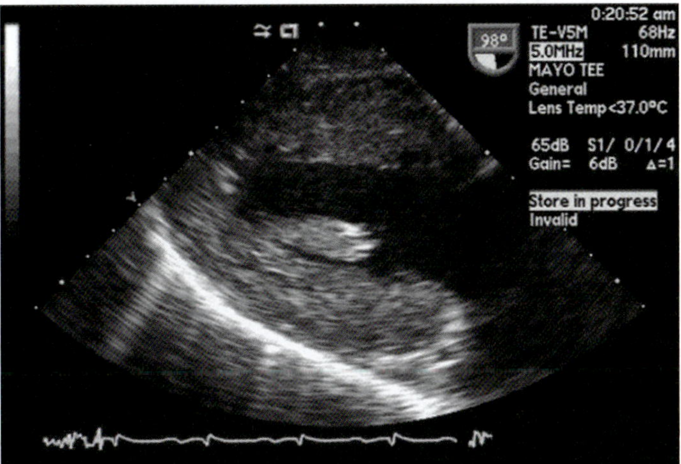

Figure 18-22 Mitral inflow velocities in amyloid restriction. In this mid-esophageal four-chamber view, a pulsed wave Doppler cursor has been placed at tips of mitral leaflets. Despite patient being in sinus rhythm, there is only a tiny A wave and a very large E wave with a very short deceleration time of 121 milliseconds.

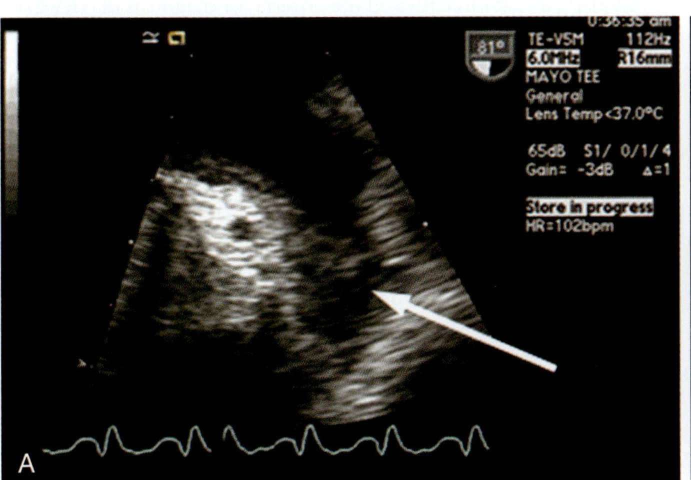

Figure 18-23 Transgastric long-axis image from cardiac amyloidosis patient undergoing cardiac transplantation. Ventricle is severely thickened. While difficult to appreciate, note granular echogenicity of myocardium, a common finding in cardiac amyloidosis.

is required for confirmation. For amyloid especially, cardiac biopsy is sensitive and specific for diagnosis and allows subtyping of the amyloid to guide future treatment decisions.

Late in the progression of RCM due to amyloid, Doppler findings (Fig. 18-22) will be consistent with those of a restrictive filling pattern, as described in Box 18-4. However, the disease is progressive such that imaging early in the disease may reveal filling patterns consistent with only impaired relaxation or pseudonormalization. Over time the ventricle will continue to thicken. Systolic function is usually maintained but may become impaired late in the disease. Oftentimes the protein deposition will lead to increased echogenicity of the myocardium, often described as a "granular" or "sparkling" appearance (Fig. 18-23 and Video 18-4) . This finding is helpful in making the diagnosis when seen, but it has relatively low sensitivity. In one series of amyloid patients, only 26% displayed this myocardial appearance.[98]

The patient with cardiac amyloidosis should be imaged closely for the appearance of thrombus within the heart. In one autopsy study including 156 patients with cardiac amyloidosis, 27% had evidence of thrombus. The bulk of the thrombi were found in the left or right atrial appendages (Video 18-5). Atrial fibrillation, decreased diastolic function, and lower LA appendage emptying velocities were associated with higher occurrence of thrombus in this series (Fig. 18-24).[99]

Newer echocardiographic techniques may be of benefit in evaluating and following patients with cardiac amyloidosis. Tissue Doppler imaging reveals decreased velocities in both lateral and septal walls in patients with restrictive filling pressures as well as those without.[100] This finding was independent of age and LV mass. Myocardial strain and strain rate measurements detect early systolic and late diastolic myocardial dysfunction before patients present with heart failure symptoms.[101]

Occasionally, and particularly earlier in the disease state, the echocardiographer may be confronted with a hypertrophied ventricle with hyperdynamic function. Given the small hyperdynamic ventricle, SAM of the mitral valve may be present as well. Given this scenario, it may be difficult to decide whether the findings are consistent with those of hypertrophy secondary to hypertension, HCM, or amyloidosis. The ECG can be extremely helpful in this situation. When LV mass is increased, one expects to find increased voltage, but this is unreliable for hypertrophy.[39] However, cardiac amyloidosis is associated with a low-voltage ECG. The finding of increased LV mass with decreased ECG voltage is unique to cardiac amyloidosis.[98,102] Other conditions with low-voltage ECGs (e.g., cardiac tamponade) do not display ventricular hypertrophy. In one series, the combination of a low-voltage ECG and a ventricular septal thickness greater than 1.98 cm was 72% sensitive and 91% specific for the diagnosis of cardiac amyloidosis.[98]

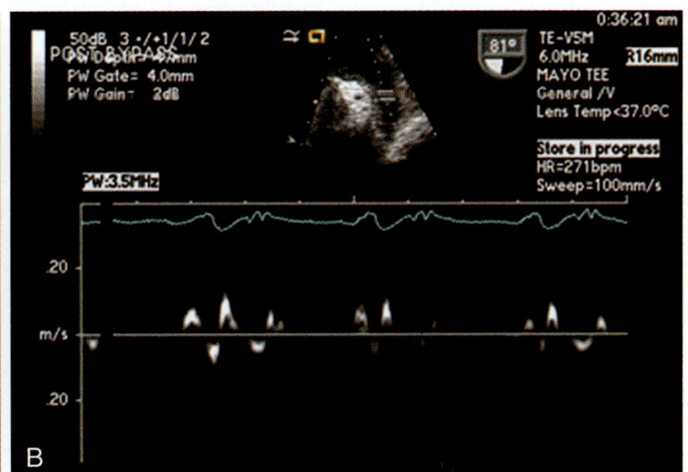

Figure 18-24 **A,** Midesophageal view with focus on left atrial appendage (LAA). Note stagnant flow with spontaneous contrast and potentially overt thrombus in LAA. **B,** Pulsed wave Doppler signal has been placed at LAA orifice. Emptying velocity of appendage is low (<20 cm/s), indicating substrate for stagnant flow.

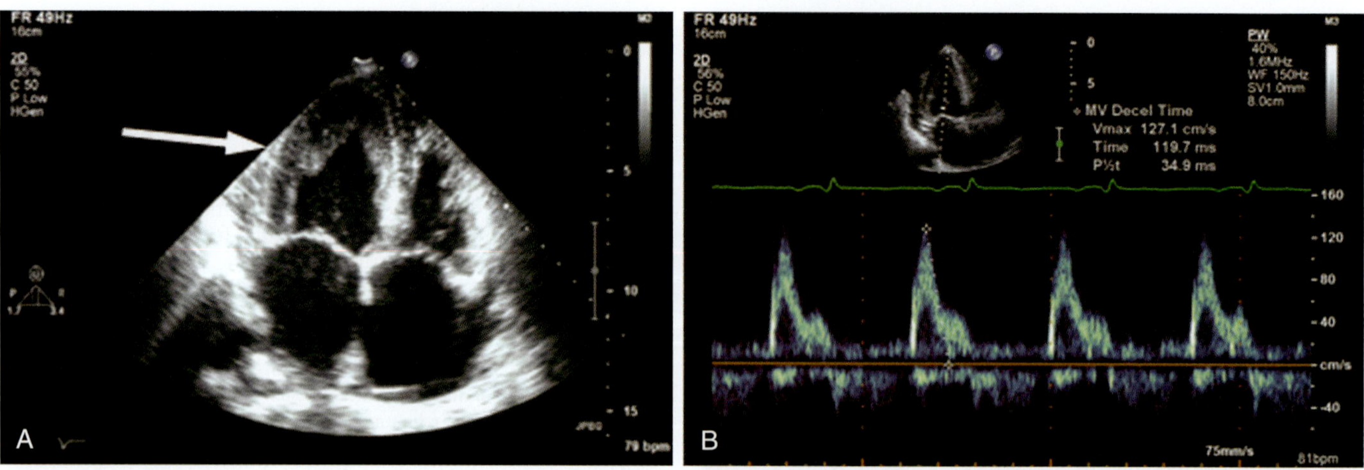

Figure 18-25   Transthoracic imaging in patient with hypereosinophilic syndrome and cardiac manifestation. **A,** Apical four-chamber two-dimensional image shows left ventricular myocardium is severely thickened *(arrow)*, with obliteration of apical portion of ventricle. **B,** Pulsed waved Doppler showing mitral inflow velocities. E wave is very steep and much larger than A wave, with a very short deceleration.

Historically, the hypereosinophilic syndrome was defined as the presence of over 1500 eosinophils/mm^3 for 6 months without an identifiable cause (i.e., parasitic infection, allergic reaction, etc.) along with end-organ involvement.[103] More recently, experts have begun to subdivide this heterogeneous group of syndromes into more disease-specific diagnoses,[104] which is beyond the scope of this discussion. Regardless, cardiac involvement in this syndrome is common and deserves consideration.

Infiltration of the myocardium with eosinophils and granular deposits results in decreased compliance and the typical Doppler findings of restrictive diastolic function. In addition, thrombus formation at the apex of the left LV is common. The appearance is that of increased echodensity at the ventricular apex with 2D imaging, or failure of the apex to fill with contrast when it is administered (Fig. 18-25). Apical obliteration may also occur in the RV. The inferior basal septal wall often becomes thickened, as does the posterior mitral leaflet, resulting in MR.[105] Rarely the hypereosinophilic syndrome results in myocarditis with a dilated ventricle and systolic dysfunction.

Arrhythmogenic Right Ventricular Cardiomyopathy/Dysplasia

Originally called *arrhythmogenic right ventricular dysplasia*, the AHA Scientific Committee defined arrhythmogenic right ventricular cardiomyopathy/dysplasia (ARVC/D) as an "uncommon form of inheritable heart muscle disease (estimated 1:5000)."[1] The definition further states that it primarily affects the RV, with a progressive loss of myocytes that turns into fatty or fibrofatty tissue causing regional or global abnormalities (Fig. 18-26). Primarily thought of as a disorder of the RV, involvement of the LV is now appreciated in a greater percentage of individuals than in the past.[1] ARVC/D is the most arrhythmogenic form of human heart disease[4] and, although rare, accounts for 20% of sudden cardiac death in the young.[106] Viral myocarditis may often be associated with ARVC/D, but it is not an inflammatory cardiomyopathy. Some of the confusion surrounding the diagnosis of ARVC/D is owed to the fact that humans are the only species that develop fat in the RV without corresponding fibrosis. Today, molecular biology has better defined ARVC/D as a developmental or structural defect that arises during embryologic development and continues into adulthood.[107]

ARVC/D is familial in 30% to 50% of persons. It is mostly autosomal dominant in inheritance, with variable expressivity; penetrance is dependent on age and gender.[9] Recent work with clinical and genetic evaluation in patients and relatives with ARVC/D is identifying the importance of phenotype diversity that is displayed as the difference in the expression of ARVC/D between the patient (proband) and relatives.[9]

Even though the ARVC/D is present embryologically, the affected individual is usually unaware of it until the onset of fatal arrhythmias in adolescence. Recently a clinical and molecular genetic evaluation was performed in 210 first-degree and 45 second-degree relatives from 100 families with ARVC/D.[9] In more than half these families, the proband presented with sudden cardiac death; most of the remainder had an arrhythmic presentation, and in only 3 living probands was the diagnosis incidental. Thirty-one percent of probands died suddenly between the ages of 14 and 20 years. In contrast to probands, first-degree relatives had milder disease expression; major structural and functional abnormalities of the RV were less common, as was LV dysfunction. Disease expression in gene-positive relatives was age related and developed in the fifth decade of life and beyond in more than 50% of affected individuals.

ARVC/D usually presents with onset of arrhythmias ranging from PVCs to ventricular fibrillation. The replacement of myocardium with fat and fibrous tissue creates an excellent environment for a fatal arrhythmia.[108] The 10-year mortality is 15%.[109] The disease is now known to proceed through four phases: (1) concealed, without symptoms or evidence of heart disease but some electrophysiologic changes that place one at risk for sudden cardiac death; (2) overt electrical disorder dysrhythmias; (3) isolated right heart failure; and (4) biventricular involvement and failure.[110]

In 2010, a task force revised the criteria for diagnosis of ARVC/D to include more genetic screening of desmosomal gene mutations as well as ECG and electroanatomic features.[111] The range of presentations of the disease and lack of a single diagnostic noninvasive test increases diagnostic difficulty. The history and physical exam may be unremarkable, yet the structural and functional changes may be present in the RV.[106] Clinical presentation may range from asymptomatic myopathic involvement to overt clinical disease with diffuse biventricular involvement.[108,112] The electrical instability characteristic of ARVC/D is not solely responsible for the natural history of the disease. Recently it has been shown that significant ventricular mechanical dyssynchrony is present in 50% of patients.[113] This leads to a more dilated RV as well as one with poorer function compared to those without it. Myocardial loss with progressive ventricular dysfunction progresses ultimately to heart failure, accounting for 20% of deaths. End-stage ARVC/D may be difficult to distinguish from DCM because of the extent of LV involvement.

Diagnosis is rare in the early stages of ARVC/D. Newer imaging techniques (e.g., cardiac magnetic resonance imaging [MRI], contrast-enhanced echocardiography, electroanatomic voltage mapping) may help, as well as updates in the diagnostic criteria for 12-lead ECG. ECG

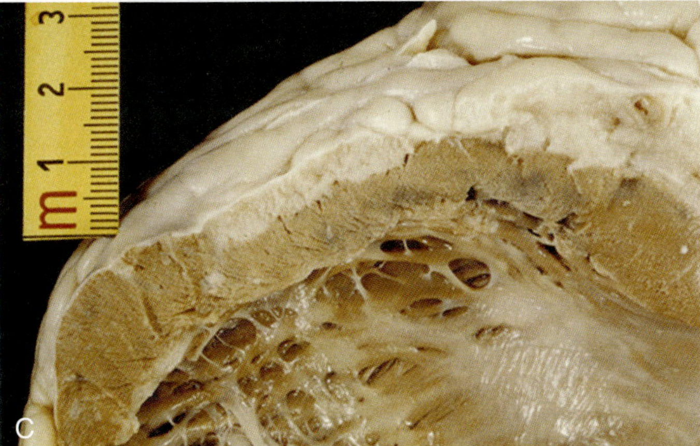

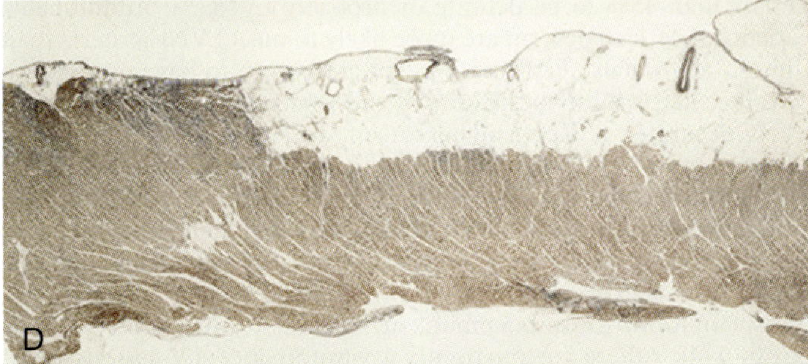

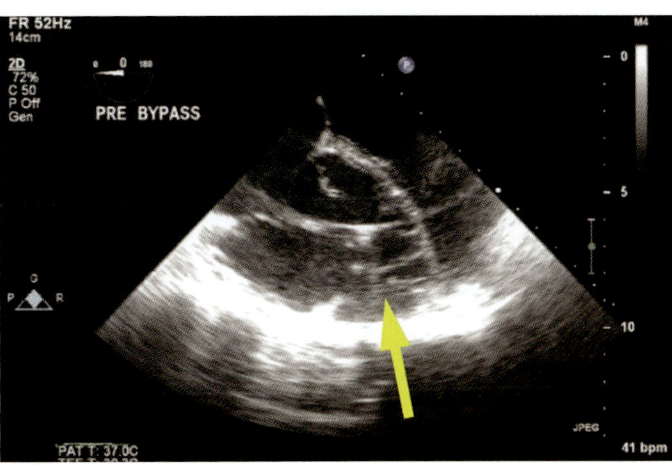

Figure 18-27 Midesophageal four-chamber view with probe rotated to focus on right ventricle. Ventricle is severely dilated and showed severe reduction in systolic function. Note prominent trabeculation in apex *(arrow)*.

TABLE 18-1	Sensitivity and Specificity of Proposed Right Ventricular Imaging Criteria		
	Value	*Sensitivity (%)*	*Specificity (%)*
Echocardiogram: Major			
PLAX RVOT (diastole)	≥32 mm	75	95
Corrected for body size (PLAX/BSA)	≥19 mm/m²		
PSAX RVOT (diastole)	≥36 mm	62	95
Corrected for body size (PSAX/BSA)	≥21 mm/m²		
Fractional area change	≤33%	55	95
Echocardiogram: Minor			
PLAX RVOT (diastole)	≥29mm	87	87
Corrected for body size (PLAX/BSA)	≥16 to < 18 mm/m²		
PSAX RVOT (diastole)	≥32 mm	80	80
Corrected for body size (PSAX/BSA)	≥18 to ≤ 20 mm/m²		
Fractional area change	≤40%	76	76

aVF, Augmented voltage unipolar left foot lead; *aVL,* augmented voltage unipolar left arm lead; *BSA,* body surface area; *PLAX,* parasternal long-axis view; *PSAX,* parasternal short-axis view; *RVOT,* right ventricular outflow tract.
Data from Marcus FI, McKenna WJ, Sherrill D, et al. Diagnosis of arrhythmogenic right ventricular cardiomyopathy/dysplasia: proposed modification of the task force criteria. *Circulation.* 2010;121:1533-1541.

Figure 18-26 Gross view **(A)** of the RV outflow tract showing severe transmural loss of the RV free wall and an infundibular parchment-like aneurysm. Histologic view **(B)** at high magnification of surviving degenerated right ventricular myocytes in the setting of extensive fatty replacement and tiny interstitial fibrosis. Gross **(C)** and histologic **(D)** sections of anterior left ventricular wall showing striking subepicardial fatty infiltration and fibrosis. *(From Corrado D, Basso C, Thiene G, et al. Spectrum of clinicopathologic manifestations of arrhythmogenic right ventricular cardiomyopathy/dysplasia: A multicenter study. J Am Coll Cardiol. 1997;30:1512.)*

changes may occur prior to any histologic changes such as loss of myocytes or RV dysfunction.[111] A new immunohistochemical analysis of a biopsy sample has proven to be highly sensitive and specific for identifying ARVC.[114] Endomyocardial biopsy may be diagnostic but also incorrect if the sample is obtained from the septal area of the myocardium, known for its lack of characteristic features.[14]

Unlike most cardiomyopathies, echocardiography is not a major component of diagnosis in ARVC/D. The perioperative transesophageal echocardiographer will rarely encounter it. A dilated RV with prominent trabeculations and/or echodense moderator bands should prompt further investigation into the potential diagnosis of ARVC/D in a perioperative patient (Fig. 18-27 and Video 18-6). 

In 2005, a report from the Multidisciplinary Study of Right Ventricular Dysplasia attempted to describe the echocardiographic structural findings in patients with ARVC/D.[115] When compared to matched controls, patients with ARVC/D had significantly increased RV dimensions and decreased RV fractional area change during systole (i.e., dilated RV with decreased systolic function). In 2010, data from 108 probands with newly diagnosed ARVC/D, age older than 12 years, were enrolled in the National Institutes of Health–supported Multidisciplinary Study of Right Ventricular Dysplasia. A task force proposed new modified criteria for the diagnosis of ARVC/D by comparing to controls.[111] These criteria contain both major and minor echocardiographic criteria to aid in the diagnosis of ARVC/D (Table 18-1). It is important to note severe tricuspid regurgitation in ARVC/D during an echocardiographic examination, because it carries an adverse prognosis in these patients.[109]

Left Ventricular Noncompaction

Left ventricular noncompaction (LVNC) is an anatomic condition of LV myocardial development. Incomplete myocardial compaction results in thickened areas of LV myocardium and prominent trabeculations separated by deep recesses on the endocardial surface (Fig. 18-28). The morphologic appearance of the LV has been characterized as "spongy."[1] The presence of a thinner "compacted" layer of myocardium adjacent to the epicardial surface gives rise to a typical two-layer appearance (Fig. 18-29). Sometimes referred to as *LV hypertrabeculation*, LVNC has been increasingly reported, most likely reflecting greater use of high-resolution noninvasive cardiac imaging modalities (including echocardiography and MRI) as well as increased awareness of the condition among physicians.[116]

Although the disease has been described at autopsy for at least 80 years, LVNC has not been widely recognized or classified. In 1995, the World Health Organization listed LVNC as an unclassified cardiomyopathy.[41] Eleven years later, a working group of the AHA defined LVNC as a primary cardiomyopathy of genetic origin (see Fig. 18-1).[1] Numerous gene mutations have only recently been found in patients expressing the LVNC phenotype,[117] and some experts recommend screening first-degree relatives for the condition.[2] Non-familial cases have also been reported, and some patients seem to have acquired LVNC, because previous echocardiographic examinations did not show the abnormality in these individuals.[116] X-linked inheritance, autosomal dominant, and autosomal recessive inheritance have been reported in families.[10] LVNC has been found together with other congenital heart defects including aortic coarctation, atrial septal defect, VSD, and complex cyanotic defects.[1] Many patients with LVNC who lack congenital heart disease findings have also been described and are considered to have isolated LVNC.

Originally considered a congenital condition, LVNC is thought to be the outcome of intrauterine arrest of the normal process by which trabecular fibers and spaces condense into myocardium and capillaries.[118] This process of condensation typically proceeds from the base to the apex of the LV. Interruption in the base-to-apex sequence of myocardial compaction may explain why noncompacted myocardial segments are most commonly found at the apex and least commonly found at the basal ventricular level.[119] However, some physicians believe LVNC develops in certain cases as an adaptive response to LV dilation, remodeling, and altered loading conditions.[120] These physicians challenge the concept that all instances of LVNC are congenital in origin and highlight cases in which prominent LV trabeculations appear and subsequently diminish on serial echocardiograms.

The reported incidence of LVNC varies widely and likely reflects both demographic variations in the populations studied and differences in diagnostic criteria used. Originally, isolated LVNC was thought to have a prevalence of 0.05% to 0.24%.[117] However, Kohli et al.[6] recently studied 190 patients referred to a heart failure clinic and reported that 24% of this group fulfilled at least one set of diagnostic criteria for LVNC, as did 8% of healthy controls. The concern was that diagnostic criteria for LVNC might be too sensitive. Echocardiographic examinations in a community hospital setting found nearly 3.7% of those with EF less than 45% to be definite or probably LVNC.[121] Additionally, patients of African descent are more likely to meet LVNC criteria than whites. Individuals of African descent are known to have more heavily trabeculated LV myocardium,[122] and whether the increased rate of LVNC accurately reflects a higher rate of cardiomyopathy in this group or rather represents an erroneous classification of a normal phenotypic variant is unknown.

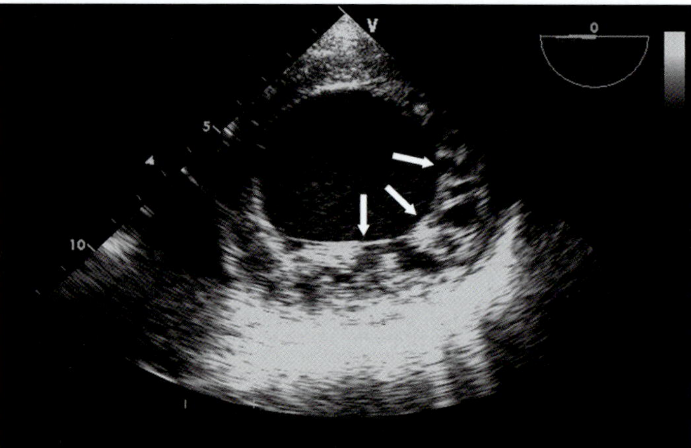

Figure 18-28   Transgastric mid–left ventricular short-axis image showing changes of noncompaction in lateral wall *(arrows)*.

The natural course of the disease has not really been defined, and the clinical outcome of patients with LVNC is highly variable. Some patients experience heart failure, cardiac death or the need for transplantation, thromboemboli, arrhythmias, and sudden cardiac death, while others are apparently asymptomatic.[1] LV systolic function may be normal or severely reduced. After reviewing the clinical course of more than 100 patients with LVNC, Saleeb et al. concluded that the clinical outcome of these patients is predicted by the degree of ventricular dysfunction and not the morphologic changes of hypertrabeculation.[120]

Clinicians most often make the antemortem diagnosis of LVNC based on echocardiographic studies, but cardiac MRI and ECG findings may be supportive. No single set of echocardiographic findings is diagnostic for LVNC; investigators frequently cite three different sets of diagnostic criteria (Table 18-2). Chin et al.[123] described a progression of trabecular prominence that increased from base to apex. By using TTE SAX and apical views at end-diastole, Chin's group measured the distance from the epicardial surface to the trough of the intertrabecular recess (distance X) as well as the distance from the epicardial surface to the trabecular peak (distance Y). An X/Y ratio of 0.5 or less was consistent with LVNC (Fig. 18-30). Jenni et al.[124] proposed a diagnostic approach using TTE parasternal SAX imaging in which a two-layer myocardium was visible, with a thinner compacted epicardial layer and a thicker trabeculated or noncompacted endocardial layer. In this scheme, the relative thickness of the two layers is

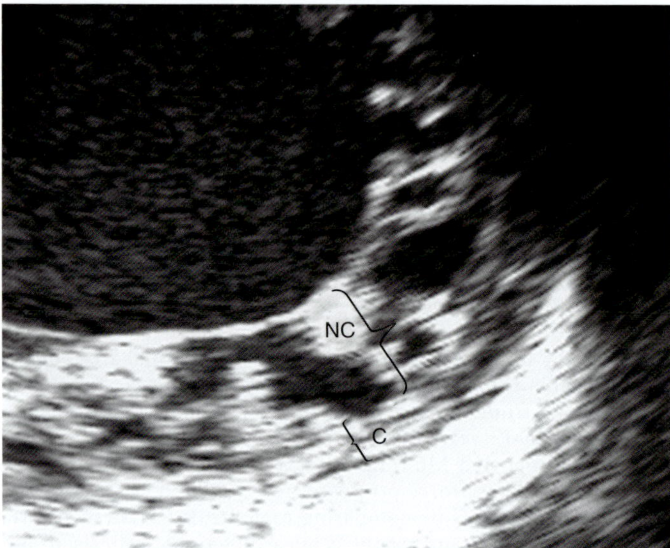

Figure 18-29   Transgastric mid–left ventricular short-axis image with focus on anterolateral wall. Typical two-layer appearance of noncompaction is evident, with both a normal "compacted" component *(C)* and a thicker noncompacted portion *(NC)*.

measured at end-systole, with the noncompacted layer measuring at least twice as thick as the compacted layer. Finally, Stollberger et al.[125] defined LVNC as the presence of more than three LV trabeculations visible in a single echocardiographic imaging plane apical to the papillary muscles. All three diagnostic schemes imply that the blood present within the intratrabecular recesses is in continuity with the LV cavity (Fig. 18-31 and Video 18-7).

TABLE 18-2	Proposed Diagnostic Criteria for Left Ventricular Noncompaction
Chin et al.[123]	End-diastolic measurements Transthoracic parasternal short-axis or apical views $X/Y \leq 0.5$ (where X = distance from epicardial surface to trough of intertrabecular recess and Y = distance from epicardial surface to peak of trabeculation)
Jenni et al.[124]	End-systolic measurements Transthoracic parasternal short-axis views $NC/C > 2$ (where NC = thickness of non-compacted layer and C = thickness of compacted layer)
Stollberger et al.[125]	Echocardiographic imaging plane apical to the papillary muscles More than three left ventricular trabeculations visible in a single echocardiographic plane

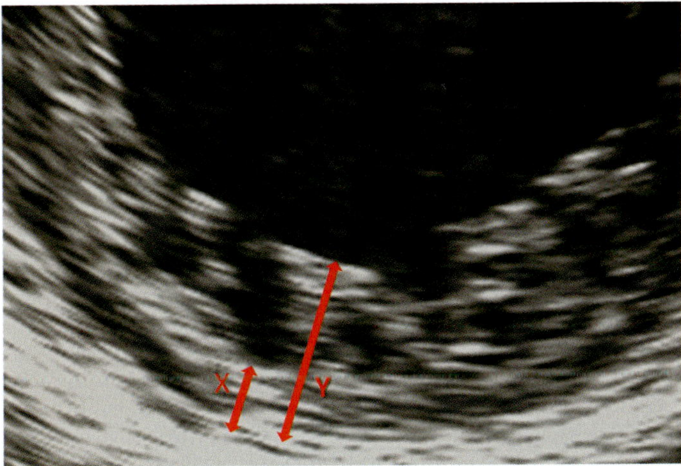

Figure 18-30 Transgastric mid–left ventricular short-axis image with focus on anterior wall. Measurement of compacted layer *(X)* and noncompacted layer *(Y)* as proposed by Chin et al. is demonstrated. *(From Chin TK, Perloff JK, Williams RG, et al. Isolated noncompaction of left ventricular myocardium. A study of eight cases. Circulation. 1990;82:507-513.)*

During echocardiographic imaging, the changes of LVNC are typically seen at the apex of the heart and rarely at the basal ventricular level (Video 18-8). At the midventricular level, the lateral and inferior walls are more likely than the anterior and septal walls to display the typical hypertrabeculated appearance.[119] Interestingly, the measurement of LV chamber dimensions and systolic function are not included in currently published diagnostic criteria. Global systolic function can range from normal to severely reduced. Sviggum et al.[116] studied 60 patients with LVNC and found that LVEF was normal in only 27% and reduced in 73%.

Given the variability in published diagnostic criteria, it is not surprising that interobserver agreement in establishing the diagnosis of LVNC is fairly low.[120] When the echocardiograms of 104 patients with previously diagnosed LVNC were subsequently reviewed by different echocardiographers, the condition was confirmed in only 67% of cases.[120] Interobserver agreement was highest (74%-79%) for establishing a noncompacted-to-compacted thickness ratio greater than 2 or less than 2. Interobserver agreement was lower (59%-73%) for determining whether three or more trabeculations were present in a given patient.

Noncompacted myocardial segments are often hypocontractile. Given the unusual appearance of noncompacted myocardium, it can be difficult to visually estimate the degree of thickening and active versus passive tissue excursion throughout the cardiac cycle. Tissue Doppler imaging has been proposed as one possible modality to assess myocardial motion in patients with LVNC.[41] In one study of children with LVNC, a tissue Doppler velocity less than 7.8 cm/s measured at the lateral mitral annulus was predictive of heart failure, cardiac death, and the need for transplantation.[126] Strain and strain rate imaging have been insightful in some types of cardiomyopathy, though studies in patients with LVNC are lacking.[41]

Although the existing echocardiographic diagnostic criteria rely on TTE imaging,[123] analogous views may be obtained with TEE. In particular, TG mid-SAX or basal SAX views may be substituted for the TTE parasternal SAX view. Additional retroflexion of the TEE probe may be used in the TG position to better visualize the LV apex (Video 18-9). Instead of apical TTE views, the ME four-chamber, two-chamber, and LAX views may be used. The TG two-chamber view may also allow visualization of affected segments (Fig. 18-32). Care must be taken to avoid foreshortening the apex, since the changes of LVNC are often most prominent in the apical segments.

Demonstration of perfusion within the intratrabecular recesses of blood derived from the LV cavity can be accomplished with color Doppler imaging (see Fig. 18-31). Because the angle between the transducer and the intracavity blood flow may not be favorable, reducing the aliasing velocity may be required to adequately demonstrate blood flow between trabeculations. Alternatively, using an intravenously injected

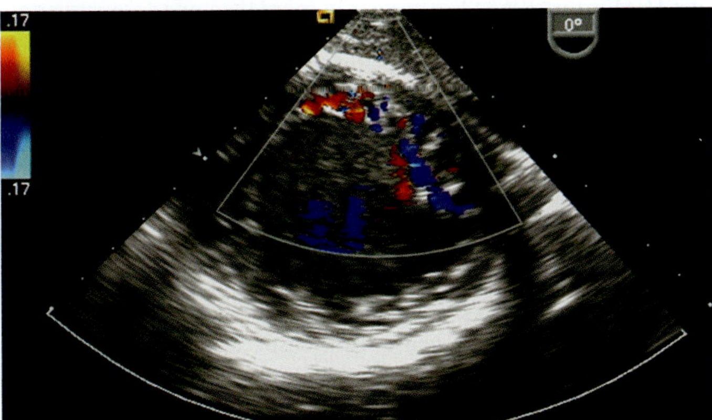

Figure 18-31 Transgastric mid–left ventricular short-axis image in patient with noncompaction. Color Doppler imaging demonstrates perfusion of intratrabecular recesses from left ventricular cavity. Note lower aliasing velocity.

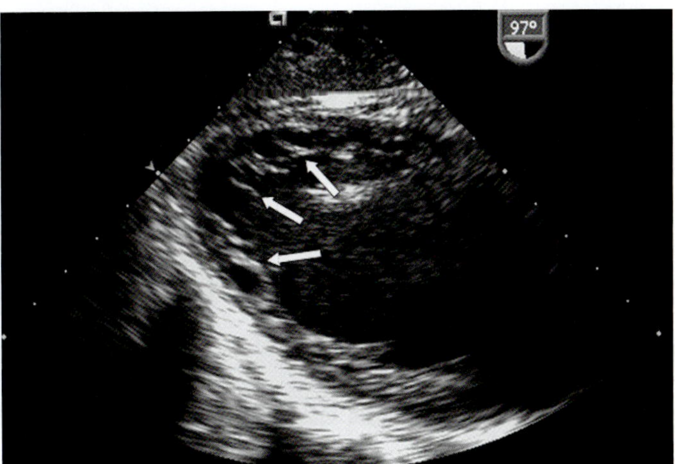

Figure 18-32 Transgastric two-chamber view demonstrating noncompaction involving left ventricular apex *(arrows)*.

contrast agent with transpulmonary passage may highlight the trabeculations and blood flow between the LV cavity and intertrabecular recesses.

The discovery of LV apical thrombi in some patients with LVNC led earlier investigators to conclude that the condition is associated with an increased risk for thromboembolic disease.[123] However, subsequent investigation has failed to confirm LVNC as an independent risk factor for intracardiac thrombus formation.[120] In fact, the risk of intracardiac thrombosis relates more to the degree of systolic dysfunction and other comorbidities than to the presence of LV trabeculations. However, if LV dysfunction is present, a comprehensive echocardiographic examination should include a search for intracardiac masses.

Takotsubo Cardiomyopathy

Takotsubo cardiomyopathy (TTCM), also known as *apical ballooning syndrome*, *stress-induced cardiomyopathy*, and *broken heart syndrome*, is increasingly recognized and reported in the literature. Japanese physicians described a series of five patients with the condition in 1991.[127] The morphology of the LV during imaging studies in which apical akinesis (Fig. 18-33) was seen together with normal or hyperdynamic basal systolic function typically resembled a traditional Japanese octopus trapping jar, hence the term *takotsubo*. Commonly, patients would present with chest pain and other typical features of acute coronary syndrome (ACS) following a physically or emotionally stressful situation. Interestingly, sudden cardiac death following intensely stressful events had been reported decades earlier by Engel,[128] and a stress-induced cardiomyopathy has been postulated to explain some deaths in believers of voodoo.[129]

At presentation, TTCM can be difficult to distinguish from ACS. Chest pain is present in 70% to 90% of TTCM patients, along with elevation of cardiac biomarkers and ECG changes including ST-segment elevation and T-wave inversion.[130] The typical TTCM patient is a postmenopausal woman who presents shortly after a physically or psychologically stressful event. In one large series, 43% of patients developed cardiac symptoms following an acute medical condition such as stroke, surgery, or an asthma exacerbation.[131] Additionally, approximately one quarter of patients presented after an emotionally or physically stressful event. Other cases have been described in the setting of cocaine use, thyrotoxicosis, and opioid withdrawal.[130] Iatrogenic cases have also been reported. Abraham et al. noted TTCM features in nine patients after infusion of either epinephrine or dobutamine.[132]

Imaging studies in patients with TTCM have classically revealed akinesis of the LV apex, with preserved systolic function in the basal segments (Videos 18-10 to 18-12). However, variants of the condition in which akinesis of the middle or basal LV segments is found together with normal apical function are increasingly reported.[130] Thus, the term *apical ballooning syndrome* (and even the term *takotsubo*) may be misleading, since not all patients present with the classic LV morphology. Diagnostic criteria for TTCM have been proposed and include transient LV wall motion abnormalities that extend beyond a single coronary distribution, lack of obstructive CAD, new ECG changes or modest elevation of cardiac biomarkers, and no evidence of myocarditis or pheochromocytoma.[133] A TTCM diagnosis technically requires visualization of coronary anatomy. Reversibility of the condition over a period of days or weeks also suggests the diagnosis. In one study, the LVEF at presentation was 41% at admission and 64% at hospital discharge.[131] Mechanical complications such as LV rupture are rare, but up to 22% of patients may experience pulmonary edema, 15% suffer cardiogenic shock, and 9% experience VT or fibrillation.[130] Since basal LV systolic function may be hyperdynamic, SAM of the mitral valve and LVOT obstruction may be noted during echocardiographic examination.

The pathophysiology of TTCM centers on acute catecholamine excess. Although coronary spasm was originally postulated as a cause of the condition, experts now doubt that spasm plays an important role in the etiology of TTCM.[130] Cardiologists rarely note coronary spasm during angiography in these patients. Furthermore, acute ECG changes are often documented in the absence of spasm. Instead, investigators believe catecholamine-induced myocyte toxicity is likely produced by a cyclic adenosine monophosphate (cAMP)-mediated calcium overload.[129] The reason why some patients suffer TTCM while others who are exposed to similar potential triggers do not may be explained by specific β-receptor polymorphisms that have been noted in affected patients.[134] Specific polymorphisms may render affected patients more susceptible to catecholamine-triggered intracellular calcium overload.

Transient LV systolic dysfunction may be noted in patients suffering subarachnoid hemorrhage, those with critical illness, and in the setting of pheochromocytoma. It seems likely that the conditions that produce a surge in circulating catecholamines share similar pathophysiologic mechanisms and exist together with TTCM on the spectrum of stress-induced cardiomyopathies.

Terms such as *apical ballooning* and *takotsubo* were applied to some patients with apparent stress-induced cardiomyopathy because of the typical appearance of the LV during dynamic studies such as angiography or echocardiography. As already noted, initial reports described patients in whom the LV apex was akinetic or "ballooning" while the basal segments remained normal or showed hyperdynamic systolic function (see Videos 18-10 to 18-12).[129] However, experts now believe that transient systolic dysfunction may affect any level of the LV. Hence, apical function may appear normal while the middle or basal segments may be akinetic. Standard echocardiographic views are used to assess regional wall motion, including two-chamber, four-chamber, LAX, and SAX imaging. Ideally, regional wall motion abnormalities (RWMA) are confirmed in more than one view. One hallmark of TTCM is that RWMA is present in more than one coronary artery distribution.

Segmental RV systolic dysfunction may be present in a subset of TTCM patients. Akinesis of the middle or apical RV free wall may be revealed by echocardiographic examination. A careful inspection of the RV should be performed in all patients with suspected TTCM. RV dysfunction, if present, may portend a higher complication rate and increased length of hospital stay.[130]

Because basal LV systolic function may be hyperdynamic, the echocardiographer should perform a careful inspection of the mitral valve and LVOT to detect the presence of SAM and LVOT obstruction. Clearly, detection of SAM (Video 18-13) has important clinical implications. Patients with hypotension and suspected LV systolic dysfunction may be treated with infusions of inotropic agents, but these agents would potentially worsen the hemodynamic profile in the setting of dynamic LVOT obstruction.

Typical mechanical complications of ischemic heart disease are not expected in patients with TTCM. Findings suggesting VSD, myocardial rupture, rapidly expanding pericardial effusion, or papillary muscle rupture most likely indicate that the patient is suffering complications

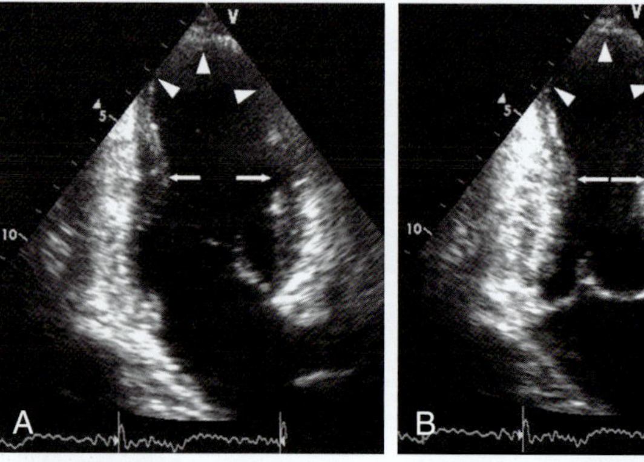

Figure 18-33   Transthoracic apical two-chamber view of patient with takotsubo cardiomyopathy. **A,** Diastolic frame. **B,** Systolic frame. Apex is akinetic *(arrowheads)* while systolic function of base and middle segments *(arrows)* is normal.

of acute coronary artery occlusive disease. A diagnosis of TTCM is much less likely in these situations.

As with any patient who is found to have an akinetic apex during echocardiographic examination, a thorough search for LV thrombus should be performed. LV apical thrombus is a potential complication in patients with TTCM, and anticoagulation may be required.

Conclusion

Genetic advancements have enabled clinicians to have a better understanding of the primary cardiomyopathies. There is hope that in the future, understanding the true molecular mechanisms responsible for disease expression will enhance development of more optimal care for affected individuals. Continued improvements in diagnostic measures will not only better define these entities, but provide future treatment strategies. The use of echocardiography will continue to be on the front line of diagnosis and management of these patients for years to come.

REFERENCES

1. Maron BJ, Towbin JA, Thiene G, et al. Contemporary definitions and classification of the cardiomyopathies: an American Heart Association Scientific Statement from the Council on Clinical Cardiology, Heart Failure and Transplantation Committee; Quality of Care and Outcomes Research and Functional Genomics and Translational Biology Interdisciplinary Working Groups; and Council on Epidemiology and Prevention. *Circulation*. 2006;113:1807-1816.
2. Hershberger RE, Lindenfeld J, Mestroni L, et al. Genetic evaluation of cardiomyopathy–a Heart Failure Society of America practice guideline. *J Cardiac Fail*. 2009;15:83-97.
3. Raju H, Alberg C, Sagoo GS, et al. Inherited cardiomyopathies. *BMJ*. 2011;343:d6966.
4. Saffitz JE. Arrhythmogenic cardiomyopathy: advances in diagnosis and disease pathogenesis. *Circulation*. 2011;124:e390-e392.
5. Elliott P, Andersson B, Arbustini E, et al. Classification of the cardiomyopathies: a position statement from the European Society Of Cardiology Working Group on Myocardial and Pericardial Diseases. *Eur Heart J*. 2008;29:270-276.
6. Kohli SK, Pantazis AA, Shah JS, et al. Diagnosis of left-ventricular non-compaction in patients with left-ventricular systolic dysfunction: time for a reappraisal of diagnostic criteria? *Eur Heart J*. 2008;29:89-95.
7. Ashrafian H, Watkins H. Reviews of translational medicine and genomics in cardiovascular disease: new disease taxonomy and therapeutic implications cardiomyopathies: therapeutics based on molecular phenotype. *J Am Coll Cardiol*. 2007;49:1251-1264.
8. Hershberger RE, Cowan J, Morales A, et al. Progress with genetic cardiomyopathies: screening, counseling, and testing in dilated, hypertrophic, and arrhythmogenic right ventricular dysplasia/cardiomyopathy. *Circ Heart Fail*. 2009;2:253-261.
9. Quarta G, Muir A, Pantazis A, et al. Familial evaluation in arrhythmogenic right ventricular cardiomyopathy: impact of genetics and revised task force criteria. *Circulation*. 2011;123:2701-2709.
10. Ackerman MJ, Priori SG, Willems S, et al. HRS/EHRA expert consensus statement on the state of genetic testing for the channelopathies and cardiomyopathies this document was developed as a partnership between the Heart Rhythm Society (HRS) and the European Heart Rhythm Association (EHRA). *Heart Rhythm*. 2011;8:1308-1339.
11. Givertz MM. Underlying causes and survival in patients with heart failure. *N Engl J Med*. 2000;342:1120-1122.
12. Luk A, Ahn E, Soor GS, et al. Dilated cardiomyopathy: a review. *J Clin Pathol*. 2009;62:219-225.
13. Aleksova A, Sabbadini G, Merlo M, et al. Natural history of dilated cardiomyopathy: from asymptomatic left ventricular dysfunction to heart failure–a subgroup analysis from the Trieste Cardiomyopathy Registry. *J Cardiovasc Med*. 2009;10:699-705.
14. Franz WM, Muller OJ, Katus HA. Cardiomyopathies: from genetics to the prospect of treatment. *Lancet*. 2001;358:1627-1637.
15. Elliott P. Cardiomyopathy. Diagnosis and management of dilated cardiomyopathy. *Heart*. 2000;84:106-112.
16. Park S-M, Park SW, Casaclang-Verzosa G, et al. Diastolic dysfunction and left atrial enlargement as contributing factors to functional mitral regurgitation in dilated cardiomyopathy: data from the Acorn trial. *Am Heart J*. 2009;157:762.e3-e10.
17. McBride BF, White CM. Acute decompensated heart failure: a contemporary approach to pharmacotherapeutic management. *Pharmacotherapy*. 2003;23:997-1020.
18. Patterson JH, Adams Jr KF. Pathophysiology of heart failure: changing perceptions. *Pharmacotherapy*. 1996;16:27S-36S.
19. Cheng V, Kazanagra R, Garcia A, et al. A rapid bedside test for B-type peptide predicts treatment outcomes in patients admitted for decompensated heart failure: a pilot study. *J Am Coll Cardiol*. 2001;37:386-391.
20. Oh JK, Seward JP, Tajik AJ. *The Echo Manual*. Journal 3rd ed. Baltimore, Md: Lippincott Williams & Wilkins; 2006.
21. Gelsomino S, van Garsse L, Luca F, et al. Impact of preoperative anterior leaflet tethering on the recurrence of ischemic mitral regurgitation and the lack of left ventricular reverse remodeling after restrictive annuloplasty. *J Am Soc Echocardiogr*. 2011;24:1365-1375.
22. Matsumoto K, Tanaka H, Okajima K, et al. Relation between left ventricular morphology and reduction in functional mitral regurgitation by cardiac resynchronization therapy in patients with idiopathic dilated cardiomyopathy. *Am J Cardiol*. 2011;108:1327-1334.
23. Sadeghpour A, Abtahi F, Kiavar M, et al. Echocardiographic evaluation of mitral geometry in functional mitral regurgitation. *J Cardiothorac Surg*. 2008;3:54.
24. La Vecchia L, Paccanaro M, Bonanno C, et al. Left ventricular versus biventricular dysfunction in idiopathic dilated cardiomyopathy. *Am J Cardiol*. 1999;83:120-122:A9.
25. Faris R, Coats AJ, Henein MY. Echocardiography-derived variables predict outcome in patients with nonischemic dilated cardiomyopathy with or without a restrictive filling pattern. *Am Heart J*. 2002;144:343-350.
26. Hunt SA. American College of Cardiology/American Heart Association Task Force on Practice Guidelines. ACC/AHA 2005 guideline update for the diagnosis and management of chronic heart failure in the adult: a report of the American College of Cardiology/American Heart Association Task Force on Practice Guidelines (Writing Committee to Update the 2001 Guidelines for the Evaluation and Management of Heart Failure). *J Am Coll Cardiol*. 2005;46:e1-e82.
27. Shivkumar K, Jafri SM, Gheorghiade M. Antithrombotic therapy in atrial fibrillation: a review of randomized trials with special reference to the Stroke Prevention in Atrial Fibrillation II (SPAF II) Trial. *Prog Cardiovasc Dis*. 1996;38:337-342.
28. Ng ACC, Sindone AP, Wong HSP, et al. Differences in management and outcome of ischemic and non-ischemic cardiomyopathy. *International Cardiol*. 2008;129:198-204.
29. Siu SC, Sole MJ. Dilated cardiomyopathy. *Curr Opin Cardiol*. 1994;9:337-343.
30. MERIT-HF Study Group. Effect of metoprolol CR/XL in chronic heart failure: Metoprolol CR/XL Randomised Intervention Trial in Congestive Heart Failure (MERIT-HF). *Lancet*. 1999;353:2001-2007.
31. Borggrefe M, Block M, Breithardt G. Identification and management of the high risk patient with dilated cardiomyopathy. *Br Heart J*. 1994;72(suppl):S42-S55.
32. Brachmann J, Hilbel T, Grunig E, et al. Ventricular arrhythmias in dilated cardiomyopathy. *PACE*. 1997;20:2714-2718.
33. O'Connell JB, Moore CK, Waterer HC. Treatment of end stage dilated cardiomyopathy. *Br Heart J*. 1994;72(suppl):S52-S56.
34. Connolly SJ, Hallstrom AP, Cappato R, et al. Meta-analysis of the implantable cardioverter defibrillator secondary prevention trials. AVID, CASH and CIDS studies. Antiarrhythmics vs Implantable Defibrillator study. Cardiac Arrest Study Hamburg. Canadian Implantable Defibrillator Study. *Eur Heart J*. 2000;21:2071-2078.
35. Kadish A, Dyer A, Daubert JP, et al. Prophylactic defibrillator implantation in patients with nonischemic dilated cardiomyopathy. *N Engl J Med*. 2004;350:2151-2158.
36. Tjang YS, van der Heijden GJMG, Tenderich G, et al. Impact of recipient's age on heart transplantation outcome. *Ann Thorac Surg*. 2008;85:2051-2055.
37. Rose EA, Moskowitz AJ, Packer M, et al. The REMATCH trial: rationale, design, and end points. Randomized Evaluation of Mechanical Assistance for the Treatment of Congestive Heart Failure. *Ann Thorac Surg*. 1999;67:723-730.
38. Romano MA, Bolling SF. Update on mitral repair in dilated cardiomyopathy. *J Card Surg*. 2004;19:396-400.
39. Maron BJ. Hypertrophic cardiomyopathy: a systematic review. *JAMA*. 2002;287:1308-1320.
40. Gersh BJ, Maron BJ, Bonow RO, et al. 2011 ACCF/AHA guideline for the diagnosis and treatment of hypertrophic cardiomyopathy: a report of the American College of Cardiology Foundation/American Heart Association Task Force on Practice Guidelines. *Circulation*. 2011;124:e783-e831.
41. Richardson P, McKenna W, Bristow M, et al. Report of the 1995 World Health Organization/International Society and Federation of Cardiology Task Force on the Definition and Classification of cardiomyopathies. *Circulation*. 1996;93:841-842.
42. Ommen SR. Hypertrophic cardiomyopathy. *Curr Probl Cardiol*. 2011;36:409-453.
43. Nishimura RA, Appleton CP, Redfield MM, et al. Noninvasive doppler echocardiographic evaluation of left ventricular filling pressures in patients with cardiomyopathies: a simultaneous Doppler echocardiographic and cardiac catheterization study. *J Am Coll Cardiol*. 1996;28:1226-1233.
44. Nagueh SF, Lakkis NM, Middleton KJ, et al. Doppler estimation of left ventricular filling pressures in patients with hypertrophic cardiomyopathy. *Circulation*. 1999;99:254-261.
45. Geske JB, Sorajja P, Nishimura RA, et al. Evaluation of left ventricular filling pressures by Doppler echocardiography in patients with hypertrophic cardiomyopathy: correlation with direct left atrial pressure measurement at cardiac catheterization. *Circulation*. 2007;116:2702-2708.
46. Geske JB, Sorajja P, Nishimura RA, et al. The relationship of left atrial volume and left atrial pressure in patients with hypertrophic cardiomyopathy: an echocardiographic and cardiac catheterization study. *J Am Soc Echocardiogr*. 2009;22:961-966.
47. Williams LK, Frenneaux MP, Steeds RP. Echocardiography in hypertrophic cardiomyopathy diagnosis, prognosis, and role in management. *Eur J Echocardiogr*. 2009;10:iii9-iii14.
48. Ommen SR, Nishimura RA. Hypertrophic cardiomyopathy. *Curr Probl Cardiol*. 2004;29:239-291.
49. Maron BJ, McKenna WJ, Danielson GK, et al. American College of Cardiology/European Society of Cardiology clinical expert consensus document on hypertrophic cardiomyopathy. A report of the American College of Cardiology Foundation Task Force on Clinical Expert Consensus Documents and the European Society of Cardiology Committee for Practice Guidelines. *J Am Coll Cardiol*. 2003;42:1687-1713.
50. Shapiro LM, McKenna WJ. Distribution of left ventricular hypertrophy in hypertrophic cardiomyopathy: a two-dimensional echocardiographic study. *J Am Coll Cardiol*. 1983;2:437-444.
51. Klues HG, Schiffers A, Maron BJ. Phenotypic spectrum and patterns of left ventricular hypertrophy in hypertrophic cardiomyopathy: morphologic observations and significance as assessed by two-dimensional echocardiography in 600 patients. *J Am Coll Cardiol*. 1995;26:1699-1708.
52. Roberts R, Sigwart U. New concepts in hypertrophic cardiomyopathies, part I. *Circulation*. 2001;104:2113-2116.
53. Maron MS, Olivotto I, Zenovich AG, et al. Hypertrophic cardiomyopathy is predominantly a disease of left ventricular outflow tract obstruction. *Circulation*. 2006;114:2232-2239.
54. Ommen SR, Shah PM, Tajik AJ. Left ventricular outflow tract obstruction in hypertrophic cardiomyopathy: past, present and future. *Heart*. 2008;94:1276-1281.
55. Kern MJ, Deligonul U. Interpretation of cardiac pathophysiology from pressure waveform analysis: III. Intraventricular pressure gradients. *Cathet Cardiovasc Diagn*. 1991;22:145-152.
56. Maron MS, Olivotto I, Betocchi S, et al. Effect of left ventricular outflow tract obstruction on clinical outcome in hypertrophic cardiomyopathy. *N Engl J Med*. 2003;348:295-303.
57. Cannon RO III, Dilsizian V, O'Gara PT, et al. Myocardial metabolic, hemodynamic, and electrocardiographic significance of reversible thallium-201 abnormalities in hypertrophic cardiomyopathy. *Circulation*. 1991;83:1660-1667.
58. Knaapen P, Germans T, Camici PG, et al. Determinants of coronary microvascular dysfunction in symptomatic hypertrophic cardiomyopathy. *Am J Physiol Heart Circ Physiol*. 2008;294:H986-H993.
59. Fifer MA, Vlahakes GJ. Management of symptoms in hypertrophic cardiomyopathy. *Circulation*. 2008;117:429-439.
60. Brown ML, Schaff HV. Surgical management of hypertrophic cardiomyopathy in 2007: what is new? *World J Surg*. 2008;32:350-354.
61. Sherrid MV, Chaudhry FA, Swistel DG. Obstructive hypertrophic cardiomyopathy: echocardiography, pathophysiology, and the continuing evolution of surgery for obstruction. *Ann Thorac Surg*. 2003;75:620-632.
62. Minakata K, Dearani JA, Nishimura RA, et al. Extended septal myectomy for hypertrophic obstructive cardiomyopathy with anomalous mitral papillary muscles or chordae. *J Thorac Cardiovasc Surg*. 2004;127:481-489.
63. Klues HG, Maron BJ, Dollar AL, et al. Diversity of structural mitral valve alterations in hypertrophic cardiomyopathy. *Circulation*. 1992;85:1651-1660.
64. Klues HG, Roberts WC, Maron BJ. Anomalous insertion of papillary muscle directly into anterior mitral leaflet in hypertrophic cardiomyopathy. Significance in producing left ventricular outflow obstruction. *Circulation*. 1991;84:1188-1197.
65. Ommen SR, Park SH, Click RL, et al. Impact of intraoperative transesophageal echocardiography in the surgical management of hypertrophic cardiomyopathy. *Am J Cardiol*. 2002;90:1022-1024.
66. Wan CKN, Dearani JA, Sundt TM III, et al. What is the best surgical treatment for obstructive hypertrophic cardiomyopathy and degenerative mitral regurgitation? *Ann Thorac Surg*. 2009;88:727-731:discussion 31–2.
67. Maron BJ, Yacoub M, Dearani JA. Controversies in cardiovascular medicine. Benefits of surgery in obstructive hypertrophic cardiomyopathy: bring septal myectomy back for European patients. *Eur Heart J*. 2011;32:1055-1058.

68. Louie EK, Edwards LC III. Hypertrophic cardiomyopathy. *Prog Cardiovasc Dis.* 1994;36:275-308.

69. Deb SJ, Schaff HV, Dearani JA, et al. Septal myectomy results in regression of left ventricular hypertrophy in patients with hypertrophic obstructive cardiomyopathy. *Ann Thorac Surg.* 2004;78:2118-2122.

70. Ommen SR, Maron BJ, Olivotto I, et al. Long-term effects of surgical septal myectomy on survival in patients with obstructive hypertrophic cardiomyopathy. *J Am Coll Cardiol.* 2005;46:470-476.

71. Biagini E, Spirito P, Leone O, et al. Heart transplantation in hypertrophic cardiomyopathy. *Am J Cardiol.* 2008;101:387-392.

72. Hagege AA, Desnos M. New trends in treatment of hypertrophic cardiomyopathy. *Arch Cardiovasc Dis.* 2009;102:441-447.

73. Maron BJ, Shen WK, Link MS, et al. Efficacy of implantable cardioverter-defibrillators for the prevention of sudden death in patients with hypertrophic cardiomyopathy. *N Engl J Med.* 2000;342:365-373.

74. Chang AC, McAreavey D, Fananapazir L. Identification of patients with hypertrophic cardiomyopathy at high risk for sudden death. *Curr Opin Cardiol.* 1995;10:9-15.

75. Maron BJ. Risk stratification and prevention of sudden death in hypertrophic cardiomyopathy. *Cardiol Rev.* 2002;10:173-181.

76. Brown ML, Schaff HV. Surgical management of obstructive hypertrophic cardiomyopathy: the gold standard. *Expert Rev Cardiovasc Ther.* 2008;6:715-722.

77. Melacini P, Maron BJ, Bobbo F, et al. Evidence that pharmacological strategies lack efficacy for the prevention of sudden death in hypertrophic cardiomyopathy. *Heart.* 2007;93:708-710.

78. Lin G, Nishimura RA, Gersh BJ, et al. Device complications and inappropriate implantable cardioverter defibrillator shocks in patients with hypertrophic cardiomyopathy. *Heart.* 2009;95:709-714.

79. Nishimura RA, Trusty JM, Hayes DL, et al. Dual-chamber pacing for hypertrophic cardiomyopathy: a randomized, double-blind, crossover trial. *J Am Coll Cardiol.* 1997;29:435-441.

80. Alam M, Dokainish H, Lakkis N. Alcohol septal ablation for hypertrophic obstructive cardiomyopathy: a systematic review of published studies. *J Interv Cardiol.* 2005;19:319-327.

81. Nagueh SF, Buergler JM, Quinones MA, et al. Outcome of surgical myectomy after unsuccessful alcohol septal ablation for the treatment of patients with hypertrophic obstructive cardiomyopathy. *J Am Coll Cardiol.* 2007;50:795-798.

82. Nishimura RA, Holmes Jr DR. Clinical practice. Hypertrophic obstructive cardiomyopathy. [Erratum appears in N Engl J Med. 2004 Sep 2;351(10):1038.]. *N Engl J Med.* 2004;350:1320-1327.

83. Ammash NM, Seward JB, Bailey KR, et al. Clinical profile and outcome of idiopathic restrictive cardiomyopathy. *Circulation.* 2000;101:2490-2496.

84. Stollberger C, Finsterer J. Extracardiac medical and neuromuscular implications in restrictive cardiomyopathy. *Clin Cardiol.* 2007;30:375-380.

85. Mogensen J, Arbustini E. Restrictive cardiomyopathy. *Curr Opin Cardiol.* 2009;24:214-220.

86. Kushwaha SS, Fallon JT, Fuster V. Restrictive cardiomyopathy. *N Engl J Med.* 1997;336:267-276.

87. Nihoyannopoulos P, Dawson D. Restrictive cardiomyopathies. *Eur J Echocardiogr.* 2009;10:iii23-iii33.

88. Chatterjee K, Alpert J. Constrictive pericarditis and restrictive cardiomyopathy: similarities and differences. *Heart Fail Monit.* 2003;3:118-126.

89. Hancock EW. Differential diagnosis of restrictive cardiomyopathy and constrictive pericarditis. *Heart.* 2001;86:343-349.

90. Nagueh SF, Appleton CP, Gillebert TC, et al. Recommendations for the evaluation of left ventricular diastolic function by echocardiography. *J Am Soc Echocardiogr.* 2009;22:107-133.

91. Ha JW, Ommen SR, Tajik AJ, et al. Differentiation of constrictive pericarditis from restrictive cardiomyopathy using mitral annular velocity by tissue Doppler echocardiography. *Am J Cardiol.* 2004;94:316-319.

92. McCall R, Stoodley PW, Richards DAB, et al. Restrictive cardiomyopathy versus constrictive pericarditis: making the distinction using tissue Doppler imaging. *Eur J Echocardiogr.* 2008;9:591-594.

93. Talreja DR, Nishimura RA, Oh JK, et al. Constrictive pericarditis in the modern era: novel criteria for diagnosis in the cardiac catheterization laboratory. *J Am Coll Cardiol.* 2008;51:315-319.

94. From AM, Maleszewski JJ, Rihal CS. Current status of endomyocardial biopsy. *Mayo Clin Proc.* 2011;86:1095-1102.

95. Wilmshurst PT, Katritsis D. Restrictive cardiomyopathy. *Br Heart J.* 1990;63:323-324.

96. Seifert FC, Miller DC, Oesterle SN, et al. Surgical treatment of constrictive pericarditis: Analysis of outcome diagnostic error. *Circulation.* 1985;72(suppl 2):II264-II273.

97. Dubrey SW, Cha K, Simms RW, et al. Electrocardiography and Doppler echocardiography in secondary (AA) amyloidosis. *Am J Cardiol.* 1996;77:313-315.

98. Rahman JE, Helou EF, Gelzer-Bell R, et al. Noninvasive diagnosis of biopsy-proven cardiac amyloidosis. *J Am Coll Cardiol.* 2004;43:410-415.

99. Feng D, Syed IS, Martinez M, et al. Intracardiac thrombosis and anticoagulation therapy in cardiac amyloidosis. *Circulation.* 2009;119:2490-2497.

100. Palka P, Lange A, Donnelly JE, et al. Doppler tissue echocardiographic features of cardiac amyloidosis. *J Am Soc Echocardiogr.* 2002;15:1353-1360.

101. Koyama J, Ray-Sequin PA, Falk RH. Longitudinal myocardial function assessed by tissue velocity, strain, and strain rate tissue Doppler echocardiography in patients with AL (primary) cardiac amyloidosis. *Circulation.* 2003;107:2446-2452.

102. Carroll JD, Gaasch WH, McAdam KP. Amyloid cardiomyopathy: characterization by a distinctive voltage/mass relation. *Am J Cardiol.* 1982;49:9-13.

103. Hardy WR, Anderson RE. The hypereosinophilic syndromes. *Ann Intern Med.* 1968;68:1220-1229.

104. Klion AD, Bochner BS, Gleich GJ, et al. Approaches to the treatment of hypereosinophilic syndromes: a workshop summary report. *J Allergy Clin Immunol.* 2006;117:1292-1302.

105. Ducharme MB, Lounsbury DS. Self-rescue swimming in cold water: the latest advice. *Appl Physiol Nutr Metab.* 2007;32:799-807.

106. Marcus FI, Zareba W, Calkins H, et al. Arrhythmogenic right ventricular cardiomyopathy/dysplasia clinical presentation and diagnostic evaluation: results from the North American Multidisciplinary Study. *Heart Rhythm.* 2009;6:984-992.

107. Fontaine GH. The multiple facets of right ventricular cardiomyopathies. *Eur Heart J.* 2011;32:1049-1051.

108. El Demellawy D, Nasr AA, Loawmi S. An updated review on the clinicopathologic aspects of arrhythmogenic right ventricular cardiomyopathy. *Am J Forensic Med Pathol.* 2009;30:78-83.

109. Pinamonti B, Dragos AM, Pyxaras SA, et al. Prognostic predictors in arrhythmogenic right ventricular cardiomyopathy: results from a 10-year registry. *Eur Heart J.* 2011;32:1105-1113.

110. Sarvari SI, Haugaa KH, Anfinsen O-G, et al. Right ventricular mechanical dispersion is related to malignant arrhythmias: a study of patients with arrhythmogenic right ventricular cardiomyopathy and subclinical right ventricular dysfunction. *Eur Heart J.* 2011;32:1089-1096.

111. Marcus FI, McKenna WJ, Sherrill D, et al. Diagnosis of arrhythmogenic right ventricular cardiomyopathy/dysplasia: proposed modification of the task force criteria. *Circulation.* 2010;121:1533-1541.

112. Corrado D, Basso C, Thiene G, et al. Spectrum of clinicopathologic manifestations of arrhythmogenic right ventricular cardiomyopathy/dysplasia: a multicenter study. *J Am Coll Cardiol.* 1997;30:1512-1520.

113. Tops LF, Prakasa K, Tandri H, et al. Prevalence and pathophysiologic attributes of ventricular dyssynchrony in arrhythmogenic right ventricular dysplasia/cardiomyopathy. *J Am Coll Cardiol.* 2009;54:445-451.

114. Asimaki A, Tandri H, Huang H, et al. A new diagnostic test for arrhythmogenic right ventricular cardiomyopathy. *New Engl J Med.* 2009;360:1075-1084.

115. Yoerger DM, Marcus F, Sherrill D, et al. Echocardiographic findings in patients meeting task force criteria for arrhythmogenic right ventricular dysplasia: new insights from the multidisciplinary study of right ventricular dysplasia. *J Am Coll Cardiol.* 2005;45:860-865.

116. Sviggum HP, Kopp SL, Rettke SR, et al. Perioperative complications in patients with left ventricular non-compaction. *Eur J Anaesthesiol.* 2011;28:207-212.

117. Pantazis AA, Elliott PM. Left ventricular noncompaction. *Curr Opin Cardiol.* 2009;24:209-213.

118. Eidem BW. Noninvasive evaluation of left ventricular noncompaction: what's new in 2009? *Pediatr Cardiol.* 2009;30:682-689.

119. Oechslin EN, Attenhofer Jost CH, Rojas JR, et al. Long-term follow-up of 34 adults with isolated left ventricular noncompaction: a distinct cardiomyopathy with poor prognosis. *J Am Coll Cardiol.* 2000;36:493-500.

120. Saleeb SF, Margossian R, Spencer CT, et al. Reproducibility of echocardiographic diagnosis of left ventricular noncompaction. *J Am Soc Echocardiogr.* 2012;25:194-202.

121. Sandhu R, Finkelhor RS, Gunawardena DR, et al. Prevalence and characteristics of left ventricular noncompaction in a community hospital cohort of patients with systolic dysfunction. *Echocardiography.* 2008;25:8-12.

122. Stollberger C, Finsterer J. A diagnostic dilemma in non-compaction, resulting in near expulsion from the Football World Cup. *Eur J Echocardiogr.* 2011;12:E8.

123. Chin TK, Perloff JK, Williams RG, et al. Isolated noncompaction of left ventricular myocardium. A study of eight cases. *Circulation.* 1990;82:507-513.

124. Jenni R, Oechslin E, Schneider J, et al. Echocardiographic and pathoanatomical characteristics of isolated left ventricular non-compaction: a step towards classification as a distinct cardiomyopathy. *Heart.* 2001;86:666-671.

125. Stollberger C, Finsterer J, Blazek G. Left ventricular hypertrabeculation/noncompaction and association with additional cardiac abnormalities and neuromuscular disorders. *Am J Cardiol.* 2002;90:899-902.

126. McMahon CJ, Pignatelli RH, Nagueh SF, et al. Left ventricular non-compaction cardiomyopathy in children: characterisation of clinical status using tissue Doppler-derived indices of left ventricular diastolic relaxation. *Heart.* 2007;93:676-681.

127. Dote K, Sato H, Tateishi H, et al. [Myocardial stunning due to simultaneous multivessel coronary spasms: a review of 5 cases]. [Article in Japanese] *J Cardiol.* 1991;21:203-214.

128. Engel GL. Sudden and rapid death during psychological stress. Folklore or folk wisdom? *Ann Intern Med.* 1971;74:771-782.

129. Richard C. Stress-related cardiomyopathies. *Ann Intensive Care.* 2011;1:39.

130. Hurst RT, Prasad A, Askew JW III, et al. Takotsubo cardiomyopathy: a unique cardiomyopathy with variable ventricular morphology. *JACC Cardiovasc Imaging.* 2010;3:641-649.

131. Tsuchihashi K, Ueshima K, Uchida T, et al. Transient left ventricular apical ballooning without coronary artery stenosis: a novel heart syndrome mimicking acute myocardial infarction. Angina pectoris-myocardial infarction investigations in Japan. *J Am Coll Cardiol.* 2001;38:11-18.

132. Abraham J, Mudd JO, Kapur NK, et al. Stress cardiomyopathy after intravenous administration of catecholamines and beta-receptor agonists. *J Am Coll Cardiol.* 2009;53:1320-1325.

133. Prasad A, Lerman A, Rihal CS. Apical ballooning syndrome (Tako-Tsubo or stress cardiomyopathy): a mimic of acute myocardial infarction. *Am Heart J.* 2008;155:408-417.

134. Spinelli L, Trimarco V, Di Marino S, et al. L41Q polymorphism of the G protein coupled receptor kinase 5 is associated with left ventricular apical ballooning syndrome. *Eur J Heart Fail.* 2010;12:13-16.

Aneurysms and Dissections

JOHN G. AUGOUSTIDES | ALBERT T. CHEUNG

Thoracic Aorta

The thoracic aorta can be comprehensively evaluated by transesophageal echocardiography (TEE).[1] Aneurysms and dissections of the aorta produce structural lesions that are readily detectable by TEE in high resolution, owing to the close anatomic relationship between the esophagus and aorta. This is limited, however, in the distal ascending aorta and proximal aortic arch because the trachea lies between the esophagus and aorta, rendering TEE blind to these aortic segments.[2] This blind spot of TEE can be eliminated with epiaortic imaging, which together with epicardial imaging complements TEE for evaluation of aortic diseases.[3-5]

TEE is a high-quality imaging modality for aortic evaluation.[6] Firstly, TEE is indispensable for emergency evaluation of clinically unstable patients with acute aortic syndromes.[6-7] Secondly, TEE, including three-dimensional (3D) imaging, can also detect complications of aortic dissection such as pericardial tamponade, aortic regurgitation, and myocardial ischemia.[8] Thirdly, TEE can guide surgical decision making before and after aortic intervention.[6-8]

Although TEE is feasible in awake patients, topical anesthesia and sedation must be adequate to prevent aortic rupture from hypertensive responses during TEE examination.[9] Although TEE is safe during general endotracheal anesthesia, giant aortic aneurysms may still render TEE hazardous. The risk of esophageal perforation during TEE examination may be higher due to extrinsic esophageal compression.[10] Furthermore, insertion of a TEE probe may aggravate pulmonary artery and/or major airway compression, precipitating severe hypoxemia from ventilation/perfusion mismatch.[11,12]

Anatomy of the Aorta

Aortic Wall

The aortic wall consists of three layers: outer adventitia, middle media, and inner intima. Under normal circumstances, TEE cannot distinguish these layers. Diseases such as dissection and atheroma alter aortic wall anatomy. In aortic dissection, the intimal layer separates from the adventitia as the false lumen develops. Aortic atherosclerosis injures the intima to cause thickening, calcification, and ulceration.

The aortic adventitia is the thin outermost collagenous layer that contains the vasa vasorum and nerves. Although it is thin, its rich collagen content gives the adventitia the greatest tensile strength of the three aortic wall layers. The aortic media is the thick middle layer between the adventitia and intima. The media normally accounts for up 80% of the aortic wall thickness and consists of elastic tissue intertwined with muscle fibers. The aortic intima is the thin inner wall layer, characterized histologically by a basement membrane lined with endothelium that is in direct contact with the blood. Because of its delicate structure, the intima is most susceptible to injury.

Aortic Segments

The aorta begins at the ventricular-aortic junction with the aortic valve and terminates in the abdomen when it bifurcates into the common iliac arteries. The major aortic segments are the aortic root, ascending aorta, aortic arch, descending thoracic aorta, and abdominal aorta.

The *aortic root* begins at the ventricular-aortic junction and terminates at the sinotubular junction. The aortic root complex consists of the aortic valve annulus, aortic valve cusps, sinuses of Valsalva (sinus segment), and sinotubular junction, where the sinus segment joins the tubular ascending aorta. The aortic root and proximal ascending aorta lie within the pericardium. The weakest area of the aortic wall is the sinus segment. These anatomic relationships are important because aortic rupture at this level will be intrapericardial and cause acute cardiac tamponade. The aortic root components are clearly demonstrated by TEE in the midesophageal (ME) aortic valve long-axis view, where their diameters can be precisely quantified (Fig. 19-1).[13] The aortic valve cusps and their corresponding sinuses of Valsalva are described by their anatomic relationship to the coronary artery ostia as follows: right coronary, left coronary, and noncoronary. The aortic root complex is also known as the *functional aortic annulus*, since alterations in one or more of its components can produce aortic regurgitation.[13]

The *ascending aorta* is defined as the tubular aorta that ascends from the sinotubular junction to join the aortic arch at the origin of the innominate artery. The ascending aorta can be imaged in both short and long axis at the level of the right pulmonary artery (Fig. 19-2). As explained earlier, TEE fails to interrogate the distal ascending aorta and proximal aortic arch owing to the attenuation of ultrasound imaging across the air-filled trachea.[2]

The *aortic arch* contains the origins of the brachiocephalic vessels— the innominate, left carotid, and left subclavian arteries (Fig. 19-3). Anatomic variations in aortic arch branch vessel anatomy have a collective incidence as high as 25%.[14] The most frequent variant pattern (with a 20% incidence) is the *bovine arch*, defined as a common origin for the innominate and left common carotid arteries.[15]

The *descending thoracic aorta* extends from the left subclavian artery to the diaphragmatic hiatus (Fig. 19-4). Its major branches are the paired intercostal arteries that contribute substantially to the spinal cord collateral network. The aortic isthmus lies just beyond the origin of the left subclavian artery at the site of the ligamentum arteriosum, a vestige of the fetal ductus arteriosus. The aortic isthmus is the most common location for aortic coarctation, patent ductus arteriosus (PDA), and traumatic intimal disruptions.

The *abdominal aorta* begins at the diaphragmatic hiatus and terminates at the aortic bifurcation where it gives rise to the common iliac arteries. Its major branches include the celiac trunk, superior mesenteric artery, renal arteries, inferior mesenteric artery, and lumbar segmental arteries.

Aortic Segmental Anatomy for Thoracic Endovascular Aortic Repair

Aortic Arch

The proximal thoracic aorta is divided into five anatomic zones that describe the landing zone for thoracic aortic endovascular repair (TEVAR) (Fig. 19-5).[16] Zone 0 is defined as the ascending aorta and proximal aortic arch to the innominate artery. Zone 1 is defined as the aortic segment between the innominate and left carotid arteries. Zone 2 is defined as the aortic segment between the left common carotid artery and the left subclavian artery. Zone 3 is defined as the curved segment of the distal aortic arch and proximal descending thoracic aorta beyond the left subclavian artery. Zone 4 is defined as the straight part of the descending thoracic aorta from the level of the 4th thoracic vertebra.

Although zones 2 through 4 are accessible landing zones for TEVAR, a zone 2 landing requires left subclavian coverage that often prompts

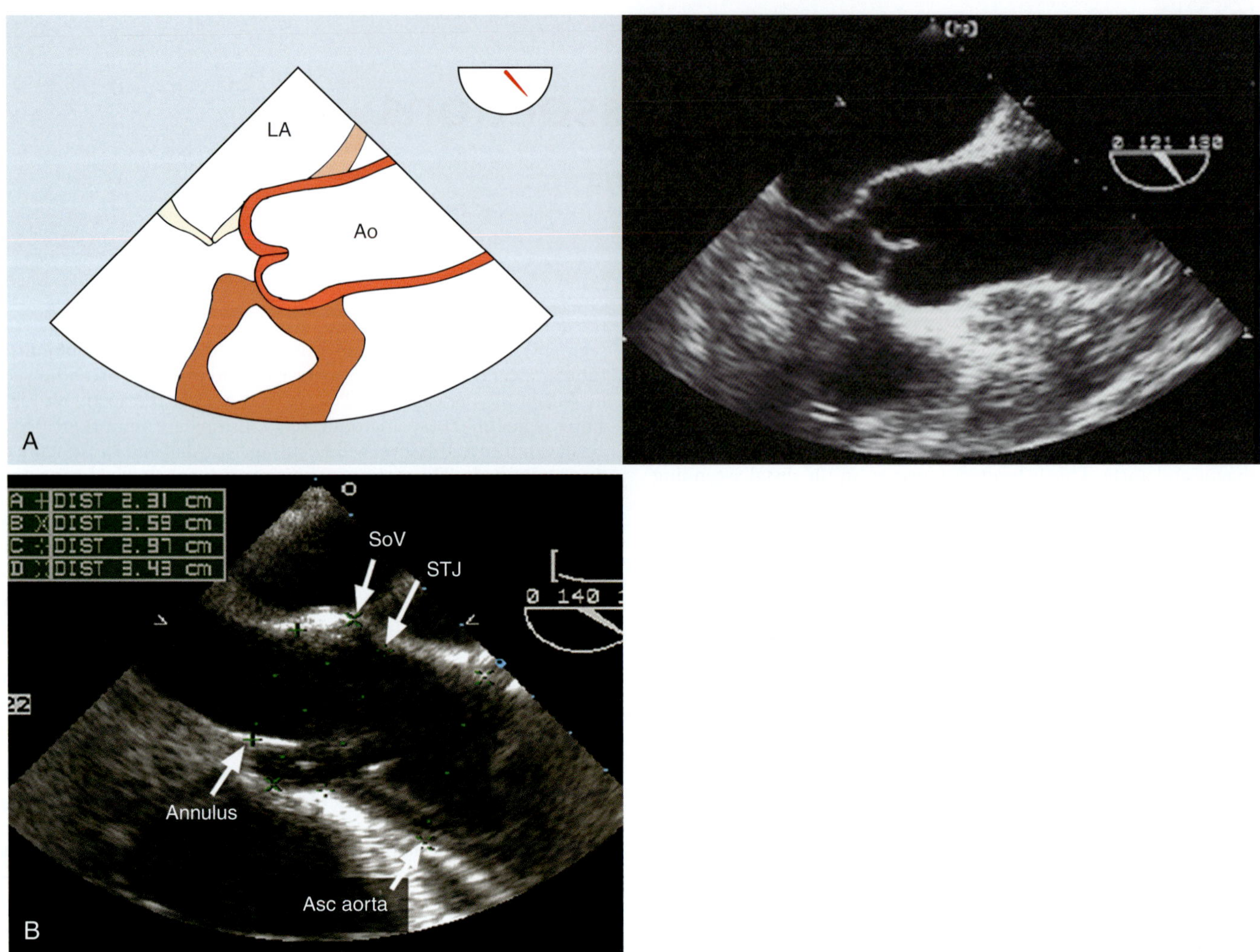

Figure 19-1   **A,** Midesophageal (ME) aortic valve long-axis view at a multiplane angle of 121 degrees. This view images aortic root in cross-section and is ideal for quantifying diameters of aortic root at the levels of aortic valve annulus, sinuses of Valsalva, and sinotubular junction. **B,** ME aortic valve long-axis image at a multiplane angle of 140 degrees. Patient has a Stanford type A aortic dissection characterized by an intimal flap originating in aortic root and extending into ascending aorta *(Asc aorta)*. Aortic diameters were quantified as follows: A, aortic valve annulus; B, sinuses of Valsalva; C, sinotubular junction; and D, ascending aorta. *Ao,* Aorta; *LA,* left atrium; *SoV,* sinuses of Valsalva; *STJ,* sinotubular junction. *(Adapted from Cheung AT, Weiss SJ. Diseases of the aorta. In: Oxorn DC, ed.* Intraoperative Echocardiography. *Philadelphia: Saunders; 2012:161-182.)*

an ancillary vascular procedure to minimize the risks of stroke and upper extremity ischemia.[17,18] Zones 0 and 1 landings require debranching of the brachiocephalic vessels prior to TEVAR to maintain cerebral perfusion.[19] These techniques are collectively termed *hybrid aortic arch repair*.[19]

Descending Thoracic Aorta

The descending thoracic aorta has also been classified into three types of coverage with respect to TEVAR.[20,21] Type A coverage extends from the left subclavian artery to the level of the 6th thoracic vertebra.[20,21] Type B coverage extends from the level of the 6th thoracic vertebra to the diaphragmatic hiatus.[20,21] Type C coverage extends from the left subclavian artery to the diaphragmatic hiatus.[20,21]

Important Anatomic Relationships of the Aorta

The anatomic relationships between the thoracic aorta and esophagus are clinically important (Fig. 19-6). The aortic root and proximal ascending aorta lie within the pericardium, explaining the risk for cardiac tamponade in acute aortic dissection (Fig. 19-7). Since these aortic segments also lie anterior to the esophagus and left atrium, they are clearly imaged by TEE, with the left atrium providing the acoustic

window (see Fig. 19-1). The right pulmonary artery courses between the esophagus and ascending aorta, providing an acoustic window and anatomic reference for TEE imaging of the ascending aorta (see Figs. 19-1 and 19-2).

Since the ascending aorta initially lies directly anterior to the esophagus, it is clearly visualized during TEE imaging. The distal trachea and left mainstem bronchus obstruct TEE imaging of the distal ascending aorta and proximal aortic arch because they course between the esophagus and these two aortic segments (see Fig. 19-6). The descending thoracic aorta is initially anterior to the esophagus, then lateral to the esophagus in the mid-thorax, then posterior to the esophagus at the diaphragmatic hiatus (see Fig. 19-6). Despite this changing anatomic relationship with the esophagus, the descending thoracic aorta can be imaged clearly by TEE throughout its entire length.

Normal Size of the Aorta

Although there are guidelines for the normal aortic segment dimensions, these normal values vary according to age, gender, and body size (Table 19-1).[6,22,23] The aortic diameter is greatest in the sinus segment and then tapers gradually beyond the sinotubular junction (see Table 19-1). Recent thoracic aortic guidelines recommend that aortic

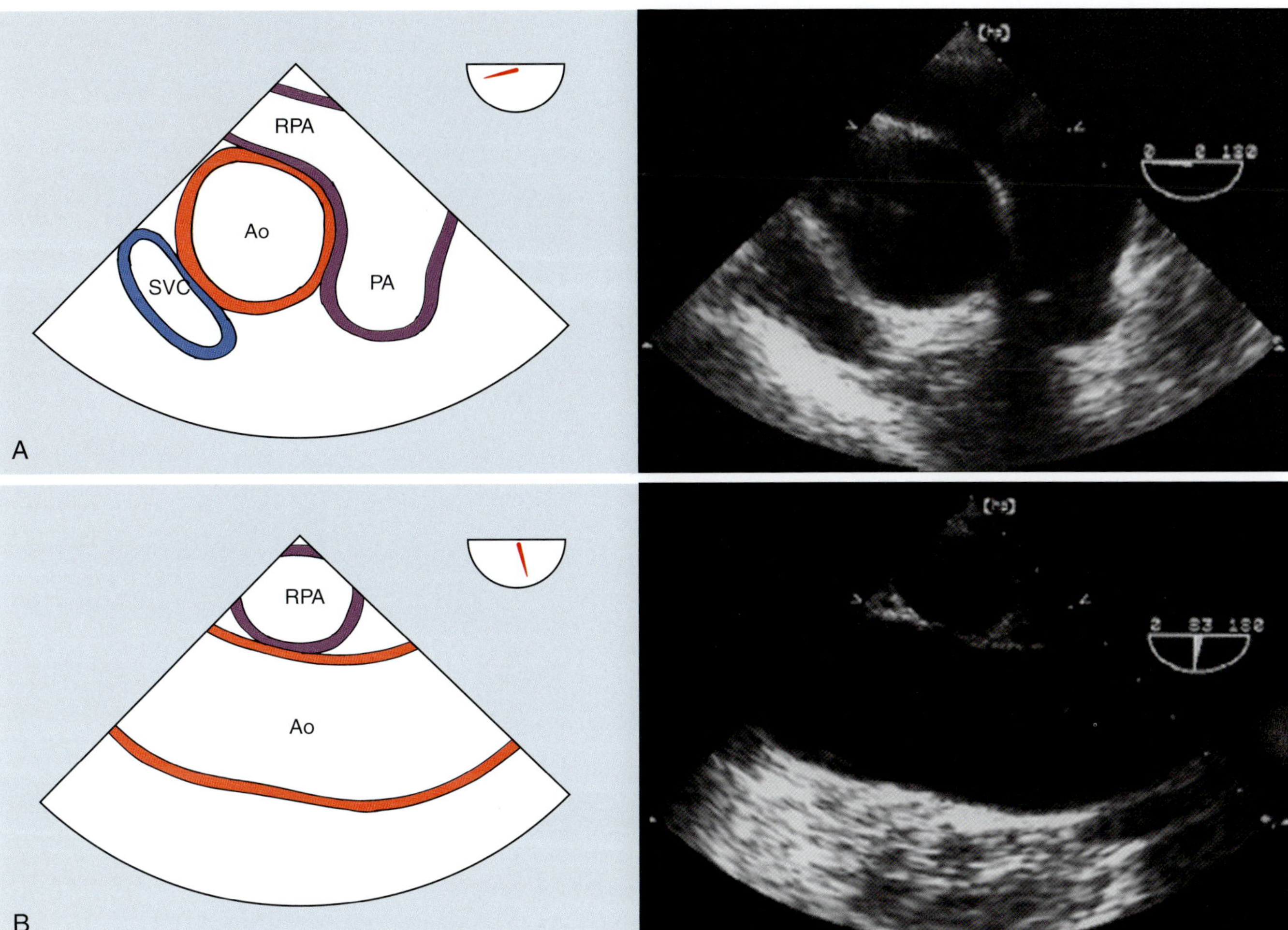

Figure 19-2 *A,* Midesophageal (ME) ascending aortic short-axis view with a multiplane angle in the 30-degree range. Ascending aorta can be clearly assessed for dissection and aneurysm. This view provides the opportunity to measure ascending aortic diameter at level of right pulmonary artery. *B,* ME ascending aortic long-axis view at a multiplane angle of 83 degrees. This view facilitates analysis of ascending aorta at level of right pulmonary artery with regard to dimensions, dissection, aneurysm, atheroma, calcification, and rupture. *Ao,* Aorta; *PA,* main pulmonary artery; *RPA,* right pulmonary artery; *SVC,* superior vena cava. (See Video 19-1.) *(Adapted from Cheung AT, Weiss SJ. Diseases of the aorta. In: Oxorn DC, ed. Intraoperative Echocardiography. Philadelphia: Saunders; 2012:161-182.)*

diameter determinations be performed perpendicular to the axis of blood flow (Class I Recommendation; Level C Evidence [Fig. 19-8]).[6] Furthermore, echocardiographic determination of aortic diameter should measure the internal diameter (intima to intima) perpendicular to the direction of blood flow (Class I Recommendation; Level C Evidence [see Fig. 19-8]).[6] At the aortic root level, the echocardiographic determination should use the widest diameter, which is typically at the mid-sinus level (Class I Recommendation; Level C Evidence).[6] Since aortic diameters measured by computed tomography (CT) are determined from adventitia to adventitia perpendicular to the axis of blood flow, aortic diameters measured by echocardiography are typically slightly smaller (see Fig. 19-8).

Definitions of Aortic Enlargement

According to recent guidelines, the spectrum of aortic enlargement is clearly defined.[6] An *aortic aneurysm* (or *true aneurysm*) is defined as a focal permanent aortic dilation with a diameter greater than 50% the normal diameter for that aortic segment.[6] Although a true aneurysm has all three aortic wall layers, the intima and media may be so attenuated in giant aneurysms that they are undetectable. An *aortic pseudoaneurysm* (or *false aneurysm*) results from aortic rupture, and its wall consists of periarterial connective tissue rather than all the aortic wall layers.[6] If a pseudoaneurysm freely communicates with the intravascular space, it is also termed a *pulsating hematoma*. *Aortic ectasia* is defined as aortic dilation less than 150% of the expected diameter for that aortic segment.[6] *Aortomegaly* is defined as aneurysmal involvement of two or more aortic segments.[6]

Thoracic Aortic Imaging with TEE

A Systematic Stepwise Approach (Box 19-1)

First, image the aortic root in the ME short-axis aortic valve view. Identify the aortic valve cusps, their calcification pattern, their mobility profiles, and measure the aortic valve area. Interrogate the aortic valve with color flow Doppler to assess for aortic regurgitation in relation to the valve cusps. Furthermore, examine the origins of the right and left coronary arteries.

Second, image the aorta in the ME long-axis aortic valve view (Fig. 19-9; also see Fig. 19-1, *A*). Measure the aortic root diameters from intima to intima (see Fig. 19-1, *B*). Analyze aortic valve cusp mobility, aortic root calcification, and the extent of sinotubular junction disease. Interrogate the aortic valve with color Doppler imaging to assess for presence and severity of aortic regurgitation.

Third, image the proximal ascending aorta in short axis at the level of the right pulmonary artery by withdrawing and anteflexing the TEE probe from the aortic valve level (see Fig. 19-2, *A*). Determine the

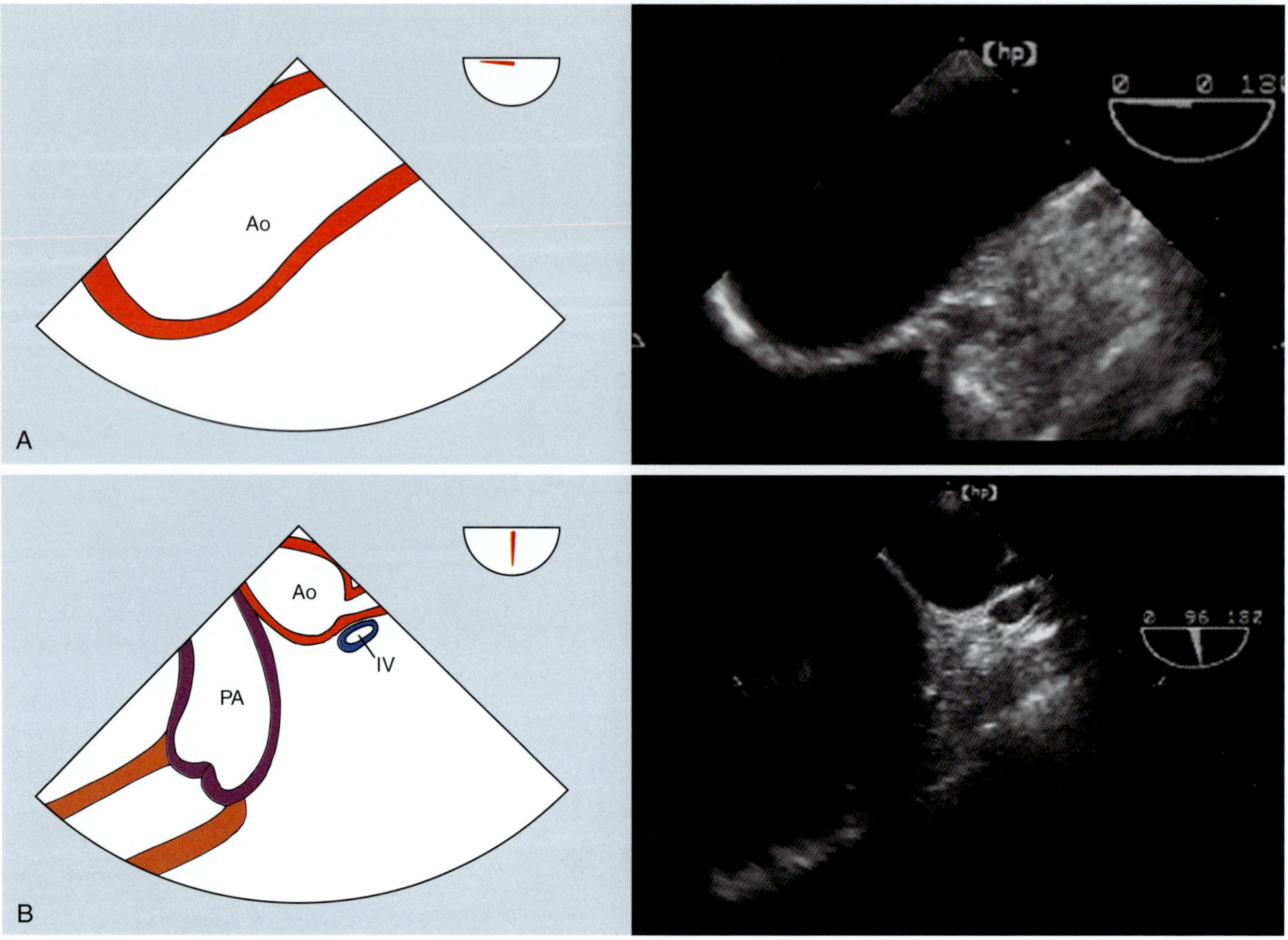

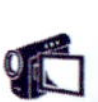

Figure 19-3   **A,** Upper esophageal (UE) aortic arch long-axis view at a multiplane angle of 0 degrees. This view interrogates distal aortic arch and facilitates detection of dissection and/or aneurysm in aortic arch. **B,** UE aortic arch short-axis view at a multiplane angle of 86 degrees. This view interrogates distal aortic arch and frequently images pulmonary artery, innominate vein, subclavian artery origin, and left carotid artery origin. This view facilitates detection of aortic arch branch involvement with dissection or aneurysm. *Ao,* Aorta; *IV,* innominate vein; *PA,* main pulmonary artery. (See Video 19-2.) *(Adapted from Cheung AT, Weiss SJ. Diseases of the aorta. In: Oxorn DC, ed.* Intraoperative Echocardiography. *Philadelphia: Saunders; 2012:161-182.)*

diameter of the ascending aorta at this level. Examine the aortic wall for signs of atheroma, calcification, and dissection. Remember that the distal ascending aorta and the proximal aortic arch lie in the blind spot of TEE.[1,2] Image the proximal ascending aorta in long axis at this level by multiplane rotation to about 90 degrees (see Fig. 19-2, *B*). Measure the ascending aortic diameter, and assess the aortic wall for signs of atheroma, calcification, and dissection.

Fourth, image the descending thoracic aorta in short axis (see Fig. 19-4, *A*). Determine the aortic diameter and assess for atherosclerosis, aneurysm, dissection, and pleural effusion (see Fig. 19-4, *A*). Image the descending thoracic aorta in long axis at this level, with multiplane rotation to approximately 90 degrees (see Fig. 19-4, *B*). This view facilitates close examination of the aortic intima for signs of disease.

Fifth, interrogate the distal descending thoracic aorta to the diaphragmatic level as the TEE probe is gradually advanced and rotated counterclockwise. The proximal descending thoracic aorta can be interrogated as the TEE probe is gradually withdrawn and rotated clockwise. In this fashion, the entire extent of this aortic segment can be examined, noting that the distal aortic arch is typically 20 to 25 cm from the incisors, the mid-descending thoracic aorta at 30 to 35 cm from the incisors, and the diaphragm at 40 to 45 cm from the incisors. As the aorta is imaged distally, its pulsatility and diameter decrease, especially in the setting of aortic valve disease.[24,25] The TEE descending

aortic short-axis views also permit detection of left pleural effusions that layer adjacent to the aorta in a supine patient.

Sixth, examine the distal aortic arch as the TEE probe is withdrawn from imaging the distal descending thoracic aorta, noting the distances from the incisors. A long-axis view of the distal aortic arch is typically depicted at a 0-degree multiplane angle (see Fig. 19-3, *A*). A short-axis view of the distal aortic arch will be displayed by multiplane rotation to 90 degrees (see Fig. 19-3, *B*). The origins of the brachiocephalic vessels (most often the left subclavian artery) can be sought by rotating the TEE probe clockwise from left to right as the aortic arch is imaged. Color flow Doppler imaging can frequently image blood flow in the brachiocephalic vessels by decreasing the Nyquist limit as needed, since flow is often laminar and off-axis to the ultrasound beam. These views allow detailed assessment of the distal aortic arch with respect to diameter, aneurysm formation, dissection, and atheroma. The upper esophageal aortic arch short-axis view may also display the long-axis view of the pulmonic valve and main pulmonary artery as well as the innominate vein in short-axis (Fig. 19-10).

Imaging Artifacts During Echocardiographic Aortic Imaging

Imaging artifacts during echocardiographic evaluation are common, especially in the lumen of a dilated ascending aorta. Since motion

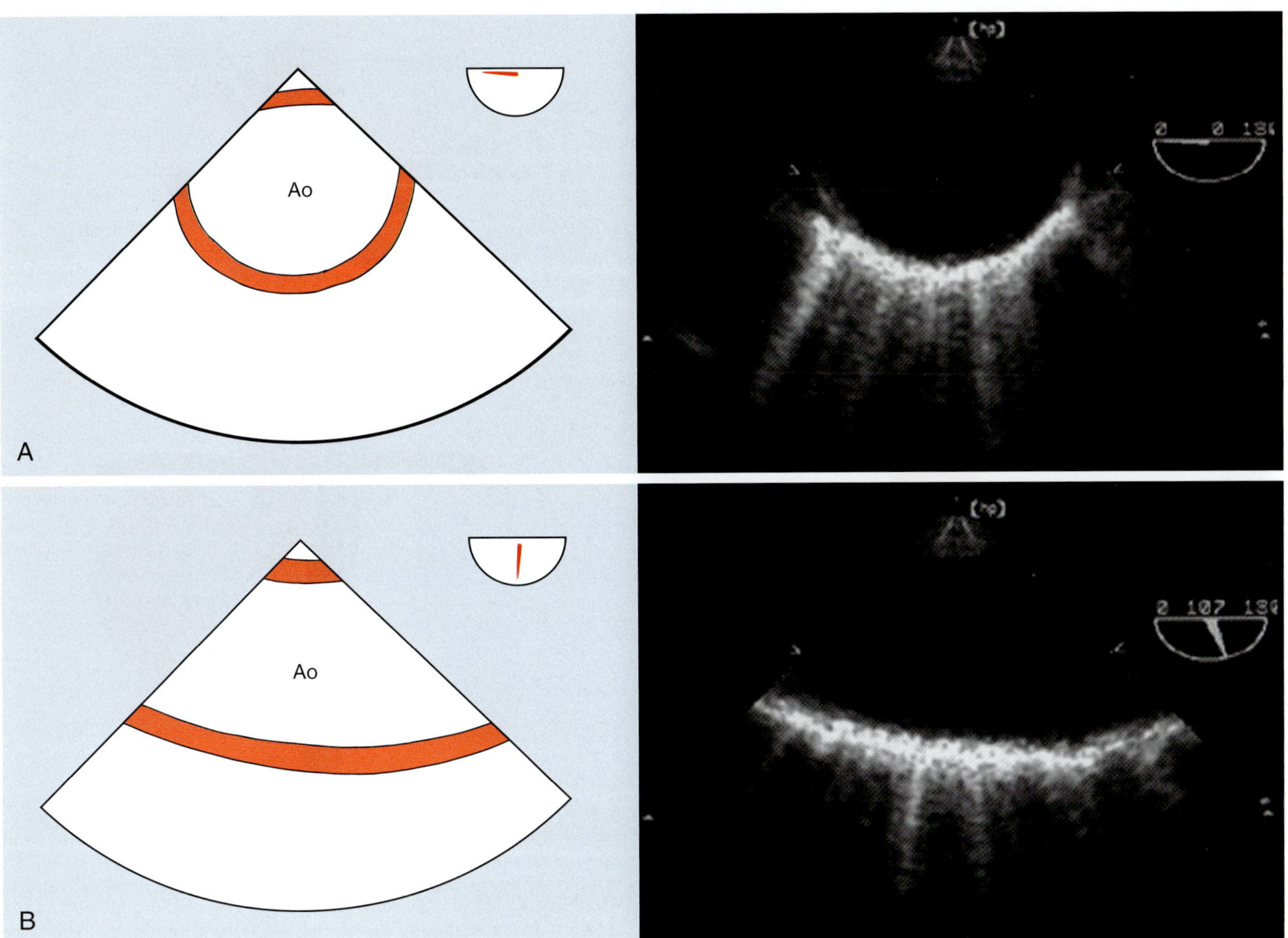

Figure 19-4 **A,** Midesophageal (ME) descending aortic short-axis view at a multiplane angle of 0 degrees. It facilitates determination of descending aortic diameter. Entire descending thoracic aorta can be evaluated for dissection and aneurysm by manipulating TEE probe along the length of this aortic segment. **B,** ME descending aortic long-axis view at a multiplane angle of 107 degrees. It provides an opportunity for detailed interrogation of intimal surface of descending thoracic aorta. *Ao,* Aorta. *(Adapted from Cheung AT, Weiss SJ. Diseases of the aorta. In: Oxorn DC, ed.* Intraoperative Echocardiography. *Philadelphia: Saunders; 2012:161-182.)*

artifacts are possible during CT aortic imaging, it is possible they, together with ultrasound imaging artifacts, may be misdiagnosed as the intimal flap of an acute aortic dissection. Artifacts can readily be recognized because they often cross anatomic boundaries and are often not visible in multiple imaging planes.

Linear artifacts result from reverberations between chamber or vessel walls. These reverberations between the walls of the left atrium and/or right pulmonary artery may create a linear artifact in the ascending aortic lumen, resembling an intimal flap of aortic dissection. Note that in Figure 19-8 the linear artifacts course outside the aortic boundaries. Linear artifacts of this type also result from reverberations between a vessel/chamber surface and an intravascular catheter, as in the example of a Swan-Ganz catheter in the pulmonary artery.

Side-lobe artifacts can be generated by calcified aortic plaques or intravascular catheters, such as a Swan-Ganz catheter. Side-lobe artifacts can produce linear artifacts within the aortic lumen. Linear artifacts from side lobes appear as curvilinear shadows at a constant depth and often extend outside the aorta.

Mirroring artifacts are generated when ultrasound is reflected by acoustic interfaces such as the aortic wall. This process results in a mirror image of the aorta adjacent to the interface of interest. A mirror-image artifact juxtaposed to the descending thoracic aorta can mimic aortic dissection. See Chapter 6 for a more detailed explanation of imaging artifacts.

Imaging Pitfalls During Echocardiographic Aortic Imaging

Vessels adjacent to the aortic wall can mimic the appearance of an aortic dissection. The innominate vein appears adjacent to the aortic arch in upper esophageal views and may mimic aortic dissection during long-axis imaging (see Fig. 19-10). The innominate vein can be readily identified by imaging in multiple views and by imaging luminal echocontrast injected into a peripheral vein of the left upper extremity.

Para-aortic effusions may also mimic aortic dissection. A left pleural effusion adjacent to the descending thoracic aorta is readily distinguished from aortic dissection during ME short-axis imaging to depict the characteristic crescent-shaped effusion in the left pleural cavity (Fig. 19-11). A right pleural effusion can be imaged by rotating the TEE probe to the right, looking for a crescent-shaped fluid collection oriented to the right.

Epiaortic Imaging of the Aorta

The aortic root, ascending aorta, and aortic arch can be imaged directly with a 5- to 7-MHz ultrasound transducer in sterile sheath against the anterior aortic wall (Fig. 19-12).[4,5] Epiaortic imaging during cardiac operations is typically feasible after sternotomy, with a systematic comprehensive examination as the standard.[3-5] To improve the image quality of near-field structures, an acoustic standoff is typically utilized by filling the mediastinum with warm sterile saline and/or filling the sterile sheath with fluid or ultrasound gel.

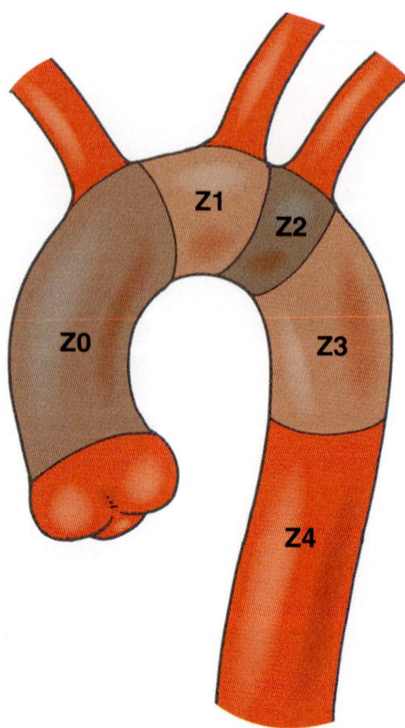

Figure 19-5 Aortic landing zones for thoracic endovascular aortic repair. Thoracic aorta is divided into five anatomic zones that relate to the landing zone for thoracic endovascular aortic repair. Zone 0, ascending aorta and proximal arch to innominate artery; Z1, segment between innominate artery and left common carotid artery; Z2, segment between left common carotid and left subclavian arteries; Z3, segment beyond left subclavian along curved portion of distal arch; Z4, straight portion of descending thoracic aorta starting at level of the 4th thoracic vertebra. *Z, Zone. (Adapted from Cheung AT, Weiss SJ. Diseases of the aorta. In: Oxorn DC, ed.* Intraoperative Echocardiography. *Philadelphia: Saunders; 2012:161-182.)*

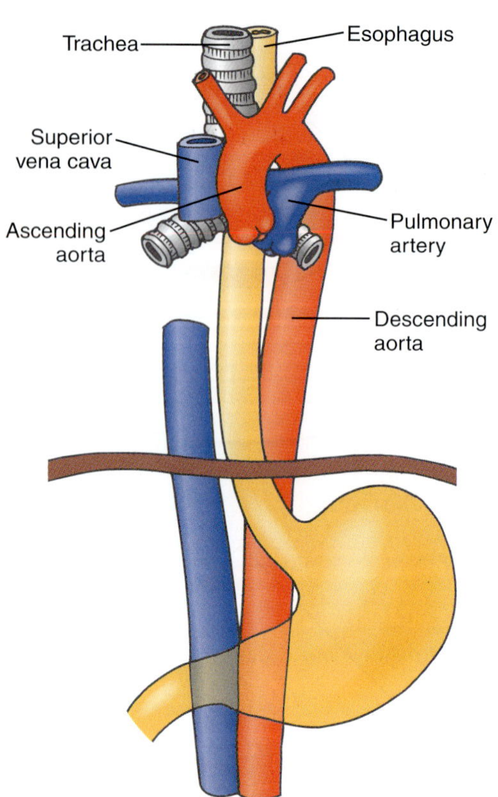

Figure 19-6 Diagram illustrating anatomic relationships between thoracic aorta *(red)*, main pulmonary artery *(blue)*, left pulmonary artery, right pulmonary artery, superior vena cava *(blue)*, inferior vena cava, esophagus *(yellow)*, and trachea *(gray)*. Descending thoracic aorta is anterior to esophagus near aortic arch, then lateral to esophagus in mid-thorax, and finally posterior to esophagus at diaphragmatic hiatus. Distal trachea and left mainstem bronchus lie between esophagus and aortic arch. *(Adapted from Cheung AT, Weiss SJ. Diseases of the aorta. In: Oxorn DC, ed.* Intraoperative Echocardiography. *Philadelphia: Saunders; 2012:161-182.)*

An important indication for epiaortic ultrasound is for assessment of ascending aortic atheroma or calcification prior to manipulation and instrumentation of the ascending aorta during cardiac surgery. Typical ascending aortic events that are associated with cerebral atheroembolism include cannulation for cardiopulmonary bypass and aortic clamping. Risk factors for significant ascending aortic atheroma include prior embolic stroke, severe peripheral vascular disease, severe aortic stenosis, aortic atheroma on preoperative radiographic imaging, and severe atherosclerosis of the descending thoracic aorta detected by TEE.[26,27] Epiaortic imaging can also assess for aneurysm and dissection in the ascending aorta and aortic arch where TEE imaging is inadequate, such as in the TEE blind spot and in patients with contraindications to TEE.[1-5]

According to recent guidelines, epiaortic imaging planes are oriented as short axis or long axis in relation to the direction of blood flow along the length of the vessel.[5] The aortic walls are designated as anterior, right lateral, left lateral, or posterior (see Fig. 19-12).[5] The proximal ascending aorta is imaged in short axis at a level proximal to the right pulmonary artery. The mid-ascending aorta short axis is imaged at the level of the right pulmonary artery. The distal ascending aorta short axis is imaged at a level distal to the right pulmonary artery and proximal to the aortic arch. The ascending aorta long axis is imaged at the level of the right pulmonary artery, showing portions of the proximal, mid-, and distal ascending aorta. The aortic arch long axis is imaged at the level of the innominate, left carotid, and left subclavian arteries.

Aortic Dissection

Aortic dissection is characterized by an intimal disruption with blood entering the medial layer and stripping the intima from the adventitia.[28] If clinical presentation is within 2 weeks of symptom onset, the dissection is classified as acute.[28] If clinical presentation is over 2 weeks from symptom onset, the dissection is classified as chronic.[29]

The diagnostic echocardiographic feature of aortic dissection is an intimal flap within the aortic lumen separating the true lumen of the vessel from the false lumen (see Figs. 19-1, *B*, 19-9, and 19-11). Color Doppler interrogation may demonstrate intimal tears by demonstrating blood flow across the intimal flap (see Fig. 19-11). Intramural hematoma (IMH) is a variant of aortic dissection characterized by separation of the intima from the adventitia, with a hematoma within the medial layer (Fig. 19-13).[30] A typical feature of IMH is that echocardiography cannot identify an intimal tear, although at times the hematoma will contain echolucent areas consistent with non-coagulated blood within the media.

The diagnostic accuracy of TEE in suspected aortic dissection is similar to helical CT and magnetic resonance imaging (MRI), with sensitivity and specificity better than 90%.[6,28-31] The clinical portability and diagnostic accuracy of TEE explain its popularity for rapid bedside evaluation of hemodynamically unstable patients with suspected acute aortic dissection (Fig. 19-14). Recent thoracic aortic disease guidelines recommend urgent and definitive aortic imaging with TEE, CT, or MRI to evaluate for aortic dissection in patients at high risk (Class I Recommendation; Level of Evidence B).[6] In surgical patients in whom the diagnosis of aortic dissection has already been confirmed, comprehensive intraoperative TEE evaluation confirms dissection extent, detects complications of aortic dissection, and guides surgical management (Fig. 19-15).

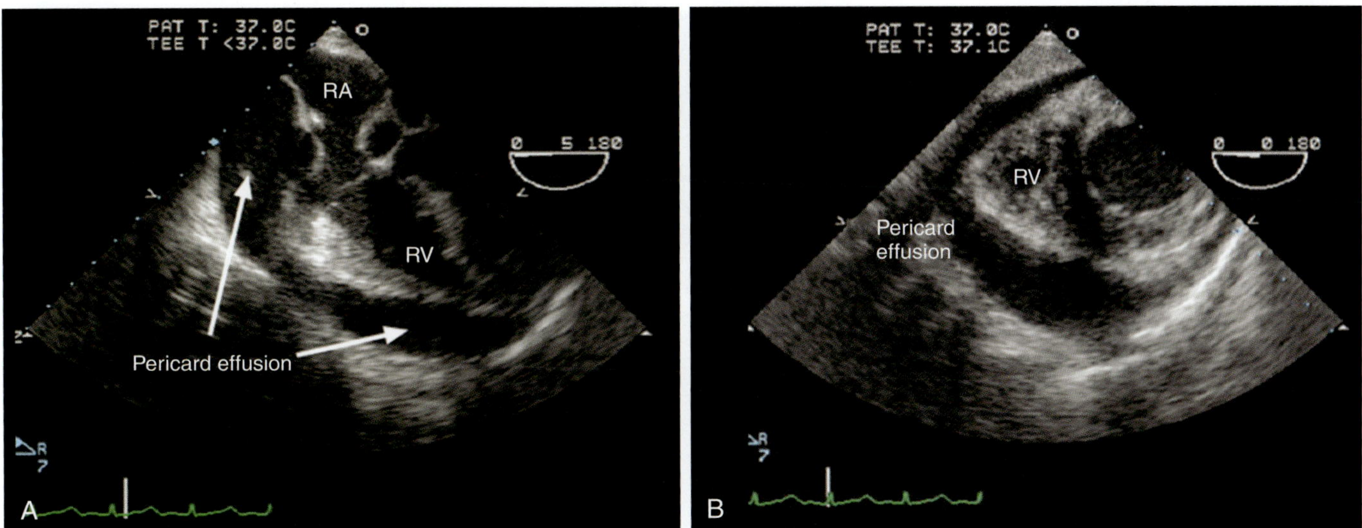

Figure 19-7 Aortic rupture with hemopericardium. This image pair demonstrate midesophageal four-chamber view **(A)** and transgastric ventricular short-axis view **(B)** in a hypotensive patient with Stanford type A aortic dissection. Circumferential pericardial effusion shown in both images was diagnostic for rupture of proximal ascending aorta causing hemopericardium. **A** demonstrates diastolic collapse of right atrium *(RA)*, indicating development of pericardial tamponade. *RV,* Right ventricle. *(Adapted from Cheung AT, Weiss SJ. Diseases of the aorta. In: Oxorn DC, ed. Intraoperative Echocardiography. Philadelphia: Saunders; 2012:161-182.)*

TABLE 19-1	Normal Adult Thoracic Aortic Diameters		
Aortic Segment	*Men: Mean ± SD (cm)*	*Women: Mean ± SD (cm)*	*Imaging Technique*
Aortic valve annulus	2.6 ± 0.3	2.3 ± 0.2	Echo
Sinuses of Valsalva	3.4 ± 0.3	3.0 ± 0.3	Echo
Sinotubular junction	2.9 ± 0.3	2.6 ± 0.3	Echo
Proximal ascending aorta	3.0 ± 0.4	2.7 ± 0.4	Echo
Mid-descending aorta	2.7 ± 0.3	2.5 ± 0.3	CT
Distal descending aorta	2.6 ± 0.3	2.4 ± 0.3	CT

CT, Computed tomography; *Echo,* echocardiography; *SD,* standard deviation.
Data from Johnston KW, Rutherford RB, Tilson MD, et al. Suggested standards for reporting on arterial aneurysms. Subcommittee on Reporting Standards for Arterial Aneurysms, Ad Hoc Committee on Reporting Standards, Society for Vascular Surgery and North American Chapter, International Society for Cardiovascular Surgery. *J Vasc Surg.* 1991;13:452-458; and Roman MJ, Devereux RB, Kramer-Fox R, et al. Two-dimensional echocardiographic aortic root dimensions in normal children and adults. *Am J Cardiol.* 1989;64:507-512.

Classification of Aortic Dissection

Aortic dissection can be classified according to intimal tear site and dissection extent (Fig. 19-16). The DeBakey scheme has three main subtypes. The Stanford scheme has two main subtypes. The classification of aortic dissection is clinically important for clinical management, including prognosis. Acute aortic dissections that involve the ascending aorta are typically surgical emergencies, since delays in surgical management are associated with high mortality risk.[32,33]

The Stanford classification emphasizes the clinical importance of ascending aortic dissection (see Fig. 19-16). Stanford type A aortic dissection is defined as any dissection involving the ascending aorta, regardless of intimal tear site (surgical repair typically recommended). Stanford type B dissection is defined as any dissection that does not involve the ascending aorta (medical management recommended unless complicated by threatened/frank aortic rupture and/or malperfusion).[28,29]

The DeBakey classification focuses on intimal tear site and dissection extent (see Fig. 19-16). DeBakey type I dissection is characterized by an intimal tear within the ascending aorta complicated by dissection involving the ascending aorta, aortic arch, and descending aorta (surgical repair recommended). DeBakey type II dissection is characterized by an intimal tear within the ascending aorta complicated by dissection confined to the ascending aorta (surgical repair recommended). DeBakey type III dissection is characterized by an intimal tear within the descending thoracic aorta complicated by dissection of the descending aorta (medical management recommended unless complicated by threatened/frank aortic rupture and/or malperfusion). If dissection in this setting is confined to the descending thoracic aorta, it is defined as DeBakey type IIIa. If dissection in this setting involves the descending aorta and abdominal aorta, it is DeBakey type IIIb.

Although ascending aortic dissection is a surgical emergency, perioperative mortality depends significantly on clinical presentation, specifically the presence of branch vessel malperfusion (regional ischemia) and/or circulatory compromise (generalized ischemia).[34,35] Recently, the Penn classification of clinical presentation in acute type A dissection has been derived and validated to focus future interventions on clinical presentations in this life-threatening disease as part of the collective effort to improve clinical outcomes yet further.[34,35] Penn Class **A** presentations are characterized by the *a*bsence of ischemia, specifically the absence of malperfusion and circulatory compromise. Penn Class **B** presentations are characterized by *b*ranch vessel malperfusion (e.g., stroke, cold pulseless upper extremity). Penn Class **C** presentations are characterized by *c*irculatory *c*ompromise including shock and/or cardiac arrest. Penn Class **B&C** presentations are characterized by both *b*ranch vessel and *c*irculatory *c*ompromise. The clinical presentation in acute type A dissection as defined by the Penn classification independently predicts perioperative mortality.[34,35] An integrated Penn classification of Stanford acute type A aortic dissection has recently been proposed to encourage a comprehensive management strategy of this acute aortic syndrome by considering Penn clinical presentation and DeBakey extent of dissection.[36] This integration of the three classifications of ascending aortic dissection will likely frame future advances in diagnosis and management of this surgical emergency.[36]

The European classification of acute aortic dissection consists of five classes and focuses on the anatomic spectrum of aortic dissection, including its variants (Fig. 19-17).[37] Class I is defined as classic aortic dissection with an intimal tear, complicated by an intimal flap separating the true and false aortic lumens. Class II is defined as IMH with hematoma formation within the medial layer. An intimal tear is not usually detected by echocardiography. Class III is defined as limited dissection confined to a short aortic segment. A partial tear of the inner

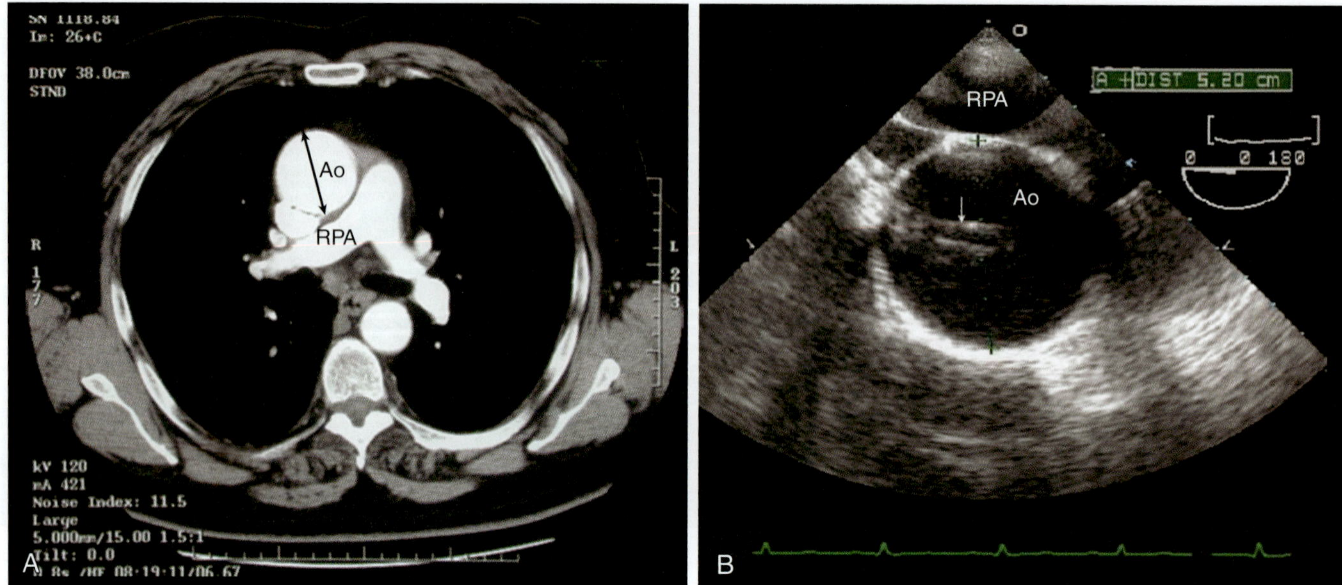

Figure 19-8   Ascending aortic aneurysm with imaging artifacts. **A,** Computed tomographic angiogram (CTA) of axial slice through ascending aorta (Ao) at level of right pulmonary artery (RPA). **B,** TEE midesophageal ascending aorta short-axis image at level of RPA. Ascending aorta is dilated. Ascending aortic diameter measured from adventitia to adventitia was 5.4 cm by CTA. Ascending aortic diameter measured from intima to intima was 5.2 cm by TEE. Note that TEE image is complicated by linear imaging artifacts (arrow) as a consequence of reverberation and side lobe artifacts. Linear imaging artifacts are common during TEE examination in patients with a dilated ascending aorta and can be distinguished from the intimal flap of an aortic dissection because they course outside boundaries of ascending aorta. (See Video 19-10 and 19-11.) (Adapted from Cheung AT, Weiss SJ. Diseases of the aorta. In: Oxorn DC, ed. Intraoperative Echocardiography. Philadelphia: Saunders; 2012:161-182.)

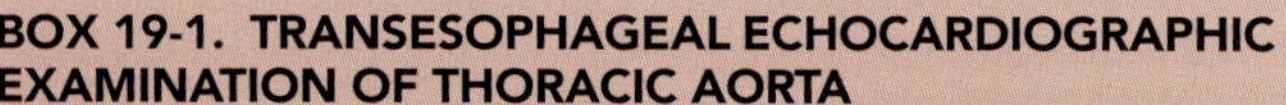

BOX 19-1.   TRANSESOPHAGEAL ECHOCARDIOGRAPHIC EXAMINATION OF THORACIC AORTA

1. Summarize pathologic findings, including a description of anatomic location and extent according to thoracic aortic segments.
2. Where possible, make all aortic measurements from intima to intima perpendicular to the axis of blood flow.
3. Report location and maximum diameter of dilated aortic segments.
4. Report diameters of the aortic valve annulus, sinus of Valsalva, sinotubular junction, ascending aorta at the level of the right pulmonary artery, distal aortic arch, and descending thoracic aorta.
5. Assess and quantify aortic valvular function by standard criteria.
6. Assess and quantify atherosclerosis by standard criteria (see Table 19-3).
7. Assess extent and location of mural thrombus.
8. Determine extent and location of aortic wall calcification.
9. Search for evidence of pleural effusion, pericardial effusion, or perivascular hematoma that may indicate aortic rupture.

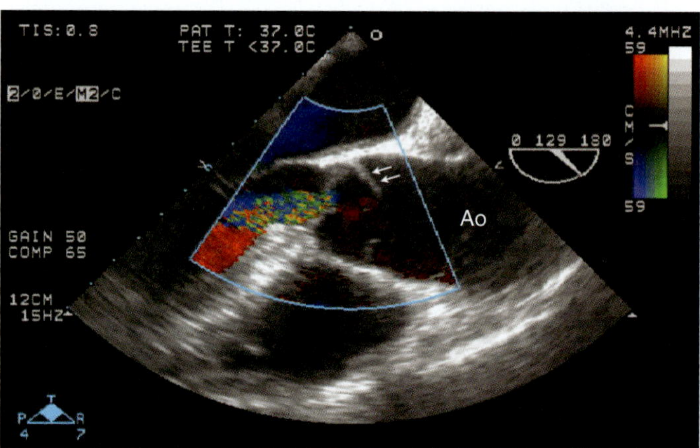

Figure 19-9   Stanford type A dissection shown in midesophageal aortic valve long-axis image at a multiplane angle of 129 degrees. An intimal flap (arrows) is present in aorta (Ao), extending to base of aortic valve cusps within aortic root. Color flow Doppler imaging reveals moderate aortic regurgitation. (See Video 19-3.) (Adapted from Cheung AT, Weiss SJ. Diseases of the aorta. In: Oxorn DC, ed. Intraoperative Echocardiography. Philadelphia: Saunders; 2012:161-182.)

aortic wall is termed a *subtle dissection*, and scar formation at this partial tear site is termed an *abortive discrete dissection*. Class IV is defined as a penetrating atherosclerotic ulcer (PAU) with localized hematoma or pseudoaneurysm. Class V is defined as traumatic or iatrogenic aortic dissection, typically associated with aortic catheterization or surgical aortic manipulation.

As a variant of aortic dissection, IMH is characterized by a medial hematoma that may also be subadventitial.[38] It accounts for up to 30% of patients presenting with an acute aortic syndrome (see Fig. 19-13), especially in Asia.[39,40] The typical patient with IMH is elderly, hypertensive, and has established peripheral vascular disease.[38,39] The genesis of IMH is still debated as to whether it is aortic dissection with a thrombosed false lumen or whether it is intramedial hemorrhage from rupture of the vasa vasorum.[38,41] The extent of IMH is classified by the Stanford approach as type A and type B. Indications for surgery in type A IMH include refractory pain, ascending aortic diameter 5 cm or greater, hematoma thickness greater than 1 cm, and hemodynamic instability.[38]

As a variant of aortic dissection, PAU is a focal atherosclerotic plaque that corrodes through the internal elastic lamina into the media.[38,39] It may be complicated by IMH or formation of a pseudoaneurysm. The typical patient with PAU is an elderly man with established atherosclerotic disease. The distribution of PAU in order of frequency is descending aorta, aortic arch, abdominal aorta, and (rarely) ascending aorta.[38,39,42] Indications for endovascular repair of PAU include refractory pain, aortic rupture, and aortic diameter larger than 55 mm.[38]

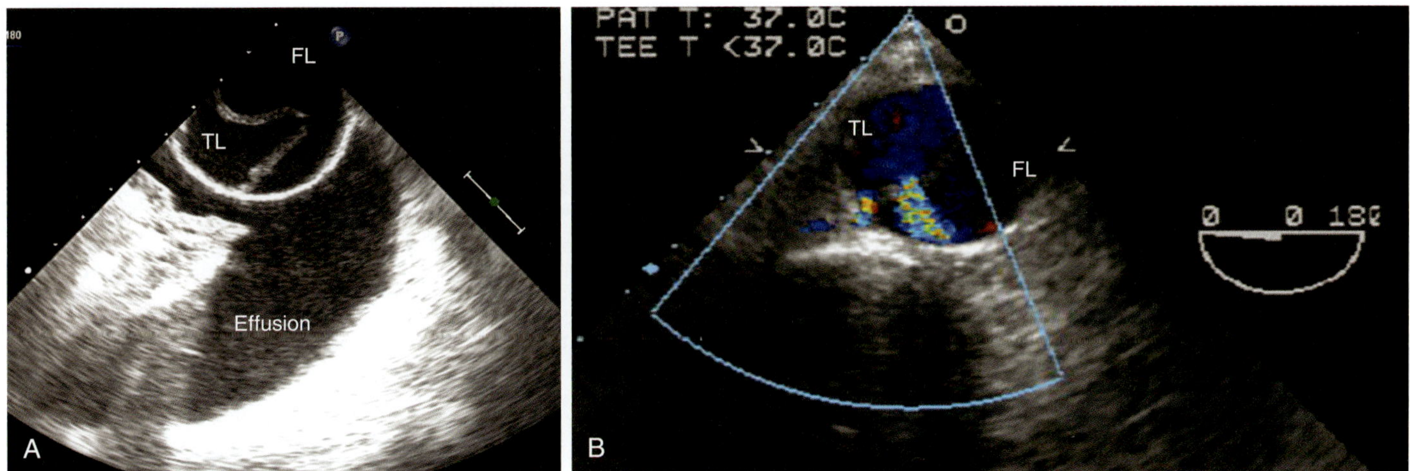

Figure 19-10 Innominate vein shown in upper esophageal aortic arch long-axis view at a multiplane angle of 0 degrees on left and aortic arch short-axis view at a multiplane angle of 88 degrees on right. From these views, it is clear that distal aortic arch *(Ao)* and innominate vein *(Innom V)* are intimately related. In long-axis view, anterior aortic wall against adjacent innominate vein mimics an intimal flap of aortic dissection. Short-axis view, however, resolves this artifact by clearly distinguishing the vessels. Imaging a structure of interest in multiple planes minimizes this kind of misinterpretation. *(Adapted from Cheung AT, Weiss SJ. Diseases of the aorta. In: Oxorn DC, ed. Intraoperative Echocardiography. Philadelphia: Saunders; 2012:161-182.)*

Figure 19-11 **A,** Dissection of descending thoracic aorta shown in midesophageal (ME) descending aorta short-axis view at a multiplane angle of 0 degrees. There is an aortic dissection, with an intimal flap separating true lumen *(TL)* from false lumen *(FL)* of aorta. Pleural effusion in left pleural cavity *(effusion)* may result from rupture of descending aorta or heart failure. **B,** ME descending aorta short-axis view at a multiplane angle of 0 degrees showing dissection of descending thoracic aorta. Aortic dissection is evident, with an intimal flap separating true lumen *(TL)* from false lumen *(FL).* Doppler color flow interrogation has demonstrated two fenestrations in intimal flap consistent with intimal tears that allow blood flow from true lumen into false lumen. (See Video 19-4 and 19-5.) *(Adapted from Cheung AT, Weiss SJ. Diseases of the aorta. In: Oxorn DC, ed. Intraoperative Echocardiography. Philadelphia: Saunders; 2012:161-182.)*

Echocardiographic Evaluation for Complications of Aortic Dissection

Hemopericardium, acute severe aortic regurgitation, coronary malperfusion, and aortic arch branch vessel malperfusion associated with aortic dissection are surgical emergencies. Cardiac tamponade often follows aortic rupture into the pericardium and is a common cause of death in acute ascending aortic dissection, regardless of extent.[28,29] Hemopericardium associated with aortic dissection appears as a circumferential pericardial effusion during echocardiographic assessment (see Fig. 19-7). Pericardial tamponade is manifested echocardiographically by features such as chamber compression, marked respiratory variation in ventricular filling, and diastolic chamber collapse.

Aortic regurgitation is a common feature of ascending aortic dissection (see Figs. 19-1, *B* and 19-9).[28,29] If severe aortic regurgitation is acute, it is often associated with heart failure, given that the left ventricle has had insufficient time to adapt. The mechanisms of aortic regurgitation include dilation of the aortic root, dissection into the aortic root with consequent malsuspension of the aortic valve cusps, and/or prolapse of the intimal flap through the aortic valve (Fig. 19-18).[43,44]

Coronary artery malperfusion due to coronary artery dissection may occur in ascending aortic dissection if the dissection extends proximally into the aortic root and coronary ostia. Echocardiographic signs of right coronary artery malperfusion include right ventricular dysfunction and left ventricular inferior wall hypokinesis. Echocardiographic signs of left coronary malperfusion include left ventricular dysfunction and regional wall motion abnormalities, depending on the extent of branch vessel compromise.[34-36]

Carotid artery malperfusion may be caused by extension of the dissection into the aortic arch branch vessels (static obstruction) or by obstruction of the origins of the aortic arch branch vessels by the intimal flap within the aortic arch (dynamic obstruction). Aortic arch branch vessel malperfusion is often associated with upper extremity

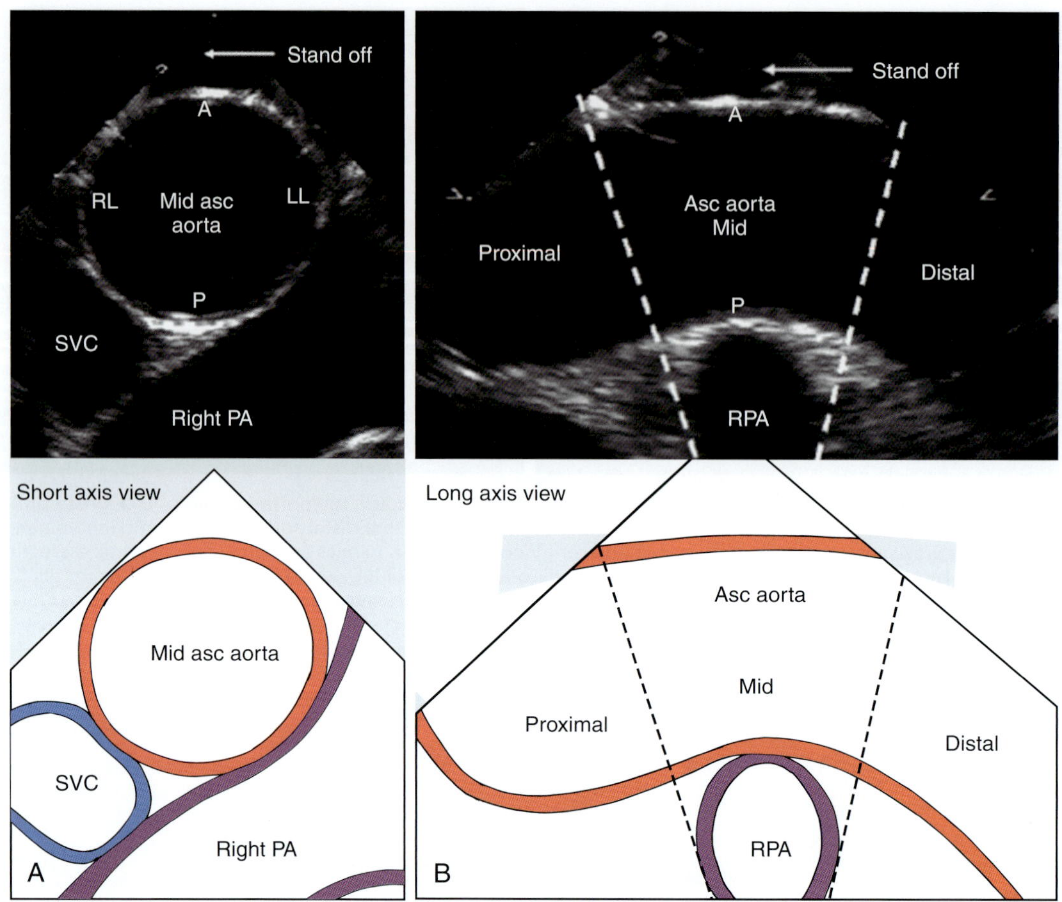

Figure 19-12 Epiaortic imaging of ascending aorta (*Asc Aorta*) in short axis (**A**) and long axis (**B**). Segments of ascending aorta are designated as proximal, mid-, and distal in relation to right pulmonary artery (*RPA*). Walls of ascending aorta are designated as anterior (*A*), posterior (*P*), right lateral (*RL*), and left lateral (*LL*). *PA*, Pulmonary artery; *SVC*, superior vena cava. (*Adapted from Glas KE, Swaminathan M, Reeves ST, et al. Guidelines for the performance of a comprehensive intraoperative epiaortic ultrasonographic examination: recommendations of the American Society of Echocardiography and the Society of Cardiovascular Anesthesiologists; endorsed by the Society of Thoracic Surgeons. J Am Soc Echocardiogr. 2007;20:1227-1235.*)

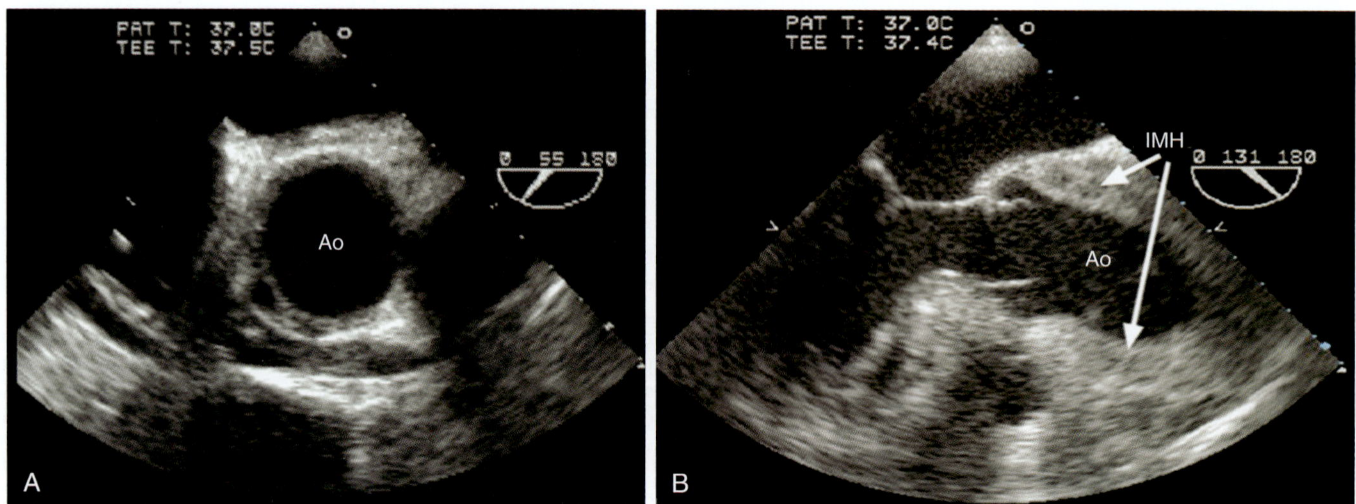

Figure 19-13 Intramural hematoma (*IMH*) shown in midesophageal views of aortic valve in short axis at a multiplane angle of 55 degrees (**A**) and in long axis at a multiplane angle of 131 degrees (**B**). **A** demonstrates IMH as a variant of aortic dissection as a circumferential or crescent-shaped thickening of aortic wall. In acute IMH, blood may appear within aortic wall as lucent cavities. **B** depicts longitudinal thickening of wall of the aortic root and ascending aorta caused by intramural hematoma. *Ao*, Aorta. (*Adapted from Cheung AT, Weiss SJ. Diseases of the aorta. In: Oxorn DC, ed. Intraoperative Echocardiography. Philadelphia: Saunders; 2012:161-182.*)

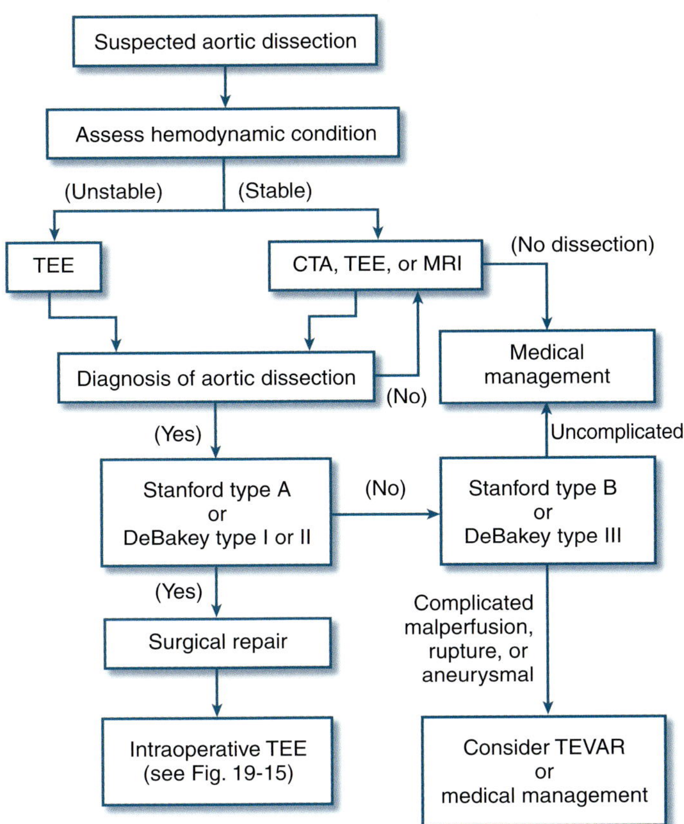

Figure 19-14 Role of transesophageal echocardiography *(TEE)* for evaluation and diagnosis of aortic dissection. *CTA,* Computed tomographic angiogram; *MRI,* magnetic resonance imaging; *TEVAR,* thoracic endovascular aortic repair. *(Adapted from Cheung AT, Weiss SJ. Diseases of the aorta. In: Oxorn DC, ed. Intraoperative Echocardiography. Philadelphia: Saunders; 2012:161-182.)*

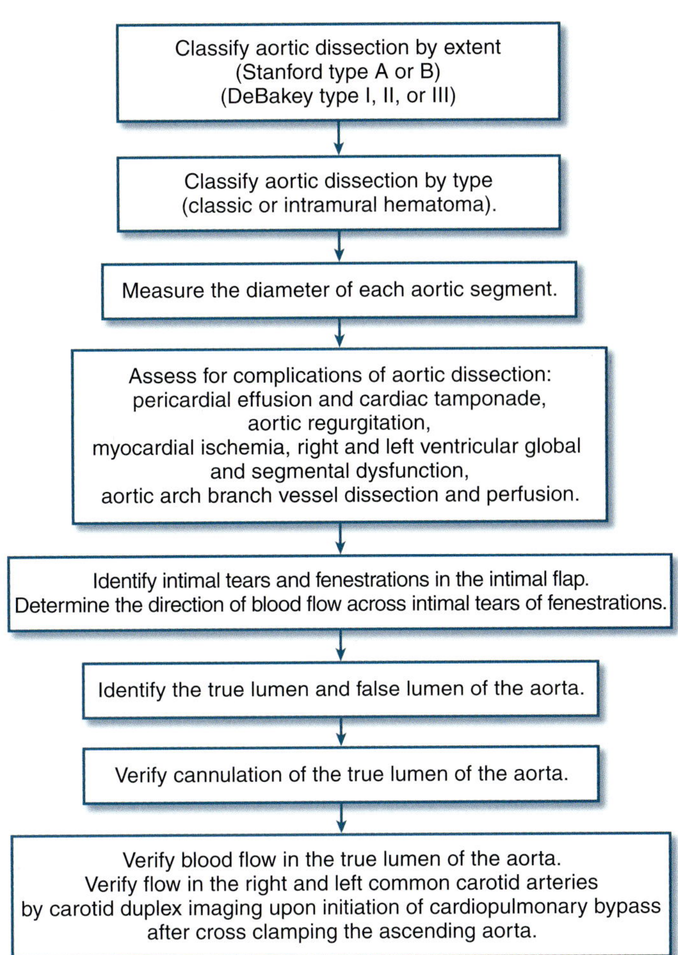

Figure 19-15 Intraoperative transesophageal echocardiography examination for aortic dissection. *(Adapted from Cheung AT, Weiss SJ. Diseases of the aorta. In: Oxorn DC, ed. Intraoperative Echocardiography. Philadelphia: Saunders; 2012:161-182.)*

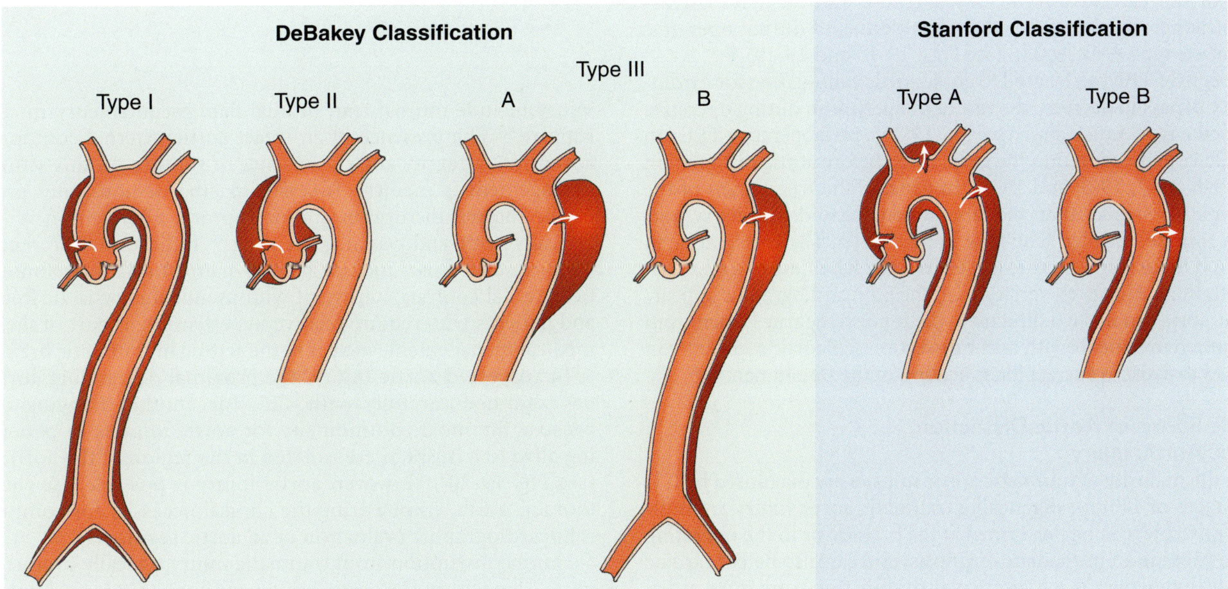

Figure 19-16 Classification of aortic dissection. Two anatomic classifications of aortic dissection focus on intimal tear site and extent of dissection: DeBakey scheme has three main subtypes, and Stanford scheme has two main subtypes. Acute aortic dissections involving ascending aorta are typically considered surgical emergencies (DeBakey I and II; Stanford type A). *(Adapted from Cheung AT, Weiss SJ. Diseases of the aorta. In: Oxorn DC, ed. Intraoperative Echocardiography. Philadelphia: Saunders; 2012:161-182.)*

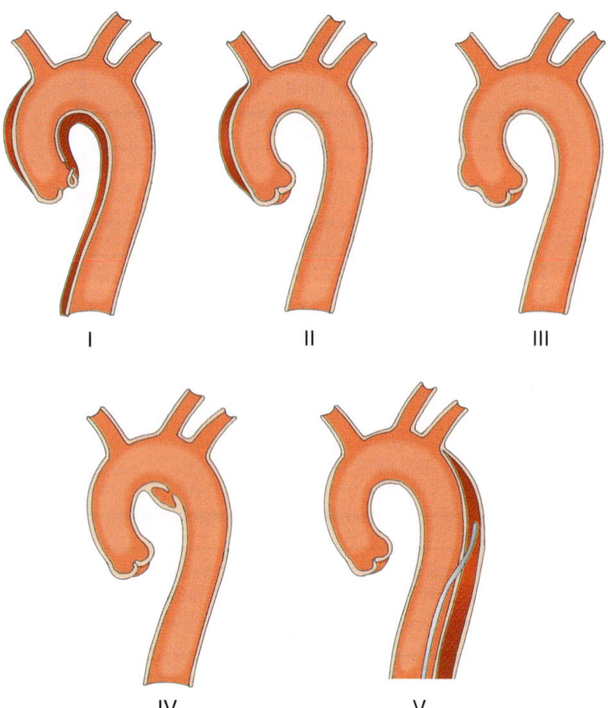

Figure 19-17   European classification for variants of aortic dissection: class I, classic aortic dissection; class II, intramural hematoma; class III, subtle discrete aortic dissection; class IV, plaque rupture or ulceration; class V, traumatic or iatrogenic aortic dissection. *(Adapted from Cheung AT, Weiss SJ. Diseases of the aorta. In: Oxorn DC, ed.* Intraoperative Echocardiography. *Philadelphia: Saunders; 2012:161-182.)*

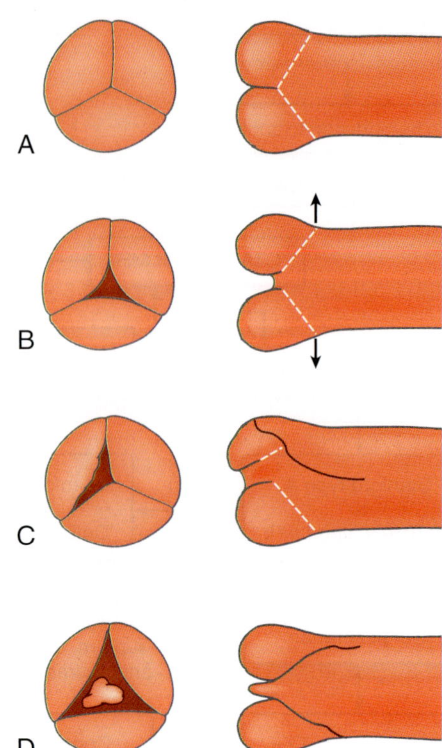

Figure 19-18   Mechanisms of aortic regurgitation in Stanford type A dissection. **A,** Normal aortic valve anatomy in midesophageal short-axis view *(left)* and long-axis view *(right)*. Dotted lines represent attachment of leaflet tips to sinotubular junction. **B,** Incomplete leaflet closure due to dilation of sinotubular junction *(arrows)*. This typically results in central aortic regurgitation on color flow Doppler imaging. **C,** Aortic leaflet prolapse due to disruption of aortic cusp attachments to aortic wall. This typically results in involved cusp prolapsing below valve plane to produce eccentric aortic regurgitation. **D,** Dissection flap prolapse that results when intimal flap prolapses through aortic valve leaflets to produce central aortic insufficiency that may be intermittent. *(Adapted from Movsowitz HD, Levine RA, Hilgenberg AD, et al. Transesophageal echocardiographic description of the mechanisms of aortic regurgitation in acute type A aortic dissection: implications for aortic valve repair.* J Am Coll Cardiol. *2000;36:884-890.)*

pulse deficits or acute ischemic stroke. Carotid Duplex examination can be used to detect a dissection flap or compromised blood flow within the common carotid artery (Fig. 19-19). Intraoperative carotid Duplex imaging can be used to verify perfusion in the common carotid arteries after aortic cannulation, start of cardiopulmonary bypass, and application of the ascending aortic cross-clamp. Surface ultrasound scanning of the carotid arteries can diagnose and facilitate correction of intraoperative brachiocephalic malperfusion during operative repair of acute type A dissection (see Figs. 19-15 and 19-19).[45,46]

Intraoperative TEE can be used to guide aortic cannulation for cardiopulmonary bypass to decrease the risk of malperfusion during operative repair of acute type A dissection (see Fig. 19-15). Intraoperative TEE can verify guidewire insertion into the true lumen before aortic cannulation (Videos 19-6, 19-7, 19-8, and 19-9). In general, the true lumen of the aorta is typically smaller than the false lumen, expands during systole, and has a rounded border. The false lumen is typically crescenteric in shape. Blood flows from the true lumen into the false lumen across intimal fenestrations. However, variations in the echocardiographic appearance of the aorta can make it difficult to distinguish the true lumen from the false lumen in patients with aortic dissection. Epiaortic scanning can also be used to assist in correct identification of the true lumen.[47,48]

Traumatic Forms of Aortic Dissection
Traumatic Aortic Injury
Although the majority of traumatic aortic injuries are diagnosed by CT, the advantages of TEE for diagnosing traumatic aortic injury are multiple: it is portable; can be performed at the bedside or in the operating room; can provide an immediate diagnosis; and can also detect cardiac tamponade, hypovolemia, or ventricular dysfunction from myocardial contusion. The frequent survivable aortic injuries result from blunt chest trauma or rapid deceleration. The most common site of injury is at the aortic isthmus between the aortic arch and descending thoracic aorta (Fig. 19-20). The echocardiographic features of traumatic aortic

injury include intimal tear, intimal flap, pseudoaneurysm, and aortic rupture.[49] The presence of an intact aortic external contour suggests adventitial integrity and the absence of rupture. In this setting, initial management is medical. If serial imaging demonstrates progression of the intimal disruption and/or rupture, intervention is indicated, typically with endovascular stenting.[49] Indications for more urgent endovascular repair include hemodynamic instability; abnormal aortic external contour consistent with pseudoaneurysm or free rupture; and patients who require relative hypertension as part of their general medical management, such as in the setting of traumatic brain injury.[49]

In suspected aortic injury, the proximal descending aorta should be examined carefully with TEE (or another imaging modality) because the most common site for aortic injuries in patients arriving alive to a hospital are isolated in the region of the aortic isthmus (see Fig. 19-20). However, aortic injury is possible elsewhere in the thoracic aorta, emphasizing the clinical necessity for comprehensive echocardiographic evaluation of all aortic segments.

Intimal disruption from traumatic injury typically produces a thick mural flap within the aortic lumen confined to a 1- to 2-cm length of the aorta (see Fig. 19-20). The mural flap is usually less mobile than the intimal flap associated with classic aortic dissection. Intimal disruption can also appear as a small defect or discontinuity along the intimal surface of the aortic lumen.

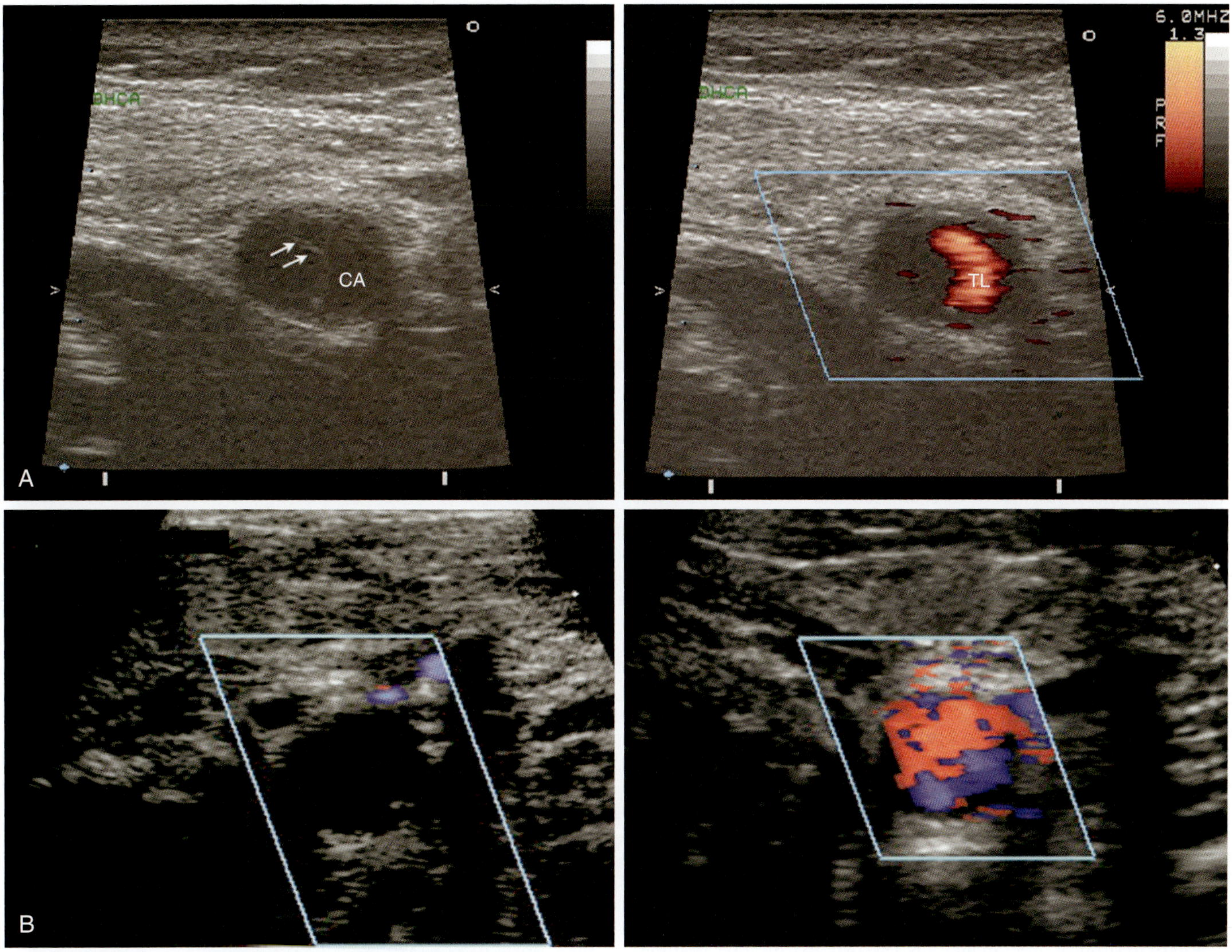

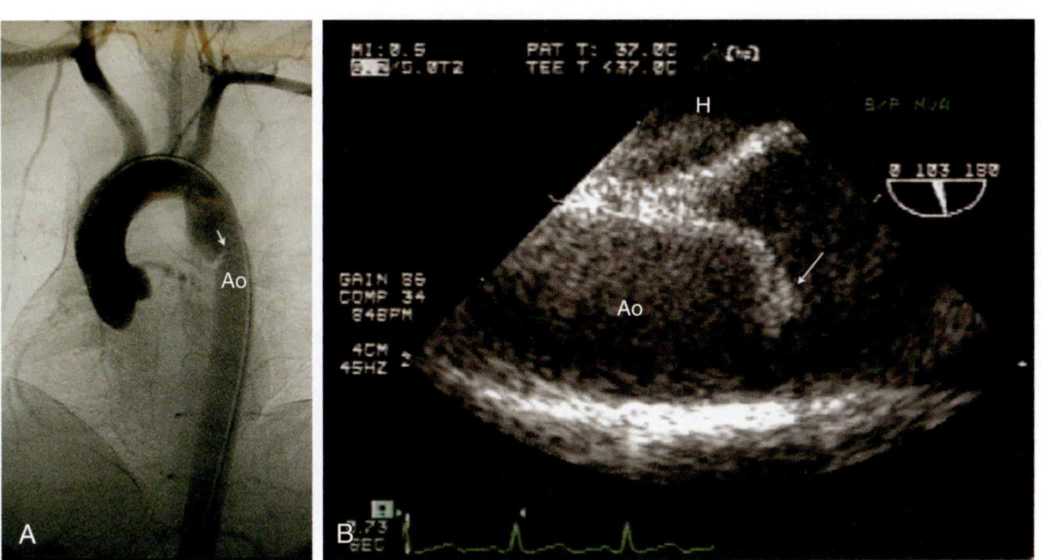

Figure 19-19 **A,** Transcutaneous scanning of carotid artery in type A dissection. Surface ultrasound imaging of right neck in patient with a Stanford type A aortic dissection and extension of dissection into innominate artery and right common carotid artery. An intimal flap *(arrows)* was imaged in right carotid artery *(CA)*. Color Doppler demonstrated flow in true lumen *(TL)* of carotid artery during cardiopulmonary bypass *(right panel)*. **B,** Transcutaneous scanning (surface ultrasound imaging) of right carotid artery in patient with a Stanford type A aortic dissection during cardiopulmonary bypass. After clamping of ascending aorta, color flow Doppler imaging demonstrated acute loss of blood flow in right carotid artery *(left panel)*, suggesting loss of false lumen perfusion across a large intimal fenestration below aortic clamp. Cardiac surgeon was immediately notified. Right panel shows immediate return of right carotid blood flow after intimal fenestration above the level of ascending aortic clamp. *(**A** Adapted from Cheung AT, Weiss SJ. Diseases of the aorta. In: Oxorn DC, ed.* Intraoperative Echocardiography. *Philadelphia: Saunders; 2012:161-182.* ***B** adapted from Augoustides JG, Kohl BA, Harris H, et al. Color-flow Doppler recognition of intraoperative brachiocephalic malperfusion during operative repair of acute type A dissection: utility of transcutaneous carotid artery ultrasound scanning.* J Cardiothorac Vasc Anesth. *2007;21:81-84.)*

Figure 19-20 Traumatic aortic injury. Aortic angiogram **(A)** and proximal descending aorta long axis at a multiplane angle of 103 degrees **(B)** both demonstrate blunt traumatic aortic injury involving aortic isthmus. Both angiogram and transesophageal echocardiography (TEE) depict a thick mural flap *(arrow)* within lumen of descending aorta *(Ao)* that indicates an aortic wall disruption with a resultant external aortic contour abnormality. TEE image also demonstrates a periaortic hematoma *(H)* in space between descending thoracic aorta and esophagus, consistent with a contained rupture. *(Adapted from Cheung AT, Weiss SJ. Diseases of the aorta. In: Oxorn DC, ed.* Intraoperative Echocardiography. *Philadelphia: Saunders; 2012:161-182.)*

IMH indicates a contained rupture at the site of aortic injury and appears as a regional thickening of the aortic wall associated with an abnormal external aortic contour. Perivascular hematoma from a contained rupture appears as a tissue density surrounding the aorta at the site of injury. Perivascular hematoma may cause a separation between the TEE probe tip in the esophagus from the posterolateral wall of the aortic isthmus or a distortion of the vessel wall (see Fig. 19-20). Frank rupture into the pleural space will produce a hemothorax that can be detected by TEE as an effusion with thrombus within the left pleural cavity (see Fig. 19-11, *A*).

Iatrogenic Aortic Injury

Iatrogenic aortic dissection is most often associated with cardiac surgery or cardiac catheterization.[50] A recent massive observational study (N = 2,219,991) documented an incidence of 0.06% for aortic dissection as a complication of cardiac surgery.[51] Although very rare, this complication had a 48% operative mortality. Independent risk factors for this devastating complication included exposure to preoperative steroids, peripheral vascular disease, and femoral arterial cannulation (odds ratio 2.67; 95% confidence interval, 1.78-3.99).[51]

The majority of iatrogenic dissections associated with cardiac surgery are Stanford type A. In contrast, the majority of aortic dissections that complicate cardiac catheterization are Stanford type B. In cardiac surgical procedures requiring TEE, the thoracic aorta should be interrogated at one or more intervals to rule out aortic injury.[52]

Aortic Aneurysm

An aortic aneurysm is defined as a permanent focal aortic dilation with a diameter at least 50% greater than the normal diameter for that aortic segment.[6] Whereas true aneurysms involve all three layers of the aorta, pseudoaneurysms are defined by their *failure* to involve all three aortic wall layers. Aortic aneurysms may be classified according to shape as fusiform or saccular. Thoracic aortic aneurysms have multiple etiologies including atherosclerotic disease, collagen vascular diseases, genetic syndromes, inflammatory diseases, infection, and trauma (Table 19-2).[6] Pseudoaneurysms arise from defects in the aortic wall secondary to surgical instrumentation, vascular anastomoses, trauma, penetrating atherosclerotic ulcer, or infection (Fig. 19-21).

The echocardiographic evaluation of aortic aneurysms should characterize their size, shape, location, and extent, since these features drive surgical decision making (see Box 19-1 and Table 19-2). Furthermore, TEE can also characterize aneurysmal features such as low flow, mural thrombus, and associated aortic dissection. The presence of spontaneous echo contrast is very suggestive of low flow within the aneurysm.

Aneurysm diameter is an important prognostic feature because it is a powerful risk factor for rupture.[53] The TEE measurement of aortic diameter typically underestimates aortic diameter by several millimeters compared to CT measurements. The explanation for this apparent difference is that TEE measurements are typically performed from intima to intima, and CT measurements are performed from adventitia to adventitia (see Fig. 19-8 and Table 19-2).

An aortic aneurysm associated with bicuspid aortic valve, collagen vascular disease, or a familial syndrome is significantly more likely to rupture at a narrower diameter (see Table 19-2).[53,54] Furthermore, saccular aneurysms and pseudoaneurysms are at significantly greater risk for rupture than fusiform aneurysms.

Giant ascending aortic or aortic arch aneurysms may cause a mediastinal mass effect, with external compression of the right pulmonary artery, left mainstem bronchus, trachea, esophagus, right ventricular outflow tract, or superior vena cava (see Fig. 19-6). TEE should be performed cautiously in patients with evidence of a mediastinal mass effect, because the volume of the TEE probe in the esophagus has the potential to cause airway obstruction or circulatory collapse.[10-12] Simultaneous compression of the right pulmonary artery and left mainstem bronchus may cause hypoxemia. The TEE probe should not be advanced into the esophagus if resistance is encountered; injury may result. Large descending thoracic aortic aneurysms may distort

TABLE 19-2	Indications for Surgical Repair for Thoracic Aortic Aneurysm
Condition	*Indication for Surgical Repair*
Degenerative aneurysm	Asc Ao ≥ 5.5 cm Asc Ao < 5.5 cm and growth rate > 0.5 cm/yr Desc Ao > 6.0 cm Desc Ao > 5.5 cm and candidate for TEVAR Saccular aneurysm Pseudoaneurysm
Marfan syndrome	Asc Ao (4.0-5.0) cm
Ehlers-Danlos syndrome	Asc Ao (4.0-5.0) cm & family history of aortic dissection
Turner syndrome	Asc Ao (4.0-5.0) cm & rapidly expanding aneurysm
Bicuspid aortic valve	Asc Ao (4.0-5.0) cm & planned pregnancy
Familial TAA	Asc Ao (4.0-5.0) cm & significant aortic regurgitation
Familial aortic dissection	Desc Ao > 5.5 cm
Loeys-Dietz syndrome	Asc Ao ≥ 4.2 cm by TEE Asc Ao ≥ 4.4 cm by CT or MRI
Aortic valve repair/ replacement	Asc Ao > 4.5 cm

Asc Ao, Ascending aortic diameter; *CT,* computed tomography; *Desc Ao,* descending aortic diameter; *MRI,* magnetic resonance imaging; *TAA,* thoracic aortic aneurysm; *TEVAR,* thoracic endovascular aortic repair; *TEE,* transesophageal echocardiography.
Data from Hiratzka LF, Bakris GL, Beckman JA, et al. ACC/AHA/AATS/ACR/ASA/SCA/SCAI/SIR/STS/SVM guidelines for the diagnosis and management of patients with thoracic aortic disease. *J Am Coll Cardiol.* 2010;55:e27-e129.

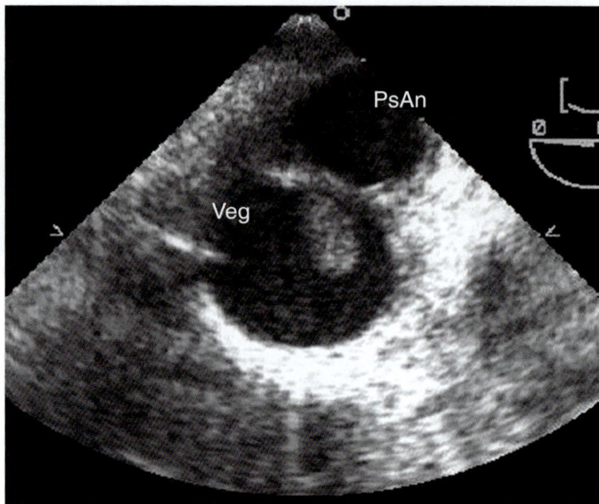

Figure 19-21 Mycotic pseudoaneurysm shown in midesophageal descending thoracic aortic short-axis view at a multiplane angle of 0 degrees. In this patient with endocarditis, a mobile vegetation *(Veg)* was imaged in lumen of descending thoracic aorta adjacent to a mycotic pseudoaneurysm *(PsAn)*. *(Adapted from Cheung AT, Weiss SJ. Diseases of the aorta. In: Oxorn DC, ed. Intraoperative Echocardiography. Philadelphia: Saunders; 2012:161-182.)*

the esophagus. In this setting, instrumentation of the esophagus could injure the esophagus or rupture the aneurysm.

Aneurysm of the aortic root or ascending aorta can contribute to aortic regurgitation as the aortic cusps are pulled apart (Figs. 19-22 to 19-25).[55] Aortic root aneurysm may be isolated to a single sinus of Valsalva (see Fig. 19-25). The complications of a sinus segment aneurysm include compression or rupture into neighboring heart chambers, such as the right atrium, left atrium, or right ventricle.[56] In this setting, TEE can localize and size the aneurysm as well as evaluate for complications such as compression, rupture, or exacerbation of aortic regurgitation. Furthermore, TEE can assess the surgical repair (see Fig. 19-25). If repair is undertaken with transcatheter intervention, TEE can also provide real-time guidance for successful occlusion of a ruptured sinus segment aneurysm.[57]

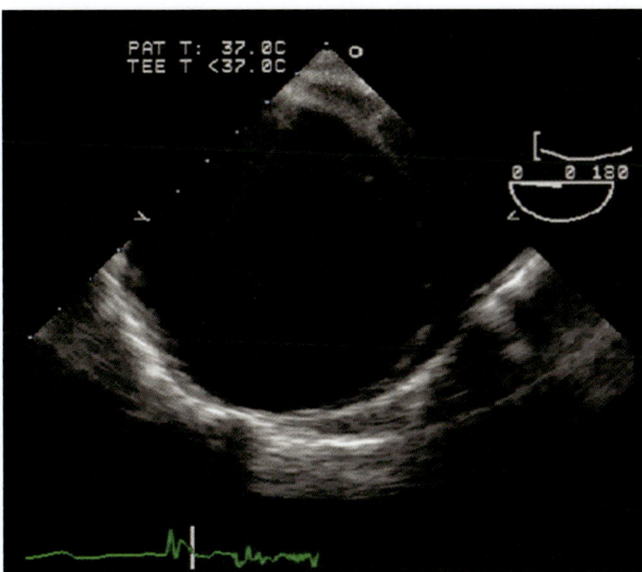
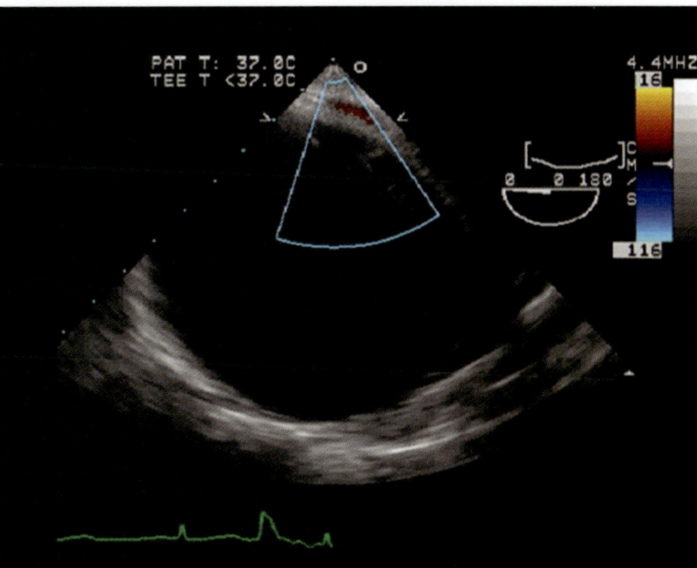
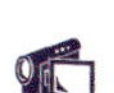

Figure 19-22 Ascending aortic aneurysm shown in midesophageal ascending aortic short-axis image at level of right pulmonary artery with a multiplane angle of 0 degrees. Note giant ascending aortic aneurysm. Giant ascending thoracic aortic aneurysms may produce a mediastinal mass effect. Color Doppler imaging *(right panel)* demonstrated that right pulmonary artery, lying directly behind ascending aorta, is compressed by aneurysm. Insertion of transesophageal echocardiography probe into esophagus directly behind right pulmonary artery has the potential to cause hypoxemia if both left mainstem bronchus and right pulmonary artery are simultaneously obstructed. (See Video 19-12.) *(Adapted from Cheung AT, Weiss SJ. Diseases of the aorta. In: Oxorn DC, ed.* Intraoperative Echocardiography. *Philadelphia: Saunders; 2012:161-182.)*

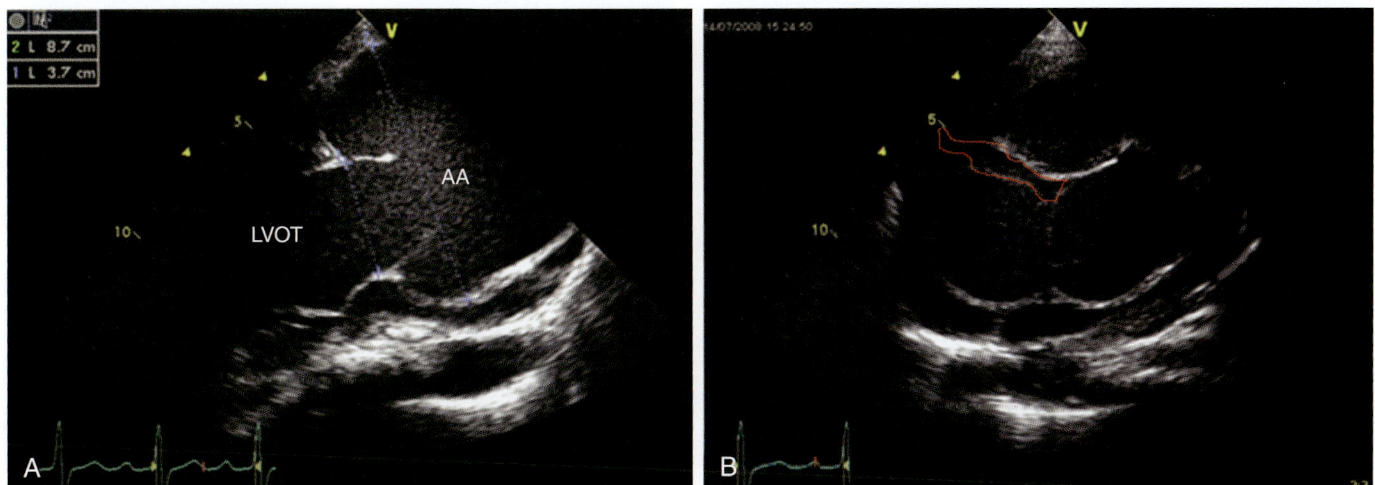

Figure 19-23 Aortic root aneurysm. **A,** Midesophageal (ME) aortic valve long-axis view in systole. Aortic annulus is dilated (diameter 3.7 cm). Sinus segment is aneurysmal (diameter 8.7 cm). **B,** ME aortic valve short-axis view in diastole. Traced area indicates clear diastolic separation of aortic valve cusps due to giant aortic root aneurysm which has pulled these cusps apart to allow development of significant aortic regurgitation. *AA,* Ascending aorta; *LVOT,* left ventricular outflow tract. *(Adapted from Myers PO, Aggom Y, Tissot C. Giant aortic root aneurysm in Marfan syndrome: a rare complication in early childhood. J Thorac Cardiovasc Surg. 2011;141:293-294.)*

A bicuspid aortic valve is associated with an increased risk for proximal thoracic aortic aneurysm due to an associated aortopathy.[58,59] The pattern of aortic dilation typically falls into one of four clusters: cluster I, aortic root; cluster II, ascending aorta; cluster III, ascending aorta and aortic arch; cluster IV, aortic root, ascending aorta, and aortic arch.[60] Cluster IV represents the most common pattern.[60] The distribution and severity of aortic dilation determines the type of surgical aortic replacement.[60,61]

TEE has a role in the conduct of thoracic aortic endovascular aortic repair for evaluation of landing zones (see Fig. 19-5) and for detection of endovascular leaks after stent-graft deployment.[62,63] An endovascular leak can be detected as blood flow within the excluded aneurysm cavity during color Doppler interrogation and/or presence of swirling spontaneous echo contrast (Fig. 19-26). An added advantage of TEE in

this setting is that it decreases the requirement for radiographic contrast agents to accomplish the procedure.

TEE also has a role in detection and evaluation of atheroma in the aortic arch and descending thoracic aorta (Table 19-3). Severe and/or mobile atheroma can put patients at risk for atheroembolic complications during endoaortic events such as wire manipulations, endovascular stenting, and transcatheter aortic valve replacement (see Fig. 19-25).[64-66]

Aortic Atheroma

The severity of atherosclerotic disease is graded according to plaque thickness and presence of mobile atheroma (see Table 19-3). In the atheromatous aorta, TEE can detect and grade the severity of atheroma lesions to estimate the risk of atheroembolism. Atheroma appears on

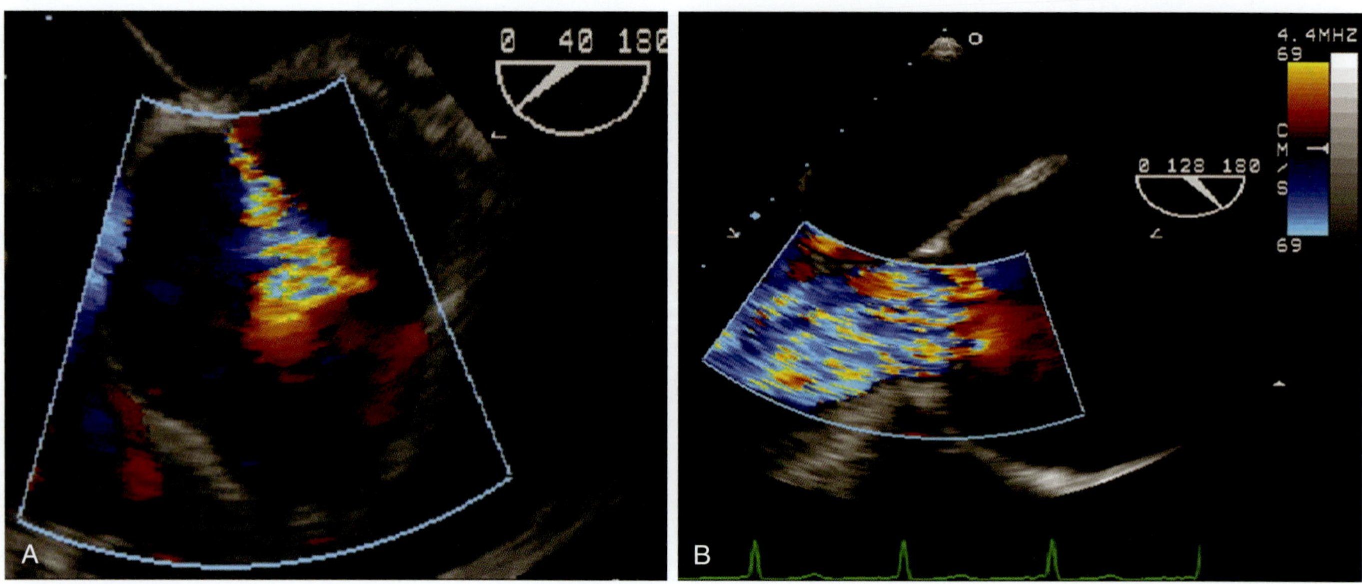

Figure 19-24   Aortic regurgitation associated with aortic root aneurysm. **A,** Midesophageal (ME) aortic valve short-axis view at a multiplane angle of 42 degrees. **B,** ME aortic valve long-axis view at a multiplane angle of 128 degrees. Color Doppler imaging demonstrates severe central aortic regurgitation associated with aortic root aneurysm. Dilation of aortic root has caused outward cusp tethering with impaired diastolic coaptation to result in a central and triangular-shaped regurgitant orifice. *(Adapted from Cheung AT, Weiss SJ. Diseases of the aorta. In: Oxorn DC, ed. Intraoperative Echocardiography. Philadelphia: Saunders; 2012:161-182.)*

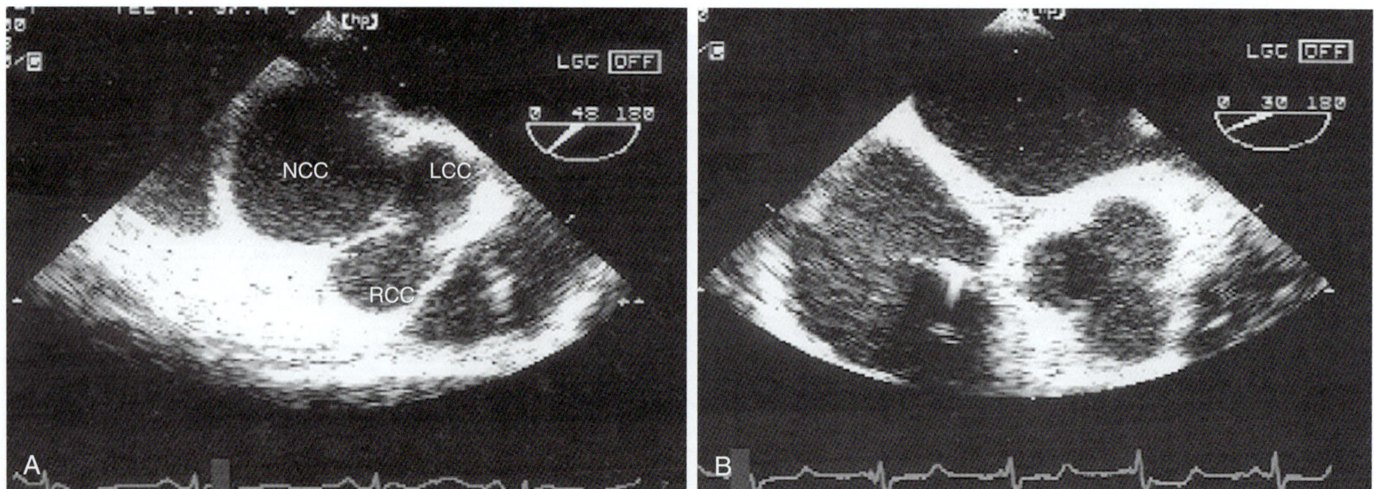

Figure 19-25   Aneurysm of sinus of Valsalva. **A,** Midesophageal (ME) aortic valve short-axis view at a multiplane angle of 48 degrees. The three sinuses of Valsalva are displayed. There is aneurysmal degeneration of noncoronary sinus of Valsalva. **B,** ME aortic valve short-axis view at a multiplane angle of 30 degrees. Noncoronary sinus of Valsalva has been restored to normal configuration through reconstruction with a prosthetic patch. *LCC,* Left coronary cusp; *NCC,* noncoronary cusp; *RCC,* right coronary cusp. *(Adapted from Hines MH, Kon ND. Sinus of Valsalva aneurysm repair with partial allograft and 10-year follow-up. Ann Thorac Surg. 2010;90:1701-1703.)*

echocardiographic examination as irregular thickening along the intimal surface of the aorta (Figs. 19-27 and 19-28). The increased density of atherosclerotic plaques cause it to appear brighter on ultrasound imaging compared to normal regions of the vessel wall. Calcified plaques will produce ultrasound shadowing (see Fig. 19-28).

Severe atherosclerosis of the aortic arch and mobile atheroma detected by TEE in the aortic arch are risk factors for perioperative stroke (see Fig. 19-27). These atheroma types are vulnerable to embolism during thoracic aortic manipulations. Furthermore, in this setting, the echocardiographer should evaluate for complications of aortic atheroma such as aneurysm and penetrating atherosclerotic ulcer with or without IMH.

Echocardiographic assessment of aortic atheroma with TEE and/or epiaortic ultrasound scanning can define the location and size of aortic atheroma. This approach can decrease the risk of stroke during cardiac surgery from maneuvers such as aortic cannulation and aortic clamping. Epiaortic ultrasound is more sensitive than manual palpation or

TEE for detecting atherosclerosis of the ascending aorta, taking into account the blind spot of TEE described earlier.[1-5] In recent guidelines, routine epiaortic ultrasound scanning of the ascending aorta during cardiac surgery was recommended to evaluate the presence, location, and severity of atheromatous plaque for reduction of atheroembolic complications (Class IIa Recommendation; Level of Evidence B).[66]

TEE can also be performed to assess the burden of atherosclerosis in the descending thoracic aorta for intraaortic balloon insertion. If TEE evaluation suggests severe aortic atheroma, alternative arterial cannulation sites for cardiopulmonary bypass should be considered.[67]

Aortic Coarctation Associated with Aortic Aneurysm

Coarctation of the aorta ranges from localized stenosis to complete interruption of the aorta. In adults, the segment of aortic coarctation is

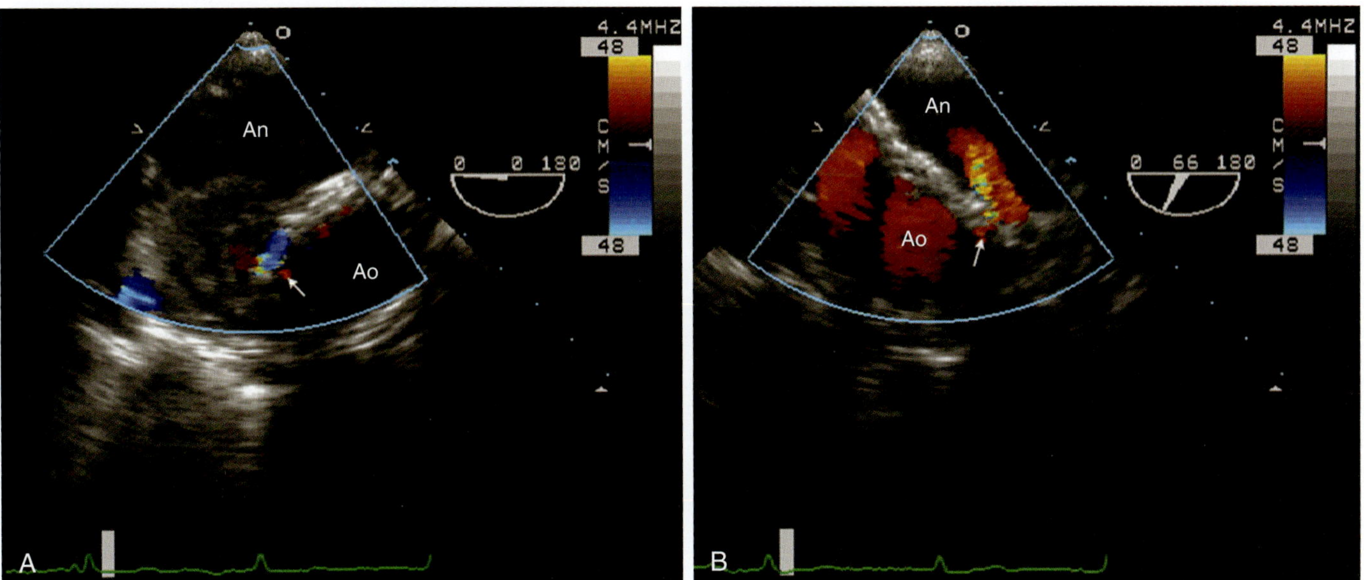

Figure 19-26 Thoracic endovascular aortic repair. Midesophageal (ME) short-axis view **(A)** and long-axis view **(B)** of descending thoracic aorta. After endovascular stent deployment, transesophageal echocardiography demonstrates aortic lumen *(Ao)* and excluded aneurysm *(An)*. Thrombus and swirling spontaneous echo contrast were imaged within excluded aneurysm cavity. Doppler color flow imaging demonstrated an endovascular leak with flow from aortic lumen into excluded aneurysm cavity *(arrow)*. *(Adapted from Cheung AT, Weiss SJ. Diseases of the aorta. In: Oxorn DC, ed. Intraoperative Echocardiography. Philadelphia: Saunders; 2012:161-182.)*

TABLE 19-3	Grading of Aortic Atherosclerosis by Transesophageal Echocardiography	
Grade	*Severity*	*Description*
I	Normal	Normal to mild intimal thickening
II	Mild	Intimal thickening ≤ 3 mm without irregularities
III	Moderate	Sessile atheroma protruding < 5 mm into lumen
IV	Severe	Sessile atheroma protruding ≥ 5 mm into lumen
V	Severe	Any size atheroma with mobile components

Data from Katz ES, Tunick PA, Rusinek H, et al. Protruding aortic atheromas predict stroke risk in elderly patients undergoing cardiopulmonary bypass: experience with intraoperative transesophageal echocardiography. *J Am Coll Cardiol.* 1992;20:70-77.

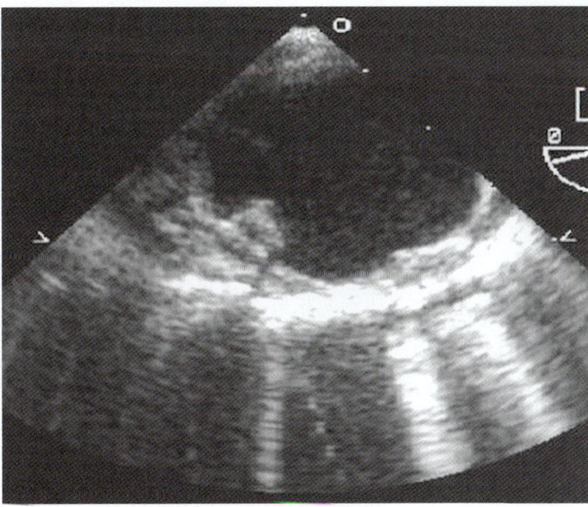

Figure 19-28 Thoracic aortic atheroma. Midesophageal descending thoracic aortic short-axis view at a multiplane angle of 15 degrees showing obvious atherosclerotic disease with an irregular intimal surface. Aortic wall is calcified, as evidenced by specular echoes and shadowing artifacts. This patient's atherosclerosis was graded as severe, since atheroma protrudes 5 mm or more into aortic lumen. Presence of mobile elements in atheroma would also qualify it as severe disease. *(Adapted from Cheung AT, Weiss SJ. Diseases of the aorta. In: Oxorn DC, ed. Intraoperative Echocardiography. Philadelphia: Saunders; 2012:161-182.)*

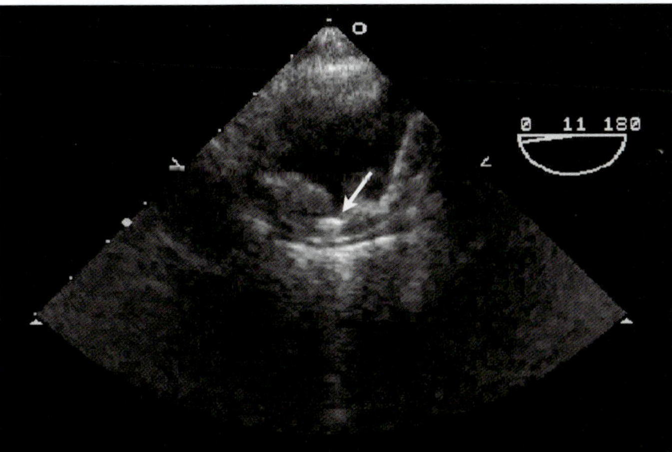

Figure 19-27 Thoracic aortic atheroma: risk for atheroembolism. Midesophageal (ME) short-axis view of proximal descending thoracic aorta in patient undergoing thoracic endovascular aortic repair. Transesophageal echocardiography (TEE) demonstrated severe atherosclerosis (grade V) with mobile atheroma at proximal landing zone for stent-graft. TEE was used to reposition a guidewire *(arrow)* to prevent atheroma dislodgement prior to endovascular stent deployment. *(Adapted from Cheung AT, Weiss SJ. Diseases of the aorta. In: Oxorn DC, ed. Intraoperative Echocardiography. Philadelphia: Saunders; 2012:161-182.)*

typically postductal, which is just beyond the origin of the subclavian artery or distal to the insertion of the ligamentum arteriosum. TEE diagnosis of this condition is typically challenging. In this setting, the proximal descending aorta appears to be interrupted as the TEE probe is withdrawn to track the descending aorta into the aortic arch. Color Doppler imaging may demonstrate high-velocity turbulent flow at the site of coarctation. Gradient estimation by spectral Doppler is typically difficult because the ultrasound beam cannot be aligned parallel to the direction of maximum flow across the stenotic aortic segment.

Aortic coarctation may be associated with thoracic aortic aneurysm because of their mutual link with the aortopathy of the bicuspid aortic valve syndrome.[68,69] Furthermore, aneurysm formation after surgical repair of aortic coarctation occurs in 10% of cases.[70-72] In this setting, endovascular repair has emerged as an attractive alternative to repeat surgical repair.[73] The presence of a bicuspid aortic valve is a reason for the echocardiographer to search diligently for aneurysm and coarctation of the thoracic aorta.

Pulmonary Artery

See also Chapter 17.

Anatomy of the Pulmonary Artery

The main pulmonary artery is the continuation of the right ventricular infundibulum, with its initial portion within the pericardium. It lies on the roof of the left atrium. At its base, the main pulmonary artery is anterior to the aorta, but as it ascends, it courses leftward and posterior to the aorta to divide into the right and left pulmonary arteries (see Fig. 19-6). Although the right pulmonary artery courses horizontally behind the ascending aorta and the superior vena cava, it lies anterior to the right mainstem bronchus (see Figs. 19-8 and 19-22).

TEE Examination of the Pulmonary Artery

The main pulmonary artery and pulmonic valve can be imaged in front and just to the left of the aorta in the TEE ME aortic valve short-axis view. The TEE upper esophageal aortic arch short-axis view also provides a long-axis image of the pulmonic valve and main pulmonary artery (see Fig. 19-3, B). The distal main pulmonary artery and its bifurcation can be imaged to the left of the ascending aorta in the ME ascending aortic short-axis and long-axis views (see Fig. 19-3). The right pulmonary artery is imaged in long axis in the ME ascending aortic short-axis view, and in short axis in the ME ascending aortic long-axis view. Pulmonary artery catheters can reflect ultrasound beams to create linear artifacts within the aortic lumen to mimic aortic dissection (Fig. 19-29). Although the proximal left pulmonary artery can be imaged in the ME ascending aortic short-axis view, it is obscured more distally by the left mainstem bronchus.

Pulmonary Artery Dissection

Although pulmonary artery dissection is rare, it is most common in patients with severe pulmonary hypertension (Fig. 19-30).[74,75] Its

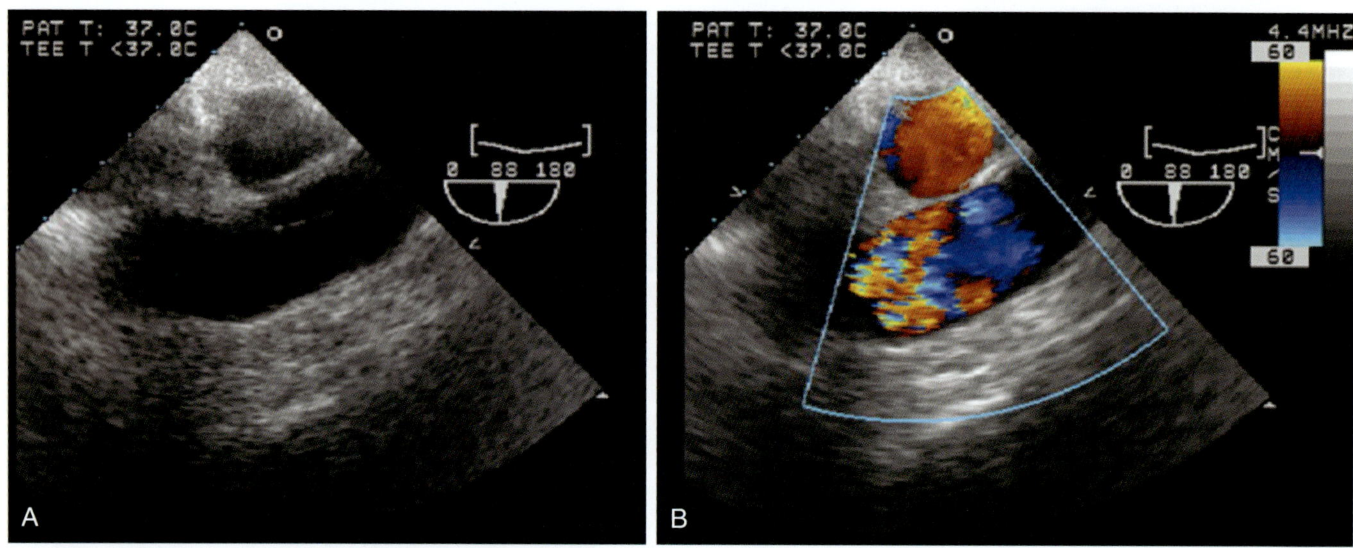

Figure 19-29   Imaging artifacts from pulmonary artery in high esophageal ascending aortic long-axis view at a multiplane angle of 88 degrees. **A** demonstrates side-lobe artifact, which appears as a linear density within aortic lumen. This artifact is created by ultrasound reflecting off a catheter within right pulmonary artery. **B,** Side-lobe artifacts appear as linear densities that can cross anatomic structures and do not cause separation of blood flow on Doppler color flow imaging. *(Adapted from Cheung AT, Weiss SJ. Diseases of the aorta. In: Oxorn DC, ed. Intraoperative Echocardiography. Philadelphia: Saunders; 2012:161-182.)*

Figure 19-30 Pulmonary artery dissection. **A,** High esophageal ascending aortic short-axis view at a multiplane angle of 0 degrees. Main pulmonary artery is aneurysmal (diameter 5.18 cm) in patient with chronic severe pulmonary hypertension. Arrow indicates intimal flap, consistent with pulmonary artery dissection. **B,** Epiarterial scan of pulmonary artery, with arrow pointing to intimal flap. *(Adapted from Rousou AJ, Haddadin AS, Badescu G, et al. Surgical repair of pulmonary artery dissection. Eur J Cardiothorac Surg. 2010;38:805.)*

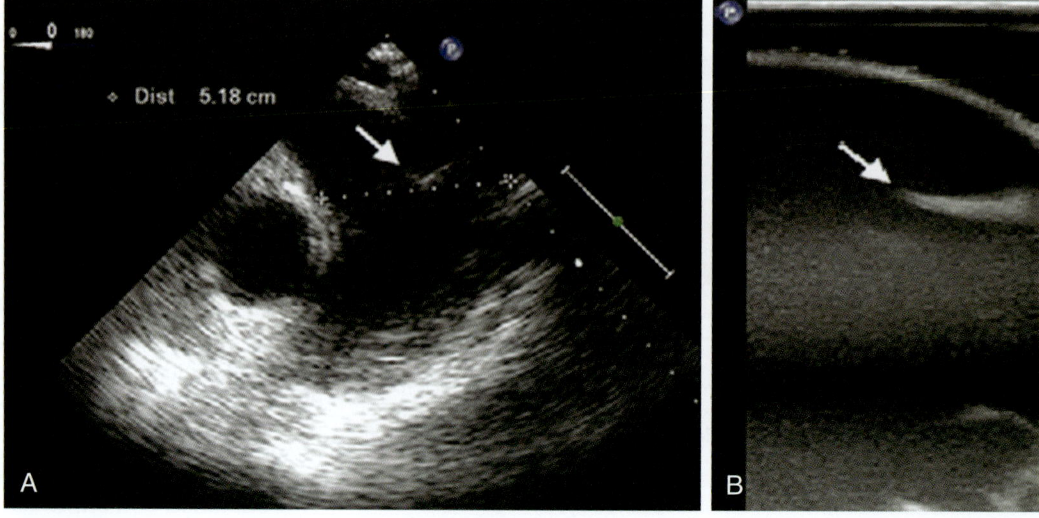

complications include rupture and pericardial tamponade.[76] Pulmonary artery dissection can also be secondary to a PDA complicated by severe pulmonary hypertension, including the Eisenmenger syndrome.[76,77]

A PDA is persistence of the ductus arteriosus, connecting the pulmonary artery to the descending aorta in the fetus (Fig. 19-31). Color Doppler imaging can demonstrate a PDA with flow from the aorta to the pulmonary artery (Fig. 19-32). If the PDA is restrictive, pressure in the aorta exceeds the pressure in the pulmonary artery throughout the cardiac cycle, resulting in high-velocity continuous flow through the PDA (Fig. 19-33). Long-standing left-to-right shunting across a PDA results in chronic pulmonary hypertension, pulmonary artery dilation, and right ventricular hypertrophy. In severe cases, the pulmonary artery may become aneurysmal and/or dissect. In long-standing cases, Eisenmenger syndrome may develop, with shunt reversal across the PDA to cause right-to-left shunting.

Pulmonary Artery Aneurysm

The normal diameter of the pulmonary artery in adults is up to 3 cm, with the right and left pulmonary arteries typically having a diameter of about 2 cm.[78] Pulmonary artery aneurysms may be idiopathic but are typically secondary to severe pulmonary hypertension, infections, and upstream stenotic disease such as infundibular stensosis.[79-81] Although rare, pulmonary artery pseudoaneurysms may result from arterial disruption secondary to malignant tumors of the pulmonary artery.[81,82] The complications of pulmonary artery aneurysms include pulmonary regurgitation, dissection, compression of neighboring structures, and rupture into the pericardium, pleural space, and airway.[79-83] A detailed echocardiographic analysis of right ventricular function in diseases of the pulmonary artery is essential, given the frequent concomitant conditions of pulmonary hypertension and pulmonary regurgitation.[84]

Left Ventricle

Left Ventricular Aneurysm

True Aneurysm

Left ventricular true aneurysms are characterized by focal ventricular dilation, with a wall that contains all three myocardial layers. The etiologies can be congenital or acquired, including infections and ischemia.[85-88] Complications of these aneurysms include arrhythmias, rupture, pericardial tamponade, pseudoaneurysm, thrombosis, thromboembolism, and mitral regurgitation.[85-88] Echocardiographic analysis of a true ventricular aneurysm should evaluate its location, shape, dimensions, wall thickness, wall motion, presence of thrombus or calcification, presence of rupture (with or without pseudoaneurysm), and any effects on valvular function.

True aneurysms of the left ventricular inferior wall typically result from right coronary ischemia (Fig. 19-34).[89] True ventricular aneurysms that result from coronary ischemia will typically have a thinned wall, a wide neck, and a degree of mural thrombus (see Fig. 19-34). The aneurysm wall gradually thins out as the necrotic myocardium develops fibrosis and at times calcifies. Frequently the diameter of the wide neck of a true aneurysm will be greater than 50% of the maximal

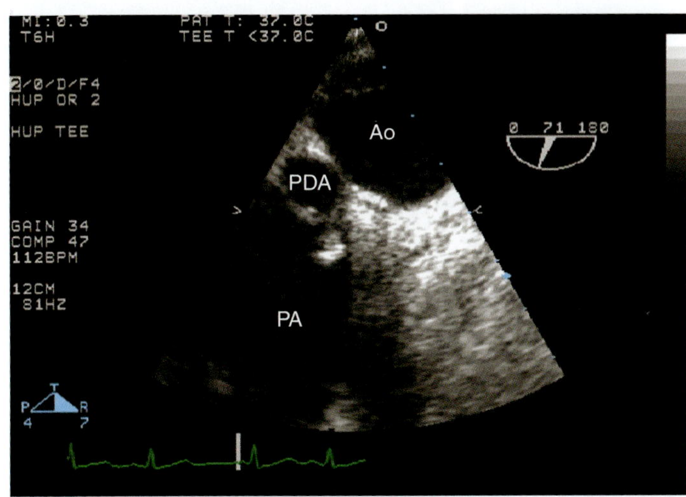

Figure 19-31 Patent ductus arteriosus *(PDA)*. Upper esophageal aortic arch short-axis view at a multiplane angle of 71 degrees. There is a PDA between aortic arch *(Ao)* in short axis and main pulmonary artery *(PA)* in long axis. *(Adapted from Cheung AT, Weiss SJ. Diseases of the aorta. In: Oxorn DC, ed. Intraoperative Echocardiography. Philadelphia: Saunders; 2012:161-182.)*

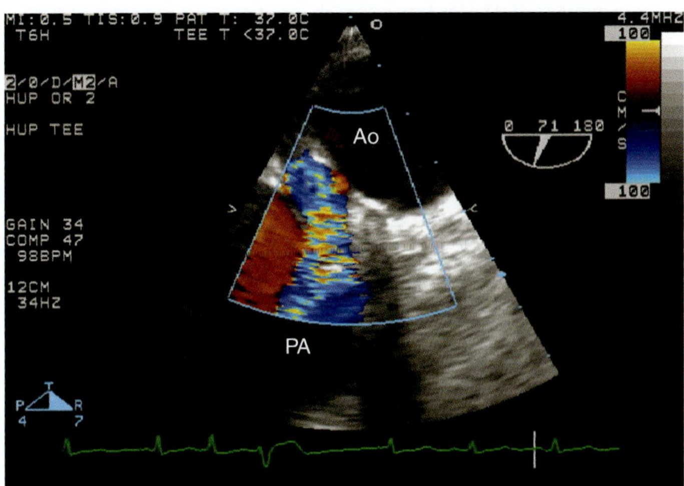

Figure 19-32 Patent ductus arteriosus (PDA). Upper esophageal aortic arch short-axis view at a multiplane angle of 71 degrees. Color flow Doppler imaging demonstrates blood flow in diastole from aortic arch *(Ao)* in short axis into main pulmonary artery *(PA)* in long axis through PDA. *(Adapted from Cheung AT, Weiss SJ. Diseases of the aorta. In: Oxorn DC, ed. Intraoperative Echocardiography. Philadelphia: Saunders; 2012:161-182.)*

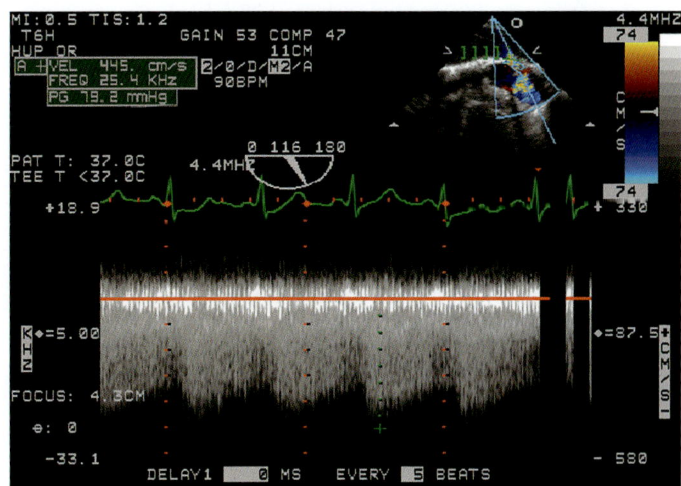

Figure 19-33 Patent ductus arteriosus (PDA). Upper esophageal aortic arch short-axis view at a multiplane angle of 116 degrees. Continuous wave Doppler demonstrated that blood flow through PDA from aorta to pulmonary artery was continuous throughout cardiac cycle, with a phasic component and a peak pressure gradient of 79.2 mmHg. *(Adapted from Cheung AT, Weiss SJ. Diseases of the aorta. In: Oxorn DC, ed. Intraoperative Echocardiography. Philadelphia: Saunders; 2012:161-182.)*

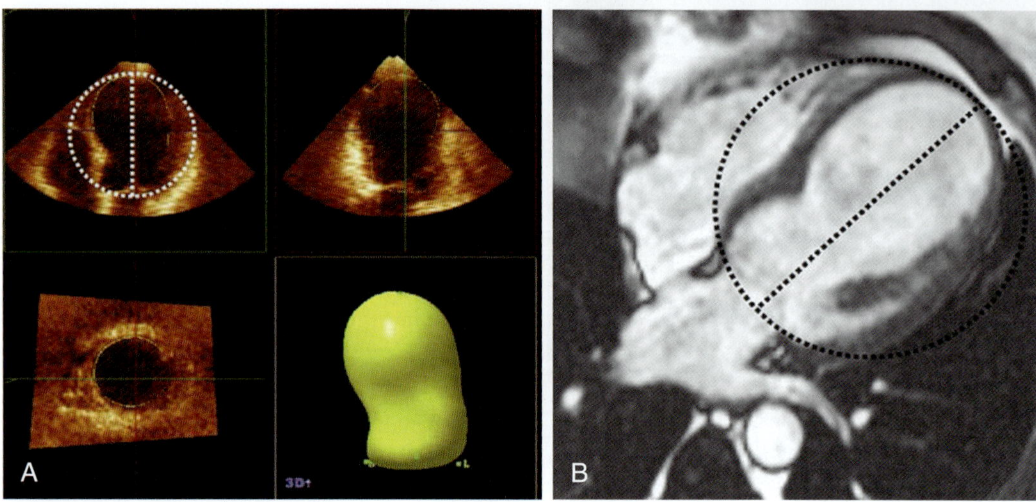

Figure 19-34 Giant left ventricular aneurysm. **A,** Mid-esophageal two-chamber view. Arrows indicate large inferior left ventricular *(LV)* true aneurysm involving basal and middle segments of inferior wall. Note layer of thrombus in aneurysm due to sluggish blood flow. **B,** Preoperative left ventriculogram depicts the considerable extent of inferior aneurysm, which was associated with a chronically occluded right coronary artery. *LA,* Left atrium. *(Adapted from Grimaldi A, Castiglioni A, De Bonis M, et al. Large left ventricular aneurysm. J Thorac Cardiovasc Surg. 2011;142:940-941.)*

Figure 19-35 Three-dimensional (3D) echocardiography for left ventricular (LV) aneurysm: shape. 3D echocardiography **(A)** and magnetic resonance imaging (MRI) **(B)** show calculation of sphericity index in the setting of LV aneurysm. *Sphericity index* is defined as LV end-diastolic volume divided by volume of a sphere whose diameter was calculated from LV long axis. Major end-diastolic LV long axis was calculated by 3D echocardiography as longest distance between center of mitral annulus and endocardial apex, optimized by cropping 3D dataset **(A)**. LV end-diastolic volume was calculated according to standard volumetric analysis of 3D full-volume dataset *(lower right-hand panel of A)*. Similar approach was followed in analysis of MRI data **(B)**. (See Video 19-13.) *(Adapted from Marsan NA, Westenberg JJM, Roes SD, et al. Three-dimensional echocardiography for the preoperative assessment of patients with left ventricular aneurysm. Ann Thorac Surg. 2011; 91(1): 113-21.)*

diameter of the aneurysm. Echocardiographic analysis of aneurysm wall motion will demonstrate severe regional wall motion abnormalities such as akinesis or dyskinesis.

MRI is currently considered the gold standard for perioperative evaluation of postinfarction left ventricular aneurysms to guide surgical therapy of these lesions.[90-92] The recent advent of 3D echocardiography has displaced MRI for evaluating left ventricular size, shape, global and regional systolic function, myocardial scar, and valvular regurgitation (Figs. 19-35 to 19-37).[91] Echocardiography offers distinct advantages over MRI for evaluation of aneurysm, including its availability, portability, ease of use, bedside and intraoperative applications, avoidance of contrast media, and safety in patients with indwelling metal devices.[91] A limitation of 3D echocardiography is that full-volume imaging requires electrocardiographic gating. A clinical consequence of this gating requirement is that this type of 3D imaging is not possible in the setting of atrial fibrillation.[91]

False Aneurysm (Pseudoaneurysm)

A left ventricular pseudoaneurysm is a contained rupture of the ventricle with a wall that typically contains pericardium. A pseudoaneurysm will usually have a narrow neck at the site of ventricular rupture.[89] In contrast to a true aneurysm, the neck diameter is less than 50% of the maximal diameter of the pseudoaneurysm. The narrow neck is connected to a large saccular echolucent chamber that is both external to the ventricular cavity and frequently filled with thrombus due to stasis (Fig. 19-38). A further characteristic feature is that Doppler interrogation of blood flow at its neck typically reveals systolic flow into and diastolic flow out of the pseudoaneurysm (Fig. 19-39).

Pseudoaneurysms are typically secondary to myocardial infarction or surgical myocardial procedures such as true aneurysm repair, apicoaortic bypass, and transapical aortic valve implantation (see Figs. 19-38 and 19-39).[93,94] Analogous to true aneurysms, left ventricular pseudoaneurysms frequently distort the mitral valve complex, resulting in surgical mitral regurgitation. The mitral valve can be repaired or replaced through the transventricular approach, allowing a single incision for both pseudoaneurysm and mitral repair.[95]

Left ventricular outpouchings such as true aneurysms and pseudoaneurysms must be distinguished from a *left ventricular diverticulum,*

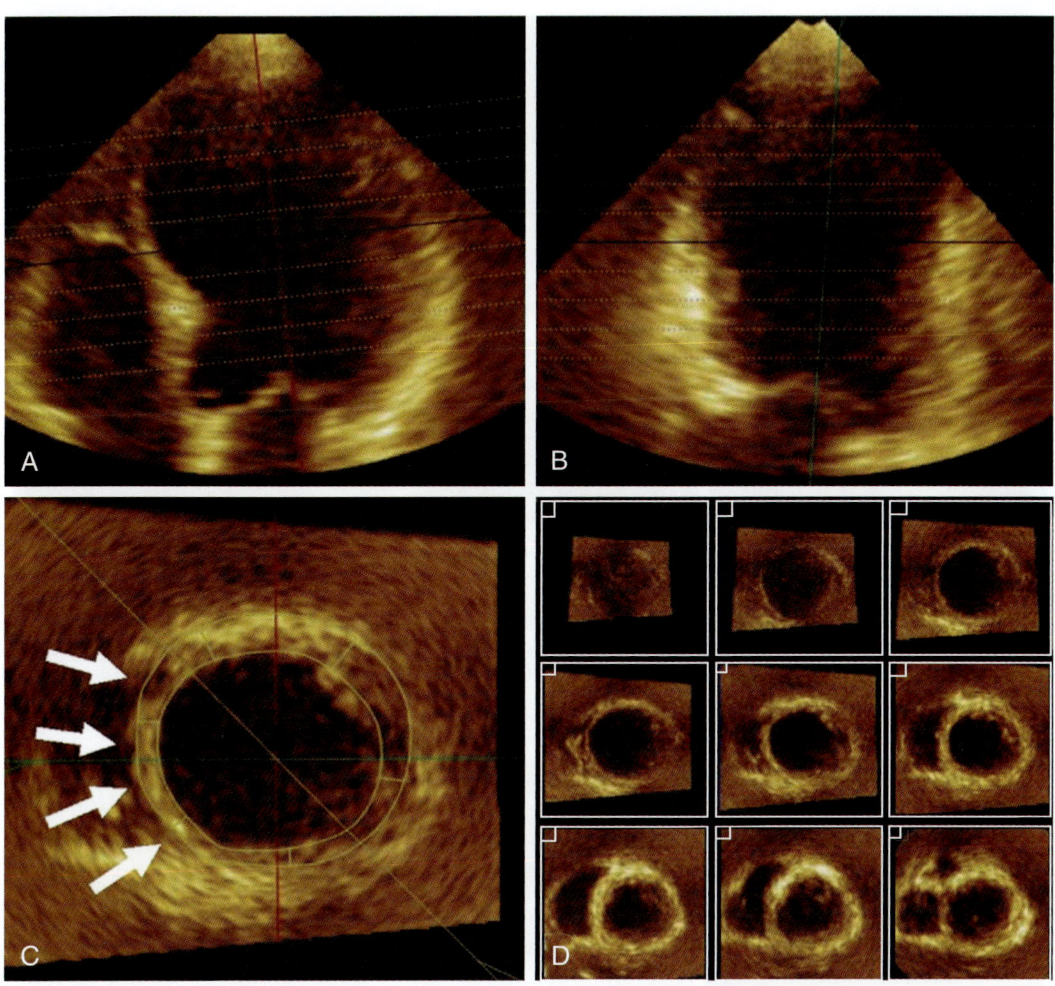

Figure 19-36 Three-dimensional (3D) echocardiography for left ventricular (LV) aneurysm: scar. Assessment of LV regional wall thickness with 3D echocardiography. Four-chamber view (**A**) and two-chamber view (**B**) demonstrate slicing of 3D dataset into 9 LV short axes (3 at basal level, 3 at midventricular level, 3 at apical level). **C** shows tracing of endocardial and epicardial borders at end-diastole at midventricular level. White arrows indicate septal thinning, consistent with transmural scar. **D** demonstrates that LV apical segments are also significantly thinned. (*Adapted from Marsan NA, Westenberg JJM, Roes SD, et al. Three-dimensional echocardiography for the preoperative assessment of patients with left ventricular aneurysm. Ann Thorac Surg. 2011;91:113-121.*)

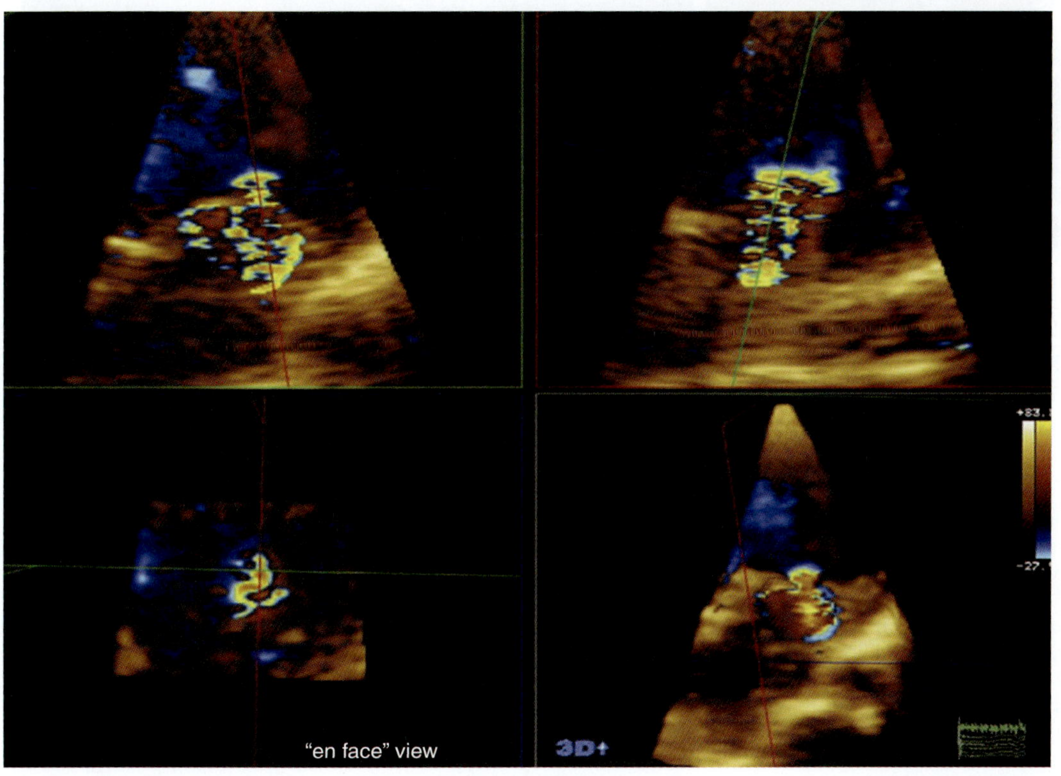

Figure 19-37 Three-dimensional (3D) echocardiography for left ventricular (LV) aneurysm: mitral valve. Assessment of mitral regurgitation with 3D echocardiography in patient with LV aneurysm. 3D dataset is manually cropped by an image plane perpendicular to regurgitant jet until narrowest cross-sectional area of jet. Image is then tilted to an "en face view" for manual planimetry of effective regurgitant orifice area, measured at 0.26 cm² and consistent with mild to moderate mitral regurgitation in this case. (*Adapted from Marsan NA, Westenberg JJM, Roes SD, et al. Three-dimensional echocardiography for the preoperative assessment of patients with left ventricular aneurysm. Ann Thorac Surg. 2011;91:113-121.*)

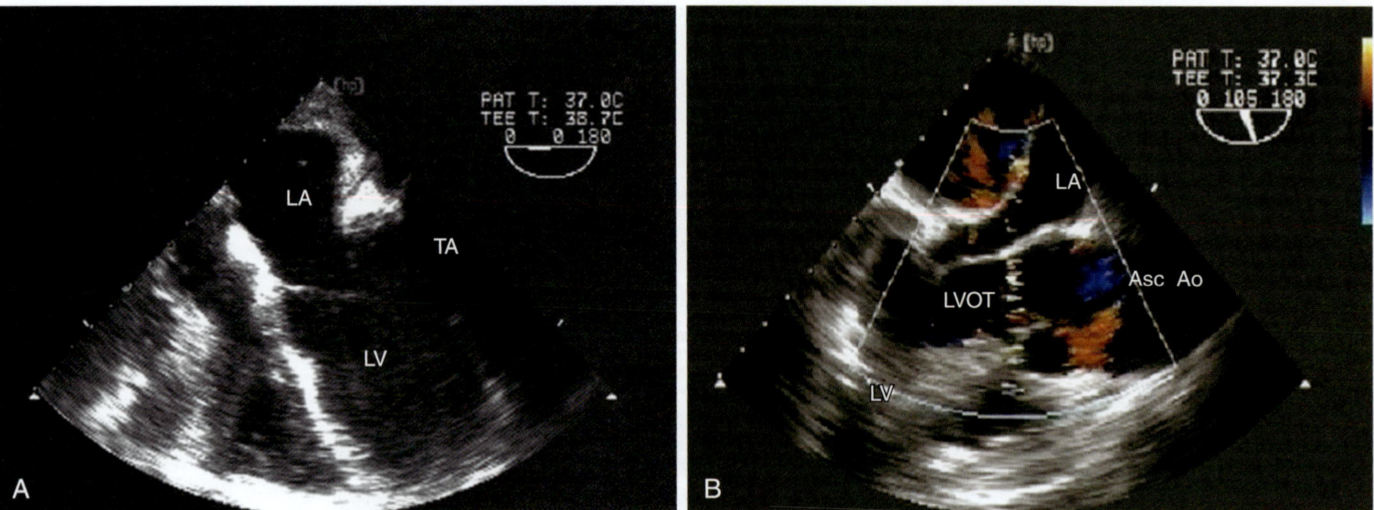

Figure 19-38   Left ventricular (*LV*) pseudoaneurysm after myocardial infarction. **A,** Midesophageal (ME) four-chamber view at a multiplane angle of 0 degrees. Note true aneurysm (*TA*) involving lateral wall of LV and thrombus formation outside wall of left atrium (*LA*). **B,** ME long-axis view of aortic valve at a multiplane angle of 105 degrees. Note echolucent cavity behind LA. Color flow Doppler imaging reveals flow in this echolucent cavity. Further imaging revealed that this cavity was continuous with TA via a thin neck. Taken together, these features are consistent with LV true aneurysm of lateral wall, complicated by rupture and pseudoaneurysm formation behind LA, with secondary thrombus. *Asc Ao,* Ascending aorta; *LVOT,* left ventricular outflow tract. (*Adapted from Sidebotham D, Lai J. An abnormal echo-free space behind the left atrium. J Cardiothorac Vasc Anesth. 2004;18:671-672.*)

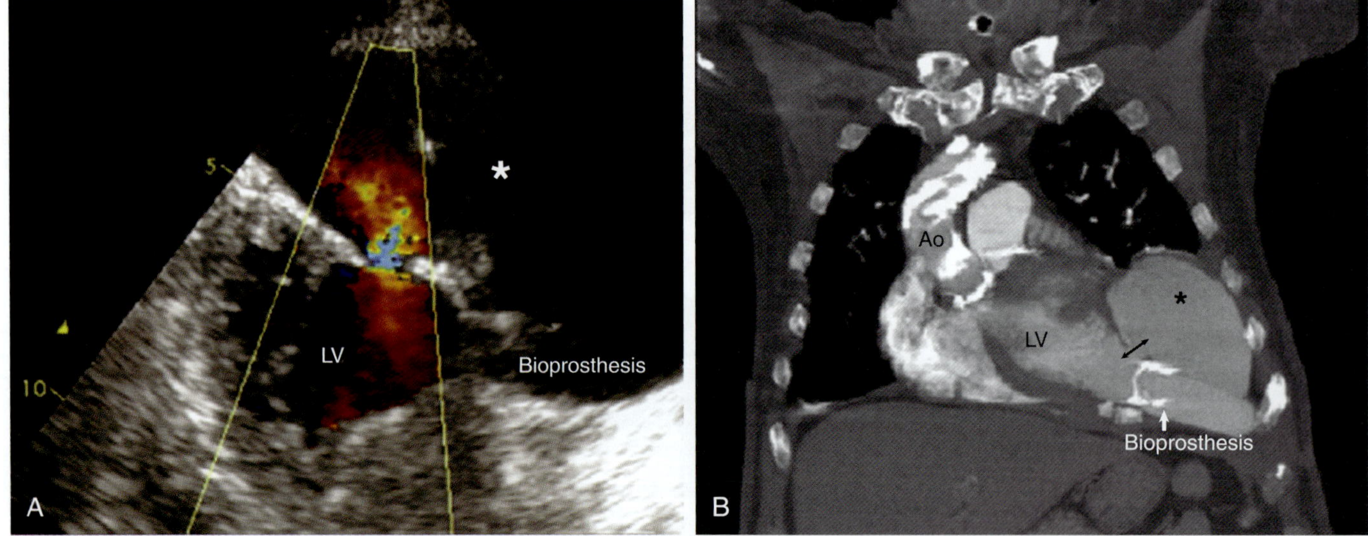

Figure 19-39   Left ventricular pseudoaneurysm after apicoaortic bypass. **A,** Transgastric short-axis view of left ventricle (*LV*) in patient who has undergone apicoaortic bypass with a tissue valve conduit for management of severe aortic stenosis. Aortic bioprosthesis is labeled. Asterisk points out echolucent cavity behind LV. Color Doppler imaging reveals systolic blood flow from LV into cavity through a narrow neck. Taken together, these features are consistent with left ventricular contained rupture and pseudoaneurysm formation after apicoaortic bypass. **B,** Computed tomographic imaging of pseudoaneurysm. Note that ascending aorta (*Ao*) is heavily calcified. This is consistent with a "porcelain aorta," the reason this patient did not undergo conventional aortic valve replacement (high stroke risk). Heavily calcified native aortic valve annulus is also evident. Apical pseudoaneurysm formation is also a described complication of transapical aortic valve replacement. (*Adapted from Chen JS, Huang JH, Chu SH, et al. Left ventricular pseudoaneurysm after apicoaortic bypass. Eur J Cardiothorac Surg. 2011;40:e132.*)

which is a benign congenital finding (Fig. 19-40).[89,96] It is important for the perioperative echocardiographer to consider this possibility in the differential diagnosis of left ventricular outpouchings to avoid unnecessary surgical intervention.[89] The diagnostic features of a ventricular diverticulum include a narrow neck, full ventricular wall thickness, preserved systolic contractility, and systolic blood flow across the neck into the ventricular cavity (see Fig. 19-40). Indications for surgical resection of a left ventricular diverticulum include rupture, severe arrhythmias, and systemic embolization. In the absence of these major complications, the management is typically medical.

Left Ventricular Thrombus

Although ventricular thrombus may be primary in patients with hypercoagulable disorders, it is typically secondary to myocardial diseases.[97] These secondary etiologies are typically characterized by low flow and include cardiomyopathies, regional wall motion abnormalities, true aneurysms, pseudoaneurysms, and diverticula. The low-flow state is the major risk factor for the associated ventricular thrombosis.[88-97] The thrombus may be mural or free-floating (Figs. 19-41 and 19-42).[98,99] Mural thrombus is typically associated with focal pathology such as

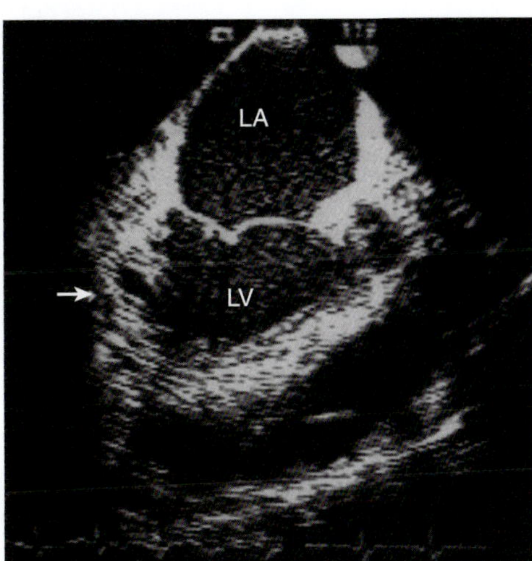

Figure 19-40 Left ventricular diverticulum. Midesophageal long-axis view of left ventricle *(LV)*. Note echolucent cavity adjacent to anteroseptal wall of LV that communicates via a narrow neck *(arrow)* with cavity of LV. Differential diagnosis of this LV outpouching included true aneurysm, pseudoaneurysm, and diverticulum. Further echocardiographic imaging revealed features consistent with pseudoaneurysm: full thickness of diverticular walls, normal contractility of diverticular walls, and systolic blood flow from diverticulum into LV. *LA,* Left atrium. *(Adapted from Boyd WC, Rosengard TK, Hartman GS. Isolated left ventricular diverticulum in an adult. J Cardiothorac Vasc Anesth. 1999;13:468-470.)*

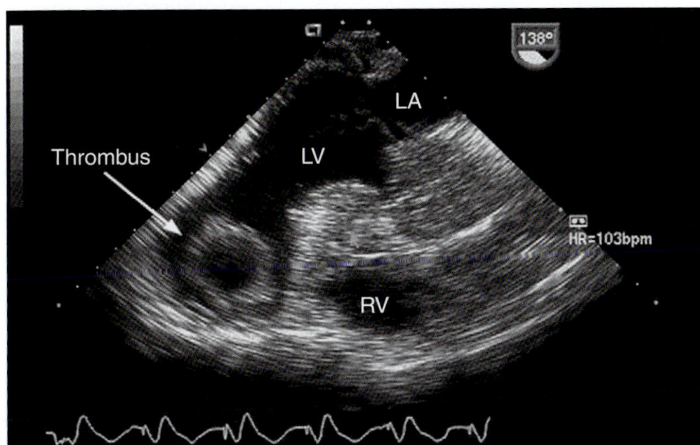

Figure 19-41 Left ventricular mobile ball thrombus. Midesophageal long-axis view of aortic valve at a multiplane angle of 138 degrees. Note large ball thrombus in left ventricular apex. Although differential diagnosis also includes left ventricular tumor, anteroapical thinning and dilation in this view suggest prior myocardial ischemia and apical aneurysm, features that support the diagnosis of thrombus. At surgery, a large ball thrombus was extracted intact through a ventriculotomy, and apical aneurysm was resected. *LA,* Left atrium; *LV,* left ventricle; *RV,* right ventricle. *(Adapted from Sharma S, Ehsan A, Couper GS, et al. Unrecognized left ventricular thrombus during reoperative coronary artery bypass grafting. Ann Thorac Surg. 2004;78:e79-80.)*

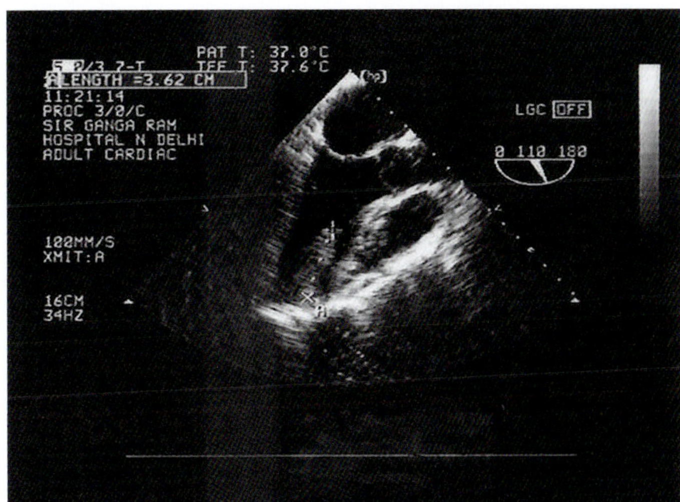

Figure 19-42 Left ventricular apical thrombus. Midesophageal long-axis view of aortic valve at a multiplane angle of 110 degrees. Note left ventricular apical pedunculated mass with a measured length of 3.62 cm. Mass was highly mobile. Ventricular systolic function was normal with no evidence of regional wall motion abnormalities. Differential diagnosis was tumor or thrombus. Owing to multiple serious embolic events, surgical resection of this apical mass was performed; histologic analysis of mass was consistent with thrombus. Subsequent investigation for a hypercoagulable state was negative. *(Adapted from Yadava OP, Yadav S, Juneja S, et al. Left ventricular thrombus sans overt cardiac pathology. Ann Thorac Surg. 2003;76:623-625.)*

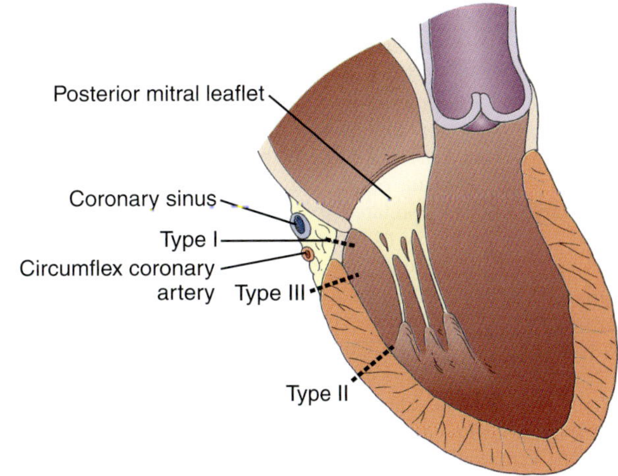

Figure 19-43 This figure illustrates the three patterns of left ventricular posterior wall rupture. Type I ruptures occur in atrioventricular (AV) groove and are the most common of the three types. Intimate anatomic relationship of coronary sinus and circumflex coronary artery to AV groove render these structures at high risk for injury during surgical repair of type I lesions. Type II ruptures occur between AV groove and papillary muscle. Type III ruptures occur at level of papillary muscle. *(Adapted from Zacharias A. Repair of spontaneous rupture of the posterior wall of the left ventricle after mitral valve replacement. Oper Tech Thor Cardiovasc Surg. 2003;8:36-41.)*

Ventricular Rupture

Atrioventricular Groove Disruption

regional wall motion abnormalities, true aneurysm, pseudoaneurysm, or diverticulum. The presenting feature of a ventricular thrombus is thromboembolism.[98,99]

The echocardiographic examination for ventricular thrombus should define the dimensions, location, mobility, consistency, and associated cardiac abnormalities. During echocardiography for left ventricular assist device placement, it is important to rule out apical thrombosis to avoid the risk of embolism during apical cannula placement.[100]

Left ventricular rupture in the region of the atrioventricular groove is most commonly associated with mitral valve surgery, since the posterior mitral annulus is intimately related to the atrioventricular groove (Fig. 19-43).[101] Additional risk factors for this complication during mitral valve procedures include excessive mitral manipulation and advanced mitral pathologies, such as annular calcification, papillary

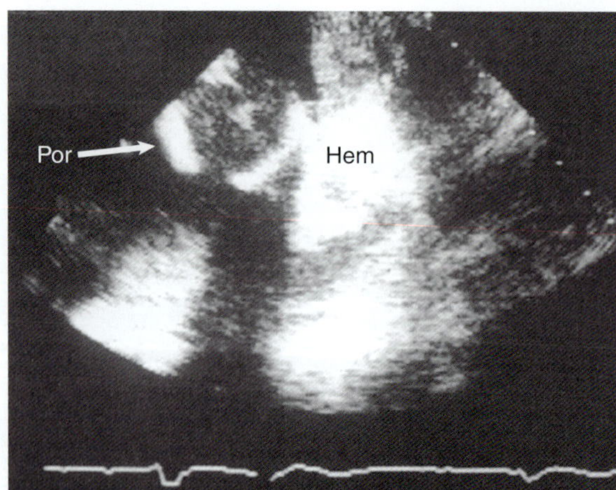

Figure 19-44 Left ventricular wall rupture: type I. Midesophageal four-chamber view at a multiplane angle of 0 degrees. Zoom function has been utilized to focus on freshly implanted porcine mitral valve prosthesis *(Por)* just after separation from cardiopulmonary bypass. Note dissecting hematoma *(Hem)* with extensive involvement of left atrial wall and lateral wall of left ventricle. Cardiopulmonary bypass was reinstituted. Surgical inspection revealed a contained rupture of posterior atrioventricular groove consistent with a type I tear. Despite surgical repair, patient was unable to be weaned from cardiopulmonary bypass. *(Adapted from Lingreen R, Eaton M, Lappas D, et al. Diagnosis by transesophageal echocardiography of atrioventricular groove dissection after mitral valve replacement. J Cardiothorac Vasc Anesth. 1991;5:61-62.)*

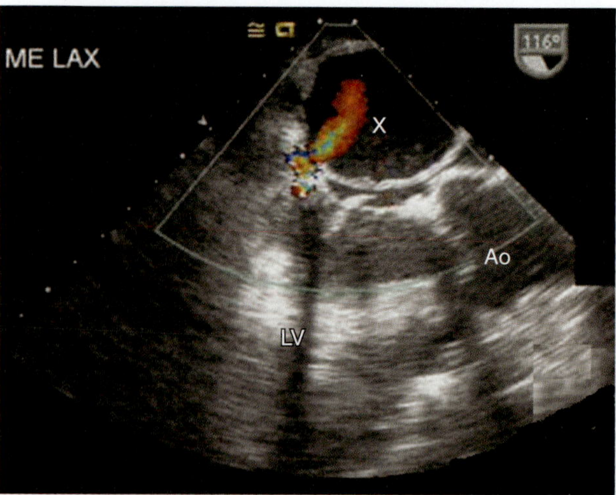

Figure 19-45 Left ventricular wall rupture: type II. Midesophageal long-axis view *(ME LAX)* of aortic valve at a multiplane angle of 116 degrees. Patient had just undergone mitral valve repair with an annuloplasty. The X indicates posterior left atrial wall hematoma with compression of left atrial lumen. Color Doppler interrogation reveals a systolic jet of blood flowing from left ventricle *(LV)* into left atrial wall hematoma, consistent with a left ventricular wall rupture above level of the papillary muscle, with extension into left atrial wall. These features are all consistent with a type II tear. After surgical repair, patient was successfully weaned from cardiopulmonary bypass and subsequently had an uncomplicated recovery. *Ao,* Aorta. *(Adapted from Milla F, Adams DH, Mittnacht AJ. Contained left ventricular rupture with left atrial dissection after mitral valve repair. J Cardiothorac Vasc Anesth. 2010;24:817-819.)*

muscle calcification, and extensive annular abscess.[102-105] There are three types of serious ventricular injury in this setting.[101] Type I ruptures are characterized by atrioventricular disruption with contained or frank rupture (Fig. 19-44; also see Fig. 19-43).

Comprehensive echocardiographic evaluation can guide surgical decision making for extent of annular resection and annular repair.[103-105] There is a risk of injury to the circumflex coronary artery and coronary sinus during repairs for type I ruptures, because these structures are intimately related to the atrioventricular groove (see Fig. 19-43). Serious injury to the circumflex coronary artery is typically associated with hypokinesis/akinesis of the left ventricular lateral wall, with or without electrocardiographic evidence of ischemia. Management options include revision of the annular repair, coronary bypass grafting, and percutaneous coronary stenting. Serious injury to the coronary sinus may result in rupture or fistula. Rupture of the coronary sinus may be evident echocardiographically as a retrocardiac dissecting hematoma. Coronary sinus fistula follows communication with the left ventricular cavity, resulting in a large acute left-to-right shunt. This is evident echocardiographically as high-pressure turbulent flow in the coronary sinus.[106] If the shunt is large, it will precipitate acute cardiac failure and require surgical repair.[107]

Type II ruptures are located between the mitral annulus and the level of the posteromedial papillary muscle (Fig. 19-45; also see Fig. 19-43). Type III ruptures occur at the level of the papillary muscle (Fig. 19-46; also see Fig. 19-43). If the rupture is contained, it leads to a dissecting hematoma due to high left ventricular pressures (see Fig. 19-45). If the rupture is complete, it will breach the left ventricular wall and present with pericardial hemorrhage (see Fig. 19-45). Although type III ruptures typically involve the inferoposterior wall, they may involve the anterior left ventricular wall if the anterolateral papillary muscle is extensively calcified (see Figs. 19-43 and 19-46). Although type II and type III lesions have become rarer (associated with preservation of the mitral chordal apparatus in mitral valve procedures), they still require urgent high-risk surgical repair.

Ventricular Septal Rupture

Ventricular septal rupture is most commonly ischemic or traumatic (Figs. 19-47 to 19-49).[108-110] Echocardiographic evaluation of an

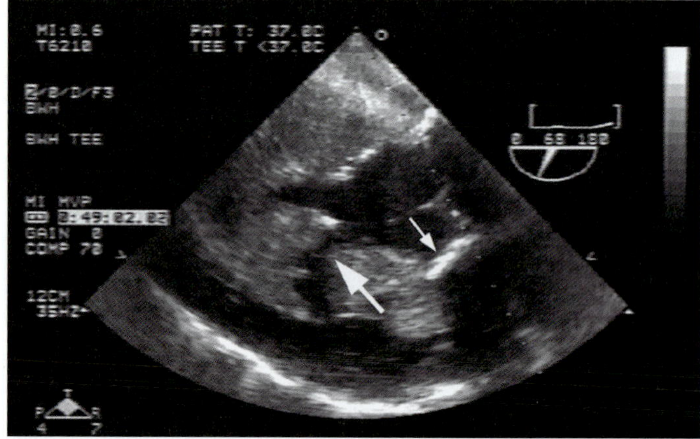

Figure 19-46 Left ventricular wall rupture: type III. Transgastric long-axis view of mitral valve *(small arrow)* at a multiplane angle of 68 degrees. Patient had just undergone mitral valve replacement. Large arrow indicates a rupture of anterior left ventricular wall at level of papillary muscle, complicated by full-thickness rupture with hemorrhage into pericardial space. Surgical repair of this rupture after mitral valve replacement was complicated by development of a pseudoaneurysm that required left thoracotomy for resection 3 months later. This type III rupture was unusual in that it involved not posterior wall but anterior wall of left ventricle. Risk factor for this unusual location may have been the calcified anterolateral papillary muscle, which had decreased tensile strength during manipulation of left ventricle to allow surgical access for mitral valve replacement on cardiopulmonary bypass. *(Adapted from Mihaljevic T, Couper GS, Byrne JG, et al. Echocardiographic localization of left ventricular free wall rupture after minimally invasive mitral valve replacement. J Cardiothorac Vasc Anesth. 2003;17:733-735.)*

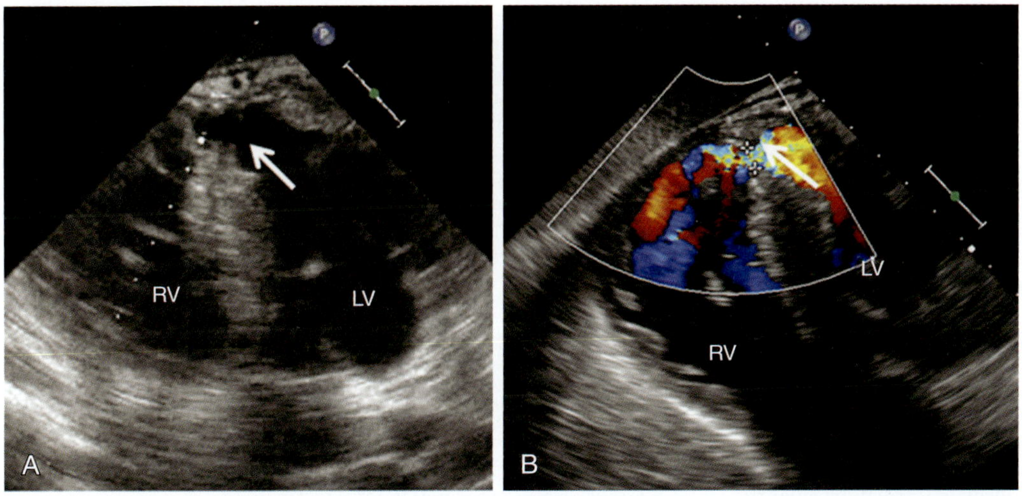

Figure 19-47 **A** and **B,** Transgastric biventricular view of ischemic ventricular septal defect (VSD) in patient with myocardial infarction. Arrow in **A** points to inferior VSD. Color flow Doppler imaging (**B**) demonstrates turbulent blood flow across VSD from left ventricle *(LV)* into right ventricle *(RV),* features consistent with transmural infarction due to right coronary artery occlusion. *(Adapted from Kulkarni M, Conte Ah, Huang A, et al. Coronary artery disease, acute myocardial infarction, and a newly developing ventricular septal defect: surgical repair or percutaneous closure. J Cardiothorac Vasc Anesth. 25:1213-1216.)*

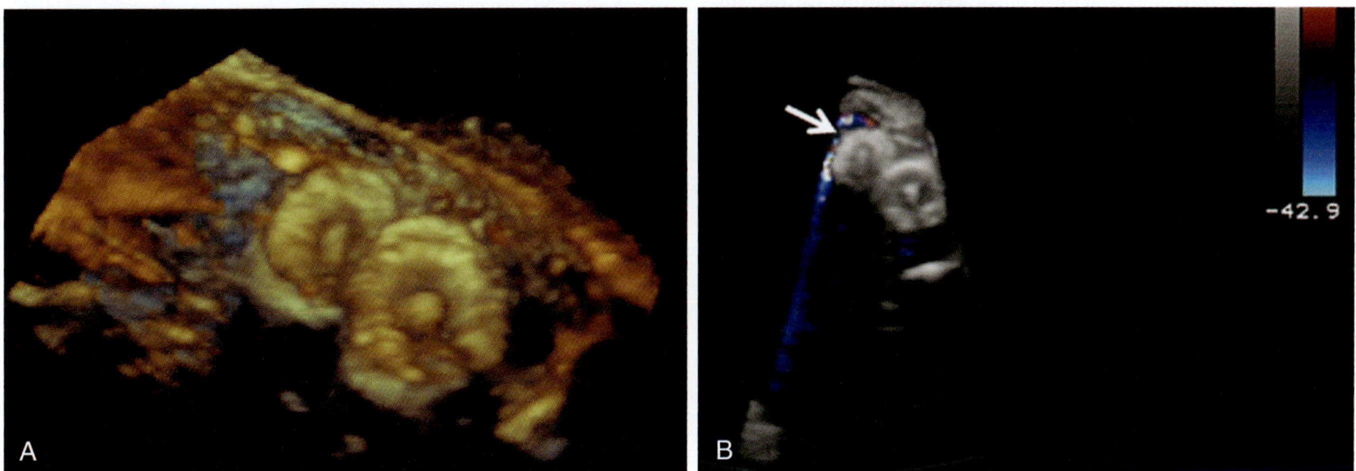

Figure 19-48 Percutaneous repair of ischemic left inferior ventricular septal defect (VSD). **A** and **B,** Three-dimensional echocardiographic views of VSD. **A** shows transcatheter septal repair with double Amplatzer occluder devices positioned under real-time echocardiographic guidance. Color flow imaging (**B**) shows small residual shunt across defect *(arrow).* *(Adapted from Kulkarni M, Conte Ah, Huang A, et al. Coronary artery disease, acute myocardial infarction, and a newly developing ventricular septal defect: surgical repair or percutaneous closure. J Cardiothorac Vasc Anesth. 25(6): 1213-16.)*

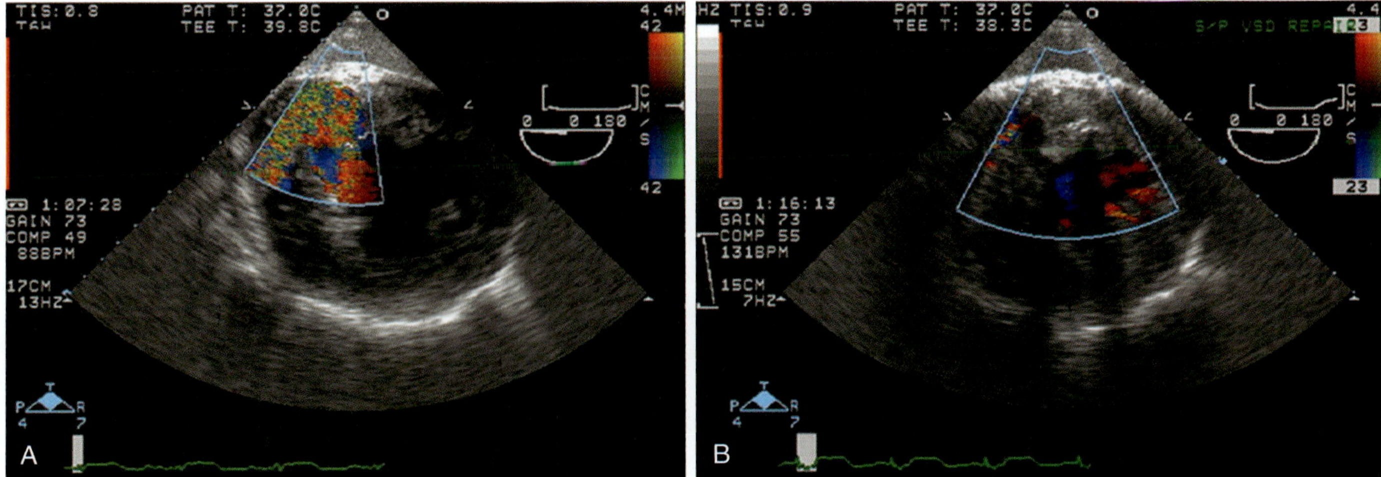

Figure 19-49 Large traumatic left inferior ventricular septal defect (VSD) in patient with stab wound to left chest: transgastric short-axis biventricular view at a multiplane angle of 0 degrees. **A,** Color flow Doppler imaging shows turbulent flow across VSD from left ventricle into right ventricle. **B,** After successful surgical repair, color flow Doppler following cardiopulmonary bypass demonstrates no blood flow across VSD. *(Adapted from Stein E, Daigle S, Weiss SJ, et al. Successful management of a complicated traumatic ventricular septal defect. J Cardiothorac Vasc Anesth. 2011;25:547-552.)*

acquired ventricular septal defect (VSD) should evaluate location, size, shape, direction of blood flow, and associated cardiac abnormalities. In ischemic septal defects, there is often associated ventricular dysfunction, regional wall motion abnormalities, and mitral regurgitation.[108,109] In traumatic VSD, a careful search should be undertaken echocardiographically to rule out valvular, myocardial, pericardial, and aortic lesions due to the cardiac trauma, whether blunt and/or sharp.[110]

Management options include medical management, transcatheter closure, and surgical repair (see Figs. 19-47 to 19-49). The indications and technology for transcatheter VSD closure are still evolving. In this setting, 3D TEE can provide real-time procedural guidance and post-procedural evaluation of septal occlusion.[108-111]

Conclusions

High-resolution images of almost the entire aorta are feasible with TEE, except for the distal ascending aorta and the proximal aortic arch that is obscured by the trachea. Transcervical, epicardial, or epiaortic ultrasound imaging can complement TEE for evaluation of the ascending aorta, aortic arch, and brachiocephalic vessels during cardiac surgery, especially when TEE is contraindicated or limited. Furthermore, TEE is the imaging modality of choice for emergency evaluation of clinically unstable patients with acute aortic syndromes, including complications such as cardiac tamponade, aortic regurgitation, hypovolemia, myocardial ischemia, ventricular dysfunction, malperfusion syndromes, and pleural effusion. Caution must be exercised when patients have a "tight mediastinum" due to the mass effect of giant aortic aneurysms, where insertion of the TEE probe into the esophagus may result in acute cardiovascular collapse due to large vessel or large airway compression.

The common sites for aortic dissection are the proximal ascending aorta or the descending thoracic aorta beyond the left subclavian artery. Aortic dissection is commonly classified using the Stanford classification into type A (involving the ascending aorta) or type B (confined to the descending aorta). The extent and presentation of dissections are described by the DeBakey and Penn classifications, respectively. Identification of a mobile intimal flap separating the aorta into true and false lumens in multiple views during the TEE examination is diagnostic for aortic dissection. Aortic IMH and penetrating atherosclerotic ulcer are variants of aortic dissection.

Aortic aneurysms that involve the aortic root often cause central aortic regurgitation as a consequence of outward tethering of the aortic valve cusps and may require aortic valve replacement, resuspension, or reimplantation. Large aortic aneurysms may cause external compression of the esophagus, making TEE hazardous. TEE detection of severe aortic atheroma is an independent predictor of stroke and death in coronary artery bypass surgery patients. Epiaortic imaging is superior to digital palpation for detecting atherosclerotic plaques in the ascending aorta. Detection of significant atheroma anywhere in the aorta by TEE suggests the presence of disease throughout the thoracic aorta.

Most traumatic aortic injuries occur around the aortic isthmus and are characterized by a thick mural flap and perivascular hematoma. Bacterial aortitis may have endothelial vegetations and mycotic aneurysms. Aortic imaging with TEE can guide precise placement of intraaortic catheters, such as the intraaortic balloon pump and endoaortic balloon clamp, as well as detect iatrogenic aortic dissection.

Pulmonary hypertension is a common risk factor for pulmonary artery aneurysm and/or dissection. A PDA is a rare but eminently treatable etiology of pulmonary hypertension. A comprehensive echocardiographic evaluation of right ventricular function is essential in diseases of the pulmonary artery, especially when surgical intervention is planned.

Left ventricular aneurysms and pseudoaneurysms are commonly secondary to ischemia or surgery. Recent evidence suggests that 3D echocardiography can be the perioperative imaging modality of choice. Left ventricular ruptures associated with mitral valve procedures are

classified into three types depending on the level of the rupture. Atrioventricular groove reconstruction has a risk of damage to the circumflex coronary artery and/or coronary sinus.

Acquired VSDs are commonly secondary to ischemia or trauma. A complete analysis of these defects is possible with TEE. If transcatheter closure is planned, 3D TEE can also provide procedural guidance.

Aneurysms and dissections of the thoracic aorta, pulmonary artery, and left ventricle collectively can be characterized in fine detail by comprehensive TEE in the perioperative period. It is likely that the advent of 3D TEE will extend even further the diagnostic and therapeutic abilities of the perioperative echocardiographer.

REFERENCES

1. Shanewise JS, Cheung AT, Aronson S, et al. ASE/SCA guidelines for performing a comprehensive intraoperative multiplane transesophageal echocardiography examination: recommendations of the American Society of Echocardiography Council for Intraoperative Echocardiography and the Society of Cardiovascular Anesthesiologists Task Force for Certification in Perioperative Transesophageal Echocardiography. *Anesth Analg.* 1999;89(4):870-884.
2. Konstadt SN, Reich DL, Quintana C, et al. The ascending aorta: how much does transesophageal echocardiography see? *Anesth Analg.* 1994;78(2):240-244.
3. Eltzschig HK, Kallmeyer IJ, Mihaljevic T, et al. A practical approach to a comprehensive epicardial and epiaortic echocardiographic examination. *J Cardiothorac Vasc Anesth.* 2003;17(4):422-429.
4. Reeves ST, Glas KE, Eltschig H, et al. Guidelines for performing a comprehensive epicardial echocardiography examination: recommendations of the American Society of Echocardiography and the Society of Cardiovascular Anesthesiologists. *Anesth Analg.* 2007;105(1):22-28.
5. Glas K, Swaminathan M, Reeves ST, et al. Guidelines for performance of a comprehensive intraoperative epiaortic ultrasonographic examination: recommendations of the American Society of Echocardiography and the Society of Cardiovascular Anesthesiologists: endorsed by the Society of Thoracic Surgeons. *Anesth Analg.* 2008;106(5):1376-1384.
6. Hiratzka LF, Bakris GL, Beckman JA, et al. 2010 ACCF/AHA/AATS/ACR/ASA/SCA/SCAI /SIR/STS/ SVM guidelines for the diagnosis and management of patients with thoracic aortic disease. A report of the American College of Cardiology Foundation/American Heart Association Task Force on Practice Guidelines, American Association for Thoracic Surgery, American College of Radiology, American Stroke Association, Society of Cardiovascular Anesthesiologists, Society for Cardiovascular Angiography and Interventions, Society of Interventional Radiology, Society of Thoracic Surgeons, and Society for Vascular Medicine. *J Am Coll Cardiol.* 2010;55(14):e27-e129.
7. Bavaria JE, Brinster D, Gorman RC, et al. Advances in the treatment of acute type A dissection: an integrated approach. *Ann Thorac Surg.* 2002;74(5):S1848-S1852.
8. Scohy TV, Geniets B, McGhie J, et al. Feasibility of real-time three-dimensional transesophageal echocardiography in type A aortic dissection. *Interact Cardiovasc Thorac Surg.* 2010;11(1):112-113.
9. Kim CM, Yu SC, Hong SJ. Cardiac tamponade using transesophageal echocardiography in circumferential aortic dissection. *J Korean Med Sci.* 1997;12(3):266-268.
10. Augoustides JG, Hosalkar HH, Milas BL, et al. Upper gastrointestinal injuries related to perioperative transesophageal echocardiography: index case, literature review, classification proposal and call for a registry. *J Cardiothorac Vasc Anesth.* 2006;20(3):379-384.
11. Nakao S, Eguchi T, Ikeda S, et al. Airway obstruction by a transesophageal echocardiography probe in an adult patient with a dissecting aneurysm of the ascending aorta and arch. *J Cardiothorac Vasc Anesth.* 2000;14(2):186-187.
12. Arima H, Sobue K, Tanaka S, et al. Airway obstruction associated with transesophageal echocardiography in a patient with a giant aortic pseudoaneurysm. *Anesth Analg.* 2002;95(3):558-560.
13. Augoustides JG, Szeto WY, Bavaria JE. Advances in aortic valve repair: focus on functional approach, clinical outcomes, and central role of echocardiography. *J Cardiothorac Vasc Anesth.* 2010;24(6):1016-1020.
14. Natsis KI, Tsitouidis IA, Didagelos MV, et al. Anatomical variations in the branches of the human aortic arch in 633 angiographies: clinical significance and literature review. *Surg Radiol Anat.* 2009;31(5):319-323.
15. Jakanani GC, Adair W. Frequency of variations in aortic arch anatomy depicted on multidetector CT. *Clin Radiol.* 2010;65(6):481-487.
16. Desai ND, Szeto WY. Complex aortic arch aneurysm and dissections: hybrid techniques for surgical and endovascular therapy. *Curr Opin Cardiol.* 2009;24(6):521-527.
17. Rizvi AZ, Murad MH, Fairman RM, et al. The effect of left subclavian artery coverage on morbidity and mortality in patients undergoing thoracic aortic interventions: a systematic review and meta-analysis. *J Vasc Surg.* 2009;50(5):1159-1169.
18. Matsumura JS, Lee WA, Mitchell RS, et al. The Society for Vascular Surgery practice guidelines: management of left subclavian artery with thoracic endovascular aortic repair. *J Vasc Surg.* 2009;50(5):1155-1158.
19. Bavaria JE, Milewski RK, Baker J, et al. Classic hybrid evolving approach to distal arch aneurysms: toward the zone zero solution. *J Thorac Cardiovasc Surg.* 2010;140(suppl 6):S77-S80.
20. Cheung AT, Pochettino A, McGarvey ML, et al. Strategies to manage paraplegia risk after endovascular stent repair of descending thoracic aortic aneurysms. *Ann Thorac Surg.* 2005;80(4):1280-1288.
21. Ullery BW, Wang GJ, Low D, et al. Neurological complications of thoracic endovascular aortic repair. *Semin Cardiothorac Vasc Anesth.* 2011;15(4):123-140.
22. Johnston KW, Rutherford RB, Tilson MD, et al. Suggested standards for reporting on arterial aneurysms. Subcommittee on Reporting Standards for Arterial Aneurysms, Ad Hoc Committee on Reporting Standards, Society for Vascular Surgery and North American Chapter, International Society for Cardiovascular Surgery. *J Vasc Surg.* 1991;13(3):452-458.
23. Roman MJ, Devereux RB, Kramer-Fox R, et al. Two-dimensional echocardiographic aortic root dimensions in normal children and adults. *Am J Cardiol.* 1989;64(8):507-512.
24. Cholley BP, Shroff SG, Korcarz C, et al. Aortic elastic properties with transesophageal echocardiography with automated border detection: validation according to regional differences between proximal and distal descending thoracic aorta. *J Am Soc Echocardiogr.* 1996;9(4):539-548.
25. Petrini J, Yousry M, Rickenlund A, et al. The feasibility of velocity vector imaging by transesophageal echocardiography for assessment of elastic properties of the descending aorta in aortic valve disease. *J Am Soc Echocardiogr.* 2010;23(9):985-992.
26. Beique FA, Joffe D, Tousignant G, et al. Echocardiography-based assessment and management of atherosclerotic disease of the thoracic aorta. *J Cardiothorac Vasc Anesth.* 1998;12(2):206-220.
27. Osranek M, Pilip A, Patel PR, et al. Amounts of aortic atherosclerosis in patients with aortic stenosis as determined by transesophageal echocardiography. *Am J Cardiol.* 2009;103(5):713-717.
28. Golledge J, Eagle KA. Acute aortic dissection. *Lancet.* 2008;372(9632):55-66.
29. Nienaber CA, Powell JT. Management of acute aortic syndromes. *Eur Heart J.* 2012;33(1):26-35.

30. Shiga T, Wajima Z, Apfel CC, et al. Diagnostic accuracy of transesophageal echocardiography, helical computed tomography, and magnetic resonance imaging for suspected thoracic aortic dissection: systematic review and meta-analysis. *Arch Intern Med.* 2006;166(13):1350-1356.

31. Moore AG, Eagle KA, Bruckman D, et al. Choice of computed tomography, transesophageal echocardiography, magnetic resonance imaging, and aortography in acute aortic dissection: International Registry of Acute Aortic Dissection (IRAD). *Am J Cardiol.* 2002;89(10):1235-1238.

32. Km Harris, Strauss CE, Eagle KA, et al. Correlates of delayed recognition and treatment of acute type A aortic dissection: the International Registry of Acute Aortic Dissection (IRAD). *Circulation.* 2011;124(18):1911-1918.

33. Bonser RS, Ranasinghe AM, Loubani M, et al. Evidence, lack of evidence, controversy and debate in the provision and performance of the surgery of acute type A dissection. *J Am Coll Cardiol.* 2011;58(24):2455-2474.

34. Augoustides JG, Geirsson A, Wy Szeto, et al. Observational study of mortality risk stratification by ischemic presentation in patients with acute type A aortic dissection: the Penn classification. *Nat Clin Pract Cardiovasc Med.* 2009;6(2):140-146.

35. Olsson C, Hillebrandt CG, Liska J, et al. Mortality in acute type A aortic dissection: validation of the Penn classification. *Ann Thorac Surg.* 2011;92(4):1376-1382.

36. Augoustides JG, Szeto WY, Desai ND, et al. Classification of acute type A dissection: focus on clinical presentation and extent. *Eur J Cardiothorac Surg.* 2011;39(4):519-522.

37. Erbel R, Alfonso F, Boileau C, et al. Diagnosis and management of aortic dissection. *Eur Heart J.* 2001;22(18):1642-1681.

38. Sl Lansman, Saunders PC, Malekan R, et al. Acute aortic syndrome. *J Thorac Cardiovasc Surg.* 2010;140(suppl 6):S92-S97.

39. Vilacosta I, Aragoncillo P, Canadas V, et al. Acute aortic syndrome: a new look at an old conundrum. *Heart.* 2009;95(14):1130-1139.

40. Pelzel JM, Braverman AC, Hirsch AT, et al. International heterogeneity in diagnosing frequency and clinical outcomes of ascending aortic intramural hematoma. *J Am Soc Echocardiogr.* 2007;20: 1260-1268.

41. Baikoussis NG, Apostolakis EE, Papakonstantinou NA, et al. The implications of vasa vasorum in surgical diseases of the aorta. *Eur J Cardiothorac Surg.* 2011;40(2):412-417.

42. Nathan DP, Boon W, Lai E, et al. Presentation, complications, and natural history of penetrating atherosclerotic ulcer disease. *J Vasc Surg.* 2012;55(1):10-15.

43. Movsowitz HD, Levine RA, Hilgenberg AD, et al. Transesophageal echocardiographic description of the mechanisms of aortic regurgitation in acute type A aortic dissection: implications for aortic valve repair. *J Am Coll Cardiol.* 2000;36(3):884-890.

44. Keane MG, Wiegers SE, Yang E, et al. Structural determinants of aortic regurgitation in type A dissection and the role of valvular resuspension as determined by intraoperative transesophageal echocardiography. *Am J Cardiol.* 2000;85(5):604-610.

45. Geirsson A, Szeto WY, Pochettino A, et al. Significance of malperfusion syndromes prior to contemporary surgical repair for acute type A dissection: outcomes and need for additional revascularizations. *Eur J Cardiothorac Surg.* 2007;32(2):255-262.

46. Augoustides JG, Kohl BA, Harris H, et al. Color-flow Doppler recognition of intraoperative brachiocephalic malperfusion during operative repair of acute type A dissection: utility of transcutaneous carotid artery ultrasound scanning. *J Cardiothorac Vasc Anesth.* 2007;21(1):81-84.

47. Inoue Y, Takahashi R, Ueda T, et al. Synchronized epiaortic two-dimensional and color Doppler echocardiographic guidance enables routine ascending aortic cannulation in type A acute aortic dissection. *J Thorac Cardiovasc Surg.* 2011;141(2):354-360.

48. Attaran S, Safar M, Saleh HZ, et al. Cannulating a dissecting aorta using ultrasound-epiaortic and transesophageal guidance. *Heart Surg Forum.* 2011;14(6):E373-E375.

49. Starnes BW, Lundgren RS, Gunn M, et al. A new classification scheme for treating blunt aortic injury. *J Vasc Surg.* 2012;55(1):47-54.

50. Jl Januzzi, Sabatine MS, Eagle KA, et al. Iatrogenic aortic dissection. *Am J Cardiol.* 2002;89(5): 623-626.

51. Williams ML, Sheng S, Gammie JS, et al. Aortic dissection as a complication of cardiac surgery: report from the Society of Thoracic Surgeons database. *Ann Thorac Surg.* 2010;90(6):1812-1816.

52. Williams JB, Andersen ND, Bhattacharya SD, et al. Retrograde ascending aortic dissection as an early complication of thoracic endovascular aortic repair. *J Vasc Surg.* 2012:[Epub ahead of print].

53. Elefteriades J. Indications for aortic replacement. *J Thorac Cardiovasc Surg.* 2010;140(suppl 6):S5-S9.

54. Augoustides JG, Palppert T, Bavaria JE. Aortic decision making in the Loeys-Dietz syndrome: aortic root aneurysm and a normal caliber ascending aorta and aortic arch. *J Thorac Cardiovasc Surg.* 2009;138(2):502-503.

55. Augoustides JG, Szeto WY, Bavaria JE. Advances in aortic valve repair: focus on functional approach, clinical outcomes, and central role of echocardiography. *J Cardiothorac Vasc Anesth.* 2010;24(6):1016-1020.

56. Guo HW, Sun XG, Xu JP, et al. A new and simple classification for the non-coronary sinus of Valsalva aneurysm.*Eur J Cardiothorac Surg.* 2011;40(5):1047-1051:2011.

57. Kerhar PG, Laniewar CP, Mishra N, et al. Transcatheter closure of ruptured sinus of Valsalva aneurysm using the Amplatz duct occluder: immediate results and mid-term follow-up. *Eur Heart J.* 2010;31(23):2881-2887.

58. Augoustides JG, Wolfe Y, Ek Walsh, et al. Recent advances in aortic valve disease: highlights from a bicuspid aortic valve to transcatheter aortic valve replacement. *J Cardiothorac Vasc Anesth.* 2009;23(4):569-576.

59. Hi Michelena, Khanna AD, MahoneyD, et al. Incidence of aortic complications in patients with bicuspid aortic valves. *JAMA.* 2011;306(10):1104-1112.

60. Fazel SS, Mallidi HR, Lee RS, et al. The aortopathy of bicuspid aortic valve disease has distinctive patterns and usually involves the transverse aortic arch. *J Thorac Cardiovasc Surg.* 2008;135(4):901-907.

61. Park CB, Kl Greason, Suri KL, et al. Fate of nonreplaced sinuses of Valsalva in bicuspid aortic valve disease. *J Thorac Cardiovasc Surg.* 2011;142(2):278-284.

62. Rouseau H, Chabbert V, Maracher MA, et al. The importance of imaging assessment before endovascular repair of thoracic aorta. *Eur J Vasc Endovasc Surg.* 2009;38(4):408-421.

63. Roselli EE, Soltesz EG, Mastracci T, et al. Antegrade delivery of stent grafts to treat complex thoracic aortic disease. *Ann Thorac Surg.* 2010;90(2):539-546.

64. Szeto WY, Augoustides JG, Desai ND, et al. Cerebral embolic exposure during transfemoral and transapical transcatheter aortic valve replacement. *J Card Surg.* 2011;26(4):348-354.

65. Gutsche JT, Cheung AT, McGarvey ML, et al. Risk factors for perioperative stroke after thoracic endovascular aortic repair. *Ann Thorac Surg.* 2007;84(4):1195-1200.

66. Hillis ID, Smith PK, Anderson JL, et al. 2011 ACCF/AHA guidelines for coronary artery bypass graft surgery: a report of the American College of Cardiology Foundation/American heart Association Task Force on Practice Guidelines. *J Thorac Cardiovasc Surg.* 2012;143(1):4-34.

67. Augoustides JG, Harris H, Pochettino A. Direct innominate artery cannulation in acute type A dissection and severe aortic atheroma. *J Cardiothorac Vasc Anesth.* 2007;21(5):727-729.

68. Oliver JM, Alonso-Gonzalez R, Gonzalez AE, et al. Risk of aortic root or ascending aorta complications in patients with bicuspid aortic valve with and without coarctation of the aorta. *Am J Cardiol.* 2009;104(7):1001-1006.

69. Borger MA, David TE. Management of the valve and ascending aorta in adults with bicuspid aortic valve disease. *Semin Thorac Cardiovasc Surg.* 2005;17(2):143-147.

70. von Kodolitsch Y, Aydin MA, Koschyk DH, et al. Predictors of aneurysmal formation after surgical correction of aortic coarctation. *J Am Coll Cardiol.* 2002;39(4):617-624.

71. von Kodolitsch Y, Aydin AM, Bernhardt AM, et al. Aortic aneurysms after correction of aortic coarctation: a systematic review. *Vasa.* 2010;39(1):3-16.

72. Perloff JK. The variant associations of the aortic isthmus coarctation. *Am J Cardiol.* 2010;106(7): 1038-1041.

73. Yazar O, Budts W, Maleux G, et al. Thoracic endovascular aortic repair for treatment of late complications after aortic coarctation repair. *Ann Vasc Surg.* 2011;25(8):1005-1011.

74. Rousou AJ, Haddadin AS, Badescu G, et al. Surgical repair of pulmonary artery dissection. *Eur J Cardiothorac Surg.* 2010;38(6):805.

75. Meng J, Qian Y, Xiao X. Eisenmenger syndrome complicated by pulmonary artery dissection*Thorac Cardiovasc Surg.* 2012:[Epub ahead of print].

76. Khush KK, Randhawa R, Israel E. A full house: complications from an uncorrected patent ducts arteriosus. *Curr Cardiol Rep.* 2005;7(4):310-313.

77. Zhao Y, Li ZA, Henein MY. PDA with Eisenmenger complicated by pulmonary artery dissection. *Eur J Echocardiogr.* 2010;11(8):E32.

78. Cohen GI, White M, Sochowski RA, et al. Reference values for normal adult transesophageal echocardiographic measurements. *J Am Soc Echocardiogr.* 1995;8(3):221-230.

79. Araujo I, Escribano P, Lopez-Gude MJ, et al. Giant pulmonary artery aneurysm in a patient with vasoreactive pulmonary hypertension: a case report. *BMC Cardiovasc Disord.* 2011;11:64.

80. Matsuo S, Sato Y, Higashida R, et al. A giant pulmonary artery aneurysm associated with infundibular pulmonary stenosis. *Cardiovasc Revasc Med.* 2008;9(3):188-189.

81. Piveta RB, Al Arruda, Rodrigues AC, et al. Rupture of a giant aneurysm of the pulmonary artery caused by schistosomiasis. *Eur Heart J.* 2012:[Epub ahead of print].

82. Terra RM, Fernandez A, Bammann RH, et al. Pulmonary artery sarcoma mimicking a pulmonary artery aneurysm. *Ann Thorac Surg.* 2008;86(4):1354-1355.

83. Koch A, Mechtersheimer G, Tochtermann U, et al. Ruptured pseudoaneurysm of the pulmonary artery–rare manifestation of a primary pulmonary artery sarcoma. *Interact Cardiovasc Thorac Surg.* 2010;10(1):120-121.

84. Muthiatu N, Raju V, Muthubaskaran V, et al. Idiopathic pulmonary artery aneurysm with pulmonary regurgitation. *Ann Thorac Surg.* 2010;90(6):2049-2051.

85. Frary G, Hasselman T, Patel P. Atypical left ventricular outflow tract aneurysm diagnosed by three-dimensional echocardiography. *Cardiol Young.* 2012:[Epub ahead of print].

86. Carod-Artal FJ, Gascon J. Chagas disease and stroke. *Lancet Neurol.* 2010;9(5):533-542.

87. Adhyapak SM, Parachuri VR. Architecture of the left ventricle: insights for optimal surgical ventricular restoration. *Heart Failure Rev.* 2010;15(1):73-83.

88. Grimaldi A, Castiglioni A, De Bonis M, et al. Large left ventricular aneurysm. *J Thorac Cardiovasc Surg.* 2011;142(4):940-941.

89. Boyd WC, Rosengard TK, Hartman GS. Isolated left ventricular diverticulum in an adult. *J Cardiothorac Vasc Anesth.* 1999;13(4):468-470.

90. Dor V, Civaia F, Alexandrescu C, et al. The postmyocardial infarction scarred ventricle and congestive heart failure: the preeminence of magnetic resonance imaging for preoperative, intraoperative, and postoperative assessment. *J Thorac Cardiovasc Surg.* 2008;136(6):1405-1412.

91. Marsan NA, Westenberg JJM, Roes SD, et al. Three-dimensional echocardiography for the preoperative assessment of patients with left ventricular aneurysm. *Ann Thorac Surg.* 2011;91(1):113-121.

92. Mukdaddirov M, Demaria RG, Perrault LP, et al. Reconstructive surgery of postinfarction left ventricular aneurysms: techniques and unsolved problems. *Eur J Cardiothorac Surgery.* 2008;34(2): 256-261.

93. Jackson BM, Gorman RC. Invited commentary. *Ann Thorac Surg.* 2011;91(1):121-122.

94. Zoffoli G, Mangino D, Venturini A, et al. Diagnosing left ventricular aneurysm from pseudoaneurysm: a case report and a review of the literature. *J Cardiothorac Surg* 4:11

95. Karas TZ, Gregoric ID, Frazier OH, et al. Delayed left ventricular pseudoaneurysms after left ventricular aneurysm repairs with the CorRestore Patch. *Ann Thorac Surg.* 2007;84(1):266-269.

96. Woo YJ, McCormick RC. Transventricular mitral valve operations. *Ann Thorac Surg.* 2011;92(4):1501-1503.

97. Makkuni P, Koller MN, Fiqueredo VM. Diverticular and aneurysmal structures of the left ventricle in adults: report of a case within the context of a literature review. *Tex Heart Inst J.* 2010;37(6): 699-705.

98. Urgesi R, Zampaletta C, Masini A, et al. A spontaneous right ventricular thrombus in a patient with ulcerative colitis and protein C deficiency: a review with a case report. *Eur Rev Med Pharmacol Sci.* 2010;14(5):455-463.

99. Kanemitsu S, Miyake Y, Okabe M. Surgical removal of a left ventricular thrombus associated with cardiac sarcoidosis. *Interact Cardiovasc Thorac Surg.* 2008;7(2):333-335.

100. Berdajs DA, Ruchat P, Tozzi PT, et al. Acute Leriche syndrome due to thrombus of the left ventricle. *Eur J Cardiothorac Surg.* 2011;39(3):423.

101. Thunberg CA, Gaitan BD, Arabia FA, et al. Ventricular assist devices today and tomorrow. *J Cardiothorac Vasc Anesth.* 2010;24(4):656-680.

102. Zacharias A. Repair of spontaneous rupture of the posterior wall of the left ventricle after mitral valve replacement. *Oper Tech Thor Cardiovasc Surg.* 2003;8(1):36-41.

103. Lawton JS, Deshpande SP, Zanaboni PB, et al. Spontaneous atrioventricular groove disruption during off-pump coronary artery bypass grafting. *Ann Thorac Surg.* 2005;79(1):339-341.

104. Turkoz R, Gulcan O, Uguz E, et al. Mitral valve replacement after application of atrial appendix flap in endocarditis with posterior annular abscess. *Eur J Cardiothorac Surg.* 2004;26(4):837-838.

105. Feindel CM, Tufail Z, David TE, et al. Mitral valve surgery in patients with extensive calcification of the mitral annulus. *J Thorac Cardiovasc Surg.* 2003;126(3):777-782.

106. Augoustides JG, Hosalkar H, Lin J. Echocardiographic-directed decision making for mitral valve endocarditis. *J Cardiothorac Vasc Anesth.* 2005;19(5):646-649.

107. Benisty J, Roller M, Sahar G, et al. Iatrogenic left ventricular–right atrial fistula following mitral valve replacement and tricuspid annuloplasty: diagnosis by transthoracic and transesophageal echocardiography. *J Heart Valve Dis.* 2005;9(5):732-735.

108. Sun X, Yang C, Zhou G, et al. Acquired left ventricular–right atrial communication following mitral valve replacement. *J Heart Valve Dis.* 2010;19(6):801-802.

109. Mahmood F, Swaminathan M. Postinfarction ventricular septal defects: surgical or percutaneous closure—between a rock and a hard place. *J Cardiothorac Vasc Anesth.* 2011;25(6):1217-1218.

110. Kulkarni M, Conte Ah, Huang A, et al. Coronary artery disease, acute myocardial infarction, and a newly developing ventricular septal defect: surgical repair or percutaneous closure. *J Cardiothorac Vasc Anesth* 25(6): 1213-16

111. Stein E, Daigle S, Weiss SJ, et al. Successful management of a complicated traumatic ventricular septal defect. *J Cardiothorac Vasc Anesth.* 2011;25(3):547-552.

112. Attia R, Blauth C. Which patients might be suitable for a septal occlude device closure of postinfarction ventricular septal rupture rather than immediate surgery? *Interactive Cardiovasc Thorac Surg.* 2010;11(5):626-629.

Endocarditis

MARTIN E. GOLDMAN

Infective endocarditis (IE) is an infection of the endothelium of the heart or blood vessels. Heart valves are particularly susceptible, but IE can occur on any endothelial lined surface, including the papillary muscles, walls of the atria or ventricles, pulmonary artery, or endothelialized surfaces of prosthetic valves or implanted devices such as catheters, pacemakers, and automatic implantable cardioverter-defibrillators (AICDs).[1,2] Structural heart disease is the most common predisposing risk factor for IE, which includes acquired valvular disease, congenital abnormalities, prosthetic heart valves, and indwelling devices.

Echocardiography is the imaging technology of choice for the diagnosis of IE and recognition of its potential complications.[3-5] Once IE is confirmed by blood cultures and echocardiography, appropriate treatment with bactericidal antibiotics and surgery (if indicated) can reduce the morbidity and mortality of IE. Unrecognized and untreated, IE is invariably fatal.[6] Perioperative echocardiography must be performed in IE to help the surgeon in the assessment and management of these patients.[7]

The American Heart Association (AHA) estimates the incidence of IE in the United States to be 10,000 to 15,000 new cases annually.[8] The pathophysiologic mechanism of IE is blood flowing from a zone of relatively high pressure to one of lower pressure. If the Reynolds number is surpassed, turbulent flow will be generated and cause endothelial damage, forming a susceptible nidus for implantation and subsequent infection with an adhering organism during bacteremia or fungemia. As part of the native immune response, adherence factors such as fibrin, platelets, and inflammatory cells are drawn to the infective surface, creating a heterogeneous irregular meshwork called *vegetation*. Vegetations are typically located on the low-pressure side of high-velocity turbulence, on the atrial side of mitral or tricuspid regurgitation, on the ventricular side of aortic or pulmonic regurgitation, on the ventricular side of mitral stenosis, or on the aortic side of aortic stenosis (Figs. 20-1 and 20-2; Videos 20-1 and 20-2). Similarly, if there is a ventricular septal defect (VSD) with left-to-right shunting, the vegetation will be on the low-pressure side, or in this specific scenario, the right ventricular side of the defect. An atrial septal defect (ASD) usually has low pressure on either side of the defect and subsequently does not create a turbulent jet, resulting in a much lower likelihood of developing endocarditis.

The definitive diagnosis of endocarditis by echocardiography is detection of a vegetation diagnosed with either transthoracic or transesophageal echocardiography (TTE, TEE). This is identified as an irregularly shaped echogenicity mass that may be sessile or pedunculated, mobile or immobile, fibrinous or multilobar and usually has a distinct separation and echogenicity (tissue density) from the underlying valve or endocardial tissue. Infection may involve the valve leaflet or its support apparatus. Any endocardial surface that is attached or adherent to an indwelling cardiac device can also become the site for formation of a vegetation (Video 20-3).

The echocardiogram can also diagnose complications of IE including abscess formation, ruptured chordae or papillary muscle, leaflet or sinus of Valsalva perforation, prosthetic valve dehiscence, development of fistulous tracts, and suppurative pericarditis (Fig. 20-3 and Video 20-4). The differential diagnosis of a vegetation includes *Libman-Sacks lesions*, which are nonbacterial thrombotic lesions found in inflammatory disorders such as systemic lupus erythematosus in up to 18% of patients.[9,10] These broad-based lesions may appear on the basilar portion of the valve leaflets (not necessarily associated with jet lesions) and are usually sessile. *Marantic endocarditis* can also occur in patients with advanced neoplasms such as melanoma and may be difficult to differentiate from endocarditis in a patient with malignancy and fever. *Lambl excrescences* are small, fibrinous, filiform lesions usually seen on aortic valve leaflet coaptation points as a result of mechanical trauma. They can also appear on the mitral valve (MV).

Duke Criteria

The Duke criteria for diagnosis of IE, originally published in 1994 and modified in 2000, includes endocardial involvement as documented by positive TTE or TEE as one of the two major criteria in the diagnosis of endocarditis, the other being positive blood cultures (Box 20-1).[3,11,12] Minor criteria include a broader range of clinical findings: predisposing cardiac conditions, elevated temperature/fever, vascular phenomena, immunologic phenomena, and certain microbiological findings. The criteria also define three diagnostic categories: (1) "definite" by pathologic or clinical criteria, (2) "possible," and (3) "rejected."[3] The category "possible IE" is defined as having at least one major criterion and one minor criterion or three minor criteria.[11]

The Duke criteria have also been validated in the intravenous drug user (IVDU) population, in whom right-sided endocarditis, especially involving the tricuspid valve, occurs much more frequently than in the non-IVDU population (Video 20-5).[13] IVDUs with definite diagnosis of IE more commonly have vascular phenomena (arterial embolism, septic pulmonary infarction, mycotic aneurysm, intracranial hemorrhage, or Janeway lesions) and multiple opacities on chest radiography than those with possible endocarditis.

Because the clinical presentation of IE can be equivocal and blood cultures may be negative in up to 30% of cases, echocardiography plays a significant role in the definitive diagnosis. Blood culture–negative endocarditis is often due to empirical antibiotic treatment before blood culture sampling or to fungal or fastidious organisms. Among 759 patients with blood culture–negative endocarditis, a causative microorganism was later identified in 62.7% (including *Streptococcus*, Q fever, and *Bartonella* infections) and a noninfective etiology in 2.5% (particularly neoplastic or autoimmune disease).[14]

Transthoracic and Transesophageal Echocardiography

With advances in technology, vegetations as small as 1 to 2 mm may be detected on native valves by TTE. However, in 20% to 40% of adult patients, TTE may be inadequate for evaluating suspected endocarditis.[6] Two-dimensional (2D) TTE has a sensitivity for detection of endocarditis of 29% to 65% and a specificity of 90% and is consequently used as an initial screening test in patients with low clinical suspicion of IE.[15] Prosthetic or indwelling devices may be difficult to fully evaluate by TTE owing to acoustic shadowing. TEE has a higher sensitivity (85% to 98%) and a specificity of better than 90% for IE detection because it uses higher transmit frequencies (7 MHz compared to TTE's 2-4 MHz) and its retrocardiac position is closer to the heart and does not require penetration through the chest wall and lungs, as does TTE. The negative predictive value of TEE is nearly 100% for patients with native valves, but vegetations may be missed with prosthetic valves owing to acoustic shadowing. In a recent study of 511 patients, TTE detected only 45% of vegetations seen by TEE.[15] As a result, TEE should be the initial screening test for all patients with prosthetic

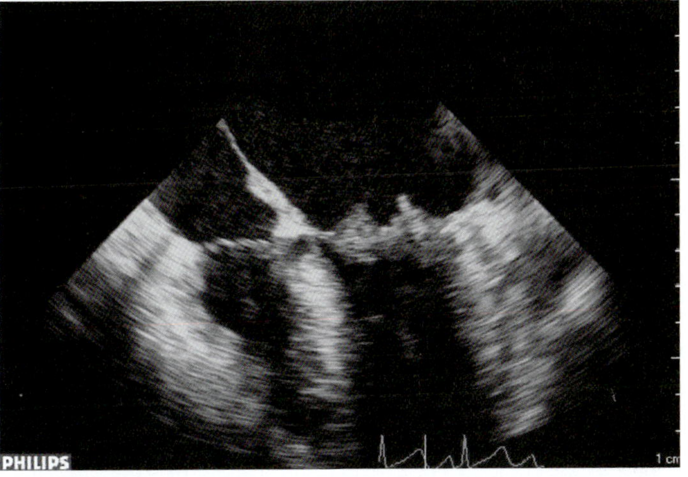

Figure 20-1 Four-chamber view showing vegetations on both anterior and posterior leaflets.

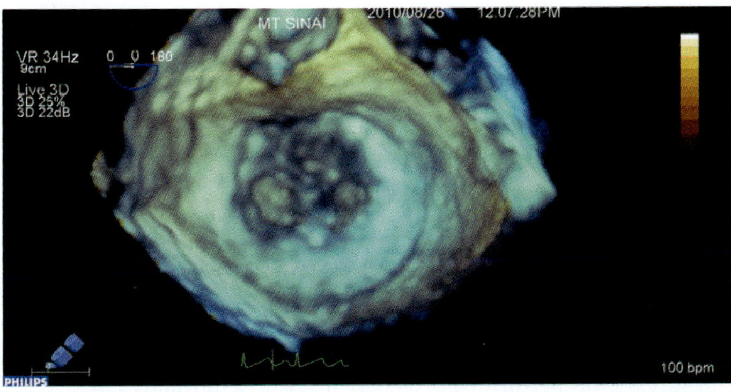

Figure 20-2 Three-dimensional en face view of same valve seen Figure 20-1 and Video 20-1. Vegetations seen in both commissures and at A2.

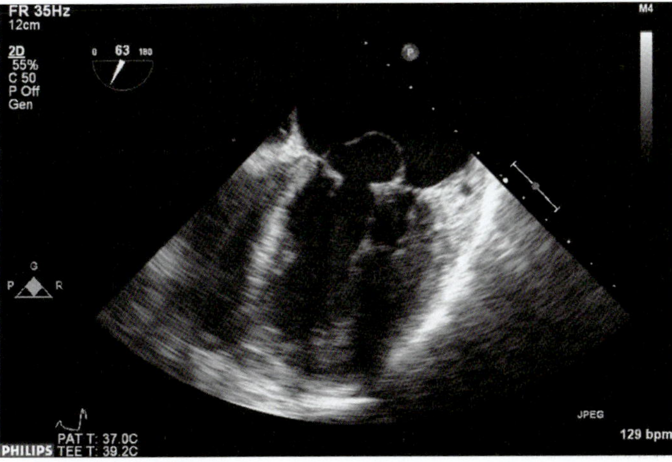

Figure 20-3 Commissure view showing aneurysm and perforation of anterior leaflet.

valves, suspected technically difficult transthoracic echocardiograms, or indwelling cardiac devices.

According to the 2011 appropriate use criteria of echocardiography guidelines, TTE received a score of 9 (the highest score possible) for initial evaluation of suspected endocarditis with positive blood cultures or a new murmur as well as reevaluation of IE at high risk of progressive complications or a change in clinical status or cardiac exam.[16] TEE also carries an appropriate use score of 9 to diagnose IE with a moderate to high test probability (*Staphylococcus* bacteremia, fungemia, prosthetic heart valve, or intracardiac device).

Patients with indwelling hemodialysis catheters, pacemakers, or AICDs can develop endocardial erosions and mural thrombi within the right atrium, tricuspid valve, or right ventricle, which then can become superinfected, producing endocarditis.[17] Additionally, mural endocarditis can occur on the right ventricular side of the interventricular septum or on the contralateral wall of a VSD jet. These structures have to be interrogated carefully when performing a TEE because they may be difficult to image by TTE.

False negatives by TEE can include fibrocalcific lesions on valves or the mitral annulus, prosthetic valves obscuring penetration of the sound wave, very small lesions, and partially treated infections. False

BOX 20-1. MAJOR AND MINOR DUKE CRITERIA FOR DIAGNOSIS OF INFECTIVE ENDOCARDITIS

Major Criteria
- Positive blood cultures for infective endocarditis. Typical microorganism for infective endocarditis from two separate blood cultures in the absence of a primary focus:
  - Viridans streptococci
  - *Streptococcus bovis*, including nutritional variant strains
  - HACEK group—*Haemophilus* spp., *Actinobacillus actinomycetemcomitans, Cardiobacterium hominis, Eikenella* spp., and *Kingella kingae*
  - Community-acquired *Staphylococcus aureus* or enterococci
- Persistently positive blood culture, defined as recovery of a microorganism consistent with infective endocarditis from:
  - Blood cultures drawn more than 12 hours apart *OR*
  - All of three or a majority of four or more separate blood cultures, with first and last drawn at least 1 hour apart
- Evidence of endocardial involvement
- Positive echocardiogram for infective endocarditis
  - Oscillating intracardiac mass on valve or supporting structures, or in the path of regurgitant jets, or on implanted material in the absence of an alternative anatomic explanation *OR*
  - Abscess *OR*
  - New partial dehiscence of prosthetic valve *OR*
  - New valvular regurgitation (increase or change in preexisting murmur not sufficient)

Minor Criteria
- Predisposition—predisposing heart condition or intravenous drug use
- Fever—38.0°C (100.4°F)
- Vascular phenomena—major arterial emboli, septic pulmonary infarcts, mycotic aneurysm, intracranial hemorrhage, conjunctival hemorrhages, Janeway lesions
- Immunologic phenomena—glomerulonephritis, Osler nodes, Roth spots, rheumatoid factor
- Microbiologic evidence—positive blood culture but not meeting major criterion as noted previously (excluding single positive cultures for coagulase-negative staphylococci and organisms that do not cause endocarditis) *OR* serologic evidence of active infection with organism consistent with infective endocarditis
- Echocardiogram—consistent with infective endocarditis but not meeting major criterion as noted previously

From Durack DT, Lukes AS, Bright DK. New criteria for diagnosis of infective endocarditis: utilization of specific echocardiographic findings. Duke Endocarditis Service. *Am J Med.* 1994;96:200-209.

positives may be due to floppy redundant MV tissue, ruptured chordae, Lambl excrescences, thrombi, and fibrocalcific degeneration of valves or annuli. TEE is cost-effective in patients considered at high risk of endocarditis.[18]

The European Society of Echocardiography recently recommended TTE as the first-line imaging modality in patients suspected of having IE and TEE in patients with high clinical suspicion of IE and a normal TTE. TEE should be considered in the majority of adult patients with suspected IE, even in cases with positive TTE, to assess for severity and potential complications. Repeat TTE/TEE within 7 to 10 days is recommended in cases of initially negative examination when clinical suspicion of IE remains high. TEE is not indicated in patients with a good-quality negative TTE and low clinical suspicion of IE.[7]

The recent paper by the Working Party of the British Society for Antimicrobial Chemotherapy provides a practical algorithm for echocardiography in the diagnosis of IE (Fig. 20-4).[19]

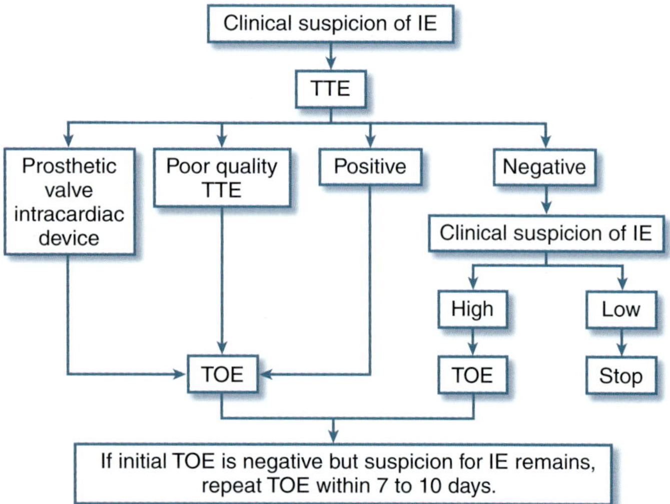

Figure 20-4 Indications for echocardiography in suspected infective endocarditis (IE). Transesophageal echocardiography *(TOE)* is not mandatory in isolated right-sided native valve IE with good-quality transthoracic echocardiography *(TTE)* examination and unequivocal echocardiographic findings. *(From Gould FK, Denning DW, Elliott TS, et al. Guidelines for the diagnosis and antibiotic treatment of endocarditis in adults: a report of the Working Party of the British Society for Antimicrobial Chemotherapy. J Antimicrob Chemother. 2012;67:269-289.)*

Complications of Infective Endocarditis

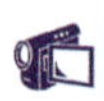

Complications of IE occur in 30% to 40% of patients with native valves and 60% to 80% of patients with prosthetic valves. The most common complication is heart failure related to valvular insufficiency, which may account for up to 90% of deaths in patients with endocarditis.[6]

Echocardiography is invaluable for detecting complications of IE such as valvular and ventricular dysfunction, heart failure, abscess formation, and emboli. The presence of a vegetation on the valve leaflet can affect coaptation, causing regurgitation, and if large enough can even obstruct forward flow, creating relative stenosis. Significant regurgitation can also lead to ventricular dysfunction and elevated intracardiac pressures, leading to pulmonary congestion. All such pathologies can be detected by echocardiography.

TEE is more sensitive than TTE for detecting an *abscess*, which is defined as a region of tissue necrosis and purulent material (Fig. 20-5 and Video 20-6). An abscess can lead to heart block, fistula formation, purulent pericarditis, dehiscence of a prosthetic valve, and pseudoaneurysm. Presence of an abscess is detected by its different echogenicity compared to the underlying myocardium, usually adjacent to an infected valve. The aortic or mitral annulus may show an increase in size or areas of liquefaction and echolucency, strongly suggestive of abscess formation. An abscess in the aortic root has a predilection for the noncoronary sinus/left atrial border, where there is less annulofibrosis support.

In a 5-year study of 115 patients with definite IE by the modified Duke criteria who underwent TEE and cardiac surgery, abscesses were found perioperatively in 44 patients (38%); only 21 of them (48%) detected by TEE.[20] In patients with a missed abscess, 61% were localized on the posterior mitral annulus and obscured by calcification. Delay for surgical treatment was significantly longer ($P = .04$) and mortality was nonsignificantly higher ($P = 0.2$) than in patients in whom the abscess was detected preoperatively.[20]

Aortocavitary fistulous tract formation is an uncommon but extremely serious complication of IE that can accelerate hemodynamic instability. In a retrospective multicenter study of 4681 episodes of IE, fistulae were found in 1.8% of cases of native valve IE and 3.5% of cases of prosthetic valve IE.[21] TTE and TEE detected the fistulous tracts in 53% and 97% of cases, respectively. Periannular abscesses were detected in 78% of cases, fistulae originated in similar rates from the three sinuses of Valsalva, and the four cardiac chambers were equally involved in the fistulous tracts. Heart failure developed in 62% of cases, and surgery was performed in 66 patients, with a mortality rate of 41% in the overall population.[21]

One of the most serious complications of IE is embolic events, which can lead to arterial occlusion and strokes, ischemic organs, or limb damage. In a multicenter prospective European study of 384

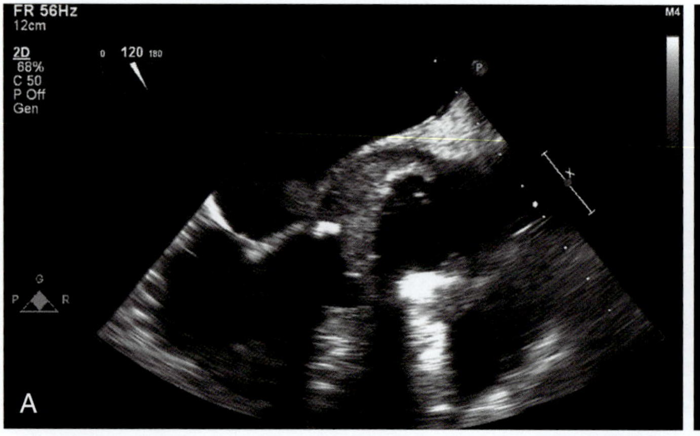
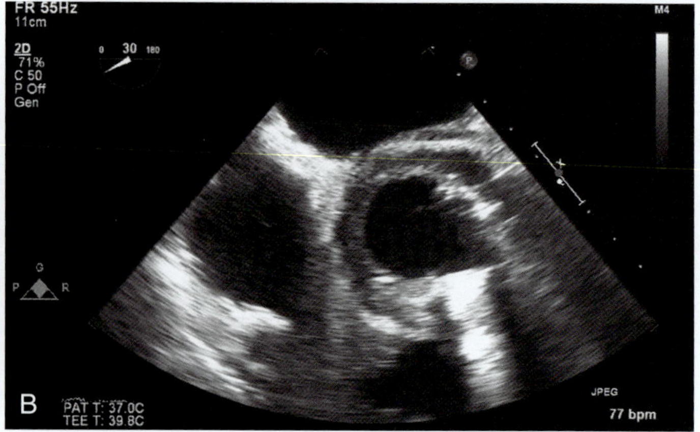

Figure 20-5 **A,** Long-axis view of bioprosthetic aortic valve endocarditis with annular abscess. Note rocking motion of valve during cardiac cycle. **B,** Short-axis view showing annular abscess.

consecutive patients (aged 57 ± 17 years) with definite IE (according to Duke criteria) who had TEE, 131 (34.1%) had an embolic event and 28 (7.3%) had an embolus after initiation of antibiotic therapy.[22] Infection with *Staphylococcus aureus* or *Streptococcus bovis* were independently associated with emboli. Vegetation length greater than 10 mm and severe mobility were predictors of new emboli, even after adjustment for *S. aureus* and *S. bovis*. One-year mortality was 20.6%. In multivariate analysis, vegetation length greater than 15 mm was a predictor of 1-year mortality (adjusted relative risk = 1.8; 95% confidence interval, 1.10-2.82; *P* = 0.02).[22] The conclusion of this analysis was that identification of a large mobile vegetation may warrant an aggressive surgical approach to prevent embolization.

In an earlier study, 66 (37%) of 178 patients with IE who underwent TEE had one or more embolic events. A significant higher incidence of embolism was present in patients with a vegetation length greater than 10 mm (60%; *P* < 0.001) and in patients with mobile vegetations (62%; *P* < 0.001). Embolism was particularly frequent among 30 patients with both severely mobile and large vegetations (>15 mm) (83%; *P* < 0.001). On multivariate analysis, the only predictors of embolism were vegetation length (*P* = 0.03) and mobility (*P* = 0.01).[23]

Patients with a vegetation diameter greater than 10 mm have a significantly higher incidence of embolization than those with a vegetation diameter of 10 mm or less, and this risk appears to be higher in patients with MV endocarditis than in those with aortic valve endocarditis.[24] However, surgery on the basis of vegetation size alone is controversial.

Leaflet perforation occurs either at the site of the primary valve as the direct result of erosion by the inflammatory process, or at a neighboring valve as the result of a high-velocity jet. This scenario is most commonly encountered in the setting of an infected regurgitant aortic valve. The high-velocity jet directed toward the anterior leaflet of the MV creates a high-pressure lesion. The transmitted infected blood leads to abscess formation and subsequent perforation of that leaflet. The size of the perforation seen by TEE, usually 2 to 7 mm, closely corresponds to surgical and pathologic findings.[25] Therefore, in the face of aortic endocarditis and regurgitation, the MV should be carefully interrogated by echocardiography and thoroughly inspected during surgery.

Prosthetic Valve Endocarditis

Prosthetic valve IE may be difficult to diagnose with standard TTE, making TEE the first-line imaging technique of choice.[26] The leaflets of a tissue prosthetic valve should be inspected for excessive regurgitation, irregularities that may represent infected thrombus or vegetation, and abscess formation. Irregular movement or uncoordinated movement of prosthetic valve discs may represent "sticking" due to endothelial pannus ingrowth or obstruction due to the presence of vegetations causing valvular regurgitation (see Video 20-6, *A*). The acceleration velocity through a prosthesis may be increased by both high cardiac output (as a result of systemic inflammation) and partial obstruction (presence of a thrombus/vegetation). Prosthetic valve endocarditis is associated with a worse prognosis than endocarditis on native valves, with a mortality rate ranging between 20% and 40%.[27] Although TTE can detect prosthetic valve irregularities, initial investigation with TEE is more expeditious in making the diagnosis and detecting complications of prosthetic valve endocarditis.

Intracardiac Device–Related Infections

With the increase in pacemaker and AICD device implantation, there has been a significant increase in documented device infections. The incidence of definite device infection is 1.9 per 1000 device-years. Patients with AICDs have a higher incidence of IE when compared to patients with standard pacemakers.[28] Diagnosis is facilitated by inspection of the pocket in which the device was implanted and echocardiographic interrogation of the wires in the superior vena cava, as well as the right atrium, right atrial appendage, tricuspid valve, right

ventricle, and the free wall of the right atrium, against which the wire may impinge as it makes a turn in the right atrium to enter through the tricuspid valve. All these serve as potential sites for vegetation formation. In a Mayo Clinic series of device-related IE, TEE detected the abnormality in all cases of valvular involvement, but only one case was diagnosed by TTE.[28] Similarly, vegetations on leads were seen by TEE in 80% of cases but in less than 10% by TTE.[28] *Staphylococcus* species were the most commonly isolated pathogens. Nearly all patients were treated with a combined approach of complete hardware removal and parenteral antibiotics (see Video 20-3). 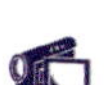

Surgical Considerations

Intraoperatively, TEE can define the extent of complications from endocarditis, which may alter the surgical procedure. Extensive deterioration of valve leaflets will warrant valve replacement, whereas a small focal vegetation may be removed in a valve-sparing operation. Extensive involvement of the valve or annular abscess may require repositioning of the sewing ring deeper into the atrium to avoid reinfection of the new valve.

According to the AHA/American College of Cardiology (ACC) recommendations for endocarditis, surgery is indicated in patients with life-threatening congestive heart failure or cardiogenic shock and should not be delayed.[29] Surgery is not indicated if complications (severe embolic cerebral damage) or comorbid conditions make the prospect of recovery remote. Surgery is recommended in patients with annular or aortic abscesses, heart block, recurrent emboli (despite being treated with appropriate antibiotic therapy), infections resistant to antibiotic therapy, and fungal endocarditis. Prosthetic valve endocarditis and native valve endocarditis due to *S. aureus* are usually surgical diseases. Early surgery for MV endocarditis due to virulent organisms (e.g., *S. aureus* or fungi) may make repair feasible. With increased surgical experience in mitral repair techniques, MV endocarditis has become more consistently treatable, with native valve preservation. There appears to be a low risk of recurrent infection or need for a prosthesis,[30] but surgery must not be delayed until extensive valve disruption has occurred.

Patients with prosthetic valves who receive warfarin anticoagulation and develop endocarditis should have their warfarin discontinued and replaced with heparin. This recommendation is less related to the possibility of hemorrhagic complications of endocarditis than to the possibility of urgent surgery. If surgery is required, the effects of warfarin will have dissipated and heparin can easily be reversed. If neurologic symptoms develop, anticoagulation should be discontinued until an intracranial hemorrhagic event is excluded by magnetic resonance imaging or computed tomographic scanning.

Surgery for Native Valve Endocarditis

Class I

1. Surgery of the native valve is indicated in patients with acute IE who present with valve stenosis or regurgitation resulting in heart failure. (Level of Evidence: B)
2. Surgery of the native valve is indicated in patients with acute IE who present with aortic regurgitation (AR) or mitral regurgitation (MR) with hemodynamic evidence of elevated left ventricular end-diastolic or left atrial pressures (e.g., premature closure of MV with AR, rapid decelerating MR signal by continuous wave Doppler (v-wave cutoff sign), or moderate or severe pulmonary hypertension). (Level of Evidence: B)
3. Surgery of the native valve is indicated in patients with IE caused by fungal or other highly resistant organisms. (Level of Evidence: B)
4. Surgery of the native valve is indicated in patients with IE complicated by heart block, annular or aortic abscess, or destructive penetrating lesions (e.g., sinus of Valsalva to right atrium, right ventricle, or left atrium fistula; mitral leaflet perforation with aortic valve endocarditis; or infection in annulus fibrosa). (Level of Evidence: B)

Class IIa

Surgery of the native valve is reasonable in patients with IE who present with recurrent emboli and persistent vegetations despite appropriate antibiotic therapy. (Level of Evidence: C)

Class IIb

Surgery of the native valve may be considered in patients with IE who present with mobile vegetations in excess of 10 mm with or without emboli. (Level of Evidence: C) Patients with left-sided native valve endocarditis complicated by congestive heart failure, systemic embolization to vital organs, or presence of a large vegetation on echocardiography have poor outcomes on medical treatment alone. A large cohort study using a multivariate model reported that valve surgery was associated with improved 6-month survival. An additional benefit of early surgery is likely to include successful valve repair as an outcome, especially for the MV. When at all possible, MV repair should be performed instead of MV replacement in the setting of active infection because of the risk of infection of prosthetic materials. Aortic valves may often be repaired as well if there are leaflet perforations, and this is preferable to aortic valve replacement for the same reasons.

Surgery for Prosthetic Valve Endocarditis

Class I

1. Consultation with a cardiac surgeon is indicated for patients with IE of a prosthetic valve. (Level of Evidence: C)
2. Surgery is indicated for patients with IE of a prosthetic valve who present with heart failure. (Level of Evidence: B)
3. Surgery is indicated for patients with IE of a prosthetic valve who present with dehiscence evidenced by cine fluoroscopy or echocardiography. (Level of Evidence: B)
4. Surgery is indicated for patients with IE of a prosthetic valve who present with evidence of increasing obstruction or worsening regurgitation. (Level of Evidence: C)
5. Surgery is indicated for patients with IE of a prosthetic valve who present with complications (e.g., abscess formation). (Level of Evidence: C)

Class IIa

1. Surgery is reasonable for patients with IE of a prosthetic valve who present with evidence of persistent bacteremia or recurrent emboli despite appropriate antibiotic treatment. (Level of Evidence: C)
2. Surgery is reasonable for patients with IE of a prosthetic valve who present with relapsing infection. (Level of Evidence: C)

Class III

Routine surgery is not indicated for patients with uncomplicated IE of a prosthetic valve caused by first infection with a sensitive organism. (Level of Evidence: C)

Summary

Postprocedure TEE is useful to determine the adequacy of surgical intervention, particularly detecting any evidence of paravalvular leak before the patient has left the operating room. The International Collaboration on Endocarditis Merged Database is a large multicenter international registry of patients with definite endocarditis by Duke criteria, including 367 patients with prosthetic valve infective endocarditis (PVIE). Clinical, microbiological, and echocardiographic variables were analyzed to determine those factors associated with use of surgery for PVIE. Surgical therapy for PVIE was performed in 148 (42%) of 367 patients. In-hospital mortality was similar for patients treated with

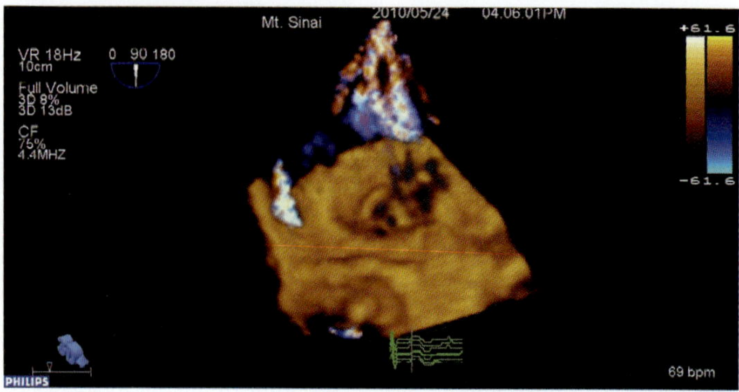

Figure 20-6   Three-dimensional (3D) view from left atrial perspective looking at a mitral valve prosthesis from anterior to posterior. Exact anatomic localization of paravalvular leaks can easily be seen with 3D transesophageal echocardiography.

surgery and those treated with medical therapy alone. Surgical therapy was independently associated with patient age, microorganism, intracardiac abscess, and congestive heart failure. After adjustment for factors related to surgical intervention, brain embolism and *S. aureus* infection were independently associated with in-hospital mortality, and a trend toward a survival benefit of surgery was evident.[31]

Introduction of three-dimensional (3D) echocardiography has several advantages over 2D echocardiography in diagnosing endocarditis[32-34] by providing planes of investigation not available by 2D echocardiography alone. Particularly, 3D TEE imaging allows better topographical localization of prosthetic valve paravalvular leaks and dehiscence (Fig. 20-6 [also see Fig. 20-2]; Video 20-7 [also see Video 20-2]). Whether this new imaging modality will help improve diagnostic accuracy is still to be determined. 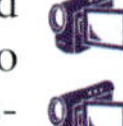

REFERENCES

1. Jain R, Kolias TJ. Three-dimensional transesophageal echocardiography of pacemaker endocarditis. *J Am Coll Cardiol.* Apr 7 2009;53(14):1241.
2. Vincelj J, Barsic B, Rudez I, Unic D, Udovicic M. Echocardiography in detecting implantable cardioverter defibrillator lead endocarditis: case report. *Acta Clin Croat.* Mar 2011;50(1):121-124.
3. Durack DT, Lukes AS, Bright DK. New criteria for diagnosis of infective endocarditis: utilization of specific echocardiographic findings. Duke Endocarditis Service. *Am J Med.* Mar 1994;96(3):200-209.
4. Santise G, D'Ancona G, Mamone G, et al. Echocardiography in acute native aortic valve endocarditis. *J Cardiothorac Vasc Anesth.* Jun 2010;24(3):516-518.
5. Ansari A, Rigolin VH. Infective endocarditis: an update on the role of echocardiography. *Curr Cardiol Rep.* May 2010;12(3):265-271.
6. Paterick TE, Paterick TJ, Nishimura RA, Steckelberg JM. Complexity and subtlety of infective endocarditis. *Mayo Clin Proc.* May 2007;82(5):615-621.
7. Habib G, Badano L, Tribouilloy C, et al. Recommendations for the practice of echocardiography in infective endocarditis. *Eur J Echocardiogr.* Mar 2010;11(2):202-219.
8. Chopra T, Kaatz GW. Treatment strategies for infective endocarditis. *Expert Opin Pharmacother.* Feb 2010;11(3):345-360.
9. Shroff H, Benenstein R, Freedberg R, Mehl S, Saric M. Mitral valve Libman-Sacks endocarditis visualized by real time three-dimensional transesophageal echocardiography. *Echocardiography.* 2012;29(4):E100-101.
10. Galve E, Candell-Riera J, Pigrau C, Permanyer-Miralda G, Garcia-Del-Castillo H. Soler- Soler J. Prevalence, morphologic types, and evolution of cardiac valvular disease in systemic lupus erythematosus. *N Engl J Med.* Sep 29 1988;319(13):817-823.
11. Li JS, Sexton DJ, Mick N, et al. Proposed modifications to the Duke criteria for the diagnosis of infective endocarditis. *Clin Infect Dis.* Apr 2000;30(4):633-638.
12. Tissieres P, Gervaix A, Beghetti M, Jaeggi ET. Value and limitations of the von Reyn, Duke, and modified Duke criteria for the diagnosis of infective endocarditis in children. *Pediatrics.* Dec 2003;112 (6 Pt 1):e467.
13. Palepu A, Cheung SS, Montessori V, Woods R, Thompson CR. Factors other than the Duke criteria associated with infective endocarditis among injection drug users. *Clin Invest Med.* Aug 2002;25(4):118-125.
14. Fournier PE, Thuny F, Richet H, et al. Comprehensive diagnostic strategy for blood culture-negative endocarditis: a prospective study of 819 new cases. *Clin Infect Dis.* Jul 15 2010;51(2):131-140.
15. Kini V, Logani S, Ky B, et al. Transthoracic and transesophageal echocardiography for the indication of suspected infective endocarditis: vegetations, blood cultures and imaging. *J Am Soc Echocardiogr.* Apr 2010;23(4):396-402.
16. Hendel RC, Berman DS, Di Carli MF, et al. ACCF/ASNC/ACR/AHA/ASE/SCCT/SCMR/SNM 2009 Appropriate Use Criteria for Cardiac Radionuclide Imaging: A Report of the American College of Cardiology Foundation Appropriate Use Criteria Task Force, the American Society of Nuclear Cardiology, the American College of Radiology, the American Heart Association, the American Society of Echocardiography, the Society of Cardiovascular Computed Tomography, the Society for Cardiovascular Magnetic Resonance, and the Society of Nuclear Medicine. *J Am Coll Cardiol.* Jun 9 2009;53(23):2201-2229.
17. Rallidis LS, Komninos KA, Papasteriadis EG. Pacemaker-related endocarditis: the value of transesophageal echocardiography in diagnosis and treatment. *Acta Cardiol.* Feb 2003;58(1):31-34.

18. Heidenreich PA, Masoudi FA, Maini B, et al. Echocardiography in patients with suspected endocarditis: a cost-effectiveness analysis. *Am J Med*. Sep 1999;107(3):198-208.
19. Gould FK, Denning DW, Elliott TS, et al. Guidelines for the diagnosis and antibiotic treatment of endocarditis in adults: a report of the Working Party of the British Society for Antimicrobial Chemotherapy. *J Antimicrob Chemother*. Feb 2012;67(2):269-289.
20. Hill EE, Herijgers P, Claus P, Vanderschueren S, Peetermans WE, Herregods MC. Abscess in infective endocarditis: the value of transesophageal echocardiography and outcome: a 5-year study. *Am Heart J*. Nov 2007;154(5):923-928.
21. Anguera I, Miro JM, Vilacosta I, et al. Aorto-cavitary fistulous tract formation in infective endocarditis: clinical and echocardiographic features of 76 cases and risk factors for mortality. *Eur Heart J*. Feb 2005;26(3):288-297.
22. Thuny F, Di Salvo G, Belliard O, et al. Risk of embolism and death in infective endocarditis: prognostic value of echocardiography: a prospective multicenter study. *Circulation*. Jul 5 2005;112(1):69-75.
23. Di Salvo G, Habib G, Pergola V, et al. Echocardiography predicts embolic events in infective endocarditis. *J Am Coll Cardiol*. Mar 15 2001;37(4):1069-1076.
24. Mugge A, Daniel WG, Frank G, Lichtlen PR. Echocardiography in infective endocarditis: reassessment of prognostic implications of vegetation size determined by the transthoracic and the transesophageal approach. *J Am Coll Cardiol*. Sep 1989;14(3):631-638.
25. De Castro S, d'Amati G, Cartoni D, et al. Valvular perforation in left-sided infective endocarditis: a prospective echocardiographic evaluation and clinical outcome. *Am Heart J*. Oct 1997;134(4):656-664.
26. Scandura S, Cammalleri V, Caggegi AM, Mignosa C, Tamburino C. Infective endocarditis in mitral mechanical prosthesis: the role of three-dimensional transoesophageal echocardiography. *Eur J Echocardiogr*. Oct 2011;12(10):801.
27. Habib G, Thuny F, Avierinos JF. Prosthetic valve endocarditis: current approach and therapeutic options. *Prog Cardiovasc Dis*. Jan-Feb 2008;50(4):274-281.
28. Sohail MR, Uslan DZ, Khan AH, et al. Infective endocarditis complicating permanent pacemaker and implantable cardioverter-defibrillator infection. *Mayo Clin Proc*. Jan 2008;83(1):46-53.
29. Bonow RO, Carabello BA, Kanu C, et al. ACC/AHA 2006 guidelines for the management of patients with valvular heart disease: a report of the American College of Cardiology/American Heart Association Task Force on Practice Guidelines (Writing Committee to Revise the 1998 Guidelines for the Management of Patients with Valvular Heart Disease): developed in collaboration with the Society of Cardiovascular Anesthesiologists: endorsed by the Society for Cardiovascular Angiography and Interventions and the Society of Thoracic Surgeons. *Circulation*. Aug 1 2006;114(5):e84-231.
30. Zegdi R, Debieche M, Latremouille C, et al. Long-term results of mitral valve repair in active endocarditis. *Circulation*. May 17 2005;111(19):2532-2536.
31. Wang A, Pappas P, Anstrom KJ, et al. The use and effect of surgical therapy for prosthetic valve infective endocarditis: a propensity analysis of a multicenter, international cohort. *Am Heart J*. Nov 2005;150(5):1086-1091.
32. Shapira Y, Weisenberg DE, Vaturi M, et al. The impact of intraoperative transesophageal echocardiography in infective endocarditis. *Isr Med Assoc J*. Apr 2007;9(4):299-302.
33. Lopez-Pardo F, Gonzalez-Calle A, Lopez-Haldon J, Acosta-Martinez J, Rangel-Sousa D, Rodriguez-Puras MJ. Real time three-dimensional transesophageal echocardiography in the anatomical assessment of complex mitral valve regurgitation secondary to endocarditis. *Rev Esp Cardiol*. Feb 2012;65(2):188-190.
34. Liu YW, Tsai WC, Lin CC, et al. Usefulness of real-time three-dimensional echocardiography for diagnosis of infective endocarditis. *Scand Cardiovasc J*. 2009;43(5):318-323.

Imaging of Cardiac Tumors and Solid and Gaseous Materials

PATRICIA M. APPLEGATE | RICHARD L. APPLEGATE II

Introduction

In many cases, the diagnosis of a mass visualized by echocardiography is not known with certainty until a tissue specimen has been obtained. Importantly, both normal variants and imaging artifacts can be mistaken for pathologic findings when seen during an echocardiographic examination.

Cardiac Pseudo-masses

Many normal variants can be misinterpreted as pathologic abnormalities and are thus "pseudo-masses." A number of intracardiac structures can be difficult to distinguish from cardiac tumors. The eustachian valve (Fig. 21-1) is an incomplete valve at the orifice of the inferior vena cava (IVC). The Chiari network is a remnant of congenital fibers that attach from the crista terminalis region to the eustachian valve. They are often mobile and may entrap a catheter or wire. The Chiari network does not typically prolapse through the tricuspid valve. The crista terminalis is a muscle ridge that extends from the right sides of the superior vena cava (SVC) and IVC and continues cephalad to the right atrial appendage.[1] The moderator band is a normal structure in the right ventricle that extends from the anterior papillary muscle to the septum and is a part of the septomarginal trabeculation.[2] The moderator band contains the right bundle branch conduction tissue. It is reported that Leonardo da Vinci first described this structure, calling it the "catena of the right ventricle."[3] Another potential confounder is a left atrial cord or free fibrous cord. Left atrial cords have been well recognized in autopsy specimens and should not be confused with a true cor triatriatum. There is one description in the literature from an autopsy case describing a cord that originated from the right atrial wall and passed through a patent foramen ovale (PFO), attached to the left atrial wall and then the mitral valve, looped up and attached to the aortic valve, and finally to the aorta.[4] Prominent papillary muscles in either the right or left ventricles may appear to be intracardiac masses in some scan planes. Similarly, apical hypertrophic cardiomyopathy[5] or prominent ventricular noncompaction[6] can appear similar to cardiac tumors. Prominent apical trabeculation or a left ventricular false tendon can also appear to be an intracardiac mass or thrombus.[7]

Atrial findings that can be confused with cardiac tumors include the ridge of tissue between the upper pulmonary vein and left atrial appendage (Fig. 21-2) and suture lines in the left atrium that are associated with cardiac transplantation. A prominent atrial septal aneurysm may be interpreted as a bulging cystic mass.[8-10] Fatty infiltrate of the atrial septum, known as *lipomatous atrial septal hypertrophy* (LASH),[11,12] can appear to be a cardiac tumor. LASH is a nonencapsulated hyperplastic accumulation of mature adipose tissue in the atrial septum (Fig. 21-3, Video 21-1). These infiltrates can be very large (up to 7 cm or more), are common in elderly obese women, and have a possible association with atrial dysrhythmias. LASH creates a dumbbell-type appearance of the atrial septum due to sparing of the fossa ovalis, with fatty infiltrate in the inferior and superior portions of the atrial septum. LASH is typically preferential to the right atrium. When there is massive infiltration of the atrial septum, the adipose tissue in other parts of the heart is generally increased, particularly the right

ventricular epicardial surface. Magnetic resonance imaging (MRI) is helpful in characterization of this abnormality if there is a clinical doubt after echocardiographic imaging. Adipose tissue has typical MRI characteristics that allow distinction from tumors or thrombus. There is no absolute diagnostic dimension established for the diagnosis of LASH, but 20 mm is often quoted. A dilated coronary sinus can bulge into the atrium as an extracardiac mass. Patients with prominent dilation of the coronary sinus should be evaluated for the presence of persistent left SVC-to–coronary sinus connection and for conditions associated with chronic elevation of right atrial pressure. Pectinate muscles in the right and left atrial appendages may be difficult to distinguish from tumor or thrombus. Similarly, a multilobed atrial appendage or an inverted left atrial appendage[13,14] can be misinterpreted as cardiac masses.

Vegetations are a type of intracardiac mass that must be distinguished from cardiac tumors. These are discussed in Chapter 20. Redundancy of the mitral valve supporting apparatus can appear to be an intracardiac mass, as can mitral annular calcification. Excess epicardial fat will appear to be an extracardiac mass; this has been associated with prolonged corticosteroid therapy.[15] A cardiac varix can occur in the right atrium[16,17] and may appear to be a cardiac mass when seen on transesophageal echocardiographic (TEE) examination.[18] Similarly, fat in the atrioventricular (AV) groove or transverse sinus may be misinterpreted as an extracardiac mass. Several imaging artifacts can give rise to the appearance of cardiac masses, including beam-width artifact, side-lobe artifact, reverberation artifact, and mirror-image artifact (see Chapter 6). Fibrin debris in pericardial fluid can appear to be extracardiac masses. Pectus excavatum may displace structures anterior to the heart, giving rise to the appearance of an extracardiac mass.[19] Finally, a hiatal hernia can be confused as a mass when imaged from either transthoracic or transesophageal windows.[20-22] This pseudo-mass will opacify when the patient ingests a carbonated beverage.

Imaging True Cardiac Masses

In assessing masses by echocardiography, the size, location, mobility, attachment, and associated clinical history are important in establishing a differential diagnosis.[23] Cardiac tumors can be benign or malignant and primary or secondary.[15,24-33] The most common primary cardiac tumors are summarized in Table 21-1.

The first premortem diagnosis of a cardiac tumor was made in 1934, when a sarcoma was identified.[34] Secondary (metastatic) tumors are up to 40 (or more) times more common than primary tumors. Of all cardiac tumors, 94% are benign and 6% are malignant. The most commonly encountered metastatic tumor at autopsy is lung carcinoma (17%). However, of malignancies, melanoma has the highest frequency of metastases to the heart (46%). According to Lam[26] in a series of 12,485 consecutive autopsies, there was an incidence of 1.23% (154) metastatic tumors and 0.056% (7) primary tumors. According to McAllister[35] in a series of 533 primary malignant cardiac tumors, angiosarcoma was the most common (31%), followed by rhabdomyosarcoma (21%), mesothelioma (15%), fibrosarcoma (11%), other sarcomas (9%), lymphoma (6%), and miscellaneous (7%). In a series of 319 primary benign cardiac tumors,[35] myxoma was the most common (40%), followed by lipoma (14%), papillary fibroelastoma (14%), rhabdomyoma (11%), fibroma (5%),

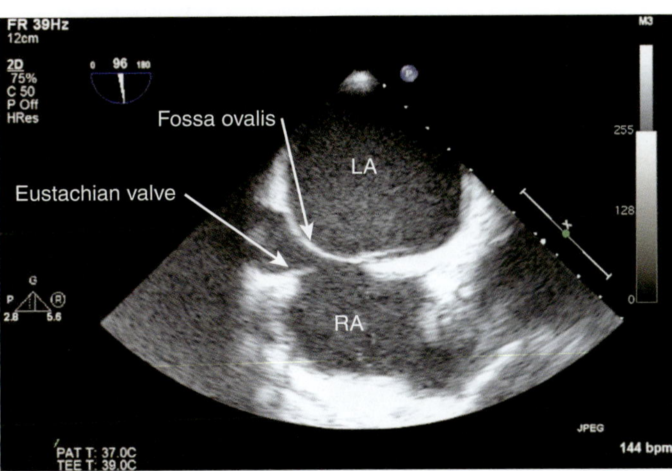

Figure 21-1 The eustachian valve is an embryologic remnant seen at junction of inferior vena cava and right atrium *(RA)*. It may be misidentified as mass or thrombus. *LA*, Left atrium.

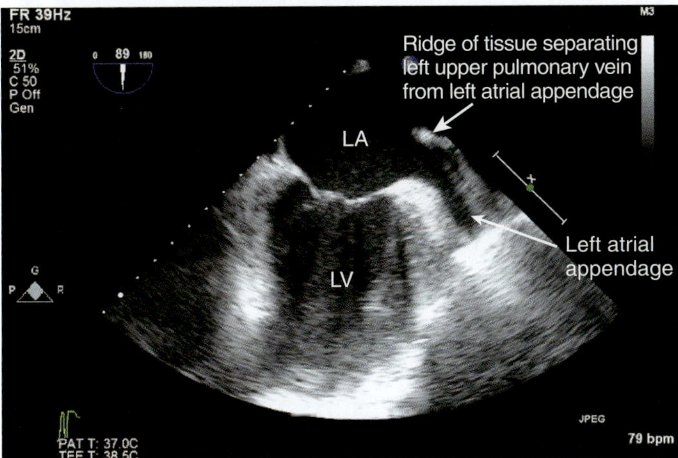

Figure 21-2 The ridge of tissue between left upper pulmonary vein and left atrial appendage can be misinterpreted as mass or thrombus. Careful imaging will allow correct identification of this structure. *LA*, Left atrium; *LV*, left ventricle.

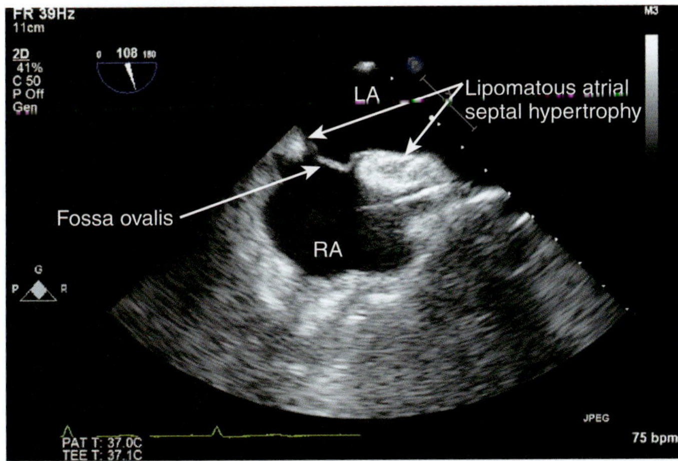

Figure 21-3 Lipomatous atrial septal hypertrophy may be misinterpreted as tumor in atrial septum. *LA*, Left atrium; *RA*, right atrium.

hemangioma (5%), teratoma (4%), and other. There is a difference with age; rhabdomyoma is the most common tumor in pediatric patients, in whom this tumor type has a strong association with tuberous sclerosis. Masses usually found on heart valves are summarized in Table 21-2.

Masses found in the AV groove or pericardium may be interpreted as being in the heart. These include pericardial cysts, which are benign masses often incidentally found with echocardiography and typically located in the right AV groove, echinococcal (hydatid) cysts, coronary artery aneurysm (Fig. 21-4), lipoma, pheochromocytoma, loculated pericardial effusion, or diaphragmatic hernia. Esophageal hiatal hernia has been misinterpreted as a cardiac mass during TEE. Abnormalities of the aorta may appear as intracardiac (Fig. 21-5, Videos 21-2 and 21-3) or extracardiac masses. 

TABLE 21-1	Tumors of the Heart	
Malignant Primary Cardiac Tumors	*Benign Primary Cardiac Tumors*	
Angiosarcoma	Myxoma	
Rhabdomyosarcoma	Lipoma	
Mesothelioma	Papillary fibroelastoma	
Fibrosarcoma	Rhabdomyoma	
Leiomyosarcoma	Fibroma	
Synovial sarcoma	Hemangioma	
Lymphoma	Teratoma	
	Mesothelioma of atrioventricular node	

TABLE 21-2	Masses on Cardiac Valves
Mass Found on Valve	*Comments*
Papillary fibroelastoma	Pedunculated, mobile
Lambl excrescence	Thin, mobile filamentous structures; single or multiple; 1 mm thick; 1-5 mm long; along closure line of valve, AV>>MV; avascular connective tissue matrix covered by single layer of endothelium; degenerative process; frequency increased with age
Fenestration	Degenerative change in valve leaflet
Cysts	Blood cyst is thin walled; multilobed; attached to valve leaflet
Immune-mediated valve disease	Nodules of Arantius and lunulae

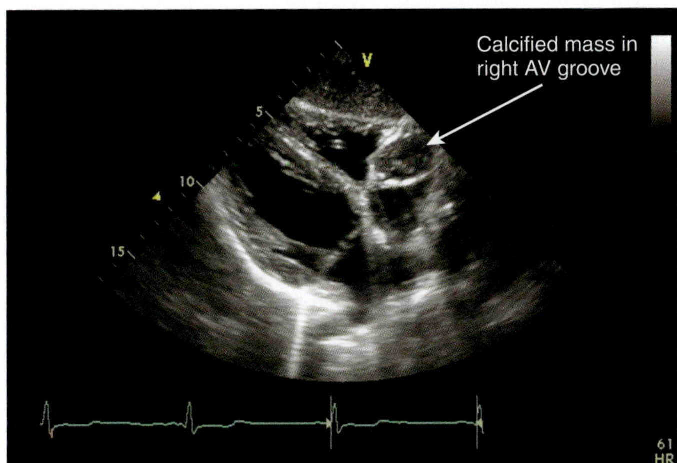

Figure 21-4 Coronary artery aneurysms can appear in the atrioventricular *(AV)* groove. In this transthoracic echocardiogram example, the coronary artery aneurysm has calcified and appears as a solid mass. Subcostal transthoracic view shows calcified coronary artery aneurysm distorting right atrium.

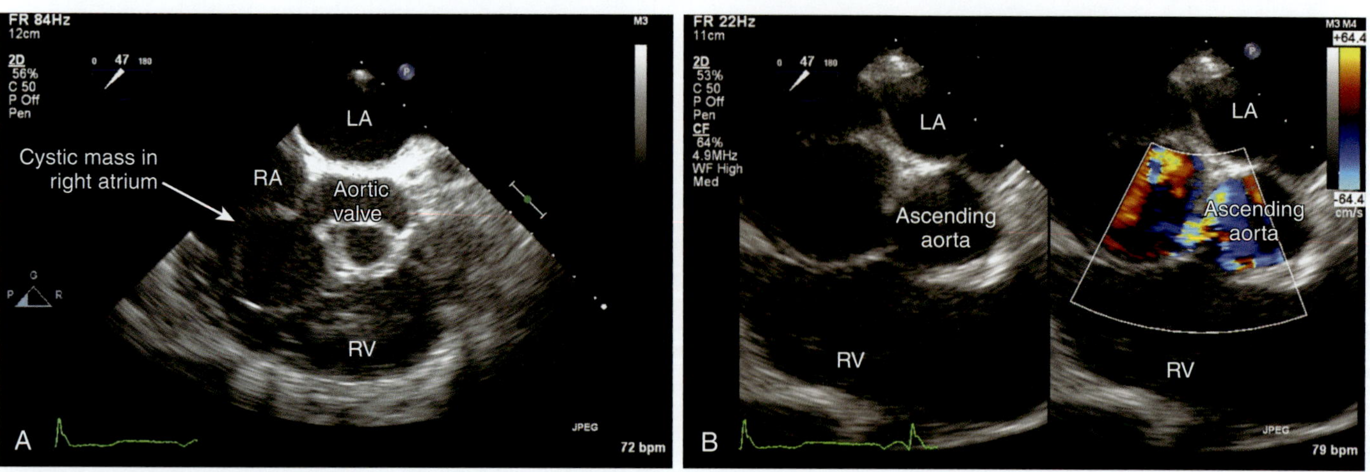

Figure 21-5   Abnormalities of the aorta may appear to be intra- or extracardiac masses. **A,** This atypical sinus of Valsalva aneurysm can be seen protruding into right atrium *(RA)* and right ventricle *(RV),* giving the appearance of a cystic mass. **B,** Color flow Doppler demonstrates flow from ascending aorta into aneurysm, giving rise to the appearance of a cystic mass in RA. *LA,* Left atrium.

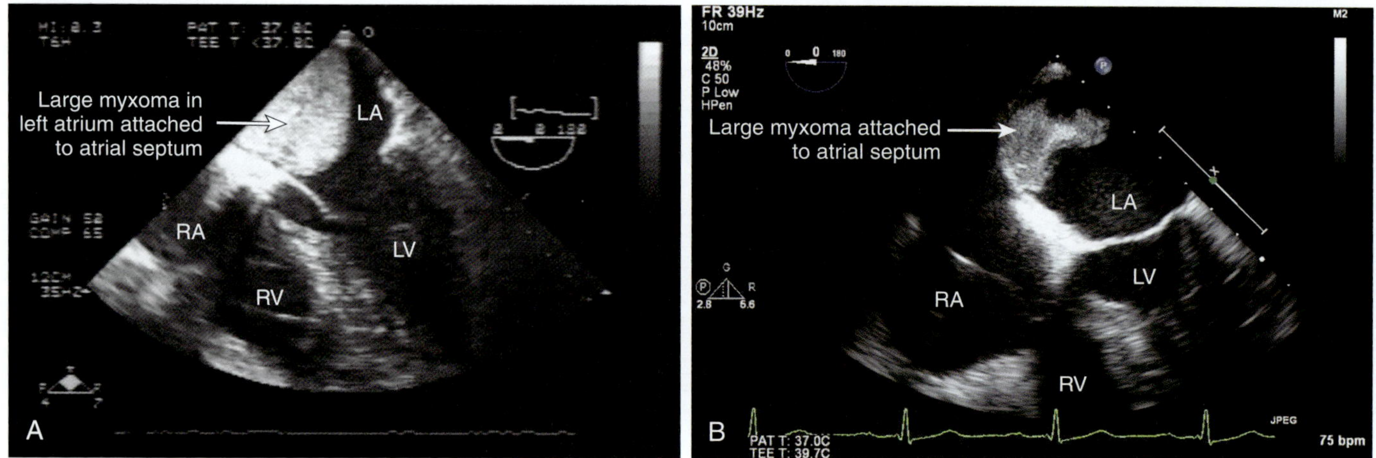

Figure 21-6   The most common site of myxoma attachment is left atrial side of atrial septum on fossa ovalis. **A,** Large smooth myxoma attached to left atrial side of atrial septum. **B,** Large pedunculated myxoma attached to left atrial side of atrial septum. *LA,* Left atrium; *LV,* left ventricle; *RA,* right atrium; *RV,* right ventricle.

Primary Benign Cardiac Tumors

Myxoma

The cell of origin of the myxoma is still unclear.[15,36-43] The most common location for myxomas (the other acceptable plural form is *myxomata*) is the left atrium, and the most common attachment is the atrial septum (Fig. 21-6, Video 21-4). The reported distribution of myxomas is 75% in the left atrium, 20% in the right atrium, and the remainder in the left or right ventricle. There are very rare case reports of myxomas on the AV valves (Fig. 21-7, Video 21-5). Myxomas may be smooth or papillary or grapelike in appearance (Fig. 21-8); these myxomas are more likely to embolize than well-encapsulated tumors. Typically, myxomas are pedunculated (although they may be sessile) and attached via a narrow stalk in the fossa ovalis region. Myxomas appear heterogeneous and may have cavitations and protruding frond-like extensions. The myxoma tumor may be large enough to prolapse through the AV valve (Fig. 21-9), causing obstruction and the associated physical exam findings (diastolic murmur or "plop"). Color flow and continuous wave Doppler allow assessment of the degree of functional stenosis/flow obstruction.

Myxomas generally present between the ages of 30 to 60 years and may be spontaneous/sporadic, familial, or complex. Complexes that include myxoma may be referred to as *syndrome myxoma, Carney syndrome, NAME syndrome* (nevi, atrial myxoma, neurofibroma, ephelides), or *LAMB syndrome* (lentigines, atrial myxoma, blue nevi). Spontaneous (sporadic) myxomas are the most common; 70% are found in women.[15,44] The familial variety[45] represents approximately 7% to 10% of myxomas, with autosomal dominant inheritance, and presents earlier in life (mean age 25). The familial form may be part of a complex syndrome that frequently presents with multiple tumors in several chambers. These are often in atypical locations (13% in the ventricular cavity), and patients require ongoing screening for a high recurrence rate that may approach 21% (usually occurring within 4 years after the initial resection). If a patient has multiple tumors, first-degree relatives should be screened. The Carney complex syndrome[46-50] is uncommon and includes myxomas of skin, mucosa, or heart. Family history will be positive because these patients have an abnormal chromosome sequence at 17q22-24 encoding the regulatory subunit 1A of protein kinase A (PRKAR1A).[51-54] There is an association with lentigenes, blue nevus, acromegaly, Cushing syndrome, thyroid cancer or nodules, melanotic schwannoma, breast ductal adenomas, and testicular tumors.

The typical clinical presentation in patients with myxoma includes syncope, dyspnea, heart failure, and possibly sudden cardiac death, which is related to obstruction of the AV valve by the myxoma. There is embolization in approximately 30% to 40% of patients. Patients with myxoma often have fever, malaise, rash, weight loss, Raynaud

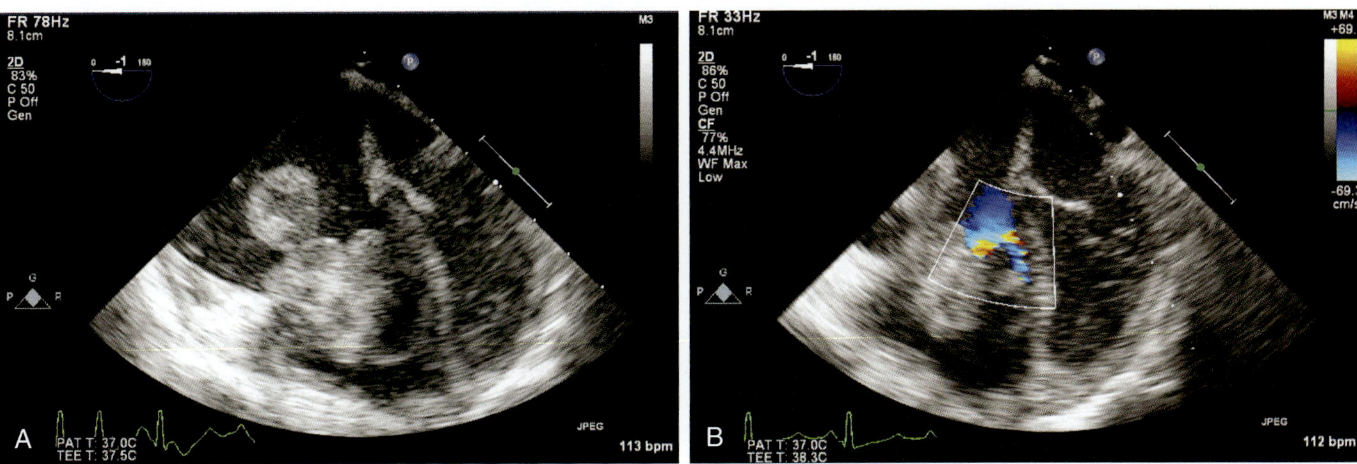

Figure 21-7 Large irregular myxoma attached to and moving with tricuspid valve. **A,** In diastole, myxoma prolapses into right ventricle, obstructing ventricular filling, as demonstrated by color flow Doppler imaging **(B)**.

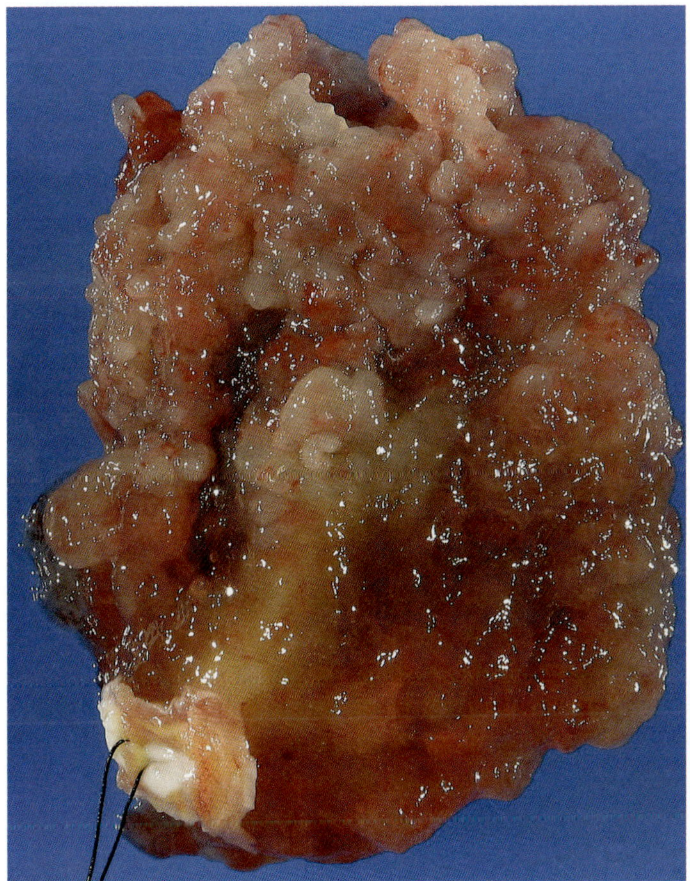

Figure 21-8 Photograph of myxoma specimen removed at surgery, demonstrating irregular surface of tumor. Suture indicates point at which this myxoma attached to valve leaflet.

phenomena, leukocytosis, thrombocytopenia, increased gamma globulins, anemia, and elevated C-reactive protein and erythrocyte sedimentation rate—all of which are nonspecific constitutional findings. Many of the symptoms associated with myxoma are thought to be due to synthesis and secretion of interleukin (IL)-6, since increased levels have been found in myxoma tissue. IL-6 is a proinflammatory cytokine that creates an acute-phase response.

Differential diagnoses of masses resembling myxoma on echocardiography include thrombus, papillary fibroelastoma, lipoma, and metastases. The management of myxomas is surgical. TEE is generally indicated preoperatively to assist in characterizing the morphology and attachment of the tumor and to evaluate for the possibility of multiple tumors. Intraoperative TEE is indicated to evaluate for any residual tumor, related valvular dysfunction, or complications related to the resection (e.g., atrial septal defect).

Papillary Fibroelastoma

Papillary fibroelastoma (PFE) are generally small (mean 8 mm; up to 40 mm), usually single (>90%), typically attached to valve surfaces, and may be pedunculated and mobile.[55-59] A study from the Cleveland Clinic[60] reported on a series of 162 patients with papillary fibroelastoma. Of these, 45% (49/162) were on the aortic valve, most often the right coronary cusp, followed by the noncoronary cusp, and least often on the left coronary cusp. Forty of 49 were on the aortic side of the aortic valve. The mitral valve was the location of 40/162 of these tumors: 23 anterior and 17 posterior leaflet; 32 of these 40 were on the atrial surface, and some attached to the supporting apparatus. Valve dysfunction or regurgitation related to PFE is uncommon. A PFE is generally round, oval, or irregular but homogeneous with well-demarcated borders. In approximately 50%, the PFE is attached via a stalk (50%) and is mobile. Embolic events secondary to PFE have been described,[61,62] with resulting stroke, transient ischemic attack (TIA), angina, sudden death, myocardial infarction (MI), pulmonary embolism, and retinal artery occlusion. PFEs smaller than 2 mm will not be visible by TTE. PFE may be difficult to differentiate from degenerative valve disease. Surgical excision may be indicated in patients with large, mobile, left-sided tumors (>1 cm), those who have had embolic events, and those in whom complications are directly related to tumor mobility, such as coronary ostial occlusion.[56,63] Tumor mobility is an independent predictor of death or nonfatal embolization, and in these patients, surgical intervention should be considered. Patients who are not surgical candidates may be given oral anticoagulants, but there are no randomized controlled data to support this.

Rhabdomyoma

Rhabdomyoma is the most common cardiac tumor in infants and children.[64-69] There has been some discussion about whether this is a true neoplasm or a hamartoma. Rhabdomyomas are usually multiple, involve both the left and right ventricular myocardium equally, generally project into the cavity, and may move freely (with some reported cases of outflow obstruction).[70,71] In certain instances of outflow obstruction, surgical intervention is indicated, but spontaneous resolution of these tumors has been described, and surgical intervention is not generally necessary in the asymptomatic patient. There is an associated increased incidence of ventricular pre-excitation or Wolff-Parkinson-White syndrome in patients with rhabdomyoma.

Studies have reported that many patients (30%-80%) with rhabdomyoma have associated tuberous sclerosis (angiofibromas on the face, fibromas around fingernails, café au lait spots, and subcutaneous nodules).[72]

Fibroma

Fibromas are generally intramural within the left ventricular wall and occur mostly in infants and children.[73-75] These tumors are histologically benign, but they may be associated with malignant dysrhythmias[76] and severe heart failure. It is estimated that 70% of patients with fibromas are symptomatic. If present, symptoms are related to obstruction, systolic dysfunction, or conduction abnormalities. Sudden death has been reported in approximately 15% of patients. Cardiac fibromas may appear as disproportional irregular hypertrophy and can be confused with thrombus or true hypertrophy. Surgical resection may help, but because these tumors may infiltrate extensively, resection will not necessarily ameliorate the problem.

Lipoma

Lipomas are mature fat cell tumors. They can occur anywhere in the heart and may be very small or massive. Most occur in the subepicardial or subpericardial space, but approximately 25% are intramuscular. The left ventricle, right atrium, and interatrial septum are the most common sites. They can also occur on the valves. MRI allows for definitive identification of these tumors. Surgical resection is indicated when tumor size or location produces symptoms.

Hemangiomas

Cardiac hemangiomas most often occur in the ventricular septum or AV node and are best diagnosed by coronary angiography by a characteristic "tumor blush." Contrast-enhanced echocardiography can also be useful in assessing the vascular nature of these tumors. These tumors may cause heart block and sudden death and generally cannot be excised completely.

Other Tumors of the Heart

Cardiac angiomas, teratomas, mesotheliomas of the AV node, and endocrine tumors are extremely rare. Cardiac teratomas occur in the pericardial space and may be associated with a pericardial effusion; the combined effect of the mass and fluid accumulation may become large enough to cause hemodynamic compromise. Teratomas arise and receive their blood supplies from the ascending aorta or pulmonary trunk through the vasa vasorum. They are found primarily in female infants and children.

Primary Cardiac Malignant Tumors

Sarcoma

Sarcomas are the most common primary malignant cardiac tumors. They commonly occur between the ages of 30 and 50 years and are unusual in children. Sarcomas occur equally in men and women and are more common in the right heart chambers. There have been some reports of sarcomas developing around Dacron grafts or prosthetic valves in the heart and in peripheral vessels.[77-79] A rat study published in 1958 suggested that plastics with long-chain polymers are carcinogenic with a long latency period.[80] More recently, it has been suggested that this may be related to reactive oxygen species.[81] Cardiac sarcomas are aggressive and associated with a rapid downhill clinical course. Death is related to widespread myocardial infiltration or extensive metastatic disease. Sarcomas may cause inflow or outflow obstruction and may invade into the pericardial space. Dysrhythmias are common.

Angiosarcoma

Angiosarcomas are the most common cardiac sarcoma and characteristically originate from the right atrium. They are more common in males. Angiosarcomas tend to be very vascular and because of this may produce a continuous murmur. About one quarter of angiosarcomas will be intracavitary and produce obstruction and right-sided heart failure.

Rhabdosarcoma

Rhabdosarcoma is the second most common cardiac sarcoma. It is also more common in males, but has no predilection for a particular cardiac chamber, so can be found in any of the four chambers.

Metastatic Cardiac Tumors

Metastatic tumors to the heart are more commonly carcinomas than sarcomas, simply because carcinomas are far more common than sarcomas. Secondary cardiac masses can reach the heart as a result of several mechanisms, which are summarized in Table 21-3.

The metastatic tumor can appear as discrete areas of enlargement in the myocardium or can present as extensive infiltration (Fig. 21-10, Videos 21-6 and 21-7). Extension of renal or liver malignancy via the IVC can sometimes be imaged using echocardiography (Fig. 21-11). Cardiac metastases should be suspected when a patient with a primary tumor in an organ other than the heart develops cardiac enlargement, dysrhythmias, or heart failure. However, only a minority (10%) of patients with cardiac metastases develop signs or symptoms of cardiac dysfunction. Of those that develop cardiac signs or symptoms, 90% result from pericardial involvement and 10% from intracavitary or

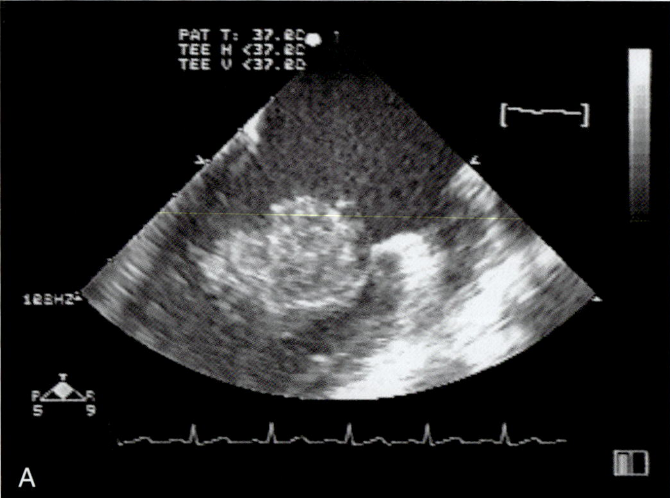

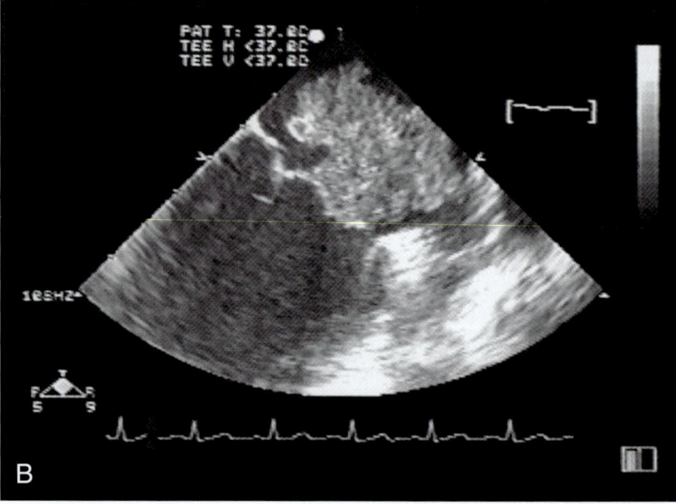

Figure 21-9   Highly mobile myxoma is seen to move between left atrium and left ventricle during cardiac cycle. Surface shape may change as myxoma moves. **A,** Diastole. **B,** Systole. A highly mobile myxoma is more likely to be associated with embolization.

intramyocardial involvement.[15] It is rare that the metastatic lesion will be limited to the heart: cardiac metastases usually indicate widespread metastases.

Primary Cancers Associated with Cardiac Metastasis

Lung carcinoma tends to invade the parietal pericardium and then the visceral pericardium, leading to pericardial effusion and/or constriction. Lung carcinoma may also invade via the pulmonary veins into the left atrium and can cause secondary left ventricular inflow obstruction.

TABLE 21-3	Metastasis to Heart
Mechanism	**Tumor Types**
Direct extension	Lung, breast, esophageal, mediastinal
Venous spread	Renal (hypernephroma) most common; up to 43% of patients with this tumor have right atrial involvement;[82] adrenal, hepatoma, thyroid, lung, leiomyosarcoma
Hematogenous	Melanoma (46%), breast, lung, genitourinary tract, gastrointestinal tract
Lymphatic	Leukemia, lymphoma

Asymptomatic neoplastic tumors may also invade the left ventricular myocardium. Breast carcinoma also tends to invade the parietal and visceral pericardium, leading to effusion and constriction. Breast and lung carcinoma may also invade the main, right, or left pulmonary artery and create pulmonary arterial obstruction.

Melanoma has the highest frequency (46%) of cardiac metastases of any neoplasm and may invade any of the four chamber walls as well as epicardium and endocardium. Cardiac metastasis of melanoma is often only found incidentally. These solid intracardiac metastases are well described but most commonly are subclinical and visually described as a "charcoal heart," with tumor studding of the pericardial surface.

Leiomyosarcomas are derived from smooth muscle cells and may originate from the smooth muscle of the pulmonary veins. Radical surgical resection is the treatment of choice and is combined with adjuvant chemotherapy and radiation therapy. Prognosis is poor, with a mean survival of less than 7 months after surgery. The majority of malignant cardiac tumors occur preferentially in the right heart, except for leiomyosarcoma, which often occurs in the left atrium.

Imaging Thrombi and Emboli

TEE is highly sensitive for detecting intracardiac thrombus or embolus and superior to transthoracic echocardiography (TTE) for evaluating many patients with intracardiac masses or thrombi.[83-86] In one report

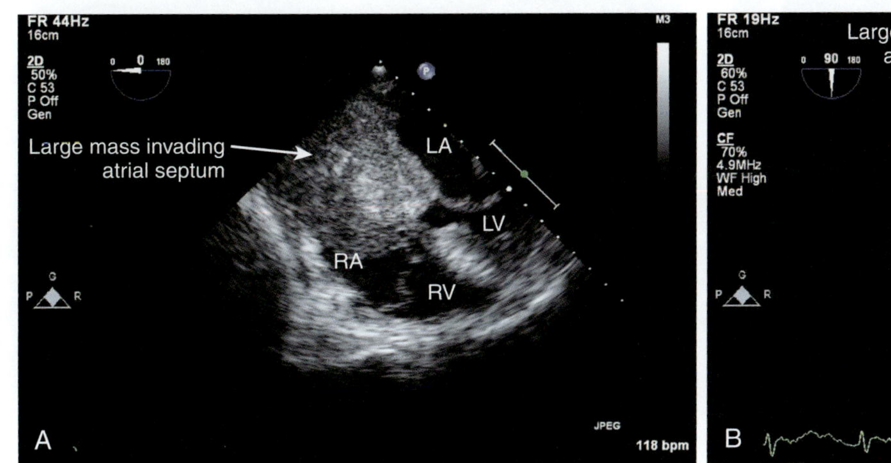

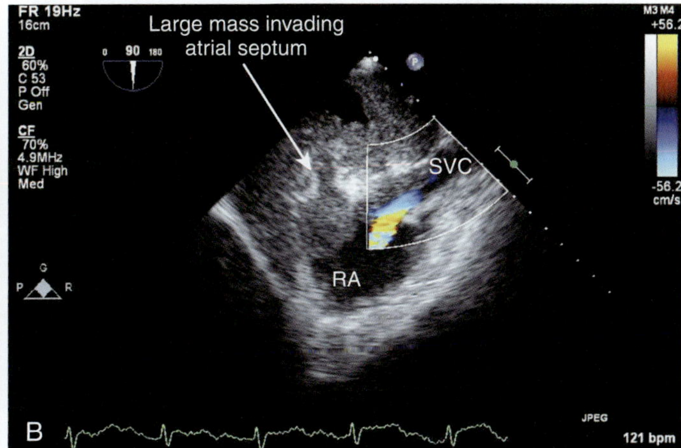

Figure 21-10 Metastatic tumor invading atrial septum. **A,** Large tumor mass nearly fills right atrium (*RA*). **B,** Color flow Doppler demonstrates flow obstruction caused by large infiltrative mass in atria. *LA,* Left atrium; *LV,* left ventricle; *RV,* right ventricle; *SVC,* superior vena cava.

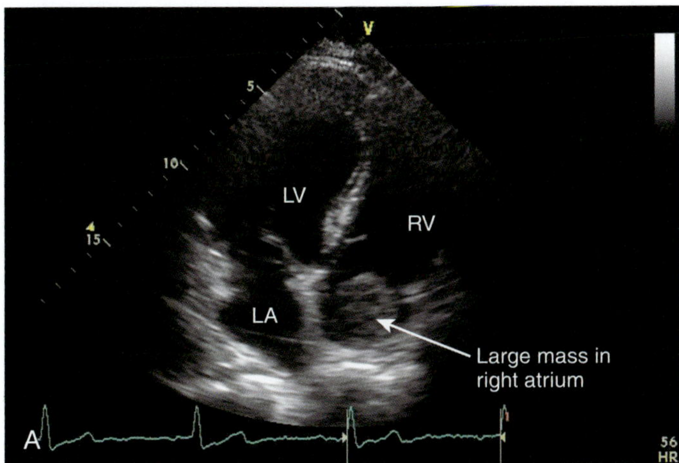

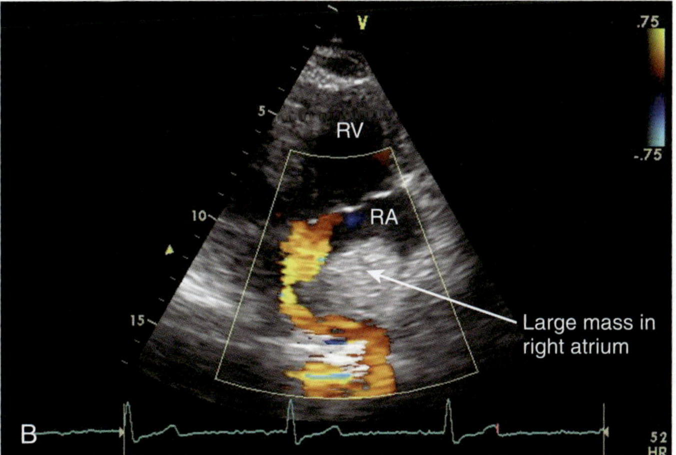

Figure 21-11 Transthoracic echocardiogram done to evaluate possible tumor extension from liver into heart. **A,** Large tumor mass nearly fills right atrium (*RA*). Imaging demonstrated mass extending from hepatic vein into inferior vena cava and into RA. **B,** Flow from RA to right ventricle (*RV*) is impeded by large tumor mass in atrium. *LA,* Left atrium; *LV,* left ventricle.

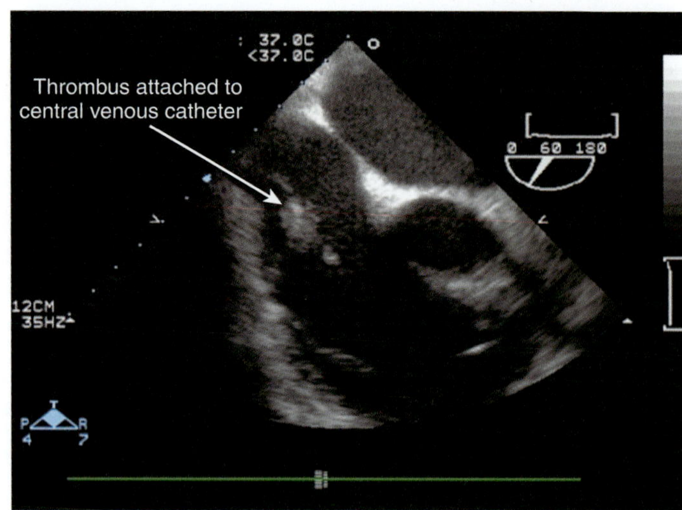

Figure 21-12 Midesophageal transesophageal view demonstrating thrombus attached to a central venous catheter in right atrium.

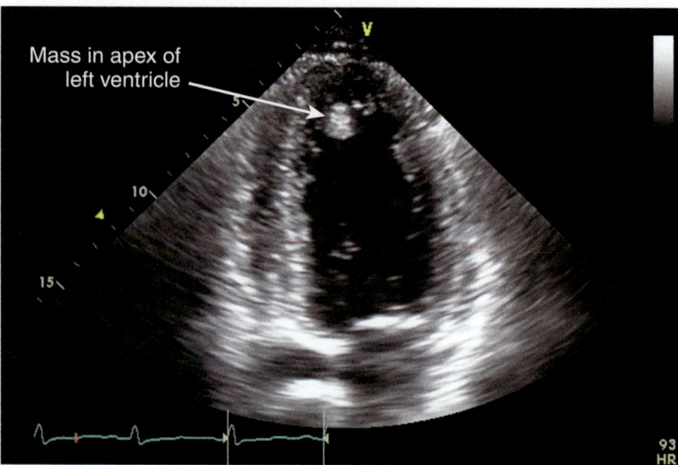

Figure 21-14 Transthoracic echocardiography often provides superior imaging of left ventricular apex. Multiple transthoracic echocardiography windows may be needed to clearly delineate size of an apical left ventricular thrombus.

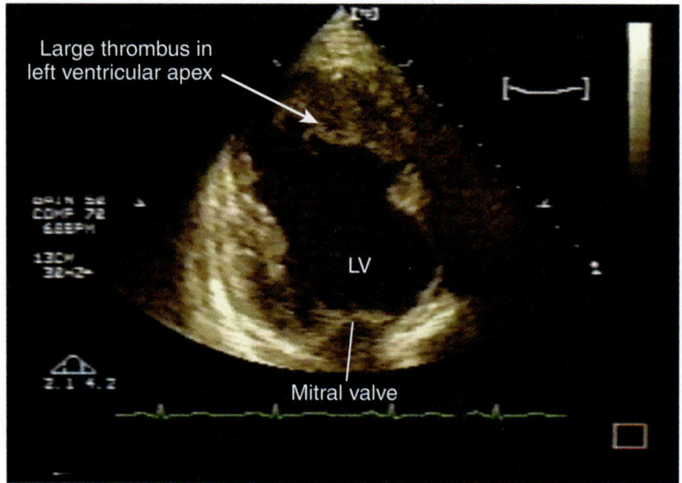

Figure 21-13 Transthoracic echocardiography often provides superior imaging of left ventricular apex. Large thrombus is seen in apex in a region of hypokinesis. Colorization may improve ability to differentiate between ventricular muscle and attached thrombus. *LV,* Left ventricle.

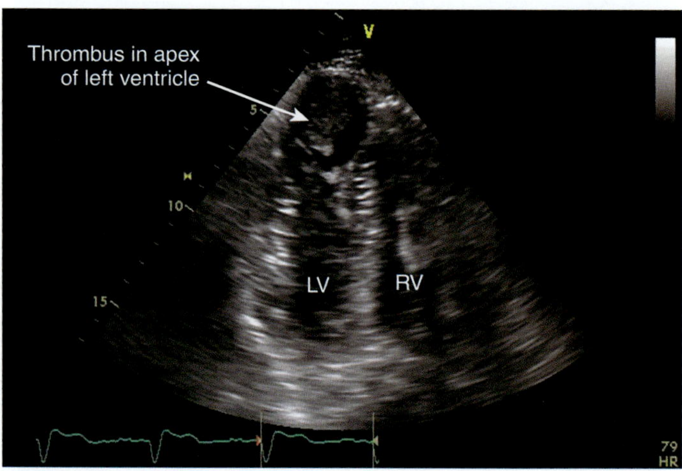

Figure 21-15 Transthoracic echocardiogram demonstrating presence of a large apical thrombus. Importance of thorough scanning is highlighted by this case, since usual mid-ventricular scan plane did not clearly demonstrate thrombus. Posterior tilt of transducer allowed visualization of large apical thrombus. *LV,* Left ventricle; *RV,* right ventricle.

of 231 patients with no preexisting indication for anticoagulation but with a recent TIA or stroke,[87] TTE and TEE were used to evaluate for a cardiac source of embolus. Over half (127) of these patients had a potential cardiac source demonstrated, but the source of embolus was demonstrated only by TEE in 90 of the 127 patients.

Thrombus can form in any cardiac chamber or vessel under certain conditions, generally associated with abnormal flow dynamics. Echocardiographic characteristics of intracardiac thrombi include distinct margins and ultrasound reflection with motion that is independent of surrounding structures and visible in more than one imaging plane.[88-91] Intracardiac thrombus is more frequently associated with abnormalities such as atrial fibrillation or flutter, mitral stenosis, and left ventricular dysfunction or acute MI. Intracardiac thrombus is also associated with foreign materials such as venous catheters (Fig. 21-12), pacemaker leads, and surgery-related materials such as patches or sutures.

Development of intraventricular thrombus is more common following acute MIs of the anterior wall (compared with other regions)[92-94] and is associated with worse outcome.[92] This appears to be true even with earlier and better percutaneous revascularization and platelet inhibitor therapy.[95,96] Thrombus in the left ventricular apex is often better seen from transthoracic imaging windows (Fig. 21-13, Video 21-8).

In the setting of thrombus formation following MI, there will be abnormal wall motion in the region underlying the thrombus (Fig. 21-14). There may be organization or calcification of a thrombus that has been present for some time following infarction (Fig. 21-15). Thrombus may also develop in aneurysmal regions of the left ventricle. Ventricular thrombus may also develop in dilated cardiomyopathy (see Chapter 18). Patients with left ventricular thrombus are at increased risk for embolic events and death.[84,92] It may be difficult to identify mural thrombus in some patients, although use of echocardiographic contrast agents is reported to improve diagnostic sensitivity.[97-100] Similarly, three-dimensional (3D) echocardiography[101-103] is reported to improve detection of mural thrombi and allow better assessment of thrombus mobility and volume. Intraoperative TEE can allow diagnosis of mural thrombi following acute MI, which may lead to important alterations of patient management.[104]

Thrombus can develop in the right atrium (Fig. 21-16) and may be associated with indwelling catheters or pacemaker leads. Left atrial thrombus is more commonly found in patients with atrial fibrillation or mitral stenosis, and less commonly in patients with mitral regurgitation. Thrombus can be difficult to differentiate from other intracardiac masses, such as myxoma,[85,105-107] or inversion of the left atrial

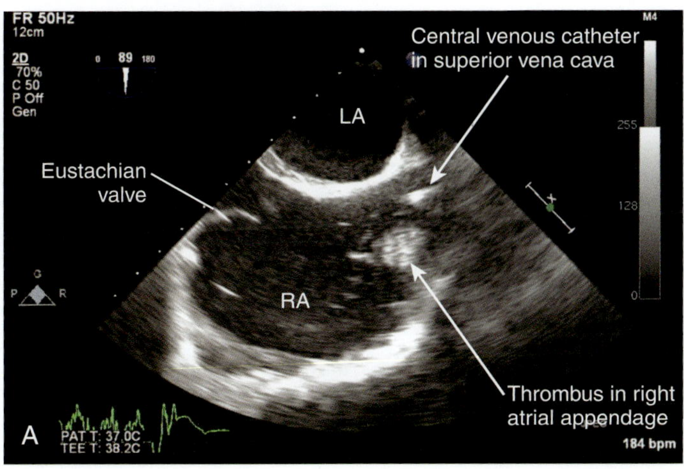

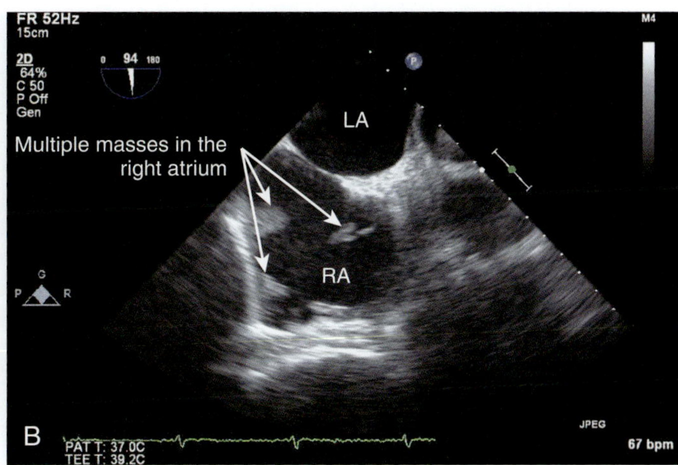

Figure 21-16 **A,** Thrombus in right atrial appendage. **B,** Multiple thrombi in right atrium *(RA). LA,* Left atrium.

appendage.[14] History of a condition known to be associated with atrial thrombi can often provide useful guidance as to the more likely type of mass present. Patients with atrial thrombi have an increased risk of embolic stroke even when treated with anticoagulants.[91,108] Thrombus may form in the left atrial appendage (Fig. 21-17) even in the absence of atrial fibrillation.[109] Use of 3D imaging may allow better delineation of thrombus size and mobility (Fig. 21-18, Video 21-9). Either the tissue separating the left upper pulmonary vein from the left atrium (see Fig. 21-2) or atrial pectinate muscles can be mistaken for atrial thrombi, as can the atrial suture line following cardiac transplantation. Imaging from several scan planes and over multiple cardiac cycles should decrease these incorrect interpretations of the echocardiogram.[90]

Spontaneous echo contrast (SEC) is visualized as swirling reflections in the cardiac chambers that are not caused by contrast agents (Fig. 21-19, Video 21-10). This imaging pattern is sometimes referred to as "smoke," since it seems to move to and fro in the currents of the atrium. Correct imaging technique is important because excessive gain can make backscatter appear similar to SEC. The severity can be graded: 0 = absent; 1 = mild (transient SEC in left atrial appendage); 2 = mild to moderate (swirling pattern in left atrial appendage); 3 = moderate (dense swirling in left atrial appendage with some swirling in the atrial cavity); 4 = severe (intense density and swirling in the left atrial appendage and left atrial chamber).[110] More simply, SEC may be graded as none, mild, or severe.[111,112] These grading systems correlate well with digital backscatter analysis. The appearance of SEC is believed to result from low-velocity blood flow in disease states such as atrial fibrillation, mitral stenosis, left atrial dilation, dilated poorly functional left ventricles, and within the false lumen of aortic dissection.[109,113] Left atrial and left atrial appendage SEC (Fig. 21-20, Video 21-11) is commonly found in patients with atrial fibrillation, even in the absence of mitral valve stenosis.[114] Conversely, SEC is uncommon in the presence of significant mitral regurgitation with the associated increase in left atrial blood flow.[113,115] The presence of SEC is associated with an increased incidence of thrombus formation[84,114] but can make the diagnosis of thrombus difficult. Evaluation of a subgroup of 744 of 1104 patients[116] with atrial fibrillation who had adequate anticoagulation for at least 3 weeks prior to study revealed mild or mild to moderate SEC in half and moderate to severe SEC in 25% prior to cardioversion. Only 5.9% of this subgroup had atrial thrombi revealed by TEE. High-grade SEC is a marker for future stroke risk but may not be a contraindication to early cardioversion if no thrombus is present.[117] On occasion, SEC will appear during the gradual return of left ventricular function with rewarming on cardiopulmonary bypass (CPB).

Embolism of blood clot, fat, marrow, amniotic fluid, and other substances can be detected by TEE. The presence of right heart thrombi is associated with an increased risk of pulmonary embolism.[118] Finding mobile thromboembolic material is not common in acute pulmonary embolism, but visualization of embolic material in the right heart is

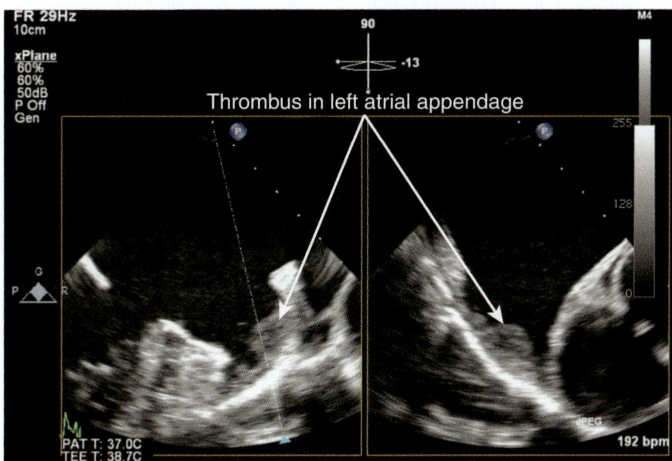

Figure 21-17 Atrial fibrillation predisposes to development of left atrial appendage thrombus, as seen here.

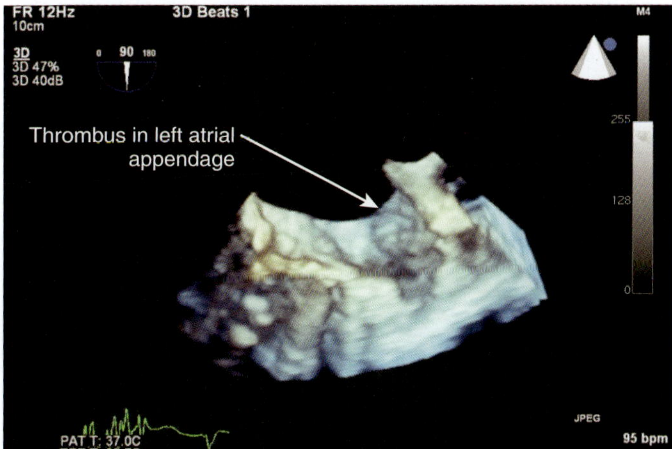

Figure 21-18 Transesophageal three-dimensional echocardiography may allow better determination of size and extent of left atrial appendage thrombus.

highly specific for pulmonary embolism (Fig. 21-21, Video 21-12). Some 4% to 12% of patients with acute pulmonary embolism have mobile right heart emboli demonstrated on baseline echocardiograms.[119,120] Patients in whom emboli are in transit are found to have greater hemodynamic instability and worse prognosis.[121-123] There

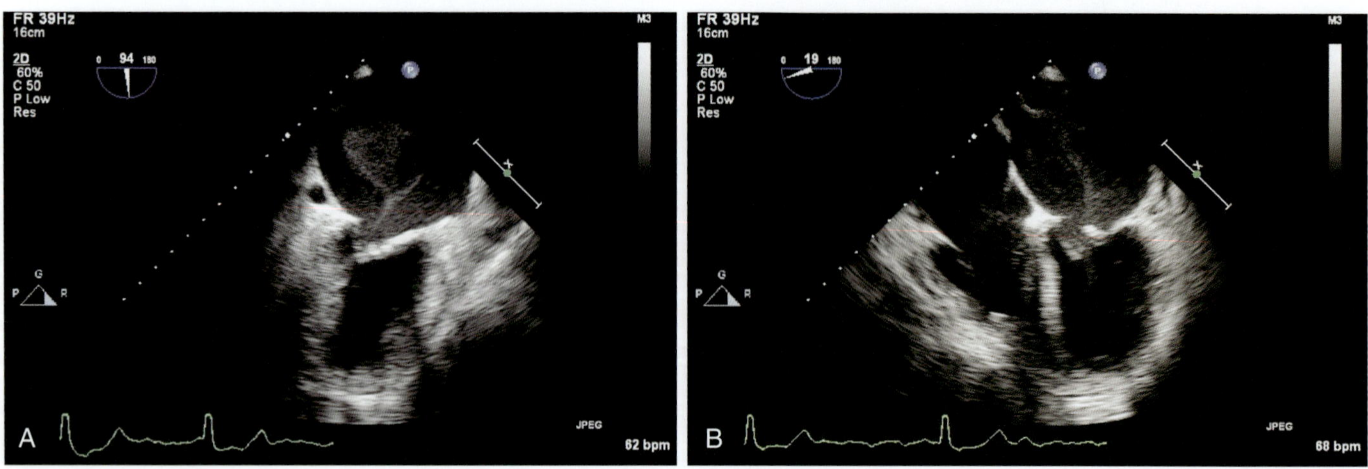

Figure 21-19 Spontaneous echo contrast (SEC) or "smoke" may be seen in areas of low blood flow velocity. SEC appears as a swirling area of reflections not caused by injected contrast agents. **A,** SEC seen in this midesophageal two-chamber view is associated with severe mitral stenosis. **B,** Appearance of spontaneous echo contrast can change over the cardiac cycle, as shown in this midesophageal four-chamber view from same patient.

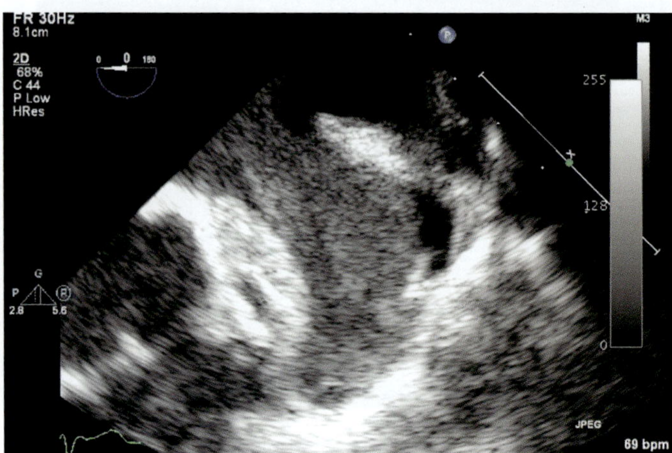

Figure 21-20 Spontaneous echo contrast (SEC) may be seen in left atrial appendage, particularly in patients with atrial fibrillation. SEC nearly fills left atrial appendage. Presence of SEC is associated with thrombus but can make diagnosis of thrombus uncertain because it may mask borders of a thrombus.

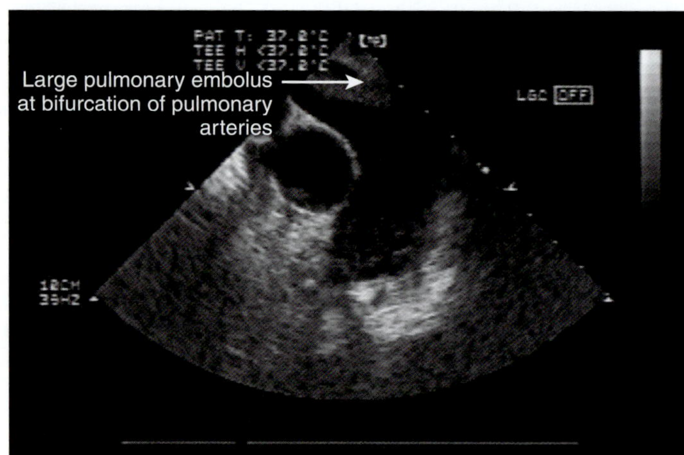

Figure 21-22 Large pulmonary embolus *(arrow)* seen at bifurcation of pulmonary artery.

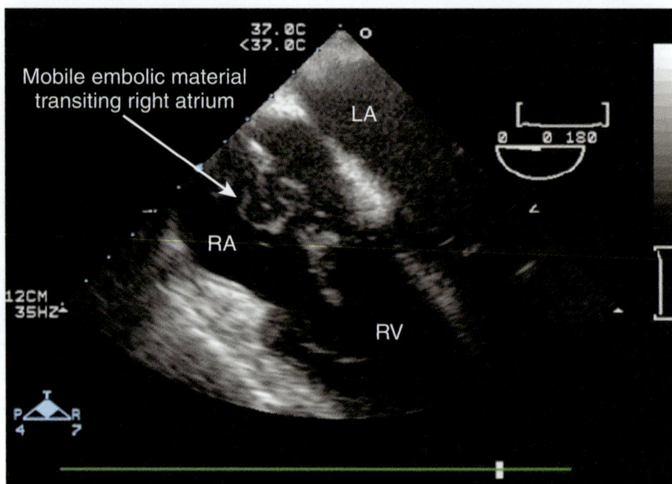

Figure 21-21 Highly mobile substances in transit may be seen during acute embolization of thrombus, tumor, fat, or other materials. Note large serpiginous collection of embolic material in right atrium *(RA)*, which later lodged in pulmonary artery. *LA,* Left atrium; *RV,* right ventricle.

are reports of echocardiographic imaging of thrombus transiting a PFO.[124] Right heart emboli of thrombus,[125-127] fat,[128,129] tumor,[130-132] cement,[133] and amniotic fluid[134] have been visualized using TEE during a variety of procedures, notably orthopedic surgery[135,136] and liver transplantation.[137] This is often in the setting of unexpected hemodynamic instability. Mobile right heart thrombi are occasionally seen in relation to central venous catheters but may be seen anywhere in the right heart or pulmonary arteries. On occasion, saddle embolism of the pulmonary artery can be visualized (Fig. 21-22). Imaging the right pulmonary artery may demonstrate the extent of large emboli (Fig. 21-23, Video 21-13). Imaging the left pulmonary artery by TEE requires additional probe manipulations because of the interposition of the left bronchus between the esophagus and left pulmonary artery.[138]

Imaging Intravascular Air

The large difference in acoustic impedance between air and blood leads to intense reflection of ultrasound and generates bright images. This property allows detection of very small quantities of air known as *microbubbles*. TEE has been reported to detect air bubbles as small as 5 μm in diameter.[139,140] These air bubbles are distinguished by their rapid movement and frequent side-lobe or ring-down acoustic artifacts. Air can be seen in the heart in quantities ranging from microbubbles to relatively large pools.[141-144] Air dissolved in intravenous (IV) fluid may

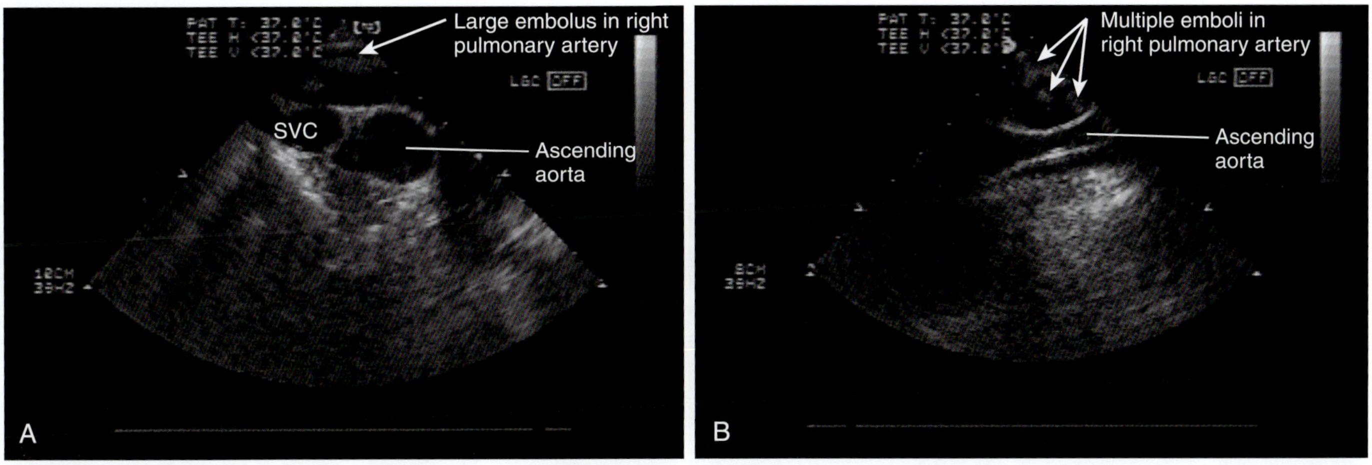

Figure 21-23 Transesophageal echocardiography can be sometimes demonstrate extensive embolization to pulmonary arteries. **A,** Large amount of embolic material is present in right pulmonary artery. **B,** Short-axis imaging of right pulmonary artery demonstrates multiple strands of embolic material in the artery. *SVC,* Superior vena cava.

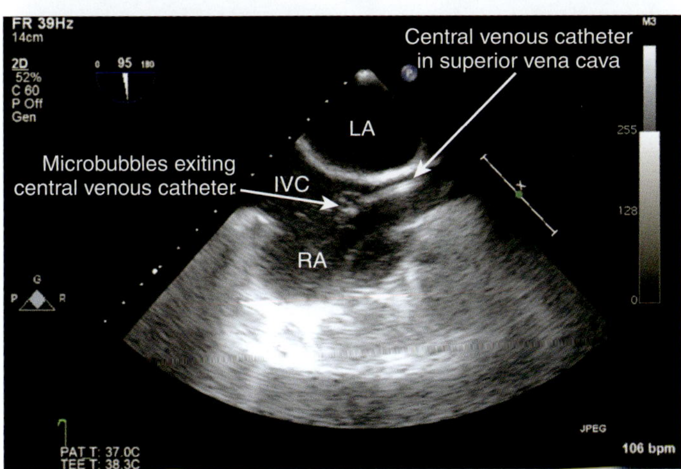

Figure 21-24 Pressurized injection of fluid through a catheter can lead to microbubble formation. Microbubbles can be seen exiting central venous catheter in right atrium *(RA)*. *IVC,* inferior vena cava; *LA,* left atrium.

be visible by echocardiography, particularly when rapid IV infusion is being administered. In some patients this presents as small numbers of microbubbles exiting the tip of a central venous catheter (Fig. 21-24, Video 21-14). Small quantities of air may be entrained from the surgical field during a variety of surgical procedures. Craniotomy in the sitting or head-elevated position poses a higher risk for this event, but venous air embolism has been detected by echocardiography in a wide range of surgical procedures.[144] During cardiac surgery, microbubbles may be seen in any cardiac chamber (Fig. 21-25, Video 21-15). The likelihood of entraining left-sided air is greater during open heart surgery through the left atrium but can occur in other settings, including isolated coronary artery bypass grafting (CABG).[145] There is conflicting evidence regarding the association between large numbers of intracardiac microbubbles and poor neurologic outcome following cardiac surgery.[142,146]

Intracardiac air may pool in the cardiac chambers. Pooled air presents as a linear undulating interface that shadows structures in the far field. Small bubbles are frequently seen bouncing off the air/blood interface of pooled air during cardiac contraction or surgical de-airing manipulation (Fig. 21-26, Video 21-16). One group has called this breaking away of small bubbles from the pool of air the "popcorn sign."[139] These pools of air can be difficult to clear using manual de-airing methods. The amount of air present can be difficult

to quantify, since the blood/air interface shadows the far-field cardiac structures. Using an in vitro model of a known cardiac size and shape, one group of investigators[147] demonstrated that the echocardiographic dimension of pooled air correlated well with the volume of air in the test chamber. This volume could easily reach 5 mL. In their model, a diameter across the air interface of 2 cm represented a pool of air larger than 1.5 mL. Application of this method to humans is limited by the inability to measure the depth of the pooled air because of acoustic shadowing induced by the air/blood interface and the lack of a known model to superimpose on the echocardiographic image to provide the depth dimension. Regardless, large-diameter intracardiac air pools present a hazard to the patient that should be addressed prior to separation from CPB.

The location of air in the heart depends on the rate of entry, surgical intervention being performed, and position of the heart chambers relative to gravity. Open cardiac procedures to repair defects, resect masses, or repair or replace valves are more frequently associated with intracardiac air than CABG. However, reports of intraventricular air during coronary grafting have been published. Further, intracardiac air has been reported during minimally invasive surgery[148] and off-pump CABG.[149] The critical times for appearance of intracardiac microbubbles are at the time of aortic cross-clamp release and during return of circulation through the pulmonary vasculature. The pulmonary veins are a frequent repository of air in procedures involving left atriotomy. Pooling of air in the pulmonary veins has been known to be a source of intracardiac air for years, but other areas of the heart may also collect air during bypass. Intracardiac air is more frequently found in some areas of the heart and great vessels than others (Table 21-4).

Echocardiography has been used to guide removal of air from the heart during surgery, using maneuvers ranging from manual compression to transmural needle aspiration.[150]

The amount of intracardiac air seen during TEE was reported to be greater in patients who develop new regional wall motion abnormalities after separation from CPB.[148] This results from air embolism to the coronary arteries, with entry into the right coronary artery more frequent because of the more superior (gravitationally) position of the right coronary orifice.[139,148] Intramyocardial contrast may be noted as an area of brightness in the distribution of the affected coronary artery.[151-154] This is usually associated with ST-segment abnormalities and is often transient if blood pressure can be supported until resolution can occur.[148,152,154] The associated wall motion abnormalities can be severe and may require inotropic drug administration, return to CPB, or other mechanical circulatory support (Fig. 21-27, Video 21-17). Scoring systems for quantifying the severity of intracardiac air based on the number or extent of microbubbles visualized in the heart have been proposed (Table 21-5).

Ultrasound imaging is very sensitive to small air bubbles, with a reported ability to detect bubbles as small as 5 μm. Microbubbles of this size can be produced by agitating saline. The injection of agitated saline provides a readily available contrast agent for imaging right-sided structures. Larger intravenously injected microbubbles created during agitation of saline are filtered out by the lung vasculature. Most of the smaller bubbles appear to collapse as a result of surface tension,[140] although a small number may appear in the left atrium. Commercially prepared contrast agents are available that contain bubbles (of air or other gases) in shells that are resistant to collapse from surface tension and can thereby transit the pulmonary vasculature and be used for left-sided contrast. Since the time course for collapse of microbubbles

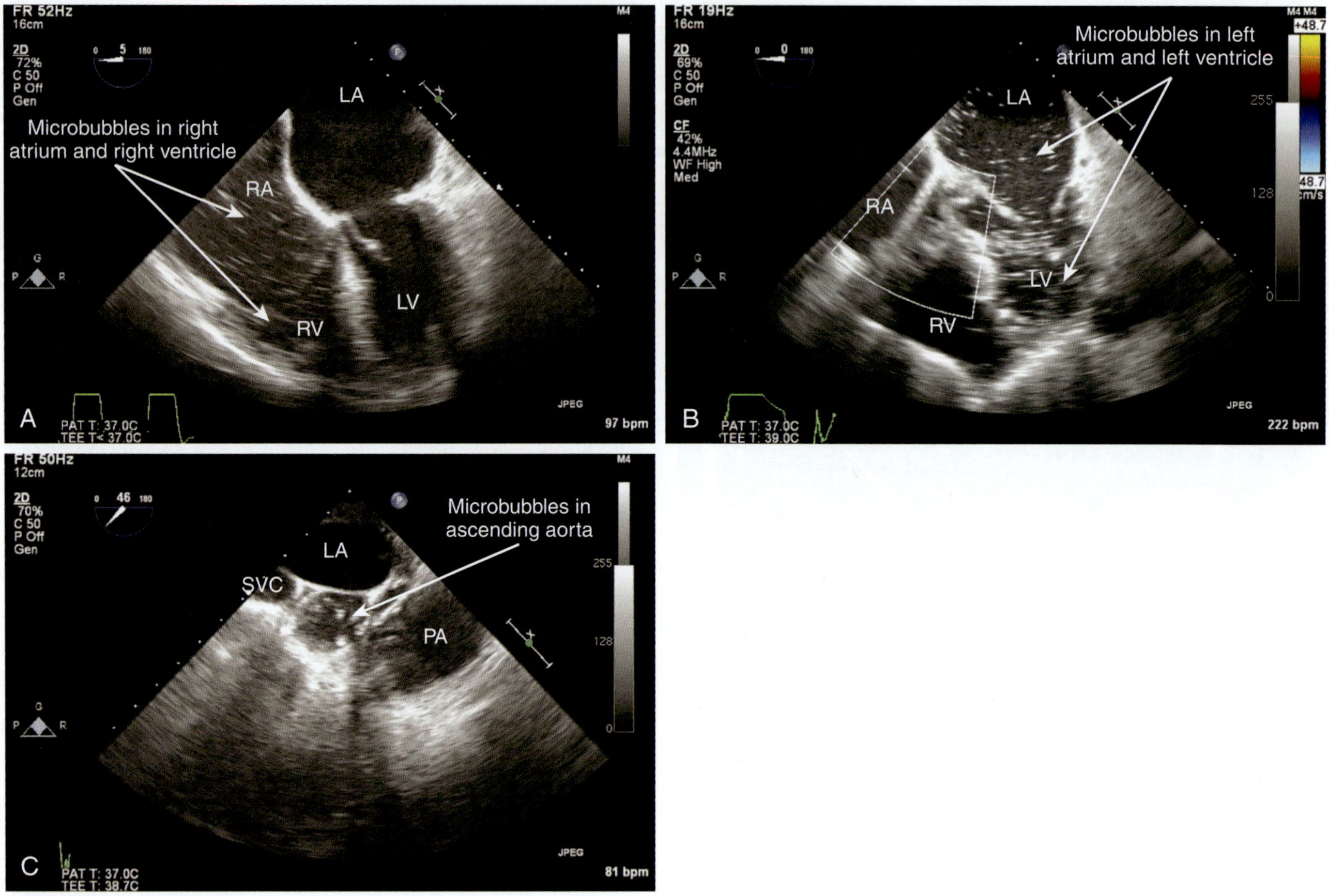

Figure 21-25   Microbubbles may be present in any cardiac chamber following open heart surgery. **A,** Moderate amounts of microbubbles in right atrium *(RA)* and right ventricle *(RV).* **B,** Microbubbles in left atrium *(LA)*, left ventricle *(LV)*, and aorta. **C,** Numerous microbubbles in ascending aorta. *SVC,* Superior vena cava.

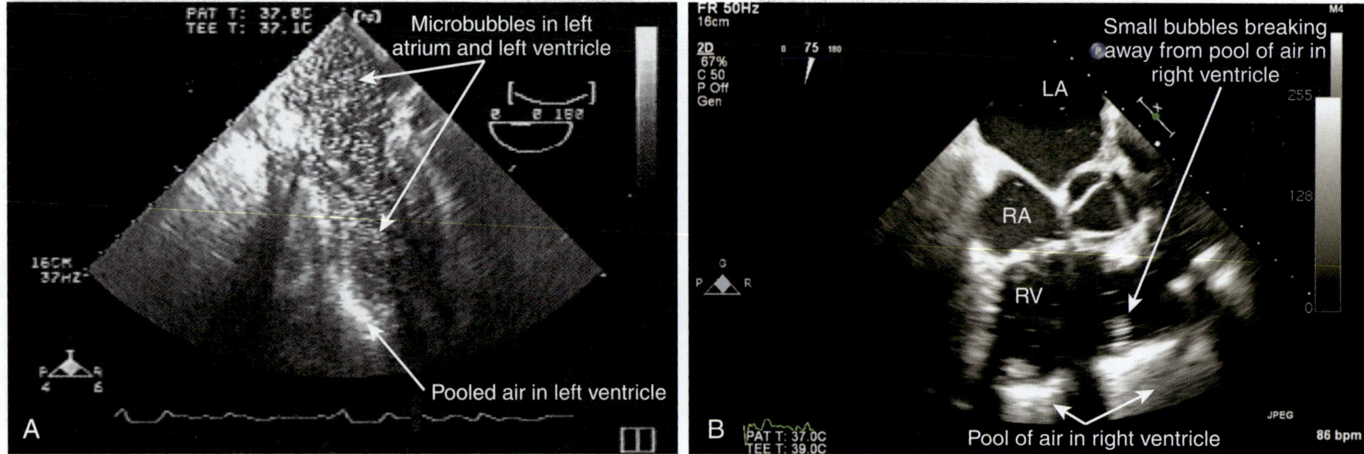

Figure 21-26   Air may pool in any cardiac chamber. A pool of air will have a bright undulating surface that shadows structures beyond the blood/air interface. **A,** Large quantity of intracardiac air in left atrium *(LA)* and left ventricle *(LV).* Note air pool in LV, from which bubbles can be seen to break away during cardiac cycle. **B,** Large pool of air is present in right ventricle *(RV)*, shadowing structures beyond blood/air interface. Small groups of air bubbles may break away from pool of air during cardiac cycle.

in agitated saline is shorter than the normal pulmonary blood transit time, microbubbles may be used as a contrast agent for detection of right-to-left shunts. A method to prepare agitated saline contrast has been described by a number of investigators.[158-161] A syringe containing 9 mL of saline is connected through a 3-way stopcock to a syringe containing 1 mL of air. Use of a small quantity of blood or colloid has

been proposed to increase the microbubbles generated. The contents are mixed by vigorously injecting the contents between the syringes until the saline appears cloudy or milky, which may take 5 to 20 forceful injections from syringe to syringe. This contrast should be injected into a free-flowing IV infusion catheter soon after preparation via the stopcock. An adequate contrast injection should completely opacify the right atrium after appropriate transit time from the injection site, which will be shorter if a central venous catheter is used for the injection rather than a peripheral IV. Applications of saline contrast injection include the diagnosis of PFO, pulmonary arteriovenous malformation (AVM) and persistent left SVC.

PFO is reported in 25% of the population in autopsy series. A similar prevalence is reported in echocardiographic investigations of patients without stroke,[162-164] with a greater prevalence in series of patients being evaluated specifically for this condition.[160,161,165] Right-to-left shunt across a PFO may occur when right atrial pressure exceeds left atrial pressure. Injection of agitated saline contrast can be used to establish the presence of this shunt flow. Adequate technique is essential to conclusively rule out PFO.[158-161] The sensitivity of saline contrast echocardiography in the presence of PFO may be increased by fluid loading[162] or making repeated injections.[166] The balance of right-to-left atrial pressure can be altered by several clinical maneuvers. In an awake patient, the Valsalva maneuver and coughing are reported to improve sensitivity of saline contrast echocardiography for detecting PFO.[160,161,167] A strong Valsalva maneuver will be accompanied by shift of the atrial septum to the left during the release

TABLE 21-4	Common Locations of Intracardiac Air	
Study	*Surgical Setting*	*Location of Air (Most to Least Frequent Site in This Report)*
Orihashi 1993[139]	Open heart surgery	Right upper pulmonary vein Left ventricle Left atrium Right sinus of Valsalva Pulmonary artery Left atrial appendage Left upper pulmonary vein
Hoka 1997[150]	Open heart surgery	Left atrium Ventricle Aortic root
Secknus 1999[148]	Minimally invasive valve surgery	Left ventricular apex Anterior left atrium Upper pulmonary veins
Svenarud 2004[151]	Single valve surgery	Left atrium Left ventricle Aorta

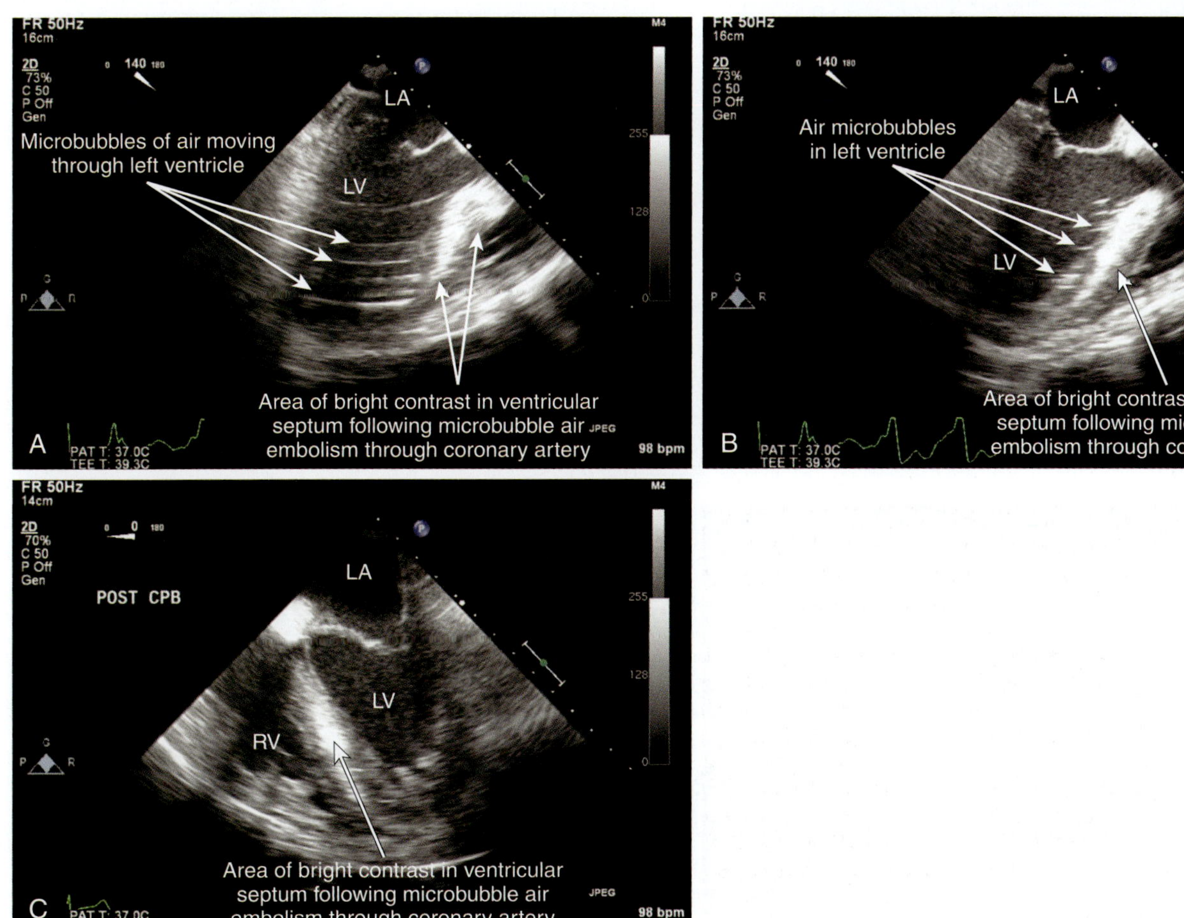

Figure 21-27 Air microbubbles can embolize through coronary arteries or bypass grafts. Bright areas of intramyocardial contrast will be seen following this. **A,** Air microbubbles are seen moving through left ventricle *(LV)*. Streaks of bright contrast are an imaging artifact generated by the moving microbubbles. **B,** Air embolization through coronary artery or graft resulted in an area of bright contrast in ventricular septum, abnormal electrocardiogram, and need for pressure support. **C,** Area of bright intramyocardial contrast is present but diminishing following clinical improvement and separation from cardiopulmonary bypass. *LA,* Left atrium; *RV,* right ventricle.

phase,[158,167] at which point right atrial pressure is higher than left, and PFO flow may be seen as microbubbles crossing the atrial septum or in the left atrium. In mechanically ventilated patients, this effect can be produced during the release phase of positive end-expiratory pressure (PEEP), sigh, or inspiratory hold.[163,168-170] Variable diagnostic criteria relating the number of microbubbles seen in the left atrium to the presence of PFO have been used. Since larger bubbles are filtered by the lungs, the appearance of any microbubbles in the left atrium early after opacification of the right atrium (within 3 to 5 beats) indicates right-to-left flow at the atrial level (Fig. 21-28, Video 21-18).[167] Delayed appearance of microbubbles (5 or more beats after right atrial opacification) is consistent with pulmonary AVM. However, various investigators have suggested using larger numbers of microbubbles in the left atrium to establish the diagnosis of PFO. Early appearance of microbubbles traveling through pulmonary AVMs to the left atrium can occur in some clinical settings.[171] Similarly, the amount of flow through the PFO has been graded differently by various investigators.[161] The appearance of echo contrast in the left atrium from pooled blood exiting the pulmonary veins on release of Valsalva or ventilator pressure should be distinguished from saline contrast microbubbles. The best management for an incidentally found PFO in a patient with no symptoms suggestive of shunt or paradoxical embolism is a matter of discussion. While some suggest closure of the PFO in settings where postoperative right-to-left shunt is likely[172-174] (e.g., cardiac transplant or placement of left ventricular assist devices), others suggest there is little evidence to support a benefit from PFO closure in the absence of preoperative symptoms.[175,176]

Since the direction of shunt is pressure dependent, some patients with PFO will have predominant left-to-right flow. This is particularly true in patients with chronic elevation of left atrial pressure, as may occur in mitral stenosis or left ventricular failure. The reported prevalence of positive contrast studies demonstrating PFO is lower in this subset of patients. In the setting of elevated left atrial pressure, an area of negative contrast in the otherwise opacified right atrium during an agitated saline contrast study may appear.[177] Because an injection of agitated saline may not demonstrate an existing PFO, several factors should be considered before asserting the contrast study was negative for shunt (Table 21-6).

TABLE 21-6	Potential Causes of False-Negative Contrast Studies in Patent Foramen Ovale Patients
Potential Cause of False-Negative Contrast Study	*Considerations*
Inadequate right atrial opacification	Repeated injections may increase diagnostic yield.
	Consider adding 1 mL blood or colloid to agitated saline contrast to improve echogenicity.
	Prominent eustachian valve may direct contrast into right ventricle; consider injection via lower extremity vein.
Elevated left atrial pressure	Review patient history for conditions associated with elevated left atrial pressure (e.g., mitral stenosis, left ventricular dysfunction).
	Evaluate image for evidence of negative contrast area in opacified right atrium, which may represent left-to-right shunt across PFO.
Inadequate increase of right atrial pressure	Awake patient: coach and practice Valsalva maneuver prior to contrast injection.
	Cough following release phase of Valsalva maneuver may increase diagnostic yield.
	Intubated patient: adequate PEEP or inspiratory hold should decrease right atrial area; atrial septum should shift toward left atrium during release of inspiratory pressure.
	Timing: release phase should start with complete right atrial opacification by agitated saline contrast.

PEEP, Positive end-expiratory pressure; *PFO,* patent foramen ovale.

TABLE 21-5	Grading of Intracardiac Air
Authors	*Scoring*
Rodigas 1982[142,155] Topol 1985[142]	0: No microbubbles seen 1: <5 per frame 2: 10-20 per frame 3: Many
Tingleff 1995[145]	0: None 1: Bubbles "do not dominate" image 2: Bubbles "dominate" image
Secknus 1999[148]	Mild: <3 bubbles per frame Moderate: >3 bubbles per frame but no chamber opacification Severe: >30 bubbles per frame OR chamber opacification
Al-Rashidi 2009,[156] 2011[157]	0: No air 1: Air in left atrium in single cardiac cycle 2: Air in left atrium and left ventricle in single cardiac cycle 3: Air in left atrium, left ventricle, and aorta in single cardiac cycle

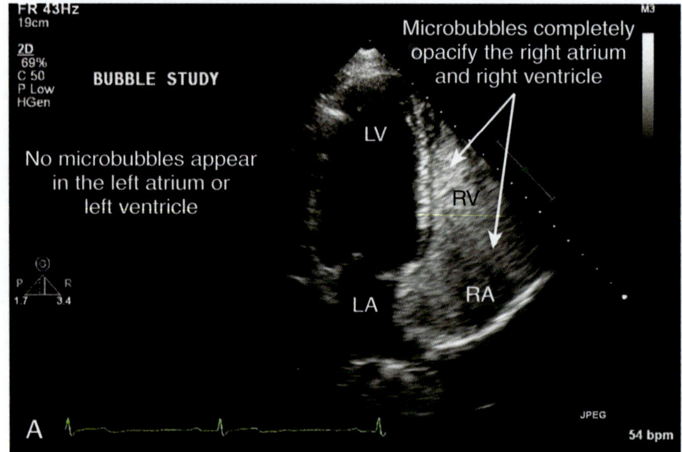

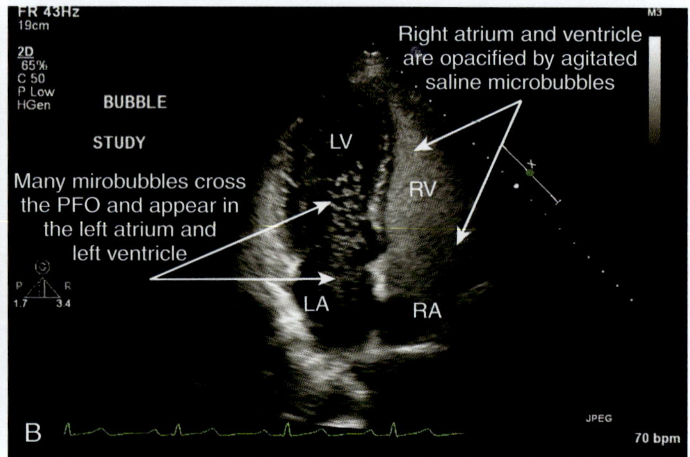

Figure 21-28 Injection of agitated saline allows use of microbubbles as a contrast agent. **A,** Transthoracic echocardiogram demonstrates a negative patent foramen ovale *(PFO)* study, since no microbubbles cross atrial septum when right atrial pressure is greater than left atrial pressure. **B,** Transthoracic echocardiogram demonstrates a positive PFO study because microbubbles cross atrial septum within first 3 beats after complete opacification of right atrium *(RA)*. *LA,* Left atrium; *LV,* left ventricle; *RV,* right ventricle.

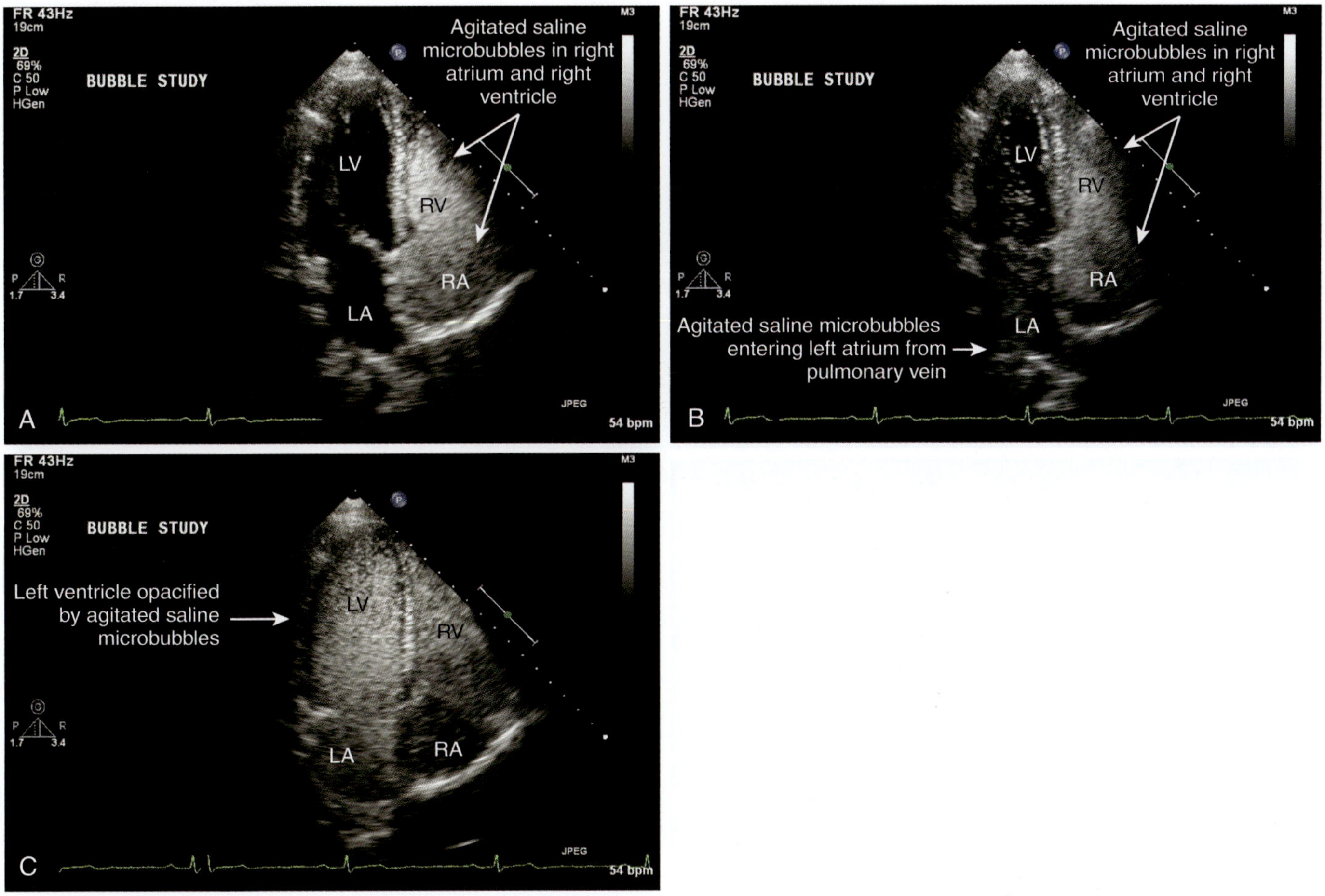

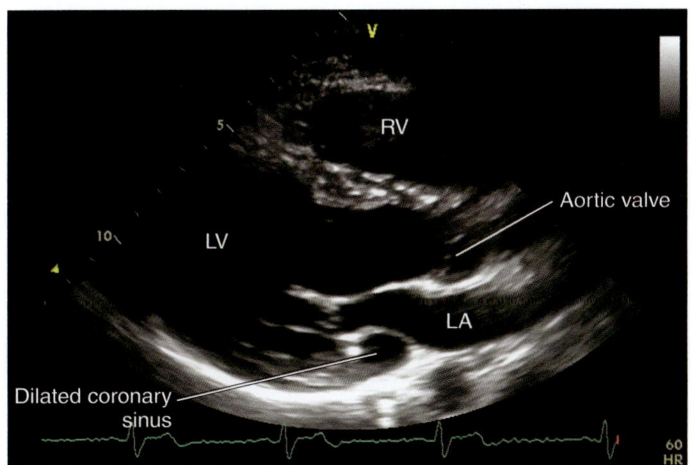

Figure 21-29 Agitated saline contrast injection shows appearance of microbubbles in left atrium (*LA*) several beats after opacification of right atrium (*RA*). **A,** Complete opacification of RA and right ventricle (*RV*), with no microbubbles crossing atrial septum. **B,** Microbubbles are seen entering LA several beats after complete opacification of RA. **C,** Flow through pulmonary arteriovenous malformation is so large, sufficient agitated saline microbubbles transit lungs to completely opacify LA and left ventricle (*LV*).

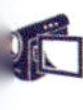

Figure 21-30 Transthoracic echocardiogram demonstrates a dilated coronary sinus. *LA,* Left atrium; *LV,* left ventricle; *RV,* right ventricle.

As discussed, the time course of appearance of microbubbles in the left atrium after injection into a systemic vein has been used as a marker for the presence of pulmonary AVM. Opacification of the left atrium 5 beats after appearance of contrast in the right atrium suggests pulmonary AVM (Fig. 21-29, Video 21-19). Of note, higher-grade pulmonary AVMs have been associated with more rapid appearance of microbubbles in the left atrium as early as 3 beats after opacification of the right atrium.[171,178] Imaging may allow demonstration of microbubbles entering the left atrium from the pulmonary veins, further establishing the diagnosis of pulmonary AVM.[179-183] TEE can provide a sensitive means of evaluating pulmonary vein inflow to the left atrium during agitated saline contrast studies. Transthoracic saline contrast echocardiography has a high sensitivity (97%) and negative predictive value (99%) when used as a screening method for pulmonary AVM.[184,185]

Persistent left SVC may be suspected when a large coronary sinus is visualized by echocardiography (Fig. 21-30). The coronary sinus can also enlarge in patients with chronic elevation of right atrial pressure, as may accompany tricuspid regurgitation or pulmonary hypertension.[186] The presence of a persistent left SVC can be confirmed by injection of agitated saline into a vein in the left arm. In normal anatomy, this injection will result in microbubbles appearing in the right atrium prior to appearing near or in the coronary sinus. In the presence of a persistent left SVC, agitated saline contrast will be visualized entering the coronary sinus before appearing in the right atrium (Fig. 21-31, Video 21-20).

Summary

A careful clinical history followed by a comprehensive echocardiographic examination will facilitate accurate identification of the general classification of masses in the heart, whether solid or gaseous. A thorough knowledge of the physics of imaging solid and gaseous materials and of the pathologies that affect the heart will guide the echocardiographer in diagnostic efforts.

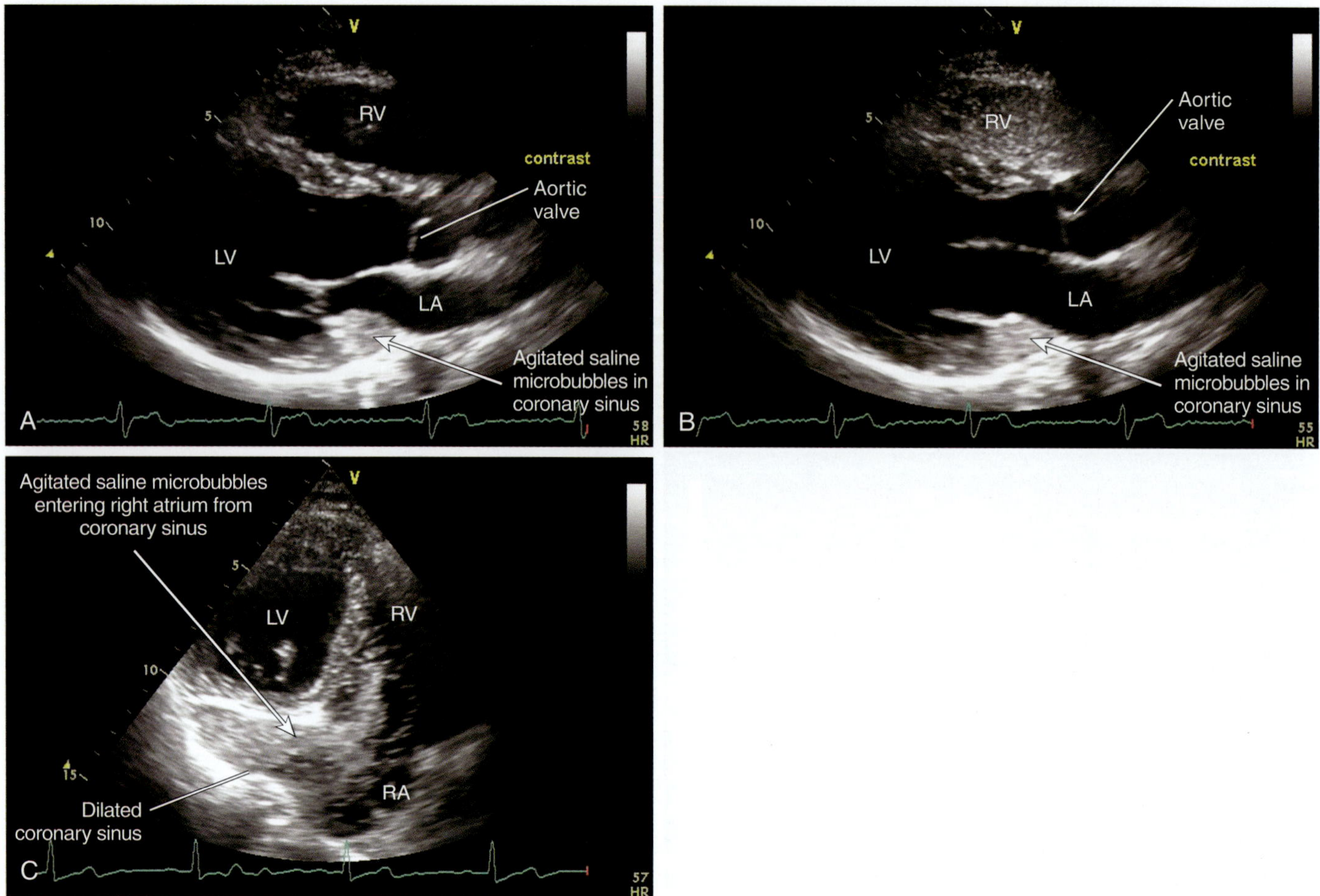

Figure 21-31   Agitated saline contrast injected into a left arm vein to demonstrate presence of a persistent left superior vena cava (SVC). **A,** Agitated saline microbubbles appear in coronary sinus before right atrium (*RA*). **B,** Agitated saline microbubbles appear in the right heart after appearing in coronary sinus. In this patient, sufficient flow is present to opacify right ventricle (*RV*). **C,** Entry of agitated saline microbubbles from coronary sinus to RA following injection of agitated saline into a left arm vein confirms presence of a persistent left SVC. *LA,* Left atrium; *LV,* left ventricle

REFERENCES

1. Pharr JR, West MB, Kusumoto FM, et al. Prominent crista terminalis appearing as a right atrial mass on transthoracic echocardiogram. *J Am Soc Echocardiogr.* 2002;15:753-755.
2. Loukas M, Klaassen Z, Tubbs RS, et al. Anatomical observations of the moderator band. *Clin Anat.* 2010;23:443-450.
3. Durant W. *Heroes of History: A Brief History of Civilization from Ancient Times to the Dawn of the Modern Age*New York: Simon & Schuster; 2001, page 211.
4. Goforth J. Unique heart anomaly: free fibrous cord passing through three heart chambers to the aorta. *JAMA.* 1926;86(21):1612-1613:2.
5. Ward RP, Weinert L, Spencer KT, et al. Quantitative diagnosis of apical cardiomyopathy using contrast echocardiography. *J Am Soc Echocardiogr.* 2002;15:316-322.
6. Agmon Y, Connolly HM, Olson LJ, et al. Noncompaction of the ventricular myocardium. *J Am Soc Echocardiogr.* 1999;12:859-863.
7. Tamborini G, Pepi M, Celeste F, et al. Incidence and characteristics of left ventricular false tendons and trabeculations in the normal and pathologic heart by second harmonic echocardiography. *J Am Soc Echocardiogr.* 2004;17:367-374.
8. Malaterre HR, Cohen F, Kallee K, et al. Giant interatrial septal aneurysm mimicking a right atrial tumor. *Int J Card Imaging.* 1998;14:163-166.
9. Mugge A, Daniel WG, Angermann C, et al. Atrial septal aneurysm in adult patients. A multicenter study using transthoracic and transesophageal echocardiography. *Circulation.* 1995;91:2785-2792.
10. Malaterre HR, Kallee K, Deharo JC, et al. Right- and left-sided interatrial septal aneurysm mimicking atrial tumor and stroke. *J Am Soc Echocardiogr.* 1998;11:829-831.
11. Shirani J, Roberts WC. Clinical, electrocardiographic and morphologic features of massive fatty deposits ("lipomatous hypertrophy") in the atrial septum. *J Am Coll Cardiol.* 1993;22:226-238.
12. O'Connor S, Recavarren R, Nichols LC, et al. Lipomatous hypertrophy of the interatrial septum: an overview. *Arch Pathol Lab Med.* 2006;130:397-399.
13. Minich LL, Hawkins JA, Tani LY, et al. Inverted left atrial appendage presenting as an unusual left atrial mass. *J Am Soc Echocardiogr.* 1995;8:328-330.
14. Aronson S, Ruo W, Sand M. Inverted left atrial appendage appearing as a left atrial mass with transesophageal echocardiography during cardiac surgery. *Anesthesiology.* 1992;76:1054-1055.
15. Roberts WC. Primary and secondary neoplasms of the heart. *Am J Cardiol.* 1997;80:671-682.
16. Trocciola SM, Yee H, Balsam LB, et al. Cardiac varix presenting as a right atrial mass. *J Card Surg.* 2011;26:164-165.
17. Okamoto Y, Matsumoto M, Inoue H. Varix of the heart. *Circ Cardiovasc Imaging.* 2009;2:e22-e24.
18. Harrity PJ, Tazelaar HD, Edwards WD, et al. Intracardiac varices of the right atrium: a case report and review of the literature. *Int J Cardiol.* 1995;48:177-181.
19. Jaroszewski DE, Warsame TA, Chandrasekaran K, et al. Right ventricular compression observed in echocardiography from pectus excavatum deformity. *J Cardiovasc Ultrasound.* 2011;19:192-195.
20. Chan J, Manning WJ, Appelbaum E, et al. Large hiatal hernia mimicking left atrial mass: a multimodality diagnosis. *J Am Coll Cardiol.* 2009;54:569.
21. Percy RF, Conetta DA, Miller AB. Esophageal compression of the heart presenting as an extracardiac mass on echocardiography. *Chest.* 1984;85:826-828.
22. Frans EE, Nanda NC, Patel V, et al. Transesophageal two-dimensional echocardiographic identification of hiatal hernia. *Echocardiography.* 2005;22:533-535.
23. Peters PJ, Reinhardt S. The echocardiographic evaluation of intracardiac masses: a review. *J Am Soc Echocardiogr.* 2006;19:230-240.
24. Bruce CJ. Cardiac tumours: diagnosis and management. *Heart.* 2011;97:151-160.
25. Shapiro LM. Cardiac tumours: diagnosis and management. *Heart.* 2001;85:218-222.
26. Lam KY, Dickens P, Chan AC. Tumors of the heart. A 20-year experience with a review of 12,485 consecutive autopsies. *Arch Pathol Lab Med.* 1993;117:1027-1031.
27. Reynen K. Frequency of primary tumors of the heart. *Am J Cardiol.* 1996;77:107.
28. Mukai K, Shinkai T, Tominaga K, et al. The incidence of secondary tumors of the heart and pericardium: a 10-year study. *Jpn J Clin Oncol.* 1988;18:195-201.
29. Maraj S, Pressman GS, Figueredo VM. Primary cardiac tumors. *Int J Cardiol.* 2009;133:152-156.
30. Elbardissi AW, Dearani JA, Daly RC, et al. Survival after resection of primary cardiac tumors: a 48-year experience. *Circulation.* 2008;118:S7-15.
31. Chan HS, Sonley MJ, Moes CA, et al. Primary and secondary tumors of childhood involving the heart, pericardium, and great vessels. A report of 75 cases and review of the literature. *Cancer.* 1985;56:825-836.
32. Cina SJ, Smialek JE, Burke AP, et al. Primary cardiac tumors causing sudden death: a review of the literature. *Am J Forensic Med Pathol.* 1996;17:271-281.
33. Simpson L, Kumar SK, Okuno SH, et al. Malignant primary cardiac tumors: review of a single institution experience. *Cancer.* 2008;112:2440-2446.
34. Barnes ARBD, Snell AM. Primary sarcoma of the heart: Report of a case with electrocardiographic and pathological studies. *Am Heart J.* 1934;9:12.
35. McAllister HAFJ. *Tumors of the cardiovascular system: Armed Forces Institute of Pathology*; 1978.
36. Malekzadeh S, Roberts WC. Growth rate of left atrial myxoma. *Am J Cardiol.* 1989;64:1075-1076.
37. Keeling IM, Oberwalder P, Anelli-Monti M, et al. Cardiac myxomas: 24 years of experience in 49 patients. *Eur J Cardiothorac Surg.* 2002;22:971-977.
38. Burke A, Virmani R. More on cardiac myxomas. *N Engl J Med.* 1996;335:1462-1463; author reply 3-4.
39. Markel ML, Waller BF, Armstrong WF. Cardiac myxoma. A review. *Medicine (Baltimore).* 1987;66:114-125.
40. St John Sutton MG, Mercier LA, Giuliani ER, et al. Atrial myxomas: a review of clinical experience in 40 patients. *Mayo Clin Proc.* 1980;55:371-376.

41. Ferrans VJ, Roberts WC. Structural features of cardiac myxomas. Histology, histochemistry, and electron microscopy. *Hum Pathol.* 1973;4:111-146.
42. Goldberg HP, Glenn F, Dotter CT, et al. Myxoma of the left atrium; diagnosis made during life with operative and post-mortem findings. *Circulation.* 1952;6:762-767.
43. Pinede L, Duhaut P, Loire R. Clinical presentation of left atrial cardiac myxoma. A series of 112 consecutive cases. *Medicine (Baltimore).* 2001;80:159-172.
44. Carney JA. Differences between nonfamilial and familial cardiac myxoma. *Am J Surg Pathol.* 1985;9:53-55.
45. van Gelder HM, O'Brien DJ, Staples ED, et al. Familial cardiac myxoma. *Ann Thorac Surg.* 1992;53:419-424.
46. Boikos SA, Stratakis CA. Carney complex: the first 20 years. *Curr Opin Oncol.* 2007;19:24-29.
47. Carney JA, Gordon H, Carpenter PC, et al. The complex of myxomas, spotty pigmentation, and endocrine overactivity. *Medicine (Baltimore).* 1985;64:270-283.
48. Mahilmaran A, Seshadri M, Nayar PG, et al. Familial cardiac myxoma: Carney's complex. *Tex Heart Inst J.* 2003;30:80-82.
49. Stratakis CA. Clinical genetics of multiple endocrine neoplasias, Carney complex and related syndromes. *J Endocrinol Invest.* 2001;24:370-383.
50. Stratakis CA, Kirschner LS, Carney JA. Clinical and molecular features of the Carney complex: diagnostic criteria and recommendations for patient evaluation. *J Clin Endocrinol Metab.* 2001;86:4041-4046.
51. Almeida MQ, Stratakis CA. Carney complex and other conditions associated with micronodular adrenal hyperplasias. *Best Pract Res Clin Endocrinol Metab.* 2010;24:907-914.
52. Rothenbuhler A, Stratakis CA. Clinical and molecular genetics of Carney complex. *Best Pract Res Clin Endocrinol Metab.* 2010;24:389-399.
53. Shetty Roy AN, Radin M, Sarabi D, et al. Familial recurrent atrial myxoma: Carney's complex. *Clin Cardiol.* 2011;34:83-86.
54. Pan L, Peng L, Jean-Gilles J, et al. Novel PRKAR1A gene mutations in Carney Complex. *Int J Clin Exp Pathol.* 2010;3:545-548.
55. Klarich KW, Enriquez-Sarano M, Gura GM, et al. Papillary fibroelastoma: echocardiographic characteristics for diagnosis and pathologic correlation. *J Am Coll Cardiol.* 1997;30:784-790.
56. Gowda RM, Khan IA, Nair CK, et al. Cardiac papillary fibroelastoma: a comprehensive analysis of 725 cases. *Am Heart J.* 2003;146:404-410.
57. Topol EJ, Biern RO, Reitz BA. Cardiac papillary fibroelastoma and stroke. Echocardiographic diagnosis and guide to excision. *Am J Med.* 1986;80:129-132.
58. Waltenberger J, Thelin S. Images in cardiovascular medicine. Papillary fibroelastoma as an unusual source of repeated pulmonary embolism. *Circulation.* 1994;89:2433.
59. Zamora RL, Adelberg DA, Berger AS, et al. Branch retinal artery occlusion caused by a mitral valve papillary fibroelastoma. *Am J Ophthalmol.* 1995;119:325-329.
60. Sun JP, Asher CR, Yang XS, et al. Clinical and echocardiographic characteristics of papillary fibroelastomas: a retrospective and prospective study in 162 patients. *Circulation.* 2001;103:2687-2693.
61. Gegouskov V, Kadner A, Engelberger L, et al. Papillary fibroelastoma of the heart. *Heart Surg Forum.* 2008;11:E333-E339.
62. Saloura V, Grivas PD, Sarwar AB, et al. Papillary fibroelastomas: innocent bystanders or ignored culprits? *Postgrad Med.* 2009;121:131-138.
63. Ngaage DL, Mullany CJ, Daly RC, et al. Surgical treatment of cardiac papillary fibroelastoma: a single center experience with eighty-eight patients. *Ann Thorac Surg.* 2005;80:1712-1718.
64. Becker AE. Primary heart tumors in the pediatric age group: a review of salient pathologic features relevant for clinicians. *Pediatr Cardiol.* 2000;21:317-323.
65. Burke A, Virmani R. Pediatric heart tumors. *Cardiovasc Pathol.* 2008;17:193-198.
66. Fenoglio Jr JJ, M, CAllister HAJ, Ferrans VJ. Cardiac rhabdomyoma: a clinicopathologic and electron microscopic study. *Am J Cardiol.* 1976;38:241-251.
67. Fesslova V, Villa L, Rizzuti T, et al. Natural history and long-term outcome of cardiac rhabdomyomas detected prenatally. *Prenat Diagn.* 2004;24:241-248.
68. Smythe JF, Dyck JD, Smallhorn JF, et al. Natural history of cardiac rhabdomyoma in infancy and childhood. *Am J Cardiol.* 1990;66:1247-1249.
69. Burke AP, Virmani R. Cardiac rhabdomyoma: a clinicopathologic study. *Mod Pathol.* 1991;4:70-74.
70. Padalino MA, Basso C, Milanesi O, et al. Surgically treated primary cardiac tumors in early infancy and childhood. *J Thorac Cardiovasc Surg.* 2005;129:1358-1363.
71. Verhaaren HA, Vanakker O, De Wolf D, et al. Left ventricular outflow obstruction in rhabdomyoma of infancy: meta-analysis of the literature. *J Pediatr.* 2003;143:258-263.
72. Bass JL, Breningstall GN, Swaiman KF. Echocardiographic incidence of cardiac rhabdomyoma in tuberous sclerosis. *Am J Cardiol.* 1985;55:1379-1382.
73. Cho JM, Danielson GK, Puga FJ, et al. Surgical resection of ventricular cardiac fibromas: early and late results. *Ann Thorac Surg.* 2003;76:1929-1934.
74. Parmley LF, Salley RK, Williams JP, et al. The clinical spectrum of cardiac fibroma with diagnostic and surgical considerations: noninvasive imaging enhances management. *Ann Thorac Surg.* 1988;45:455-465.
75. Williams DB, Danielson GK, McGoon DC, et al. Cardiac fibroma: long-term survival after excision. *J Thorac Cardiovasc Surg.* 1982;84:230-236.
76. Wong JA, Fishbein MC. Cardiac fibroma resulting in fatal ventricular arrhythmia. *Circulation.* 2000;101:E168-E170.
77. Ben-Izhak O, Vlodavsky E, Ofer A, et al. Epithelioid angiosarcoma associated with a Dacron vascular graft. *Am J Surg Pathol.* 1999;23:1418-1422.
78. Fyfe BS, Quintana CS, Kaneko M, et al. Aortic sarcoma four years after Dacron graft insertion. *Ann Thorac Surg.* 1994;58:1752-1754.
79. Okada M, Takeuchi E, Mori Y, et al. An autopsy case of angiosarcoma arising around a woven Dacron prosthesis after a Cabrol operation. *J Thorac Cardiovasc Surg.* 2004;127:1843-1845.
80. Oppenheimer BS, Oppenheimer ET, Stout AP, et al. The latent period in carcinogenesis by plastics in rats and its relation to the presarcomatous stage. *Cancer.* 1958;11:204-213.
81. Okada F. Beyond foreign-body-induced carcinogenesis: impact of reactive oxygen species derived from inflammatory cells in tumorigenic conversion and tumor progression. *Int J Cancer.* 2007;121:2364-2372.
82. Almassi GH. Surgery for tumors with cavoatrial extension. *Semin Thorac Cardiovasc Surg.* 2000;12:111-118.
83. Mugge A, Daniel WG, Haverich A, et al. Diagnosis of noninfective cardiac mass lesions by two-dimensional echocardiography. Comparison of the transthoracic and transesophageal approaches. *Circulation.* 1991;83:70-78.
84. Corrado G, Klein AL, Santarone M. Echocardiography in atrial fibrillation. *J Cardiovasc Med (Hagerstown).* 2006;7:498-504.
85. Alam M, Rosman HS, Grullon C. Transesophageal echocardiography in evaluation of atrial masses. *Angiology.* 1995;46:123-128.
86. Pop G, Sutherland GR, Koudstaal PJ, et al. Transesophageal echocardiography in the detection of intracardiac embolic sources in patients with transient ischemic attacks. *Stroke.* 1990;21:560-565.
87. de Bruijn SF, Agema WR, Lammers GJ, et al. Transesophageal echocardiography is superior to transthoracic echocardiography in management of patients of any age with transient ischemic attack or stroke. *Stroke.* 2006;37:2531-2534.
88. Kronik G, Stollberger C, Schuh M, et al. Interobserver variability in the detection of spontaneous echo contrast, left atrial thrombi, and left atrial appendage thrombi by transoesophageal echocardiography. *Br Heart J.* 1995;74:80-83.
89. Stollberger C, Chnupa P, Kronik G, et al. Transesophageal echocardiography to assess embolic risk in patients with atrial fibrillation. ELAT Study Group. Embolism in Left Atrial Thrombi. *Ann Intern Med.* 1998;128:630-638.
90. Schneider B, Stollberger C. Diagnosis of left atrial appendage thrombi by multiplane transesophageal echocardiography: interlaboratory comparative study. *Circ J.* 2007;71:122-125.
91. Bernhardt P, Schmidt H, Hammerstingl C, et al. Atrial thrombi-a prospective follow-up study over 3 years with transesophageal echocardiography and cranial magnetic resonance imaging. *Echocardiography.* 2006;23:388-394.
92. van Dantzig JM, Delemarre BJ, Bot H, et al. Left ventricular thrombus in acute myocardial infarction. *Eur Heart J.* 1996;17:1640-1645.
93. Nayak D, Aronow WS, Sukhija R, et al. Comparison of frequency of left ventricular thrombi in patients with anterior wall versus non-anterior wall acute myocardial infarction treated with antithrombotic and antiplatelet therapy with or without coronary revascularization. *Am J Cardiol.* 2004;93:1529-1530.
94. Nihoyannopoulos P, Smith GC, Maseri A, et al. The natural history of left ventricular thrombus in myocardial infarction: a rationale in support of masterly inactivity. *J Am Coll Cardiol.* 1989;14:903-911.
95. Rehan A, Kanwar M, Rosman H, et al. Incidence of post myocardial infarction left ventricular thrombus in the era of primary percutaneous intervention and glycoprotein IIb/IIIa inhibitors. A prospective observational study. *Cardiovasc Ultrasound.* 2006;4:20.
96. Osherov AB, Borovik-Raz M, Aronson D, et al. Incidence of early left ventricular thrombus after acute anterior wall myocardial infarction in the primary coronary intervention era. *Am Heart J.* 2009;157:1074-1080.
97. Mansencal N, Nasr IA, Pilliere R, et al. Usefulness of contrast echocardiography for assessment of left ventricular thrombus after acute myocardial infarction. *Am J Cardiol.* 2007;99:1667-1670.
98. Weinsaft JW, Kim RJ, Ross M, et al. Contrast-enhanced anatomic imaging as compared to contrast-enhanced tissue characterization for detection of left ventricular thrombus. *JACC Cardiovasc Imaging.* 2009;2:969-979.
99. Siebelink HM, Scholte AJ, Van de Veire NR, et al. Value of contrast echocardiography for left ventricular thrombus detection postinfarction and impact on antithrombotic therapy. *Coron Artery Dis.* 2009;20:462-466.
100. Mansencal N, Revault-d'Allonnes L, Pelage JP, et al. Usefulness of contrast echocardiography for assessment of intracardiac masses. *Arch Cardiovasc Dis.* 2009;102:177-183.
101. Anwar AM, Nosir YF, Ajam A, et al. Central role of real-time three-dimensional echocardiography in the assessment of intracardiac thrombi. *Int J Cardiovasc Imaging.* 2010;26:519-526.
102. Puskas F, Cleveland Jr JC, Singh R, et al. Detection of left ventricular apical thrombus with three-dimensional transesophageal echocardiography. *Semin Cardiothorac Vasc Anesth.* 2011;15:102-104.
103. Lo CI, Chang SH, Hung CL. Demonstration of left ventricular thrombi with real-time 3-dimensional echocardiography in a patient with cardiomyopathy. *J Am Soc Echocardiogr.* 2007;20(905):e9-13.
104. Maslow A, Lowenstein E, Steriti J, et al. Left ventricular thrombi: intraoperative detection by transesophageal echocardiography and recognition of a source of post CABG embolic stroke: a case series. *Anesthesiology.* 1998;89:1257-1262.
105. Yadava OP, Yadav S, Juneja S, et al. Left ventricular thrombus sans overt cardiac pathology. *Ann Thorac Surg.* 2003;76:623-625.
106. Robinson NM, Desai J, Monaghan MJ. Atrial and pulmonary mass: intracardiac thrombus mimicking myxoma on multiplane transesophageal echocardiography. *J Am Soc Echocardiogr.* 1997;10:93-96.
107. Deluigi CC, Meinhardt G, Ursulescu A, et al. Images in cardiovascular medicine. Noninvasive characterization of left atrial mass. *Circulation.* 2006;113:e19-e20.
108. Fagan SM, Chan KL. Transesophageal echocardiography risk factors for stroke in nonvalvular atrial fibrillation. *Echocardiography.* 2000;17:365-372.
109. DeRook FA, Pearlman AS. Transesophageal echocardiographic assessment of embolic sources: intracardiac and extracardiac masses and aortic degenerative disease. *Crit Care Clin.* 1996;12:273-294.
110. Fatkin D, Loupas T, Jacobs N, et al. Quantification of blood echogenicity: evaluation of a semiquantitative method of grading spontaneous echo contrast. *Ultrasound Med Biol.* 1995;21:1191-1198.
111. Ito T, Suwa M, Kobashi A, et al. Integrated backscatter assessment of left atrial spontaneous echo contrast in chronic nonvalvular atrial fibrillation: relation with clinical and echocardiographic parameters. *J Am Soc Echocardiogr.* 2000;13:666-673.
112. Klein AL, Murray RD, Black IW, et al. Integrated backscatter for quantification of left atrial spontaneous echo contrast. *J Am Coll Cardiol.* 1996;28:222-231.
113. Cavalcante JL, Al-Mallah M, Arida M, et al. The relationship between spontaneous echocontrast, transesophageal echocardiographic parameters, and blood hemoglobin levels. *J Am Soc Echocardiogr.* 2008;21:868-872.
114. Black IW. Spontaneous echo contrast: where there's smoke there's fire. *Echocardiography.* 2000;17:373-382.
115. Ozkan M, Kaymaz C, Kirma C, et al. Predictors of left atrial thrombus and spontaneous echo contrast in rheumatic valve disease before and after mitral valve replacement. *Am J Cardiol.* 1998;82:1066-1070.
116. Maltagliati A, Galli CA, Tamborini G, et al. Incidence of spontaneous echocontrast, 'sludge' and thrombi before cardioversion in patients with atrial fibrillation: new insights into the role of transesophageal echocardiography. *J Cardiovasc Med (Hagerstown).* 2009;10:523-528.
117. Patel SV, Flaker G. Is early cardioversion for atrial fibrillation safe in patients with spontaneous echocardiographic contrast? *Clin Cardiol.* 2008;31:148-152.
118. Ogren M, Bergqvist D, Eriksson H, et al. Prevalence and risk of pulmonary embolism in patients with intracardiac thrombosis: a population-based study of 23 796 consecutive autopsies. *Eur Heart J.* 2005;26:1108-1114.
119. Torbicki A, Galie N, Covezzoli A, et al. Right heart thrombi in pulmonary embolism: results from the International Cooperative Pulmonary Embolism Registry. *J Am Coll Cardiol.* 2003;41:2245-2251.
120. Pierre-Justin G, Pierard LA. Management of mobile right heart thrombi: a prospective series. *Int J Cardiol.* 2005;99:381-388.
121. Casazza F, Bongarzoni A, Centonze F, et al. Prevalence and prognostic significance of right-sided cardiac mobile thrombi in acute massive pulmonary embolism. *Am J Cardiol.* 1997;79:1433-1435.
122. Ferrari E, Benhamou M, Berthier F, et al. Mobile thrombi of the right heart in pulmonary embolism: delayed disappearance after thrombolytic treatment. *Chest.* 2005;127:1051-1053.
123. Chartier L, Bera J, Delomez M, et al. Free-floating thrombi in the right heart: diagnosis, management, and prognostic indexes in 38 consecutive patients. *Circulation.* 1999;99:2779-2783.
124. Shah DP, Min JK, Raman J, et al. Thrombus-in-transit: two cases and a review of diagnosis and management. *J Am Soc Echocardiogr.* 2007;20(1219):e6-e8.
125. Langeron O, Goarin JP, Pansard JL, et al. Massive intraoperative pulmonary embolism: diagnosis with transesophageal two-dimensional echocardiography. *Anesth Analg.* 1992;74:148-150.
126. Rastogi S, Abraham M, Geelani MA, et al. Anaesthetic considerations in a patient with right heart thrombi-in-transit. *Acta Anaesthesiol Scand.* 2005;49:117-121.
127. Nicoara A, Assaad S, Geirsson A. Unexpected intraoperative diagnosis of pulmonary embolism by transesophageal echocardiography. *J Cardiothorac Vasc Anesth.* 2010;24:639-640.
128. Issack PS, Lauerman MH, Helfet DL, et al. Fat embolism and respiratory distress associated with cemented femoral arthroplasty. *Am J Orthop (Belle Mead NJ).* 2009;38:72-76.
129. Akhtar S. Fat embolism. *Anesthesiol Clin.* 2009;27:533-550:table of contents.
130. Boorjian SA, Sengupta S, Blute ML. Renal cell carcinoma: vena caval involvement. *BJU Int.* 2007;99:1239-1244.

131. Sharma V, Cusimano RJ, McNama P, et al. Intraoperative migration of an inferior vena cava tumour detected by transesophageal echocardiography. *Can J Anaesth.* 2011;58:468-470.

132. Schallner N, Wittau N, Kehm V, et al. Intraoperative pulmonary tumor embolism from renal cell carcinoma and a patent foramen ovale detected by transesophageal echocardiography. *J Cardiothorac Vasc Anesth.* 2011;25:145-147.

133. Donaldson AJ, Thomson HE, Harper NJ, et al. Bone cement implantation syndrome. *Br J Anaesth.* 2009;102:12-22.

134. Gist RS, Stafford IP, Leibowitz AB, et al. Amniotic fluid embolism. *Anesth Analg.* 2009;108:1599-1602.

135. Koessler MJ, Fabiani R, Hamer H, et al. The clinical relevance of embolic events detected by transesophageal echocardiography during cemented total hip arthroplasty: a randomized clinical trial. *Anesth Analg.* 2001;92:49-55.

136. Hagio K, Sugano N, Takashina M, et al. Embolic events during total hip arthroplasty: an echocardiographic study. *J Arthroplasty.* 2003;18:186-192.

137. Warnaar N, Molenaar IQ, Colquhoun SD, et al. Intraoperative pulmonary embolism and intracardiac thrombosis complicating liver transplantation: a systematic review. *J Thromb Haemost.* 2008;6:297-302.

138. Nowak M, Shernan SK, Eltzschig HK, et al. A novel view for visualizing a left pulmonary artery thromboembolus with intraoperative transesophageal echocardiography. *J Clin Anesth.* 2008;20:136-138.

139. Orihashi K, Matsuura Y, Hamanaka Y, et al. Retained intracardiac air in open heart operations examined by transesophageal echocardiography. *Ann Thorac Surg.* 1993;55:1467-1471.

140. Meltzer RS, Tickner EG, Popp RL. Why do the lungs clear ultrasonic contrast? *Ultrasound Med Biol.* 1980;6:263-269.

141. Oka Y, Inoue T, Hong Y, et al. Retained intracardiac air. Transesophageal echocardiography for definition of incidence and monitoring removal by improved techniques. *J Thorac Cardiovasc Surg.* 1986;91:329-338.

142. Topol EJ, Humphrey LS, Borkon AM, et al. Value of intraoperative left ventricular microbubbles detected by transesophageal two-dimensional echocardiography in predicting neurologic outcome after cardiac operations. *Am J Cardiol.* 1985;56:773-775.

143. Webb WR, Harrison Jr LH, Helmcke FR, et al. Carbon dioxide field flooding minimizes residual intracardiac air after open heart operations. *Ann Thorac Surg.* 1997;64:1489-1491.

144. Mirski MA, Lele AV, Fitzsimmons L, et al. Diagnosis and treatment of vascular air embolism. *Anesthesiology.* 2007;106:164-177.

145. Tingleff J, Joyce FS, Pettersson G. Intraoperative echocardiographic study of air embolism during cardiac operations. *Ann Thorac Surg.* 1995;60:673-677.

146. Neville MJ, Butterworth J, James RL, et al. Similar neurobehavioral outcome after valve or coronary artery operations despite differing carotid embolic counts. *J Thorac Cardiovasc Surg.* 2001;121:125-136.

147. Orihashi K, Matsuura Y. Quantitative echocardiographic analysis of retained intracardiac air in pooled form: an experimental study. *J Am Soc Echocardiogr.* 1996;9:567-572.

148. Secknus MA, Asher CR, Scalia GM, et al. Intraoperative transesophageal echocardiography in minimally invasive cardiac valve surgery. *J Am Soc Echocardiogr.* 1999;12:231-236.

149. Akhtar S, Lluberes V, Allen K, et al. Unexpected, transesophageal echocardiography-detected left ventricular microbubbles during off-pump coronary artery bypass graft surgery. *J Cardiothorac Vasc Anesth.* 2001;15:131-133.

150. Hoka S, Okamoto H, Yamaura K, et al. Removal of retained air during cardiac surgery with transesophageal echocardiography and capnography. *J Am Soc Echocardiogr.* 1996;9:457-461.

151. Svenarud P, Persson M, van der Linden J. Effect of CO2 insufflation on the number and behavior of air microemboli in open-heart surgery: a randomized clinical trial. *Circulation.* 2004;109:1127-1132.

152. Chandraratna A, Ashmeg A, Chamsi Pasha H. Detection of intracoronary air embolism by echocardiography. *J Am Soc Echocardiogr.* 2002;15:1015-1017.

153. Orihashi K, Matsuura Y, Sueda T, et al. Pooled air in open heart operations examined by transesophageal echocardiography. *Ann Thorac Surg.* 1996;61:1377-1380.

154. Lamm G, Auer J, Punzengruber C, et al. Intracoronary air embolism in open heart surgery–an uncommon source of myocardial ischaemia. *Int J Cardiol.* 2006;112:e85-e86.

155. Rodigas PC, Meyer FJ, Haasler GB, et al. Intraoperative 2-dimensional echocardiography: ejection of microbubbles from the left ventricle after cardiac surgery. *Am J Cardiol.* 1982;50:1130-1132.

156. Al-Rashidi F, Blomquist S, Hoglund P, et al. A new de-airing technique that reduces systemic microemboli during open surgery: a prospective controlled study. *J Thorac Cardiovasc Surg.* 2009;138:157-162.

157. Al-Rashidi F, Landenhed M, Blomquist S, et al. Comparison of the effectiveness and safety of a new de-airing technique with a standardized carbon dioxide insufflation technique in open left heart surgery: a randomized clinical trial. *J Thorac Cardiovasc Surg.* 2011;141:1128-1133.

158. Attaran RR, Ata I, Kudithipudi V, et al. Protocol for optimal detection and exclusion of a patent foramen ovale using transthoracic echocardiography with agitated saline microbubbles. *Echocardiography.* 2006;23:616-622.

159. Clarke NR, Timperley J, Kelion AD, et al. Transthoracic echocardiography using second harmonic imaging with Valsalva manoeuvre for the detection of right to left shunts. *Eur J Echocardiogr.* 2004;5:176-181.

160. Lam YY, Yu CM, Zhang Q, et al. Enhanced detection of patent foramen ovale by systematic transthoracic saline contrast echocardiography. *Int J Cardiol.* 2011;152:24-27.

161. Soliman OI, Geleijnse ML, Meijboom FJ, et al. The use of contrast echocardiography for the detection of cardiac shunts. *Eur J Echocardiogr.* 2007;8:S2-12.

162. Afonso L, Kottam A, Niraj A, et al. Usefulness of intravenously administered fluid replenishment for detection of patent foramen ovale by transesophageal echocardiography. *Am J Cardiol.* 2010;106:1054-1058.

163. Greim CA, Trautner H, Kramer K, et al. The detection of interatrial flow patency in awake and anesthetized patients: a comparative study using transnasal transesophageal echocardiography. *Anesth Analg.* 2001;92:1111-1116.

164. Hagen PT, Scholz DG, Edwards WD. Incidence and size of patent foramen ovale during the first 10 decades of life: an autopsy study of 965 normal hearts. *Mayo Clin Proc.* 1984;59:17-20.

165. Thanigaraj S, Valika A, Zajarias A, et al. Comparison of transthoracic versus transesophageal echocardiography for detection of right-to-left atrial shunting using agitated saline contrast. *Am J Cardiol.* 2005;96:1007-1010.

166. Johansson MC, Helgason H, Dellborg M, et al. Sensitivity for detection of patent foramen ovale increased with increasing number of contrast injections: a descriptive study with contrast transesophageal echocardiography. *J Am Soc Echocardiogr.* 2008;21:419-424.

167. Woods TD, Patel A. A critical review of patent foramen ovale detection using saline contrast echocardiography: when bubbles lie. *J Am Soc Echocardiogr.* 2006;19:215-222.

168. Jaffe RA, Pinto FJ, Schnittger I, et al. Aspects of mechanical ventilation affecting interatrial shunt flow during general anesthesia. *Anesth Analg.* 1992;75:484-488.

169. Koroneos A, Politis P, Malachias S, et al. End-inspiratory occlusion maneuver during transesophageal echocardiography for patent foramen ovale detection in intensive care unit patients. *Intensive Care Med.* 2007;33:1458-1462.

170. Naqvi TZ, Rafie R, Daneshvar S. Original Investigations. Potential faces of patent foramen ovale (PFO). *Echocardiography.* 2010;27:897-907.

171. Freeman JA, Woods TD. Use of saline contrast echo timing to distinguish intracardiac and extracardiac shunts: failure of the 3- to 5-beat rule. *Echocardiography.* 2008;25:1127-1130.

172. Sukernik MR, Bennett-Guerrero E. The incidental finding of a patent foramen ovale during cardiac surgery: should it always be repaired? A core review. *Anesth Analg.* 2007;105:602-610.

173. Argenziano M. PRO: The incidental finding of a patent foramen ovale during cardiac surgery: should it always be repaired? *Anesth Analg.* 2007;105:611-612.

174. Flachskampf FA. CON: The incidental finding of a patent foramen ovale during cardiac surgery: should it always be repaired? *Anesth Analg.* 2007;105:613-614.

175. Krasuski RA, Hart SA, Allen D, et al. Prevalence and repair of intraoperatively diagnosed patent foramen ovale and association with perioperative outcomes and long-term survival. *JAMA.* 2009;302:290-297.

176. Lo TT, Jarral OA, Shipolini AR, et al. Should a patent foramen ovale found incidentally during isolated coronary surgery be closed? *Interact Cardiovasc Thorac Surg.* 2011;12:794-798.

177. Lindeboom JE, van Deudekom MJ, Visser CA. Traditional contrast echocardiography may fail to demonstrate a patent foramen ovale: negative contrast in the right atrium may be a clue. *Eur J Echocardiogr.* 2005;6:75-78.

178. Parra JA, Bueno J, Zarauza J, et al. Graded contrast echocardiography in pulmonary arteriovenous malformations. *Eur Respir J.* 2010;35:1279-1285.

179. Ahmed S, Nanda NC, Nekkanti R, et al. Contrast transesophageal echocardiographic detection of a pulmonary arteriovenous malformation draining into left lower pulmonary vein. *Echocardiography.* 2003;20:391-394.

180. Gudavalli A, Kalaria VG, Chen X, et al. Intrapulmonary arteriovenous shunt: diagnosis by saline contrast bubbles in the pulmonary veins. *J Am Soc Echocardiogr.* 2002;15:1012-1014.

181. Margreiter J, Dessl A, Mair P, et al. Pulmonary arteriovenous fistula detected with transesophageal contrast echocardiography. *J Cardiothorac Vasc Anesth.* 2001;15:755-757.

182. Duch PM, Chandrasekaran K, Mulhern CB, et al. Transesophageal echocardiographic diagnosis of pulmonary arteriovenous malformation. Role of contrast and pulsed Doppler echocardiography. *Chest.* 1994;105:1604-1605.

183. Jassal DS, Qureshi A, Neilan TG, et al. Pulmonary arteriovenous malformations in hereditary hemorrhagic telangiectasia: an echocardiographic perspective. *J Am Soc Echocardiogr.* 2006;19:e5-e7; 229.

184. Gazzaniga P, Buscarini E, Leandro G, et al. Contrast echocardiography for pulmonary arteriovenous malformations screening: does any bubble matter? *Eur J Echocardiogr.* 2009;10:513-518.

185. van Gent MW, Post MC, Luermans JG, et al. Screening for pulmonary arteriovenous malformations using transthoracic contrast echocardiography: a prospective study. *Eur Respir J.* 2009;33:85-91.

186. Kolski BC, Khadivi B, Anawati M, et al. The dilated coronary sinus: utility of coronary sinus cross-sectional area and eccentricity index in differentiating right atrial pressure overload from persistent left superior vena cava. *Echocardiography.* 2011;28:829-832.

Intracardiac Devices, Catheters, and Cannulas

MARC E. STONE | CESAR RODRIGUEZ-DIAZ

General Concepts

The close anatomic relationship between the esophagus and the mediastinal contents (as well as the descending aorta) allows for transesophageal echocardiographic (TEE) imaging of the various intracardiac devices inherent to the practice of modern cardiac surgery and anesthesiology. The following is a non-exhaustive list of potential applications of TEE in this regard for confirmation of the desired position of:

- Cannulas (including those used for bypass and the guidewires sometimes used to introduce those cannulas):
  - Superior vena cava (SVC)
  - Inferior vena cava (IVC)
  - Right atrium (RA)
  - Aorta
- Catheters:
  - Retrograde cardioplegia catheter in coronary sinus (CS)
  - Pressure-monitoring lines
  - Pulmonary artery (PA) catheter
  - Left atrial (LA) pressure catheter
  - Central venous catheters (e.g., in pediatric population)
- "Vents": left ventricular (LV) vent
- Devices (positioning and function):
  - Intraaortic balloon pump
  - Aortic stents
  - Ventricular assist devices
- Occluders:
  - Used to close a patent foramen ovale
  - Used to close a paravalvular leak
  - Used to close a persistent ductus arteriosus
- Pacing leads: LV lead in CS

TEE can also be helpful in detecting obstruction of cannulas and conduits and ensuring the presence of adequate blood flow in the aortic arch during bypass when alternative arterial cannulation sites (e.g., axillary artery) are used.

Ultrasound imaging depends critically on the angle of intercept between the structure or device of interest and the ultrasound beam, with the best visualization obtained when the object of interest lies directly perpendicular to the ultrasound beam. Objects that lie parallel to the beam are poorly visualized because of the lack of reflectivity back to the transducer of ultrasound waves intercepting objects at parallel angles. However, flow through such parallel objects can be detected and quantitated with Doppler methodologies, including color flow mapping.

As with other "tubes" (e.g., aorta), if the ultrasound beam cuts perpendicularly through a cannula in its short axis, that section will be displayed as a circular "donut," and if the ultrasound beam cuts perpendicularly through a cannula in its long axis, a longitudinal "pipe" consisting of two parallel lines is displayed. An oblique angle of intercept will result in at least partial deflection of the beam at an oblique angle away from the transducer, resulting in poor image resolution. For this reason, if the beam intersects a cannula at an oblique angle, an oblique section with a variable appearance will be displayed.

Most medical devices are made of high-density plastic or metal, which, while highly echogenic, tends to create artifacts in addition to the echocardiographic image of the device itself. On occasion, devices themselves are not well visualized, and only the presence of artifacts suggests that something is present in that location. The most commonly seen artifacts associated with echocardiography of medical devices are shadowing, side lobes and grating lobes, and reverberations. Such artifacts can be mistaken for abnormalities of the cardiac chambers, valves, or great vessels, and the echocardiographer must be aware of this possibility.

- Shadowing occurs when the ultrasound beam fails to penetrate a strong reflector, resulting in an absence of signal in the far field beyond the structure or object. It appears on the echo image as a dark area (shadow) past a bright structure.
- Reverberations occur when a strong reflector causes ultrasound waves to bounce back and forth between the structure or object of interest and the transducer face, creating multiple signals at evenly spaced intervals. On the echo image, they look like comet tails or a series of copies of an object into the far field of the image.
- Side lobe and grating lobe artifacts occur when laterally directed ultrasound emanations return from real structures in the periphery with the main lobe, causing central misplacement of a signal from an actual peripheral structure (e.g., a curvilinear line across the display). The intensity of such reflections is generally far less than those of the main lobe signals, and the artifacts can often be identified when they appear to cross through cardiac structures. Grating lobes are unique to phased-array transducers but are relatively uncommon given the design of modern transducers. Both side lobes and grating lobes can create diagnostic confusion.

Owing to the likelihood of artifacts, it is best to confirm the position of devices in at least two different views to ensure proper placement; three-dimensional (3D) imaging can also be helpful. The easiest way to obtain a different view without changing the position of the probe is by advancing/rotating the multiplane angle. Cannulas imaged in their long axis (tubular appearance) will be imaged in the short axis (circular appearance) or vice versa when the multiplane angle is changed by 90 degrees.

Cannulas

Cannulation for Cardiopulmonary Bypass

Typically, the aortic cannula is the first one placed by cardiac surgeons when cannulating for cardiopulmonary bypass (CPB). The aortic cannula is commonly placed in the distal part of the ascending aorta, often reaching the proximal arch, but it is generally not possible to visualize it by TEE because this segment of the aorta is coursing anterior to the left bronchus, and the large difference in acoustic impedance between blood/tissue and the air in the bronchus results in reflection of ultrasound waves. In some patients with slightly differing anatomy (or when the cannula is very long or placed very high), it might be possible to image the routine aortic cannula (Fig. 22-1), and one could certainly use epiaortic scanning if necessary.

Atheromatous plaques have been correlated with strokes and cognitive dysfunction.[1] The ME aortic valve long-axis (LAX) view and upper esophageal (UE) aortic arch LAX view provide an idea of the degree of atheromatous burden near the cannulation site, but only visualization of the actual cannulation and cross-clamp sites with epiaortic scanning by the surgeon can rule out significant disease in those sites, and it is important to do so.[2]

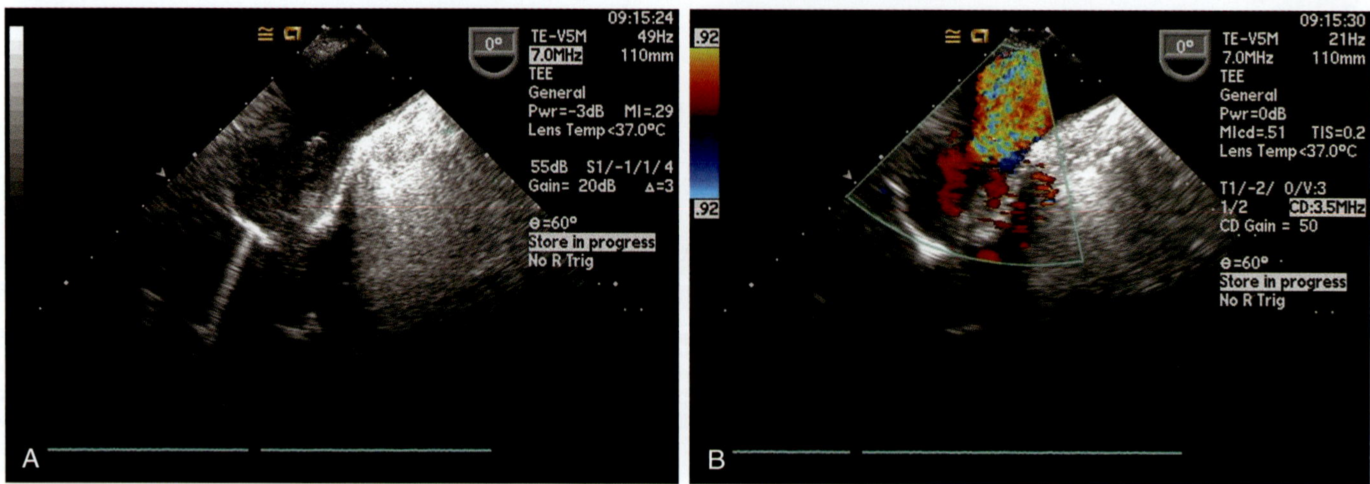

Figure 22-1 **A,** Proximal aortic arch showing tip of aortic cannula in upper esophageal aortic arch long-axis view. **B,** Color flow Doppler used to confirm flow on bypass.

TEE also allows for assessment of the aorta for the presence of dissection after cannulation. An aortic dissection might extend proximally into the ascending aorta or distally into the arch or descending aorta. The ME aortic valve LAX view, UE aortic arch LAX view, and ME aortic arch short axis (SAX) view allow imaging of the aorta proximal and distal to the aortic cannula. Once CPB is commenced, assessing the aorta for the presence of flow in the aortic arch and descending aorta is recommended to avoid the possible catastrophic outcome of malperfusion, especially when a non-central cannulation has been performed (e.g., cannulation of axillary or femoral artery). This is typically done in the aortic arch LAX view and descending aorta LAX view using color Doppler. The presence of laminar flow might require the Nyquist limit to be adjusted to visualize flow.

Venous Cannulation

For procedures not involving opening of the heart chambers (e.g., aortocoronary bypass), a two-stage venous cannula is generally inserted through the right atrial appendage (RAA), with the distal orifice directed into the IVC and the proximal orifice positioned in the RA. It is ideal for the tip of the IVC cannula to be located within the IVC, but one does not want it entering a hepatic vein (Fig. 22-2). It is convenient to image the cannula and locate the tip starting from the ME bicaval view. One follows the cannula from its entrance through the RAA into the IVC. Advancement and slight rotation of the probe to the right will optimize the image of the cannula within the IVC. Non-standard views of the IVC and hepatic veins at whatever multiplane angle is optimal can be used to determine the location of the IVC cannula tip. Ideally, the tip should reside in the lumen of the IVC. If the tip of the cannula enters a hepatic vein, it should be repositioned to avoid poor venous drainage and potential abdominal distention.

For procedures where heart chambers are opened (e.g., valve surgery), the SVC and IVC are often each cannulated directly with two separate cannulas (bicaval technique). The SVC can usually be visualized in its long axis to the right of the display in the ME bicaval view and also in its short axis in the ME aortic valve SAX view. Figure 22-3 shows a cannula in the SVC.

An alternate site of venous cannulation of the RA is through the femoral vein, using a Seldinger technique. Femoral vein cannulation requires a long multistaged cannula that courses from the IVC to the SVC. Correct placement into the SVC begins first by imaging the guidewire as it comes up the IVC, crosses the RA (use ME bicaval view), and enters the SVC (Fig. 22-4). The cannula is then advanced over the wire. Care should be taken when there is a patent foramen ovale (PFO) to ensure the wire does not inadvertently enter the LA.

For optimal venous drainage, it is necessary to confirm the tip of the cannula ultimately lies in the SVC.

Cannulas for Partial Cardiopulmonary Bypass

Partial left heart bypass used for repair of descending aortic aneurysms requires placement of a venous inflow cannula in the LA (often from a left pulmonary vein) (Fig. 22-5) and a femoral arterial (FA) outflow cannula. In this "LA-FA bypass," the heart and lungs maintain oxygenation of the blood in the body, the native cardiac output from the LV perfuses only the upper body, and the outflow from the LA-FA bypass provides what is called *distal perfusion* (oxygenated blood is drained from the LA and returned to the lower body distal to the aneurysm to perfuse the spinal cord and viscera from below). The conduct of the partial bypass then requires a balancing of the upper and lower circulations by the perfusionist. For example, if the upper pressure is too high, a higher flow is used to drain the upper body and perfuse the lower until the pressures equalize. If the upper body pressure is too low, lower flows are used until the pressure in the circulations are optimally balanced.

The ME four-chamber and ME two-chamber views are used to confirm proper position of the LA cannula. Improper positioning of the LA cannula tip into a right pulmonary vein will restrict the amount of blood that can be perfused into the lower body and will also volume overload the upper body circulation. The LA cannula can also be improperly positioned into the LV through the mitral valve, with the possibility of inducing severe mitral regurgitation and reduced cardiac output to the upper body.

Cannulas for Cardioplegia

Unless there is significant aortic insufficiency, antegrade cardioplegia is generally given via a small catheter positioned in the root of the aorta proximal to the cross-clamp. Although the cardioplegia cannula is not commonly imaged, TEE is helpful in evaluating and assessing the degree of ventricular distention that occurs during infusion of antegrade cardioplegia in the setting of aortic regurgitation (which will also result in poor cardioplegia distribution down the coronaries). When the ventricle is distended, the cardioplegia is not fully distributed in the endocardium, and the wall tension is increased in the LV (which increases the myocardial oxygen demand), rendering myocardial protection suboptimal. The ME LAX view allows visualization of the degree of cardioplegia regurgitation and the volume inside the ventricle. The TG midpapillary SAX view is used to assess the degree of LV distention.

An LV vent can be placed (typically via a pulmonary vein) to decompress the ventricle while cardioplegia is being administered if

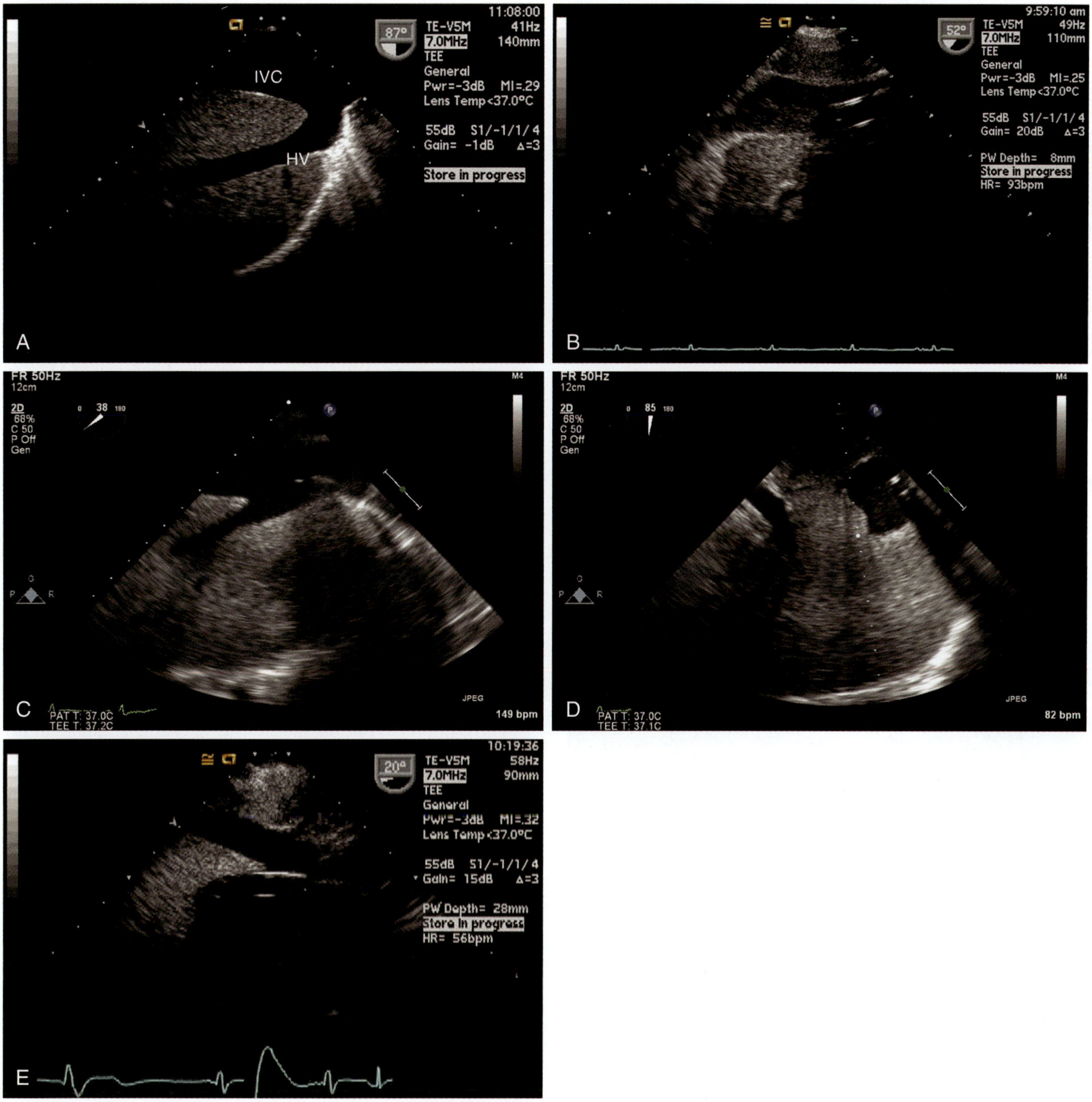

Figure 22-2 **A,** Long-axis view of inferior vena cava (IVC) and left hepatic vein (HV) obtained via transgastric view with probe rotated to right and multiplane angle advanced to nearly 90 degrees. **B,** Typical appearance of IVC cannula in a reasonable position. **C,** Venous cannula in IVC. This view is sometimes difficult to develop, but information obtained can be of paramount importance in confirming correct position of venous cannula. **D,** Short-axis view of cannula is obtained by advancing multiplane angle. **E,** Malpositioned IVC venous cannula seen entering a hepatic vein. Cannula has to be repositioned into IVC to avoid improper drainage and risk of abdominal distention.

needed. ME views of the mitral valve and LV can be used to ensure that the LV vent actually crosses the mitral valve and that the tip resides in the LV. Alternatively, the surgeon can stop the administration of cardioplegia, open the cardioplegia cannula to air, and manually decompress the LV, forcing the cardioplegia solution inside the ventricle to exit through the aortic valve into the cardioplegia cannula.

Retrograde cardioplegia is administered through a catheter placed via the RAA into the CS. This is typically a blind procedure, but confirmation of correct placement can be verified by TEE. Slight advancement of the probe from the ME four-chamber view will reveal the CS just above the septal leaflet of the tricuspid valve in almost all patients (Fig. 22-6, *A*; Video 22-1).[3] Slight posterior flexion of the probe tends to improve visualization of the CS. The CS can also be visualized in the ME bicaval view close to the IVC. Confirmation of correct placement of the catheter can also be accomplished by visualization of the catheter inside the CS in the ME two-chamber view (Fig. 22-6, *B* and *C*). Many CS cardioplegia catheters have a characteristic self-inflating balloon that makes them easily

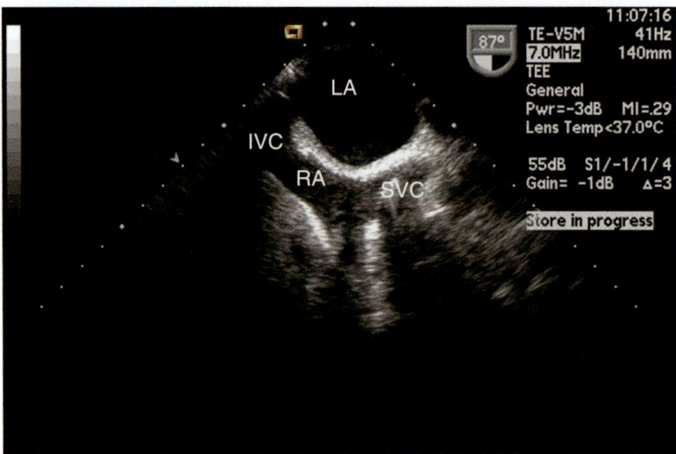

Figure 22-3   Cannula seen entering right atrium into superior vena cava in midesophageal bicaval view. *IVC,* Inferior vena cava; *LA,* left atrium; *RA,* right atrium; *SVC,* superior vena cava.

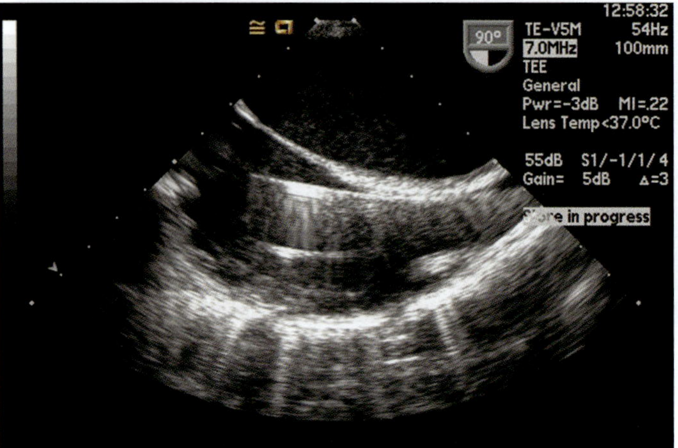

Figure 22-4   Guidewire for femoral venous cannulation of the right atrium. Wire was introduced into a femoral vein and is seen entering superior vena cava in midesophageal bicaval view. Lower linear reflector is the pulmonary artery catheter. *IVC,* Inferior vena cava; *LA,* left atrium; *RA,* right atrium; *SVC,* superior vena cava.

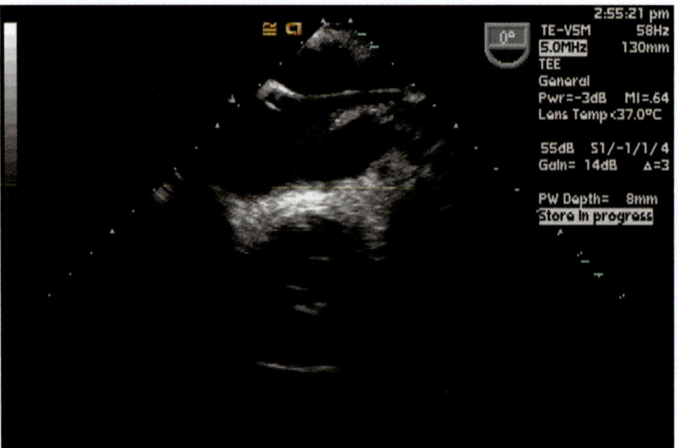

Figure 22-5   Left atrial cannula used for left heart bypass seen entering left atrium from left upper pulmonary vein in a modified midesophageal four-chamber view.

recognizable (Fig. 22-6, *D-F*). Visual confirmation that the balloon is not partially in the RA is essential because the cannula might slip out during the procedure, and administration of retrograde cardioplegia will be rendered ineffective. However, a cannula placed too deep into the CS will not provide adequate cardioplegia to the right ventricle, since its venous drainage tends to be close to the os of the CS. Percutaneous placement of the retrograde cardioplegia catheter (via the right internal jugular vein) is sometimes performed for minimally invasive procedures.[4] In such a case, the ME bicaval view will allow visualization of the catheter through the SVC and entering the CS.

A dilated CS (typically >1.5cm) should prompt the echocardiographer to rule out the presence of a persistent left superior vena cava (PLSVC) draining into the CS (Fig. 22-7).[5] In the presence of PLSVC, attempted retrograde cardioplegia does not optimally perfuse the myocardium as the cardioplegia enters the systemic veins, and this should be avoided. Injection of agitated saline into a left upper extremity vein will allow opacification and/or visualization of turbulent flow in the CS in this scenario. A PLSVC can be visualized in modified ME aortic valve SAX view with the probe slightly withdrawn and slightly anteflexed. The PLSVC courses between the left atrial appendage and the left lower pulmonary vein.

Intraaortic Balloon Pump

The intraaortic balloon pump (IABP) consists of a ballooned catheter that is typically inserted percutaneously in a Seldinger fashion via the femoral artery into the descending thoracic aorta, but it can also be placed via the subclavian artery or ascending aorta.[6,7] The IABP inflates during diastole, augmenting coronary perfusion pressure, and rapidly deflates just before systole, decreasing ventricular afterload and favoring enhanced stroke volume. The most commonly placed IABP size in an average-height adult is a 40-mL, 8F, 70-cm catheter. Table 22-1 outlines the role of TEE where an IABP is concerned and suggests views with regard to IABP placement and use.

TEE is helpful to rule out the presence of contraindications to IABP placement and/or use and to confirm correct catheter placement. Generally accepted contraindications to IABP use include aortic insufficiency (which will decrease the efficacy of the augmentation of coronary perfusion pressures and will cause LV distention once the IABP is functioning), mobile atheromas in the proximal descending aorta and arch (greatly increasing the risk of embolization), and thoracic aortic aneurysm. Relative contraindications include severe atheromatous disease in the descending aorta (increasing the risk of embolization), abdominal aortic aneurysm (increasing the risk of rupture and embolization), pregnancy, and the presence of aortic dissections.[8] However, IABPs have been placed successfully in these cases, often under TEE guidance.[9]

In general, the descending aorta should be evaluated for significant atheromatous burden and mobile plaques from the arch to as far down as one can visualize prior to inserting the device. During a standard insertion from the femoral artery, the wire over which the device is placed should be visualized in the thoracic aorta, with the tip near the left subclavian artery. Failure of the wire to appear in the correct location should prompt consideration of where the wire actually went *prior to* attempted introduction of the device itself. The IABP tip should come to rest 2 to 4 cm distal to the left subclavian artery.[10] An IABP placed too distal will fail to decrease the afterload that is decreasing myocardial oxygen demand with balloon deflation, and may obstruct flow to the celiac axis and renal arteries.[11] The aorta should be reevaluated after device placement (especially if placement was difficult) to rule out complications (e.g., presence of a new dissection). Once support by the IABP is engaged, the balloon should be assessed for completeness of inflation and filling of the aorta during diastole, as well as for the completeness of deflation to allow forward blood flow during systole. Figure 22-8 shows the appearance of a deployed IABP. Balloon rupture can easily be detected by the appearance of bubbles in the aorta with attempted inflation (the inflation gas is helium because of its low viscosity), and unusual motions or apparent mismatch of sizing of the device should prompt immediate discussion with the proceduralist placing the device.

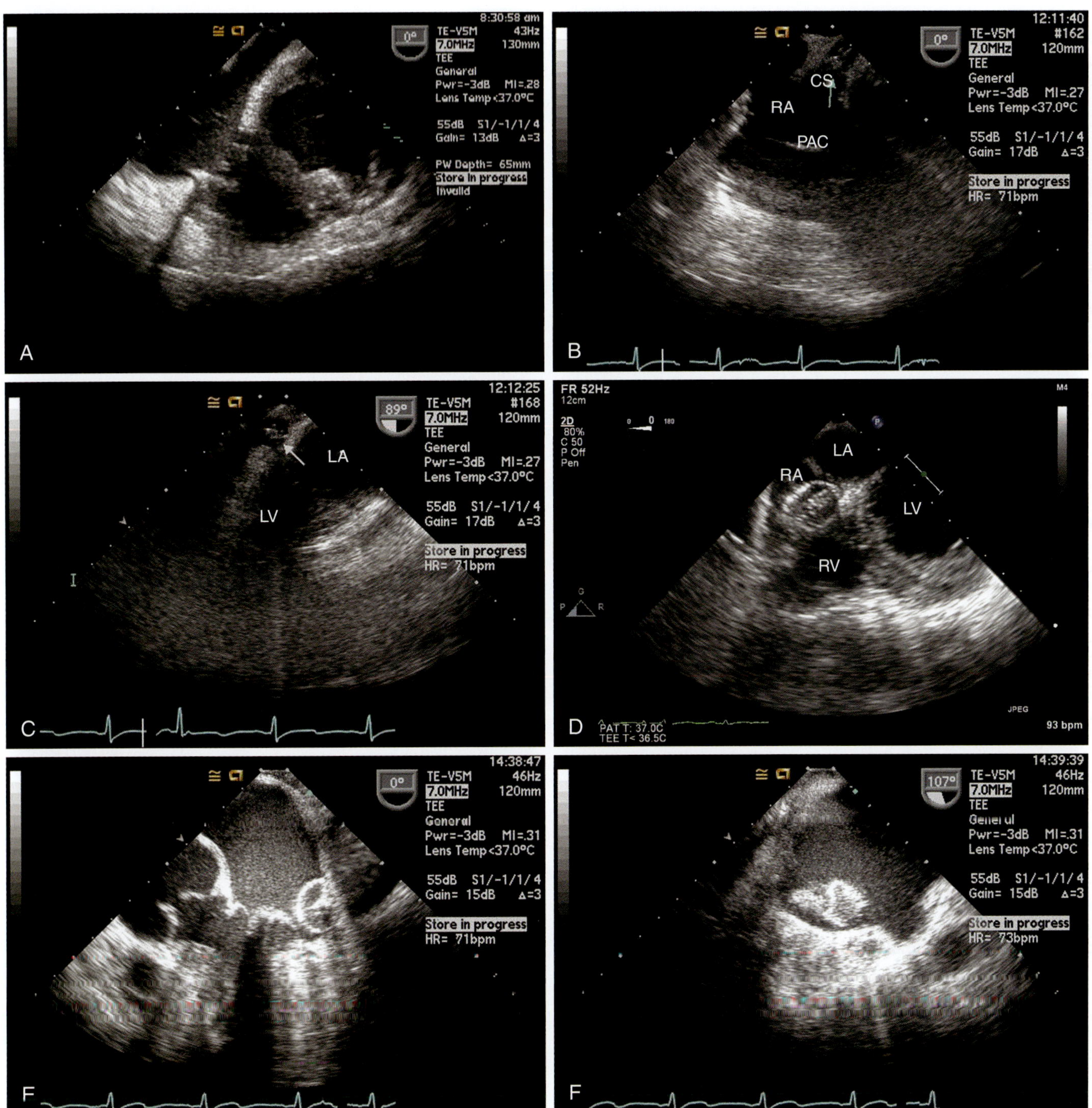

Figure 22-6 **A,** Coronary sinus (CS) is visualized via a modified midesophageal (ME) four-chamber view, with probe advanced until CS comes into view just above septal leaflet of tricuspid valve, often by retroflexing probe tip. **B,** Retrograde cardioplegia catheter *(arrow)* is seen in long axis in good position in CS in a modified ME four-chamber view. **C,** Retrograde cardioplegia catheter *(arrow)* is seen in short axis in CS in a modified ME two-chamber view. **D,** Self-inflating balloon of a retrograde cardioplegia catheter can be seen in right atrium (RA). **E,** Malpositioned retrograde cardioplegia catheter is seen in left atrium (LA) in ME four-chamber view. **F,** Multiplane angle advanced 100 degrees shows that catheter seen in LA is not likely an artifact. *LV,* Left ventricle; *PAC,* pulmonary artery catheter; *RV,* right ventricle.

Ventricular Assist Devices

Mechanical circulatory support (MCS) with ventricular assist devices (VADs) has become the routine management of refractory cardiogenic shock of any etiology. In acute situations (e.g., intractable low cardiac output syndrome following cardiotomy, myocardial infarction, viral myocarditis, etc.), certain VADs can be used as a "bridge to immediate survival," a "bridge to next decision," and/or a "bridge to recovery." In more chronic situations (e.g., the patient with end-stage cardiomyopathy requiring transplantation), certain VADs can be used as a "bridge to transplantation," or even as a "bridge to improved candidacy" for transplantation. Transplant-ineligible patients with end-stage failure may receive certain VADs as a permanent management solution in lieu of transplantation ("destination therapy").

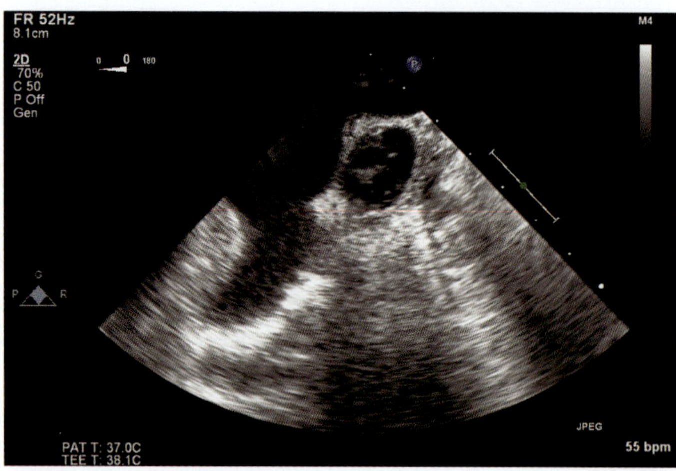

Figure 22-7 Persistent left superior vena cava (PLSVC) is present in center of image. Left atrium can be seen to immediate left of PLSVC, and left atrial appendage to left and below PLSVC. Structure above PLSVC is a left pulmonary vein.

The VADs most commonly used in the United States at the time of this writing are the Heartmate II LVAS (Thoratec Corporation, Woburn, Mass.; Fig. 22-9) and the CentriMag (Thoratec Corporation, Woburn, Mass.; Fig. 22-10). Members of the Impella platform (Abiomed, Danvers, Mass.; Fig. 22-11) and the TandemHeart (Cardiac Assist Inc., Pittsburgh, Pa.; Fig. 22-12) are increasingly being used as a "bridge to immediate survival" and "bridge to a bridge" in patients with acute cardiogenic shock. The Impella is increasingly used in elective situations in high-risk patients where an IABP might have been used in prior years (e.g., high-risk percutaneous coronary interventions, noncardiac surgery in high-risk patients, etc.). Other devices (e.g., the Abiomed AB5000 Ventricle, the Thoratec pVAD, etc.) may still be in use in some U.S. centers, and there are certainly many different devices available and in common use in other countries around the world.

A complete description of all such devices is beyond the scope of this chapter, but there are many similarities from the perspective of an echocardiographic examination, because regardless of manufacturer, VADs are simply pumps that divert blood from the heart and return it downstream of the failing ventricle. Cannulas are required within the heart and great vessels to accomplish this, and it is helpful to understand the cannulation strategy in use when performing an echocardiographic examination of the VAD-supported patient.

The inflow to an LVAD is most often from the LV apex (Fig. 22-13), with the outflow generally directed into the ascending aorta (Fig. 22-14), though it can be returned to the descending aorta with some devices. The inflow to an RVAD is generally from the RA, with the outflow generally directed into the main PA (but it can be returned to one of the branch PAs) (see Fig. 22-15). A complete TEE examination is always recommended, but a knowledge of the cannulation strategy in use will define the most important potential issues in a given patient and help focus the TEE exam. In some cases, the echocardiographic exam will have to address issues specific to a certain device in use, and to focus the exam the examiner will need to familiarize him- or herself with the details of that device and understand the clinical issue requiring evaluation. Echocardiography plays an important role in:

- Assessment of ventricular (dys)function that defines the indication for mechanical circulatory support
- Assisting surgical decision making regarding whether the left, right, or both ventricles require support (LVAD, RVAD, or Bi-VAD, respectively)
- Identification of existing pathologies that may impede VAD filling or effective emptying
- Identification of atherosclerotic disease in the ascending aorta and potential intracardiac thrombus, both of which may increase the risk of stroke in the perioperative period

TABLE 22-1	Role of TEE in the Presence of Intraaortic Balloon Pump	
Role	*Suggested Views*	*Comments*
Preplacement		
Assessment of LV function	ME four-chamber view ME commisural view ME two-chamber view ME AV LAX view TG mid-SAX view TG two-chamber view	
Aortic insufficiency	ME AV SAX view ME AV LAX view Deep TG view TG LAX view	
Atheromatous disease in aorta	Descending aorta LAX view Descending aorta SAX view UE aortic arch LAX view	Mobile plaques are of particular concern. Small sessile plaques usually pose little risk.
During Placement		
Wire	Descending aorta LAX view Descending aorta SAX view UE aortic arch LAX view	Failure of guidewire to appear in descending aorta should prompt consideration of where wire actually went.
Catheter	Descending aorta LAX view Descending aorta SAX view UE aortic arch LAX view	Catheter tip should be located 2-4 cm distal to takeoff of left subclavian artery.
Once Support Is Engaged		
Location	Descending aorta LAX view Descending aorta SAX view UE aortic arch LAX view	Device position should be rechecked to ensure there has been no proximal or distal migration.
Device function	Descending aorta LAX view Descending aorta SAX view	Balloon should fill aorta when inflated and should deflate sufficiently to allow for forward blood flow.
LV function	ME four-chamber view ME commisural view ME two-chamber view ME AV LAX view TG mid-SAX view TG two-chamber view	LV function should be reassessed once support is engaged.

AV, Aortic valve; *LAX*, long-axis; *LV*, left ventricular; *ME*, midesophageal; *SAX*, short-axis; *TG*, transgastric; *UE*, upper esophageal.

- Identification of intracardiac shunts and valvular pathology that will complicate patient management once VAD support is engaged
- De-airing of the device and the heart prior to engaging VAD support
- Assessment of the adequacy of VAD function and detection of complications
- Postoperative decision making with regard to fluid management, inotropic support, and vasoactive medications
- Assessment of ventricular recovery that may allow for potential weaning from VAD support (where applicable)

The Patient Receiving a Left Ventricular Assist Device

Before LVAD Placement

The echocardiographic examination preceding LVAD placement seeks to identify and rule out pathologies that may prevent the device from functioning as intended (e.g., will impair VAD filling or emptying) or may result in potentially preventable complications. Where present, such findings must be surgically addressed prior to engaging VAD support. Table 22-2 outlines these factors in detail regarding an LVAD and suggests those standard midesophageal (ME), transgastric (TG), and non-standard views in which to evaluate for potential pathology. Patients

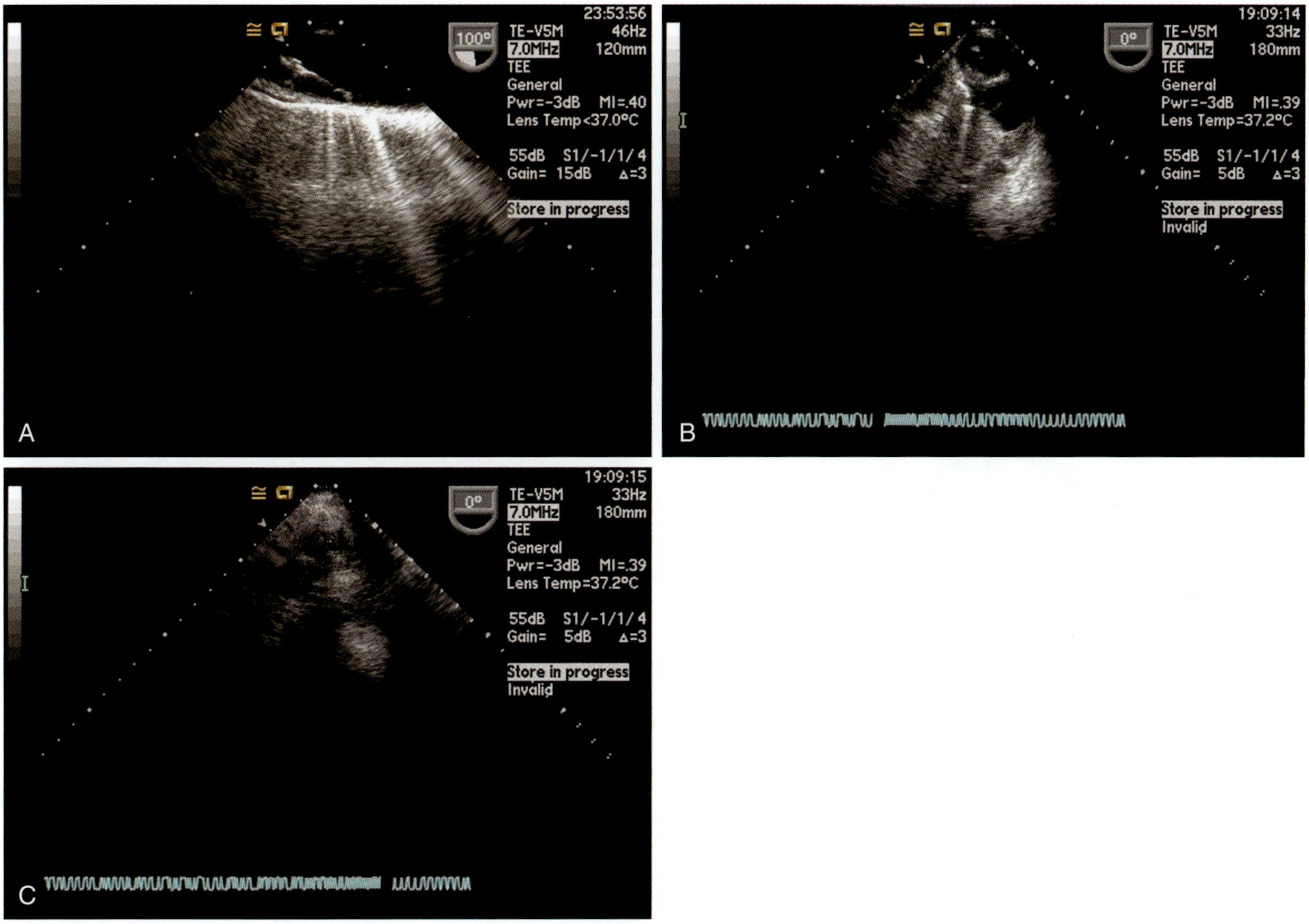

Figure 22-8 **A,** Tip of balloon pump catheter is seen approaching aortic arch from descending aorta. **B,** Short-axis view of balloon pump when it is deflated. **C,** Short-axis view of balloon when it is inflated. Note artifacts created by helium in inflated balloon.

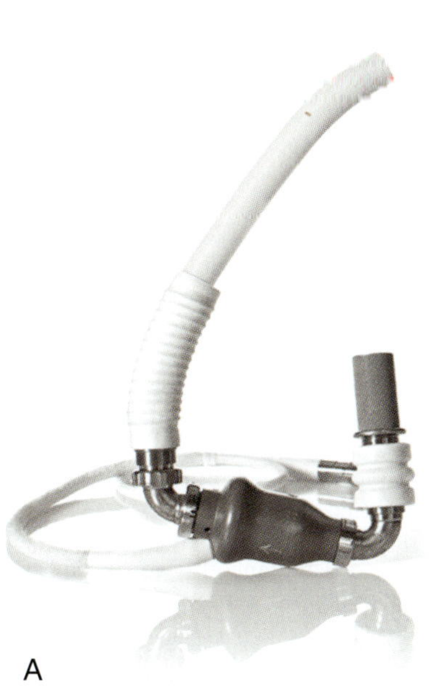

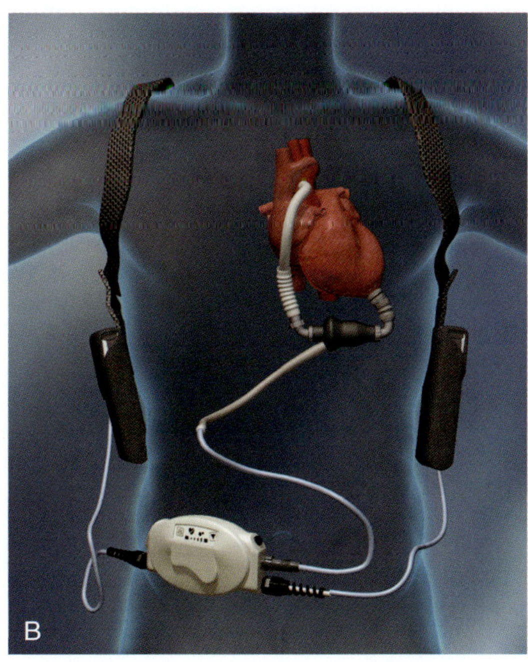

Figure 22-9 **A** and **B,** HeartMate II LVAS. Note cannulation strategy in use. Inflow to left ventricular assist device comes from apex of left ventricle, and outflow is directed into ascending aorta. *(Reprinted with permission from Thoratec Laboratories.)*

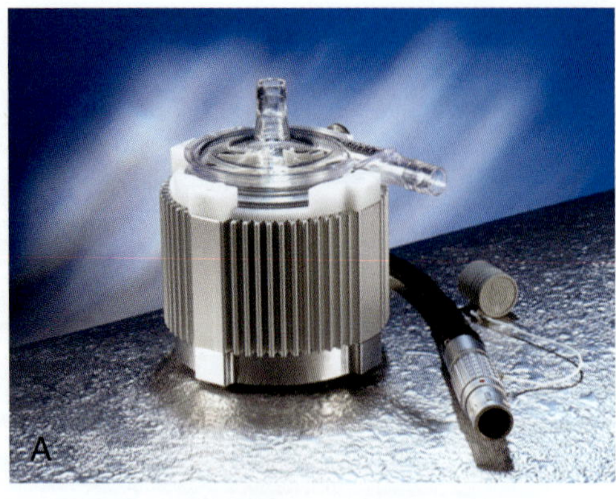

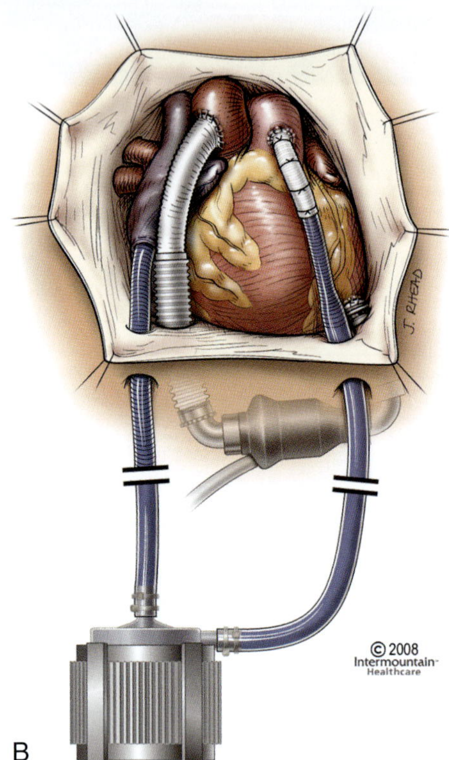

Figure 22-10   **A** and **B**, CentriMag. Note cannulation strategies in use in **B**. CentriMag is being used as right ventricular assist device, with inflow from right atrium and outflow directed into main pulmonary artery. There is a HeartMate II left ventricular assist device, with inflow coming from apex of left ventricle and outflow directed into ascending aorta. *(Reprinted with permission from Thoratec Laboratories.)*

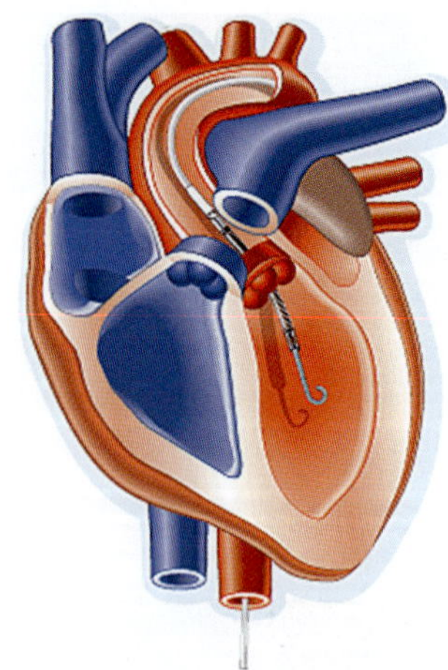

Figure 22-11   Impella LP 2.5. *(Courtesy Abiomed.)*

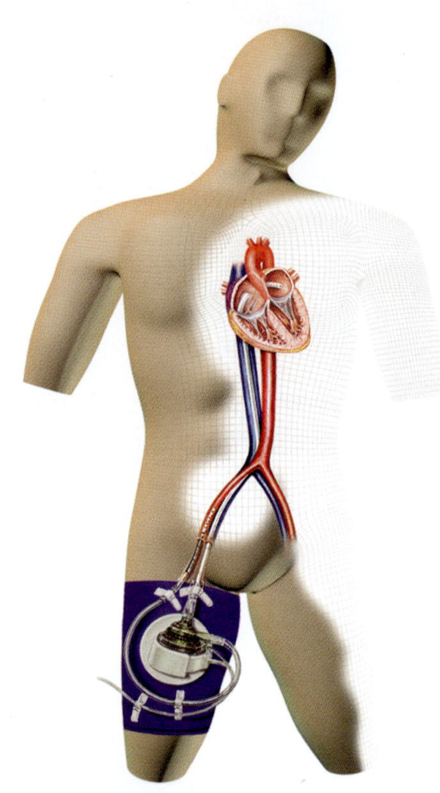

Figure 22-12   TandemHeart. *(Reproduced with permission from CardiacAssist, Inc.)*

with dilated hearts (as well as congenital anomalies) often require slight modifications of standard views to obtain optimal visualization of specific structures, owing to rotation of the mediastinal contents and altered chamber geometry. Current methodologies used to qualitatively and quantitatively evaluate the factors under consideration are described in detail in the relevant chapters throughout this textbook and elsewhere.

During LVAD Placement

TEE is used to:

- Ensure proper inflow cannula position in the LV. Often, an LV apical inflow cannula is best viewed in its long axis somewhere between the ME two-chamber view and the ME LAX view (see Fig. 22-13; Video 22-2). One can generally also see a SAX view of the inflow cannula in the ME four-chamber view, but there is generally little information provided from this view. An optimally positioned cannula points directly into the chamber toward the mitral valve (as opposed to

toward the interventricular septum or other LV wall), but it must be remembered that two-dimensional (2D) TEE is not revealing the 3D orientation of devices, and a cannula that is apparently aimed at an LV wall by 2D TEE may not actually be obstructed by that wall when there is adequate volume in the LV.
- Ensure adequate de-airing of device. Evidence of residual air in the VAD or VAD cannulas can be detected by viewing the ascending aorta SAX view and the ascending aorta LAX view.

The Impella is inserted retrograde across the aortic valve into the LV, and its position can be verified using the ME AV LAX view (Fig. 22-16; Video 22-3 and 22-4).

The TandemHeart inflow cannula is percutaneously advanced from a femoral vein up the IVC, through the RA, and into the LA across the interatrial septum at the fossa ovalis (Fig. 22-17). The ME bicaval view is used to ensure appropriate placement of the inflow cannula to this device across the fossa ovalis and into in the LA.

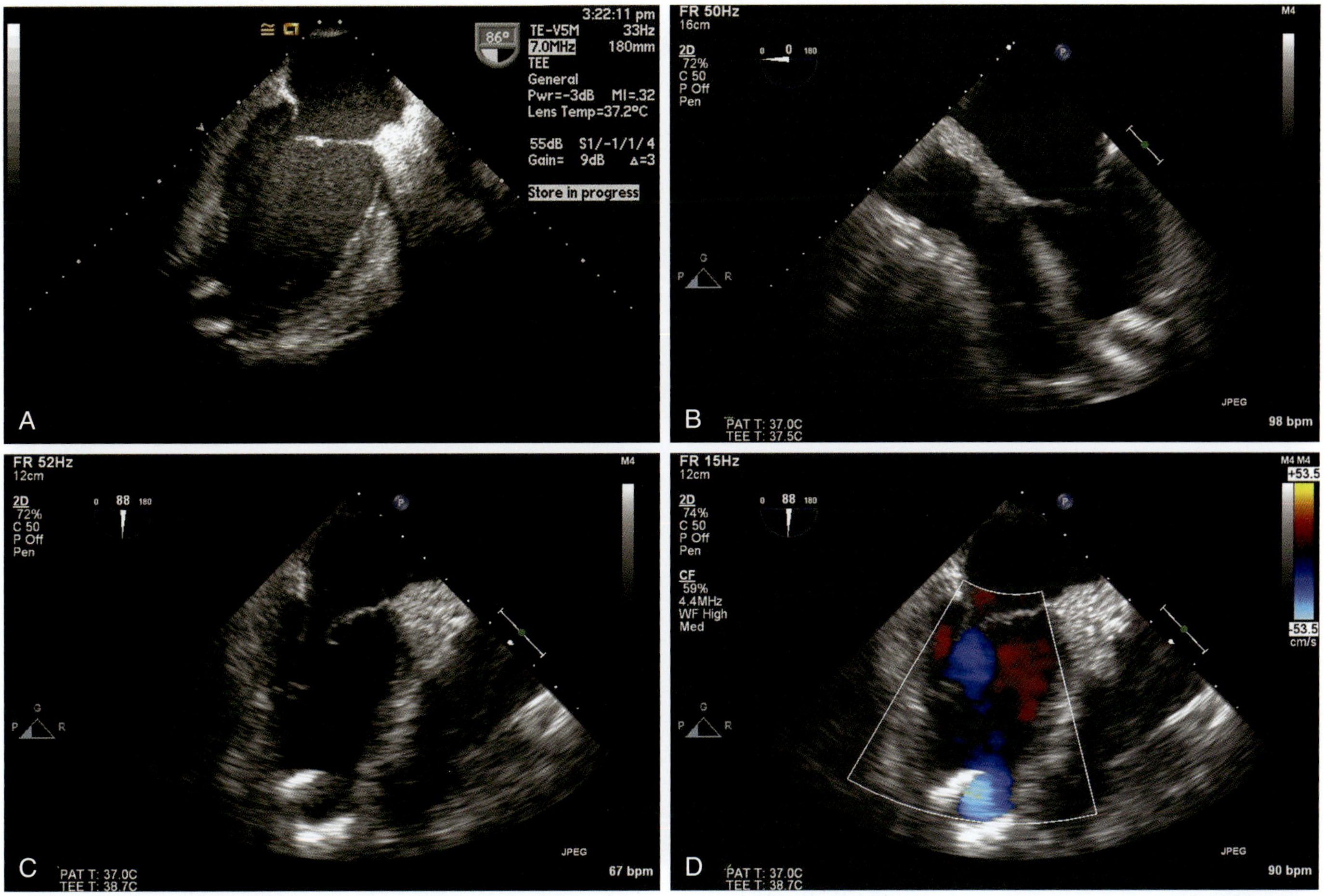

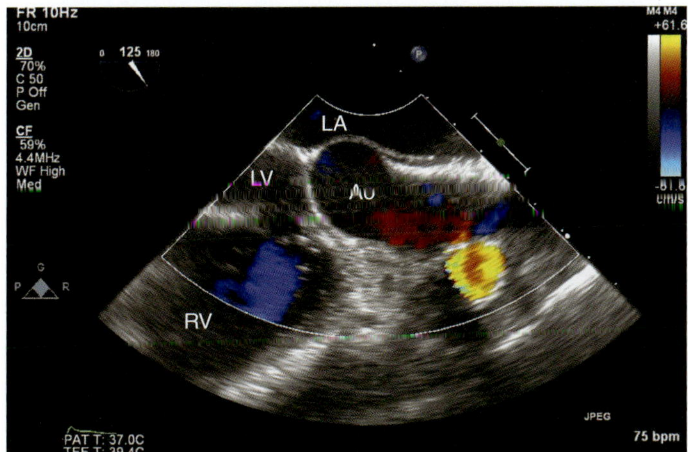

Figure 22-13   **A, B,** and **C,** Left ventricular assist device (LVAD) inflow cannulas. Typical appearance of LVAD inflow cannulas in LV apex. **D,** Unobstructed flow to LVAD inflow cannula by color flow mapping.

Figure 22-14   Left ventricular assist device (LVAD) outflow to ascending aorta. Color flow mapping can sometimes be helpful when exact position of LVAD outflow cannula or conduit is difficult to locate or to help determine whether there is obstruction of outflow. In this patient, LVAD outflow *(yellow)* can be seen within corrugated appearance of outflow conduit as it approaches ascending aorta. *Ao,* Aorta; *LA,* left atrium; *LV,* left ventricle; *RV,* right ventricle.

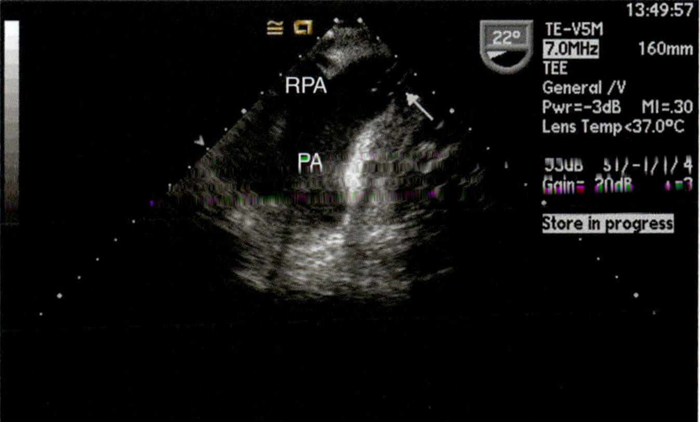

Figure 22-15   Right ventricular assist device outflow cannula is seen in left branch pulmonary artery (PA). *RPA,* Right pulmonary artery.

TABLE 22-2	Role of TEE During Left Ventricular Assist Device Placement		
Role	**Suggested Views**		**Comments**
Factors That May Impair LVAD Filling			
Mitral stenosis	ME four-chamber view ME commisural view ME two-chamber view ME AV LAX view Deep TG view		
Tricuspid regurgitation	ME four-chamber view RV inflow-outflow view Non-standard ME view of TV TG RV inflow view TG SAX view of TV		More than mild TR should be addressed. A non-standard ME view can be helpful when there is significant aortic calcification or lipomatous hypertrophy of interatrial septum.
Significant RV dysfunction	ME four-chamber view ME RV inflow-outflow view TG basal and mid-SAX views with probe rotated to right to focus on RV TG RV inflow view		It should be noted that appearance of RV free wall often has little predictive value with regard to ultimate function of RV once VAD support is engaged. Septal function often allows for RV output.
Factors That May Decrease Efficacy of LVAD Ejection and LV Decompression			
Significant aortic regurgitation	ME AV SAX view ME AV LAX view Deep TG view TG LAX view		
Intracardiac thrombus	ME four-chamber view ME commisural view ME two-chamber view Any multiplane angle that allows visualization of apex Deep TG view TG two-chamber view		Must evaluate multiple views of LV. Thrombus generally forms on akinetic walls and in apex.
Factors That May Cause Complications Once LVAD Is Functioning			
Patent foramen ovale	ME bicaval view (and modifications thereof as necessary to best view anatomy)		
Atrial septal defect	ME four-chamber view ME bicaval view (and modifications thereof as necessary to best view anatomy)		
Ascending and transverse aortic atherosclerosis and mobile plaques	Epiaortic scanning ME AV LAX view ME asc aorta SAX view ME asc aorta LAX view UE aortic arch SAX view UE aortic arch LAX view		
Intracardiac thrombus	ME four-chamber view ME commisural view ME two-chamber view Any multiplane angle that allows visualization of apex Deep TG view TG two-chamber view		Must evaluate multiple views of LV. Thrombus generally forms on akinetic walls and in apex.

asc, Ascending; *AV,* aortic valve; *LAX,* long-axis; *LV,* left ventricle; *ME,* midesophageal; *RV,* right ventricle; *SAX,* short-axis; *TG,* transgastric; *TR,* tricuspid regurgitation; *TV,* tricupid valve; *UE,* upper esophageal.

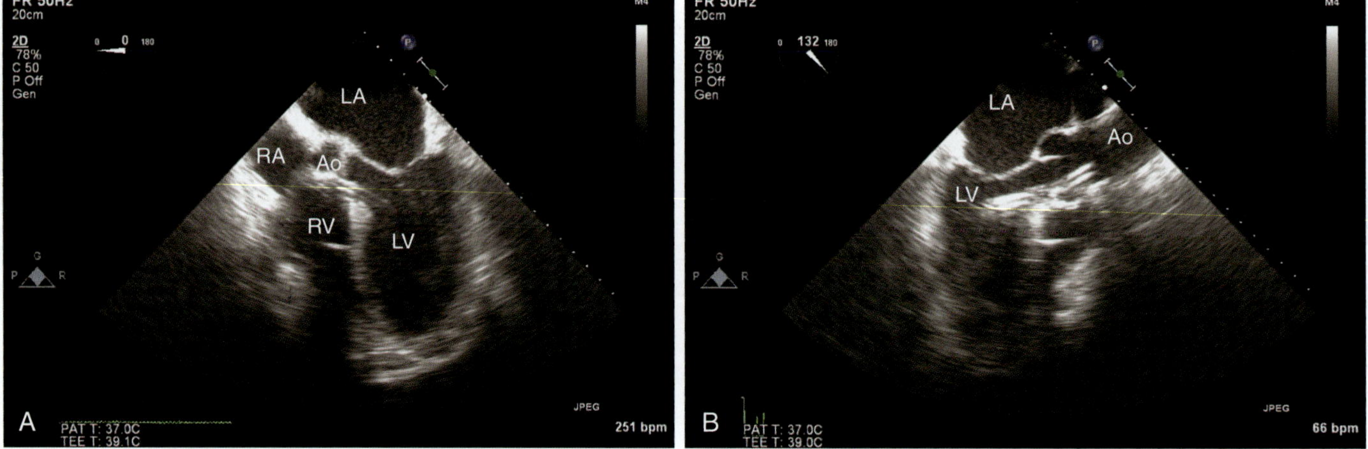

Figure 22-16   An Impella can be seen crossing aortic valve in modified midesophageal (ME) four-chamber **(A)** and ME LAX **(B)** views. Impella LP 2.5 is a miniaturized axial flow device percutaneously placed retrograde across aortic valve. Once support is engaged, 2.5 LPM of flow can be impelled from left ventricle to ascending aorta. *Ao,* Aorta; *LA,* left atrium; *LV,* left ventricle; *RA,* right atrium; *RV,* right ventricle.

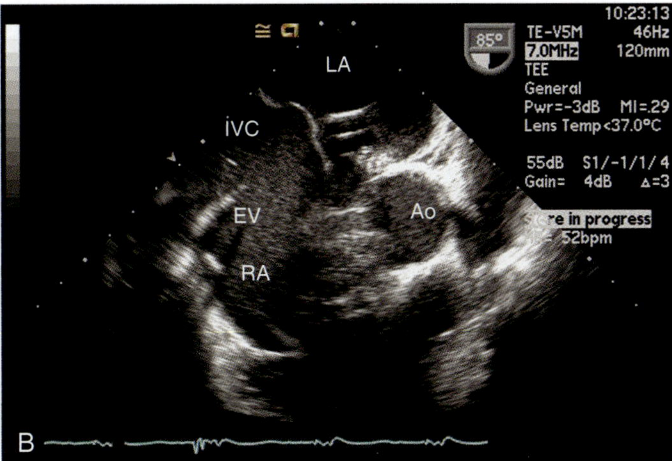

Figure 22-17 Transseptal inflow cannula of a TandemHeart can be seen approaching **(A)** then crossing **(B)** fossa ovalis. TandemHeart is a centrifugal pump that provides left atrial–femoral artery bypass via interatrial septal inflow cannula. *Ao,* Aorta; *EV,* eustachian valve; *IVC,* inferior vena cava; *LA,* left atrium; *RA,* right atrium.

An LA VAD inflow cannula to be placed through an interatrial approach from behind the heart should be evaluated using the ME bicaval and ME four-chamber views to ensure the cannula has not been inadvertently passed through the RA and across the interatrial septum into the LA.

After LVAD Placement

TEE is used to:
- Assess LV filling and function. All ME and TG views of the LV are useful to evaluate LV decompression and apparent recovery. One generally wants to see the interventricular septum in a midline neutral position because an interventricular septum bowing to the left implies underfilling of the LV. The TG basal and mid-SAX views and the ME four-chamber view are helpful in this regard.
- Ensure RV function does not deteriorate. Views in which RV function can be assessed include the ME four chamber view, ME RV inflow-outflow view, TG basal and mid-SAX views with the probe rotated to the right to focus on the RV, and the TG RV inflow view.
- Ensure tricuspid regurgitation does not worsen (or assess the need for a tricuspid valve annuloplasty in retrospect). Views in which tricuspid regurgitation can potentially be evaluated include the ME four-chamber view, RV inflow-outflow view, non-standard ME view of the tricuspid valve, TG RV inflow view, and TG SAX view of the tricuspid valve.
- Reevaluate for patent foramen ovale (must be closed if right to-left shunting is detected). Often the ME bicaval view is most helpful.
- Detect obstruction of inflow or outflow cannulas. The inflow cannula is often best imaged (and interrogated) somewhere between the ME two-chamber view and the ME LAX view. Imaging of the outflow cannula in the ascending aorta generally requires some imagination and a multiplane probe, but often one can locate the cannula in 2D imaging using the ME AV LAX view and the ME ascending aorta LAX views. Color flow mapping of the ascending aorta can also help locate the approximate location of the outflow cannula anastomosis.
- Detect pericardial effusion and/or pericardial tamponade. TG basal and mid-SAX views of the LV are helpful in this regard, as are all ME views of the heart.

Right Ventricular Assist Devices

Patients receiving RVADs require evaluation of the right-sided cardiac structures insofar as there may be interference with VAD function, filling, or emptying.

- The RVAD inflow cannula is most often placed in the RA, and the tip is often advanced into the IVC. One can usually locate the tip of an IVC cannula by starting from the ME bicaval view and following the IVC retrograde by advancing the TEE probe and rotating the probe as needed to keep the IVC in view.
- Pulmonic insufficiency (that will impede effective RVAD emptying to the PA) can be assessed using the UE aortic arch SAX view. The ME ascending aorta SAX view can also be helpful.
- An RVAD outflow cannula cannot always be seen, but the flow from the cannula can usually be detected in the PA using the UE aortic arch SAX view and the ME ascending aorta SAX view.

Pulmonary Artery Catheters

Although the benefit of pulmonary artery catheters (PACs) remains a matter of controversy and debate at the moment and their routine use is waning, PACs are still commonly placed to monitor and assist with the management of patients in the cardiac operating room and intensive care unit. PACs can prove difficult to float in certain circumstances, including when there is significant tricuspid or pulmonic regurgitation, severe tricuspid or pulmonic stenosis, following tricuspid annuloplasty, in the presence of pacing leads, when there is a dilated RA, when there is dilated cardiomyopathy with poor cardiac output, and sometimes in those with anomalies of the RA (e.g., Chiari network).

TEE guidance can facilitate placement of a PAC into the PA, and the tip of the device is easily visualized when the balloon is inflated. One can visualize the entire intended course of the PAC from either the SVC or IVC to either of the branch PAs with the following sequence of TEE views (Fig. 22-18).

The ME bicaval view will allow visualization of the PAC as it enters the RA from either the SVC or IVC and turns toward the tricuspid valve (see Fig. 22-18, *A*). Catheters that do not float easily into the ventricle typically either get stuck in the RAA or traverse the atrium angled toward the septum and enter the IVC (or possibly the CS).[12]

With the balloon inflated, the catheter is advanced to mid-atrium (see Fig. 22-18, *B*), and it is sometimes helpful to rotate the catheter slightly while advancing to make the tip angle into the tricuspid valve. If coiling is noted or if the tip gets stuck in the RAA, one should withdraw the catheter until the tip is noted to be in the middle of the RA. Once withdrawn into the middle of the RA, slight rotation of the catheter and slow advancement under TEE guidance is necessary.

The ME right ventricular inflow-outflow view will allow visualization of the PAC (see Fig. 22-18, *C*) as it enters and traverses the RV and floats across the pulmonic valve into the main PA. Catheters that do not enter the PA can be seen hitting the RV free wall and coiling. Patient, slow advancement with appropriate catheter rotation will

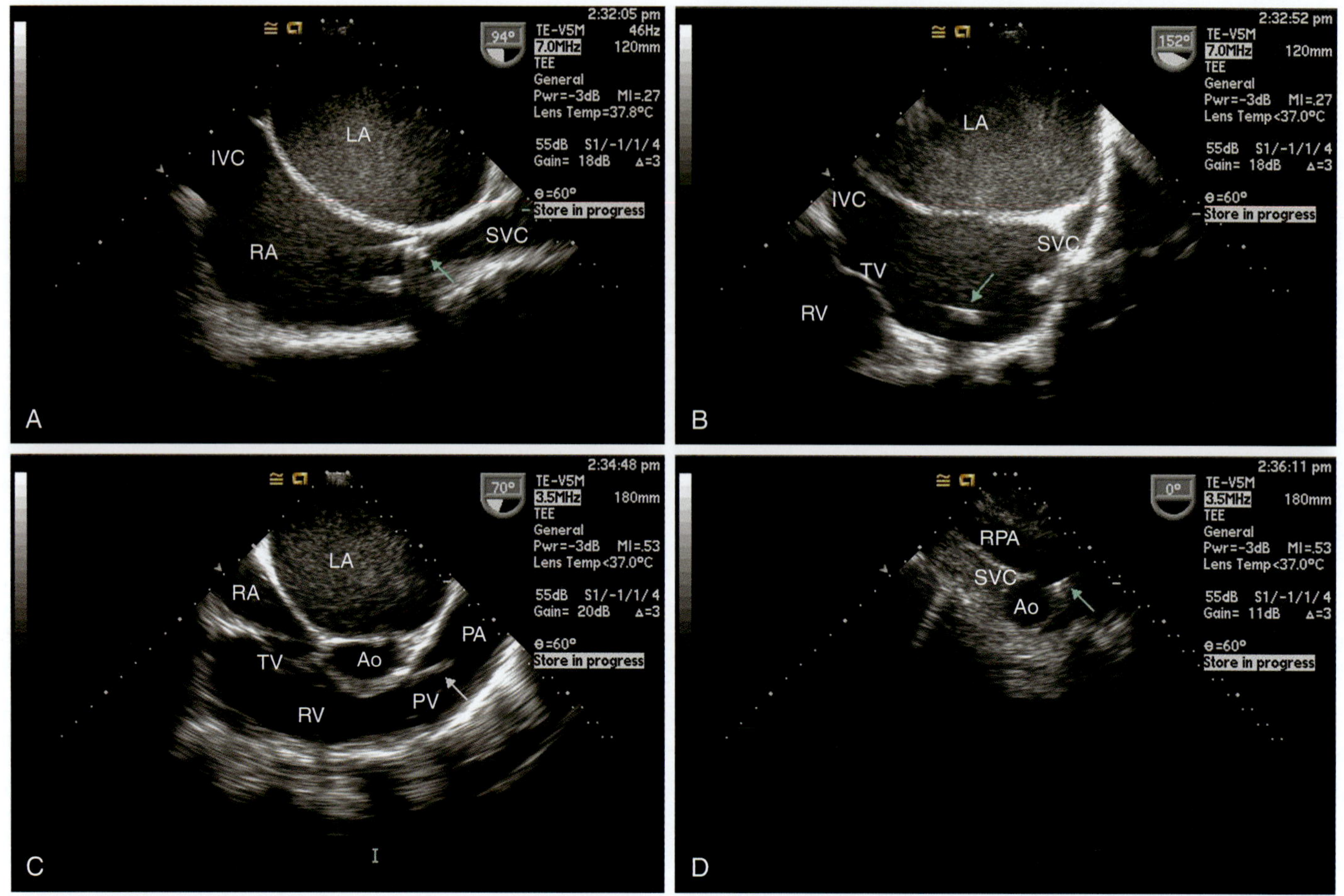

Figure 22-18   **A,** Pulmonary artery (PA) catheter *(arrow)* seen entering right atrium from superior vena cava (SVC) in midesophageal (ME) bicaval view. **B,** PA catheter *(arrow)* approaching tricuspid valve in modified ME bicaval view. **C,** PA catheter *(arrow)* seen coursing through right ventricle (RV) toward pulmonic valve in ME RV inflow-outflow view. **D,** PA catheter *(arrow)* seen at junction of right and left branch PA in ME ascending aorta short-axis view. This view is ideal for positioning tip of PA catheter. *Ao,* Aorta; *IVC,* inferior vena cava; *LA,* left atrium; *PV,* pulmonic valve; *RA,* right atrium; *RV,* right ventricle; *TV,* tricuspid valve.

direct the PAC into the PA. If coiling is noted, one should deflate the balloon and withdraw the catheter until the tip is noted to be in the middle of the RV chamber.

The ME ascending aorta SAX view will allow visualization of the catheter tip as it floats into either the right or left branch PA. Use of this view will also ensure that the PAC is not advanced so far that an increased risk of PA rupture is incurred (see Fig. 22-18, *D*). The ideal maintenance position for a PAC is likely just behind the bifurcation of the main PA in the ME ascending aorta SAX view, but the catheter may have to be advanced slightly to "wedge" it if desired.

REFERENCES

1. Hartman GS, Yao FS, Bruefach M, et al. Severity of aortic atheromatous disease diagnosed by transesophageal echocardiography predicts stroke and other outcomes associated with coronary artery surgery: a prospective study. *Anesth Analg.* 1996;83:701-708.
2. Zingone B, Rauber E, Gatti G, et al. The impact of epiaortic ultrasonographic scanning on the risk of perioperative stroke. *Eur J Cardiothorac Surg.* 2006;29:720-728.
3. Kronzon, Tunick PA, Jortner R, et al. Echocardiographic evaluation of the coronary sinus. *J Am Soc Echocardiogr.* 1995;8:518-526.
4. Plotkin IM, Collard CD, Aranki SF, Rizzo RJ, Shernan SK. Percutaneous coronary sinus cannulation guided by transesophageal echocardiography. *Ann Thorac Surg.* 1998;66:2085-2087.
5. Gonzalez-Juanatey C, Test A, Vidan J, et al. Persistent left superior vena cava draining into the coronary sinus: Report of 10 cases and literature review. *Clin Cardiol.* 2004;27:515-518.
6. Rehfeldt KH, Click RL. Intraoperative transesophageal imaging of an intra-aortic balloon pump placed via the ascending aorta. *J Cardiothorac Vasc Anesth.* 2003;17:736-739.
7. Raman J, Loor G, London M, Jolly N. Subclavian artery access for ambulatory balloon pump insertion. *Ann Thorac Surg.* 2010;90:1032-1034.
8. Krilekval KHV, Mason RA, Newton GB, Angnostopoulous CE, Vlay SC, Giron F. Complications of percutaneous intra-aortic balloon pump use in patients with peripheral vascular disease. *Arch Surg.* 1991;126(5):621-623.
9. Nakatani S, Beppu S, Tanaka N, Andoh M, Miyatake K, Nimura Y. Application of abdominal and transesophageal echocardiography as a guide for insertion of intraaortic balloon pump in aortic dissection. *Am J Cardiol.* 1989;64:1882-1883.
10. Klopman, Matthew A. Positioning an intraaortic balloon pump using intraoperative transesophageal echocardiogram guidance. *Anesth Analg.* July 2011;113(1):40-43.
11. Rastan AJ, Tillmann E, Subramanian S, et al. Visceral arterial compromise during intra-aortic balloon counterpulsation therapy. *Circulation.* 2010;122:s92-s99.
12. Matyal R, Mahmood F, Panzica P, et al. Inadvertent placement of a flow-directed pulmonary artery catheter in the coronary sinus, detected by transesophageal echocardiography. *Anesth Analg.* 2006;102:363-365.

23

Echocardiographic Evaluation of Pericardial Disease

JOHN C. KLICK | JAFER ALI | EDWIN G. AVERY IV

Pericardial Anatomy and Physiology

Pericardial Anatomy

The simplest description of the pericardium is that of a bilayered sack surrounding the heart, its appendages, and its proximal vascular connections. The pericardium measures roughly 2 mm in thickness, and its two layers are separated by a potential space containing 5 to 50 mL of fluid under normal physiologic conditions. The translucent visceral pericardium comprises the inner layer and is in direct continuity with the epicardium at its basal lamina. The opaque thicker outer layer is termed the *parietal pericardium*. The two layers fuse together at various points where they form reflections that give rise to the pericardial space and the two pericardial sinuses. Pericardial reflections surrounding the venae cavae and pulmonary veins give rise to the oblique sinus, and the transverse sinus is formed by pericardial reflections around the proximal portions of the pulmonary artery and ascending aorta (Fig. 23-1). The transverse pericardial sinus is frequently imaged with transesophageal echocardiography (TEE) in the midesophageal long-axis view (Fig. 23-2).[1,2]

Each pericardial layer is composed of loose connective tissue and an interdigitated monolayer of serosal mesothelial cells, all of which have characteristic microvillous projections. The pericardial connective tissue contains nerves, arteries, lymph nodes, and lymphatics. The same

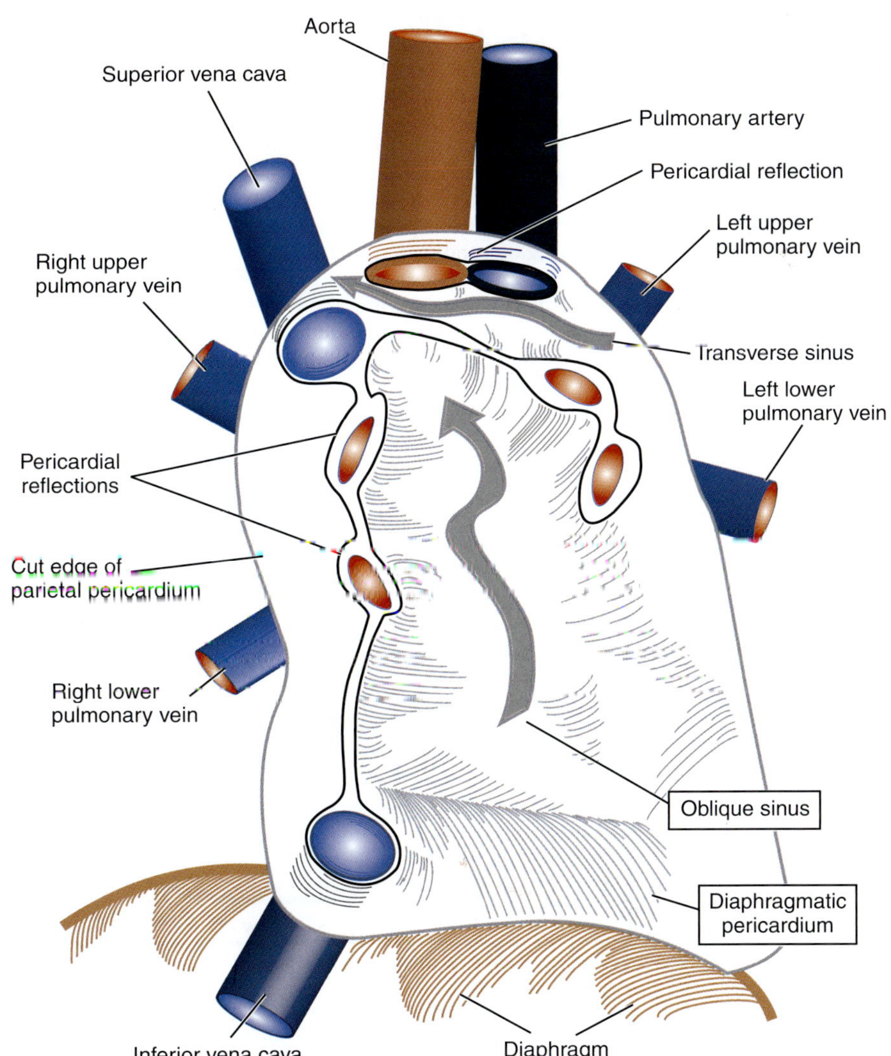

Figure 23-1 Schematic showing how visceral and parietal pericardial tissues meet to create reflections that give rise to pericardial space and two pericardial sinuses (*wide gray arrows*). (*From Savage RM, Aronson S. Comprehensive Textbook of Perioperative Transesophageal Echocardiography. Philadelphia: Lippincott Williams & Wilkins; 2010.*)

mesothelial layer that is a portion of the visceral pericardium is continuous with the parietal pericardium. However, the parietal pericardium is distinct in that its outer covering contains the fibrosa, a grouping of fibrocollagenous tissue lending thickness, increased density, and strength to the pericardium (Fig. 23-3). The microvilli-lined mesothelial cells produce a plasma ultrafiltrate that is the pericardial fluid.[1,2]

Pericardial Microphysiology

The exact microphysiologic function of the pericardium remains to be fully elucidated. The mesothelial microvilli produce the pericardial fluid and are also thought to contribute to regulating epicardial coronary vascular tone via the secretion of certain biochemical mediators such as prostacyclin. Other biochemical mediators secreted into the pericardial fluid serve a fibrinolytic function to limit clotting of any

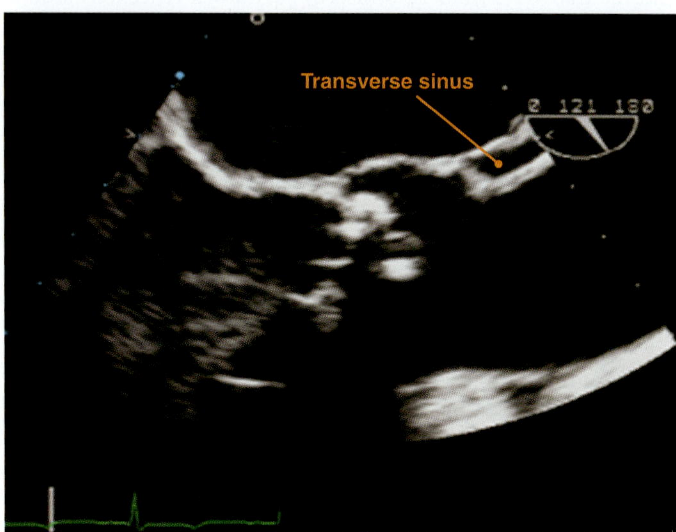

Figure 23-2   Transesophageal echocardiographic image obtained in midesophageal long-axis view. Orange marker indicates echolucency representing a small amount of pericardial fluid within transverse sinus just posterior to proximal ascending aorta. *(From Savage RM, Aronson S. Comprehensive Textbook of Perioperative Transesophageal Echocardiography. Philadelphia: Lippincott Williams & Wilkins; 2010.)*

blood that enters the pericardial space; yet other mediators may affect myocardial contractility.

Reorganization and hypertrophy of mesothelial cells permits slow accumulation of a relatively large volume of fluid in the pericardial space. However, rapid accumulation of fluid on the order of minutes or hours to days does not allow adequate time for mesothelial reorganization, and tamponade physiology may occur in this clinical scenario. Pressure-volume curves with a characteristic "J" shape can be used to characterize both acute and chronic accumulation of pericardial fluid (Fig. 23-4).[3]

Pericardial Macrophysiology

The parietal pericardium is believed to contribute to maintaining the characteristic heart-shaped morphology of the organ. In individuals whose hearts have undergone pericardiectomy or pericardiotomy, the organ is commonly observed to assume a more globular shape, although cardiac function does not appear to change grossly in such individuals. Further, a number of tendinous intersections arise from the parietal pericardium that attach at various points within the mediastinum and serve to stabilize the heart in the chest during various movements of the body. The central tendon of the diaphragm coalesces with the diaphragmatic parietal pericardium to contribute to anchoring the organ in the mediastinum (see Fig. 23-1).[1,2]

Introducing and understanding the concept of respirophasic variation is a prerequisite to understanding how echocardiography can be used to evaluate pericardial physiology. *Respirophasic variation* is the term used to describe changes in blood flow within the heart in relation to pressure dynamics in the intrapleural and intrapericardial cavities. During normal spontaneous respiration, changes in intrapleural pressures are nearly equally transmitted to the pericardial space and intracardiac chambers; thus, the pericardial pressure typically approximates the intrapleural pressure and will vary with the respiratory cycle. Pericardial pressures are typically about −6 mmHg at end-inspiration and −3 mmHg at end-expiration. During spontaneous inspiration, it is the lowering of intrathoracic and pericardial pressures that augments venous return and allows increased filling of the right-sided chambers. Transmural pressure determines the true filling pressure of the heart and is calculated by subtracting the pericardial pressure from the intracardiac pressure (Fig. 23-5, *A*). Negative inspiratory intrapleural pressure also causes blood pooling in the lower-compliance pulmonary venous circulation, which in turn causes a reduction in left atrial (LA)

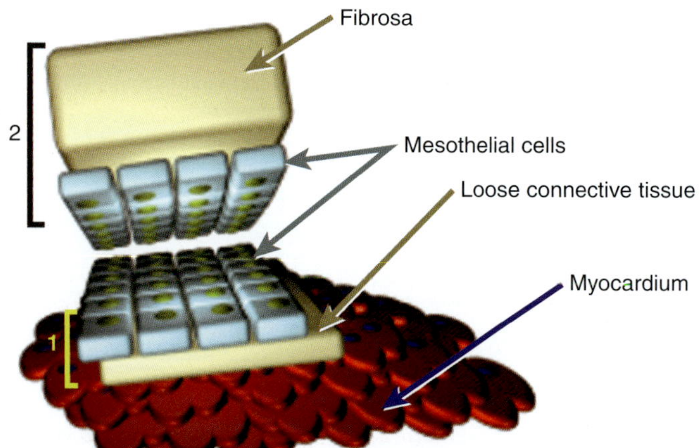

Figure 23-3   Schematic of gross composition and relationship of *1,* visceral pericardial *(yellow bracket)* and *2,* parietal pericardial *(black bracket)* tissues. Parietal pericardium is notably thicker owing to presence of fibrosa. *(From Savage RM, Aronson S. Comprehensive Textbook of Perioperative Transesophageal Echocardiography. Philadelphia: Lippincott Williams & Wilkins; 2010.)*

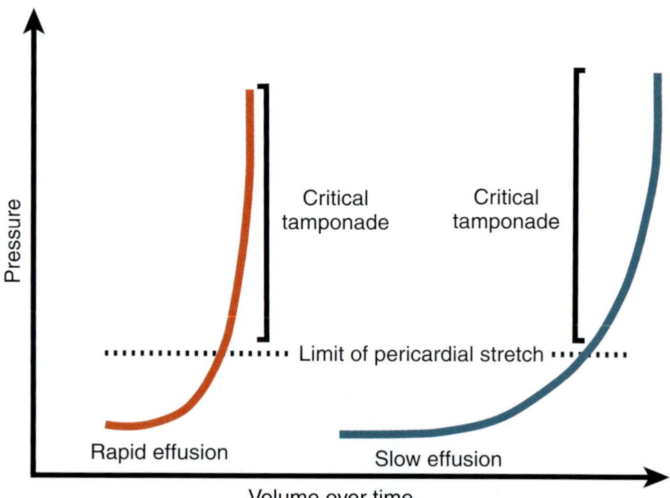

Figure 23-4   "J-shaped" pressure-volume curves represent temporal relationship between rapidly *(red line)* and slowly *(blue line)* accumulating pericardial fluid and accompanying simultaneous changes in developed intrapericardial pressure. *(From Spodick DH. Acute cardiac tamponade. N Engl J Med. 2003;349:684-690.)*

True RA Filling Pressure = RAP – Pericardial Pressure
(at end-inspiration)

RAP = 5 mmHg (directly measured)
Pericardial Pressure $\cong$ Intrapleural Pressure = -8 cm H_2O
X cm H_2O / 1.36 = mmHg   (allows conversion of cm H_2O to mmHg)

$$= 5\ mmHg\ -\ (-8\ cm\ H_2O = -6\ mmHg)$$
$$= 5\ mmHg\ -\ (-6\ mmHg)$$

A True RA Filling Pressure = 11 mmHg

True LV Afterload = DBP – Pericardial Pressure
(at end-inspiration)

DBP = 90 mmHg (directly measured)
Pericardial Pressure $\cong$ Intrapleural Pressure = -8 cm H_2O
X cm H_2O / 1.36 = mmHg   (allows conversion of cm H_2O to mmHg)

$$= 90\ mmHg\ -\ (-8\ cm\ H_2O\ /\ 1.36\ = -6\ mmHg)$$
$$= 90\ mmHg\ -\ (-6\ mmHg)$$

B True LV Afterload = 96 mmHg

Figure 23-5   Sample calculations that permit determination of **(A)** true filling pressure of right heart and **(B)** true left ventricular afterload. *(From Savage RM, Aronson S. Comprehensive Textbook of Perioperative Transesophageal Echocardiography. Philadelphia: Lippincott Williams & Wilkins; 2010.)*

filling. The decrease in LA venous return causes a drop in both left ventricular (LV) stroke volume and cardiac output. In addition, the drop in intrathoracic pressure during spontaneous inspiration in relation to the higher extrathoracic systemic arterial pressures results in a reduction of left heart output due to a relatively higher afterload secondary to the negative intrapleural pressure (Fig. 23-5, *B*). Changes in systemic vascular resistance are the primary determinants of LV afterload, but the relative differences between intrapericardial and intrathoracic pressures do affect this parameter. Respiratory cycle–related intrapericardial pressure dynamics are reflected in Doppler assessments of changes of the transatrioventricular valvular velocities. During the inspiratory phase of spontaneous respiration, transtricuspid velocities typically increase by 20% (Fig. 23-6, *A*). Conversely, transmitral velocities typically decrease by roughly 10% during spontaneous inspiration (Fig. 23-6, *B*).

Opposite changes in these transvalvular velocities are produced by the use of intermittent positive pressure ventilation (IPPV). The increased pericardial pressure that accompanies IPPV results in a decrease in both right heart filling and output which is reflected in the observed decreased transtricuspid diastolic velocities. The magnitude of the relative decrease in transtricuspid velocities during IPPV will depend on the amount of positive pressure transmitted to the right heart as well as the intravascular volume status (Fig. 23-6, *C*). The rise in intrathoracic pressure in relation to extrathoracic systemic pressure during IPPV inspiration leads to an increase in left heart output. In addition, increased intrathoracic pressure during IPPV propels blood from the lower-compliance pulmonary veins into the LA and LV, boosting left heart output. The increase in left heart inflow is manifested as an observed increase of approximately 30% in transmitral

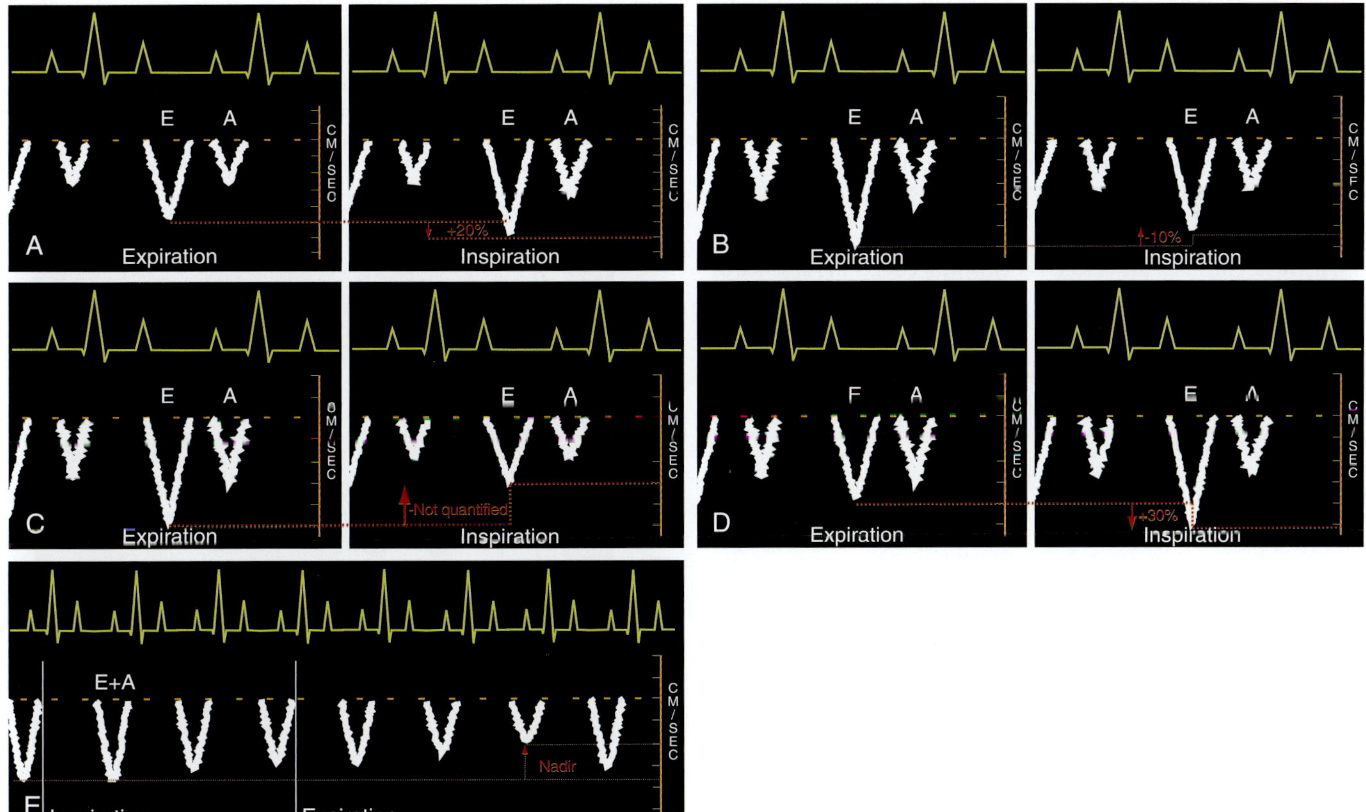

Figure 23-6   Idealized transesophageal echocardiographic imaging of transtricuspid pulsed wave Doppler (PWD) profiles during **(A)** spontaneous respiration and **(C)** intermittent positive pressure ventilation (IPPV). Idealized transmitral PWD tracings are also presented for **(B)** spontaneous respiration, **(D)** IPPV, and **(E)** intermittent positive pressure in a hypovolemic patient. *A,* Late diastolic filling associated with atrial contraction; *E,* early diastolic ventricular filing; *E+A,* fused waveforms of the early (*E*) and late (*A*) diastolic filling velocities. *(From Savage RM, Aronson S. Comprehensive Textbook of Perioperative Transesophageal Echocardiography. Philadelphia: Lippincott Williams & Wilkins; 2010.)*

valvular velocities (Fig. 23-6, *D*). An alternative pattern of transmitral flow has been observed in a canine model that is characterized by a decrease in transmitral flow velocities, which reach the nadir during expiration (Fig. 23-6, *E*). The authors of this work attributed these unexpected findings to a significant degree of intravascular depletion. *Respirophasic variation* is the term used to describe these changes in transatrioventricular valvular velocities.[1,4]

Physiologic variables such as age, heart rate, rhythm, preload, volume flow rate, ventricular systolic function, diastolic function, and atrial contractility all contribute to the observed velocities. Certain pericardial pathologies may blunt transmission of intrathoracic pressures to intrapericardial structures (e.g., pericarditis or pericardial tamponade), leading to reduced transatrioventricular velocities that are often observed under these clinical conditions.[1,2,4]

Pericardial Pathology

Evaluation of pericardial disease is performed with echocardiography to rule out specific pathologies that can directly impact myocardial function. A multiwindow, multiplane TEE or transthoracic echocardiographic (TTE) examination is necessary to thoroughly evaluate the pericardium. Box 23-1 presents the five basic categories of pericardial pathology.[1]

Congenital Pericardial Defects

Congenital pericardial defects are exceedingly rare and may consist of partial or total absence of the pericardium.[5,6] However, Mulibrey nanism, an autosomal recessive disorder primarily found in the Finnish population, is a congenital pericardial disorder that does not involve any degree of pericardial absence. Instead, it is partially characterized by development of constrictive pericarditis (CP) in later life among some afflicted patients. If the degree of CP becomes significant, these individuals can present with diastolic heart failure. CP is discussed in a later section.[7]

Most patients with any degree of pericardial absence are clinically asymptomatic (Table 23-1).[8] One small observational study found that paroxysmal stabbing chest pain that mimicked coronary ischemia was the most common clinical presentation. The putative mechanism for the observed chest pain is a temporary kinking and obstruction of coronary vessels local to the pericardial defect as a portion of the myocardium herniates through the defect. Patients with congenital absence of

the pericardium are at increased risk for additional congenital abnormalities in that up to 30% of these patients will have other pathology (e.g., septal defects).[9]

Using echocardiography, the most common findings associated with partial pericardial absence are cardiac hypermobility, paradoxical motion or flattening of the ventricular septum during systole, an exaggerated posterior LV wall, and the possible appearance of a dilated right ventricle (RV) together with a reduced dimension of the right atrium (RA). Cardiac magnetic resonance imaging (MRI), computed tomography (CT), and plain chest films (to a lesser extent) are the imaging modalities most useful in making the definitive diagnosis of congenital absence of the pericardium (Fig. 23-7). Electrocardiographic (ECG) findings in these patients may include bradycardia, right bundle branch block, poor R-wave progression in the precordial transition leads, and prominent P waves in the mid-precordial leads.[9]

Pericarditis

Pericarditis refers to inflammation of the pericardium due to various pathologies. It may present as either an acute or chronic process and is often associated with development of a pericardial effusion. Acute pericarditis may progress to chronic CP, which may induce severe diastolic dysfunction. The classic clinical triad of pericarditis consists of chest pain, diffuse ST-segment elevations on ECG, and a pericardial rub on auscultation. Table 23-2 lists the various clinical etiologies of pericarditis.[8]

Echocardiographically, the pericardium is inspected for any evidence of thickening. This typically appears as an increase in brightness (echogenicity) of the ultrasound signal. Normal pericardial thickness is approximately 2 to 3 mm. M-mode may prove useful to discern and quantify any degree of pericardial thickening; it reveals multiple parallel ultrasound reflections (Fig. 23-8). Multiple echo windows must be obtained to verify the diffuse or localized nature of pericarditis. Unfortunately, echocardiography lacks adequate fidelity to consistently quantify the degree and anatomic extent of pericarditis and thus has inadequate sensitivity and specificity for detecting the disorder when compared to other higher-fidelity imaging modalities (e.g., cardiac MRI, 64-slice CT). Figure 23-9 presents an MRI image of focally thickened pericardium.

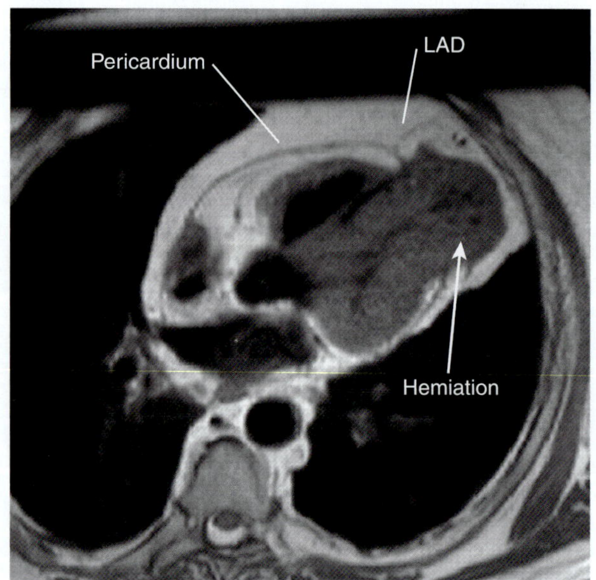

Figure 23-7   Cardiac magnetic resonance image showing herniation of ventricular myocardium *(arrow)*. *LAD*, Left anterior descending coronary artery. *(From Chassaing S, Bensouda C, Bar O, et al. A case of partial congenital absence of pericardium revealed by MRI. Circ Cardiovasc Imaging. 2010;3:632-634.)*

BOX 23-1.   GENERAL CATEGORIES OF PERICARDIAL PATHOLOGY

Congenital pericardial defects
Pericarditis
Pericardial effusion
Pericardial tamponade
Pericardial masses

TABLE 23-1	Pathologic Characteristics of Forms of Pericardial Absence	
Form	*Incidence**	*Clinical Significance*
Total bilateral absence	Rare	Mostly asymptomatic
Partial left absence	70%	Increased risk for aortic dissection if augmented heart mobility; possible herniation/strangulation of heart structures through defect, with chest pain, shortness of breath, syncope
Partial right absence	17%	Increased risk for aortic dissection if augmented mobility as a result of defect
Overall	0.01%	

*Incidence values represent a percentage of the overall incidence of 0.01%.

Pericardial Effusion and Tamponade

A *pericardial effusion* is a collection of fluid within the pericardial sac. It can be either diffusely distributed or localized (i.e., loculated) within the pericardial space. Different patterns of fluid distribution may be seen depending on patient position and fluid volume within the space. Echocardiographically, the effusion appears as an echolucent signal immediately adjacent to the epicardium. Table 23-3 presents general guidelines on pericardial effusion size and fluid distribution patterns.[8] Epicardial fat may appear similar to a pericardial fluid collection. Close observation of epicardial fat demonstrates a weak echogenic signal compared to the more echolucent signal of a pericardial fluid collection. Figure 23-10, *A* presents a gross surgical image of epicardial fat, and Figure 23-10, *B* presents its corresponding appearance with TEE.

The clinical significance of a pericardial effusion is in direct proportion to the amount of fluid in the pericardial space and the time course over which it accumulates. Large chronic effusions are frequently associated with the "swinging heart" clinical scenario, characterized by excessive anteroposterior motion of the heart along with counterclockwise rotation in the horizontal plane. This motion of the heart within the pericardial space creates the ECG finding of *electrical alternans* (Fig. 23-11), seen on the ECG as repetitive alternating heights of the QRS complex that may also involve the P, T, and U waves as well as the ST segments. It is important to note that this finding is not specific to pericardial effusions.[10]

In the postoperative cardiac surgical population, the presence of a pericardial effusion is extremely common (85%), and the incidence generally peaks by the tenth postoperative day.[11] The clinical implications of a postoperative pericardial effusion relate to the volume of fluid that accumulates and the rate at which it accumulates (Fig. 23-12).[8] Rapid accumulation of fluid in the pericardial space leads to an acute rise in pressure within the space, which may eventually reach a point where the intrapericardial pressure exceeds cardiac chamber pressure(s).

Tamponade physiology results when intrapericardial pressure has increased to the point where it compromises cardiac chamber filling; at this point, the patient manifests the clinical finding of *pericardial tamponade*. Accumulation of pericardial fluid may result in an extreme rise in intrapericardial pressure that is accompanied by *ventricular interdependence*, a clinical phenomenon characterized by respiratory cycle–related alternating left and right heart pressures related to extreme shifting of the interventricular septum.[12] Right heart filling is augmented in a spontaneously breathing patient during inspiration; as the RV fills during diastole, the interventricular septum will shift toward the LV, resulting in compromised LV filling and a decrease in LV and cardiac output along with a decrease in systemic blood pressure

TABLE 23-2	Clinical Disorders Related to Development of Pericarditis	
Category	**Detailed Causes**	
Immune/inflammation related	Rheumatoid arthritis, systemic lupus erythematosus, acute rheumatic fever, dermatomyositis, Wegener granulomatosis, mixed collagen vascular disease, post myocardial infarction (Dressler syndrome), uremia, post cardiac surgery (inflammation related)	
Infection related	Bacterial infections (e.g., tuberculosis), post viral	
Neoplasm related	Primary mesothelioma, fibrosarcoma, secondary metastatic disease (e.g., melanoma, lymphoma, leukemia, or direct extension of pulmonic or breast tumor)	
Intracardiac/ pericardial communication related	Chest trauma, post percutaneous catheter interventional procedures (e.g., cardiac valve replacement or valvulopathy, coronary interventions, arrhythmia-related procedures)	

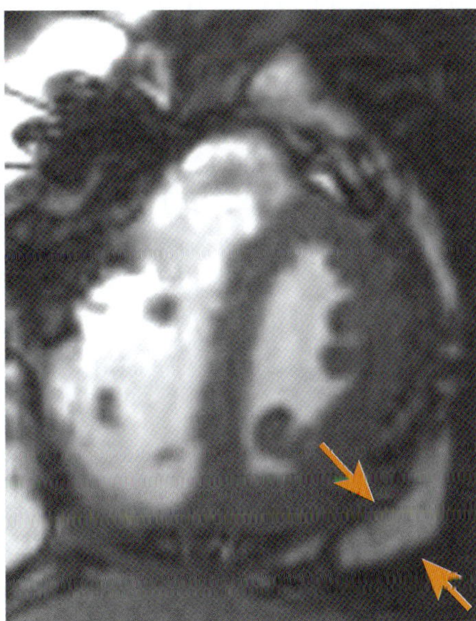

Figure 23-9 Cardiac magnetic resonance image of apparent focally thickened pericardium between orange arrowheads. (*From Savage RM, Aronson S. Comprehensive Textbook of Perioperative Transesophageal Echocardiography. Philadelphia: Lippincott Williams & Wilkins; 2010.*)

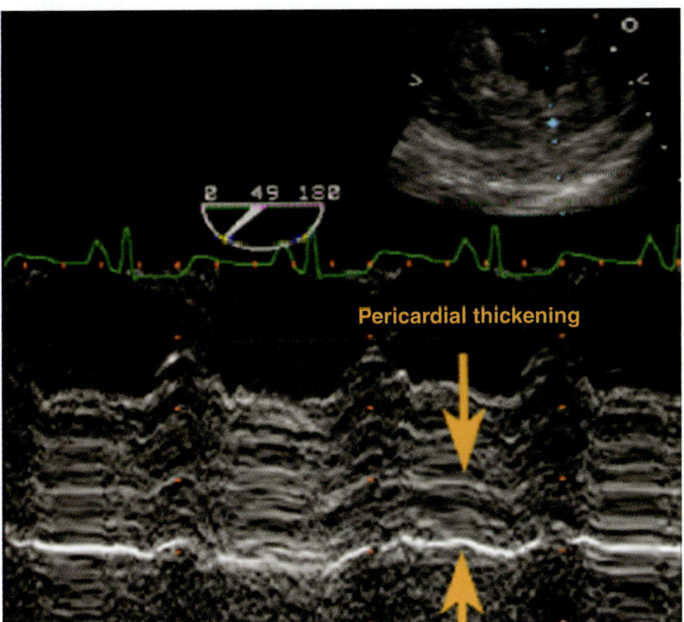

Figure 23-8 Transesophageal echocardiographic image, transgastric short-axis view using M-mode. Severely thickened pericardium is denoted between orange arrowheads. (*From Savage RM, Aronson S. Comprehensive Textbook of Perioperative Transesophageal Echocardiography. Philadelphia: Lippincott Williams & Wilkins; 2010.*)

TABLE 23-3	Pericardial Effusion Characteristics		
Severity	**Width by Echo**	**Volume (mL)**	**Localization Region**
Small	<5 mm	<100	Behind posterior left ventricle wall
Moderate	5-20 mm	100-150	Expand laterally and apically
Large	>20 mm	>500	Evenly distributed around heart

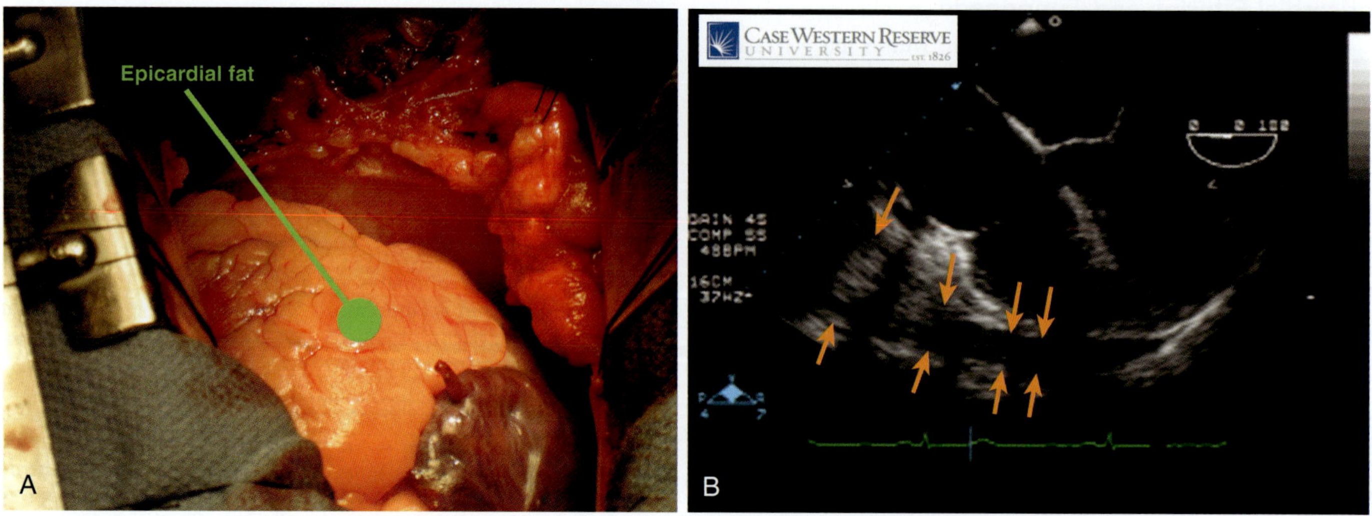

Figure 23-10   **A,** Gross surgical image showing parietal pericardium incised and retracted so apparent epicardial fat *(green marker)* enclosed within visceral pericardium is visible. **B,** Transesophageal echocardiographic midesophageal four-chamber image (same patient) reveals weak echogenic signal of epicardial fat between orange arrowheads. *(From Savage RM, Aronson S. Comprehensive Textbook of Perioperative Transesophageal Echocardiography. Philadelphia: Lippincott Williams & Wilkins; 2010.)*

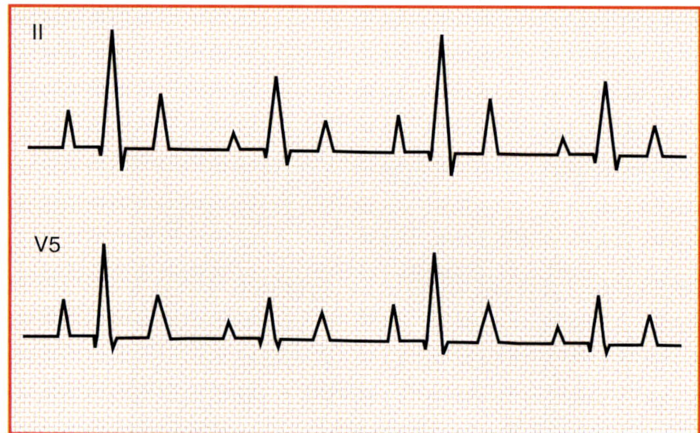

Figure 23-11   Idealized electrocardiogram of clinical finding of electrical alternans that may accompany a large pericardial effusion or cardiac tamponade. *(From Savage RM, Aronson S. Comprehensive Textbook of Perioperative Transesophageal Echocardiography. Philadelphia: Lippincott Williams & Wilkins; 2010.)*

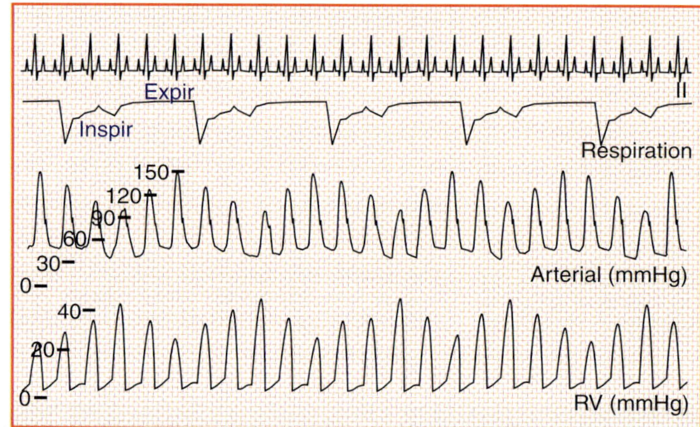

Figure 23-13   Electrocardiogram, respiratory cycle, and associated hemodynamic tracings in patient with pericardial tamponade, demonstrating ventricular interdependence as arterial pressure decreases during inspiration (pulsus paradoxus) while corresponding right ventricular pressure increases as interventricular septum shifts toward the left. *Expir,* Expiration during spontaneous respiration; *Inspir,* inspiration during spontaneous respiration; *RV,* right ventricular (pressure). *(From Savage RM, Aronson S. Comprehensive Textbook of Perioperative Transesophageal Echocardiography. Philadelphia: Lippincott Williams & Wilkins; 2010.)*

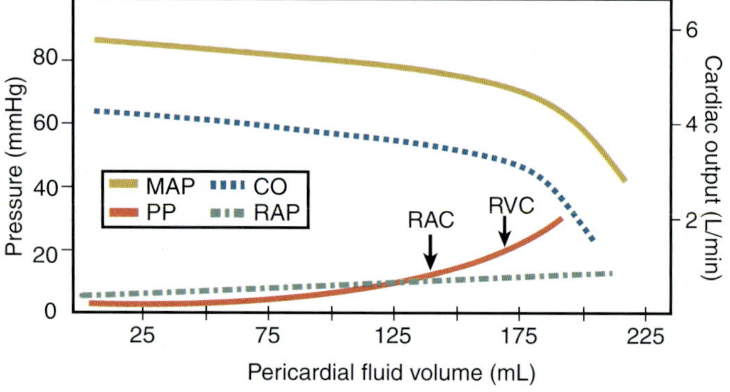

Figure 23-12   Relationship between acute accumulation of pericardial fluid and progressive development of pericardial tamponade with cardiovascular collapse. *CO,* Cardiac output; *MAP,* mean arterial pressure; *PP,* pericardial pressure; *RAC,* right atrial collapse; *RAP,* right atrial pressure; *RVC,* right ventricular collapse. *(From Savage RM, Aronson S. Comprehensive Textbook of Perioperative Transesophageal Echocardiography. Philadelphia: Lippincott Williams & Wilkins; 2010.)*

(Fig. 23-13).[12] Concurrent with the increase in right heart filling during spontaneous inspiration is a transient increase in RV pressures. Loss of the y-descent in the RA pressure tracing is also characteristic of tamponade.

It must be noted that the pericardium is highly adaptive to very slow accumulation of pericardial fluid (see Fig. 23-4).[3] Pericardial mesothelial cells have the capability to hypertrophy, thus allowing accommodation of greater amounts of pericardial fluid over time, provided the rate of accumulation is slow enough for this adaptation to occur.

With tamponade physiology, pericardial pressure exceeds cardiac chamber pressure, resulting in collapse of the chambers and ultimately total cardiovascular collapse when the cardiac output is interrupted. The lower pressure chambers, such as the RA during systole, will be affected first, eventually followed by the other cardiac chambers if the pericardial pressure continues to climb (see Fig. 23-12). In fully

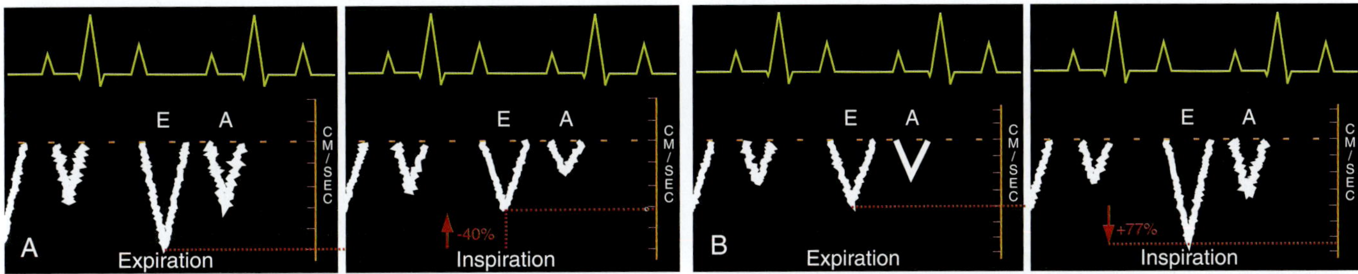

Figure 23-14   Transesophageal echocardiographic images showing (**A**) transgastric short-axis view of hemopericardium and (**B**) midesophageal four-chamber view of hemopericardium with hostile biatrial compression. Orange arrows depict clot in each image; left and right atria are the small echolucent slits at end of round green markers in **B**. *LA*, Left atrium; *LV*, left ventricle; *RA*, right atrium. (*A from Savage RM, Aronson S. Comprehensive Textbook of Perioperative Transesophageal Echocardiography. Philadelphia: Lippincott Williams & Wilkins; 2010.*)

Figure 23-15   A, Idealized pulsed wave transmitral Doppler tracing in spontaneously breathing patient with pericardial tamponade. B, Simultaneously observed transtricuspid Doppler tracings in same patient. A, Late diastolic filling associated with atrial contraction; E, early diastolic ventricular filling. (*From Savage RM, Aronson S. Comprehensive Textbook of Perioperative Transesophageal Echocardiography. Philadelphia: Lippincott Williams & Wilkins; 2010.*)

developed pericardial tamponade, all four cardiac chambers will have elevated and equal diastolic pressures. In the cardiac surgical population, loculated effusions can create tamponade physiology with a significantly smaller volume of fluid than a diffuse effusion if the fluid collection is strategically located near a low-pressure cardiac chamber such as the LA or RA. Solid matter such as a clot or a tumor in the pericardial space may also elicit tamponade physiology. Examination with two-dimensional (2D) echocardiography must incorporate multiple windows to rule out the presence of one or more loculations within the pericardial space.

Echocardiographic findings associated with pericardial effusions include:

- An echolucent signal of variable width (see Table 23-3) adjacent to the pericardium. The echolucent signal can brighten if the pericardial space contains clotted blood (as may be seen with hemopericardium). Figure 23-14, *A* presents a TEE image of a postoperative cardiac surgical patient with a large collection of thrombus in the pericardial space adjacent to the LV lateral wall. Figure 23-14, *B* presents another example of early postoperative hemopericardium that is remarkable for hostile biatrial compression.
- In patients with longstanding pericardial disease, fibrinous stranding  within the pericardial fluid may be seen (Video 23-1).
- Regional septal wall motion abnormalities
- Mitral and tricuspid valve prolapse
- Systolic anterior motion (SAM) of the anterior mitral leaflet
- Early systolic closure of the aortic valve
- Mid-systolic notching (partial closure) of either the aortic valve or pulmonic valve

When pericardial effusions have grown to the point of causing tamponade physiology, the following host of echocardiographic findings can be observed:

- Systolic collapse or inversion of the RA. Inversion for greater than one third of systole has a 94% sensitivity and 100% specificity for tamponade (Video 23-2).
- RV diastolic collapse has a sensitivity of 60% to 90% and a specificity of 85% to 100% for the diagnosis of tamponade (Video 23-3).
- Reciprocal respiratory changes in RV and LV volumes may occur. During spontaneous inspiration, the increase in RV volume causes a shift of the interventricular septum toward the LV in diastole. The reverse occurs during expiration, resulting in the phenomenon of *pulsus paradoxus* (see Fig. 23-13) on the arterial pressure waveform.
- Plethora of the inferior vena cava (IVC) may be observed in which the IVC appears dilated with less than 50% reduction in diameter near the IVC-RA junction during inspiration. This has a 97% sensitivity for tamponade but is relatively nonspecific.[5]

In the spontaneously breathing patient, Doppler echocardiography can also provide useful information to confirm the diagnosis of pericardial tamponade. As discussed, during spontaneous inspiration, the normal transmitral valve Doppler profile shows a decrease in the velocity of transmitral flow (see Fig. 23-6, *B*). This decrease is exaggerated in severe tamponade and can be as much as 37% (Fig. 23-15, *A*). Although an increase in transtricuspid valve velocities on the order of approximately 20% is expected during spontaneous respiration, one can anticipate observing an increase of up to 77% with tamponade physiology (Fig. 23-15, *B*).[13] During the tamponade state, the heart is insulated by the collected fluid or clot in the pericardial space from the intrathoracic pressure changes normally associated with the respiratory cycle. This insulation of the heart from intrapleural pressures results in accentuation of normal respirophasic variation during spontaneous respiration, along with reduction in the absolute magnitude of the transatrioventricular valvular velocities. In effect, the large effusion insulating the heart from intrapleural pressures creates a gradient between the intrapleural chest cavity and the heart that results in a gradient manifested by more dramatic changes in flow during the respiratory cycle. Video 23-4 demonstrates how RV filling is augmented during the inspiratory phase of spontaneous respiration in a patient with tamponade; the interventricular septum is noted to shift to the left and encroach upon LV filling.

As noted earlier, under normal physiologic conditions, transmitral valve velocities are characterized by an increase in flow velocity during IPPV (see Fig. 23-6, D). Because the left heart is more anatomically isolated from exposure to intrapleural pressure, the magnitude of observed respirophasic variation is smaller than observed in the right heart. The exaggerated respirophasic variation in transatrioventricular velocities seen during tamponade when spontaneously breathing is no longer seen during IPPV (Fig. 23-16). However, there will still be an overall decrease in the magnitude of flow velocities during mechanical ventilation when compared to patients without tamponade, similar to the pattern seen in spontaneously breathing patients with tamponade.[4]

Hepatic vein flow profiles assessed with pulsed wave Doppler (PWD) can also provide useful information in spontaneously breathing patients suspected of having tamponade physiology. Under normal conditions, the hepatic veins show a bimodal flow profile. Systolic forward flow equals or exceeds diastolic forward flow throughout the respiratory cycle (Fig. 23-17, A). Systolic and diastolic forward velocities normally increase during spontaneous inspiration. With tamponade physiology, systolic and diastolic forward flow velocities

also increase during spontaneous inspiration, but there is a significant decrease or reversal of both the S and D waves not seen with normal patients (Fig. 23-17, B).[13] Unfortunately, no good data on the respirophasic changes in hepatic vein Doppler profiles during IPPV are currently available, so evaluation of hepatic vein profiles with TEE during IPPV is not encouraged.

Measurement of the isovolemic relaxation time (IVRT) is yet another quantitative Doppler echo method used to assess pericardial tamponade. Based on TTE data, patients with tamponade demonstrate a marked prolongation (i.e., >100 milliseconds) of the IVRT compared to normal patients. In most age groups, the IVRT is normally less than 100 milliseconds. Changes in IVRT in patients with pericardial tamponade undergoing IPPV have yet to be described.[13]

Constrictive Pericarditis

A subtype of pericarditis termed *constrictive pericarditis* is also important when evaluating pericardial disease states. The most common cause of constriction is previous cardiac surgery, followed by various other pathologies (e.g., pericarditis, an episode of pericardial effusion, radiotherapy).[1] Imazio et al. found that CP is a relatively rare complication of viral or idiopathic acute pericarditis but, in contrast, relatively frequent for specific etiologies such as bacterial pericarditis.[14] CP can be described as a chronic and more severe form of acute pericarditis. From a clinical standpoint, CP can impair ventricular filling and easily be confused with cardiomyopathies causing restrictive diastolic dysfunction (see Chapter 18). The pathophysiologic features of CP include fibrotic pericardium, inflamed pericardium, calcific thickening of the pericardium, abnormal diastolic filling, narrow RV pulse pressure (i.e., systolic RV pressure is normal, but diastolic RV pressure is elevated), and a prominent early diastolic RV pressure dip and later plateau called the *square root sign* (Fig. 23-18). The diastolic pressure plateau is related to the fact that the RV reaches its maximal volume quickly. Since it cannot expand to accept any additional volume (related to the pericardial constriction), the pressure then plateaus. The RA pressure is usually elevated and exhibits a pronounced systolic drop (rapid y-descent followed by an increase and then an apparent postsystolic plateau). This appears as an "M-like" wave on the central venous pressure tracing (see Fig. 23-18).[1,15]

The diagnosis of CP is quite challenging and most commonly obtained by combining 2D echocardiographic analysis, Doppler echocardiographic assessment (i.e., provides dynamic assessment of diastolic function), and high-fidelity imaging modalities (e.g., cardiac MRI or 64-slice CT). The 2D echocardiographic exam can reveal a thickened pericardium and a number of other possible features presented in Box 23-2.[11] The thickened pericardium can be appreciated with TEE, but 64-slice CT and cardiac MRI provide a more accurate measurement and extent of pericardial thickening (see Figs. 23-8 and 23-9).

Doppler assessment of patients with CP is complex and requires multiple Doppler modalities to accurately diagnose this pathology. Doppler

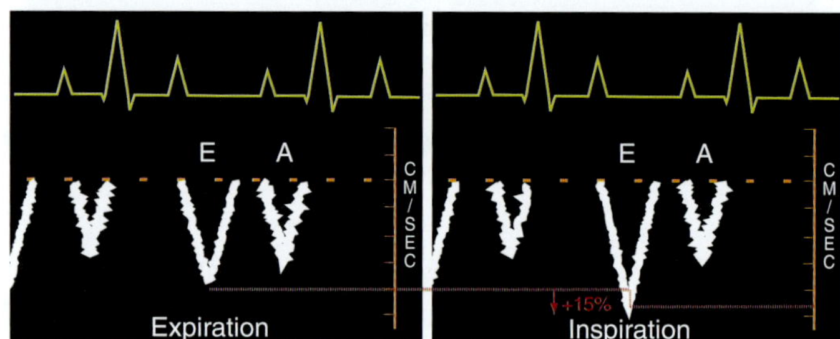

Figure 23-16 Idealized transesophageal echocardiographic transmitral pulse wave Doppler tracings obtained during intermittent positive pressure ventilation in patient with pericardial tamponade; exaggerated respirophasic variation is absent. *A,* Late diastolic filling associated with atrial contraction; *E,* early diastolic ventricular filling. *(From Savage RM, Aronson S. Comprehensive Textbook of Perioperative Transesophageal Echocardiography. Philadelphia: Lippincott Williams & Wilkins; 2010.)*

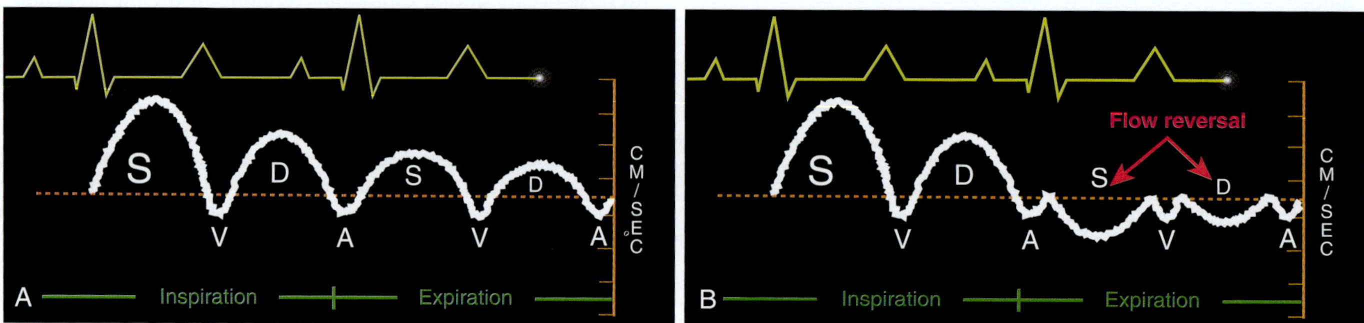

Figure 23-17 Idealized pulsed wave Doppler hepatic vein trace from spontaneously breathing patient in normal pericardial physiology **(A)** and pericardial tamponade **(B)**, which is distinguished by expiratory flow reversal *(fuchsia arrows)*. *A,* Transient hepatic flow reversal during atrial contraction; *D,* diastolic flow; *S,* systolic flow; *V,* transient hepatic flow reversal associated with tricuspid valve recoil. *(From Savage RM, Aronson S. Comprehensive Textbook of Perioperative Transesophageal Echocardiography. Philadelphia: Lippincott Williams & Wilkins; 2010.)*

modalities used to assess CP include PWD transtricuspid and transmitral tracings, PWD pulmonary vein tracings, tissue Doppler imaging of the lateral or septal mitral annulus, and color Doppler M-mode (flow propagation velocity, Vp) of transmitral inflow. Tricuspid and/or mitral regurgitation may be seen with color Doppler evaluation in patients with CP. As seen with pericardial tamponade, the transmitral PWD profile of spontaneously breathing patients with CP will demonstrate exaggerated respirophasic variation (i.e., decrease of ≈ 25% with inspiration). This characteristic should be easier to visualize with the sweep speed set at higher settings (100-150 cm/s). Figure 23-19 is a TTE image of a transmitral PWD profile in a spontaneously breathing patient with CP that shows a 30% decrease in velocity with inspiration (recall that a 10% decrease in transmitral velocity is normally observed in this setting). The echocardiographer should also realize that 20% to 50% of patients with CP will not demonstrate this classic Doppler finding, and the application of preload reducing maneuvers (e.g., reverse Trendelenburg or intravenous nitroglycerin administration) can be useful to amplify the transmitral velocity respiratory variation.[16] The

pathophysiologic mechanism for the amplified respirophasic variation is that the thickened pericardium insulates the intrapericardial structures from the intrathoracic pressure changes associated with the respiratory cycle, and this physiologic change produces an exaggerated respirophasic variation, seen in both CP and pericardial tamponade. The pericardial pathology is effectively insulating the intrapericardial structures from the influence of the intrapleural pressures, which creates a gradient between extra- and intracardiac flow that translates into exaggerated respirophasic variation. CP patients also display exaggerated respirophasic variation in the pulmonary veins, and the systolic-to-diastolic ratios are comparable to those with restrictive myocardial pathology (e.g., pulmonary vein diastolic flow velocity will be greater than systolic flow velocity in patients with a restrictive LV filling pattern, or S:D ratio <1).[17] It is unique to CP (in contrast to restrictive cardiomyopathy [RCM]) (Table 23-4) that the peak amplitude of the pulmonary venous D wave has been noted to exhibit pronounced respiratory variation (i.e., >18% increase upon inspiration in patients on IPPV).[18] Figure 23-20 shows an idealized transesophageal pulmonary vein PWD profile in a patient with CP on IPPV (S:D ratio <1 and a 20% increase in the D wave can be seen with inspiration).

The distinction between spontaneous ventilation and IPPV must be made to accurately diagnose CP using echocardiography. The exaggerated respirophasic variation seen with spontaneously breathing patients will also be seen in IPPV patients, except that the direction of

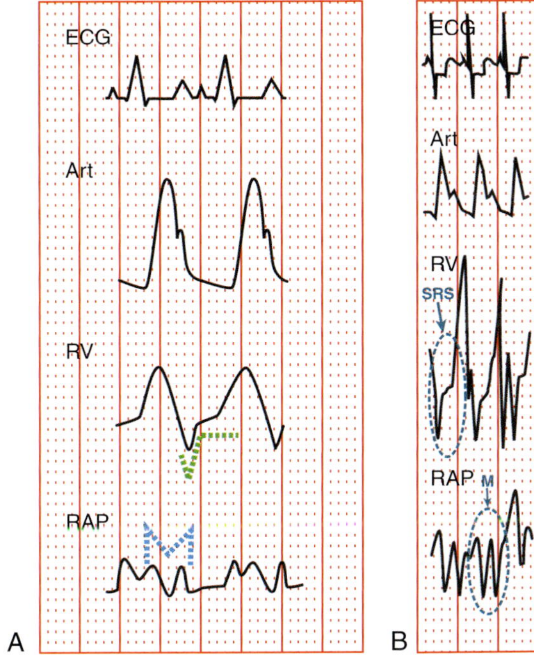

Figure 23-18 Characteristic hemodynamic tracings associated with constrictive pericarditis. Note "square root sign" *(SRS)* in right ventricular waveform *(green in A, circled in B)* and "M sign" *(M)* in right atrial pressure waveform *(blue in A, circled in B)*. Waveforms shown both idealized **(A)** and what is observed clinically **(B)**. *Art,* Arterial pressure waveform; *ECG,* electrocardiogram; *RAP,* right atrial pressure waveform; *RV,* right ventricular pressure waveform. *(B from Savage RM, Aronson S. Comprehensive Textbook of Perioperative Transesophageal Echocardiography. Philadelphia. Lippincott Williams & Wilkins; 2010.)*

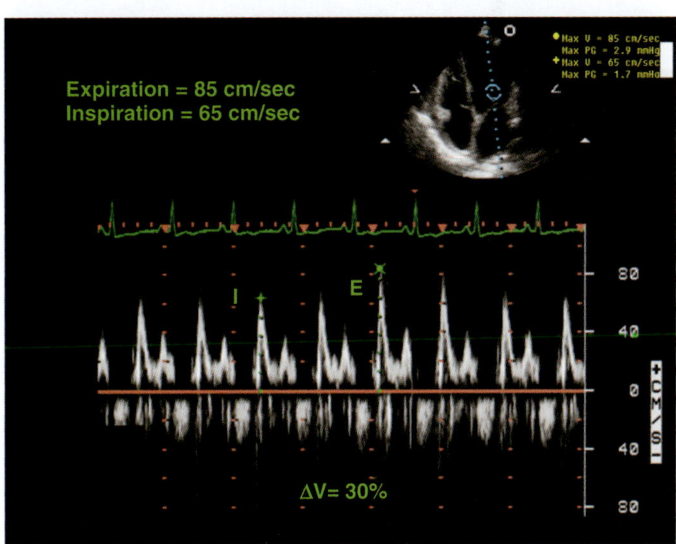

Figure 23-19 Transthoracic echocardiographic transmitral pulsed wave Doppler assessment during spontaneous respiration, showing characteristic exaggerated (30%) respirophasic variation associated with constrictive pericarditis. *E,* Expiration; *I,* inspiration. *(From Savage RM, Aronson S. Comprehensive Textbook of Perioperative Transesophageal Echocardiography. Philadelphia: Lippincott Williams & Wilkins; 2010.)*

BOX 23-2. TWO-DIMENSIONAL ECHOCARDIOGRAPHIC FINDINGS ASSOCIATED WITH CONSTRICTIVE PERICARDITIS

Paradoxical ventricular septal motion
Ventricular septal "bounce"
Diastolic flattening of posterior left ventricle
Premature mid-diastolic pulmonary valve opening
Spontaneous inspiratory leftward shift of atrial and ventricular septa
Enlarged hepatic veins
Dilated inferior vena cava without variation in size during respiration
Normal ventricular size
Normal or enlarged atria with reduced wall excursion

TABLE 23-4 Relative Sensitivities and Specificities of Various Doppler Techniques to Distinguish Between Constrictive Pericarditis and Restrictive Cardiomyopathy

Doppler Modality	Sensitivity	Specificity
Transmitral peak E-wave pulsed wave Doppler (PWD) velocity (respiratory variation ≥ 10%)	84	91
Pulmonary vein peak D-wave PWD velocity (respiratory variation ≥ 18%)	79	91
Transmitral color M-mode (Vp) slope ≥ 100 cm/s	74	91
Tissue Doppler imaging of lateral mitral annulus demonstrating E_m ≥ 8 cm/s	89	100

E_m, Early diastolic recoil of mitral annular tissue; *Vp,* flow propagation velocity.

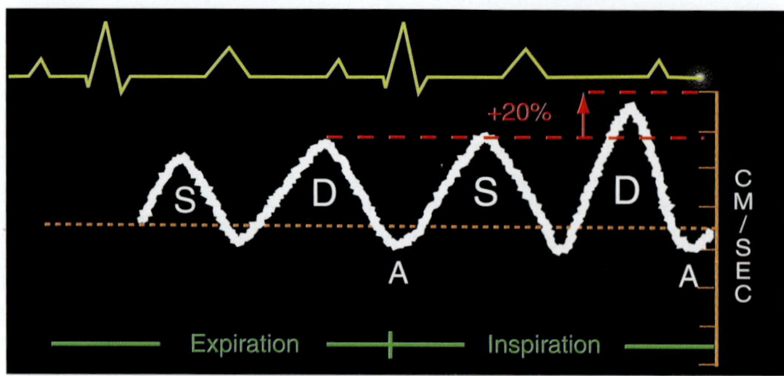

Figure 23-20 Idealized Doppler pulmonary vein tracing obtained with transesophageal echocardiography, depicting increased (20%) diastolic velocity that develops during inspiration with positive pressure ventilation. *A,* Atrial flow reversal; *CM/SEC,* centimeters per second; *D,* diastolic flow; *S,* systolic flow. *(From Savage RM, Aronson S. Comprehensive Textbook of Perioperative Transesophageal Echocardiography. Philadelphia: Lippincott Williams & Wilkins; 2010.)*

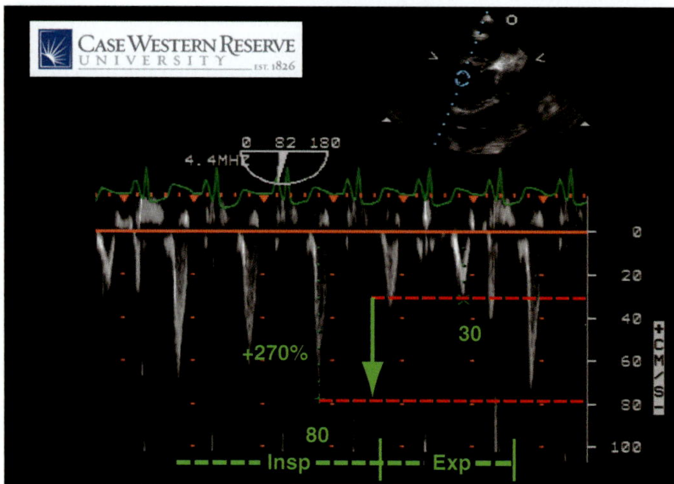

Figure 23-21 Transesophageal echocardiographic pulsed wave Doppler tracing showing constrictive pericarditis in patient on intermittent positive pressure ventilation. Note profoundly exaggerated respirophasic variation. *Exp,* Expiration; *Insp,* inspiration. *(From Savage RM, Aronson S. Comprehensive Textbook of Perioperative Transesophageal Echocardiography. Philadelphia: Lippincott Williams & Wilkins; 2010.)*

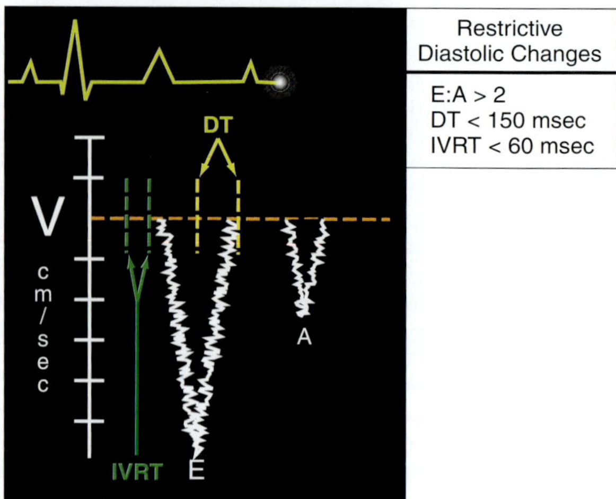

Figure 23-22 Idealized transesophageal echocardiographic transmitral pulse wave Doppler assessment representing expected findings in a heart with restrictive diastolic physiologic changes. *A,* Late diastolic flow associated with atrial contraction; *DT,* deceleration time; *E,* early diastolic flow; *IVRT,* isovolemic relaxation time; *V,* velocity. *(From Savage RM, Aronson S. Comprehensive Textbook of Perioperative Transesophageal Echocardiography. Philadelphia: Lippincott Williams & Wilkins; 2010.)*

the change in velocity is opposite.[15,18,19] This observation is explained in part by the fact that the increase in intrathoracic pressure expels blood from the low-compliance extrapericardial pulmonary veins into the LA, with a subsequent rise in transmitral blood flow (Fig. 23-21). Again, the exaggerated respirophasic variation observed in CP patients is from the thickened pericardium that insulates the intracardiac chambers (LA in this case) from the changes in intrathoracic pressure. This shielding allows an increase in the filling gradient between the pulmonary veins and the LA during inspiration, which is reflected as a relative exaggeration of the normally observed transmitral PWD flow velocities.

Despite the exaggerated respirophasic variation observed in both CP and pericardial tamponade patients, the absolute amplitude of these velocities will be reduced in both pathologies. Patients with CP have limited diastolic filling secondary to the noncompliant pericardium surrounding the heart, which effectively prevents full diastolic expansion and filling of the ventricles. Since CP limits the volume of both ventricular chambers, the previously described inspiratory increase relative to the expiratory velocity in transmitral E-wave velocity with IPPV will be accompanied by a simultaneous decrease in transtricuspid E- and A-wave velocities. There are two main reasons for this echocardiographic finding. First, the increase in intrathoracic pressure limits right-sided filling as described in Figure 23-6, *C.* Video 23-5 demonstrates how left heart filling is augmented during the inspiratory phase of IPPV while right heart filling is simultaneously impeded as the interventricular septum is noted to shift to the right. Secondly, the increased filling velocity and increased amount of blood in the LV will result in a shift of the interventricular septum to the right and compromise RV filling (i.e., the concept of ventricular interdependence is demonstrated). These changes in transmitral velocities appear to be reversible with surgical treatment (pericardial stripping or pericardiectomy), but in some cases, this therapy has been associated with LV dilatation and transient ventricular diastolic dysfunction.[20]

Making the clinical distinction between CP and RCM is an important task for the perioperative echocardiographer. Both clinical entities share the common pathophysiology of decreased LV compliance, but each has its own unique mechanism. In CP, the decreased compliance is secondary to the restrictive nature of the thickened pericardium. In RCM, the decreased compliance is secondary to pathology intrinsic to the myocardium (e.g., infiltrative disease like amyloidosis or myocardial hypertrophy). Severely decreased LV compliance can present with a restrictive LV filling pattern and is not expected to be consistently useful in differentiating CP from RCM, since CP may demonstrate some restrictive physiologic features (Fig. 23-22).

The differentiation of CP from RCM is best achieved using a combination of 2D echocardiography, high-fidelity imaging modalities, and Doppler echocardiographic assessments. With regard to pericarditis, 2D echocardiography and high-resolution CT/cardiac MRI may both reveal a thickened pericardium, but not all patients with a thickened pericardium will demonstrate constrictive physiology (see Fig. 23-9). Doppler techniques should be used to assess for exaggerated respirophasic variation in the transmitral (see Fig. 23-21) and pulmonary venous Doppler flow velocity profiles (i.e., S:D ratio <1 with a >18% variation in the D wave on inspiration during IPPV [see Fig. 23-20]). This exaggerated respirophasic variation has been previously demonstrated using TEE in anesthetized patients.[18]

Newer echocardiographic modalities to help differentiate CP from RCM include color M-mode flow propagation velocity (Vp), Doppler tissue imaging (DTI) at the level of the lateral mitral annulus, and Doppler myocardial velocity gradients (MVGs).[19,21,22] DTI provided a highly sensitive and specific means to differentiate CP from RCM

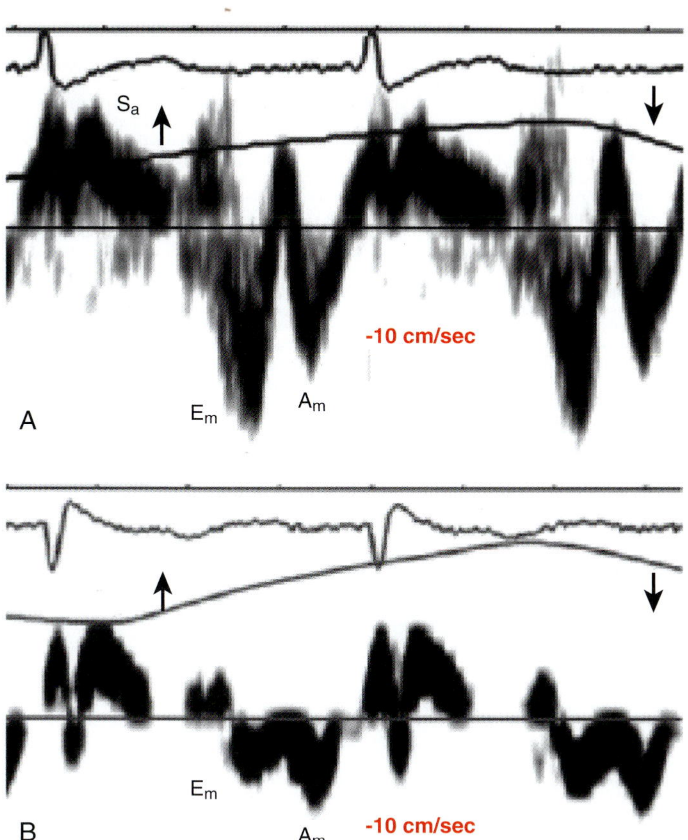

Figure 23-23 Transthoracic echocardiographic tissue Doppler imaging of lateral mitral annulus in **(A)** a patient with constrictive pericarditis and **(B)** another patient with restrictive cardiomyopathy. A_m, Late diastolic recoil associated with atrial contraction; E_m, early diastolic recoil of mitral annular tissue; S_a, systolic myocardial motion. *(From Savage RM, Aronson S. Comprehensive Textbook of Perioperative Transesophageal Echocardiography. Philadelphia: Lippincott Williams & Wilkins; 2010.)*

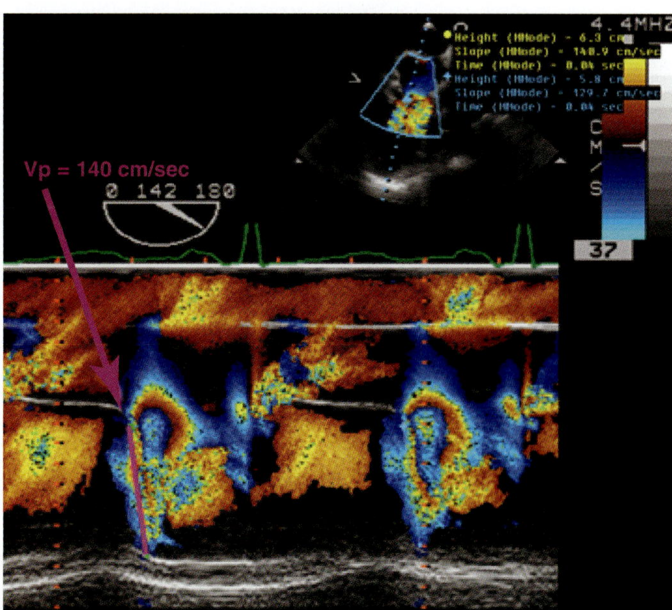

Figure 23-24 Transesophageal echocardiographic image obtained using flow propagation (Vp) in a patient with constrictive pericarditis. *(From Savage RM, Aronson S. Comprehensive Textbook of Perioperative Transesophageal Echocardiography. Philadelphia: Lippincott Williams & Wilkins; 2010.)*

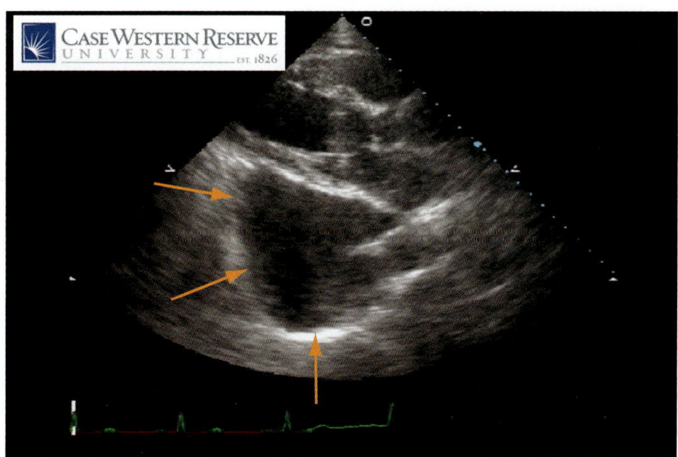

Figure 23-25 Transthoracic echocardiographic parasternal long-axis view demonstrating a large pericardial cyst *(orange arrows)* adjacent to left atrium and ventricle. *(From Savage RM, Aronson S. Comprehensive Textbook of Perioperative Transesophageal Echocardiography. Philadelphia: Lippincott Williams & Wilkins; 2010.)*

in one study of a homogenous CP patient population.[19] A distinct advantage of DTI is that it is less sensitive to preload alterations while differentiating CP from RCM. DTI at the level of the mitral annulus with both TTE and TEE allows a reproducible means to align the PWD cursor with the longitudinal axis of myocardial excursion during relaxation. With regard to peak early diastolic mitral annular velocity (E_m, also denoted as E′), patients with CP will generally have preserved myocardial diastolic function and normal myocardial velocities ($E_m >$ 8 cm/s). The reverse is true for patients with RCM in that the muscle is inherently pathologic and unable to relax adequately ($E_m <$ 8 cm/s) (Fig. 23-23) (also see Chapter 12).

Color M-mode flow propagation velocity (Vp) should also be used to assess patients suspected of having CP; Vp appears to be less preload dependent and provides excellent spatial and temporal resolution of diastolic mitral inflow. One of its drawbacks is that Vp results are not as reproducible as those of DTI, likely related to the higher degree of interoperator variability associated with Vp use. CP patients will typically demonstrate high values of flow propagation toward the LV apex (Vp > 100 cm/s), whereas those with RCM will have much lower values (Vp < 45 cm/s) (Fig. 23-24).

Pericardial Masses

Pericardial masses include benign pericardial cysts, pericardial neoplasms (e.g., mesothelioma, sarcoma, teratomas), and tumors that invade the pericardium secondary to increased regional spread (e.g., breast or lung cancer). Pericardial cysts are usually round in shape and

patients are typically asymptomatic, but presenting symptoms may include chest pain, dyspnea, cough, arrhythmias, and compression of the LA or pulmonary vein(s). Figure 23-25 presents an example of a pericardial cyst from a TTE examination. If the pericardial cyst cannot be imaged adequately with echocardiography, cardiac MRI offers a strong alternative solution. From a clinical standpoint, any of these masses can inhibit cardiac chamber filling and result in hemodynamic compromise. Pericardial thrombus is another type of pericardial mass, most commonly seen in the postsurgical state. Hemopericardium (see Fig. 23-14) can result from a number of different pathologies, including postoperative cardiac surgical bleeding, aortic dissection with extravasation of blood into the transverse sinus, percutaneous catheter interventions, and postinfarction myocardial necrosis with rupture (see Chapter 21).[1]

REFERENCES

1. Avery EG, Shernan SK. Echocardiographic Evaluation of Pericardial Disease. In: Savage RM, Aronson S, Shernan SK, eds. *Comprehensive Textbook of Perioperative Transesophageal Echocardiography.* 2nd ed. Philadelphia: Lippincott Williams and Wilkins; 2011:725-740.

2. Spodick DH. Macrophysiology, microphysiology and anatomy of the pericardium: a synopsis. *Am Heart J.* 1992;124(4):1046-1051.

3. Spodick DH. Acute cardiac tamponade. *N Engl J Med.* 2003;349(7):684-690.

4. Faehnrich JA, Noone RB, White WD, et al. Effects of positive pressure ventilation, pericardial effusion, and cardiac tamponade on respiratory variation in transmitral flow velocities. *J Cardiothorac Vasc Anesth.* 2003;17(1):45-50.

5. Gatzoulis MA, Munk MD, Merchant N, et al. Isolated congenital absence of the pericardium: clinical presentation, diagnosis, and management. *Ann Thorac Surg.* 2000;69(4):1209-1215.

6. Maisch B, Seferovic PM, Ristic AD, et al. Guidelines on the diagnosis and management of pericardial diseases executive summary. *Eur Heart J.* 2004;25(7):587-610.

7. Kivisto S, Lipsanen-Nyman M, Kupari M, et al. Cardiac involvement in Mulibrey nanism: characterization with magnetic resonance imaging. *J Cardiovasc Magn Reson.* 2004;6(3):645-652.

8. Otto C. Pericardial disease. *Textbook of Clinical Echocardiography.* 3rd ed. Philadelphia: Elsevier Health Sciences; 2004:259-275.

9. Abbas AE, Appleton CP, Liu PT, et al. Congenital absence of the pericardium: case presentation and review of literature. *Int J Cardiol.* 2005;98(1):21-25.

10. Goldschlager N, Goldman MJ. *Principles of Clinical Electrocardiography.* 13th ed. East Norwalk: Appleton and Lange; 1989. 203-213.

11. Shernan SK. Echocardiographic evaluation of pericardial disease. In: Konstadt SN, Shernan S, Oka Y, eds. *Clinical Transesophageal Echocardiography: A Problem-Oriented Approach.* 2nd ed. Philadelphia: Lippincott Williams and Wilkins; 2003:203-213.

12. Hoit BD. Pericardial disease. In: Fuster V, O'Rourke RA, Walsh RA, eds. *Hurst's The Heart.* 12th ed. China: McGraw-Hill Professional; 2007:1951-1974.

13. Burstow DJ, Oh JK, Bailey KR, et al. Cardiac tamponade: characteristic Doppler observations. *Mayo Clin Proc.* 1989;64(3):312-324.

14. Imazio M, Brucato A, Maestroni S, et al. Risk of constrictive pericarditis after acute pericarditis. *Circulation.* 2011;124(11):1270-1275.

15. Skubas NJ, Beardslee M, Barzilai B, et al. Constrictive pericarditis: intraoperative hemodynamic and echocardiographic evaluation of cardiac filling dynamics. *Anesth Analg.* 2001;92(6):1424-1426.

16. Oh JK, Tajik AJ, Appleton CP, et al. Preload reduction to unmask the characteristic Doppler features of constrictive pericarditis. A new observation. *Circulation.* 1997;95(4):796-799.

17. Klein AL, Cohen GI, Pietrolungo JF, et al. Differentiation of constrictive pericarditis from restrictive cardiomyopathy by Doppler transesophageal echocardiographic measurements of respiratory variations in pulmonary venous flow. *J Am Coll Cardiol.* 1993;22(7):1935-1943.

18. Abdalla IA, Murray RD, Awad HE, et al. Reversal of the pattern of respiratory variation of Doppler inflow velocities in constrictive pericarditis during mechanical ventilation. *J Am Soc Echocardiogr.* 2000;13(9):827-831.

19. Rajagopalan N, Garcia MJ, Rodriguez L, et al. Comparison of new Doppler echocardiographic methods to differentiate constrictive pericardial heart disease and restrictive cardiomyopathy. *Am J Cardiol.* 2001;87(1):86-94.

20. Senni M, Redfield MM, Ling LH, et al. Left ventricular systolic and diastolic function after pericardiectomy in patients with constrictive pericarditis: Doppler echocardiographic findings and correlation with clinical status. *J Am Coll Cardiol.* 1999;33(5):1182-1188.

21. Palka P, Lange A, Donnelly JE, et al. Differentiation between restrictive cardiomyopathy and constrictive pericarditis by early diastolic Doppler myocardial velocity gradient at the posterior wall. *Circulation.* 2000;102(6):655-662.

22. Garcia MJ, Thomas JD, Klein AL. New Doppler echocardiographic applications for the study of diastolic function. *J Am Coll Cardiol.* 1998;32(4):865-875.

Adult Congenital Heart Disease

DOMINIQUE A. BETTEX | MARCO BOSSHART | MATTHIAS GREUTMANN

Introduction

Congenital heart disease (CHD) affects an estimated 0.5% to 1% of all live births.[1-3] Thanks to major advances in congenital cardiac surgery made over the past few decades, the majority of these patients now survive to adulthood, even those with complex CHD lesions. The number of adult survivors with CHD has thus constantly increased over the past decades, and their number now exceeds the number of affected children.[4] It is, however, important to realize that after childhood repair of CHD, the majority of these adult survivors are not "cured"; many of them remain at risk for complications and the need for reoperations.

There are three groups of "grown-up CHD" (GUCH) patients that may be encountered:

1. **Patients after intracardiac repair of congenital cardiac defects in childhood.** Only a few of these patients (i.e., repair of atrial septal defects [ASDs] or patent ductus arteriosus in early childhood) can be regarded as cured. The majority of these patients, particularly those after repair of moderate or complex forms of CHD, are at risk for late complications due to residual hemodynamic lesions and myocardial scars.
2. **Patients with unrepaired CHD amenable to intracardiac repair in adulthood.** This group consists mainly of simple lesions such as different forms of ASDs, isolated aortic or pulmonary valve disease, or coarctation of the aorta. This group, however, also includes patients with more complex diseases such as Ebstein anomaly of the tricuspid valve, unrepaired tetralogy of Fallot (TOF), or corrected congenital transposition of the great arteries (TGA).
3. **Patients with complex defects without prior surgery or patients after palliative surgery for complex congenital cardiac malformations.** This group includes patients after Fontan palliation for single-ventricle physiology and patients after systemic-to-pulmonary shunt operations (i.e., Blalock-Taussig shunts) in the setting of complex CHD.

These patients may be encountered in the setting of a new intervention or redo cardiac surgery in adulthood, as well as in the setting of intensive care management. Their complex cardiac physiology may also affect non-cardiac surgery.

Five factors have been found to have an independent prognostic value for perioperative complications: pulmonary hypertension, cyanosis, reoperation, arrhythmias, and ventricular dysfunction.

In this chapter, we will focus on the role of transesophageal echocardiography (TEE) in intraoperative and intensive care settings. We will outline the specific concepts of classification of CHD, principals of echocardiographic estimations of shunts, propose a standardized sequence for a comprehensive echocardiographic examination, and then discuss some of the most important congenital cardiac defects requiring cardiac interventions in adulthood. The complexity and diversity of CHD does not allow a comprehensive description of all types of CHD in this chapter. We will focus on three particular aspects:

1. Evaluation of complex CHD, particularly in patients in whom the preoperative evaluation is incomplete by transthoracic echocardiography (TTE)
2. Assessment of anatomic abnormalities and their surgical repair during cardiac interventions
3. Management of hemodynamics during cardiac and non-cardiac surgery, extending into the postoperative intensive care unit (ICU)

TEE allows for a comprehensive evaluation of cardiac anatomy and function. It is superior to TTE in the evaluation of ASDs and pulmonary venous return because in most instances, it offers better visualization of the anatomy and function of the cardiac valves.

Indications for TEE

TEE during cardiac surgery for CHD is considered a category I indication.[5,6] The principal uses of TEE in the perioperative or peri-interventional setting may be classified under three headings (Box 24-1):

1. In the catheterization laboratory, TEE is often used to guide catheter-based intracardiac procedures. It is particularly useful for guidance of device closure in patients with secundum-type ASDs. TEE provides precise information on location, geometry, and number of ASDs, as well as the extent of surrounding tissue and location of adjacent structures.[7] It allows delineation of pulmonary venous return and allows exclusion of interatrial defects not amenable to device closure (i.e., sinus venosus defects). It is important to emphasize that periprocedural TEE should not stand alone as the sole diagnostic study, since there are inherent limitations in imaging certain important structures that are best identified by TTE.[8] In case of discrepant findings from the preinterventional diagnosis, mutual assessment with colleagues from cardiology is advisable.
2. In the operating room, TEE is helpful during all stages of cardiac surgery.
3. In the ICU, it is particularly important in the assessment of hemodynamically unstable patients.

The echocardiographer needs to pay attention to the hemodynamic status prior to and during the procedure. For example, mitral valve function is highly dependent on left ventricular afterload; when assessing severity of mitral regurgitation, it is of utmost importance to reestablish normal systemic vascular resistance, if necessary by administration of arterial vasopressors. Assessment of the magnitude of residual intracardiac shunting may be difficult. First, the pulmonary arterial pressure, if elevated preoperatively, may not fall immediately after separation from cardiopulmonary bypass (CPB), resulting in underestimation of the severity of a potential residual left-to-right shunt. Second, many patients require increased inspired oxygen concentration during the evaluation, which may provide a spurious error in shunt calculations. Third, although color Doppler is an excellent tool for localizing residual shunt lesions, it is unreliable for determining absolute shunt size, particularly when it is located in the muscular ventricular septum.[9]

Impact of TEE

The impact of TEE in cardiac surgery for CHD has been mostly studied in the pediatric population. The rate of new findings and/or surgical management alterations based on intraoperative TEE ranges between 3% and 39%.[10-15] Sensitivity and specificity of TEE to determine the necessity for reoperation reaches 89% and 100%, respectively.[16,17]

A major impact of TEE, defined as new information altering the planned procedure or leading to a revision of the initial repair, occurs in 13% to 16% of cases[12,13] and is most frequently seen during reoperations, valve repairs, complex AV discordances, and complex outflow tract reconstructions.[11,12] Patients who leave the operating room with

BOX 24-1. INDICATIONS FOR TEE

In the Cardiac Catheterization Laboratory:
- Reduction of fluoroscopy time and contrast load
- Continuous assessment of results and detection of potential complications
- Standard imaging modality during atrial septal defect closure, when intracardiac echocardiography (ICE) is not available
- Guiding ventricular septal defect closure
- Guiding left atrial appendage closure
- Facilitating manipulation of catheters used for complex procedures, such as device closure of paravalvular leaks after prosthetic heart valve replacement
- Optional to enhance safety for transseptal access to the left atrium

In the Operating Room Before Cardiopulmonary Bypass:
- Additional diagnostic information: TEE may confirm, exclude, or modify preoperative findings
- Assessment of hemodynamic and ventricular function
- Selection of anesthetic agents and use of inotropic support
- Assistance in placement of central venous catheters
- Control of position of venous and arterial cannulae, especially in minimally invasive cardiac surgical procedures

In the Operating Room During Cardiopulmonary Bypass:
- Assessment of dilation of cardiac chambers
- Assessment of intracardiac air and de-airing procedures

In the Operating Room After Cardiopulmonary Bypass:
- Detection of significant and potentially treatable residual defects before weaning off bypass or before sternal closure
- Assessment of cardiac function and volume status, potential aid in diagnosis of hemodynamic alterations

In the Intensive Care Unit:
- Evaluation of the critically ill postoperative patient with limited TTE views
- Assessment of ventricular function and volume status
- Assistance in determining appropriate timing and hemodynamic effects of sternal closure or discontinuation of ventricular assist devices or extracorporeal membrane oxygenation
- Assessment of the etiology of refractory hemodynamic alterations (i.e., pericardial effusion, tamponade, valve dysfunction)

TEE, Transesophageal echocardiography; *TTE,* transthoracic echocardiography.

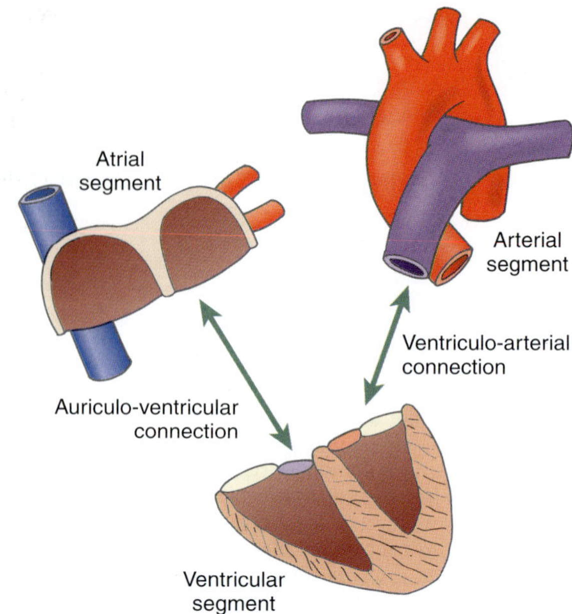

Figure 24-1 Schema of segmental approach: heart is divided into three segments (atria, ventricles, and arterial trunks) and two junctions (atrioventricular and ventriculo-arterial junctions). *(Modified from Bettex D, Chassot PG. Transesophageal echocardiography in congenital heart disease. In: Bissonnette B, ed. Pediatric Anesthesia: Basic Principles—State of the Art—Future. Shelton, CT: People's Medical Publishing House-USA; 2011, with permission.)*

significant residual defects or decreased ventricular performance tend to have a poorer outcome.[13,18,19] It has been recognized that residual anatomic or functional lesions are the main determinants of morbidity and mortality after repair of congenital cardiac defects.[19,20] Therefore, intraoperative TEE is used more and more frequently in congenital cardiac surgery to assess operative results.

Assessing the immediate result of surgical repair is of great importance. Return to CPB based on findings from intraoperative TEE is reported in 5% to 11% of cases.[10,11,14,16,21-24] After weaning from CPB, a return to bypass is always a difficult decision for the surgical team, particularly after a long and complicated procedure. It is thus essential to keep in mind that the goal of surgery is to obtain a good clinical result but not a perfect echocardiographic image. The echocardiographer must understand all the implications of a return to bypass. The decision may be easy in the case of hemodynamic compromise, but it requires careful consideration in the absence of hemodynamic instability. Optimal collaboration and communication between the echocardiographer and the surgical team in making the best decision regarding management of an individual patient is important.[9] The intraoperative surgical revision rate may decrease over time with experience, as has been shown by Ungerleider et al., who reported a decrease in rate from 8.5% to 3% to 4% over a 7-year period with the same surgeon.[18] It supports the notion that institutional surgical skill and echocardiographic experience will directly affect the impact of TEE. On the other hand, the rate of return to bypass for incomplete repair decreases from 9.6% to 0% when an experienced perioperative echocardiographer is replaced by a poorly trained echocardiographer, and the rate of missed residual problems after bypass rises from 21% to 74%[25]; these findings reinforce the importance of good collaboration between echocardiographer and surgical team and particularly the need for a well-trained and experienced echocardiographer.

Anatomic Nomenclature: The Segmental Approach

The diversity of GUCH requires a structural classification. The most useful concept is the segmental approach[26,27]: the heart is divided into three segments (atria, ventricles, and arterial trunks) connected via two junctions (atrioventricular and ventriculo-arterial) (Fig. 24-1). The definition of the segments is based on their intrinsic morphology, because the usual criteria (e.g., size, position of cardiac chambers) may be altered in CHD. Although most patients entering the operating room have been previously assessed and a diagnosis made, it is important to understand the principles of this classification to allow unambiguous communication between the echocardiographer and the surgical team. Sequential analysis of the heart includes five steps to describe cardiac anatomy.[28]

Define Atrial Situs or Atrial Arrangement

Atrial situs describes the morphology and arrangement of the atria. It can be normal (situs solitus), mirror imaged (situs inversus), or ambiguous in the setting of right or left atrial isomerism. Most often but not universally, abdominal and thoracic situs follows cardiac situs. The most important features in distinguishing the right and left atria are their appendages. Apart from its broad-based appendage, the right atrium (RA) has several morphologic characteristics that allow its differentiation from the left atrium (LA). The inferior vena cava (IVC) is almost uniquely connected to the RA. The eustachian valve boards this connection. Another typical and unique structure of the RA is the crista terminalis, separating the smooth-walled sinus

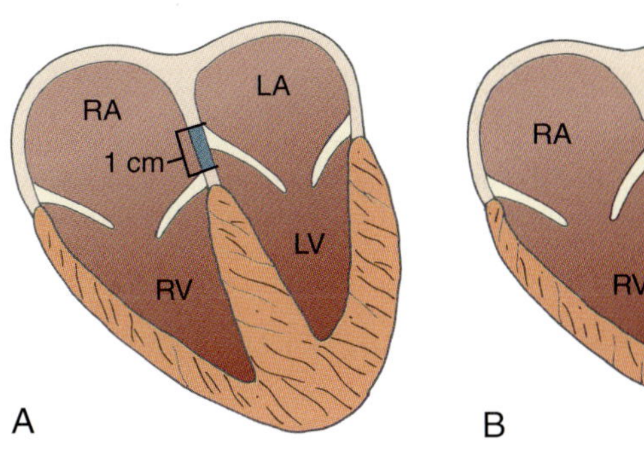
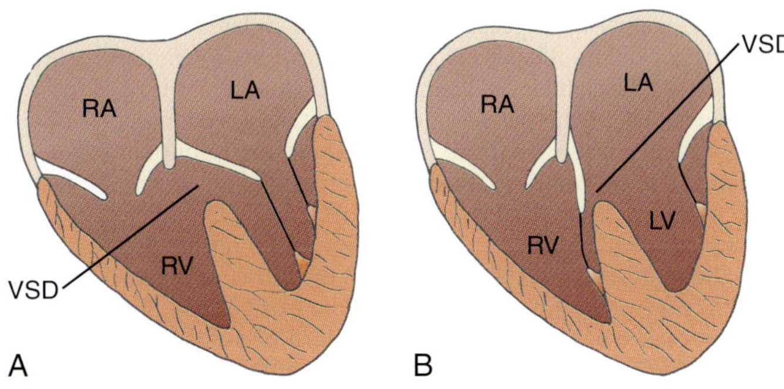

Figure 24-2 Schema of implantation of mitral and tricuspid valves. **A,** Normal anatomy: tricuspid valve is inserted lower than mitral valve at level of interventricular septum. **B,** Atrioventricular canal: mitral and tricuspid valves are inserted at same level of interventricular septum. *LA,* Left atrium; *LV,* left ventricle; *RA,* right atrium; *RV,* right ventricle. (*Courtesy PG Chassot.*)

Figure 24-3 Schema of an overriding and straddling mitral valve. **A,** Overriding mitral valve: atrioventricular valve opens less than 50% into contralateral ventricle. **B,** Straddling mitral valve: a straddling valve has chordal attachments crossing through an interventricular septal defect and inserting into opposite ventricle. *LA,* Left atrium; *LV,* left ventricle; *RA,* right atrium; *RV,* right ventricle; *VSD,* ventricular septal defect. (*Courtesy PG Chassot.*)

venarum (entry of the IVC, superior vena cava [SVC], and coronary sinus [CS] into the RA) from the trabeculated RA. The LA has very few characteristic structures other than a typically finger- or hook-shaped appendage bordered by pectinate muscles, which should not be confused with a thrombus.

Define Ventricular Chambers

The left ventricle (LV) is defined by the presence of one or two papillary muscles, fine apical trabeculations, usually a bicuspid mitral valve, and a partially fibrous outlet. The mitral valve is in fibrous continuity with the outflow tract, and there is no infundibulum. The right ventricle (RV) is defined by three or several papillary muscles (one of which inserts into the interventricular septum), a tricuspid valve with its septal leaflet inserted more apically than the anterior mitral valve leaflet (Fig. 24-2), coarse apical trabeculations, and a completely muscular outlet or infundibulum.

Define Arterial Trunks

The main pulmonary trunk is defined by its bifurcation into the right and left branch pulmonary arteries, whereas the aorta has no branches before the aortic arch. The coronary arteries usually arise from the aorta except in the case of anomalous origin of the coronary arteries from the pulmonary trunk. A *common arterial trunk* is defined as a single large arterial trunk that gives rise to the branch pulmonary and coronary arteries.

Define Atrioventricular and Ventriculo-arterial Connections

Concordant atrioventricular (AV) connection means that the RA is connected to the RV and the LA to the LV. In the case of *discordant AV connection*, the RA is connected to the LV and the LA to the RV. Variants include a common AV junction in the setting of atrioventricular septal defects (AVSDs) (see later), overriding of one of the AV valves (<50% of the valve opens into the contralateral ventricle) (Fig. 24-3), or a double inlet ventricle (>50% opens into the contralateral ventricle). *Straddling* of the AV valve is defined by the presence of chordal attachments crossing through an interventricular septal defect and inserting into the contralateral ventricle (see Fig. 24-3). This has important implications for surgical repair because it usually does not allow biventricular repair.

The *ventriculo-arterial connection* describes the relationship between the ventricles and the large arterial trunks. It can also be concordant or discordant (TGA). In the presence of a ventricular septal defect (VSD), there can be overriding of an arterial trunk (<50% connection to the opposite ventricle) (Video 24-1) or a double outlet ventricle

(>50% overriding). In the case of a double outlet right ventricle (DORV), bilateral muscular infundibula are often found, with loss of fibrous continuity between the mitral and the aortic valve.

Associated Anomalies

In a last step, we need to define all associated abnormalities, such as hypoplastic heart chambers, septal defects, obstructive lesions, and valve abnormalities. Given the principles of sequential anatomy outlined earlier, a comprehensive TEE examination in patients with CHD is recommended in a systematic and logical sequence:[29]

- Atrial segment: situs, location, arrangement, identity, venous connections
- Four-chamber view: relative size, shape, and position of each cardiac cavity
- AV connection: valvular status, univentricular, uniatrial, single-inlet
- Ventricular segment: number, size, orientation, identity
- Ventriculo-arterial connection: double outlet, single outlet, outflow tract, valvular status
- Arterial segment: great vessels orientation, identity
- Presence and direction of intracardiac and extracardiac shunts

Each TEE examination should begin with an overview of all four cavities to appreciate the relative development and remodeling of each of the cardiac chambers. In case of atresia or stenosis of a valve, structures situated downstream do not receive sufficient blood to develop normally and become involuted and hypoplastic. Conversely, the structures situated upstream sustain a volume and pressure overload. Volume overload results also from a shunt or regurgitation and induces dilation of the downstream chamber(s); pressure overload due to an obstruction or high vascular resistance leads to hypertrophy; both phenomena can occur together.

Shunt and Pressure Gradient

Intracardiac shunts may be located at the level of the interatrial septum (ASDs), interventricular septum (VSDs), or between the aorta and atria (aorto-atrial fistula) (Video 24-2). Shunts may also be located at the level of the great arteries (aorto-pulmonary window, patent ductus arteriosus) or be caused by partial or complete anomalous pulmonary venous drainage into the RA. A shunt flow can be defined by three characteristics:

1. Direction and timing of the flow: left to right (L-R), right to left (R-L), or bidirectional. The shunt flow can be systolic, diastolic, or continuous systolo-diastolic. Both flow direction and timing are determined by the pressure difference between the two affected cardiac chambers and/or vessels, which changes over the cardiac cycle.
2. Dimension of the defect: a shunt of small size generates a high-pressure gradient and turbulent flow; a large shunt does not impede blood flow, resulting in low or no gradient and laminar flow.

3. Enlargement of the receiving chambers: isolated defects situated upstream of the AV valves (ASD, anomalous pulmonary venous return) cause right-sided chamber dilation, whereas lesions located downstream of the AV junctions (VSD, ductus arteriosus) induce left-sided chamber dilation. In both cases, the pulmonary artery is dilated and pulmonary blood flow is increased.

On two-dimensional (2D) echocardiography, a septal defect appears as a loss of continuity of a septal barrier, although it can be missed when the septum is parallel to the axis of the ultrasound beam or when the defect is buried among trabeculations. The confirmation is based on the presence of an abnormal flow pattern by color Doppler. Color M-mode, pulsed, and continuous wave Doppler examination can be used to precisely assess the timing of complex or bidirectional shunts. Contrast echocardiography studies increase sensitivity and are very helpful in detecting small R-L shunts.

L-R shunt size is usually quantified as the ratio between pulmonary blood flow (Qp) and systemic blood flow (Qs): Qp/Qs. It is calculated by diagnostic catheterization or echocardiography. Echocardiographic calculation of shunt ratios is often imprecise, however, and estimation of cardiac chamber size as a measure of hemodynamic relevance of a given L-R shunt seems to be more appropriate.

Using the simplified Bernoulli formula, TEE makes it possible to noninvasively evaluate pressure gradients between cardiac chambers or between chambers and vessels. This allows for estimation of intracavitary pressures:

$$\text{Simplified Bernoulli formula: } \Delta P = 4\,(Vmax)^2$$

Systolic pulmonary artery pressure (PAPs) can be estimated from the tricuspid regurgitation (TR) jet velocity (Fig. 24-4). In the absence of pathology in the right ventricular outflow tract (RVOT), systolic RV pressure is identical to the PAPs. It equals the pressure gradient between RV and RA, which can be calculated by the simplified Bernoulli equation with the addition of the RA pressure (RAP):

$$PAPs = 4\,(Vmax^2)_{TR} + RAP$$

One should be cautious in the presence of a VSD, because flow through it may contaminate TR flow. In this case, the gradient will measure the pressure difference between LV and RA, not between RV and RA. In the case of a VSD, the right ventricular systolic pressure (RVPs) may also be calculated by the difference between systolic arterial pressure (SAP) and the pressure difference across the VSD shunt:

$$RVPs = SAP - 4\,(Vmax^2)_{VSD}$$

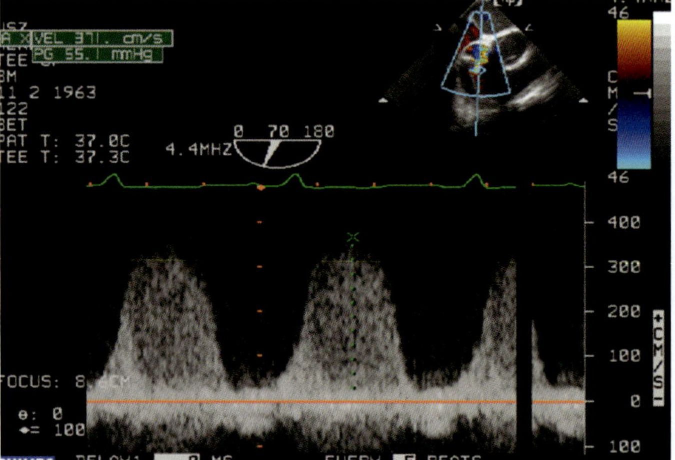

Figure 24-4   Continuous wave Doppler spectrum of tricuspid valve regurgitation. Using Bernoulli equation, peak velocity gives us peak gradient between right atrium (RA) and right ventricle (55 mmHg). Assuming RA pressure of 14, pulmonary systolic pressure, in absence of any right ventricular outflow tract pathology, would be: 55 + 14 = 69 mmHg.

This formula may be used if there is no obstruction within the left ventricular outflow tract (LVOT); the systolic arterial pressure is then roughly equivalent to the maximal LV systolic pressure.

If pulmonary regurgitation (PR) is present, the end-diastolic pulmonary artery pressure (PAPd) can be estimated from the jet velocity of the PR at end-diastole. Admitting that the RV diastolic pressure is equal to the RAP, the following formula is used to estimated end-diastolic PA pressure:

$$PAPd = 4\,(Vmax^2)_{PR} + RAP$$

Specific Congenital Cardiac Defects

The Right Ventricle in Congenital Heart Disease

In GUCH, the RV may be the subpulmonic ventricle, supporting pulmonary circulation, but in the setting of transposition complexes, it may be the subaortic ventricle, supporting systemic circulation. In these patients, anatomy and function of the RV has been of interest for quite some time. Before starting to delineate individual congenital cardiac lesions, it may be useful to give a few specific considerations to RV anatomy and physiology.[30]

The complex more triangular shape of the RV contrasts with the more conical shape of the LV (Fig. 24-5). The muscular wall of the normal RV is thin, usually 3 to 5 mm in thickness, but in cases of pressure overload, its thickness may even exceed that of the LV. Contraction of the RV myocardium relies more heavily on longitudinal shortening, and as a subpulmonary ventricle pumping into a low-resistance vascular bed, RV mechanics are quite different from LV mechanics. Although a morphologic RV seems inherently incapable of functioning as a subaortic systemic ventricular pump, it has a remarkable capacity for adaptation and may function at systemic pressures for decades (i.e., congenitally corrected transposition, Senning or Mustard repair for complete TGA). Under these circumstances, RV mechanics resemble those of an LV.

Precise and reproducible echocardiographic measurements of the RV are challenging because of its complex shape.[31] It must be imaged in multiple planes, and a qualitative visual assessment is usually applied on TEE. To define the size of the RV, its relative size compared to the LV on four-chamber view is often used as a qualitative measure. Similarly, the systolic RV function is usually characterized as normal, mildly, moderately, or severely abnormal. Rapid advancements in the field of magnetic resonance imaging (MRI) have established this technique as the reference standard for quantitative assessment of RV volumes, mass, and systolic function, regardless of whether the RV is in subpulmonic or subaortic position.

The most useful transesophageal views to assess the RV are:[32]
- Midesophageal (ME) four-chamber view: visualization of the RV lateral wall and measurement of RV internal dimensions and RV fractional area change
- ME RV inflow-outflow view (30-60 degrees): visualization of the coronary sinus, assessment of TR
- Upper esophageal (UE) views: visualization of the RVOT, assessment and quantification of pulmonary stenosis or regurgitation
- Transgastric (TG) views (0-120 degrees): short-axis views of the RV, anterior and inferior walls of the RV, the septum as well as the RV inflow and outflow tract, the IVC, and the hepatic veins
- Deep TG views: visualization of the inflow and outflow tract of the RV, tricuspid annular tissue Doppler signals

Volume-based indices of RV function have limitations because of geometrical assumption and load dependency. Other Doppler measurements may add insights into RV function, such as dP/dt of the TR velocity, as well as the index of myocardial performance, or Tei index, of the RV.[33] Other measurements include tissue Doppler imaging (TDI) of the tricuspid annulus and myocardial acceleration during isovolumic contraction, which measure intrinsic contractility but are not used routinely.[30]

We differentiate two broad contexts of RV adaptation to CHD: the volume-loaded RV and the pressure-loaded RV. The three most

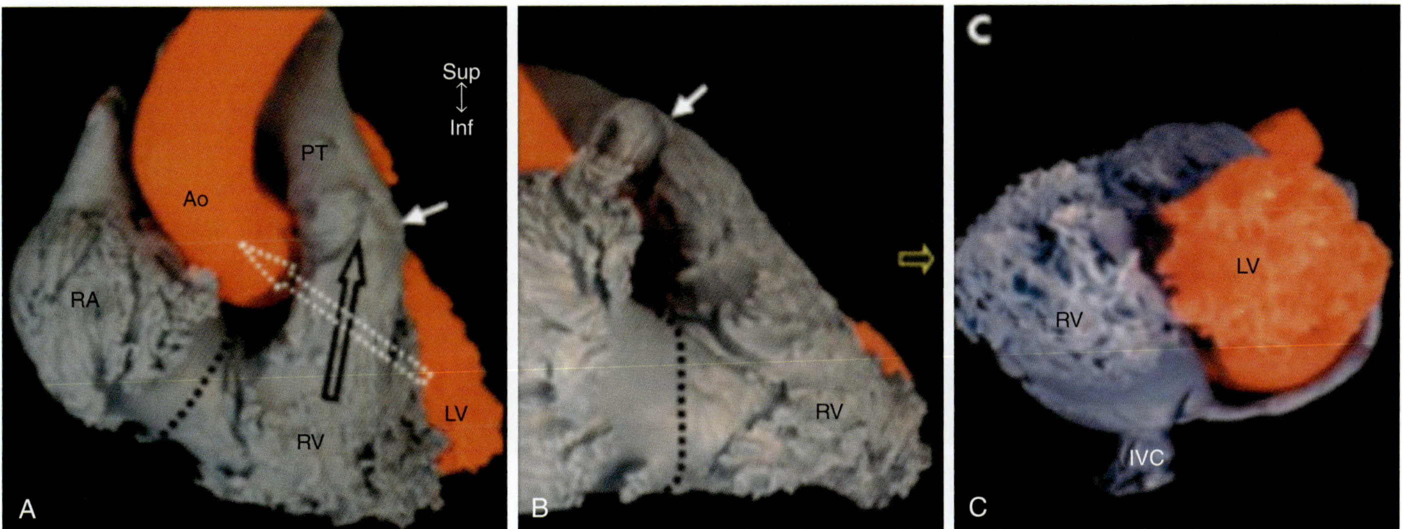

Figure 24-5 Anatomy of right ventricle *(RV)*. Endocast of a normal right heart with right heart chambers colored blue and left heart chambers colored red is viewed from different perspectives to display spatial relationships between cardiac chambers. **A,** Anterior aspect with crossover of left and right ventricular outflow tracts; pulmonary valve *(PV)* is situated more superiorly. **B,** From right and anterior: triangular shape. **C,** From apex: crescentic form, wrapping around left ventricle *(LV)*. *Ao,* Aorta; *Inf,* inferior; *IVC,* inferior vena cava; *PT,* pulmonary tract; *RA,* right atrium; *Sup,* superior. *(Modified from Ho SY, Nihoyannopoulos P. Anatomy, echocardiography, and normal right ventricular dimensions. Heart 2006;92:i2-i13, with permission.)*

common lesions associated with RV volume overload are the different types of ASDs, significant PR, and TR. The two most common lesions associated with RV pressure overload are different forms of RVOT obstruction and cases in which the RV serves as the subaortic systemic ventricle.

Individual Congenital Cardiac Lesions

Within the following sections, we will provide an overview of congenital cardiac lesions, their usual surgical treatment, and their potential complications in adulthood, with a special focus on the role of peri-interventional TEE.

Anomalous Venous Return
Anomalous Systemic Veins

Persistence of the left superior vena cava (LSVC) is the most common anomaly of the systemic venous connection, and in the absence of associated defects may be considered a variant of normal. It is found in 0.5% of the general population and up to 10% of GUCH patients.[34] The LSVC usually drains into the coronary sinus (CS) but may enter the LA directly, leading to a "right-to-left" shunt. When the LSVC drains into the CS, its hallmark on echocardiography is enlargement of the CS. (Fig. 24-6). On the transverse plane, the LSVC lies close to the lateral wall of the LA between the left upper pulmonary vein and the left atrial appendage. A microbubble injection into an upper left-sided vein follows the drainage into the anomalous system. The right SVC and innominate vein may be absent. Other etiologies may also dilate the CS, like an anomalous connection of the left pulmonary veins to the CS, a coronary fistula, or any lesion producing a marked increase in RA pressure, such as pulmonary hypertension or severe TR; they should be excluded before diagnosing a persistent LSVC. While a LSVC usually is an incidental finding without clinical implications, it may be important in the perioperative setting because it may change central venous or pacemaker accesses as well as, during CPB, the technique for venous cannulation or cardioplegia (retrograde cardioplegia is not possible).

In cases of cannulation of the venae cavae, stenosis at the site of cannulation should be excluded after bypass. With the use of color Doppler, acceleration at the level of the stenosis might be visualized (Fig. 24-7, A); the normal biphasic pulsed wave Doppler flow through the SVC is then replaced by a continuous flow without return to baseline and with a relatively high velocity (>1.5 m/s) (Fig. 24-7, B).

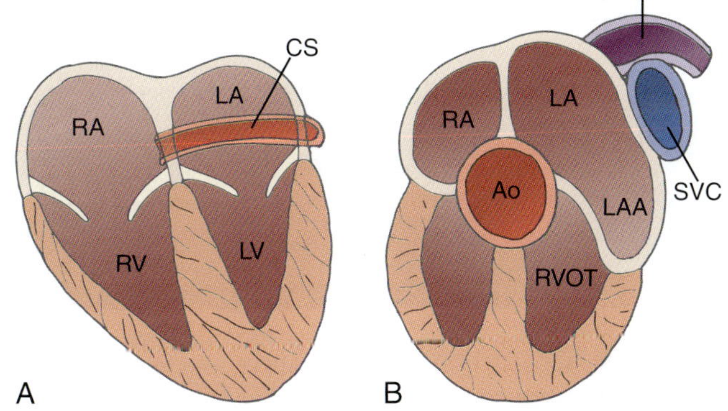

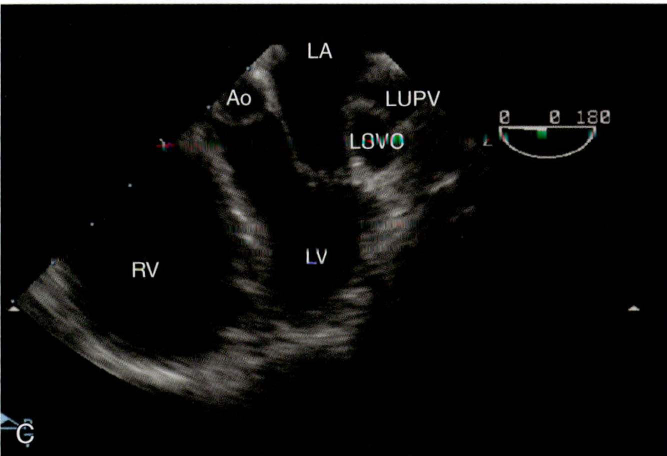

Figure 24-6 **A,** Schema of left superior vena cava *(LVSC)*. Coronary sinus is dilated and visualized in long axis at level of eso-gastric junction. **B,** Schema of LVSC. In midesophageal (ME) view, dilated vena cava may be seen between left atrial appendage *(LAA)* and superior pulmonary vein. **C,** Bidimensional imaging of LVSC in ME view. *Ao,* Aorta; *CS,* coronary sinus; *LA,* left atrium; *LUPV,* left upper pulmonary vein; *LV,* left ventricle; *RA,* right atrium; *RV,* right ventricle; *RVOT,* right ventricular outflow tract. *(A and B courtesy PG Chassot.)*

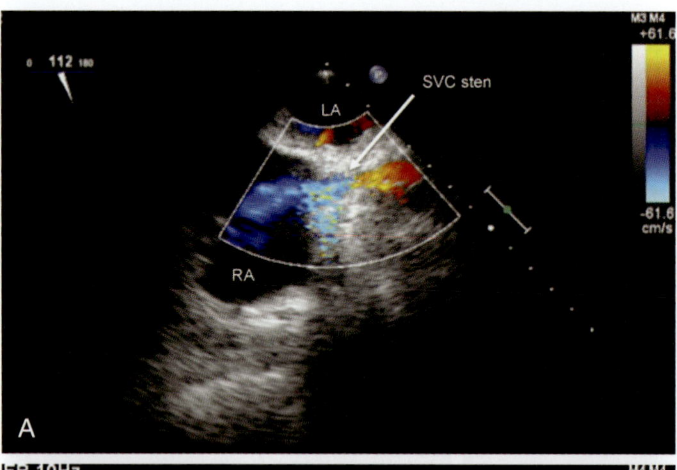

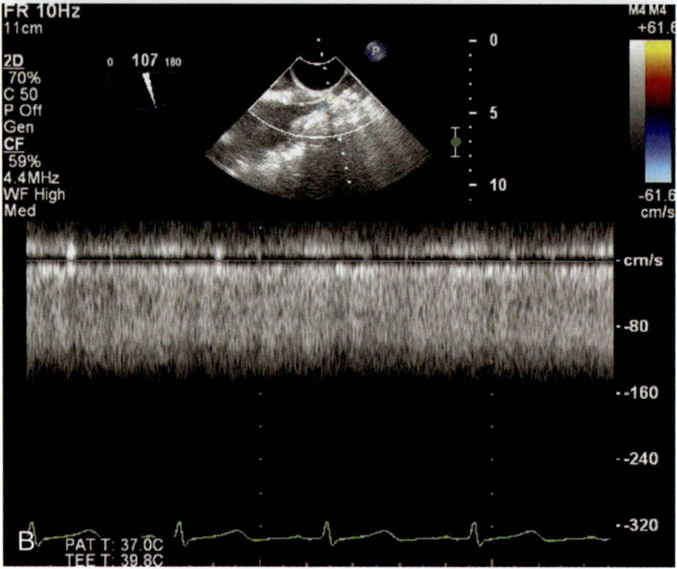

Figure 24-7   Superior vena cava stenosis *(SVC sten)*. **A,** Color Doppler of SVC: accelerated flow at entrance of SVC into right atrium *(RA)*. **B,** Continuous accelerated pulsed wave Doppler flow. *LA,* Left atrium.

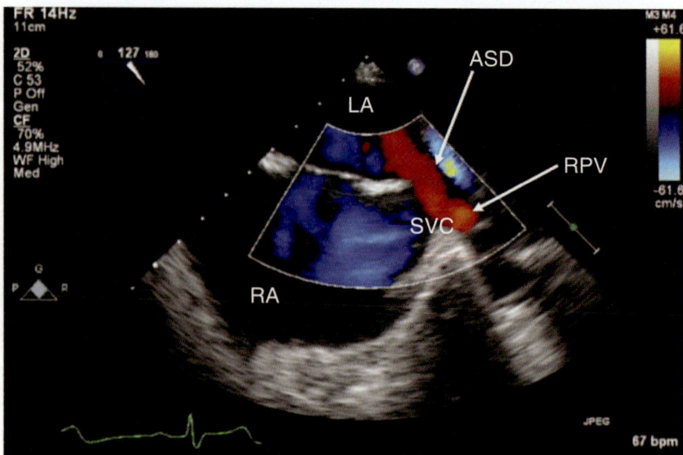

Figure 24-8   Superior sinus venosus defect. Midesophageal bicaval view: this type of atrial septal defect *(ASD)* is mostly associated with a partial anomalous pulmonary vein return. *In red,* inflow of right ventricle (RV) into superior vena cava *(SVC)*. *LA,* Left atrium; *RA,* right atrium; *RPV,* right pulmonary vein.

left-sided veins in particular may drain together into the LA. Identification of pulmonary venous connections is usually obtained from multiple views. The normal entry of pulmonary veins will be found in the UE four-chamber view at 0 and 90 degrees. If the entry of all the pulmonary veins into the LA are not visualized, anomalous connections should be searched for, especially in the case of an otherwise unexplained dilation of the IVC, SVC, RA, or RV. The exact anatomy and site of drainage of anomalous left pulmonary veins may be missed on TEE because of acoustical interference from the left bronchial tree.

Postoperative Evaluation

After surgical repair of anomalous venous connections, venous flow must be present with a biphasic systolo-diastolic pattern on spectral Doppler (Fig. 24-9), with a low maximal velocity (usually below 1 m/s) and a return to the baseline between the systolic and diastolic peaks. A continuous nonphasic pattern and a peak velocity of 1.5 m/s or more are indicative of significant residual stenosis (see Fig. 24-7, *B*).[36]

Atrial Septal Defects
General Considerations and Preoperative Evaluation

ASDs represent about 7% of all CHD and 30% of GUCH. Because these defects often cause few symptoms, diagnosis in adulthood is not uncommon.[37] *Ostium secundum*–type defects located in the fossa ovalis are most common and account for 60% to 75% of all cases. *Ostium primum*–type defects are part of the spectrum of AVSDs and account for about 15% of cases. *Sinus venosus* defects are typically associated with partially anomalous right pulmonary venous connections and account for about 10% of cases. *Coronary sinus defects* (also named *unroofed coronary sinus*) are rare defects (Fig. 24-10). The volume overload secondary to the L-R shunt is proportional to the size of the defect and the ratio between left and right atrial pressures. With progressive stiffening of the LV, a physiologic occurrence of aging resulting in increased LA pressure, the shunt flow usually increases. In large defects, volume load of the RA and RV leads to dilation of these chambers and enlargement of the size of the pulmonary artery.

The diagnosis by echocardiography is made with 2D imaging (echo dropout area in the interatrial septum) (Fig. 24-11, *A*; Video 24-3, *A*) and, importantly, with demonstration of shunt flow by color flow Doppler (Fig. 24-11, *B*; Video 24-3, *B*). Three-dimensional (3D) imaging may also be used to assess the precise localization and size of the defect (Fig. 24-11, *C*). Ostium primum and secundum defects are best identified in ME transverse (0 degrees) (Fig. 24-12) or longitudinal (90 degrees) planes (see Fig. 24-11, *A*). To delineate the size and tissue rims of these defects, careful assessment in multiple planes, as well as in 3D

Anomalous Pulmonary Venous Connections
General Considerations and Preoperative Evaluation

Some or all of the pulmonary veins may be falsely connected to the RA instead of the LA. Without surgery, patients with total anomalous pulmonary venous return do not survive to adulthood, and the unoperated patient is therefore not encountered in adulthood. In contrast, partial anomalous pulmonary venous return (PAPVR) drainage is encountered in adults, either as an isolated lesion or in combination with other defects (i.e., sinus venosus defects). The most common form is anomalous drainage of the right upper and middle pulmonary vein into the RA or into the base of the SVC. Figure 24-8 depicts PAPVR in the setting of a superior sinus venosus defect. The right lower pulmonary vein may anomalously drain into the IVC, as in Scimitar syndrome. In this case, the interatrial septum is usually intact. Isolated left pulmonary veins may connect through a left-sided vertical vein to the innominate vein or directly to the CS. PAPVR causes L-R shunting that leads to volume overload and dilation of the right-sided heart chambers.

Since the pulmonary veins return posteriorly into the atria, TEE is superior to TTE for evaluating PAPVR. It is possible to see the veins beyond their left atrial site of connection as far as the hilum of each lung.[9] At least four pulmonary veins draining into the LA must be documented to exclude significant PAPVR. In some patients, even more than four veins may be present (five in 10% of cases[35]); in others,

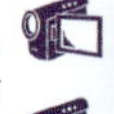

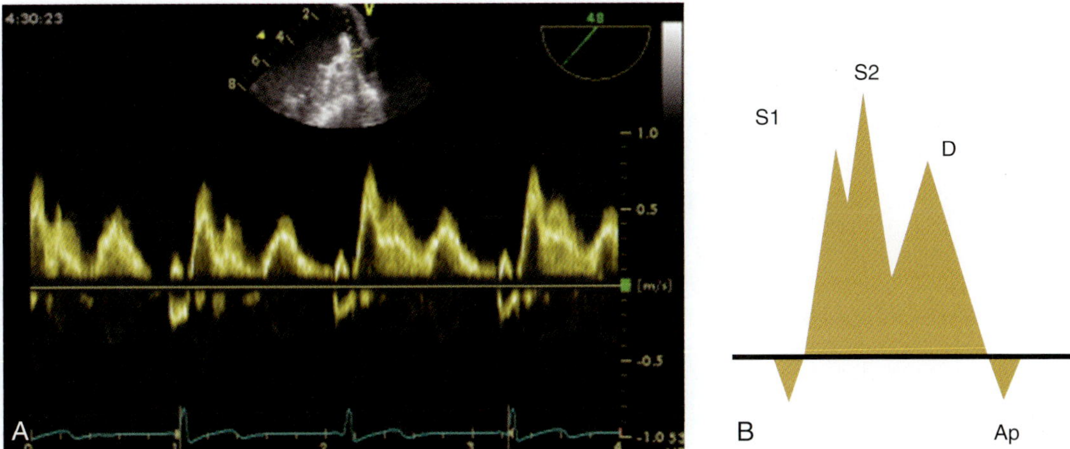

Figure 24-9 Pulmonary venous spectrum Doppler. **A,** Normal pulsed wave Doppler (PWD) of left superior pulmonary vein (PV). **B,** Schema of a normal PWD of PV. PV flow has three different parts: systolic component (which might be bifidous), with S1 simultaneous to atrial relaxation and S2 to mitral annulus descent; diastolic component *(D)* simultaneous to passive filling through mitral valve; and reverse A-wave *(Ap)* simultaneous to contraction of atrium. Maximal velocity does not exceed 1 cm/s, and flow reaches baseline between systolic and diastolic peaks.

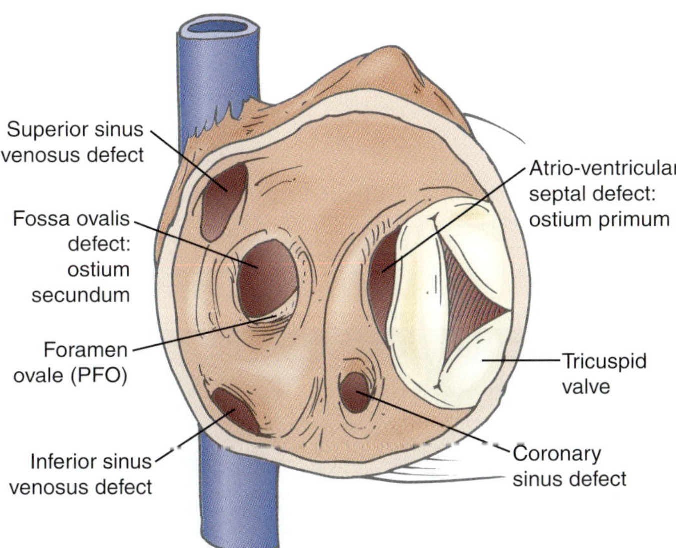

Figure 24-10 Schema of different atrial septal defects. Interatrial septum may present four types of defects: ostium secundum, situated at level of fossa ovalis; ostium primum in atrioventricular septum; sinus venosus at entry sites of venae cavae, frequently associated with abnormal pulmonary venous connection; and coronary sinus defect, an unroofing of coronary sinus into left atrium. *(Modified from Bettex D, Chassot PG. Transesophageal echocardiography in congenital heart disease. In: Bissonnette B, ed.* Pediatric Anesthesia: Basic Principles— State of the Art—Future. *Shelton, CT: People's Medical Publishing House-USA; 2011, with permission.)*

when available, is necessary. Ostium primum ASD, as a form of AVSD, is usually associated with a cleft in the left-sided AV valve. The sinus venosus defect is best detected in longitudinal planes (90-110 degrees) (Fig. 24-13) and often requires slight retraction of the ultrasound probe.[14,38] In the presence of this defect, careful search for anomalous pulmonary venous drainage using color Doppler is mandatory (Video 24-4; also see Fig. 24-8). The inferior sinus venosus defect is rare.

Since the pressure difference between both atria is usually small, the maximal blood flow velocity across the defect usually varies between 0.5 and 1.5 m/s. The L-R flow presents as a typical biphasic cyclic pattern on spectral Doppler (Fig. 24-14). Variations of the flow are related to the cardiac cycle: one peak of L-R flow occurs during late systole and early

diastole (synchronous with "v" wave), and one peak during the atrial contraction (synchronous with "a" wave). A short period of R-L shunting can usually be recorded during early systole and mid-diastole.[39,40] This flow pattern is consistent with the instantaneous cyclic pressure differences between the left and right atria (Fig. 24-15).[41] The most important shunt flow reversal is observed in protosystole when the mitral annulus descent abruptly increases the LA volume and therefore decreases its pressure.[42] Positive-pressure ventilation (PPV) and positive end-expiratory pressure (PEEP) increase the R-L components of the shunt by augmenting RV afterload. Because of the slower frame rates observed with color flow Doppler, the R-L component of the atrial shunt is usually not detectable on color flow, although it is easily identified on pulsed wave Doppler or with use of agitated saline contrast. The inflow of the IVC may sometimes be confused with an interatrial shunt, particularly in the case of a prominent eustachian valve.

Postoperative Evaluation

If a residual shunt is observed after surgical repair of an ASD, it raises two critical questions: How large is the shunt? Does it justify reoperation? Minimal residual shunting across the suture line, appearing as a little flame-like jet, is without significance; it disappears frequently after heparin reversal by protamine (Video 24-5). A large dehiscence is an indication for immediate surgical revision. An increase of more than 20% in pulmonary artery oxygen saturation compared to the value in the SVC and IVC will confirm the indication for surgical revision. The tricuspid valve function as well as the function of both ventricles might be altered after repair.[9]

After surgical closure of an ASD, TEE is performed to confirm the following:[43]
- ASD patch is intact, there is no residual shunt.
- IVC and SVC are draining correctly into the RA (see Video 24-4, *B*).
- There is no turbulent flow from the SVC or IVC.
- Pulmonary veins are all (re-)routed to the LA, and pulmonary venous flow is without turbulence if there was associated PAPVR. Confirmation by pulsed wave Doppler of normal pulmonary vein flow is required.

When technically feasible, an ostium secundum defect is currently most often treated with a percutaneous device closure. Echocardiographic guidance of this procedure, either by TEE or intracardiac echocardiography, is of paramount importance (Video 24-6).

Patent Foramen Ovale

A patent foramen ovale (PFO) is a remnant of fetal circulation characterized by an open passageway between the superior limb of the septum secundum on the RA side and the septum ovale or septum

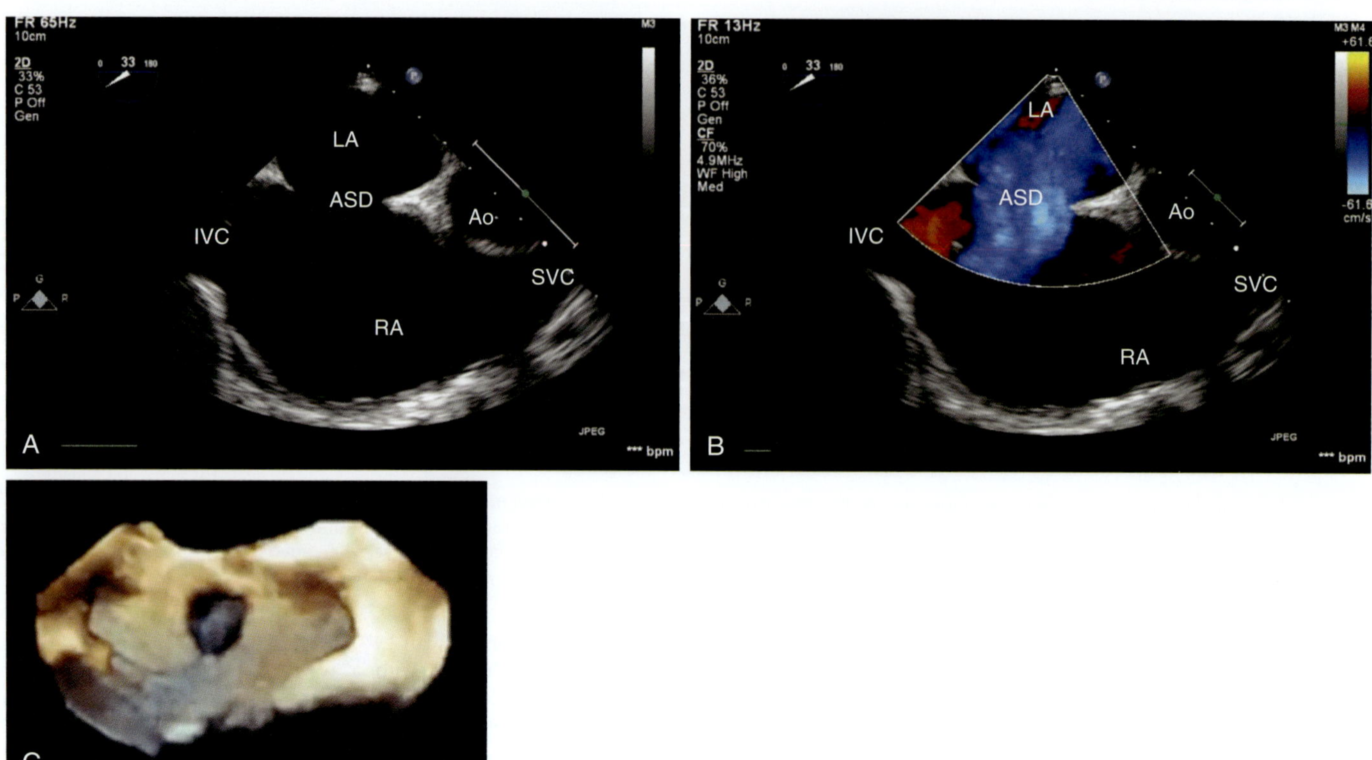

Figure 24-11   Ostium secundum defect. **A,** Bicaval midesophageal view of an atrial septal defect *(ASD)* secundum: echo-dropout in middle of interatrial septum. **B,** Same view with color Doppler: laminar color flow Doppler through ASD secundum, typical of a nonrestrictive defect. **C,** Three-dimensional imaging of ostium secundum ASD. Tricuspid valve is situated on right side of image. *Ao,* Ascending aorta; *IVC,* inferior vena cava; *LA,* left atrium; *RA,* right atrium; *SVC,* superior vena cava.) *(C courtesy PG Chassot.)*

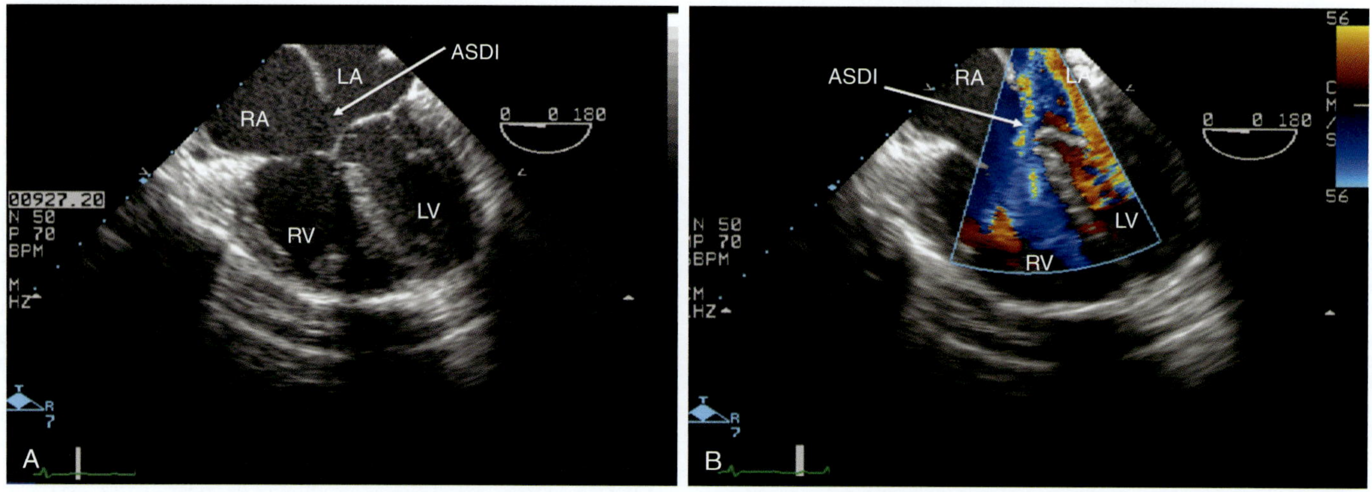

Figure 24-12   **A,** Midesophageal four-chamber view of ostium primum atrial septal defect *(ASDI)*: echo dropout at base of interatrial septum. **B,** Same image with color Doppler: laminar color flow typical of nonrestrictive shunt. *LA,* Left atrium; *LV,* left ventricle; *RA,* right atrium; *RV,* right ventricle.

primum on the LA side. Competence of the foramen ovale depends on the degree of overlapping of these two septa and the pressure gradient between the RA and LA. The flaplike opening of the foramen ovale fuses with the interatrial septum within the first few years of life in about two thirds of all people, but remains patent in the other third. When associated with the presence of a so-called interatrial septal aneurysm, epidemiologic studies suggest an increased risk of cryptogenic strokes.[44-46]

 The PFO is diagnosed by color flow (Fig. 24-16; Video 24-7, *A*) and contrast study with agitated saline (Video 24-7, *B*). Injection of microbubbles, best performed through a central or femoral line, must be synchronous with the release of endothoracic pressure after a short period of high PEEP (equivalent to the release of a Valsalva maneuver).[47] The normal pressure gradient between the atria is reversed, and the bubbles, even in small number, appear in the left-sided heart chambers within the next four cardiac cycles.[48] Their appearance after five or more cardiac cycles is suggestive of an intrapulmonary shunt. This test detects 92% of all PFOs.[44]

If there is an indication for closure of the PFO, it is usually performed by percutaneous device closure. Peri-interventional echocardiography

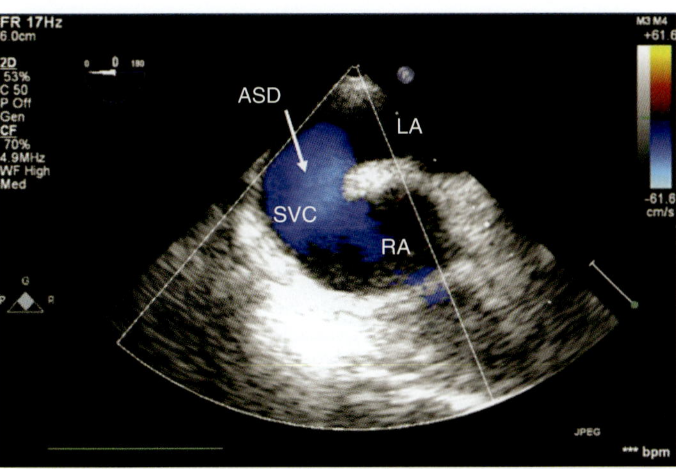

Figure 24-13 Upper esophageal basal view of superior sinus venosus defect: color flow Doppler shows communication between both atria at entrance of the superior vena cava (*SVC*) into right atrium (*RA*). Flow is laminar, shunt is nonrestrictive. *ASD*, Atrial septal defect; *LA*, left atrium.

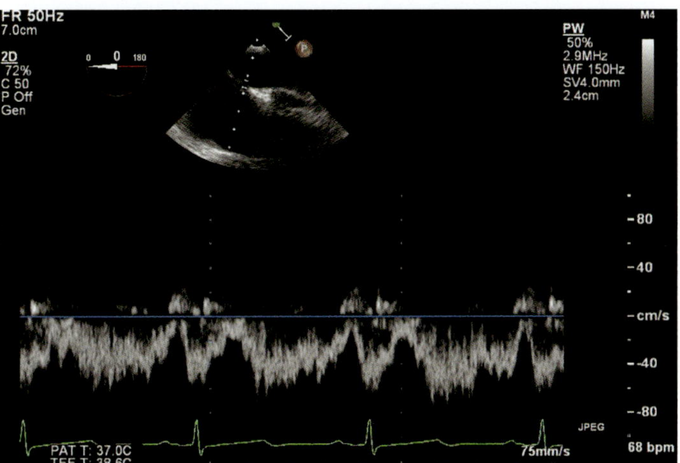

Figure 24-14 Pulsed wave Doppler (PWD) of left-to-right (L-R) shunt. Systolo-diastolic PWD flow of L-R shunt through atrial septal defect secundum. Since pressure difference between both atria is small, Vmax through shunt is in the range of 0.5 to 1.5 m/s.

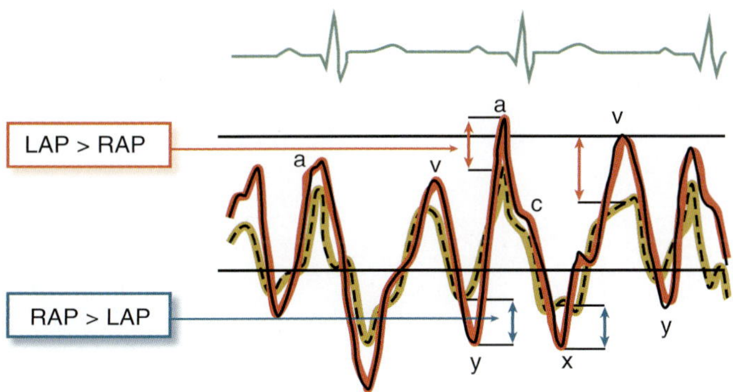

Figure 24-15 Schema of left and right atrial pressures (*LAP and RAP*). Variations of shunt flow through atrial septal defect are related to cardiac cycle: one peak of left-to-right flow occurs during late systole and early diastole (synchronous with "v" wave), and one peak during atrial contraction (synchronous with "a" wave). A short period of right-to-left shunt can usually be recorded during early systole and mid-diastole. This flow pattern is consistent with the instantaneous cyclic pressure differences between left and right atria. c, Tricuspid valve closure; x, drop of pressure during right atrial pressure and tricuspid annulus displacement in direction of apex of the heart; y, tricuspid valve opening. (*Modified from Bettex D, Chassot PG. Transesophageal echocardiography in congenital heart disease. In: Bissonnette B, ed. Pediatric Anesthesia: Basic Principles—State of the Art—Future. Shelton, CT: People's Medical Publishing House-USA; 2011, with permission.*)

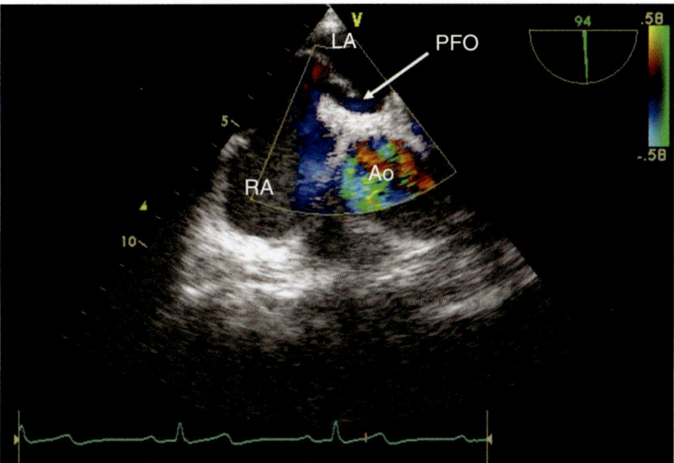

Figure 24-16 Midesophageal bicaval view with color flow Doppler on patent foramen ovale (*PFO*). Ao, Ascending aorta; *LA*, left atrium; *RA*, right atrium.

is usually not necessary. If the PFO is closed during cardiac surgery for other reasons, postoperative TEE may be useful to document complete PFO closure.

Atrioventricular Septal Defects
General Considerations and Preoperative Evaluation
An endocardial cushion defect or AVSD is caused by a lack of central septation during development of the heart. It is the most frequent cardiac defect found in patients with Down syndrome (trisomy 21) but can also occur sporadically. It results in a distinctive malformation of the internal cardiac crux (Fig. 24-17, *A*; Video 24-8, *A*). In the complete form, the AVSD includes an ostium primum defect, an inlet VSD, and a common AV valve with five distinct leaflets. There may be various degrees of AV valve regurgitation (Fig. 24-17, *B*; Video 24-8, *B*).[49] Inherent to this common AV junction is an anterior unwedged position of the aorta, with a resultant elongated LVOT with an increased risk for development of LVOT stenosis.[50,51]

If complete AVSD is not repaired in early childhood, most patients develop secondary pulmonary hypertension with Eisenmenger syndrome. Complete AVSD amenable to intracardiac repair is thus not encountered in adult patients.

Most common complications after surgical repair in childhood are progressive left-and/or right-sided AV valve regurgitation (these valves should not be called "mitral" and "tricuspid" valves, because they are morphologically very different from normal valves) (Video 24-9).  Prediction of reparability of such valves is difficult and requires careful interdisciplinary evaluation by dedicated cardiologists and cardiac surgeons. 3D TEE may be helpful in decision making because it may delineate mechanism(s) of regurgitation and thus may allow planning of repair. In addition, preoperative TEE should detect residual shunt lesions between the ventricles or the atria. If such shunts are present, depending on size and localization, the cardiosurgical team has to decide whether their closure is necessary and technically feasible.

Partial AVSDs present pathophysiologically as ASDs. Abnormal left AV valves with a "cleft" between the bridging leaflets are part of the defect. At the time of surgical patch repair of the primum ASD, the cleft is often closed by direct sutures. The physiologic consequences of a partial AV canal will mostly be dilation of the right cavities. The size of the LV is usually normal unless marked regurgitation of the mitral valve develops.

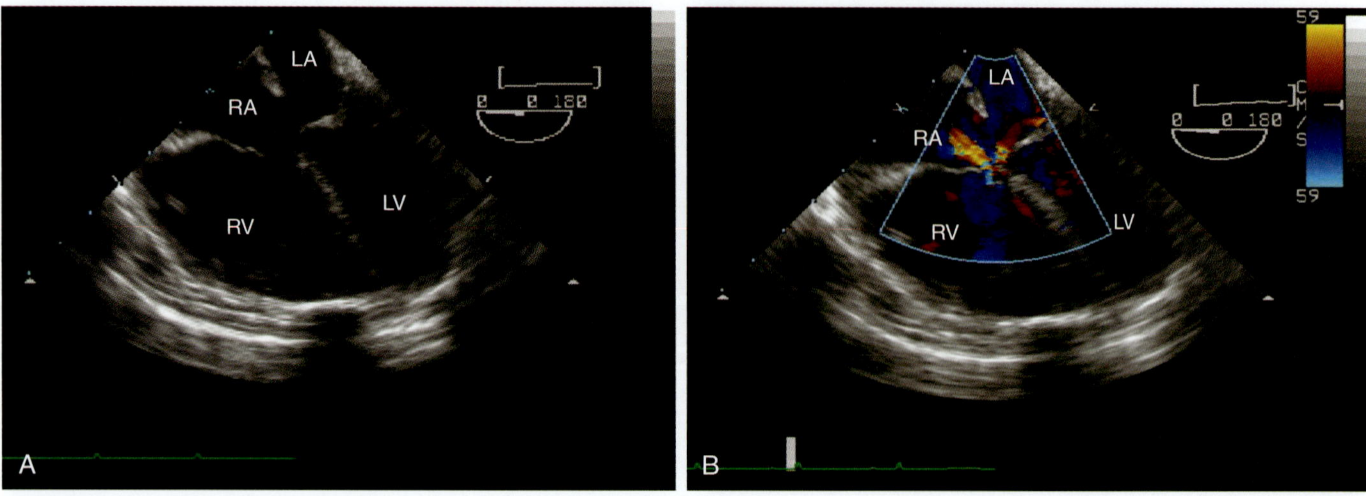

Figure 24-17 Atrioventricular septal defect (ASD). **A,** Midesophageal four-chamber view of complete ASD. Note insertion of atrioventricular valves at same level on interventricular septum. **B,** Same view with color flow Doppler in systole. Color flow may show variable degrees of shunts and regurgitations. In this case, there is a mild mitral insufficiency and tricuspid insufficiency. *LA,* Left atrium; *LV,* left ventricle; *RA,* right atrium; *RV,* right ventricle.

Postoperative Evaluation

The postoperative evaluation should address the presence of residual interatrial or interventricular shunts, the competence of the AV valves, and the presence of LVOT obstructions. Given the specific anatomy of the AV valves in the setting of AVSDs, particular attention has to be paid to residual stenosis after valve repair. The dense and echogenic prosthetic patch material often leads to suboptimal visualization of the RV cavity on ME imaging. Deep TG transverse and longitudinal planes offer better views to detect residual shunts and assess LVOT flow velocities. Small residual shunts or minimal or mild residual valve regurgitations occur frequently and may be tolerated. Small residual shunts often disappear after protamine administration and hemodynamic stabilization.[52]

Abnormalities of the Mitral Valve

Although a complete review of mitral valve pathology and function is outside the scope of this chapter, it is worthwhile mentioning some of the congenital mitral valve abnormalities. The most frequent are mitral valve prolapse and isolated cleft of the mitral valve, which will mostly be associated with mitral regurgitation (Fig. 24-18, Video 24-10). In the case of double orifice mitral valves, the valve function may be normal, and the valve can be regurgitant, stenotic, or a combination of both. Parachute mitral valves or supravalvular mitral membranes usually lead to restriction of LV inflow. TEE plays an important role in evaluating reparability of these valves.

Ebstein Anomaly
General Considerations and Preoperative Evaluation

Ebstein anomaly of the tricuspid valve is a relatively rare congenital heart defect. It is caused by abnormal development of the RV myocardium, with failure of delimitation of the tricuspid valve from the myocardial mass. It is characterized by an apical displacement of the insertion of the septal and posterior tricuspid valve leaflets. The anterior leaflet is usually large but may be dysplastic; it has been described as sail-like when it is freely mobile (Fig. 24-19, *A;* Video 24-11, *A*). The linear distance between the septal insertion of mitral and tricuspid leaflets can be measured and divided by the patient's body surface area to obtain a displacement index.[53] A displacement index greater than 8 mm/m[2] is invariably associated with Ebstein anomaly.[54,55] In patients with Ebstein anomaly, the right heart is divided into three components: the true RA, the atrialized RV, and the functional RV. The spectrum of this disease is enormous. It can present as end-stage heart failure in newborns, or in mild cases it can be found as an incidental finding in elderly persons. ASDs (PFOs or secundum-type ASDs) are common and occur

in up to 80% of cases. These defects often lead to cyanosis caused by R-L shunting across the interatrial septum. In extreme cases, the atrialized portion of the RV may occupy more than half of the RV volume, and RV dilation may be so pronounced that the ventricular septum shifts leftward, compressing the LV (Video 24-12). The tricuspid valve is typically regurgitant, rarely stenotic (Fig. 24-19, *B;* Video 24-11, *B*). Not well recognized is the accompanying RV cardiomyopathy that adds to the propensity for RV dysfunction in addition to that posed by TR.[55] The RV is usually very thin walled and vulnerable to progressive dilation and dysfunction. The tricuspid leaflets progressively display impaired mobility due to chordae shortening, tethering, or fibrosis. The functional RV cavity is reduced and its inlet portion atrialized; its function is significantly impaired.

TEE findings with potential implications for surgical repair include leaflet size and mobility, presence or absence of restriction, and size and function of the functional RV. Leaflet mobility is critical for the success of valve repair.[55]

Postoperative Echocardiography

After surgical repair, tricuspid anterograde flow should be unrestricted (mean gradient <5 mmHg); mild residual regurgitation (grade ≤II) can be tolerated. Postoperative RV dysfunction is frequent and poorly tolerated. Echocardiographically, it will manifest as a reduction of the RV ejection fraction, with dilation of the RV and paradoxical movement or dyskinesia of the interventricular septum (Video 24-13).

Ventricular Septal Defects
General Considerations and Preoperative Evaluation

VSDs occur in 20% to 25% of infants with CHD and are the most common form of CHD during the first year of life, excluding bicuspid aortic valves. The prevalence decreases progressively to 10% in adulthood, since more than 40% of VSDs close spontaneously during childhood.[28,56]

The interventricular septum is mainly muscular, with the exception of a small membranous segment located at its superior border just beneath the right and noncoronary cusps of the aortic valve and adjacent to the septal leaflet of the tricuspid valve. There are four types of VSDs (Fig. 24-20):
- *Membranous or perimembranous VSDs* (Fig. 24-21, Video 24-14). These represent the most common types of VSDs. During childhood, these defects often become smaller or close completely by interposition of redundant tricuspid valve tissue (Fig. 24-21, *A* and *C*).[57] The proximity of membranous defects to the tricuspid and aortic valves may cause progressive regurgitation even if the defect is small.

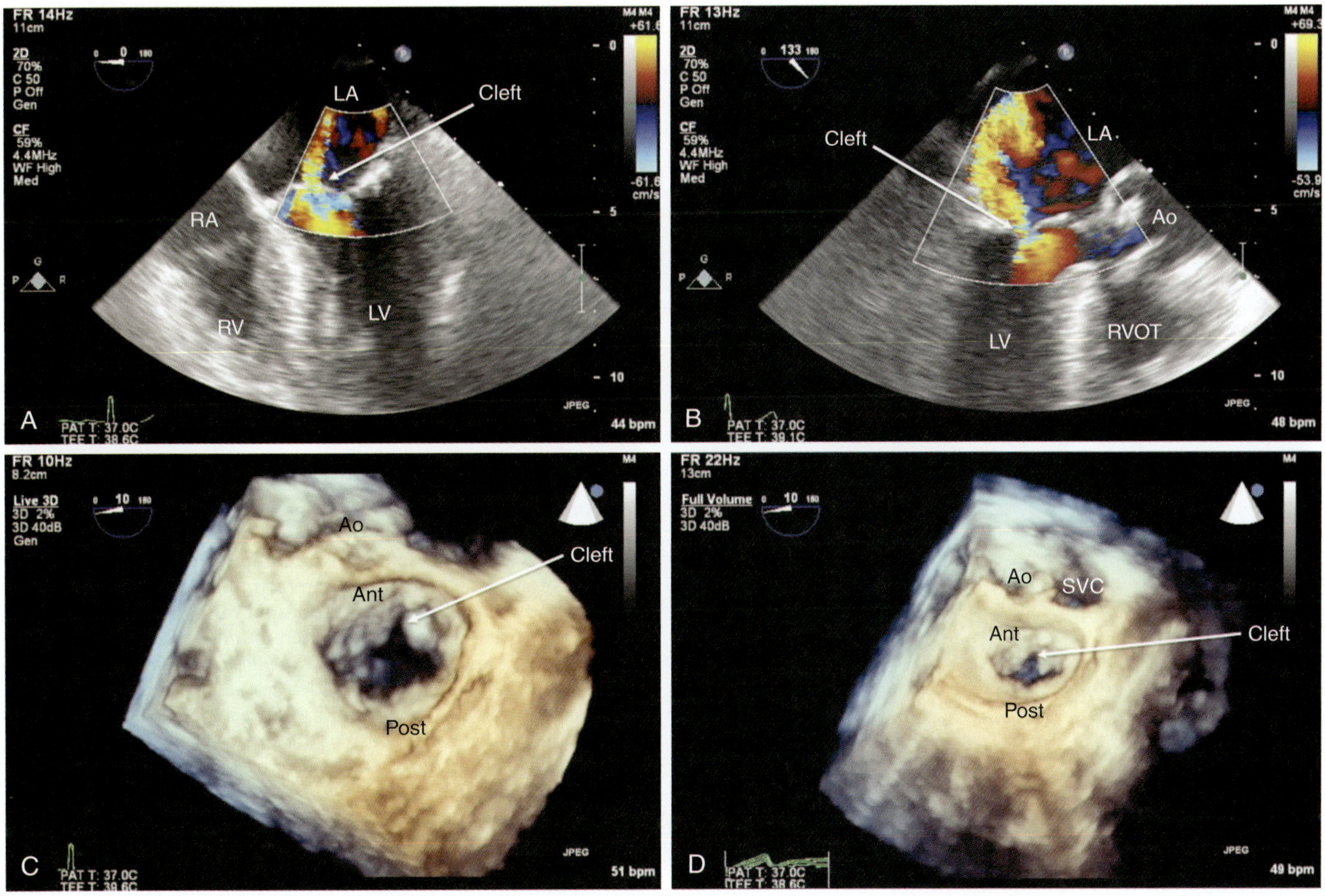

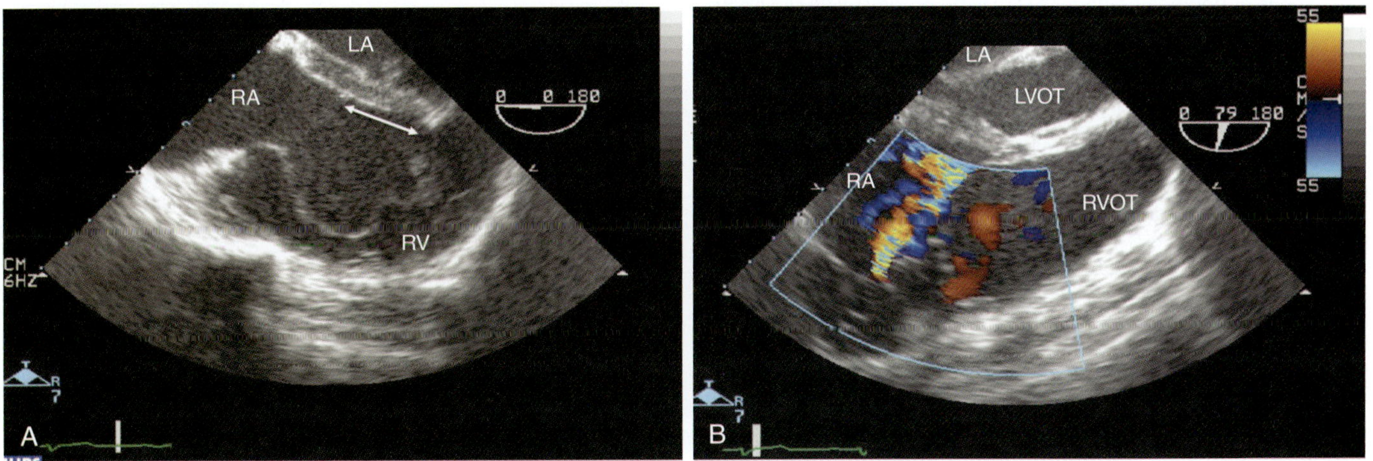

Figure 24-18 **A,** Midesophageal (ME) four-chamber view of mitral cleft. Note eccentric jet that seems to cross anterior mitral leaflet. **B,** ME long-axis view of mitral cleft. Again, note eccentric jet; its origin is difficult to localize. **C,** Three-dimensional (3D) zoom helps localize cleft in middle of anterior leaflet (*Ant*). **D,** Same view in 3D full volume. *Ao,* Ascending aorta; *LA,* left atrium; *LV,* left ventricle; *Post,* posterior; *RA,* right atrium; *RV,* right ventricle; *RVOT,* right ventricular outflow tract; *SVC,* superior vena cava.

Figure 24-19 **A,** Ebstein anomaly. Anterior leaflet is typically large and dysplastic; septal leaflet has a deep insertion at level of interventricular septum; double arrows define atrialized right ventricle (*RV*). **B,** Midesophageal inflow-outflow view of Ebstein anomaly with color Doppler: moderate tricuspid regurgitation. *LA,* Left atrium; *LVOT,* left ventricular outflow tract; *RA,* right atrium; *RVOT,* right ventricular outflow tract.

- *Inlet VSDs* are part of AVSDs (see earlier).
- *Supracristal, infundibular, or doubly committed VSDs.* These are rare defects located in the outlet septum immediately below the pulmonary and aortic valves at the base of the heart (Video 24-15). They are frequently associated with aortic regurgitation due to prolapse of the right coronary cusp, which often restricts the functional size of the

VSD; L-R shunt volumes are usually small. Given the risk of rapid progression of aortic regurgitation, repair of these VSDs is often advocated even if the L-R shunt is small.

- *Muscular VSDs.* Frequently multiple, usually located in the apical two thirds of the septal myocardium (Fig. 24-22, Video 24-16), they are less frequent among GUCH patients than in acquired cases. 

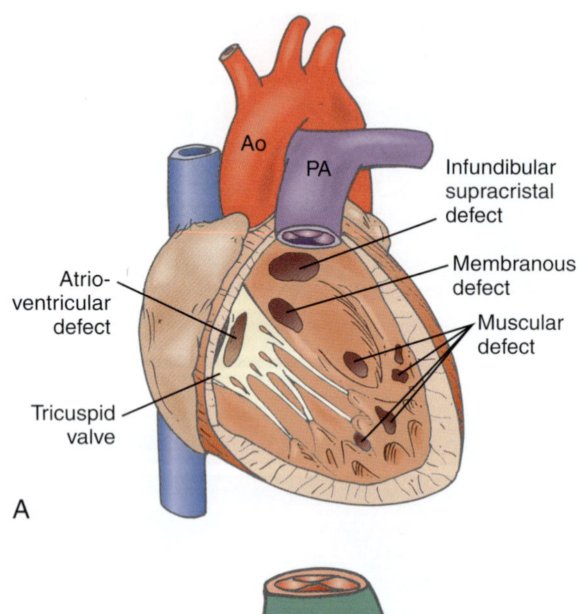

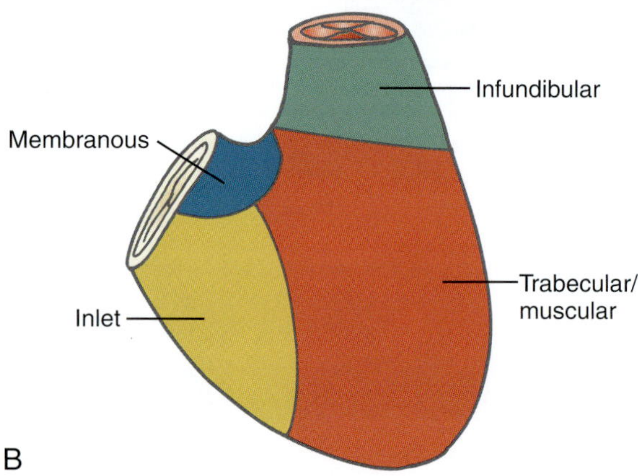

Figure 24-20　**A,** Schema of different ventricular septal defects (VSDs). Defect may supervene in four different parts of interventricular septum: muscular VSD usually located in apical two thirds of septal myocardium; membranous or perimembranous VSD may be progressively closed by septal hypertrophy surrounding defect or by redundancy of tricuspid valve septal leaflet; inlet VSD is part of an endocardial cushion defect and appears between mitral and tricuspid leaflets; and supracristal or infundibular VSD is located in outlet septum immediately below pulmonary and aortic valves at base of heart. **B,** Schema of interventricular septum viewed from right ventricle *(RV)*. *Ao,* Ascending aorta; *PA,* pulmonary artery. (**A** *modified from Bettex D, Chassot PG. Transesophageal echocardiography in congenital heart disease. In: Bissonnette B, ed. Pediatric Anesthesia: Basic Principles—State of the Art—Future. Shelton, CT: People's Medical Publishing House-USA; 2011, with permission.);* **B** *courtesy PG Chassot.)*

These defects often spontaneously close during early childhood. They are remote from any valve and thus not associated with valve dysfunction.

Large VSDs are usually diagnosed in early childhood. If spontaneous defect closure does not occur, most patients will undergo timely surgical repair in early childhood. If large defects are not repaired during childhood, development of progressive secondary pulmonary hypertension is common, and most adults with such defects are no longer amenable to intracardiac repair.

A persistent VSD creates an L-R shunt that overloads the pulmonary circulation and the LV. Anatomically, most of the congenital defects are situated close to the RV admission chamber and outflow tract in such a way that the shunted blood bypasses the RV cavity. The pressure and volume work is performed by the LV, which is chronically overloaded by the excess of volume shunted through the lungs; LV failure may ensue. The RV hypertrophies only when pulmonary hypertension

supervenes. The most important criterion to assess the severity of a VSD is to associate it with secondary LV dilation.

Adults with small defects in the perimembranous or supracristal locations are at risk of progressive aortic regurgitation due to prolapse of the aortic valve cusps. This may be an indication for surgical repair even in the absence of a large shunt.

In patients with perimembranous defects, progressive midventricular RV obstruction can occur by growth of abnormal muscle bundles ("double chambered RV"). This may be an indication for surgical repair in adulthood.

Adult patients with a VSD can be divided into four different groups:
1. Spontaneously or surgically closed VSD and no or minimal residual shunt
2. Small VSD, small shunts, and normal pulmonary pressure
3. Moderate shunt and elevated pulmonary pressures; RV is hypertrophied but pulmonary vasculature is still reactive.
4. Large shunt and Eisenmenger syndrome. *Eisenmenger syndrome* is defined as severe nonreactive pulmonary hypertension (pulmonary vascular resistance >800 dynes/s/cm^5) and progressive equalization of right and left ventricular pressures. The shunt becomes bidirectional and the RV dilates and fails, with venous stasis and TR.

The interventricular septum is a complex 3D structure. Its comprehensive assessment requires careful multiplane analysis. In perimembranous defects, redundant tricuspid valve tissue that partially or completely occludes the defect is often found. This tissue often bulges toward the RV and is also called a *membranous septal aneurysm* (see Fig. 24-21, *A to C*). A supracristal defect is characterized by a superior margin formed by fibrous continuity between both arterial valves. Prolapse of the right coronary cusp of the aortic valve is often present and may lead to aortic incompetence; this is best delineated in longitudinal planes (90-120 degrees) (see Video 24-15). Trabecular muscular VSDs are mostly antero-apical and less well visualized (see Fig. 24-22, *A and B*). In the four-chamber view, the apex is often truncated; to assess the apical part of the interventricular septum, the probe may be advanced more deeply into the fundus of the stomach with maximal retroflection. These defects are often better seen by transthoracic imaging.

The echocardiographic diagnosis of a VSD requires visualization of shunt flow by color flow Doppler. Small VSDs are often only detected by color flow Doppler and may be missed by 2D echocardiography; the presence of a proximal converging flow field (proximal isovelocity surface area, or PISA) is a good estimate for the size of the VSD: the larger the radius of the PISA shell, the more significant the VSD (see Fig. 24-21, *B*).[58] Continuous wave Doppler examination of VSD jet velocity is important. High jet velocity is typically found in small defects and is indicative of normal RV systolic pressures (Fig. 24-23). With very large defects and RV pressures approximating systemic values, the systolic velocities of the shunt may be low (<2.5 m/s) or not recorded at all.[59] Although L-R shunting occurs throughout systole in most small or moderate-sized VSDs, in some small muscular VSDs, the systolic jet occupies only a short portion of early systole, presumably because the muscular defect closes in midsystole with ventricular contraction. A low-velocity flow is usually seen during diastole because LV diastolic pressure exceeds RV diastolic pressure. The L-R diastolic shunt will disappear if there are associated lesions such as severe TR or PR causing an elevation of RV diastolic pressures.

Postoperative Echocardiography

After surgical repair of a VSD, small residual shunts located at the suture line of the patch are frequently found (Fig. 24-23, *A;* Video 24-17, *A*). Only large dehiscence (>2 mm) of the patch, with significant flow convergence on the LV side, is an indication for immediate surgical revision, or at least for assessment of shunt size by oximetry (Fig. 24-23, *B;* Video 24-17, *B*).[60,61] Tricuspid valve function should be thoroughly studied after VSD repair; tethering of the septal leaflet is sometimes found after closure of a perimembranous VSD, particularly when the tricuspid valve requires a transient detachment during repair.[43] Assessment of aortic valve function is mandatory after repair of a VSD, particularly after supracristal VSD repair. The presence and

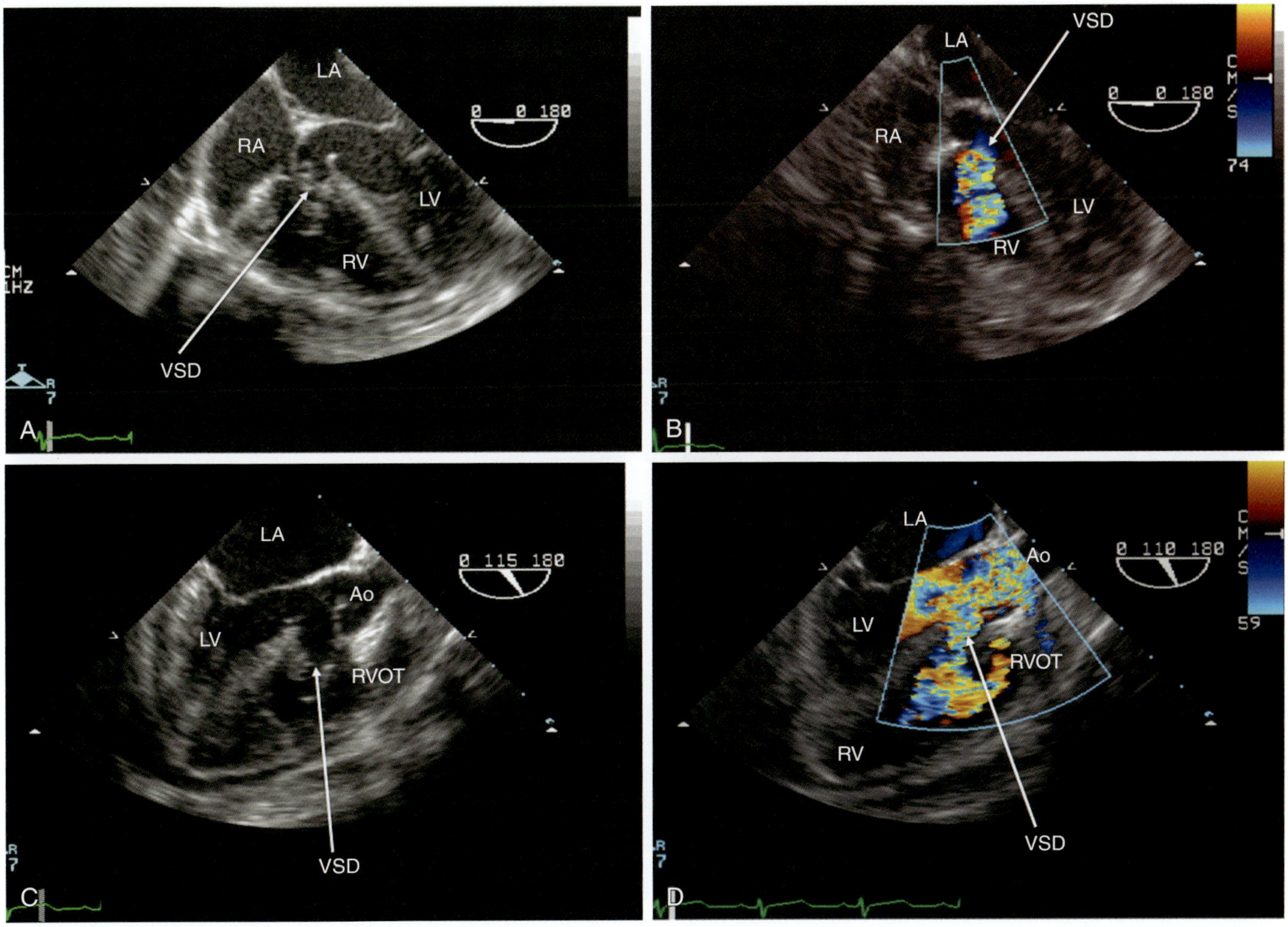

Figure 24-21 Membranous ventricular septal defect *(VSD)*. **A,** Midesophageal (ME) four-chamber view: echo dropout in proximity of tricuspid and aortic valves, partially closed by septal leaflet of tricuspid valve. **B,** Same view with color Doppler: left-to-right (L-R) shunt with proximal isovelocity surface area (PISA) effect on left ventricular side. **C,** Same patient, ME long-axis view. Note proximity of defect to aortic valve. **D,** Long-axis view with color Doppler: L-R shunt with turbulent flow in both outflow tracts. *Ao,* Ascending aorta; *LA,* left atrium; *LV,* left ventricle; *RA,* right atrium; *RV,* right ventricle; *RVOT,* right ventricular outflow tract.

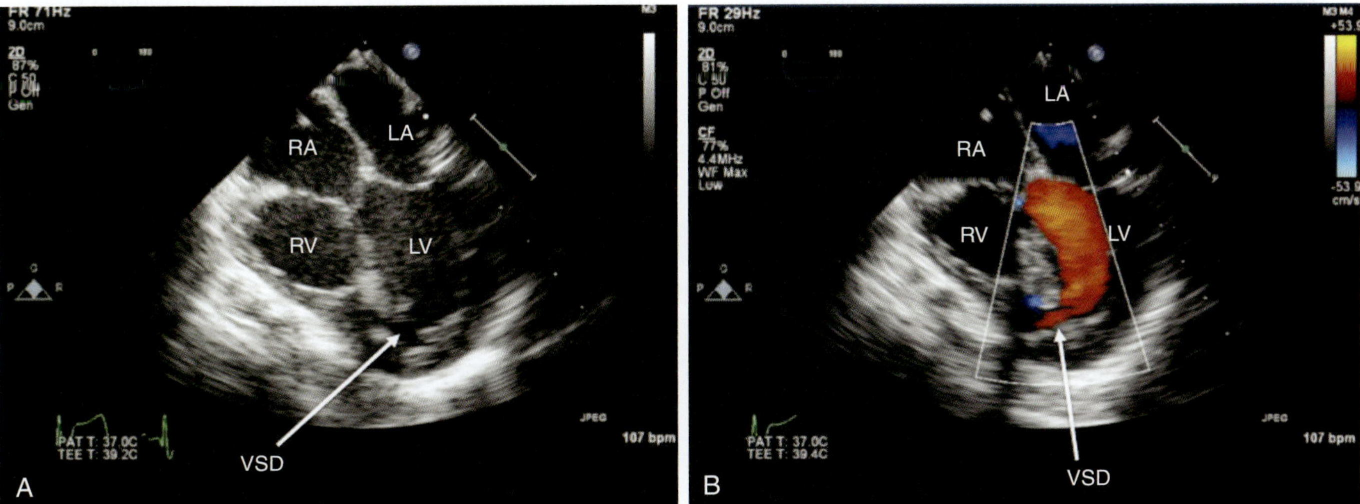

Figure 24-22 Muscular ventricular septal defect *(VSD)*. **A,** Midesophageal four-chamber view: echo dropout in apical third of interventricular septum. **B,** Same view with color Doppler: left-to-right shunt apical with laminar flow, sign of a nonrestrictive VSD with possible severe pulmonary hypertension (no left ventricle–right ventricle *[LV-RV]* gradient). *LA,* left atrium; *RA,* right atrium.

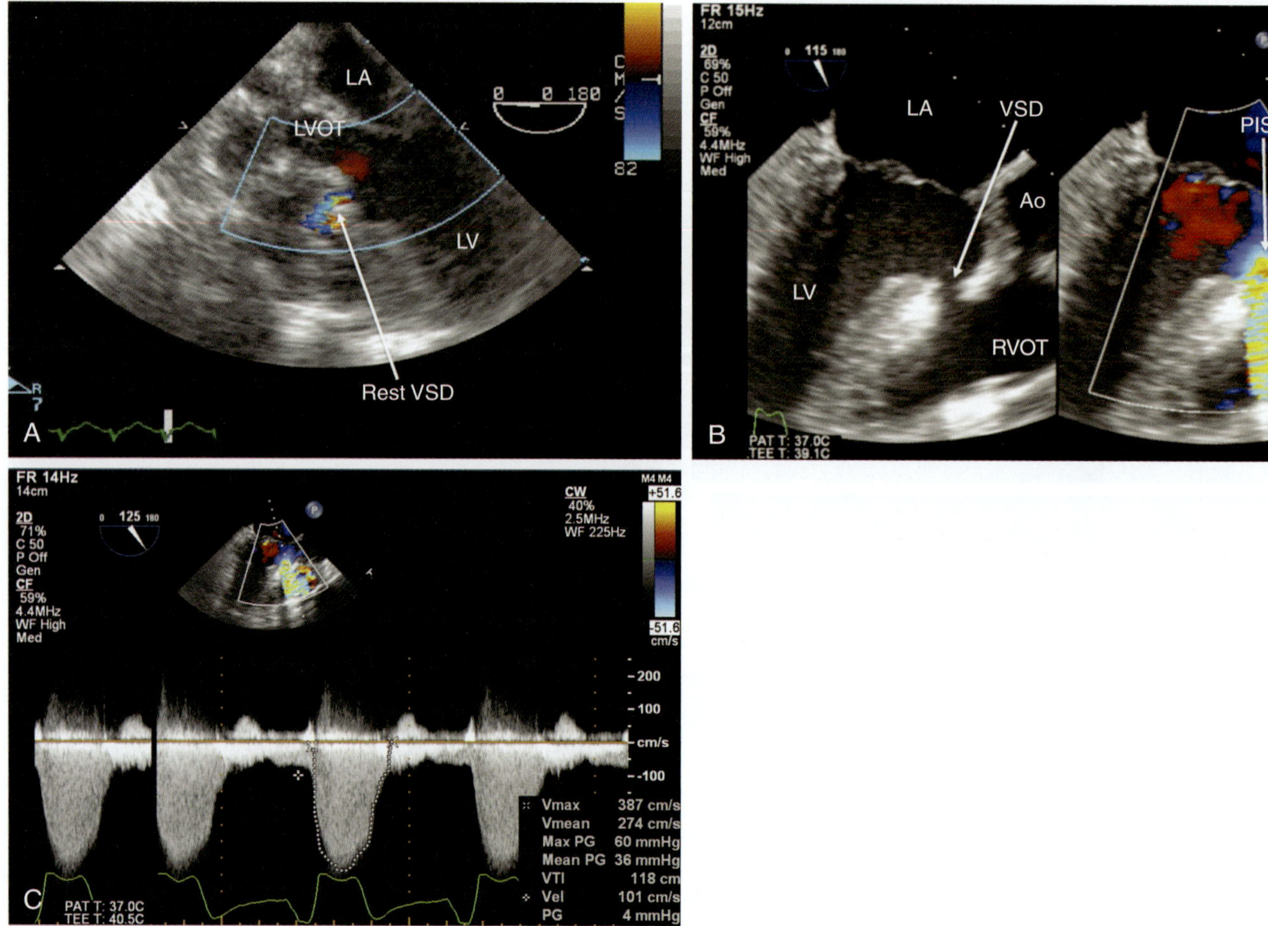

Figure 24-23   Residual ventricular septal defect *(VSD)*. **A,** Color Doppler flow on interventricular septum after patch closure of VSD shows a minimal rest VSD (<2 mm). **B,** Midesophageal long-axis color compare view of residual membranous VSD 10 years after patch repair. Note acceleration (proximal isovelocity surface area *[PISA]*) on left ventricular *(LV)* side of heart. Use of color compare view (simultaneous two-dimensional and color Doppler flow) helps precisely localize residual defect. **C,** Continuous wave Doppler through VSD: LV–right ventricle gradient of 60 mmHg, defect is restrictive, RV pressure is normal. *Ao,* Aorta; *LA,* left atrium; *LVOT,* left ventricular outflow tract; *RVOT,* right ventricular outflow tract.

degree of residual RV obstruction must be evaluated after VSD closure. Finally, an assessment of mitral and pulmonary valve flow profiles should be undertaken to exclude the presence of small obstructions that could be masked by prior increased pulmonary venous return.[9]

In particular cases, VSDs are nowadays treated with percutaneous device closure. Echocardiography guidance of these procedures is of utmost importance (Video 24-18).

Single Ventricle–Atrioventricular Connections and Fontan Circulation

Two groups of anatomic variables leading to single-ventricle physiology may be defined:

1. One of the two ventricles is too small to function as a circulatory pump. The ventricular segment may present with variable degrees of hypoplasia with marked asymmetry up to the absence of one ventricle. An anteriorly positioned accessory chamber is a rudimentary RV, whereas a posteriorly positioned one is a remnant of the LV (Fig. 24-24). A large proportion of patients with hypoplastic left heart syndrome have discordant ventriculo-arterial connections. The great vessels are aligned in parallel as in TGA.
2. The coexistence of different lesions makes it impossible to reestablish the two circulations surgically (i.e., major straddling of an AV valve in case of AV canal, severe Ebstein anomaly).

Single-ventricle hearts are among the most complex congenital heart defects, and a comprehensive discussion is beyond the scope of this chapter.

Surgically uncorrected patients with favorable physiology that allowed them to survive into adulthood are rarely encountered. These patients are cyanotic and may or may not have pulmonary hypertension. They are rarely candidates for cardiac surgery in adulthood but may have to be cared for in cases of non-cardiac surgery. Careful assessment of each patient's unique physiology prior to an elective operation is mandatory. During non-cardiac surgery, TEE may offer monitoring of cardiac function or volume status and may thus be an important tool to enhance safety in this complex patient group.

Most patients with functionally single-ventricle hearts have undergone modified Fontan procedures that offer good palliation for the first few decades of life. Fontan procedures consist in rerouting the systemic venous return directly into the pulmonary arteries, bypassing the single ventricular chamber (Fig. 24-25).[62] This operation has undergone a number of important modifications since its first description in 1968. Currently, most adult patients still undergo modified atriopulmonary-type procedures, but over the next years we expect to see more patients being palliated with lateral tunnel-type or extracardiac Fontan procedures.

In patients with recurrent atrial arrhythmias after atriopulmonary Fontan procedures, conversion to a "modern"-type Fontan anatomy is sometimes considered. During these complex operations, TEE may play a role in assessing AV valve function, assessment of fenestration and shunts, and to monitor ventricular myocardial function, volume status, and ventilation pattern of these patients.[9,63,64]

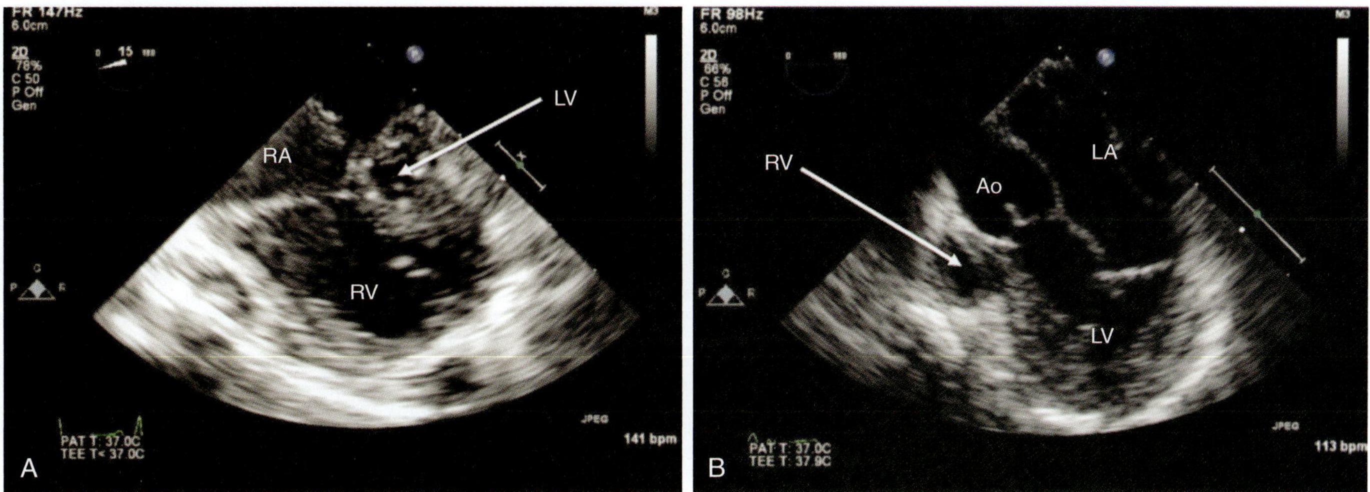

Figure 24-24 **A,** Left ventricular *(LV)* hypoplasia; posterior accessory chamber, remnant of LV. **B,** Right ventricular *(RV)* hypoplasia with tricuspid atresia; anterior accessory chamber, rudimentary RV. *Ao,* Ascending aorta; *LA,* left atrium; *RA,* right atrium.

After a Fontan procedure, the pulmonary flow drive relies entirely on the pressure gradient between central venous pressure and LA pressure; a gradient of 8 to 10 mmHg is generally considered necessary to provide adequate transpulmonary flow. The flow profile through the venopulmonary anastomosis or in the conduit shows two distinct patterns:[65] a biphasic forward flow with peak velocities during systole and diastole of 0.2 to 0.5 m/s, or a forward flow with flow reversals.[34] Patients demonstrating flow reversals show significantly reduced fractional shortening (26.5 ± 2.1 vs. 35.5 ± 6.3%) and larger pressure gradients between the RA and LA (10.8 ± 1.3 vs. 8.0 ± 09 mmHg) compared to those without flow reversal.[65] An increased flow velocity (>1.5 m/s) without cyclic variations and not reaching the baseline during the cardiac and/or respiratory cycle is suggestive of a significant obstruction.[63] The flow pattern is highly dependent on respiration: flow attenuation or even reversal has been demonstrated during the positive-pressure phase of intermittent positive-pressure ventilation (IPPV); flow is maximally increased during spontaneous inspiration (Fig. 24-26).[66]

Because patients post atriopulmonary Fontan procedures often have a very large RA with marked stasis of blood flow, they are at high risk of intracardiac clot formation even if they are on therapeutic anticoagulation.

Tetralogy of Fallot
General Considerations and Preoperative Evaluation
TOF is the most common form of cyanotic CHD. It occurs in 4% to 9% of children with CHD and is the third most common lesion encountered in adults.[53] TOF comprises four anomalies: membranous VSD, overriding aorta, RVOT and/or pulmonary valve stenosis, and RV hypertrophy. The RV hypertrophy is secondary to increased afterload due to outflow tract obstruction and to the connection to the systemic circulation through the VSD. The subvalvular muscular narrowing has an important dynamic component associated with variable degrees of pulmonary valvular stenosis and thickening and/or hypoplasia of the pulmonary arteries. Pulmonary arterial flow and pressures are generally low. The aortic valve is enlarged and competent in young children, but progressive aortic dilation may occur with age, mostly in uncorrected patients, leading to mild aortic regurgitation (grade I-II) in 75% of adults.[67] In 25% of cases, an ostium secundum ASD creates a *pentalogy*. Coronary anomalies are found in 18% to 35% of cases.[68,69] Patients are cyanotic because of the mixing of venous blood at the level of the VSD and because of the decrease in pulmonary arterial blood flow due to infundibular or pulmonary valve stenosis.

Survival without intervention is poor. Uncorrected patients have a survival rate of 30% at 10 years and less than 3% at 40 years.[70] With the advent of modern cardiac surgery, survival to adulthood has become the expectation. Surgical repair has evolved over the last few decades, both in timing and type of surgical repair techniques. Nowadays, at most centers the preferred repair technique is direct repair, without prior palliation, between 3 and 12 months of age. Repair typically includes patch closure of the VSD, resection of the infundibular RVOT obstruction, and relief of the pulmonary valve stenosis if required.

In the transverse ME plane, the large aortic valve is a striking feature (Fig. 24-27, *A*; also see Video 24-1). It opens to both ventricles by a large subaortic defect located between the right and non-coronary cusps. Blood flows through the VSD from both ventricular chambers toward the aorta; there is no clear-cut shunt from the LV to the RV. With color Doppler, the stenotic area of the RVOT is detected by an intense turbulent flow that might be at the subvalvular level (dynamic or membranous stenosis), valvular level (fibrosis and stenosis of the pulmonary valve), or supravalvular level (combined stenoses and membranes of the pulmonary tree) (Fig. 24-27, *B-C*; Video 24-19). Usually the maximal velocity (≈3 m/s) peaks in early systole in cases of fibrous stenosis, whereas it appears later in systole in cases of dynamic muscular obstruction (Fig. 24-27, *D*). Shunts and collateral circulations appear as continuous systolo-diastolic turbulent flow images in the posterior mediastinum; they may be traced from the aorta to a pulmonary vessel.

Most adult patients, after correction in childhood, do well. Residual hemodynamic lesions after childhood repair are common, however, and may predispose to atrial and ventricular arrhythmias. The single most common residual hemodynamic lesion in adults is PR, which is often severe, particularly after repair with a transannular patch in the case of a severely hypoplastic pulmonary valve annulus (Fig. 24-28, Video 24-20).

When PR becomes severe, the RV sustains volume overload, dilates, and finally fails; however, it can maintain normal systolic function for an extended time unless there is an added hemodynamic burden such as peripheral pulmonary stenosis that impedes forward flow or another volume lesion such as a residual VSD. Severe RV enlargement and dysfunction can antedate the onset of symptoms. An unfavorable ventriculo-ventricular interaction has been described in cases of severe RV enlargement; if right ventricular ejection fraction (RVEF) was impaired, left ventricular ejection fraction (LVEF) was also decreased. Cutoff values for RV volumes have been described beyond which RV size will never normalize: end-diastolic RV volume 150 mL/m^2 or less (Video 24-21).[2,30] Despite normalization of RV volume status after pulmonary valve replacement (PVR), no study has been able to show that RVEF improved. Although MRI is considered the gold-standard for PR quantification and RV volumetric analysis,

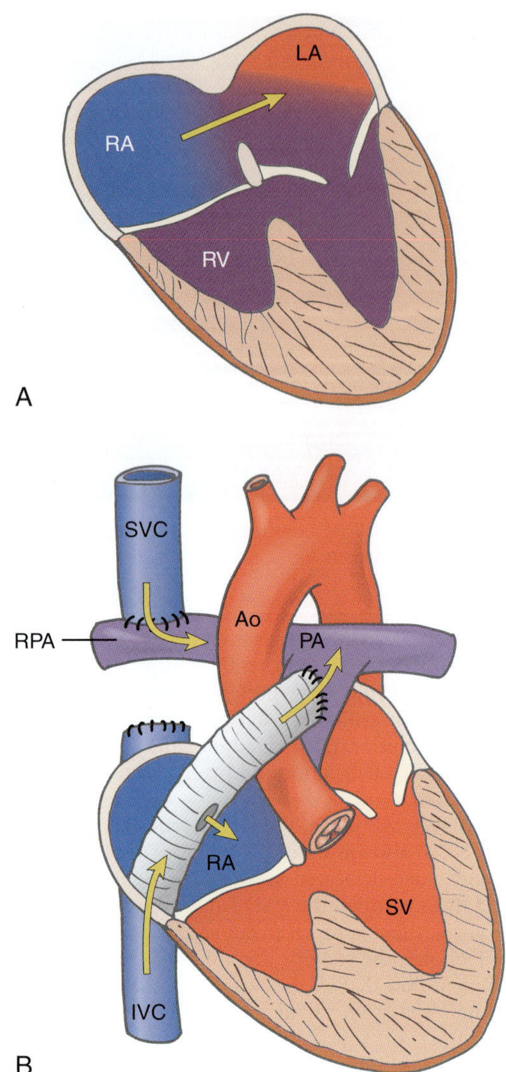

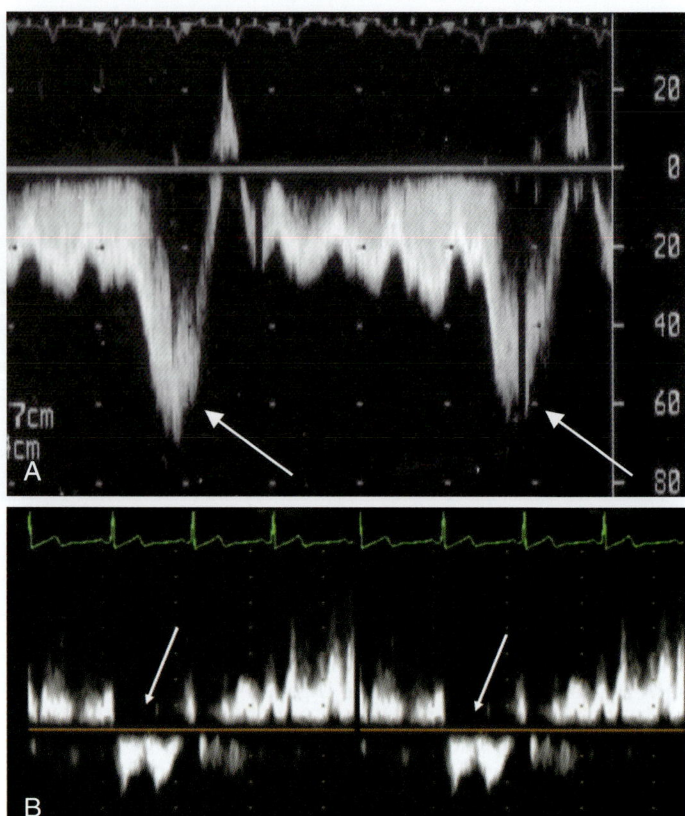

Figure 24-26 Pulsed wave Doppler flow through a Fontan circulation. **A,** Under spontaneous ventilation, flow is clearly increased during inspiration *(arrows)* and is maintained during expiration. **B,** Under intermittent positive-pressure ventilation (IPPV), flow is absent or may be reversed during inspiration *(arrows)* and maintained exclusively during expiration, explaining why Fontan patients tolerate PPV so poorly. (**A** *from Bettex D, Chassot PG. Transesophageal echocardiography in congenital heart disease. In: Bissonnette B, ed. Pediatric Anesthesia: Basic Principles—State of the Art—Future. Shelton, CT: People's Medical Publishing House-USA; 2011, with permission.)*

Figure 24-25 Schemas of tricuspid atresia and Fontan operation. **A,** Tricuspid atresia with hypoplastic right ventricle *(RV):* venous blood flows directly into left atrium *(LA)* through atrial septal defect; RV is hypoplastic. Venous blood is mixed with arterial blood in LA then ejected from systemic ventricle. **B,** Fontan operation: rerouting of systemic venous return directly into pulmonary arteries *(PA),* bypassing right heart. Bidirectional Glenn anastomosis (end-to-side anastomosis of superior vena cava *(SVC)* to right pulmonary artery *(RPA),* and an extracardiac or lateral tunnel conduit from inferior vena cava *(IVC)* redirects blood directly into PA. *Ao,* Ascending aorta; *RA,* right atrium; *SV,* systemic ventricle. *(Courtesy PG Chassot.)*

Doppler is a useful alternative for semiquantitative PR assessment using the Pulmonary Regurgitation Index (PRi): the ratio of PR duration to diastolic duration. A PRi less than 0.77 yields 100% sensitivity and 85% specificity for identifying patients with significant PR.[71] A PR pressure half-time less than 100 milliseconds is also a good indicator of significant PR (Fig. 24-29).

In the case of late pulmonary stenosis after correction of TOF, PVR is usually needed. Nowadays, interventional PVR is preferred for patients with a stenotic conduit. However, most patients who undergo re-do surgery in adulthood will have bioprosthetic PVR. Indications for this operation are controversial, and there are no prospective data to guide optimal management strategies for these patients. At times of surgical PVR, the role of TEE is to assess potential concomitant lesions such as TR, aortic regurgitation, or residual interventricular shunts.

Postoperative TEE Assessment

After bioprosthetic PVR, assessment of the prosthesis by TEE is sometimes difficult. In longitudinal views of the RVOT (ME views, 60 to 110 degrees), there may be some shadowing, but one should always try to visualize the prosthesis, since this view is best at showing leaflet motion and function. Pressure gradients are often better obtained from deep TG or UE basal views.

In the case of residual dynamic subvalvular RVOT obstruction after re-do surgery, indications to go back on CPB are sometimes difficult and require careful evaluation. These dynamic gradients often resolve with time and regression of muscular hypertrophy and may be amenable to medical treatment with β-blockers. Assessment of the patency of branch pulmonary arteries is important but may be difficult for the left branch pulmonary artery, which may be hidden by the bronchotracheal tree.[72] Although in most instances, postoperative TEE accurately quantifies residual RVOT obstruction, in 13% of cases, gradients are overestimated. Possible contributing factors include alterations in loading conditions, cardiac function, hemoglobin levels, variation in postoperative inotropic support, or the effect of the hypertrophied RV muscle bundles.

Residual septal defects are often seen after repair of TOF, but they are rarely hemodynamically significant (Video 24-22). Most of these residual shunts will spontaneously close with endothelialization of the patch. Another type of shunt reported is a coronary artery–to–right ventricular fistula.[73] These defects may not be seen preoperatively with 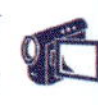

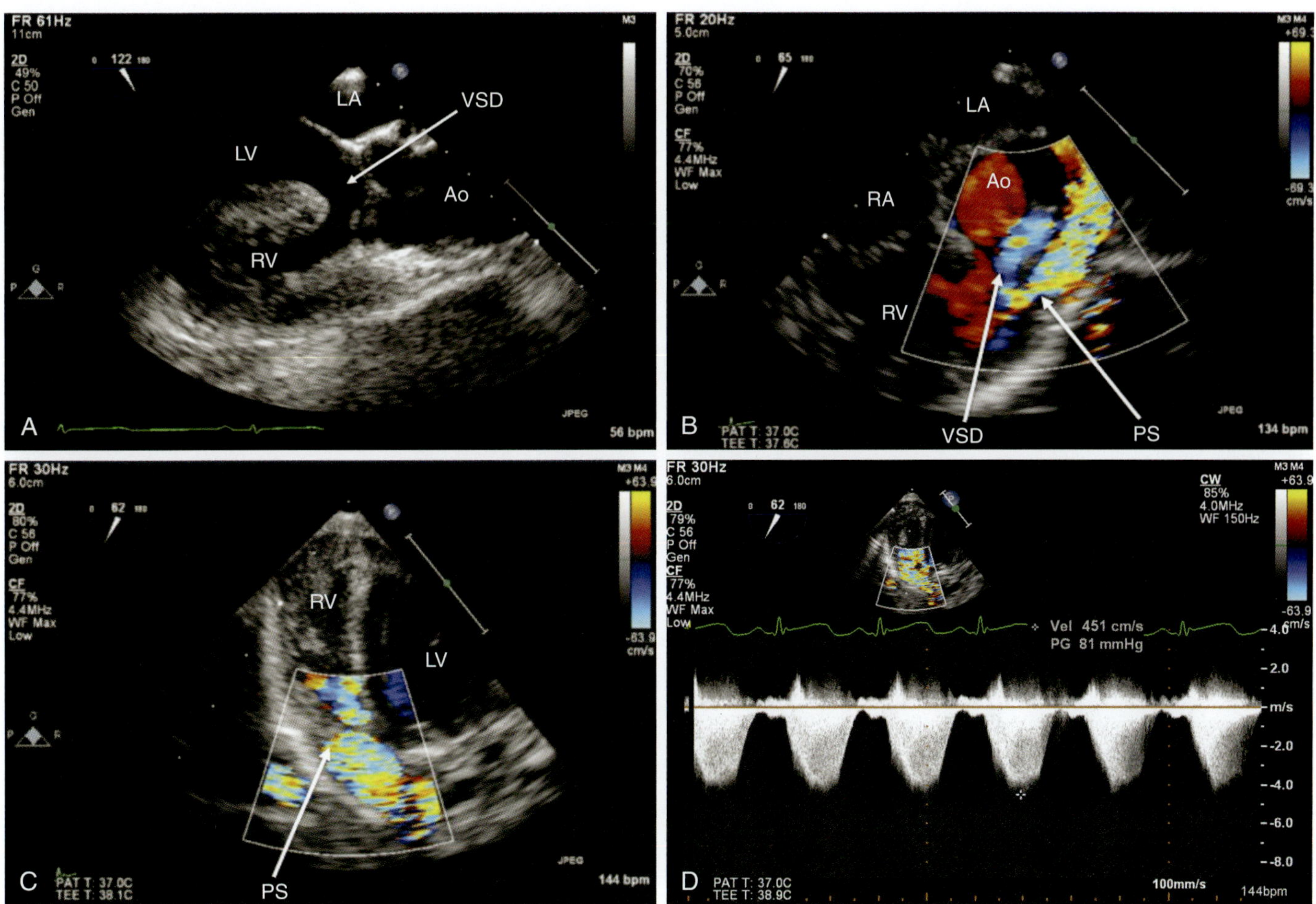

Figure 24-27 Tetralogy of Fallot. **A,** Overriding aorta with membranous ventricular septal defect *(VSD)* in long-axis midesophageal (ME) view. **B,** Color Doppler flow through pulmonary and infundibular stenosis in inflow-outflow ME view. **C,** Color Doppler flow through pulmonary and infundibular stenosis in deep transgastric long-axis view. **D,** Continuous wave Doppler flow through pulmonary and infundibular stenosis, showing a peak gradient of 81 mmHg. *Ao,* Aorta; *LA,* left atrium; *LV,* left ventricle; *PS,* pulmonary stenosis; *RA,* right atrium; *RV,* right ventricle.

color Doppler because of the systemic pressure in the RV. Postoperatively, with the decrease in RV pressure, color flow Doppler will show a continuous high-velocity turbulent jet through the fistula. Besides being congenital, these fistulas may occur as a result of RV infundibular resection.[51]

Doppler detection of forward and laminar late-diastolic pulmonary blood flow, coinciding with atrial systole and associated with a prominent retrograde SVC flow, defines "restrictive RV physiology" (Fig. 24-30).[74] A noncompliant hypertrophied RV, along with low pulmonary arterial diastolic pressures, results in partial presystolic opening of the pulmonary valve during right atrial contraction, which contributes to forward flow. This physiology is frequently present early after TOF repair, is associated with a low cardiac output state, and leads to prolonged ICU stay.[75-77] In contrast, restrictive physiology late after repair counteracts the effects of chronic PR and is associated with smaller RV size, shorter QRS duration, and better exercise capacity.[77,78]

Pulmonary Stenosis

Some degree of pulmonary stenosis is found in 10% of adult patients with CHD.[1] Anatomically, the image closely resembles what is seen in TOF but without a VSD and an overriding aorta. These patients are not cyanotic at rest and are frequently described as "pink Fallot." If major collateral arteries can preserve sufficient pulmonary blood flow, children with severe pulmonary stenosis or atresia may survive into adulthood. Isolated stenosis at the valve level represents 80% to 90% of PS cases.[77] Regardless of the level of obstruction, the RV exerts a hypertrophic response. Echocardiography is the diagnostic method of choice,

using continuous wave Doppler for estimating pressure gradients across the RVOT. Evaluation of pulmonary valve stenosis has focused on the corrected maximal instantaneous gradient until recently,[79] where mean gradients seem to be preferred for the assessment of mild to moderate pulmonary or conduit stenoses.[80,81] In the presence of low cardiac output, Doppler gradients are decreased or vanished. Outflow stenosis must then be graded morphologically.

It is a misconception that the RV dilates and fails when exposed to high pressure.[30] As long as sinus rhythm is preserved and there is no additional volume lesion, the RV may maintain good function until the fifth decade. However, when the RV pressure exceeds 50% of the systemic pressure, many patients develop symptoms.

The therapy of PS is closed or open valvotomy and a transannular patch in the case of a small pulmonary annulus. These operations always result in PR, which is well tolerated for years. Initially the RV compensates by dilation but maintains contractility and stroke volume. Often decades later, RV systolic function deteriorates, making a PVR necessary.

Left Ventricular Outflow Tract Obstruction
General Considerations and Preoperative Evaluation
The most frequent LVOT obstruction (after aortic stenosis) is isolated subaortic stenosis (SAS). It may be classified into three different types: discrete, tunnel, and dynamic.[53] In *discrete SAS,* a more or less circular fibrous thickening is present in the middle of the outflow tract; this ridge or diaphragm of fibromuscular tissue extends from the interventricular septum to the anterior leaflet of the mitral valve (Fig. 24-31,

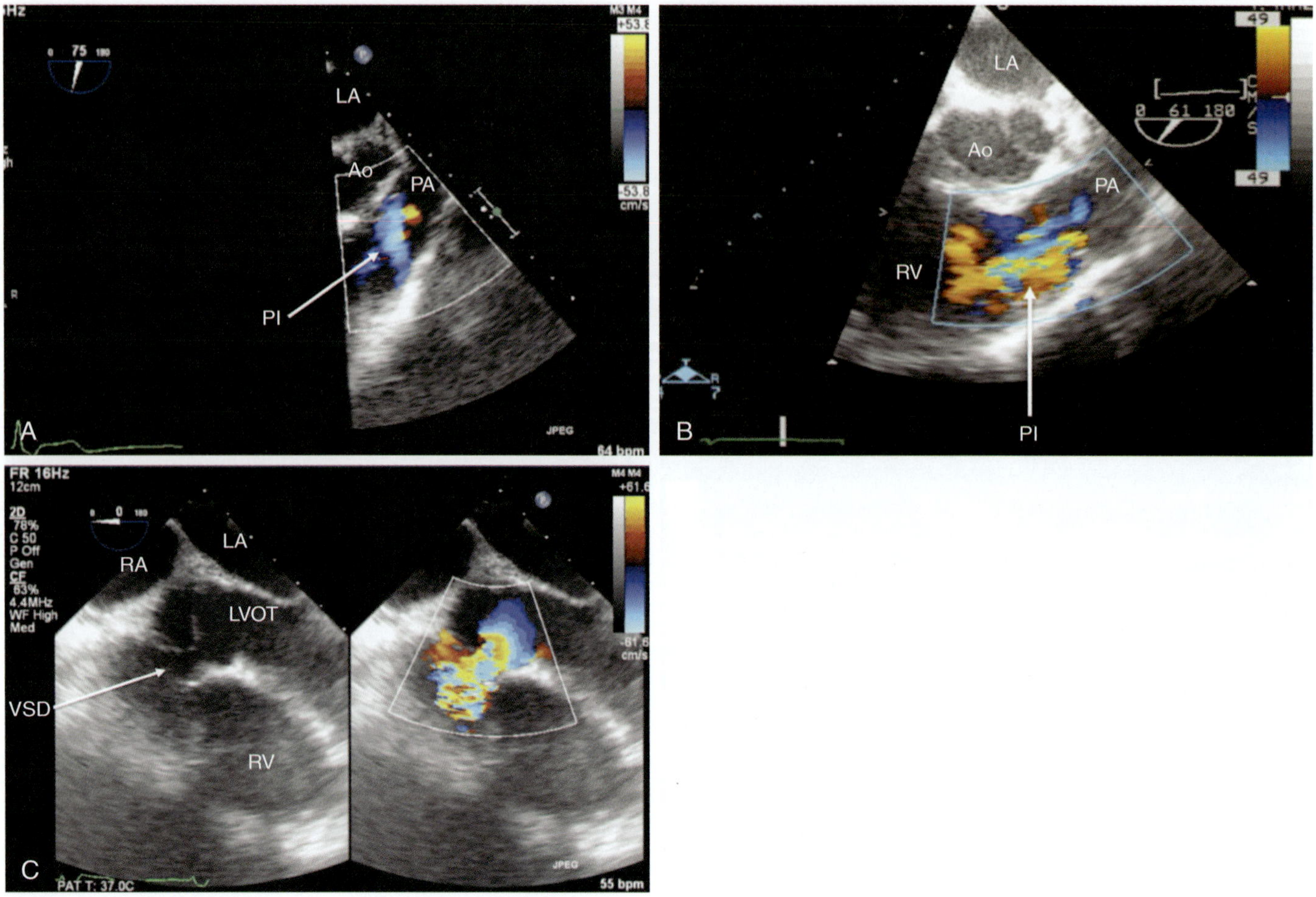

Figure 24-28   Residual defect after repair of tetralogy of Fallot. **A,** Midesophageal (ME) inflow-outflow view: residual mild pulmonary insufficiency after transannular patch. **B,** ME inflow-outflow view: residual moderate to severe pulmonary insufficiency after transannular patch. **C,** ME five-chamber view with color compare: residual severe membranous ventricular septal defect (*VSD*). *Ao,* Aorta; *LA,* left atrium; *LV,* left ventricle; *LVOT,* left ventricular outflow tract; *PA,* pulmonary artery; *PI,* pulmonary insufficiency; *RA,* right atrium; *RV,* right ventricle.

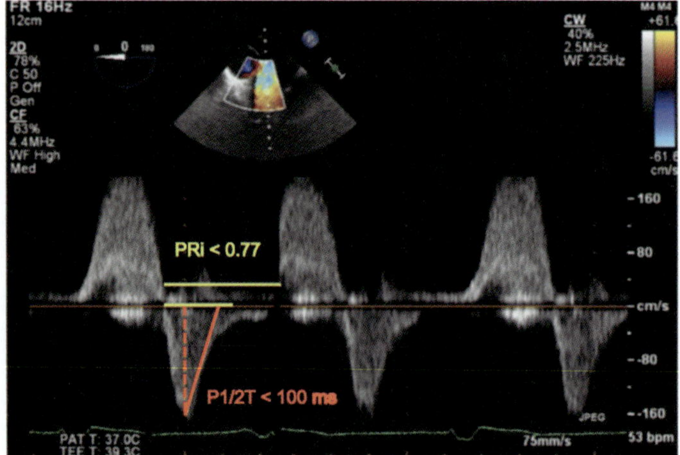

Figure 24-29   Transpulmonary pulsed wave Doppler for semiquantitative pulmonary regurgitation (*PR*) assessment. Pressure half-time (P$_{1/2}$t) less than 100 milliseconds and Pulmonary Regurgitation Index (PRi = PR$_{dur}$/Diast$_{dur}$) less than 0.77 are good indicators of significant PR. *Diast$_{dur}$,* Duration of diastole; *PR$_{dur}$,* duration of pulmonary regurgitation.

Video 24-23). Aortic regurgitation is frequently associated with this defect. *Tunnel SAS* includes diffuse hypoplasia of the LVOT with pronounced septal thickening. The aortic valve is frequently hypoplastic. These first two categories produce a fixed obstruction, with the highest gradient occurring in early systole. *Dynamic SAS* is analogous to LVOT obstruction in the setting of hypertrophic cardiomyopathy with dynamic obstruction (Fig. 24-32, Video 24-24). The obstruction progressively increases during the ejection period so that the highest gradients occur in late systole.

On TEE, quantification of LVOT obstruction can be difficult. Best alignment is usually achieved from deep TG views at 0 or 120 degrees.

Surgical treatment consists in resection of the membrane and/or myectomy of parts of the basal interventricular septum.

Postoperative TEE Evaluation

Major complications after resection of SAS are an accidental VSD due to excessive resection (Fig. 24-33, Video 24-25) or a residual stenosis due to incomplete resection. During the postoperative TEE examination, care must thus be taken to exclude any iatrogenic VSD or an injury of the mitral or aortic valves. An important impact of TEE examinations on surgical results of LVOT reconstruction has been reported: in 12% to 55% of the cases, an immediate surgical revision is indicated by the post-bypass examination in children.[16,24] This occurred significantly more frequently in complex LVOT obstruction than in discrete ones. TEE assessment of postoperative LVOT obstruction is accurate in 96% of cases.[16]

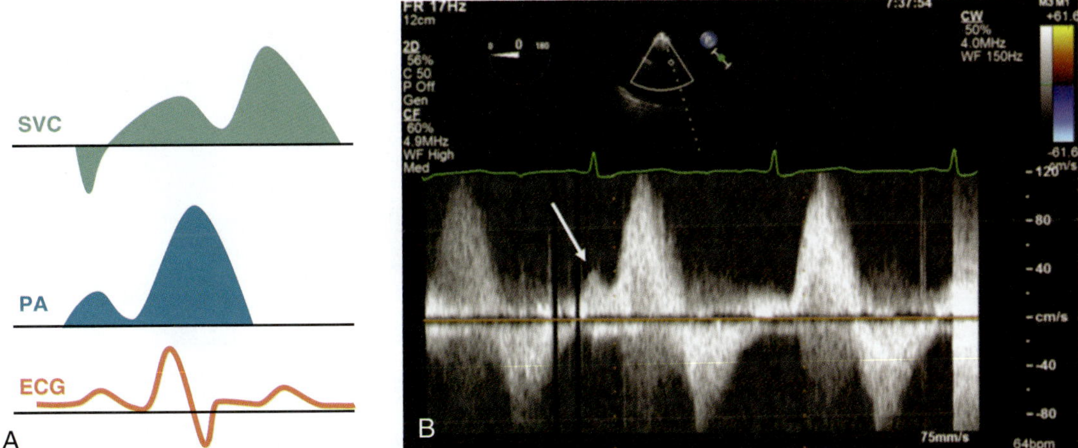

Figure 24-30 Restrictive right ventricle (RV) physiology. Forward and laminar late diastolic pulmonary blood flow coincides with atrial systole in electrocardiography *(ECG)* and is associated with prominent retrograde flow in superior vena cava *(SVC)*. **A,** Schema of restrictive RV physiology assessment: timing of Doppler through pulmonary artery *(PA)* and SVC with ECG. **B,** Spectrum transpulmonary Doppler of restrictive RV physiology after tetralogy of Fallot repair. White arrow points to forward late diastolic flow.

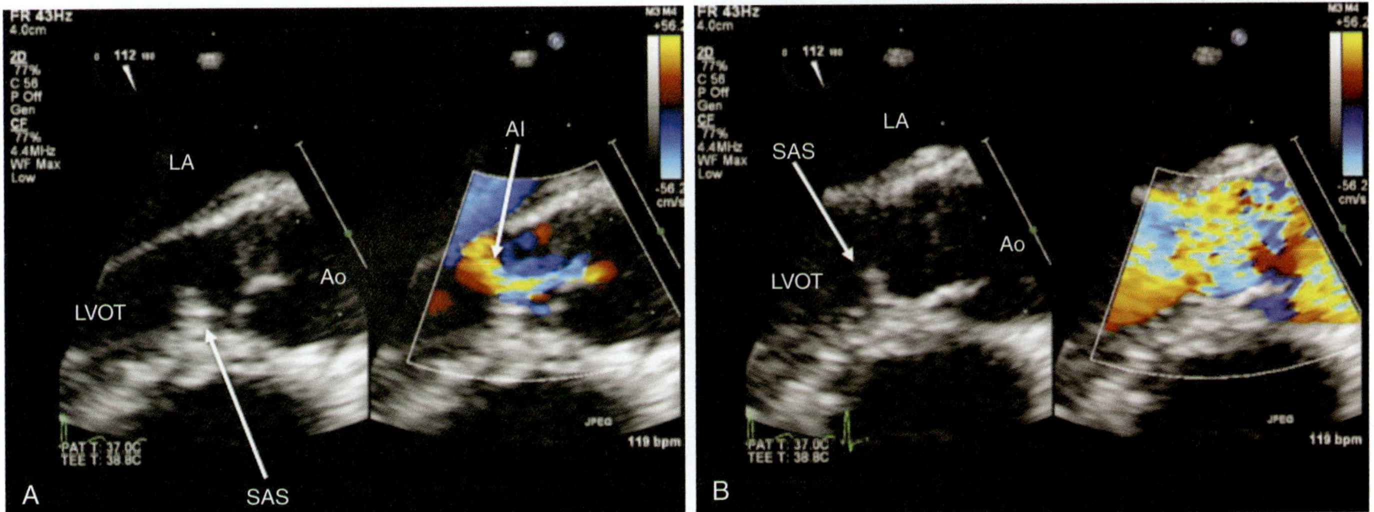

Figure 24-31 Subaortic stenosis *(SAS)*. Midesophageal long-axis color compare view of left ventricular outflow tract *(LVOT)* obstruction. **A,** In diastole, color Doppler on LVOT shows mild aortic insufficiency, often associated with SAS. **B,** In systole, obvious acceleration in LVOT secondary to subaortic membrane. *AI,* Aortic insufficiency; *Ao,* ascending aorta; *LA,* left atrium; *LV,* left ventricle.

Bicuspid Aortic Valves

Bicuspid aortic valve is the most common congenital cardiac anomaly; its incidence is reported at 2% in the general population.[82] It is characterized by having two instead of three cusps, which may be of unequal size. If asymmetric, the larger cusp often shows a fibrous raphe at the site of fusion. In systole, the shape of the valve opening looks like a fish mouth (Fig. 24-34, Video 24-26). Bicuspid aortic valves tend to degenerate 1 or 2 decades earlier than tricuspid aortic valves. Valves may become stenotic or regurgitant. Associated malformations include dilation of the ascending aorta, coarctation of the aorta, and VSDs.

The Ross procedure consists of replacement of the aortic valve by the pulmonary valve, reimplantation of the coronary arteries, and reconstruction of the RVOT with a homograft or bioprosthetic conduit. Preoperative assessment by TEE should assess the origin of the coronary arteries and particularly exclude their anomalous origin. In addition, the difference in annular size between the aortic and the pulmonary valve annulus may be of technical importance to the surgeon. TEE should also identify the function and morphology of the pulmonary valve (tricuspid or bicuspid) and the thickness of the septal portion of the muscular RVOT. Directly after unclamping of the aorta, the echocardiographer should monitor for possible dilation of the LV, which would be suggestive of significant aortic regurgitation and may lead to subendocardial ischemia. Once the patient is separated from CPB, the imager should rule out new regional wall motion abnormalities, which could be a result of technically poorly implanted coronary arteries, and document normal function of the prosthetic pulmonary valve and absence of significant aortic regurgitation.

Transposition of the Great Arteries

Complete TGA is a common congenital cardiac defect. Survival to adulthood without surgical repair or palliation is almost impossible. It is characterized by an AV concordance and a ventriculo-arterial discordance: the aorta arises from the anatomic RV (subaortic ventricle), and the pulmonary artery originates from the anatomic LV (subpulmonic ventricle). The great arteries arise in parallel at the base of the heart. The aortic valve is anterior, to the right, and slightly superior to the pulmonary valve (D-transposition). The pulmonary artery originates directly above the LVOT. This condition creates two circulations in parallel instead of in series. A VSD is present in 30% to 40%

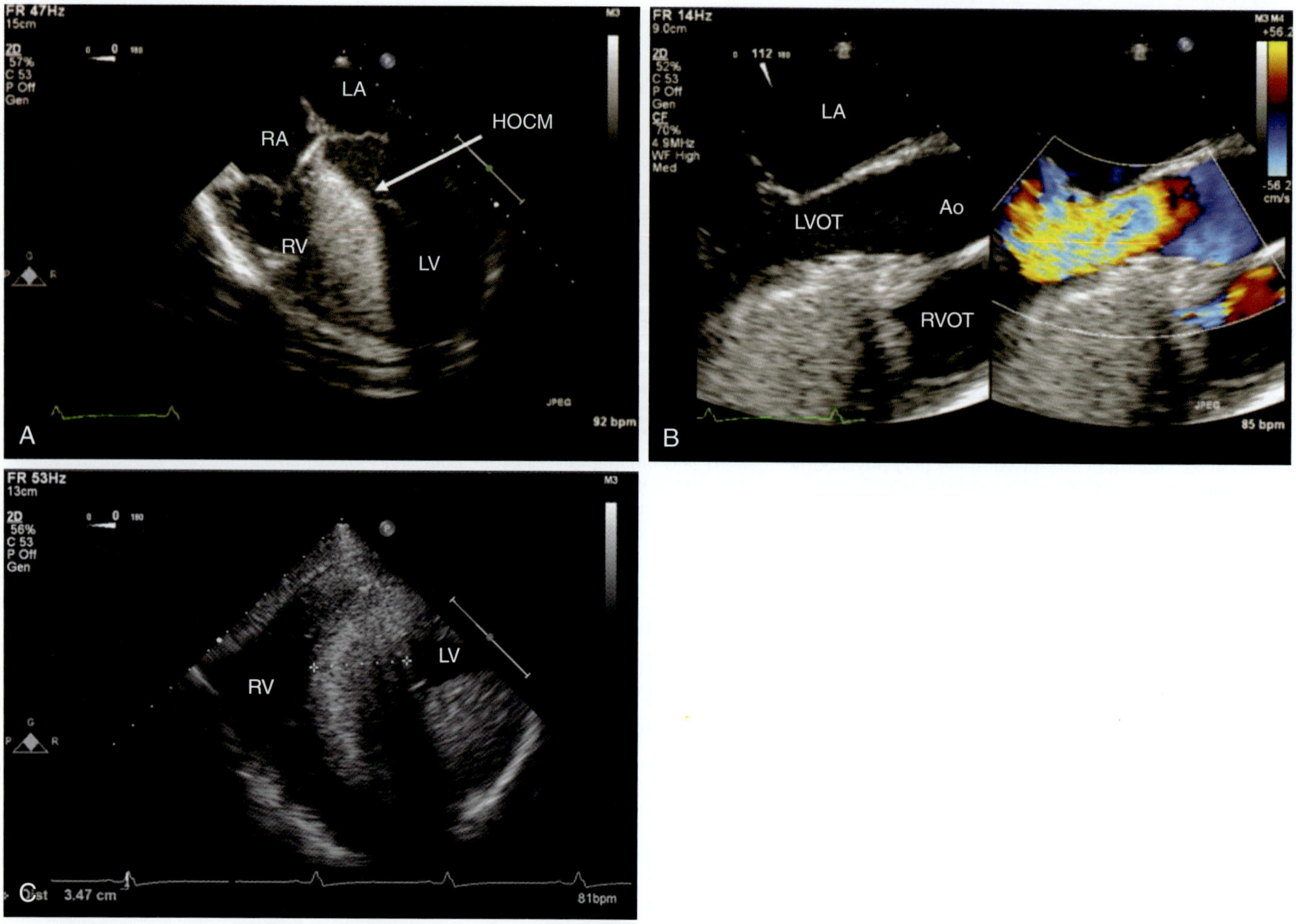

Figure 24-32 Hypertrophic obstructive cardiomyopathy. **A,** Midesophageal (ME) four-chamber view: obvious bulging of interventricular septum into left ventricular outflow tract *(LVOT)*. **B,** ME long-axis color compare view: in systole, color flow Doppler shows acceleration through LVOT. **C,** Transgastric view of severe septal hypertrophy; septum thickness 3.47 cm. *Ao,* Ascending aorta; *HOCM,* hypertrophic obstructive cardiomyopathy; *LA,* left atrium; *LV,* left ventricle; *RV,* right ventricle; *RVOT,* right ventricular outflow tract.

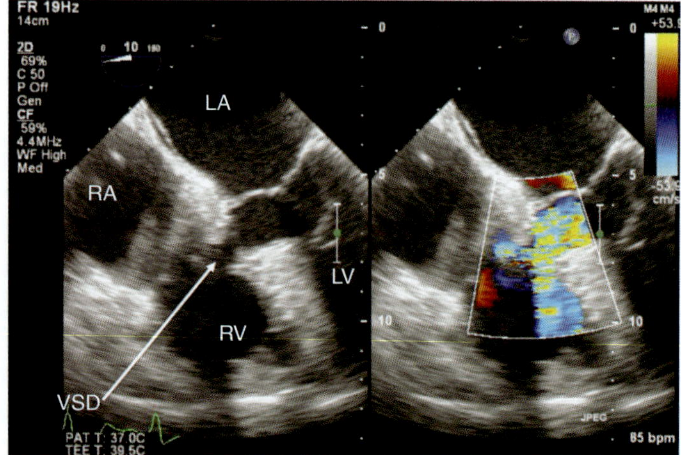

Figure 24-33 Residual ventricular septal defect (VSD) post hypertrophic obstructive cardiomyopathy *(HOCM)* resection. Midesophageal four-chamber color compare view after septal resection of HOCM: echo dropout on left image; color Doppler showing left-to-right shunt through a VSD on right image. *LA,* Left atrium; *LV,* left ventricle; *RA,* right atrium; *RV,* right ventricle.

of patients; it is generally located in the outlet septum and associated with an overriding pulmonary artery. Abnormalities of the coronary arteries are also frequently present and may increase the risk of an arterial switch procedure, especially in the case of an intramural coronary artery (6% of D-TGA).[83-85]

In the longitudinal plane (90-120 degrees), the great arteries arise in parallel at the base of the heart instead of being coiled around one another (Fig. 24-35). The entire muscular septum is much straighter than is found in a normal heart. In the transverse view (0-20 degrees), both semilunar aortic and pulmonary valves appear in the same cross-sectional plane, whereas in the normal heart, a cross-sectional view of the aorta provides a longitudinal view of the PA and vice versa. The aortic valve is anterior, to the right, and slightly superior to the pulmonary valve (D-transposition). The pulmonary artery originates directly above the LVOT, with fibrous continuity between mitral and pulmonary valves. Visualization of a posterior great artery that bifurcates is supportive evidence of TGA. An ASD allows for mixing between the pulmonary and systemic circulations.

Until the arterial switch operation became the standard of care, most patients underwent atrial switch operations (Mustard or Senning procedures), after which failure of the subaortic RV and progressive systemic tricuspid valve regurgitation have been common complications. The cause of RV dysfunction is unclear. The single right coronary artery supplies the morphologic RV, making it vulnerable to perfusion mismatch and ischemia in the context of severe

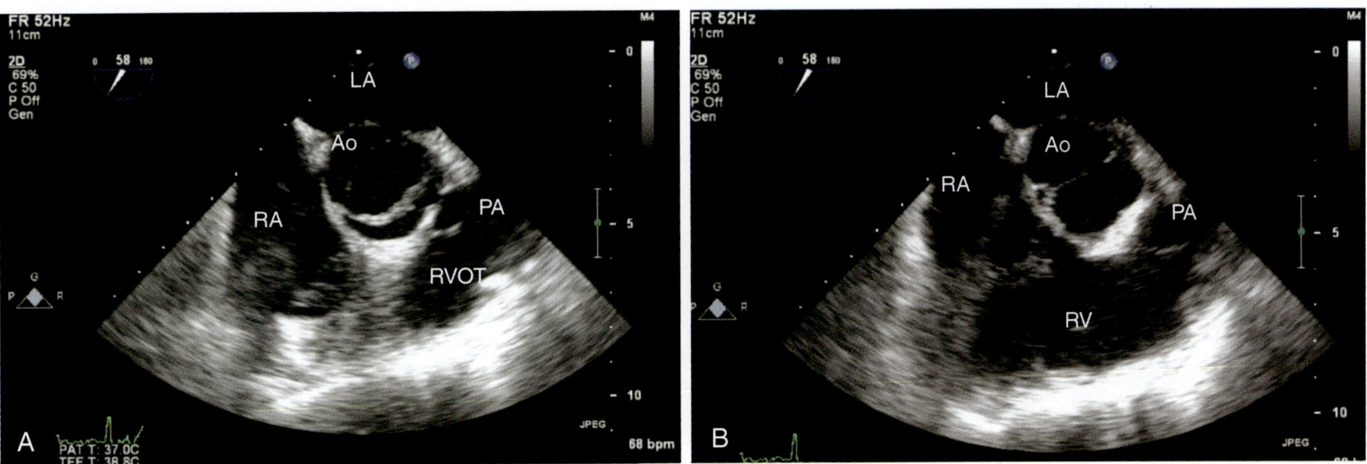

Figure 24-34 Bicuspid aortic valve. **A**, In systole, typical fish-mouth opening. **B**, In diastole, both leaflets without raphe are visualized. *Ao*, Aortic valve; *LA*, left atrium; *PA*, pulmonary artery; *RA*, right atrium; *RV*, right ventricle; *RVOT*, right ventricular outflow tract.

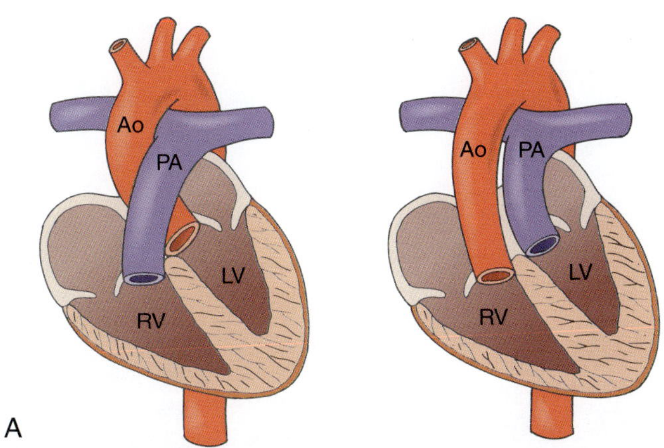

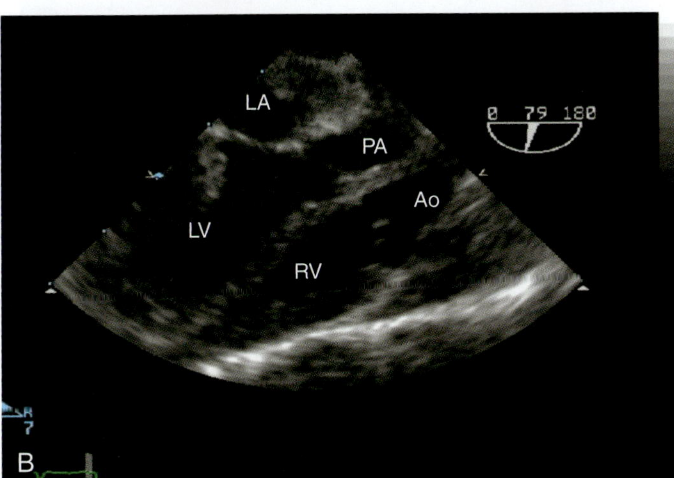

Figure 24-35 Transposition of the great arteries (TGA). **A**, *Left*, schema of normal anatomy of great arteries of heart; pulmonary artery *(PA)* is crossing aorta *(Ao)* anteriorly. *Right*, schema of TGA; Ao and PA are parallel, with Ao anteriorly displaced. **B**, Long-axis midesophageal view of TGA: Ao and PA are parallel and Ao is anterior. *LA*, Left atrium; *LV*, left ventricle; *RV*, right ventricle. *(A courtesy PG Chassot.)*

RV hypertrophic response to systemic pressure loading. Focal fibrosis has been shown by MRI with late gadolinium enhancement.[86] Hypertrophy might be associated with fibrosis in some patients and correlates inversely with RV systolic performance. Although accurate assessment of RVEF is important, the definition of normal systemic RVEF remains problematic. RVEF above 50% in the absence of significant valve regurgitation is considered normal.[77,87] The LV is small and compressed by the RV because of septum encroachment by the LV cavity. A dynamic LVOT obstruction, most frequently encountered in patients with an intact septum, may occur progressively with advancing age because of the low-resistance pulmonary arterial bed being connected to an anatomic LV chamber. Restriction to systemic or pulmonary venous return due to baffle obstruction may occur. In cases of baffle obstruction, Doppler analysis reveals turbulent flow on color mapping, loss of the phasic pattern, and increased flow velocity (>1.5 m/s) on spectral Doppler.

Although these patients are rarely considered candidates for re-do surgery in adulthood, they may be encountered in the ICU setting or for non-cardiac surgery.

A cohort of adult survivors of the arterial switch operation is just evolving. Long-term complications during adulthood will have to be defined in the future. However, two complications seem to dominate long-term survival: regurgitation of the neoaortic valve (25%) (Video 24-27) and myocardial ischemia caused by coronary ostial lesions.[88,89] RVOT or LVOT obstruction, possible residual shunts, and LV dysfunction might also be found.[90,91]

Congenitally Corrected Transposition of the Great Arteries

If an AV discordance is added to a ventriculo-arterial discordance, the circulation is physiologically corrected because the great arteries and the ventricles are inverted; systemic and pulmonary circulation are in series. Blood flows from the RA to the LV, then to the PA and to the lungs; it returns to the LA, then to the RV and to the aorta. Since the anatomic RV is in a left-sided position, and the anatomic LV stays on the right side of the heart, each ventricle is recognized by its anatomic features. In the four-chamber view, the normal RA is followed by a bileaflet high-inserted mitral valve connected to a more or less triangular ventricle with two papillary muscles and fine trabeculations (anatomic LV). On the left side, the LA is connected to a tricuspid low-inserted AV valve and a round-shaped ventricle with coarse trabeculations and three papillary muscles (anatomic RV) (Fig. 24-36, Video 24-28). In the absence of other abnormalities, these patients are not cyanotic, and the condition may not be diagnosed until adolescence or adulthood. Survival to the seventh and eighth decade has been reported.

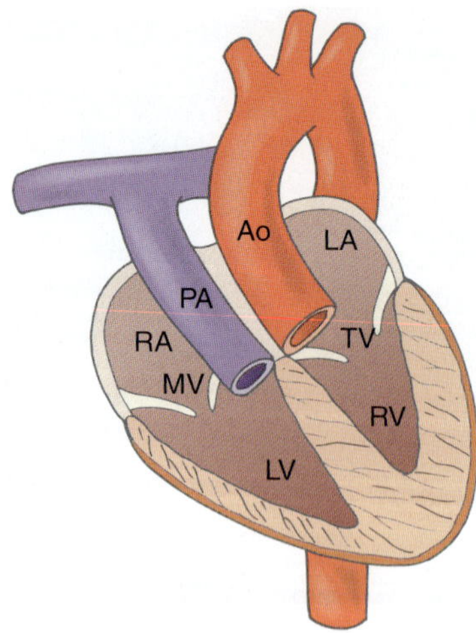

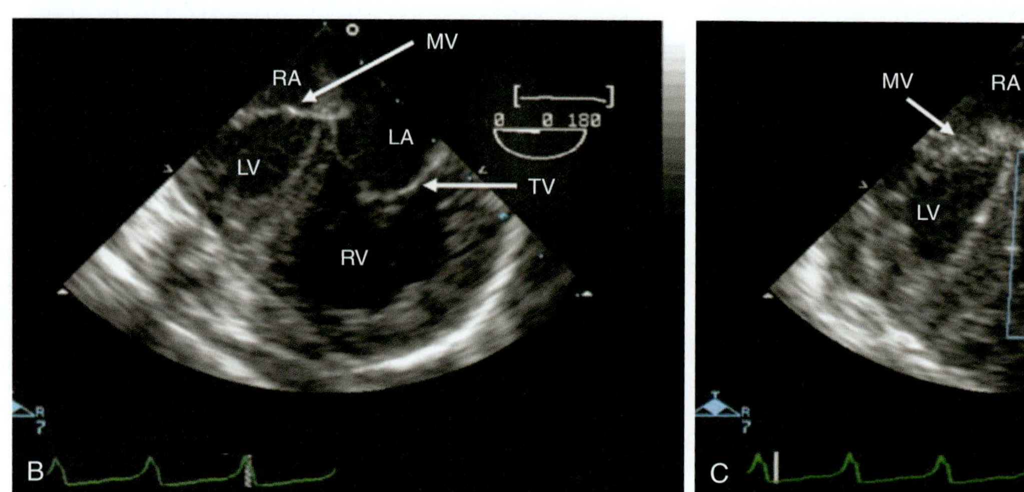

Figure 24-36   Congenitally corrected transposition of the great arteries (TGA). **A,** Schema: aorta *(Ao)* and pulmonary artery *(PA)* are parallel, with Ao anteriorly displaced and generally on left side of PA (L-TGA). Tricuspid valve *(TV)* with its ventricle (anatomic right ventricle *[RV],* functional systemic ventricle) is on left side of heart, and mitral valve *(MV)* and its ventricle (anatomic left ventricle *[LV],* functional pulmonary ventricle) on right side of heart. **B,** Midesophageal four-chamber view: lowest implanted atrioventricular valve, meaning TV is on left side of heart. **C,** Same view with color Doppler: severe tricuspid regurgitation. *LA,* Left atrium; *LV,* left ventricle; *RA,* right atrium; *TI,* tricuspid insufficiency. (**A** *courtesy PG Chassot.*)

Congenitally corrected transposition demonstrates the remarkable ability of the RV to adapt to systemic pressure. If the normal-functioning RV has a very thin wall (usually 3-5 mm) and relies more heavily on longitudinal shortening, it has a remarkable adaptation capacity when exposed to systemic pressure; the RV may become thicker than the LV and its free wall will progressively rely mostly on circumferential instead of longitudinal shortening but without any difference in interventricular septal shortening. Consequently, the systemic RV contraction pattern resembles that of the normal LV, although without its ventricular torsion. Strain rate has been shown to be significantly decreased in the systemic RV when compared to the normal LV.[92] The predominant circumferential over longitudinal free wall contraction might represent an adaptive response to the systemic load, while the lack of torsion and reduced strain rate may suggest incipient myocardial dysfunction.[92]

Any added volume lesion will precipitate ventricular dysfunction and failure of the morphologic RV. An important marker for poor survival is a depressed systemic EF and severe TR. TR strongly relates to RV dysfunction, raising the question whether TR leads to RV dysfunction or vice versa.[30,77,93] If systemic AV valve replacement (repair does not seem to work) is performed before the EF starts to decline, systemic ventricular function may be maintained even in older patients.[77]

Echocardiographically, the great arteries are positioned similarly to the TGA and run parallel; the aorta arises anteriorly but to the left of the PA (L-TGA). A VSD is present in 70% of these patients and is usually perimembranous; mitral abnormalities are found in 50% and TR in 30% of all cases. LVOT obstruction occurs in around 40% of cases, usually due to a subvalvular diaphragmatic ring or an aneurysm of the fibrous tissue that protrudes into the LVOT.[51] RVOT obstruction is less frequent and occurs in only 10% of cases. The tricuspid valve might be abnormally displaced toward the apex of the ventricle (Ebstein-like anomaly).

Arterial Anomalies
Coarctation of the Aorta

The prevalence of coarctation of the aorta is 0.2% of live births,[94] but it accounts for up to 8% of all patients with CHD. The physiology of the coarctation varies depending on the age at presentation, severity of stenosis, and presence of associated lesions.[53] Nearly 50% of young children presenting with a coarctation have associated intracardiac lesions: VSD, aortic valve stenosis, SAS, or AVSDs. Coarctation of the aorta is also frequently associated with a bicuspid aortic valve (50% of cases) or a ductus arteriosus (20% of cases). Anatomically, a posterior

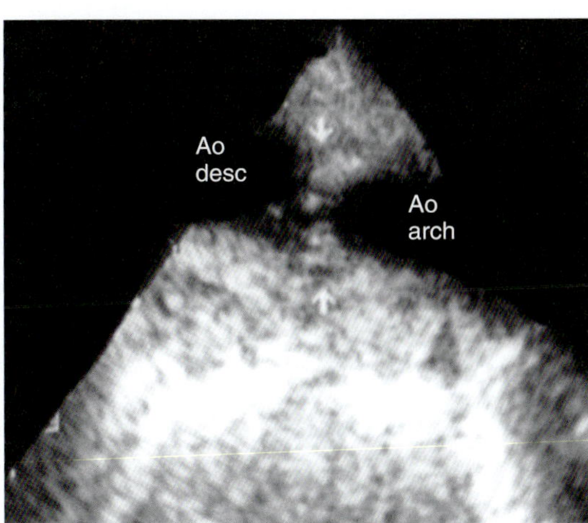

Figure 24-37   Coarctation of the aorta. Bidimensional imaging of descending aorta (*Ao desc*), with narrowing of aortic lumen right below aortic arch (*Ao arch*); arrows point to stenosis.

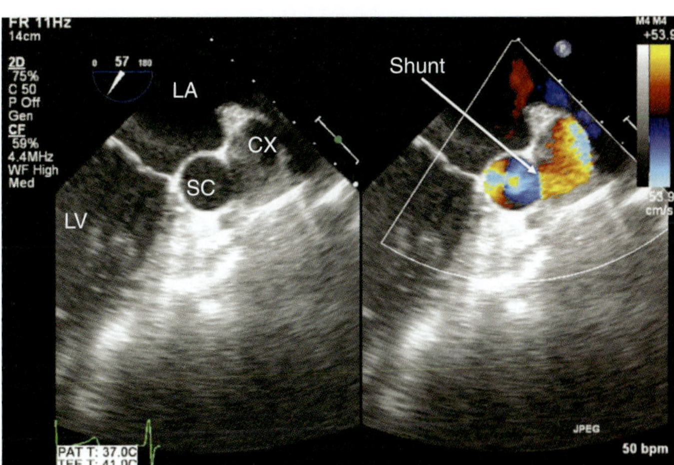

Figure 24-38   Coronary fistula. Fistula of circumflex artery (*CX*) into coronary sinus (sinus coronarius [*SC*]). Note dilation of CX and SC. Color Doppler shows left-to-right shunt (turbulent flow) at entrance of CX into SC. *LA*, left atrium; *LV*, left ventricle.

ridge of dense tissue narrows the lumen of the aorta at the level of the isthmus (Fig. 24-37). The stenotic segment can be discrete or segmental and long. An aortic arch hypoplasia may be present and tends to complicate the surgical approach. The aortic arch above the lesion is dilated and highly pulsatile, whereas the descending aorta distal to the coarctation is much less expanding in systole. The color flow map through the stenotic area is turbulent. The pressure overload imposed on the LV may induce LV hypertrophy.

After surgical repair, TEE examination should determine the degree of residual narrowing.

Coronary Anomalies

Anomalous origin of the left coronary artery (LCA) from the pulmonary artery, or ALCAPA, is a rare CHD. In this syndrome, the LCA usually arises from the lateral or posterior wall of the pulmonary artery. After birth, blood flow in the LCA depends on collateral flow from the right coronary artery (RCA) because of the fall of pulmonary arterial pressure; this leads to myocardial ischemia in infancy. In cases of sufficient collateral flow, the pulmonary origin of the LCA functions as an L-R shunt into the pulmonary artery, leading to a coronary steal phenomenon and myocardial ischemia later in life.[95] The anomalous connection is usually seen in ME 60- to 120-degree view. Color flow Doppler will show diastolic turbulent flow in the pulmonary artery at the site of the LCA connection. Retrograde flow in the LCA may also be detected. A markedly dilated RCA is usually present. Abnormal LV function with dilation is a universal feature. Segmental wall motion abnormalities may or may not be present.

The surgical repair consists in reimplantation of the LCA into the aorta. TEE will be useful for monitoring LV function as well as for demonstrating the corrected anterograde laminar flow through the LCA. It is relatively simple to determine the patency of a coronary artery by TEE, but more difficult to evaluate a stenosis. Mild increased velocities are frequently encountered after surgical manipulation of the coronary arteries.[9]

Coronary arteries may also present with anomalous origins from different aortic coronary sinuses or from a single common trunk, with possible myocardial ischemia in the case of an anomalous course between the great arteries (slitlike ostium). They may also present with an anomalous termination into the RV, pulmonary artery, or coronary sinus (Fig. 24-38, Video 24-29). This situation leads to a fistula or shunt between the LV and RV. The effective shunt ratio (Qp/Qs) is usually around 1.6.[96] Biventricular dysfunction is frequently present.

These anomalous origins of coronary arteries may be particularly relevant in the case of procedures like arterial switch or Ross operations, which require coronary artery reimplantation, as well as in the case of Fallot correction, where anomalous course of a coronary artery

anteriorly to the RVOT may prevent traditional surgical techniques of infundibulum widening.

Conclusions

With increasing numbers of adult survivors with CHD, more adult patients will need reoperations or admission to adult ICUs for noncardiac issues in the future. Echocardiography, particularly peri-interventional and perioperative TEE, is an important tool to enhance safety and efficacy of interventions in this group of patients.

The practice of TEE requires extensive training and unrestricted availability. Because of the complexity of CHD, a systematic approach for the TEE examination is required. A sequential analysis is best and allows the most precise assessment of challenging cardiac anomalies. It is of utmost importance that the echocardiographer be able to recognize the different structures and abnormalities inherent in adult CHD to better inform decisions about management and surgical repair. A multidisciplinary team approach remains essential.

REFERENCES

1. Brickner EM, Hillis LD, Lange RA. Congenital heart disease in adults. First of two parts. *N Engl J Med.* 2000;342:1-12.
2. Wren C, Richmond S, Donaldson L. Temporal variability in birth prevalence of cardiovascular malformations. *Heart.* 2000;83:414-419.
3. Ou P, Iserin L, Raisky O, et al. Post-operative cardiac lesions after cardiac surgery in childhood. *Pediatr Radiol.* 2010;40:885-894.
4. Webb GD. Care of adults with congenital heart disease – a challenge for the new millennium. *Thorac Cardiovasc Surg.* 2001;49:30-34.
5. American Society of Anesthesiologists. Practice guidelines for perioperative transesophageal echocardiography. *Anesthesiology.* 1996;84:986-1006.
6. An updated report by the American Society of Anesthesiologists and the Society of Cardiovascular Anesthesiologists. Practice guidelines for perioperative transesophageal echocardiography. *Anesthesiology.* 2010;112:1084-1096.
7. Rigby ML. Transoesophageal echocardiography during interventional cardiac catheterisation in congenital heart disease. *Heart.* 2001;86(suppl 2):II23-II29.
8. Ayres NA, Miller-Hance W, Fyfe DA, et al. Indications and guidelines for performance of transesophageal echocardiography in the patient with pediatric acquired or congenital heart disease: report from the Task Force of the Pediatric Council of the American Society of Echocardiography. *J Am Soc Echocardiogr.* 2005;18:91-98.
9. Smallhorn JF. Intraoperative transesophageal echocardiography in congenital heart disease. *Echocardiography.* 2002;19:709-723.
10. Ungerleider RM, Greeley WJ, Sheikh KH, et al. Routine use of intraoperative epicardial echocardiography and Doppler color flow imaging to guide and evaluate repair of congenital heart lesions. A prospective study. *J Thorac Cardiovasc Surg.* 1990;100:297-309.
11. Li Bezold, Pignatelli R, Altman CA, et al. Intraoperative transesophageal echocardiography in congenital heart surgery. The Texas Children's Hospital experience. *Tex Heart Inst J.* 1996;23:108-115.
12. Randolph GR, Hagler DJ, Connolly HM, et al. Intraoperative transesophageal echocardiography during surgery for congenital heart defects. *J Thorac Cardiovasc Surg.* 2002;124:1176-1182.
13. O'Leary PW, Hagler DJ, Seward JB, et al. Biplane intraoperative transesophageal echocardiography in congenital heart disease. *Mayo Clinic Proc.* 1995;70:317-326.
14. Muhiudeen-Russel IA, Miller-Hance WC, Silverman NH. Intraoperative transesophageal echocardiography for pediatric patients with congenital heart disease. *Anesth Analg.* 1998;87:1058-1076.
15. Wienecke M, Fyfe DA, Kline CH, et al. Comparison of intraoperative transesophageal echocardiography to epicardial imaging in children undergoing ventricular septal defect repair. *J Am Soc Echocardiogr.* 1991;4:607-614.

16. Rosenfeld HM, Gentles TL, Wernkovsky G, et al. Utility of intraoperative echocardiography in the assessment of residual cardiac defects. *Ped Cardiol.* 1998;19:346-351.

17. Stevenson JG, Sorensen GK, Gartman DM, et al. Left ventricular outflow tract obstruction: An indication for intraoperative transesophageal echocardiography. *J Am Soc Echocardiogr.* 1993;6:525-535.

18. Ungerleider RM, Kisslo JA, Greeley WJ, et al. Intraoperative echocardiography during congenital heart operations: Experience from 1000 cases. *Ann Thorac Surg.* 1995;60:S539-S542.

19. Ungerleider RM, Greeley WJ, Sheikh KH. The use of intraoperative echo with Doppler color flow imaging to predict outcome after repair of congenital cardiac defects. *Ann Surg.* 1989;210:526-533.

20. Muhiudeen IA, Roberson DA, Silverman DH, et al. Intraoperative echocardiography in infants and children with congenital cardiac shunt lesions: transesophageal versus epicardial echocardiography. *J Am Coll Cardiol.* 1990;16:1687-1695.

21. Bengur AR, Li JS, Herlong JR, et al. Intraoperative transesophageal echocardiography in congenital heart disease. *Semin Thorac Cardiovasc Surg.* 1998;10:255-264.

22. Stevenson JG. Role of intraoperative transesophageal echocardiography during repair of congenital cardiac defects. *Acta Paediatr Suppl.* 1995;410:23-33.

23. Bettex DA, Schmidlin D, Bernath MA, et al. Intraoperative transesophageal echocardiography in pediatric congenital heart surgery: A two-center observational study. *Anesth Analg.* 2003;97:1275-1282.

24. Stevenson JG, Sorensen GK, Gartman DM, et al. Transesophageal echocardiography during repair of congenital cardiac defects: identification of residual problems necessitating reoperation. *J Am Soc Echocardiogr.* 1993;6:356-365.

25. Stevenson JG. Adherence to physician training guidelines for pediatric transesophageal echocardiography affects the outcome of patients undergoing repair of congenital cardiac defects. *J Am Soc Echocardiogr.* 1999;12:165-172.

26. Shinebourne EA, MacCartney FJ, Anderson RH. Sequential chamber localization. Logical approach to diagnosis in congenital heart diseases. *Brit Heart J.* 1976;38:327-340.

27. Van Praagh R. Terminology of congenital heart disease. Glossary and commentary. *Circulation.* 1977;56:139-143.

28. Dupuis C, Kachaner J, Payot M. *Cardiologie pédiatrique.* Paris: Flammarion; 1991, pp 137-142.

29. Weyman AE. Complex congenital heart disease I: Diagnostic approach. In: Weyman AE, ed. *Principles and Practice of Echocardiography.* Philadelphia: Lea & Febiger; 1994:979-1001.

30. Warnes CA. Adult congenital heart disease. Importance of the right ventricle. *J Am Coll Cardiol.* 2009;54:1903-1910.

31. Lang RM, Bierig M, Devereux RB, et al. Recommendations for chamber quantifications. *Eur J Echocardiogr.* 2006;7:79-108.

32. Haddad F, Couture P, Tousignant C. DenaultAY. The right ventricle in cardiac surgery, a perioperative perspective: I Anatomy, physiology and assessment. *Anesth Analg.* 2009;108:407-421.

33. Eidem BW, O'Leary PW, Tei C, Seward JB. Usefulness of the myocardial performance index for assessing right ventricular function in congenital heart disease. *Am J Cardiol.* 2000;86:654-658.

34. Stümper O, Sutherland GR. *Transesophageal echocardiography in congenital heart disease.* London: Edward Arnold; 1994, pp 37-38.

35. Tausig A, Karch M, Schreiber K, et al. Darstellung der individuellen Pulmonalvenen-Anatomie vor und Detektion von Stenosen nach RF-Ablation von Vorhofflimmern: Ist die MRA der CTA ebenbürtig? *Fortschr Röntgenstr.* 2005;177:S1.

36. Vick GW. Pulmonary venous and systemic ventricular inflow obstruction in patients with congenital heart disease: Detection by combined two-dimensional and Doppler echocardiography. *J Am Coll Cardiol.* 1987;9:580-584.

37. Brecker SJD, Redington A, Shore D, et al. Atrial septal defects. In: Redington A, ed. *Congenital heart disease in adults. A practical guide.* London: WB Saunders Co Ltd; 1994:104-110.

38. Weintraub R, Shiota T, Elkadi T, et al. Transesophageal echocardiography in infants and children with congenital heart disease. *Circulation.* 1992;86:711-722.

39. Jaffe RA, Pinto PJ, Schnittger I, et al. Aspects of mechanical ventilation affecting interatrial shunt flow during general anesthesia. *Anesth Analg.* 1992;75:484-488.

40. Lin FC, Fu M, Yeh SH, et al. Doppler atrial flow patterns in patients with secundum atrial septal defects. Determinants, limitations and pitfalls. *J Am Soc Echocardiogr.* 1988;1:141-145.

41. Levin AR. Atrial pressure-flow dynamics in atrial septal defects (secundum type). *Circulation.* 1968;37:476-479.

42. Louie EK, Konstadt SN, Rao TL. Transesophageal echocardiographic diagnosis of the right to left shunting across the foramen ovale in adults without prior stroke. *J Am Coll Cardiol.* 1993;21:1231-1237.

43. Garg R, Murthy K, Rao S, Muralidhar K. Intra-operative transesophageal echocardiography in congenital heart disease. *Ann Cardiac Anaesth.* 2009;12:173-175.

44. Agoustides JG, Weiss SJ, Weiner J, et al. Diagnosis of patent foramen ovale with multiplane transesophageal echocardiography in adult cardiac surgical patients. *J Cardiothorac Vasc Anesth.* 2004;18:725-730.

45. Konstadt SN, Louie EK, Black S. Intraoperative detection of foramen ovale by transesophageal echocardiography. *Anesthesiology.* 1991;74:212-216.

46. Schneider B, Zienkiewicz T, Jansen V, et al. Diagnosis of patent foramen ovale by transesophageal echocardiography and correlation with autopsy findings. *Am J Cardiol.* 1996;77:1202-1209.

47. Stollberger C, Schneider B, Abzieher F, et al. Diagnosis of patent foramen ovale by transesophageal contrast echocardiography. *Am J Cardiol.* 1993;71:604-606.

48. Nacht A, Kronzon I. Intracardiac shunts. *Crit Care Clinics.* 1996;12:295-319.

49. Piccoli GP. Morphology and classification of complete atrioventricular defects. *Brit Heart J.* 1979;42:633-639.

50. Ebels T, Meijboom EJ, Anderson RH, et al. Anatomic and functional "obstruction" of the outflow tract in atrioventricular septal defects with separate valve orifices ("ostium primum atrial septal defect"): an echocardiographic study. *Am J Cardiol.* 1984 Oct 1;54(7):843-847.

51. Snider AR, Serwer GA, Ritter SB. Defects in cardiac septation. In: Snider AR, Serwer GA, Ritter SB, eds. *Echocardiography in pediatric heart disease.* 2nd ed. St Louis: Mosby; 1997:235-296.

52. Mc Grath LB, Gonzalez-Lavin L. Actuarial survival, freedom from reoperation, and other events after repair of atrioventricular septal defects. *J Thorac Cardiovasc Surg.* 1987;94:582-590.

53. Fjr Cetta, Seward JB, O'Leary PW. Echocardiography in congenital heart disease: An overview. In: Oh JK, Seward JB, Tajik AJ, eds. *The Echo Manual.* Philadelphia: Lippincott Williams & Wilkins; 2007:332-367.

54. Shiina A, Seward JB, Edwards WD, et al. Two-dimensional echocardiography spectrum of Ebstein's anomaly: detailed anatomic assessment. *J Am Coll Cardiol.* 1984;3:356-370.

55. Gussenhoven EJ, Stewart PA, Becker AE, et al. Offsetting" of the septal tricuspid leaflet in normal hearts and in hearts with Ebstein's anomaly. Anatomic and echographic correlation. *Am J Cardiol.* 1984;54:172-176.

56. Perloff JK. Survival patterns without cardiac surgery or interventional catheterization: a narrowing base. In: Perloff JK, Child JS, eds. *Congenital heart disease in adults.* 2nd ed. Philadelphia: WB Saunders; 1998:pp15-pp53.

57. Flanagan MF, Foran RB, Van Praagh R, et al. Tetralogy of Fallot with obstruction of the ventricular septal defect: Spectrum of echocardiographic findings. *J Am Coll Cardiol.* 1988;11:386-392.

58. Moises VA, Maciel BC, Homberger LK, et al. A new method for non-invasive estimation of ventricular septal defect shunt flow by color Doppler flow mapping: imaging of the laminar flow convergence region on the left septal surface. *J Am Coll Cardiol.* 1991;18:824-832.

59. Murphy Jr DJ, Ludomirsky A, Huhta JC. Continuous-wave Doppler in children with ventricular septal defect: noninvasive estimation of interventricular pressure gradient. *Am J Cardiol.* 1986;57:428-432.

60. Tee SDG, Shiota T, Weintraub R, et al. Evaluation of ventricular septal defect by transesophageal echocardiography: Intraoperative assessment. *Am Heart J.* 1994;127:585-592.

61. Dodge-Khatami A, Knirsch W, Tomaske M, et al. Spontaneous closure of small residual ventricular septal defects after surgical repair. *Ann Thorac Surg.* 2007;83:902-905.

62. Disessa TG, Child JS, Perloff JK, et al. Systemic venous and pulmonary arterial flow patterns after Fontan's procedure for tricuspid atresia or single ventricle. *Circulation.* 1984;70:898-902.

63. Stümper O, Sutherland GR. Congenital heart disease in adolescents and adults. In: Sutherland GR, ed. *Transesophageal echocardiography in clinical practice.* London: Gower Medical Publishing; 1991:14.1-14.15.

64. Frommelt PC, Lewis DA, Pelech AN. Intraoperative transgastric echo assessment during left ventricular outflow tract surgery: a reliable predictor of residual obstruction. *Echocardiography.* 1998;15:581-588.

65. Kawahito S, Kitahata H, Tanaka K, et al. Intraoperative evaluation of pulmonary artery flow during the Fontan procedure by transesophageal Doppler echocardiography. *Anesth Analg.* 2000;91:1375-1380.

66. Fyfe DA, Kline CH, Sade RM, et al. The utility of transesophageal echocardiography during and after Fontan operations in small children. *Am Heart J.* 1991;122:1403-1415.

67. Marelli AJ, Perloff JK, Child JS, et al. Pulmonary atresia with ventricular septal defect in adults. *Circulation.* 1994;89:243-251.

68. Berry Jr JM, Einzig S, Krabill KA, et al. Evaluation of coronary artery anatomy in patients with tetralogy of Fallot by two-dimensional echocardiography. *Circulation.* 1988;78:149-156.

69. Jureidini SB, Appleton RS, Nouri S. Detection of coronary artery abnormalities in tetralogy of Fallot by two-dimensional echocardiography. *J Am Coll Cardiol.* 1989;14:960-967.

70. Bertranou EG, Blackstone EH, Hazelrig JB, et al. Life expectancy without surgery in tetralogy of Fallot. *Am J Cardiol.* 1978;42:458-466.

71. Li W, Davlouros PA, Kilner PJ, et al. Doppler-echocardiographic assessment of pulmonary regurgitation in adults with repaired tetralogy of Fallot: comparison with cardiovascular magnetic resonance imaging. *Am Heart J.* 2004;147:165-172.

72. Joyce JJ, Hwang EY, Hb Wiles, et al. Reliability of intraoperative transesophageal echocardiography during tetralogy of Fallot repair. *Echocardiography.* 2000;17:319-327.

73. Swensson RE, Sahn DJ, Valdes-Cruz LM, et al. Left coronary artery to right ventricular fistula after total repair for tetralogy of Fallot. *Am J Cardiol.* 1987;59:713-714.

74. Gatzoulis MA, Clark AL, Cullen S, et al. Right ventricular diastolic function 15 to 35 years after repair of tetralogy of Fallot. Restrictive physiology predicts superior exercise performance. *Circulation.* 1995;91:1775-1781.

75. Cullen S, Shore D, Redington A. Characterization of right ventricular diastolic performance after complete repair of tetralogy of Fallot. Restrictive physiology predicts slow postoperative recovery. *Circulation.* 1995;91:1782-1789.

76. Rathore KS, Gupta N, Kapoor A, et al. Assessment of right ventricular diastolic function: does it predict post-operative course in tetralogy of Fallot. *Indian Heart J.* 2004;56:220-224.

77. Davlouros PA, Niwa K, Webb G, Gatzoulis MA. The right ventricle in congenital heart disease. *Heart.* 2006;92:i27-i38.

78. Norgard G, Gatzoulis MA, Josen M, et al. Does restrictive right ventricular physiology in the early postoperative period predict subsequent right ventricular restriction after repair of tetralogy of Fallot? *Heart.* 1998;79:481-484.

79. Currie PJ, Hagler DJ, Seward JB, et al. Instantaneous pressure gradient: a simultaneous Doppler and dual catheter correlative study. *J Am Coll Cardiol.* 1986;7:800-806.

80. Silvilairat S, Cabalka AK, Cetta F, et al. Outpatient echocardiographic assessment of complex pulmonary outflow stenosis: Doppler mean gradient is superior to the maximum instantaneous gradient. *J Am Soc Echocardiogr.* 2005;18:1143-1148.

81. Silvilairat S, Cabalka AK, Cetta F, et al. Echocardiographic assessment of isolated pulmonary valve stenosis: which outpatient Doppler gradient has the most clinical validity? *J Am Soc Echocardiogr.* 2005;18:1137-1142.

82. Friedman WF. Aortic stenosis. In: Emmanoulides GC, ed. *Moss and Adam's Heart Disease in Infants, Children and Adolescents Including Fetus and Young Adult.* Baltimore: Williams & Wilkins; 1995:1087.

83. Pasquini L, Parness IA, Colan SD, et al. Diagnosis of intramural coronary artery in transposition of the great arteries using two-dimensional echocardiography. *Circulation.* 1993;88:1136-1141.

84. Pasquini L, Sanders SP, Parness IA, et al. Diagnosis of coronary artery anatomy by two-dimensional echocardiography in patients with transposition of the great arteries. *Circulation.* 1987;75:557-564.

85. Pasquini L, Sanders SP, Parness IA, et al. Coronary echocardiography in 406 patients with D-loop transposition of the great arteries. *J Am Coll Cardiol.* 1994;24:763-768.

86. Babu-Narayan SV, Goktekin O, Moon JC, et al. Late-gadolinium enhancement cardiovascular magnetic resonance of the systemic right ventricle in adults with previous atrial redirection surgery for transposition of the great arteries. *Circulation.* 2005;111:2091-2098.

87. Hornung TS, Derrick GP, Deanfield JE, et al. Transposition complexes in the adult: a changing perspective. *Cardiol Clin.* 2002;20:405-420.

88. Formigari R, Toscano A, Giardini A, et al. Prevalence and predictors of neoaortic regurgitation after arterial switch operation for transposition of the great arteries. *J Thorac Cardiovasc Surg.* 2003;126:1753-1759.

89. Tanel RE, Wernovsky G, Landzberg MJ, et al. Coronary artery abnormalities detected at cardiac catheterization following the arterial switch operation for transposition of the great arteries. *Am J Cardiol.* 1995;76:153-157.

90. Tobler D, Williams WG, Jegatheeswaran A, et al. Cardiac outcomes in young adult survivors of the arterial switch operation for transposition of the great arteries. *J Am Coll Cardiol.* 2010;56:58-64.

91. Miller-Hance WC, Silverman NH. Transesophageal echocardiography (TEE) in congenital heart disease with focus on the adult. *Cardiol Clinics.* 2000;18:861-892.

92. Petersen E, Helle-Valle T, Edvardsen T, et al. Contraction pattern of the systemic right ventricle shift from longitudinal to circumferential shortening and absent global ventricular torsion. *J Am Coll Cardiol.* 2007;49:2450-2456.

93. Prieto LR, Hordof AJ, Secic M, et al. Progressive tricuspid valve disease in patients with congenital corrected transposition of the great arteries. *Circulation.* 1998;98:997-1005.

94. Kaemmerer H. Aortic coarctation and interrupted aortic arch. In: Gatzoulis MA, et al, ed. *Diagnosis and management of adult congenital heart disease.* Edinburgh: Churchill-Livingstone; 2003pp 253-26.

95. Backer CL, Stout MJ, Zales VR, et al. Anomalous origin of the left coronary artery. A twenty-year review of surgical management*J Thorac Cardiovasc Surg.* 1992;103:1049-1057:Discussion 1057-8.

96. Bishop A. Coronary artery anomalies. In: Redington A, ed. *Congenital Heart Disease in Adults. A practical guide.* London: WB Saunders Co Ltd; 1994:153-160.

25

Pulmonary Hypertension

TIMOTHY MAUS | DALIA A. BANKS

Introduction

Historically, the pulmonary circulation and right ventricle (RV) have not been given the same degree of attention as the left heart circulation. The increasing attention devoted to researching pulmonary hypertension (PH) and right heart failure have led to a profound increase in our understanding of pulmonary vasculature and right heart physiology. Together with advances in echocardiography, these efforts have enabled us to better characterize PH and right heart failure. This chapter will focus on the anatomy of the RV, the pathophysiology of PH, and the echocardiographic evaluation of the pulmonary hypertensive patient.

Pulmonary Hypertension and Right Heart Failure

PH is a disorder where flow to the pulmonary arterial circulation is restricted related to increased pulmonary vascular resistance (PVR), ultimately leading to right heart failure. The pulmonary circulation is normally a low-pressure, low-resistance circulation. Mild PH is generally defined as a mean pulmonary artery pressure (mPAP) above 25 mmHg at rest and PVR greater than 300 dynes·sec·cm^{-5} (>3.75 Wood units), whereas severe PH constitutes mPAP above 50 mmHg and PVR greater than 600 dynes·sec·cm^{-5} (>7.5 Wood units).[1]

At the recent 4th World Conference on Pulmonary Hypertension held by the World Health Organization, PH was classified into five groups:
1. Idiopathic pulmonary arterial hypertension (IPH), familial pulmonary hypertension (FPH), and PH associated with conditions such as connective tissue disorders, portal hypertension, pulmonary veno-occlusive disease, HIV, and anorexigens
2. PH with left heart disease
3. PH with lung diseases and/or hypoxemia
4. PH due to chronic thromboembolic disease
5. Miscellaneous[2]

Regardless of the primary pathologic mechanisms, once PH exists, the effects on the right heart and pulmonary arteries are similar.

Pathophysiology

PH is a panvasculopathy, mostly affecting small and medium-sized arterial vessels with a wide range of abnormalities, including intimal hyperplasia, medial hypertrophy, adventitial proliferation, and plexiform arteriopathy. Multiple pathogenic pathways have been implicated in the development of PH. There is a vasoconstriction phase, starting with altered vascular endothelial and smooth muscle function, leading to vasoconstriction and localized thrombosis. With progression of the disease, vascular remodeling, proliferation, and formation of plexiform lesions[3] result in increased PVR and end with right heart failure and death. The plexiform lesion, a histologic hallmark of FPH and IPH, is a result of monoclonal proliferation of endothelial cells and migration and proliferation of smooth muscle cells.[4] The basis for current medical therapies is that endothelial dysfunction leads to an imbalance between vasoconstrictors (endothelin 1, thromboxane A$_2$) and vasodilators (prostacyclin, nitric oxide).[5]

The endothelium releases thromboxane A$_2$, which is a potent vasoconstrictor, cell proliferator, and powerful platelet activator, in addition to prostacyclin, a potent vasodilator and inhibitor of platelet aggregation.[6] This mediator imbalance results in pulmonary vasoconstriction, disordered endothelial cell proliferation, and proliferation of intimal cells, leading to the characteristic plexiform lesions.

Clinical Manifestations

The most common presenting symptom in PH is dyspnea. Other symptoms may include angina, fatigue, weakness, and syncope. The first step in diagnosing PH is recognizing patients at high risk. Insidious and nonspecific onset of shortness of breath often results in delayed diagnosis. Symptoms of the disease are first noted when the RV is unable to increase contractility sufficiently to augment left ventricular (LV) preload and cardiac output during exercise.

Physical examination focuses on signs of both PH and right heart failure. Accentuation of the pulmonic component of the second heart sound and an early systolic murmur reflecting tricuspid regurgitation (that enhances with spontaneous inspiration) might be the only findings on physical exam. Jugular venous distention, hepatojugular reflux, peripheral edema, hepatomegaly, and ascites are signs of advanced PH.[7,8] Correct evaluation is essential for appropriate management, and echocardiography is the most appropriate next step. Findings such as RV hypertrophy and/or dilation, LV filling impairment, or paradoxical interventricular septal motion are indicative of right heart failure. To confirm the diagnosis, a right heart catheterization (RHC) assessment of PVR, right atrial (RA) and RV pressures, and LV pressures is required.

Right Ventricle and Pathophysiology of Right Heart Failure

The RV is a unique and complex structure. Its primary function is to pump the venous return into the pulmonary arteries. When ventricular function and loading conditions are normal, the RV is triangular in shape when viewed from the side in the midesophageal four-chamber view and crescent shaped when viewed in cross-section; the LV is ellipsoid in shape. The RV is divided into three portions: (1) the inflow, consisting of the tricuspid valve (TV), chordae tendineae, and papillary muscles; (2) the trabeculated apical myocardium; and (3) the outflow, corresponding to the smooth myocardial infundibulum and ending with the pulmonic valve (PV).

An encircling muscular band separates the RV into the inflow portion, the sinus, and the outflow portion (or conus). This muscular band is referred to as the *crista supraventricularis* and is made up of the infundibular septum and the parietal band. Two other muscular bands are present in the RV: the septal and moderator bands. The moderator band is an important landmark of the RV that is well visualized by echocardiography. It is attached to the right ventricular outflow tract (RVOT) and runs from the septum to the anterior RV wall.[9,10]

The RV contracts in a fashion resembling peristalsis, beginning with contraction of the inlet portion, followed by the apex, and ending with contraction of the infundibulum. It pumps on average the same stroke volume as the LV but generates only about 25% of the stroke work, owing to the low-pressure, low-resistance, and high-compliance nature of the pulmonary circulation.[11] As a result, the normal RV's wall thickness is half that of the LV and accordingly more compliant. Because of the RV's reduced contractile reserve compared to the LV's, it is much more sensitive to increases in afterload. Functionally and anatomically, the RV is adapted for generation of sustained low-pressure perfusion.[12] The dissimilarity in ventricular afterload is responsible for the difference in ventricular pressure-volume loops between the two ventricles. The LV has a square-shaped pressure-volume loop, whereas the RV pressure-volume loop is triangular. The triangular shape depicts the shorter pre-ejection period that is due to the RV systolic pressure, which rapidly exceeds pulmonary artery diastolic pressure. This means the normal RV has a longer period of ejection and shorter periods of isovolumic contraction and relaxation.[13] The RV pressure-volume loop becomes more square shaped with increases in RV afterload. In addition, the orientation of the interventricular septum (IVS) and geometry of the ventricles change with any increase in RV volume or pressure overload.[14]

Ventricular interdependence results from the close anatomic association between the LV and RV; they share the IVS and are enclosed within the same pericardial sac. The IVS contributes to both LV and RV function[15,16] and is responsible for approximately one third of the RV stroke work under normal conditions; it is a major determinant of overall RV performance.[17] Ventricular interdependence is mediated mainly through the IVS and plays an essential part in the pathophysiology of RV dysfunction. In the setting of RV infarction and loss of RV free wall contractility, it is the septum that continues to generate RV systolic pressure. RV ejection fraction (RVEF) is very sensitive to increases in RV afterload (i.e., pulmonary artery pressures); high afterload leads to increased RV wall tension and oxygen demand and RV ischemia. As the RV enlarges to accommodate the increase in pressure, this results in dilation of the tricuspid annulus and creates tricuspid regurgitation (TR). Eventually this results in a rise in RV end-diastolic and RA pressures, with associated clinical signs of RV failure.[18] Whereas the RV is normally perfused during both diastole and systole, the systolic component becomes compromised with raised chamber pressures.[19] Thus, maintaining perfusion pressure is essential, especially when RV systolic pressure is elevated. Vlahakes et al. examined the mechanism of RV failure in dogs under anesthesia and the importance of maintaining perfusion pressure. After producing RV failure with increasing PA pressures, infusion of phenylephrine raised aortic pressure, thereby increasing myocardial perfusion pressure and reversing RV failure, as shown by the increase in cardiac output.[20]

Normally the IVS is shifted toward the RV free wall during systole and diastole, which contributes to RV ejection. However, in conditions with increased RV pressure or volume overload, the IVS paradoxically shifts toward the LV. The shifted septum alters LV geometry, leading to decreased LV preload, increased LV end-diastolic pressure, low cardiac output, and a diminished contribution to RV ejection.[21] As noted earlier, systemic vasoconstrictors and maintenance of perfusion pressure can be used to restore RV ejection and blood supply.[22,23]

Echocardiography is extremely valuable in the diagnosis, assessment, and perioperative management of the pulmonary hypertensive patient.

◼ Echocardiographic Examination of the Pulmonary Hypertensive Patient

Echocardiographic evaluation of patients with PH includes a complete exam with particular focus on the right side of the heart. This includes examining the anatomy and function of the RA and RV (including their influence on left heart function), the TV and PV, and connecting vascular structures (superior and inferior venae cavae [SVC, IVC], pulmonary artery [PA]). The following is a brief description of the standard echocardiographic views required for evaluation of the right heart, as well as detailed descriptions of evaluating these structures in patients

with PH. In addition, Kasper et al. have described five additional views of the right heart, of which three specifically increase visualization of the RV myocardium and evaluation of the PV.[24] Use of echocardiography in estimating right heart hemodynamics will also be discussed.

Standard Transesophageal Echocardiographic Views

- **Transgastric (TG) mid-papillary short-axis view** demonstrates the anterolateral position of the RV in relation to the LV, as well as ventricular interdependence.
- **TG RV inflow view** shows a "two-chamber" view of the right heart with a focus on the TV, subvalvular apparatus, and RV free wall.
- **Midesophageal (ME) four-chamber view** displays both the RA and RV in relation to the left atrium (LA) and LV and allows for evaluation of chamber sizes, function, and anatomic variants.
- **ME RV inflow-outflow view** demonstrates the "wrapping" nature of the RA, RV, and PA in relation to the left heart. This view allows assessment of the RA, TV, RV, PV, and PA.
- **ME bicaval view** displays the LA, RA, and their separation, the interatrial septum. The SVC and IVC, as well as RA appendage, are in view in the standard bicaval view, and a modified view can reveal the coronary sinus and TV.
- **ME ascending aortic short-axis view** shows the relationship of the main and right PA to the ascending aorta and SVC, useful in identifying PA dilation and PA thrombus.
- **ME ascending aortic long-axis view** is similar to the short-axis view, with a focus on of the right PA and ascending aorta.
- **Upper esophageal (UE) aortic arch short-axis view** demonstrates the main PA, PV, and the distal RVOT in some patients. These structures are often in parallel alignment with the ultrasound beam, ideal for Doppler interrogation.

Additional Transesophageal Echocardiographic Views

- **TG RV basal short-axis view** demonstrates an en face view of the TV as well as the basal septal and free wall portions of the RV.
- **TG RV apical short-axis view** demonstrates a short-axis cross-section of the RV including apical septal and free wall portions.
- **TG RV inflow-outflow view** provides an orientation of the pulmonary valve that is ideal for Doppler interrogation.
- **Deep TG RV inflow-outflow view** provides another parallel view of the pulmonary valve for Doppler interrogation and often provides a portion of the TV annulus for M-mode or tissue Doppler interrogation.
- **Deep TG RV outflow view** demonstrates the RVOT, often with a parallel orientation for Doppler interrogation.

Right Ventricle

The RV, unlike the LV, possesses an asymmetric shape often described as a crescent that appears to "wrap" around the lateral and anterior aspects of the LV while sharing the septal wall with the LV. The RV, which is designed to facilitate the movement of blood volume from the RA through the normally low-pressure circuit of the pulmonary arterial bed, is a thin-walled structure often divided into inflow, apical, and outflow portions. Often the RV is depicted with smooth inflow and outflow portions and trabeculated apical portions. These portions are divided by a muscular band with a portion often visualized in echocardiography, the moderator band.

In response to chronically elevated RV afterload, the RV exhibits several changes readily identified by echocardiography. The responses are generally seen as volume-accommodating dilatory changes and pressure-related changes such as RV enlargement, hypertrophy, and abnormal septal motion. With increasing severity and chronicity of PH, RV failure ensues, and this is evident on echocardiography as RV systolic failure. The adaptive changes of the RV are described next.

Right Ventricular Enlargement

Chronic pressure and volume overload of the RV leads to a dilated chamber that is rapidly and easily appreciated on echocardiography. RV size is typically qualitatively assessed in the ME four-chamber view via comparison with LV size. At end-diastole, the normal RV typically occupies two thirds of the cross-sectional area of the LV area. With mild enlargement, the RV increases in size greater than two thirds of the LV area. With moderate enlargement, the RV is equal in cross-sectional area. Severe enlargement yields an RV that is larger in cross-sectional area than the LV (Fig. 25-1 and Video 25-1). RV size may be rapidly assessed via the appearance of the cardiac apex in the ME four-chamber view. Typically, the LV forms the cardiac apex. With RV enlargement, however, the RV may share the cardiac apex. With severe enlargement, the RV may completely occupy the cardiac apex in that echocardiographic view.

Quantitatively, the RV is difficult to assess owing to its asymmetric shape, and its size is frequently underestimated. Although specific normal RV dimensions have not been established for transesophageal echocardiography (TEE), the American Society of Echocardiography (ASE) has suggested a transthoracic apical four-chamber measurement of the RV basal dimension (within the basal third of the RV) with an upper reference limit of 4.2 cm (Fig. 25-2).[24] For longitudinal measurements, the suggested upper reference limit is 8.6 cm.

Right Ventricular Hypertrophy

In response to chronically elevated RV afterload, the RV myocardium hypertrophies. This may be demonstrated on echocardiography as RV free wall thickness greater than 5 mm at end-diastole (Fig. 25-3). Long-standing severe chronic PH may result in RV hypertrophy exceeding 10 mm. This measurement may be obtained in the ME four-chamber view, the ME RV inflow-outflow view, or the TG mid-papillary view, often aided by the use of M-mode echocardiography. Hypertrophy of the RV includes the encircling bands, yielding an often easily identified hypertrophied moderator band near the RV apex (Fig. 25-4 and Video 25-2).

Right Ventricular Function

As explained earlier, the normal RV is adapted to ejecting into a low-pressure pulmonary circuit. Both acute and chronic elevations in pulmonary arterial pressure may lead to RV systolic dysfunction that may be identified with routine echocardiography. As with chamber measurements, the asymmetric nature of the RV creates challenges in assessing RV systolic function. Unlike the LV, which contracts in both circumferential and longitudinal planes, the RV has a peristaltic-like contraction that aids in the movement of blood from the inflow portion through the apical segment and toward the outflow (infundibular) portion. Several modalities have been suggested for evaluating RV

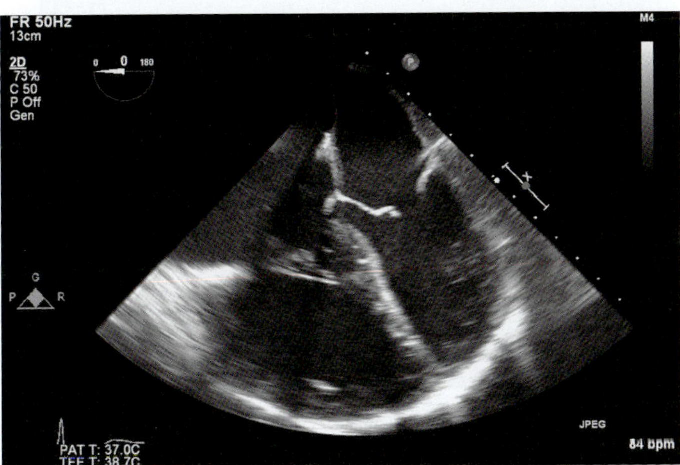

Figure 25-1 Midesophageal four-chamber view of patient with chronic thromboembolic pulmonary hypertension (CTEPH) and resulting severe right ventricular (RV) enlargement. Note that cross-sectional area of RV exceeds cross-sectional area of left ventricle. (See Video 25-1.)

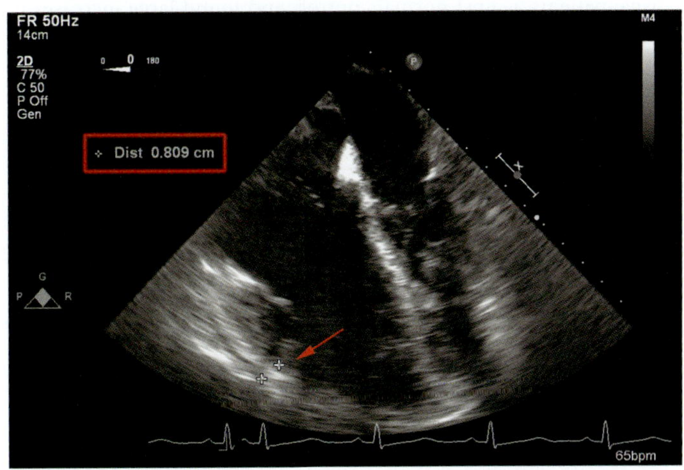

Figure 25-3 Measurement of right ventricular (RV) free wall thickness *(red arrow)* in midesophageal four-chamber view, demonstrating severe RV hypertrophy.

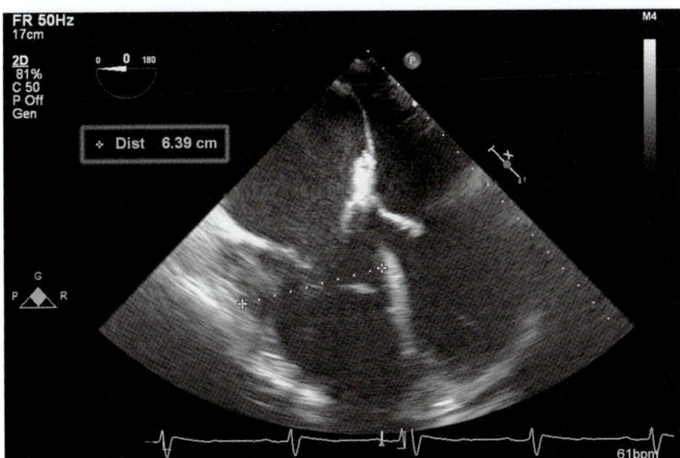

Figure 25-2 Measurement of basal dimension of right ventricle (RV) in midesophageal four-chamber view, demonstrating significant RV enlargement.

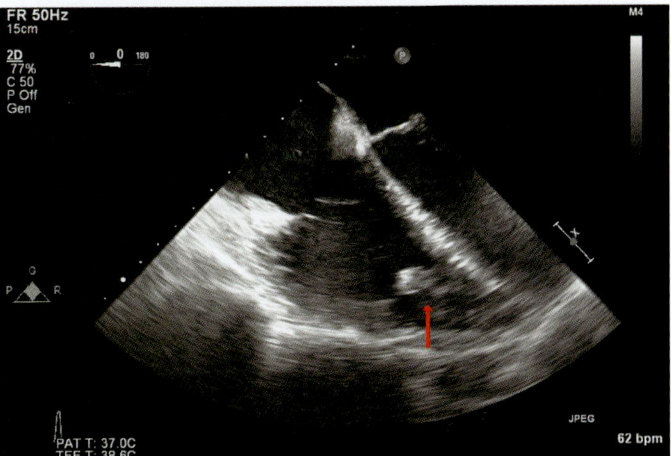

Figure 25-4 Midesophageal four-chamber view of patient with long-standing pulmonary hypertension with resultant right ventricular hypertrophy and a prominent moderator band *(red arrow)*. (See Video 25-2.)

systolic function, often validated for use with transthoracic echocardiography (TTE) and extrapolated for use with TEE.[25]

Two-Dimensional Methods

One of the most widely used measurement tools, tricuspid annular plane systolic excursion (TAPSE), is based on the longitudinal contraction of the tricuspid base toward the apex during systole. Because the septal portion of the tricuspid annulus is attached to the base of the heart, the bulk of basal RV function involves the hinge-like movement of the lateral annulus toward the apex. Two-dimensional (2D) measurements (often with the assistance of an M-mode cursor) in the ME four-chamber view quantitates the longitudinal displacement of the annulus (Fig. 25-5).[26,27] A lower reference value for TAPSE (16 mm) is a cutoff value that suggests RV dysfunction.[25]

Similar to the LV, RV fractional area of change (RV FAC) is the percentage change in ventricular area between systole and diastole. This measurement is typically obtained in the ME four-chamber view, tracing from the lateral tricuspid annulus along the RV free wall to apex and returning along the IVS to the septal tricuspid annulus. Owing to the complex geometry of the RV, the view must be optimized to prevent foreshortening of the ventricle. Anavekar et al. evaluated the RV FAC (among other 2D echocardiographic parameters of RV function) against RVEF as calculated by magnetic resonance imaging (MRI), finding that RV FAC correlated best with RVEF by cardiac MRI.[28] Hinderliter et al. compared TTE findings in primary pulmonary hypertensive patients against normal controls and found large increases in RV end-diastolic area, with associated reduced RV FACs.[29] Current guidelines suggest a lower reference limit of 35% for RV FAC.[25]

Often, 2D estimates of RV volume employ similar methods to LV volume estimates, such as disk summation techniques. Compared with MRI measurements, these often underestimate RV volumes due to the complex geometry of the RV.[25] Here, three-dimensional (3D) echocardiography appears promising in overcoming this shortcoming of 2D exams (see later discussion).

Doppler-Based Methods

Similar to its use in the LV, the rate in rise of pressure (dP/dt) of the RV has been evaluated as a marker of RV function. A continuous wave Doppler signal of TR provides the opportunity for the simplified Bernoulli equation to be applied at 0.5 and 2 m/s on the ascending portion of the envelope, allowing computation of the rate of RV pressure change over time. This measurement, however, is influenced by pulmonary artery systolic pressure,[30] so its usefulness in pulmonary hypertensive patients is yet to be determined.

The development of Doppler tissue imaging has allowed evaluation of RV myocardial motion, allowing global and regional assessments of function. A less load-dependent pulsed wave Doppler (PWD) tissue profile of the lateral tricuspid annulus yields several velocity and time measurements that can be used in evaluating RV function (Fig. 25-6). These measurements form the basis of peak systolic velocity (S′), myocardial performance index (MPI), and isovolumic acceleration.

PWD tissue imaging allows evaluation of S′ of the basal RV free wall in the ME four-chamber view (Fig. 25-7). Difficulty in aligning the Doppler beam with the path of tricuspid annular motion may exist in the ME four-chamber view, so David et al. suggested using a modified TG RV inflow view to better align the tissue Doppler sample volume.[31] Pavlicek et al. found that peak systolic velocity correlated well with RVEF determined by MRI, and most accurately distinguished between normal and reduced RVEF compared with other echocardiographic parameters.[32] However, Hsiao et al. demonstrated that the relationship between S′ and RVEF may be altered in the setting of severe TR.[33] It has also been demonstrated that S′ determined by TEE is lower than S′ determined by TTE, either due to technical differences in Doppler measurements or regional differences in RV myocardial motion.[34]

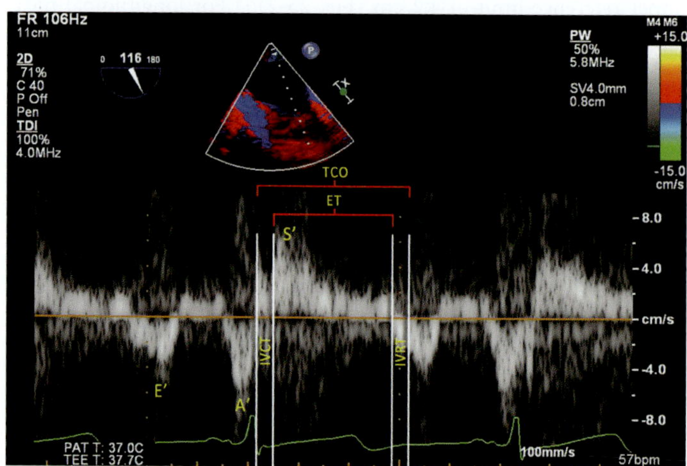

Figure 25-6 Doppler tissue imaging with pulsed wave Doppler evaluation of the inferior right ventricular (RV) wall and tricuspid annulus in a modified TG RV inflow view. *A′*, Atrial tricuspid velocity; *E′*, early tricuspid diastolic velocity; *ET*, ejection time; *IVCT*, isovolumic contraction time; *IVRT*, isovolumic relaxation time; *S′*, peak tricuspid systolic velocity; *TCO*, tricuspid closure opening time. Myocardial performance index (MPI) is calculated as (TCO − ET)/ET.

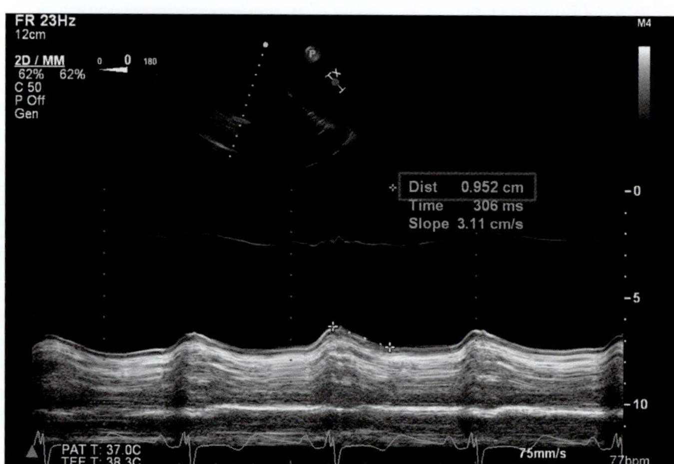

Figure 25-5 M-mode echocardiography through lateral annulus of tricuspid valve in ME four-chamber view in patient with chronic pulmonary hypertension and right ventricular failure. Tricuspid annular plane systolic excursion (TAPSE) may be determined by distance moved by lateral annulus during systole.

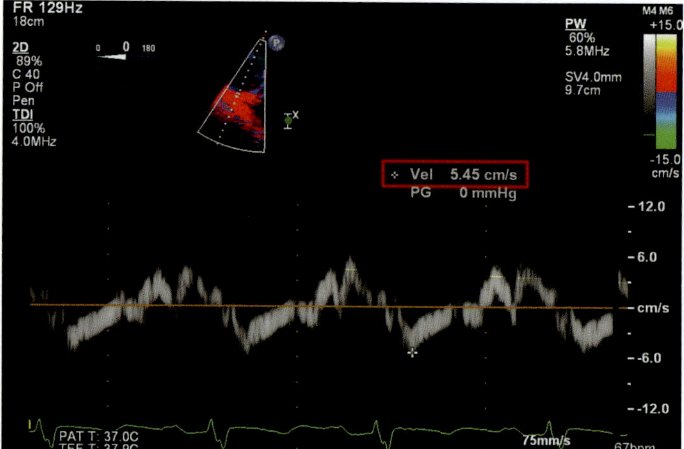

Figure 25-7 Doppler tissue imaging with pulsed wave Doppler evaluation of basal right ventricular (RV) free wall, demonstrating reduced RV systolic function.

Identification of S′ carries the same advantage of TAPSE in that it is relatively easy to employ, but with the same disadvantage of assuming that evaluating one regional segment of the RV is representative of global RV function. An S′ less than 10 cm/s suggests abnormal RV function.[25]

Myocardial performance index, synonymous with the Tei index, has been used to evaluate global (both systolic and diastolic) RV function. Being entirely Doppler derived, the MPI determination is not affected by RV geometry. Tei et al. initially described the MPI for the LV and subsequently described use of the Tei index for the RV in primary pulmonary hypertensive versus control patients.[35,36] The right-sided MPI (also known as *RIMP*) is a measurement of global function based on the work of the heart during both ejecting and nonejecting periods, and is obtained by dividing isovolumic time (isovolumetric relaxation time plus isovolumetric contraction time) by ejection time [(IVRT + ICVT)/ET]. Traditionally, the Tei index is obtained via the pulsed Doppler method using two separate cardiac cycles. Measurements include the ET, measured as the duration of flow in the RVOT, and the tricuspid closure-opening (TCO) time, measured as the duration between closure and opening of the TV (time from end of transtricuspid A wave to beginning of E wave).[25] TCO time includes IVRT, ICVT and ET; thus, MPI may be calculated as the (TCO-ET)/ET. With TEE, obtaining the views required for the pulsed Doppler method may include the ME four-chamber view for the TCO and the UE aortic arch short-axis view to evaluate RVOT flow for measurement of ET (Fig. 25-8). The Doppler tissue method, however, can determine RIMP with a single beat, which is helpful in avoiding the confounding effect of heart rate variability that occurs with the pulsed Doppler method. In the Doppler tissue method, a tissue Doppler profile is obtained at the lateral tissue annulus, demonstrating S′, E′, and A′. ET is determined as the duration of S′, whereas TCO is determined as the duration from the end of A′ to the beginning of E′ (see Fig. 25-6).

Pavlicek et al. evaluated several echocardiographic methods of RV systolic function in a cohort of patients that included those with normal RV function as well as varying degrees of RV dysfunction as determined by RVEF via cardiac MRI. It was demonstrated that several methods, including RV FAC, TAPSE, S′, and MPI, correlated with RVEF by MRI. An MPI greater than 0.50 correlated best with the presence of severely reduced RV function (RVEF ≤ 30%).[32] Blanchard

et al. evaluated the RV Tei index preoperatively and postoperatively in patients undergoing pulmonary thromboendarterectomy for chronic thromboembolic PH. They reported that the RV Tei index correlated directly with mPAP, PVR, and indirectly with cardiac output, thereby identifying the Tei index as helpful in this patient population.[37] Current guidelines note different reference ranges for MPI determined by pulsed Doppler versus tissue Doppler methods, with upper reference limits of 0.40 and 0.55, respectively.[25]

Isovolumic acceleration (IVA) measures the linear velocity change of the tricuspid annular motion during isovolumic contraction. This measurement also uses tissue Doppler imaging as described earlier, utilizing the peak isovolumic myocardial velocity divided by the time required to reach peak velocity from baseline (Fig. 25-9). Similar to other modalities that were first evaluated for LV function and subsequently validated for RV function, Vogel et al. described IVA in an animal model. They reported that the measurement adequately assessed RV contractile function and appeared unaffected by preload and afterload changes but was affected by heart rate.[38] In their evaluation of seven Doppler echocardiographic parameters (inclusive of RV IVA) against RVEF by cardiac MRI, Pavlicek et al. confirmed that all correlated significantly. However, RV IVA demonstrated an intermediate rank among the seven variables and did not correlate as strongly as S′ or MPI.[32] While others have confirmed its independence from preload, normal values have been reported with wide variability and also exhibit age dependency.[25,39] Current ASE guidelines do not offer reference ranges.[25]

RV strain and strain rate (the change in myocardial deformation and its rate of deformation over time, respectively) involve using a color-coded tissue Doppler mode. Current guidelines do not offer reference ranges, owing to lack of normative data and high variability. The complexity of the measurement requires offline analysis.[25] Additional research and evaluation is necessary to evaluate strain and strain rate's potential use in perioperative settings.

Three-Dimensional Evaluation

A relatively new method for evaluating RV function involves a commercially available offline analysis software package, 4D RV-function (TomTec Imaging Systems, Germany), which allows volume rendering of the RV with displays of RV end-diastolic and end-systolic volumes, stroke volume, and ejection fraction. The software analyzes 3D echocardiography (3DE) data sets derived from either TTE or TEE. Although cardiac MRI remains the most accurate modality, 3DE of the RV with volume-rendered imaging appears promising for assessing RV

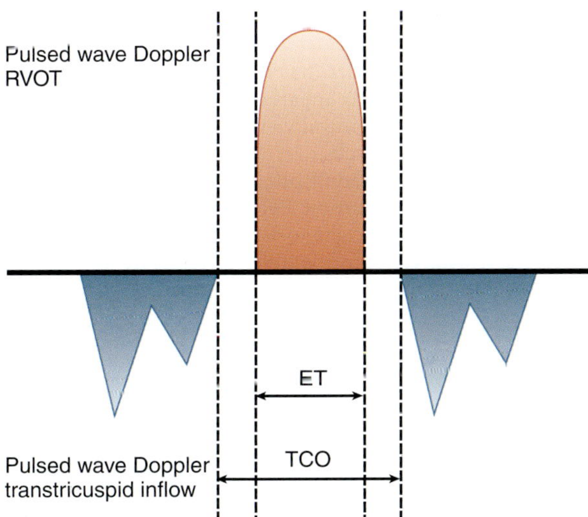

Figure 25-8 Schematic diagram of time intervals from separate Doppler-derived interrogations of right ventricular outflow tract (*RVOT*) and transtricuspid flow. Above baseline represents transesophageal echocardiographic (TEE)-based Doppler of RVOT (e.g., from UE aortic arch short-axis view); below baseline represents TEE-based Doppler measurement of transtricuspid inflow (e.g., from ME four-chamber view). *ET*, Ejection time; *TCO*, tricuspid closure opening time. Myocardial performance index (MPI) is calculated as TCO − ET.

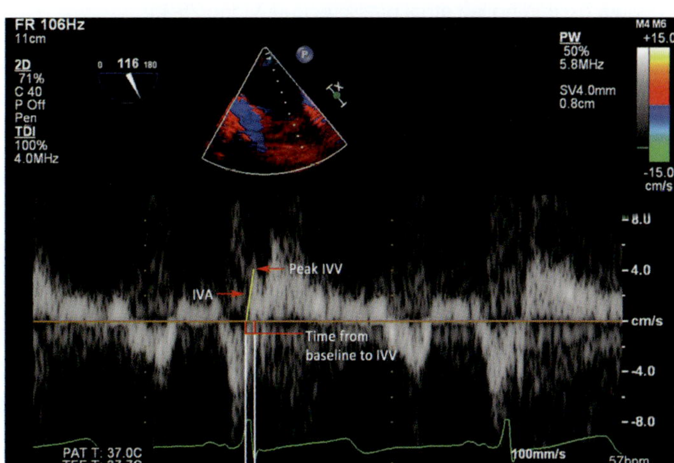

Figure 25-9 Isovolumic contraction acceleration (*IVA*) measurement. Doppler tissue imaging with pulsed wave Doppler evaluation of inferior right ventricular (RV) wall and tricuspid annulus in a modified transgastric RV inflow view. IVA, indicated by yellow slope, identifies rate of myocardial motion. *Peak IVV,* Peak isovolumic contraction velocity. IVA is calculated as peak IVV divided by time from baseline to IVV.

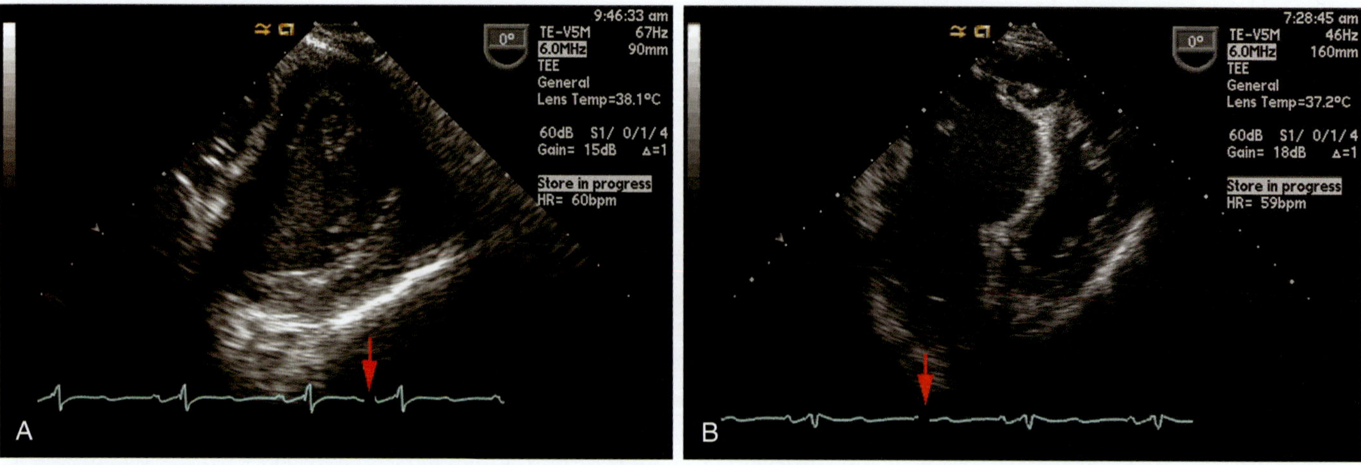

Figure 25-10   Right ventricular (RV) overload is identified by the timing of septal flattening in transgastric mid-papillary short-axis view. **A,** D-shaped interventricular septum is identified at end-systole, demonstrating RV pressure overload. Red arrow at end of T wave on electrocardiogram (ECG) marks end-systole. **B,** Septal bowing is noted at end-diastole, identifying RV volume overload. Red arrow at end of P wave on ECG marks end-diastole. (See Video 25-3.)

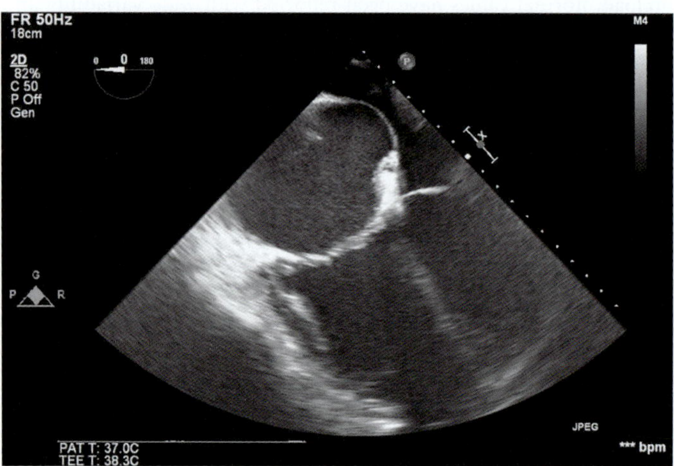

Figure 25-11   Midesophageal four-chamber view demonstrating significant right atrial (RA) enlargement in patient with chronic pulmonary hypertension. Note significant interatrial septal shift, identifying RA pressure exceeding left atrial pressure. (See Video 25-4.)

volume and RVEF.[27,40-43] Further evaluation of perioperative use of RV 3D analyses in pulmonary hypertensive patients is necessary.

Right Ventricular Overload

In its anterolateral positioning relative to the LV, the RV shares the IVS. RV overload as well as underfilling of the LV due to poor RV cardiac output may cause distortion of the IVS that is often identified and characterized echocardiographically. This septal distortion or flattening is most easily identified in the TG mid-papillary short-axis view as a leftward deviation of the septum yielding a "D-shaped" LV chamber. The timing of the deviation lends additional information to the identification of RV pressure or volume overload. RV pressure overload is identified as septal flattening at end-systole, whereas RV volume overload is identified at end-diastole (Fig. 25-10 and Video 25-3).[26]

Long-standing PH and overt RV failure may ultimately lead to a dilated RV, exhibiting either RV pressure overload or RV volume overload. In the case of severe chronic thromboembolic PH and severe RV failure, both pressure and volume overload may coexist with a deviated septum throughout most of the cardiac cycle.

Right Atrium

In addition to RV enlargement with chronic PH, the RA also becomes enlarged. Normally the RA is a thin-walled structure that accommodates blood from the systemic venous return via the SVC and IVC during ventricular systole and as a conduit to the RV via the TV during diastole. In the setting of PH, several factors may play a role in RA dilation. The failing RV with its decreased cardiac output leads to increased right-sided volume and diastolic pressure, which is transmitted to the RA. Additionally, a dilated RV often exhibits a dilated TV annulus with significant regurgitation, leading to further RA dilation (Fig. 25-11 and Video 25-4).

The RA is most often measured in the ME four-chamber view in its major and minor axes. The major axis extends from the superior aspect of the RA to the center of the tricuspid annulus, whereas the minor axis is measured from the mid-RA lateral wall to the interatrial septum. The ASE suggests upper reference limits of 4.4 and 5.3 cm, respectively, for major and minor axes dimensions.[25]

Interatrial Septum

Patients with PH and RV failure may have RA pressure exceeding that in the LA. This is often visually apparent in the ME four-chamber, ME RV inflow-outflow, or ME bicaval views as septal bowing toward the LA throughout the cardiac cycle.

An estimated 25% of the adult population exhibits a probe patent foramen ovale (PFO), and chronic PH and elevated RA pressure may "open" the PFO, leading to right-to-left intracardiac shunting.[44] This may be detected with echocardiography using color flow Doppler or agitated saline, most commonly in the ME bicaval view (Fig. 25-12 and Video 25-5).

Tricuspid Valve

As already noted, the RV and RA of patients with PH are often dilated, affecting TV anatomy such that coaptation failure results in varying degrees of TR. The echocardiographic evaluation of the PH patient should include an assessment of TR.

The TV is a trileaflet valve that may be visualized in the ME four-chamber, ME RV inflow-outflow, and modified ME bicaval views, and variably in short-axis orientation in a TG mid-papillary short-axis view. The severity of TR may be assessed via multiple modalities. Visual assessment of the ratio of jet area relative to RA size provides an estimation of TR, with greater than 50% indicating severe TR. However, this is subject to gain settings and color scales. A rapid assessment

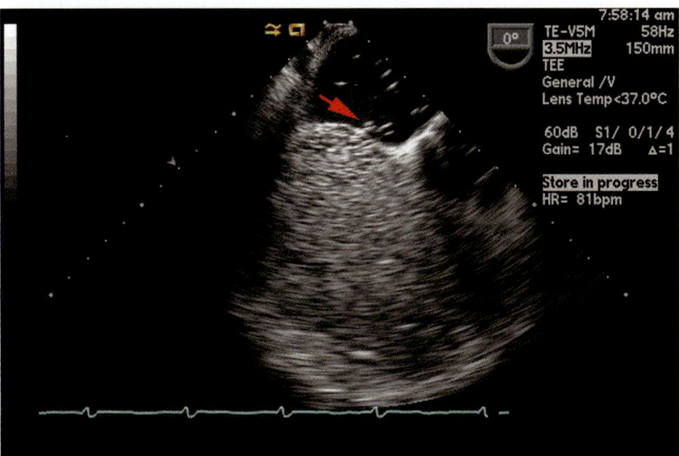

Figure 25-12   Midesophageal bicaval view with agitated saline study identifying patent foramen ovale in patient with long-standing pulmonary hypertension undergoing pulmonary thromboendarterectomy. Red arrow indicates area of intracardiac shunt. (See Video 25-5.)

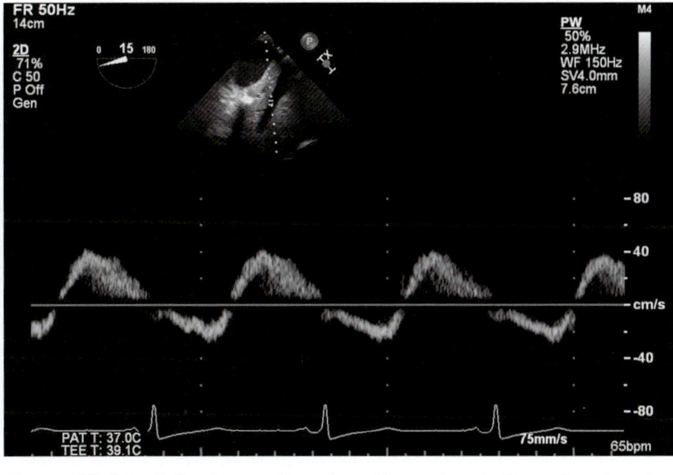

Figure 25-14   Pulsed wave Doppler of hepatic vein flow of patient imaged in Figure 25-10, demonstrating systolic flow reversal indicative of severe tricuspid regurgitation.

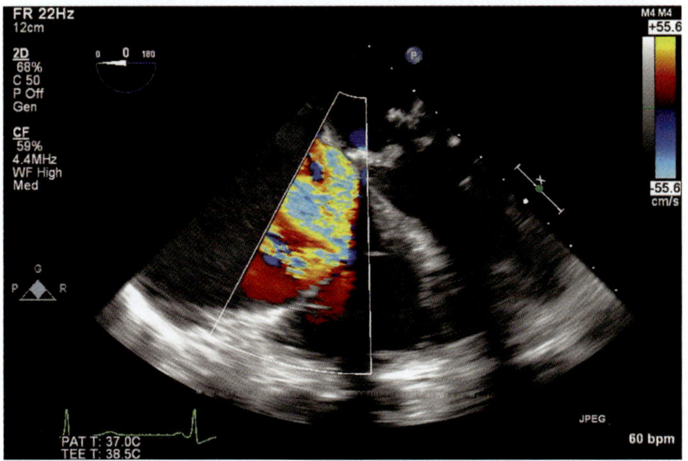

Figure 25-13   Color flow Doppler of tricuspid valve (TV) in midesophageal four-chamber view, demonstrating significant tricuspid regurgitation (TR) in patient scheduled for TV repair after prior mitral valve repair. Patient's TR was caused by annular dilation due to long-standing pulmonary hypertension and resultant right atrial enlargement. (See Video 25-6.)

of severity includes a vena contracta measurement, with greater than 0.7 cm indicating severe TR (Fig. 25-13 and Video 25-6). Additionally, PWD evaluation of hepatic vein flow pattern indicates TR severity. Normally, there is a large antegrade flow envelope identified during systole as blood flows toward the RA during atrial relaxation. Moderate TR causes a blunting of forward systolic flow, and severe TR is identified by systolic flow reversal (Fig. 25-14).

Pulmonary Artery

Along with RA, RV, and tricuspid annular dilation, the pulmonary artery may also dilate in response to long-standing PH. The main pulmonary artery is often visualized in the ME ascending aortic short-axis or UE aortic arch short-axis views. The right pulmonary artery is displayed in long and short axis in the ME ascending aortic short-axis and long-axis views, respectively. The upper reference value for the diameter of a normal-sized main pulmonary artery is 2.1 cm.[45]

Thrombus in Transit

Chronic thromboembolic pulmonary hypertension (CTEPH) is defined by PH caused by thromboembolic disease, but patients with other causes of chronic PH are at potential increased risk of venous thromboembolism due to low-flow states in the venous circulation and right heart.[46-48] Echocardiographic evaluation of the pulmonary hypertensive patient should include an evaluation for intracardiac thrombi. The thrombi may be found anywhere within the venous circulation or right heart, from the vena cava, RA, paradoxically crossing a PFO, TV-associated, attached to intracardiac catheters or pacemaker leads, as well as in the main or pulmonary artery (Fig. 25-15 and Video 25-7).

Hemodynamic Pressure Estimations

Pulmonary pressures can be estimated with Doppler echocardiography and may be helpful in evaluation of the pulmonary hypertensive patient. A continuous wave Doppler beam may be passed through TR to evaluate the peak regurgitation velocity. Applying the modified Bernoulli equation ($\Delta P = 4v^2$) with the addition of central venous pressure (CVP) yields an estimate of pulmonary artery systolic pressure (Fig. 25-16) (see Chapter 4).[25,26] Although there is potential inaccuracy, and pulmonary artery catheters can measure PA systolic pressure directly, TEE estimation retains its clinical usefulness for less invasive estimation and trending.[49,50]

Utilizing a similar technique with a pulmonary insufficiency (PI) continuous Doppler profile, pulmonary artery mean pressure (PAMP) and pulmonary artery diastolic pressure (PADP) may be estimated. PAMP is estimated by applying the Bernoulli equation with addition of CVP to the early PI velocity, whereas PADP is estimated by applying the Bernoulli equation with the addition of CVP to the end-diastolic PI velocity (Fig. 25-17).[25] Table 25-1 offers a summary of hemodynamic estimations.

Conclusion

Right heart function is increasingly identified as prognostically important. Being a complex structure and active conduit to the low-pressure, low-resistance pulmonary circuit, the right heart undergoes several changes in response to PH. In the perioperative setting, echocardiography plays a critical role in diagnosis, evaluation, and management of the pulmonary hypertensive patient.

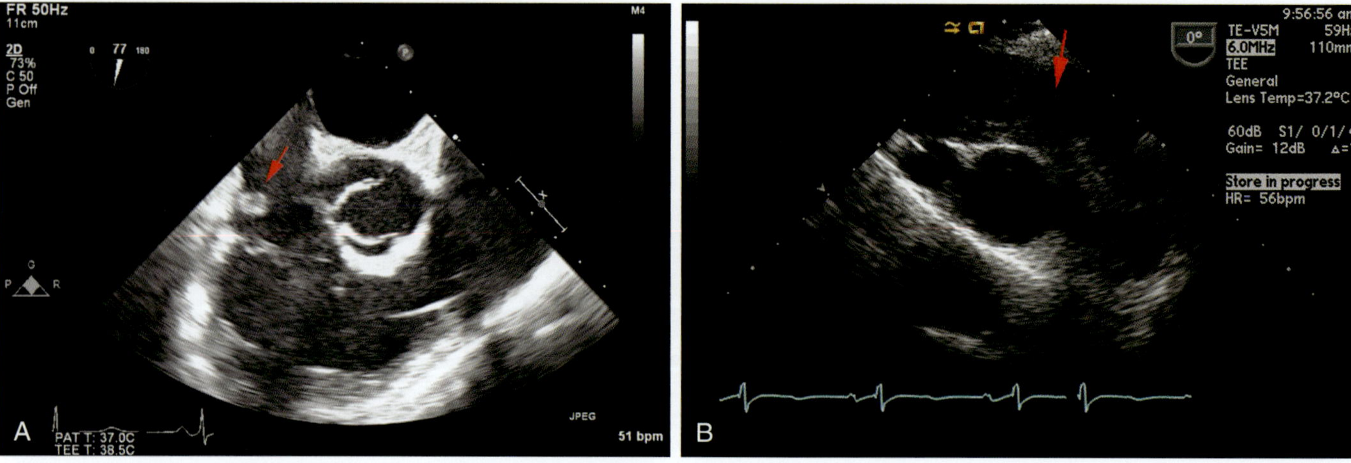

Figure 25-15 Thrombi identified in patients with chronic thromboembolic pulmonary hypertension undergoing pulmonary thromboendarterectomy. **A**, Midesophageal (ME) right ventricular inflow-outflow view demonstrating right atrial thrombus *(red arrow)*. **B**, ME ascending aortic short-axis view demonstrating dilated right pulmonary artery with occluding thrombus *(red arrow)*. (See Video 25-7.)

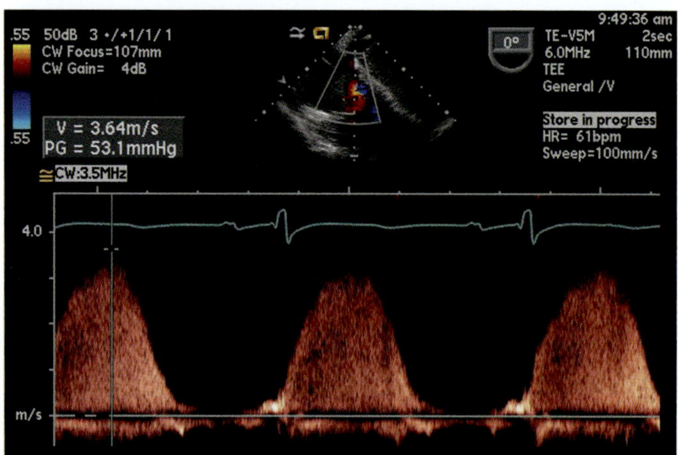

Figure 25-16 Midesophageal four-chamber view with continuous wave Doppler through tricuspid regurgitation jet in patient with long-standing pulmonary hypertension.

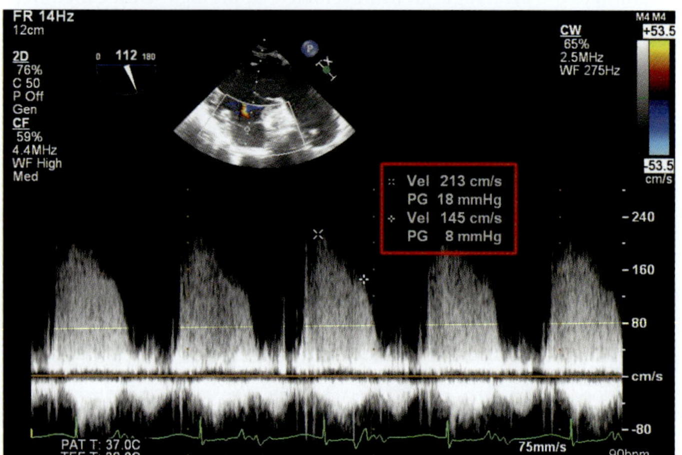

Figure 25-17 Slight rightward probe rotation and increased omniplane angle from transgastric (TG) right ventricular (RV) inflow view yielded a non-standard TG RV inflow-outflow view, allowing parallel alignment of continuous wave Doppler beam with a pulmonary insufficiency jet. Hemodynamic estimations demonstrate reduced pulmonary artery mean and diastolic pressures immediately post pulmonary thromboendarterectomy.

TABLE 25-1	Echocardiographically Derived Hemodynamic Estimations of Pulmonary Artery Pressures
PASP	$4(v_{[TR\,jet\,peak]})^2 + CVP$
PAMP	$4[v_{(PI\,jet\,early)}]^2 + CVP$
PADP	$4[v_{(PI\,jet\,late)}]^2 + CVP$

CVP, Central venous pressure; *PADP*, pulmonary artery diastolic pressure; *PAMP*, pulmonary artery mean pressure; *PASP*, pulmonary artery systolic pressure, *PI*, pulmonary insufficiency; *TR*, tricuspid regurgitation.

REFERENCES

1. Badesch DB, Champion HC, Sanchez MA, et al. Diagnosis and assessment of pulmonary arterial hypertension. *J Am Coll Cardiol.* 2009;54:S55-S66.
2. McLaughlin VV, Archer SL, Badesch DB, et al. ACCF/AHA 2009 expert consensus document on pulmonary hypertension a report of the American College of Cardiology Foundation Task Force on Expert Consensus Documents and the American Heart Association developed in collaboration with the American College of Chest Physicians; American Thoracic Society, Inc.; and the Pulmonary Hypertension Association. *J Am Coll Cardiol.* 2009;53:1573-1619.
3. Cool CD, Kennedy D, Voelkel NF, Tuder RM. Pathogenesis and evolution of plexiform lesions in pulmonary hypertension associated with scleroderma and human immunodeficiency virus infection. *Hum Pathol.* 1997;28:434-442.
4. Runo JR, Loyd JE. Primary pulmonary hypertension. *Lancet.* 2003;361:1533-1544.
5. Budhiraja R, Tuder RM, Hassoun PM. Endothelial dysfunction in pulmonary hypertension. *Circulation.* 2004;109:159-165.
6. Galie N, Manes A, Branzi A. The new clinical trials on pharmacological treatment in pulmonary arterial hypertension. *Eur Respir J.* 2002;20:1037-1049.
7. Mikhail GW, Gibbs JS, Yacoub MH. Pulmonary and systemic arterial pressure changes during syncope in primary pulmonary hypertension. *Circulation.* 2001;104:1326-1327.
8. Blaise G, Langleben D, Hubert B. Pulmonary arterial hypertension: pathophysiology and anesthetic approach. *Anesthesiology.* 2003;99:1415-1432.
9. Ho SY, Nihoyannopoulos P. Anatomy, echocardiography, and normal right ventricular dimensions. *Heart.* 2006;92(suppl 1):i2-13.
10. Farb A, Burke AP, Virmani R. Anatomy and pathology of the right ventricle (including acquired tricuspid and pulmonic valve disease). *Cardiol Clin.* 1992;10:1-21.
11. Lee FA. Hemodynamics of the right ventricle in normal and disease states. *Cardiol Clin.* 1992;10:59-67.
12. Bronicki RA, Baden HP. Pathophysiology of right ventricular failure in pulmonary hypertension. *Pediatr Crit Care Med.* 2010;11:S15-S22.
13. Redington AN, Gray HH, Hodson ME, Rigby ML, Oldershaw PJ. Characterisation of the normal right ventricular pressure-volume relation by biplane angiography and simultaneous micromanometer pressure measurements. *Br Heart J.* 1988;59:23-30.
14. Haddad F, Hunt SA, Rosenthal DN, Murphy DJ. Right ventricular function in cardiovascular disease, part I: Anatomy, physiology, aging, and functional assessment of the right ventricle. *Circulation.* 2008;117:1436-1448.
15. Kaul S. The interventricular septum in health and disease. *Am Heart J.* 1986;112:568-581.
16. Lindqvist P, Morner S, Karp K, Waldenstrom A. New aspects of septal function by using 1-dimensional strain and strain rate imaging. *J Am Soc Echocardiogr.* 2006;19:1345-1349.
17. Klima U, Guerrero JL, Vlahakes GJ. Contribution of the interventricular septum to maximal right ventricular function. *Eur J Cardiothorac Surg.* 1998;14:250-255.
18. Ribeiro A, Lindmarker P, Juhlin-Dannfelt A, Johnsson H, Jorfeldt L. Echocardiography Doppler in pulmonary embolism: right ventricular dysfunction as a predictor of mortality rate. *Am Heart J.* 1997;134:479-487.
19. Goldstein JA. Right heart ischemia: pathophysiology, natural history, and clinical management. *Prog Cardiovasc Dis.* 1998;40:325-341.
20. Vlahakes GJ, Turley K, Hoffman JI. The pathophysiology of failure in acute right ventricular hypertension: hemodynamic and biochemical correlations. *Circulation.* 1981;63:87-95.
21. Santamore WP, Dell'Italia LJ. Ventricular interdependence: significant left ventricular contributions to right ventricular systolic function. *Prog Cardiovasc Dis.* 1998;40:289-308.

22. Goldstein JA. Pathophysiology and management of right heart ischemia. *J Am Coll Cardiol.* 2002;40:841-853.

23. Piazza G, Goldhaber SZ. The acutely decompensated right ventricle: pathways for diagnosis and management. *Chest.* 2005;128:1836-1852.

24. Kasper J, Bolliger D, Skarvan K, Buser P, Filipovic M, Seeberger MD. Additional cross-sectional transesophageal echocardiography views improve perioperative right heart assessment. *Anesthesiology.* 2012;117:726-734.

25. Rudski LG, Lai WW, Afilalo J, et al. Guidelines for the echocardiographic assessment of the right heart in adults: a report from the American Society of Echocardiography, endorsed by the European Association of Echocardiography, a registered branch of the European Society of Cardiology, and the Canadian Society of Echocardiography. *J Am Soc Echocardiogr.* 2010;23:685-713, quiz 86–88.

26. Perrino AC, Reeves ST. *A Practical Approach to Transesophageal Echocardiography.* 2nd ed. Philadelphia: Wolters Kluwer Health/Lippincott Williams & Wilkins; 2008.

27. Cacciapuoti F. Echocardiographic evaluation of right heart function and pulmonary vascular bed. *Int J Cardiovasc Imaging.* 2009;25:689-697.

28. Anavekar NS, Gerson D, Skali H, Kwong RY, Yucel EK, Solomon SD. Two-dimensional assessment of right ventricular function: an echocardiographic-MRI correlative study. *Echocardiography.* 2007;24:452-456.

29. Hinderliter AL, PWt Willis, Barst RJ, et al. Effects of long-term infusion of prostacyclin (epoprostenol) on echocardiographic measures of right ventricular structure and function in primary pulmonary hypertension. Primary Pulmonary Hypertension Study Group. *Circulation.* 1997;95:1479-1486.

30. Pai RG, Bansal RC, Shah PM. Determinants of the rate of right ventricular pressure rise by Doppler echocardiography: potential value in the assessment of right ventricular function. *J Heart Valve Dis.* 1994;3:179-184.

31. David JS, Tousignant CP, Bowry R. Tricuspid annular velocity in patients undergoing cardiac operation using transesophageal echocardiography. *J Am Soc Echocardiogr.* 2006;19:329-334.

32. Pavlicek M, Wahl A, Rutz T, et al. Right ventricular systolic function assessment: rank of echocardiographic methods vs. cardiac magnetic resonance imaging. *Eur J Echocardiogr.* 2011;12:871-880.

33. Hsiao SH, Lin SK, Wang WC, Yang SH, Gin PL, Liu CP. Severe tricuspid regurgitation shows significant impact in the relationship among peak systolic tricuspid annular velocity, tricuspid annular plane systolic excursion, and right ventricular ejection fraction. *J Am Soc Echocardiogr.* 2006;19:902-910.

34. Tousignant CP, Bowry R, Levesque S, Denault AY. Regional differences in color tissue Doppler-derived measures of longitudinal right ventricular function using transesophageal and transthoracic echocardiography. *J Cardiothorac Vasc Anesth.* 2008;22:400-405.

35. Tei C, Ling LH, Hodge DO, et al. New index of combined systolic and diastolic myocardial performance: a simple and reproducible measure of cardiac function–a study in normals and dilated cardiomyopathy. *J Cardiol.* 1995;26:357-366.

36. Tei C, Dujardin KS, Hodge DO, et al. Doppler echocardiographic index for assessment of global right ventricular function. *J Am Soc Echocardiogr.* 1996;9:838-847.

37. Blanchard DG, Malouf PJ, Gurudevan SV, et al. Utility of right ventricular Tei index in the noninvasive evaluation of chronic thromboembolic pulmonary hypertension before and after pulmonary thromboendarterectomy. *JACC Cardiovasc Imaging.* 2009;2:143-149.

38. Vogel M, Schmidt MR, Kristiansen SB, et al. Validation of myocardial acceleration during isovolumic contraction as a novel noninvasive index of right ventricular contractility: comparison with ventricular pressure-volume relations in an animal model. *Circulation.* 2002;105:1693-1699.

39. Kjaergaard J, Snyder EM, Hassager C, Oh JK, Johnson BD. Impact of preload and afterload on global and regional right ventricular function and pressure: a quantitative echocardiography study. *J Am Soc Echocardiogr.* 2006;19:515-521.

40. Sugeng L, Mor-Avi V, Weinert L, et al. Multimodality comparison of quantitative volumetric analysis of the right ventricle. *JACC Cardiovasc Imaging.* 2010;3:10-18.

41. Calcutteea A, Chung R, Lindqvist P, Hodson M, Henein MY. Differential right ventricular regional function and the effect of pulmonary hypertension: three-dimensional echo study. *Heart.* 2011;97:1004-1011.

42. Tamborini G, Brusoni D, Torres Molina JE, et al. Feasibility of a new generation three-dimensional echocardiography for right ventricular volumetric and functional measurements. *Am J Cardiol.* 2008;102:499-505.

43. Grapsa J, Gibbs JS, Dawson D, et al. Morphologic and functional remodeling of the right ventricle in pulmonary hypertension by real-time three-dimensional echocardiography. *Am J Cardiol.* 2011.

44. Manecke Jr GR. Anesthesia for pulmonary endarterectomy. *Semin Thorac Cardiovasc Surg.* 2006;18:236-242.

45. Lang RM, Bierig M, Devereux RB, et al. Recommendations for chamber quantification: a report from the American Society of Echocardiography's Guidelines and Standards Committee and the Chamber Quantification Writing Group, developed in conjunction with the European Association of Echocardiography, a branch of the European Society of Cardiology. *J Am Soc Echocardiogr.* 2005;18:1440-1463.

46. Manecke Jr GR, Wilson WC, Auger WR, Jamieson SW. Chronic thromboembolic pulmonary hypertension and pulmonary thromboendarterectomy. *Semin Cardiothorac Vasc Anesth.* 2005;9:189-204.

47. McGoon MD, Kane GC. Pulmonary hypertension: diagnosis and management. *Mayo Clin Proc.* 2009;84:191-207.

48. Johnson SR, Granton JT, Mehta S. Thrombotic arteriopathy and anticoagulation in pulmonary hypertension. *Chest.* 2006;130:545-552.

49. Attaran RR, Ramaraj R, Sorrell VL, Movahed MR. Poor correlation of estimated pulmonary artery systolic pressure between echocardiography and right heart catheterization in patients awaiting cardiac transplantation: results from the clinical arena. *Transplant Proc.* 2009;41:3827-3830.

50. Ben-Dor I, Kramer MR, Raccah A, et al. Echocardiography versus right-sided heart catheterization among lung transplantation candidates. *Ann Thorac Surg.* 2006;81:1056-1060.

Recent Advances

MANISH BANSAL | PARTHO P. SENGUPTA

Speckle Tracking Echocardiography

The ability to measure myocardial contractile function has always been the "Holy Grail" of echocardiography. A number of parameters and indices (e.g., fractional shortening, ejection fraction, etc.) have been developed to achieve this goal, but each one of them is significantly influenced by the loading conditions and is not really a true measure of myocardial contractility. Tissue velocity imaging, developed in 1989, allowed measurement of myocardial motion directly and was rapidly embraced as a tool for assessment of myocardial systolic and diastolic function.[1] However, it too was an imperfect measure of myocardial contractility because it could only measure displacement of myocardium relative to the transducer, not the actual contraction. With further advancements in Doppler techniques, an innovative approach was developed to quantify actual myocardial deformation. This technique, known as *myocardial strain imaging*, involved simultaneous recording of velocities from two adjacent myocardial regions, and the difference between the two was the rate at which myocardial shortening or lengthening occurred (*strain rate*). Integration of these instantaneous velocity gradients over time provided the net extent of myocardial shortening or lengthening taking place during a specific phase of the cardiac cycle (*strain*).[2,3]

Although Doppler-based strain imaging represented a major technical advancement in echocardiographic assessment of myocardial function, it still had considerable challenges.[3] Being a Doppler-based technique, it was highly dependent on the insonation angle and therefore allowed measurement of myocardial contraction only in the direction parallel to the ultrasound beam. Consequently, only longitudinal strain and strain rate could be measured, with virtually no information about the radial, circumferential, rotational, and torsional components of the complex multidirectional process of myocardial contraction.

Speckle tracking echocardiography is a newer alternative technique for characterizing myocardial motion and contraction.[4,5] Unlike the Doppler-based technique, speckle tracking echocardiography relies on grayscale imaging and thereby permits angle-independent measurement of myocardial contraction. Speckle tracking software identifies natural acoustic reflectors, or speckles, within the myocardium and then uses an algorithm (sum of absolute differences) to track these speckles frame by frame throughout the cardiac cycle. The data are then analyzed to derive information about myocardial motion in three-dimensional (3D) space, from which the displacement, velocity, and deformation in any direction can be computed (Fig. 26-1). Longitudinal and transverse strain can be calculated from the apical views, whereas short-axis views are used for deriving circumferential strain, radial strain, rotation, and torsion. The technique has been shown to have a high degree of reproducibility and a much better signal-to-noise ratio than Doppler-based strain imaging techniques.[6]

Since its advent, speckle tracking echocardiography has rapidly evolved into a useful modality for quantifying myocardial function in a wide variety of clinical conditions.[5,7,8] The greatest advantage of this technique is that it provides a quantitative and objective measure of myocardial contraction and therefore can be used for identifying subtle changes in myocardial function that cannot be detected otherwise with conventional measures such as ejection fraction. The technique

can accurately estimate global left ventricular ejection fraction, quantify the extent of myocardial damage in patients with coronary artery disease, and differentiate a subendocardial infarct from a transmural infarct.[9-13] When used as an adjunct to dobutamine echocardiography, it has been shown to have incremental value over wall motion analysis for detection of myocardial ischemia and viability.[14,15] It has also been successfully used for detecting subclinical left ventricular systolic dysfunction in patients with valvular heart disease, cardiomyopathies, pericardial diseases, congenital heart diseases, and also in patients receiving chemotherapeutic drugs.[16-25] It can help differentiate physiologic from pathologic hypertrophy and restrictive cardiomyopathy from constrictive pericarditis.[26,27] Radial dyssynchrony identified on speckle tracking echocardiography appears to be a more robust measure of intraventricular dyssynchrony than the conventionally used Doppler-based parameters.[28,29] The technique has also been employed for evaluating left atrial and right ventricular function, with initial studies showing great promise.[30-32]

Despite the rapidly unfolding array of potential clinical applications for speckle tracking echocardiography, there are several limitations associated with this technique.[4,5] The accuracy of speckle tracking is highly dependent on grayscale image quality and frame rates. The best results can be obtained at frame rates between 50 and 70 frames/s; lower frame rates compromise tracking the speckles across frames, and higher frame rates adversely affect image resolution. Out-of-plane motion produced by heart movement during the cardiac cycle is another major limitation of two-dimensional (2D) speckle tracking echocardiography and is particularly relevant for short-axis views. Fortunately, 3D speckle tracking echocardiography, which is currently being developed, seems to overcome this limitation to a large extent.[33-35]

Another important problem with speckle tracking echocardiography relates to inter-vendor variability. Different speckle tracking echocardiographic systems use different proprietary algorithms for measurement of strain. This introduces an important source of error and precludes comparisons among studies done using different platforms.

Finally, even though speckle tracking echocardiography has been shown to have good accuracy and reproducibility for overall left ventricular function, there is still a large degree of variability at the segmental level.[36]

Cardiovascular Flow Visualization

For decades it was believed that blood flow through the cardiovascular system was predominantly laminar and unidirectional. However, recent insights gained from in vitro and in vivo experiments, fuelled largely by rapid advancements in imaging techniques, have revealed that blood flow through the cardiac chambers is actually multidirectional, nonlaminar, and vortical.[37] As the bloodstream moves through the cardiac chambers, multiple fluid layers are created that slide against each other and against the myocardial wall and tend to curl or spin to produce spiral streamlines known as *vortices*. Such vortices are formed as a consequence of the contrasting influences of the pressure head driving the forward flow, and the viscosity and shear stress between the fluid layers and containing boundaries trying to slow down the blood

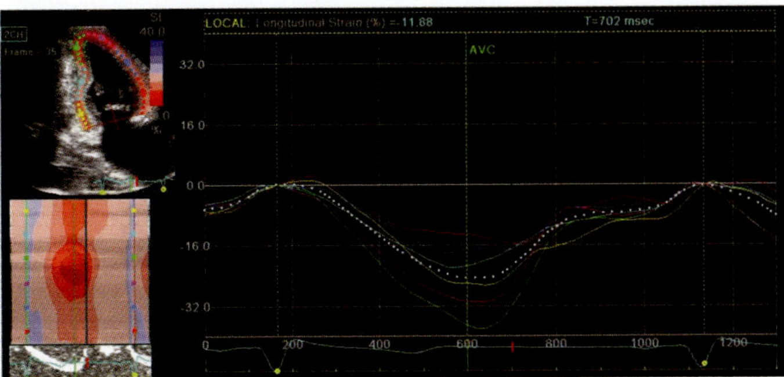

Figure 26-1   Measurement of longitudinal strain from apical two-chamber view using speckle tracking echocardiography. Lower-left segment of image shows parametric display of segmental strain values; right side of display shows graphic depiction of same.

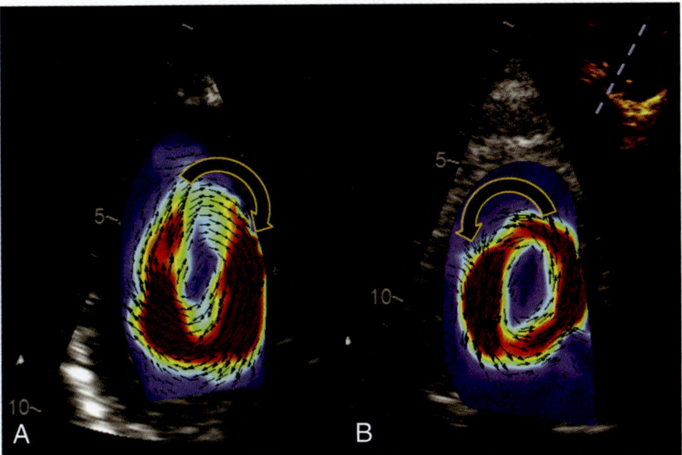

Figure 26-2   Cardiovascular flow visualization. **A,** Normal flow across mitral valve results in asymmetric vortex ring formation with clockwise rotation *(arrows)* that redirects flow toward ventricular outflow tract. Echo contrast particles have been tracked to compute two-dimensional flow. Kinetic energy is derived from bubble velocity measurements; regions of higher energy are shown in red. **B,** Flow across mitral bioprosthesis inclined toward interventricular septum *(inset)*. Abnormal orientation of prosthesis reverses flow in ventricle, generating a counterclockwise vortex *(arrows)*. Abnormal vortex formation is associated with energy dissipation that may adversely affect ventricular remodeling.

flow. This phenomenon is greatest at places where the bloodstream separates from the wall, as typically occurs when blood enters the heart cavity from a vein or through a valve. A similar phenomenon takes places in blood vessels when a relatively narrow vascular segment transitions to a dilated segment (e.g., carotid sinus) or at the site of vascular stenoses. Formation of these vortices is not merely a reflection of altered cardiovascular anatomy preventing "normal" laminar flow to continue. Rather, such multidirectional blood flow patterns are fundamental to maintenance of circulation under a wide range of physiologic and nonphysiologic conditions by allowing a delicate balance between energy conservation, conversion, and dissipation.[37]

In vivo visualization and characterization of blood flow patterns has remained a major challenge so far. However, recent technical innovations have enabled us for the first time to analyze, measure, and display these flow patterns in vivo. Velocity-encoded cardiac magnetic resonance imaging (MRI), color Doppler echocardiography, and echocardiographic contrast particle imaging velocimetry (Fig. 26-2) are the main modalities being evaluated for the purpose of cardiovascular flow characterization.[37-43] Although cardiac MRI allows complete 3D characterization of blood flow with good spatial resolution, it is limited by

longer scan time, lower temporal resolution, necessity of breath-holding, and problems associated with implanted metallic devices. Echocardiographic techniques are faster and have much higher temporal resolution but can resolve blood flow patterns only in limited directions and planes. Irrespective of these differences, all these techniques are still in their infancy, and considerable technologic advancements will be required before they can be incorporated into clinical practice.

Although routine in vivo blood flow characterization is still not feasible in clinical practice, the ability to understand and quantify alterations in blood flow patterns appears to have several potential clinical applications.[37] In various disease states, abnormalities in blood flow motion tend to develop much earlier than the disease process becomes apparent on conventional imaging techniques. This offers an opportunity to diagnose disease at an early subclinical stage, which may have significant therapeutic and prognostic implications. Formation of vortices is crucial to ensure optimum systolic and diastolic performance of the left ventricle, so an inability to produce a normal vortical flow pattern can serve as a sensitive measure of abnormal cardiac function in conditions such as dilated cardiomyopathy and those characterized by diastolic dysfunction.[37,44] Blood flow pattern analysis is also helpful in defining pathologic mechanisms involved in hypertrophic cardiomyopathy, evaluating valvular diseases, guiding surgical repair of valve regurgitation, assessing myocardial dyssynchrony, and optimizing resynchronizing devices.[45-47] Similarly, applying these blood flow visualization techniques to the atria may provide insights into atrial function/dysfunction in various congenital and acquired cardiac illnesses and help stratify risk of clot formation in these disease states.[48,49] Finally, knowledge of abnormalities of blood flow patterns in the great arteries may be helpful for quantifying risk of developing aortic dilatation, aortic dissection, pulmonary thromboembolism, pulmonary hypertension, and other problems.[40,50]

REFERENCES

1. Isaaz K, Thompson A, Ethevenot G, Cloez JL, Brembilla B, Pernot C. Doppler echocardiographic measurement of low velocity motion of the left ventricular posterior wall. *Am J Cardiol.* 1989; 64:66-75.
2. Gilman G, Khandheria BK, Hagen ME, Abraham TP, Seward JB, Belohlavek M. Strain rate and strain: a step-by-step approach to image and data acquisition. *J Am Soc Echocardiogr.* 2004;17:1011-1020.
3. Marwick TH. Measurement of strain and strain rate by echocardiography: ready for prime time? *J Am Coll Cardiol.* 2006;47:1313-1327.
4. Blessberger H, Binder T. Non-invasive imaging: Two-dimensional speckle tracking echocardiography: basic principles. *Heart.* 2010;96:716-722.
5. Geyer H, Caracciolo G, Abe H, et al. Assessment of myocardial mechanics using speckle tracking echocardiography: fundamentals and clinical applications. *J Am Soc Echocardiogr.* 2010;23:351-369:quiz 453-5.
6. Becker M, Bilke E, Kuhl H, et al. Analysis of myocardial deformation based on pixel tracking in two-dimensional echocardiographic images enables quantitative assessment of regional left ventricular function. *Heart.* 2006;92:1102-1108.
7. Blessberger H, Binder T. Two-dimensional speckle tracking echocardiography: clinical applications. *Heart.* 2010;96:2032-2040.
8. Mor-Avi V, Lang RM, Badano LP, et al. Current and evolving echocardiographic techniques for the quantitative evaluation of cardiac mechanics: ASE/EAE consensus statement on methodology and indications endorsed by the Japanese Society of Echocardiography. *J Am Soc Echocardiogr.* 2011;24:277-313.
9. Brown J, Jenkins C, Marwick TH. Use of myocardial strain to assess global left ventricular function: a comparison with cardiac magnetic resonance and 3-dimensional echocardiography. *Am Heart J.* 2009;157(102):e1-e5.
10. Bertini M, Mollema SA, Delgado V, et al. Impact of time to reperfusion after acute myocardial infarction on myocardial damage assessed by left ventricular longitudinal strain. *Am J Cardiol.* 2009;104:480-485.
11. Gjesdal O, Hopp E, Vartdal T, et al. Global longitudinal strain measured by two-dimensional speckle tracking echocardiography is closely related to myocardial infarct size in chronic ischaemic heart disease. *Clin Sci (Lond).* 2007;113:287-296.
12. Bansal M, Leano RL, Marwick TH. Clinical assessment of left ventricular systolic torsion: effects of myocardial infarction and ischemia. *J Am Soc Echocardiogr.* 2008;21:887-894.
13. Chan J, Hanekom L, Wong C, Leano R, Cho GY, Marwick TH. Differentiation of subendocardial and transmural infarction using two-dimensional strain rate imaging to assess short-axis and long-axis myocardial function. *J Am Coll Cardiol.* 2006;48:2026-2033.
14. Hanekom L, Cho GY, Leano R, Jeffriess L, Marwick TH. Comparison of two-dimensional speckle and tissue Doppler strain measurement during dobutamine stress echocardiography: an angiographic correlation. *Eur Heart J.* 2007;28:1765-1772.
15. Bansal M, Jeffriess L, Leano R, Mundy J, Marwick TH. Assessment of myocardial viability at dobutamine echocardiography by deformation analysis using tissue velocity and speckle-tracking. *JACC Cardiovasc Imaging.* 2010;3:121-131.
16. Miyazaki S, Daimon M, Miyazaki T, et al. Global longitudinal strain in relation to the severity of aortic stenosis: a two-dimensional speckle-tracking study. *Echocardiography.* 2011;28:703-708.
17. Meimoun P, Elmkies F, Benali T, et al. Assessment of left ventricular twist mechanics by two-dimensional strain in severe aortic stenosis with preserved ejection fraction. *Ann Cardiol Angeiol (Paris).* 2011;60:259-266.
18. Delgado V, Tops LF, van Bommel RJ, et al. Strain analysis in patients with severe aortic stenosis and preserved left ventricular ejection fraction undergoing surgical valve replacement. *Eur Heart J.* 2009;30:3037-3047.

19. Carasso S, Cohen O, Mutlak D, et al. Relation of myocardial mechanics in severe aortic stenosis to left ventricular ejection fraction and response to aortic valve replacement. *Am J Cardiol.* 2011;107:1052-1057.

20. Kim MS, Kim YJ, Kim HK, et al. Evaluation of left ventricular short- and long-axis function in severe mitral regurgitation using 2-dimensional strain echocardiography. *Am Heart J.* 2009;157:345-351.

21. Meluzin J, Spinarova L, Hude P, et al. Left ventricular mechanics in idiopathic dilated cardiomyopathy: systolic-diastolic coupling and torsion. *J Am Soc Echocardiogr.* 2009;22:486-493.

22. Carasso S, Yang H, Woo A, et al. Systolic myocardial mechanics in hypertrophic cardiomyopathy: novel concepts and implications for clinical status. *J Am Soc Echocardiogr.* 2008;21:675-683.

23. Tanaka H, Oishi Y, Mizuguchi Y, et al. Contribution of the pericardium to left ventricular torsion and regional myocardial function in patients with total absence of the left pericardium. *J Am Soc Echocardiogr.* 2008;21:268-274.

24. Tzemos N, Harris L, Carasso S, et al. Adverse left ventricular mechanics in adults with repaired tetralogy of Fallot. *Am J Cardiol.* 2009;103:420-425.

25. Hare JL, Brown JK, Leano R, Jenkins C, Woodward N, Marwick TH. Use of myocardial deformation imaging to detect preclinical myocardial dysfunction before conventional measures in patients undergoing breast cancer treatment with trastuzumab. *Am Heart J.* 2009;158:294-301.

26. Richand V, Lafitte S, Reant P, et al. An ultrasound speckle tracking (two-dimensional strain) analysis of myocardial deformation in professional soccer players compared with healthy subjects and hypertrophic cardiomyopathy. *Am J Cardiol.* 2007;100:128-132.

27. Sengupta PP, Krishnamoorthy VK, Abhayaratna WP, et al. Disparate patterns of left ventricular mechanics differentiate constrictive pericarditis from restrictive cardiomyopathy. *JACC Cardiovasc Imaging.* 2008;1:29-38.

28. Gorcsan 3rd J, Tanabe M, Bleeker GB, et al. Combined longitudinal and radial dyssynchrony predicts ventricular response after resynchronization therapy. *J Am Coll Cardiol.* 2007;50:1476-1483.

29. Suffoletto MS, Dohi K, Cannesson M, Saba S, Gorcsan 3rd J. Novel speckle-tracking radial strain from routine black-and-white echocardiographic images to quantify dyssynchrony and predict response to cardiac resynchronization therapy. *Circulation.* 2006;113:960-968.

30. Cameli M, Caputo M, Mondillo S, et al. Feasibility and reference values of left atrial longitudinal strain imaging by two-dimensional speckle tracking. *Cardiovasc Ultrasound.* 2009;7:6.

31. Sebag IA, Dohi K, Onishi K, et al. Reversible right ventricular regional non-uniformity quantified by speckle-tracking strain imaging in patients with acute pulmonary thromboembolism. *J Am Soc Echocardiogr.* 2009;22:1353-1359.

32. Pirat B, McCulloch ML, Zoghbi WA. Evaluation of global and regional right ventricular systolic function in patients with pulmonary hypertension using a novel speckle tracking method. *Am J Cardiol.* 2006;98:699-704.

33. Nesser HJ, Mor-Avi V, Gorissen W, et al. Quantification of left ventricular volumes using three-dimensional echocardiographic speckle tracking: comparison with MRI. *Eur Heart J.* 2009;30:1565-1573.

34. Maffessanti F, Nesser HJ, Weinert L, et al. Quantitative evaluation of regional left ventricular function using three-dimensional speckle tracking echocardiography in patients with and without heart disease. *Am J Cardiol.* 2009;104:1755-1762.

35. Reant P, Barbot L, Touche C, et al. Evaluation of global left ventricular systolic function using three-dimensional echocardiography speckle-tracking strain parameters. *J Am Soc Echocardiogr.* 2012;25:68-79.

36. Sjoli B, Orn S, Grenne B, Ihlen H, Edvardsen T, Brunvand H. Diagnostic capability and reproducibility of strain by Doppler and by speckle tracking in patients with acute myocardial infarction. *JACC Cardiovasc Imaging.* 2009;2:24-33.

37. Sengupta PP, Pedrizzetti G, kilner PJ, et al. Emerging trends in CV flow visualization. *JACC Cardiovasc Imaging.* 2012;5:305-316.

38. Roes SD, Hammer S, van der Geest RJ, et al. Flow assessment through four heart valves simultaneously using 3-dimensional 3-directional velocity-encoded magnetic resonance imaging with retrospective valve tracking in healthy volunteers and patients with valvular regurgitation. *Invest Radiol.* 2009;44:669-675.

39. Ebbers T. Flow imaging: cardiac applications of 3D cine phase-contrast MRI. *Curr Cardiovasc Imaging Rep.* 2011;4:127-133.

40. Markl M, Kilner PJ, Ebbers T. Comprehensive 4D velocity mapping of the heart and great vessels by cardiovascular magnetic resonance. *J Cardiovasc Magn Reson.* 2011;13:7.

41. Hong GR, Pedrizzetti G, Tonti G, et al. Characterization and quantification of vortex flow in the human left ventricle by contrast echocardiography using vector particle image velocimetry. *JACC Cardiovasc Imaging.* 2008;1:705-717.

42. Garcia D, Del Alamo JC, Tanne D, et al. Two-dimensional intraventricular flow mapping by digital processing conventional color-Doppler echocardiography images. *IEEE Trans Med Imaging.* 2010;29:1701-1713.

43. Swillens A, Segers P, Torp H, Lovstakken L. Two-dimensional blood velocity estimation with ultrasound: speckle tracking versus crossed-beam vector Doppler based on flow simulations in a carotid bifurcation model. *IEEE Trans Ultrason Ferroelectr Freq Control.* 2010;57:327-339.

44. Carlhall CJ, Bolger A. Passing strange: flow in the failing ventricle. *Circ Heart Fail.* 2010;3:326-331.

45. Lefebvre XP, Yoganathan AP, Levine RA. Insights from in-vitro flow visualization into the mechanism of systolic anterior motion of the mitral valve in hypertrophic cardiomyopathy under steady flow conditions. *J Biomech Eng.* 1992;114:406-413.

46. Dyverfeldt P, Kvitting JP, Carlhall CJ, et al. Hemodynamic aspects of mitral regurgitation assessed by generalized phase-contrast MRI. *J Magn Reson Imaging.* 2011;33:582-588.

47. Pedrizzetti G, Domenichini F, Tonti G. On the left ventricular vortex reversal after mitral valve replacement. *Ann Biomed Eng.* 2010;38:769-773.

48. Fyrenius A, Wigstrom L, Ebbers T, Karlsson M, Engvall J, Bolger AF. Three dimensional flow in the human left atrium. *Heart.* 2001;86:448-455.

49. Markl M, Geiger J, Kilner PJ, et al. Time-resolved three-dimensional magnetic resonance velocity mapping of cardiovascular flow paths in volunteers and patients with Fontan circulation. *Eur J Cardiothorac Surg.* 2011;39:206-212.

50. Hope MD, Meadows AK, Hope TA, et al. Clinical evaluation of aortic coarctation with 4D flow MR imaging. *J Magn Reson Imaging.* 2010;31:711-718.

SECTION III

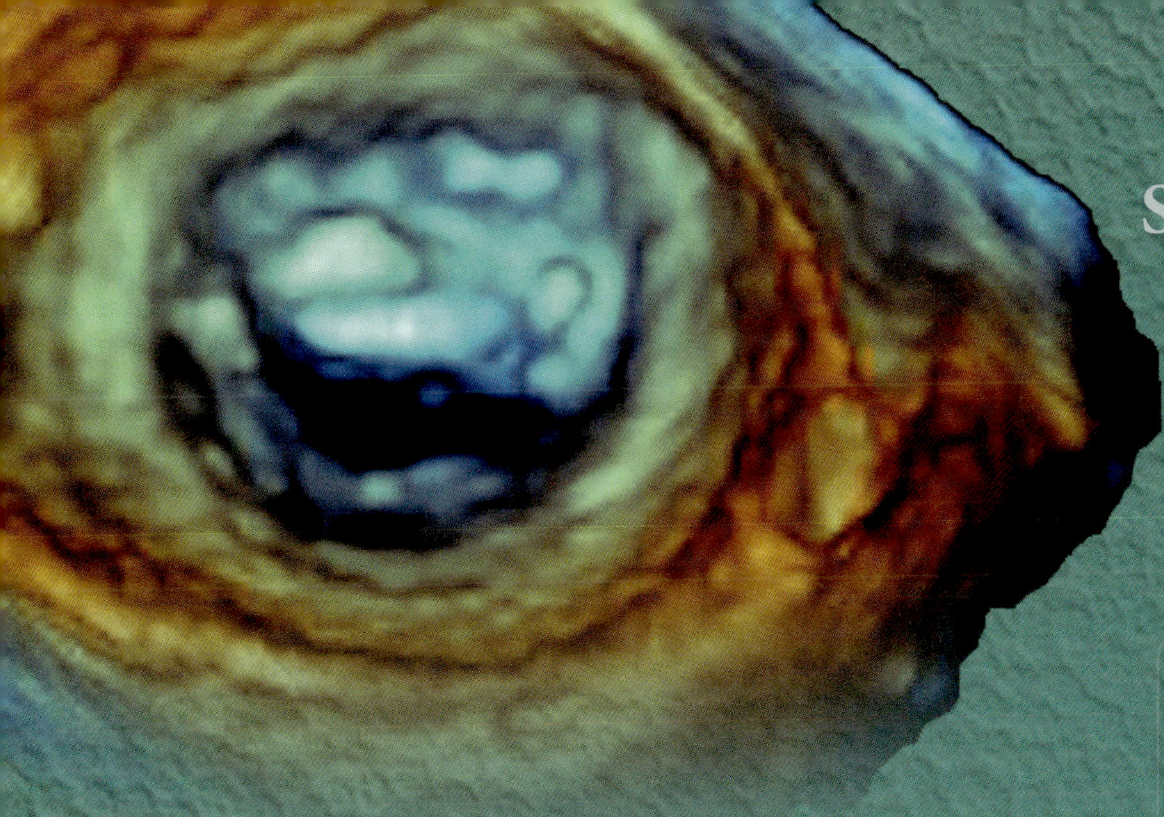

Maintaining Quality of Perioperative Echocardiography

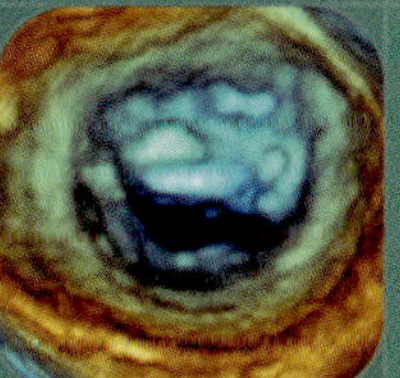

Indications for Transesophageal Echocardiography

DANIEL M. THYS | DIANA ANCA | SANFORD M. LITTWIN

Introduction

Transesophageal echocardiography (TEE) has made many strides in the 30 years since it was first introduced to aid anesthesiologists and surgeons during open heart procedures. Initially, assessments of left ventricular function were made by what would now be considered crude or ill-defined methods for assessing this function. Over the years, modern echocardiography has evolved greatly in a process analogous to what has happened in photography. Photography has moved from black-and-white film that had to be processed in a laboratory after taking pictures to the new digital age in which not only pictures are immediately viewable, but much of the postprocessing can be done by the camera itself. In a similar manner, echocardiography (echo) has evolved in its technologic abilities as well as its uses. Techniques that were not available even 5 or 10 years ago are now being incorporated into echo scanners used in clinical practice and in the software installed on them. Color flow Doppler, automatic border detection, and tissue Doppler are being supplemented with even newer technologies such as three-dimensional (3D) and real-time 3D imaging.

Echocardiography is firmly implanted in the cardiac operating room (OR), where its use allows performance of ever more complex cardiac operations, but it also reaches far beyond this domain. It is intrinsic to the success of nonsurgical cardiac interventions in the so-called hybrid OR where cardiology and cardiac surgery come together for percutaneous valve replacements. Outside the cardiac OR, TEE is used more and more often as a substitute for the pulmonary artery catheter. In noncardiac surgery and in the intensive care unit (ICU), it allows for monitoring cardiac function, detecting myocardial ischemia, and managing inotropic support and fluid replacement.

The specific indications for and details of TEE use will follow in subsequent sections of this chapter. As use of TEE has grown, so has the interest and expertise of anesthesiologists for the technique. Education in TEE is now part of the curriculum of anesthesiology residencies and is in part responsible for an upsurge in the popularity of postgraduate fellowship training in cardiothoracic anesthesiology. Fellowship training is now a requirement for certification in advanced TEE.

Who Gets TEE?

In 2010, the American Society of Anesthesiology (ASA) and the Society of Cardiovascular Anesthesiologists (SCA) updated the guidelines that define the usefulness of TEE. The criteria for recommending whether or not TEE should be utilized were evidence-based and determined by the availability of randomized trials that support the rationale for performing the procedure and the impact of TEE's use on outcomes.[1]

The findings of an exhaustive literature review and input from experts resulted in the following guidelines:
1. **Cardiac and thoracic aortic surgery:** For adult patients without contraindications, TEE should be used in all open heart (e.g., valvular procedures) and thoracic aortic surgical procedures and should be considered in coronary artery bypass graft (CABG) surgeries as well to (1) confirm and refine the preoperative diagnosis, (2) detect new or unsuspected pathology, (3) adjust the anesthetic and surgical plan accordingly, and (4) assess results of the surgical

intervention. In small children, use of TEE should be considered on a case-by-case basis because of risks unique to these patients (e.g., bronchial obstruction).
2. **Catheter-based intracardiac procedures:** For patients undergoing transcatheter intracardiac procedures, TEE may be used.
3. **Noncardiac surgery:** TEE may be used when the nature of the planned surgery or the patient's known or suspected cardiovascular pathology might result in severe hemodynamic, pulmonary, or neurologic compromise. If equipment and expertise are available, TEE should be used when unexplained life-threatening circulatory instability persists despite corrective therapy.
4. **Critical care:** For critical care patients, TEE should be used when diagnostic information that is expected to alter management cannot be obtained by transthoracic echocardiography (TTE) or other modalities in a timely manner.

It is important to state that the ASA/SCA guidelines were intended for anesthesiologists and other physicians (e.g., cardiologists, surgeons, intensivists) who actually use TEE in the perioperative setting. Recommendations to perform TEE are not applicable when the procedure cannot be performed properly or safely, nor do they apply when TEE equipment or skilled examiners are unavailable. The recommendations in the guidelines were based on consideration of the risk/benefit ratio for individual patients. Although complications from TEE are infrequent, they can and do occur. This must be considered by the anesthesiologist performing the TEE examination and the surgeon or other medical provider who is requesting the information.

Indications for Specific Procedures

For open heart operations, there is empirical evidence that TEE is helpful in intraoperative decision making in a number of specific operations. Patients who undergo valvular operations often undergo extensive preoperative evaluation by the referring cardiologists. Nonetheless, intraoperative echocardiography can add critical information during valvular surgery. It is useful to assess the evolution of the disease, to highlight findings that may have been missed in the preoperative assessment, and most importantly, it will allow the surgeon to assess the intervention while the patient is still anesthetized and in the OR. If necessary, cardiopulmonary bypass (CPB) can be reinstituted and corrective changes made. In one study, 10% to 15% of open heart procedures for valve regurgitation or stenosis were altered based on information from the intraoperative TEE evaluation that was different enough from the preoperative findings to change the course of the operation.[2]

Nonvalvular cardiac operations that benefit from intraoperative TEE are intracardiac masses, congenital cardiac operations, and hypertrophic cardiac myopathy (HCM).

Valvular Surgery

During valvular surgery, TEE provides specific views of the valvular lesions (aortic and mitral) as well as heart function. TEE examination prior to CPB evaluates the mechanism and severity of valvular dysfunction; immediately after CPB, TEE assesses the repair (residual regurgitation, presence of systolic anterior motion, or restriction of leaflet motion). TEE also provides an ongoing picture of the heart function pre- and post-correction of the valvular defect.[3] In 205 patients undergoing posterior mitral leaflet quadrangular resection as treatment for mitral regurgitation, TEE revealed immediate failures in 24 patients (11%) and in 20 of those patients, identified the mechanism of failure and guided immediate correction.[4] Another study on 437 patients who underwent various techniques of mitral valve repair showed that successful initial repair as evidenced by intraoperative TEE was the most important predictor of repair durability.[5] In a study of 2076 patients undergoing mitral valve repair, TEE identified systolic anterior motion (SAM), a known complication of this type of surgery, in 174 patients (8.4%), and 4 of these patients required immediate reoperation for severe SAM; the others were managed medically.[6] Although mitral valve repair is a well-established procedure, it is imperative that a correct assessment of the repair be accomplished to reduce future need for reoperation. Kawano et al. reported great accuracy in evaluation of mitral valve repair, in which only 5 of 34 patients showed grade 1+ mitral regurgitation (MR) on postoperative ventriculogram, and only 1 patient had recurrent MR on follow-up TTE.[7] In a 5-year prospective review of the impact of intraoperative TEE on surgical management, new information was found before CPB in 15% of patients, directly affecting surgery in 14% of them; new information after CPB was found in 6% of patients. The most common finding was valvular dysfunction, with return to CPB for further repair or replacement.[8]

In the post-CPB period, TEE evaluation of valve repair/replacement can show perivalvular leak and possible strain on the cardiac system from the repair itself, leading to volume or pressure changes that cannot be handled by the heart. In another large series by Stewart et al. studying 6340 patients undergoing cardiac surgery, return to CPB was required in 7% of the 2226 mitral valve procedures, based on the intraoperative TEE assessment.[9]

Intraoperative TEE is recommended for valve replacement (with a stentless xenograft, homograft, or autograft) as well as repair. TEE is considered reasonable for all cardiac valve surgery to detect valvular malfunction (abnormal leaflet motion) and paravalvular regurgitation. For mitral valve surgery (repair or replacement), TEE can assess the risk to left ventricular function due to possible injury/occlusion of circumflex artery during replacement.[10] Shapira et al. retrospectively studied 417 patients who underwent valve replacement (mitral valve, 237; aortic valve, 221; tricuspid valve, 43) during a 5-year period in a single institution. Intraoperative TEE was performed in 352 patients, and unexpected pathologic findings were noted on post-bypass TEE. Immediate surgical correction was required in 15 patients (3.6%), and perivalvular leak, immobilized leaflets, coronary obstruction by an aortic bioprosthesis, and an incompetent xenograft were found in 47 patients (11.3%). Post-bypass TEE contributed to evaluation of difficulty weaning from CPB and guided management in these patients.[11]

TEE provides a very reliable assessment of the cause of aortic regurgitation (AR) and predicts the reparability of the valve and postoperative outcome. In a study by Waroux et al., 163 patients undergoing AR surgery underwent TEE assessment to categorize the mechanism of AR. Compared with surgical inspection, TEE correctly predicted the final surgical approach in 93% of patients undergoing replacement and 86% of patients undergoing repair. The TEE classification of AR lesions was the determinant of valve reparability and postoperative outcome (4-year freedom from > grade 2 AR, reoperation, or death; $P = 0.04$).[12]

Although the acquisition cost of TEE is high, the value of the information results in a favorable cost/benefits ratio. Ionescu et al. studied the clinical impact and cost-saving implications of routine use of intraoperative TEE for elective valve replacement in a prospective study of 300 patients. In two patients undergoing aortic valve replacement, significant mitral regurgitation led to additional mitral valve replacement, and one patient scheduled for mitral valve replacement was found to have significant AR and required aortic valve replacement as well. The calculated savings by routine intraoperative TEE use were

$109 per patient per year.[13] Based on this figure, the potential costs for reoperative exploration or need for additional surgical correction after the initial surgery would far outpace the nominal cost of TEE performed on a routine basis.

CABG Surgery

Coronary artery bypass operations can be performed on and off CPB. TEE use in the intraoperative setting can guide the operative process. Practice guidelines for perioperative TEE by the ASA and the SCA Task Force recommend that in adults without contraindications, TEE should be considered in CABG surgeries.[14] TEE has become the mainstay of cardiac operations, with actual proven beneficial use for determining other potential pathologies that may be present, such as valve lesions, abnormal loading conditions, or regional wall motion abnormalities. TEE has been shown to be the single most important factor in guiding therapies such as fluid administration, antiischemic therapy, antiarrhythmic therapy, and vasodilator or inotropic therapy in 98 instances out of 584 intraoperative interventions (17%).[15] Savage et al. observed that intraoperative TEE led to at least one major surgical management change in 33% of patients, and in 51%, at least one anesthetic/hemodynamic alteration took place based on TEE findings. These findings show just how integrated TEE is in operative management.[16] Similar numbers have been shown in off-pump CABG (OPCAB), where 16% of 744 patients studied by Gurbuz et al. required a major modification of operative strategy.[17]

Masses

An intracardiac mass is a relatively infrequent operative lesion with a reported incidence between 0.0017% and 0.19%.[18] A very unique and practical use for intraoperative TEE is the ability to visualize a mass prior to surgical excision, as well as determine its pathologic implications, such as hindering valve function. TEE can also be used to determine if the mass has embolized before its surgical excision.

Congenital Lesions

The use of TEE for intraoperative repair of congenital lesions is performed for evaluation of flow pattern(s), stenosis, and regurgitation of the lesions. TEE probes are used in infants as small as 3 kg. Given the nature and intricacy of these lesions, TEE helps develop a clearer picture of the lesion and a view of the corrective process that helps alleviate the pathology. More children survive to adulthood when they may present for cardiac or other types of surgeries. Russell et al. offer an updated review of TEE use in the adult patient with congenital heart disease (congenitally corrected heart disease).[19]

Hypertropic Cardiomyopathy

Hypertrophic cardiomyopathy exists as a progressive disorder that is best followed by TTE and TEE. In the perioperative setting, TEE allows for determination of the gradient across the hypertrophied outflow tract and the morphology of the myocardium. Afonso et al. posit that with evolution of newer technologies (tissue Doppler, strain imaging, 3D echo), assessment has moved from ejection fraction evaluation to mechanisms of appraising cardiac performance.[20]

Great Vessels

Disease involving the great vessels, specifically pathology of the aorta, is often diagnosed by TEE, a highly sensitive and specific method of detecting injury to the thoracic aorta. It is a quick and safe test in critically injured patients with suspected traumatic rupture of the aorta and compares favorably with arch aortography.[21] Through the use of TEE, the extent, location and valvular involvement can all be ascertained for managing dissections operatively. Data from the International Registry of Acute Dissection showed that TEE's sensitivity for detection of aortic dissection (88%) is comparable to computed tomography (93%) and aortography (87%).[22] TEE can reveal the mechanism and severity of AR associated with aortic dissection, even though one of its limitations is poor image quality secondary to the superimposed trachea. The ability of TEE to detect aortic atheromas can allow for directing cannulation techniques, site, and hemodynamic management during CPB to decrease the incidence of stroke.[23]

Catheter-Based Intracardiac Procedures and Percutaneous Valve Replacement Devices

Catheter-based intracardiac procedures, such as atrial and ventricular defects closure and percutaneous valve replacement, have become routine procedures at major institutions in hybrid ORs that provide both catheterization laboratory and OR functions. TEE is playing a central role in managing such cases.

Intraoperative TEE roles include confirmation of interatrial septal anatomy, pre- and post-closure assessment of adjacent cardiac structures, and direct visualization of device position and efficacy, as well as potential complications, such as pericardial tamponade, device erosion, embolization, thrombosis, or residual shunt. In recent years, intracardiac echocardiography has also been established as an alternative imaging modality.[24] Percutaneous aortic valve implantation is an emerging technique with the potential to revolutionize treatment of aortic valve disease. Moss et al. have assessed the role of perioperative echocardiography in case selection, guiding device placement, and detecting complications. In a series of 50 patients, 37 (74%) underwent intraoperative TEE. TEE helped successfully guide device implantation in 97% of patients in whom the native valve was crossed with the percutaneous valve. TEE was used for early detection of paravalvular aortic insufficiency and aided fluoroscopy in detection of complications. Additional balloon dilation of a percutaneous heart valve was performed in 12 patients who had significant paravalvular aortic insufficiency.[25]

Cortes et al. demonstrated the usefulness of TEE in percutaneous transcatheter repairs of paravalvular mitral regurgitation, specifically in assessing the site and severity of paravalvular mitral regurgitation before closure and guiding transseptal puncture.[26] The role of two-dimensional (2D) TTE and TEE during the assessment and management of atrial septal defect (ASD) and patent foramen ovale (PFO) has been demonstrated. Percutaneous therapy is now the preferred strategy in the absence of complicated anatomy.

■ TEE Outside the Cardiac Operating Room

TEE's use in major surgical procedures has allowed for intraoperative assessment of patients' fluid status (intravascular volume), possible causes of hypotension, ischemic detection, and more subtle findings such as tamponade. As physicians become more familiar with TEE and more adept at the advantages TEE holds in multiple settings, TEE is becoming an expected diagnostic modality both in the operating arena and outside.

Noncardiac uses of TEE are now playing a more important role in medicine than ever, and the ASA/SCA guidelines (mentioned earlier) define the utility of TEE for noncardiac surgery and critical care settings.

Studies show a greater impact of TEE performed by anesthesiologists on clinical management for category I compared to categories II and III indications in the noncardiac OR surgical setting and ICU. In a study by Denault et al., 214 patients underwent TEE assessment according to the ASA guidelines, and for each examination it was noted whether TEE altered management, thereby (1) changing medical therapy, (2) changing surgical therapy, (3) confirming a diagnosis, (4) positioning an intravascular device, or (5) was used as a substitute for pulmonary artery catheterization. The impact was more significant in category I, where TEE altered therapy 60% of the time, compared with 31% and

21% for categories II and III, respectively ($P < 0.001$). The most frequent impact was a change in medical therapy in 45% of cases.[27]

Perioperative outcomes are affected adversely by hemodynamic complications such as myocardial ischemia, cardiac tamponade, thromboembolism, and hypovolemia. Perioperative echocardiography can support improved outcomes as it becomes more widely used in noncardiac surgery, especially for those patients who have cardiovascular disease and are expected to require inotropes or vasopressor drug treatment.[28]

The usefulness of perioperative echocardiography to aid clinical decision making during a variety of noncardiac surgeries (e.g., vascular, endovascular, transplant, trauma, orthopedics) has been reported in several studies.[29] It is true especially in patients with increased risk for myocardial ischemia and hemodynamic instability. A prospective observational case series on 98 patients strongly suggests that objective measurements by intraoperative TEE led to useful changes in intraoperative management (e.g., administration of fluids, pressors, vasodilators) in patients undergoing noncardiac surgery.[30] In hemodynamic assessment, TEE reveals changes in left ventricular preload better than filling pressures, as well as assesses left ventricular function. Though there are several quantitative measurements available for both preload and function, they can be time consuming and tedious, so often a subjective determination is made by the trained eye and experience of the echocardiographer.[31] For the use of TEE in noncardiac surgery, the official guidelines recommend echocardiography for investigation of major hemodynamic disturbances.[32] This affords the anesthesiologist with critical information that can be used to guide management of these patients.

Intensive Care Unit

The new setting for echocardiography is the ICU. For the critical patient, there is no better diagnostic modality than TEE to ascertain information at the bedside that will both give pertinent information as to cause as well as direct treatment. The most prevalent ICU pathology, cardiorespiratory system failure, is the very reason TEE is the new modality of choice to make decisions in this setting. Again, volume status of the patient, detection of ischemic changes to the myocardium, and frank failure of the heart as a pump are all seen in real time. Furthermore, the consequences of goal-directed therapy are seen in improvement that would not otherwise have been known in the ICU setting. Detection of valve abnormalities (e.g., regurgitation), or hypertrophy of the myocardium, or dilation of the intracardiac chamber can give clues to possible treatment regimens. In the ICU setting, TEE is safe and well tolerated in the management of patients with shock, unexplained and severe hypoxemia, or suspected endocarditis when TTE is inconclusive. TEE is probably underutilized in the ICU because of cost of equipment, lack of training of ICU physicians, and/or lack of 24-hour availability of equipment and qualified personnel.[33]

Transplantation

The unique challenges posed by transplant recipients because of their pathophysiology lend themselves to TEE's ability to circumnavigate processes that cannot be corrected and direct therapy to processes that can be more readily changed. Transplantation is an area of medicine that is both complex in the derangements suffered by a patient who is in need of transplantation, yet relatively simplistic in that once the old organ is removed, the new one is expected to start functioning and perform well. The ability of the anesthesiologist to bridge this divide comes with many uncertainties. Most stem from the systemic derangements of the patient being transplanted. The patient is most often at risk for multisystem failure because of volume problems or issues pertaining to the ability of the patient to survive the stresses of the operation. Ischemic changes and the myocardium at risk can all be determined by what is seen on TEE during transplantation surgery. Prah et al. showed that TEE used as a monitor improved hemodynamic management and had an impact on overall perioperative care in 11% of patients.[34]

Its use in liver transplantation and neurosurgical procedures shows just how often TEE is used in specialties far removed from cardiac surgery. In liver transplantation, TEE can guide anesthesiologists in decisions regarding intravascular volume, as well as cardiac performance during the different stages of transplantation. A retrospective study by Suriani et al. explored the use of TEE in patients undergoing liver transplantation. The medical records of 346 patients and the videotapes of 100 intraoperative TEE examinations were reviewed. Indications for TEE ranged from the need for intraoperative monitoring (62 patients, of whom 41 had pertinent findings) to diagnostic purposes (38 patients, in 14 of whom the expected diagnosis was verified). TEE revealed information (e.g., intracardiac defects, valvular regurgitation, ventricular function, embolization during allograft reperfusion) that would not have been detected intraoperatively by other methods and resulted in a major impact on patient management in 11% of cases. Complications were minor and rare (two patients experienced sinus bradycardia and upper gastrointestinal [GI] bleeding). It appears from this study that TEE is safe and efficacious in patients undergoing liver transplantation.[35]

During certain types of neurosurgical operations, detection of venous air embolism is key for patient safety and treatment. The use of TEE to ascertain risk based on intracardiac pathology (e.g., presence of PFO) allows for early, effective detection and treatment.

New Technologies

Over the last 3 decades, 3D echocardiography has evolved from a rotational approach with sequential data acquisition and cropping of the reconstructed 3D volume sets to display the area and structures of interest (which were time consuming and required offline processing) to the recent introduction of a new class of piezoelectric crystals with enhanced electromagnetic properties that enable real-time (4D) imaging.[36]

An increased body of literature points to the added value of 3D echocardiography in imaging and assessing cardiac structures and function, especially valvular lesions.[37,38] For visualizing and assessing the mitral valve in particular, 3D TEE has proved particularly useful, allowing for more accurate identification of its anatomy, function, and pathology.[39] The value of 3D color Doppler echocardiography in determining effective regurgitant orifice area shapes for assessing the severity of mitral regurgitation was documented in several studies.[40,41]

Grewal et al. demonstrated in a study of 42 patients undergoing mitral valve repair for mitral regurgitation that real-time intraoperative 3D TEE is superior to 2D TEE imaging in the diagnosis of P1, A2, and A3 bileaflet disease.[42] Langerveld et al. showed that 3D TEE has additional value over 2D TEE in patients with mitral stenosis undergoing percutaneous mitral balloon valvulotomy in a series of 21 cases, allowing for a better description of the mitral anatomy, especially post valvulotomy.[43]

Also, 3D echocardiography provides superior left ventricular mass and function assessment.[44] Recently, 3D echocardiography is establishing an ever-growing place in guiding percutaneous cardiac interventions.[45] Cao et al. showed the usefulness of 2D and 3D TEE in transcatheter closure of multiple ASDs using two devices and that 3D echocardiography enhanced the ability to image ASD anatomy.[46]

Safety of TEE

Since its introduction in the OR, TEE has been considered relatively safe and minimally invasive, although it is not without some risks. Hogue et al. found that age of the patient and length of intubation after surgery, as well as intraoperative use of TEE, are highly significant predictors ($P < 0.003$) of swallowing dysfunction.[47]

Lennon et al. found that compared with a group of 343 cardiac surgical patients in whom TEE was not performed, patients in whom intraoperative TEE was performed had a higher incidence of major

GI complications (1.2% vs. 0.29%).[48] Insertion and manipulation of the TEE probe can cause oropharyngeal, esophageal, or gastric trauma. In a case series of 7200 cardiac surgical patients, Kallmeyer et al. reported the morbidity was 0.2% and mortality 0%, comparable with GI endoscopy. Trauma to the GI tract may be secondary to blind insertion and advancement of the probe, large probe size relative to the esophagus, the wide range of tip flexion required to obtain certain images, and the presence of unknown esophageal or gastric pathology.[49] In a comprehensive review of TEE safety, Hilberath et al. found that the rate of major TEE-related complications in nonoperative settings is 0.2% to 0.5%, comparable with the rate associated with gastroscopy and esophagogastroduodenoscopy (0.08% to 0.13%). Intraoperative TEE carries a different risk profile because patients are intubated under general anesthesia, with TEE-related morbidity of 0.2% to 1.2%.[50]

TEE-related injuries are:
- *Oropharyngeal:* lip laceration, teeth injury, pharyngeal laceration or perforation
- *Esophageal:* odynophagia, dysphagia, perforation, Mallory-Weiss tear
- *Gastric:* laceration, perforation, hemorrhage
- *Other:* compression of mediastinal structures, airway compromise, tongue necrosis

Contraindications

- *Absolute:* perforated viscus, esophageal pathology stricture, scleroderma, Mallory-Weiss tear, active upper GI bleeding, recent upper GI surgery, esophagectomy
- *Relative:* severe cervical spine arthritis or atlantoaxial joint disease, prior radiation to the chest, severe symptomatic hiatal hernia, esophagitis, Barrett esophagus, thoracic aortic aneurysm

Risks and benefits must be weighed and appropriate precautions applied. Proceeding with caution and having a low threshold for abandoning the procedure should resistance be encountered during insertion or advancement is the prudent and appropriate approach. Also, obtaining a GI consultation, using a smaller probe, limiting manipulation of the probe, or limiting the examination should be considered, as well as considering the use of intraoperative epicardial and epiaortic techniques.[51] Epicardial and epiaortic examination are viable alternatives in patients with esophageal or GI pathology or in patients where TEE probe placement or advancement is difficult. Guidelines for performing a comprehensive epicardial and epiaortic examination have been recently published (see Chapter 28).[52,53]

Summary

In cardiac anesthesia, practice guidelines for examination and accreditation for echocardiography have been well established. Recently these educational initiatives have been extended to include noncardiac practice and ICU settings. In the near future, improvements in education, affordable basic equipment, and smaller devices will lead to more widespread use of echocardiography by anesthesiologists. Practice guidelines developed by professional organizations classify indications for perioperative TEE based on the strength of the supporting scientific evidence or expert opinion. TEE indications have expanded with the newer techniques, such as catheter-based intracardiac procedures (percutaneous valve replacements/repairs and intracardiac defects closures), which are becoming routine in major centers. Complex procedures outside of cardiac ORs have led to expansion of TEE use for noncardiac surgery, as well as in the critical care setting, and guidelines have been developed for a basic TEE exam and certification.

Despite a generally good safety record (TEE probe insertion and manipulation has very low morbidity and virtually no mortality), in patients at risk for oropharyngeal, esophageal, or GI complications, alternative modalities (e.g., epicardial and epiaortic echocardiography) should be considered.

REFERENCES

1. Practice guidelines for perioperative transesophageal echocardiography. An updated report by the American Society of Anesthesiologists and Society of Cardiovascular Anesthesiologists Task Force on Transesophageal Echocardiography. *Anesthesiology*. 2010 May;112(5):1084-1096.
2. Click RL, Abel MD, Schaff HV. Intraoperative transesophageal echocardiography: 5-year prospective review of impact on surgical management. *Mayo Clin Proc*. 2000 Mar;75(3):241-247.
3. Cheitlin MD, Alpert JS, Armstrong WF, et al. ACC/AHA Guidelines for the clinical application of echocardiography. A report of the American College of Cardiology/American Heart Association Task Force on Practice Guidelines (Committee on Clinical Application of Echocardiography). Developed in collaboration with the American Society of Echocardiography. *Circulation*. 1997 Mar 18;95(6):1686-1744.
4. Agricola E, Oppizzi M, Maisano F, et al. Detection of mechanism of immediate failure by transesophageal echocardiography in quadrangular resection mitral valve repair technique for severe mitral regurgitation. *Am J Cardiol*. 2003 Jan;91(2):175-179.
5. Shin HJ, Lee YJ, Choo SJ, et al. Analysis of recurrent mitral regurgitation after mitral valve repair. *Asian Cardiovasc Thorac Ann*. 2005 Sep;13(3):261-266.
6. Brown ML, Abel MD, Click RL, et al. Systolic anterior motion after mitral valve repair: Is surgical intervention necessary? *J Thorac Cardiovasc Surg*. 2007 Jan;133(1):136-143.
7. Kawano H, Mizoguchi T, Ayoagi S. Intraoperative transesophageal echocardiography for evaluation of mitral valve repair. *J Heart Valve Dis*. 1999 May;8(3):287-293.
8. Click RL, Abel MD, Schaff HV. Intraoperative transesophageal echocardiography: 5-year prospective review of impact on surgical management. *Mayo Clin Proc*. 2000 Mar;75(3):241-247.
9. Stewart WJ, Thomas JD, Klein AL, et al. Ten year trends in utilization of 6340 intraoperative echocardiographies. *Circulation*. 1995;92(suppl):2453.
10. Bonow RO, Carabello BA, Chatterjee K, et al. ACC/AHA 2006 guidelines for the management of patients with valvular heart disease: a report of the American College of Cardiology/American Heart Association Task Force on Practice Guidelines (writing Committee to Revise the 1998 guidelines for the management of patient with valvular heart disease) developed in collaboration with the Society of Cardiovascular Anesthesiologists endorsed by the Society for Cardiovascular Angiography and Interventions and the Society of Thoracic Surgeons. *J Am Coll Cardiol*. 2006 Aug 1;48(3):e1-e148.
11. Shapira Y, Vaturi M, Weisenberg DE, et al. Impact of intraoperative transesophageal echocardiography in patients undergoing valve replacement. *Ann Thorac Surg*. 2004 Aug;78(2):579-583.
12. le Polain de Waroux JB, Pouleur AC, Goffinet C, et al. Functional anatomy of aortic regurgitation: accuracy, prediction of surgical repairability and outcome implications of transesophageal echocardiography. *Circulation*. 2007 Sep 11;116:1264-1269.
13. Ionescu AA, West RR, Proudman C, et al. Prospective study of routine perioperative transesophageal echocardiography for elective valve replacement: clinical impact and cost-saving implications. *J Am Soc Echocardiogr*. 2001 Jul;14(7):659-667.
14. Practice guidelines for perioperative transesophageal echocardiography. An updated report by the American Society of Anesthesiologists and Society of Cardiovascular Anesthesiologists Task Force on transesophageal echocardiography. *Anesthesiology*. 2010 May;112(5):1084-1096.
15. Bergquist BD, Bellows WH, Leung JM. Transesophageal echocardiography in myocardial revascularization: influence on intraoperative decision-making. *Anesth Analg*. 1996 Jun;82(6):1139-1145.
16. Savage RM, Lytle BW, Aronson S, et al. Intraoperative echocardiography is indicated in high-risk coronary artery bypass grafting. *Ann Thorac Surg*. 1997 Aug;64(2):368-373.
17. Gurbuz AT, Hecht ML, Arslan AH. Intraoperative transesophageal echocardiography modifies strategy in off-pump coronary artery bypass grafting. *Ann Thorac Surg*. 2007 Mar;83(3):1035-1040.
18. Kwong RY. Cardiovascular magnetic resonance imaging (contemporary cardiology) In: *Cardiac and Pericardial Tumors*. Totowa, NJ: Humana Press, Inc.; 2009:429-465.
19. Russell IA, Rouine-Rapp K, Stratman G, et al. Congenital heart disease in the adult: a review with Internet-accessible transesophageal echocardiographic images. *Anesth Analg*. 2006 Mar;102(3):694-723.
20. Afonso LC, Bernal J, Bax JJ, et al. Echocardiography in hypertrophic cardiomyopathy: the role of conventional and emerging technologies. *JACC Cardiovasc Imaging*. 2008 Nov;1(6):787-800.
21. Smith M, Cassidy JM, Souther S, et al. Transesophageal echocardiography in the diagnosis of traumatic rupture of the aorta. *N Engl J Med*. 1995 Feb 9;332(6):356-362.
22. Moore AG, Eagle KA, Bruchman D, et al. Choice of computed tomography, transesophageal echocardiography, magnetic resonance imaging, and aortography in acute aortic dissection. International Registry of Acute Aortic Dissection (IRAD). *Am J Cardiol*. 2002 May 15;89(10):1235-1238.
23. Gold JP, Torres KE, Maldarelli W, et al. Improving outcomes in coronary surgery: the impact of echo-directed aortic cannulation and perioperative hemodynamic management in 500 patients. *Ann Thorac Surg*. 2004 Nov;78(5):1579-1585.
24. Yared K, Baggish AL, Solis J, et al. Echocardiographic assessment of percutaneous patent foramen ovale and atrial septal defect closure complications. *Circ Cardiovascular Imaging*. 2009 Mar;2(2):141-149.
25. Moss RR, Ivens E, Pasupati S, et al. Role of echocardiography in percutaneous aortic valve implantation. *JACC Cardiovasc Imaging*. 2008 Jan;1(1):15-24.
26. Cortes M, Garcia E, Garcia-Fernandez MA, et al. Usefulness of transesophageal echocardiography in percutaneous transcatheter repairs of paravalvular mitral regurgitation. *Am J Cardiol*. 2008 Feb 1; 101(3):382-386.
27. Denault AY, Couture P, McKenty S, et al. Perioperative use of transesophageal echocardiography by anesthesiologists: impact in noncardiac surgery and in the intensive care unit. *Can J Anaesth*. 2002 Mar;49(3):287-293.
28. Ng A, Swanevelder J. Perioperative echocardiography for non-cardiac surgery: what is its role in routine hemodynamic monitoring? *Br J Anaesth*. 2009 Jun;102(6):731-734.
29. Mahmood F, Christie A, Matyal R. Transesophageal echocardiography and non-cardiac surgery. *Semin Cardiothoracic Vasc Anesth*. 2008 Dec;12(4):265-289.
30. Schulmeyer MC, Santelices E, Vega R, et al. Impact of intraoperative transesophageal echocardiography during noncardiac surgery. *J Cardiothorac Vasc Anesth*. 2006 Dec;20(6):768-771.
31. Click RL, Abel MD, Schaff HV. Intraoperative transesophageal echocardiography: 5-year prospective review of impact on surgical management. *Mayo Clin Proc*. 2000 Mar;75(3):241-247.
32. Cheitlin MD, Armstrong WF, Aurigemma GP, et al. ACC/AHA/ASE 2003 guideline update for the clinical application of echocardiography: summary article. A report of the American College of Cardiology/American Heart Association Task Force on Practice Guidelines (ACC/AHA/ASE Committee to Update the 1997 Guidelines for the Clinical Application of Echocardiography). *J Am Soc Echocardiogr*. 2003 Oct;16(10):1091-1110.
33. Slama MA, Novara A, Van De Putte P, et al. Diagnostic and therapeutic implications of transesophageal echocardiography in medical ICU patients with unexplained shock, hypoxemia, or suspected endocarditis. *Intensive Care Med*. 1996 Sep;22(9):916-922.
34. Prah GN, Lisman SR, Maslow AD, et al. Transesophageal echocardiography reveals an unusual cause of hemodynamic collapse during orthotopic liver transplantations–two case reports. *Transplantation*. 1995 Mar 27;59(6):921-925.
35. Suriani RJ, Cutrone A, Feierman D, et al. Intraoperative transesophageal echocardiography during liver transplantation. *J Cardiothorac Vasc Anesth*. 1996 Oct;10(6):699-707.
36. Mackensen GB, Swaminathan M, Mathew JP. PRO editorial: PRO: three-dimensional transesophageal echocardiography is a major advance for intraoperative clinical management of patients undergoing cardiac surgery. *Anesth Analg*. 2010 Jun 1;110(6):1574-1578.
37. Sugeng L, Shernan SK, Weinert L, et al. Real-time three-dimensional transesophageal echocardiography in valve disease: comparison with surgical findings and evaluation of prosthetic valves. *J Am Soc Echocardiogr*. 2008 Dec;21(12):1347-1354.
38. Abraham TP, Warner Jr JG, Kon ND, et al. Feasibility, accuracy and incremental value of intraoperative three-dimensional transesophageal echocardiography in valve surgery. *Am J Cardiol*. 1997 Dec 15;80(12):1577-1582.
39. Agricola E, Oppizzi M, Pisani M, et al. Accuracy of real-time 3D echocardiography in the evaluation of functional anatomy of mitral regurgitation. *Int J Cardiol*. 2008 Jul 21;127(3):342-349.
40. Little SH, Igo SR, Pirat B, et al. In vitro validation of real-time three-dimensional color Doppler echocardiography for direct measurement of proximal isovelocity surface area in mitral regurgitation. *Am J Cardiol*. 2007 Aug;99(10):1440-1447.
41. Kahlert P, Plicht B, Schenk IM, et al. Direct assessment of size and shape of noncircular vena contracta area in functional versus organic mitral regurgitation using real-time three-dimensional echocardiography. *J Am Soc Echocardiogr*. 2008 Aug;21(18):912-921.
42. Grewal J, Mankad S, Freeman WK, et al. Real-time three-dimensional transesophageal echocardiography in the intraoperative assessment of mitral valve disease. *J Am Soc Echocardiogr*. 2009 Jan;22(1):34-41.
43. Langerveld J, Valocik G, Plokker HW, et al. Additional value of three-dimensional transesophageal echocardiography for patients with mitral valve stenosis undergoing balloon valvuloplasty. *J Am Soc Echocardiogr*. 2003 Aug;16(8):841-849.
44. Mor-Avi V, Sugeng L, Weinert L, et al. Fast measurement of left ventricular mass with real-time three-dimensional echocardiography: comparison with magnetic resonance imaging. *Circulation*. 2004 Sep 28;110(13):1814-1818.
45. Balzer J, Kühl H, Rassaf T, et al. Real-time transesophageal three-dimensional echocardiography for guidance of percutaneous cardiac interventions: first experience. *Clin Res Cardiol*. 2008 Sep;97(9):565-574.
46. Cao Q, Rdatke W, Berger F, et al. Transcatheter closure of multiple atrial septal defects. Initial results and value of two- and three-dimensional transesophageal echocardiography. *Eur Heart J*. 2000 Jun;21(11):941-947.
47. Hogue Jr CW, Lappas GD, Creswell LL, et al. Swallowing dysfunction after cardiac operations. Associated outcomes and risk factors including intraoperative transesophageal echocardiography. *J Thorac Cardiovasc Surg*. 1995 Aug;110(2):517-522.
48. Lennon MJ, Gibbs NM, Weightman WM, et al. Transesophageal echocardiography-related gastrointestinal complications in cardiac surgical patients. *J Cardiothorac Vasc Anesth*. 2005 Apr;19(2):141-145.
49. Kallmeyer IJ, Collard CD, Fox JA, et al. The safety of intraoperative transesophageal echocardiography: a case series of 7200 cardiac surgical patients. *Anesth Analg*. 2001 May;92(5):1126-1130.
50. Hilberath JN, Oakes DA, Shernan SK, et al. Safety of transesophageal echocardiography. *J Am Soc of Echocardiogr*. 2010 Nov;23(11):1115-1127.
51. Hilberath JN, Oakes DA, Shernan SK, et al. Safety of transesophageal echocardiography. *J Am Soc of Echocardiogr*. 2010 Nov;23(11):1115-1127.
52. Glas KE, Swaminathan M, Reeves ST, et al. Guidelines for the performance of a comprehensive intraoperative epiaortic ultrasonographic examination: recommendations of the American Society of Echocardiography and the Society of Cardiovascular Anesthesiologists; endorsed by the Society of Thoracic Surgeons. *J Am Soc Echocardiogr*. 2007 Nov;20(11):1227-1235.
53. Reeves ST, Glas Ke, Eltzschig H, et al. Guidelines for performing a comprehensive epicardial echocardiography examination: recommendations of the American Society of Echocardiography and the Society of Cardiovascular Anesthesiologists. *J Am Soc Echocardiogr*. 2007 Apr;20(4):427-437.

Complications of Transesophageal Echocardiography

SANDEEP KRISHNAN | JENNIE Y. NGAI | MARC KANCHUGER

Introduction

Transesophageal echocardiography (TEE) is widely used to diagnose and monitor cardiac function. This essential imaging modality is now found in practically all cardiac surgical operating rooms, delivering pertinent information to guide surgical interventions (e.g., myocardial revascularization, valvular competence, and repair of congenital heart defects) and pharmacologic support and/or fluid administration during the perioperative period.[1] Over time, TEE's applications have developed considerably, and its safety has been evaluated by many studies over the years; it is considered relatively safe and noninvasive. The reported risk of complications associated with TEE is 0.2% to 0.5% in the nonoperative setting, while reported mortality is 0.01%.[2-5] When examining the subpopulation of cardiac surgery patients, the risk of morbidity ranges from 0.05% to 1.2%, and the risk of mortality has been reported as high as 0.02%.[6-9] The goal of this chapter is to describe potential complications of TEE that can be encountered during everyday practice (Table 28-1).

Oropharyngeal Complications

Dental trauma, pharyngeal abrasions and hemorrhage,[10] and temporomandibular joint subluxation[11,12] can occur with TEE insertion. These complications can vary with blind placement versus placement under direct vision. Rigid laryngoscope–assisted insertion of the TEE probe reduces the incidence of oropharyngeal mucosal injury (55% vs. 5%), odynophagia (32.5% vs. 2.5%), and the number of insertion attempts.[13] Variations in experience and technical skill can contribute to difficulty in placement.

Insertion of the TEE probe can also be complicated by neoplasms in the oropharynx, edema or inflammatory changes, and even cervical spondylosis.[14] Difficult placement can stem from a stenotic entrance to the proximal esophagus, a Zenker diverticulum, or even hypertrophy of the cricopharyngeal muscle.[15] Other disorders, including achalasia, esophageal strictures, Schatzki rings, esophageal webs, scleroderma, and diffuse esophageal spasm can make TEE probe placement more difficult as well. Even normal anatomic variations such as a large left atrium, a large left mainstem bronchus, and esophageal cysts can hinder TEE insertion into the esophagus.[13] Double aortic arch[16] and mucosal abnormalities such as prior radiation exposure, decreased saliva production, and prior tracheostomy can also make TEE insertion more challenging.[15] These issues can lead to hypopharyngeal perforation.[17] In one series of 159 adults, optically guided TEE probe placement with transnasal videoendoscopic monitoring of the hypopharynx resulted in significantly fewer hypopharyngeal injuries than traditional blind probe placement.[18] Larger multiplane probes have also been shown to increase the difficulty of placement.[14]

Increased duration of placement has also been seen to cause tongue necrosis and ischemia. The pathophysiologic mechanism of this injury includes prolonged glossal compression with venous congestion, edema, and ischemia.[19] Presence of the TEE probe may also increase the endotracheal cuff pressure more than is generally recommended.

One study showed that mean intracuff pressure increased from 27.7 (±1.5) to 36.2 (±6.4) cm H_2O and was over 35 cm H_2O in 45% of patients. This increase in tracheal cuff pressure can be associated with reduced mucosal blood flow in the trachea and postoperative sore throat.[20]

Odynophagia and Dysphagia

Odynophagia and dysphagia are the most common complaints after TEE probe placement. Some studies have reported that the incidence of swallowing dysfunction can be as high as 7.9%. Long-standing controversy exists about whether TEE is an independent risk factor for postoperative dysphagia and recurrent laryngeal nerve injury. In a study enrolling 1245 patients, 217 receiving TEE, there was no difference in the incidence of dysphagia between those who were monitored with TEE and those who were not.[21] A study enrolling 81 patients prospectively (40 patients with TEE for cardiac surgery and 41 patients without TEE for cardiac surgery) and 200 patients retrospectively (all 200 with TEE during cardiac surgery) found that the incidence of postoperative gastroesophageal symptoms were comparable in the three groups.[22] On the other hand, an examination of 869 patients noted a 4% incidence of swallowing dysfunction, and this was associated with pulmonary aspiration (90%), increased frequency of pneumonia, increased frequency of tracheostomy, and increased length of stay in the intensive care unit.[23] The incidence of recurrent laryngeal nerve palsy and concomitant dysphagia has also been attributed to TEE in some patients. However, Kawahito et al. looked at 116 patients undergoing cardiovascular surgery and concluded that placement of the TEE probe was not responsible for postoperative recurrent laryngeal nerve palsy. It was likely the surgical manipulation, duration of surgery, cardiopulmonary bypass (CPB), and tracheal intubation were related to the palsy.[24] A case of intramural esophageal hematoma and odynophagia was reported in a patient undergoing atrial fibrillation ablation under general anesthesia with TEE. In this particular case, the TEE was advanced after induction of general anesthesia for evaluation of the heart and then removed. After removal of the TEE probe, there was some difficulty advancing the esophageal temperature probe, indicating a change in tissue integrity.[25] A recent study of 200 patients investigated whether modifying the TEE probe placement protocol could reduce the incidence of postoperative dysphagia. In the first group (n = 100), the TEE probe was inserted after anesthetic induction and remained in place for the duration of the surgery. In the second group (n = 100), the TEE probe was inserted after anesthetic induction and then removed after the cardiac exam. The probe was reinserted again before weaning from CPB and then immediately removed after the post-CPB examination. The incidence of dysphagia was significantly higher in patients who had the probe in place for the duration of the surgery (51.1% vs. 28.6%). Multivariate regression analysis showed that the length of time the TEE probe was in the esophagus was an independent predictor of dysphagia.[26] Although there are opposing sides to the argument over whether TEE causes postoperative dysphagia and odynophagia, it is clear that care must be taken when using or deciding to use TEE in any patient.

TABLE 28-1	**TEE-Related Injuries**
Site	*Injury*
Oropharynx	Dental/lip trauma, pharyngeal abrasions/hemorrhage, temporomandibular joint pain, tongue injury, hypopharyngeal perforation, tracheal intubation/vocal cord trauma
Esophageal	Dysphagia, odynophagia, perforation/laceration, hemorrhage
Gastric	Perforation/laceration, hemorrhage
Other	Splenic laceration, airway compromise, arrhythmias, vascular compression, burns/thermal injury, infection

TEE, Transesophageal echocardiography.

Esophageal Perforation

Esophageal perforation, a rare but life-threatening event, is the most feared complication of TEE. Studies report the risk to be anywhere from 0.01%[6] to 0.38%.[7] Many factors can predispose a patient to esophageal perforation: poor patient cooperation, inadequate technical skills of the clinician, a large calcified lymph node,[27] spasm or hypertrophy of the cricopharyngeal sphincter, cervical arthritis, forward and left lateral bending of the distal esophagus, and esophageal disease such as inflammation or neoplasm to name a few.[28] Increased risk for perforation from TEE may occur in patients with gastroesophageal pathology (Zenker diverticulum, esophageal stricture or obstructing mass, fibrosis secondary to prior chest radiation) and distorted anatomy (massive cardiomegaly,[29] tracheoesophageal fistula or atresia, and resistance to probe insertion).[30] Some authors have even suggested that small stature, longer procedures, congestive heart failure, low cardiac output prior to CPB,[31] advanced age,[32] and chronic steroid or bisphosphonate use[2] can translate into increased risk for esophageal perforation.

The site of esophageal perforation also varies. One study reported that the most common site of perforation is in the abdominal portion of the esophagus (57.3%), followed by the intrathoracic (33.3%) and cervical (9.3%) portions.[33]

The mechanism of injury with the TEE probe may be multifactorial. Local pressure effects, vascular insufficiency, thermal injury, and impaired mucosal blood supply during CPB may all be involved.[7] Urbanowicz et al. studied whether the pressure produced by contact between a TEE probe and the esophagus was sufficient to cause esophageal damage. The authors concluded that the maximum surface contact pressure between the esophagus and a fully flexed TEE probe is low in dogs and in most humans and not associated with histologic esophageal damage even with prolonged exposure. They also stated that potentially dangerous pressures (>60 mmHg) could be generated in some cases in humans. The authors suggested that the TEE probe not be left in a flexed position for prolonged periods of time.[34]

Direct trauma from placing the TEE probe (blind vs. direct visualization), advancing the probe, flexion, extension, lateral movement, and the general manipulation required to generate clearer images may also contribute to esophageal injury (Fig. 28-1). Kharasch et al. have theorized that the vibration of the piezoelectric crystal that produces the ultrasound wave can actually heat the tip of the TEE probe itself and cause thermal injury to gastrointestinal (GI) tissues. They stated that underlying tissue ischemia may prevent dissipation of the produced heat, increasing the susceptibility to thermal injury.[35] O'Shea et al.,[36] however, were unable to see any pathologic evidence of thermal injury to the esophageal mucosa in animals after prolonged CPB.

Symptoms of esophageal perforation can vary greatly from immediate and severe discomfort to delayed-onset symptoms even weeks after the time of TEE placement. The most common presentation of esophageal perforation include hemorrhage, subcutaneous emphysema, and the appearance of the TEE probe in the surgical field. Perforation can present in a much more insidious manner and can often be masked by general anesthesia during cardiac surgery.[37] Patients may

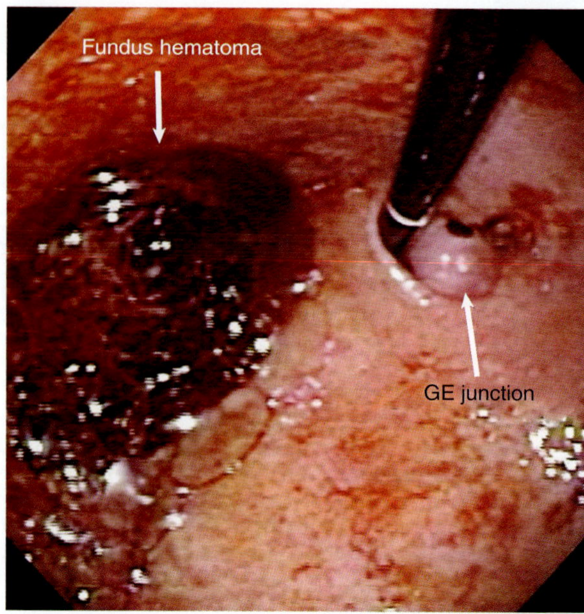

Figure 28-1 Upper endoscopy on 55-year-old man following mitral valve repair shows a medium-sized fundal hematoma. Endoscopy probe is retroflexed for the view. This hematoma was likely caused by retroflexion from TEE probe intraoperatively. *GE,* gastroesophageal.

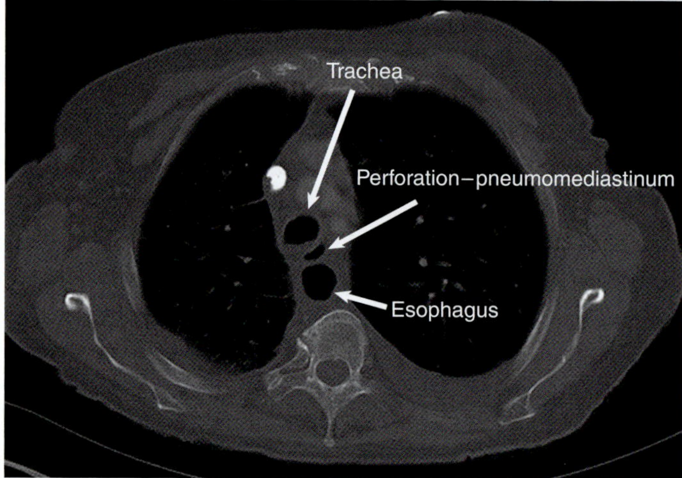

Figure 28-2 Axial image from computed tomography of chest, bone window. Normal air-filled trachea and esophagus can be seen. The third focus of air between the two, which is abnormal, is likely pneumomediastinum.

present much later with nonspecific signs such as dyspnea, agitation, fever, or bloody nasogastric aspirates. Symptoms relating to spontaneous esophageal perforation, such as Meckler's triad of vomiting, pain, and subcutaneous emphysema, are rarely present. According to one study looking at esophageal perforation from any cause, up to 33% of initial chest radiographs are within normal limits.[22,30] Some studies have even suggested that late presentations were as common or more common than early presentation (Fig. 28-2). Lennon et al. reported that in their study of 859 patients, all of the esophageal perforations (2) presented more than 48 hours after surgery (day 11 and day 4). In fact, one patient was discharged home on full anticoagulation only to return 5 days later with vague symptoms of lightheadedness and anemia. Esophagogastroduodenoscopy revealed a large amount of fresh blood in the stomach.[7] Cote et al. evaluated all reported cases of esophageal perforation after TEE procedures and found that 11/30 perforations

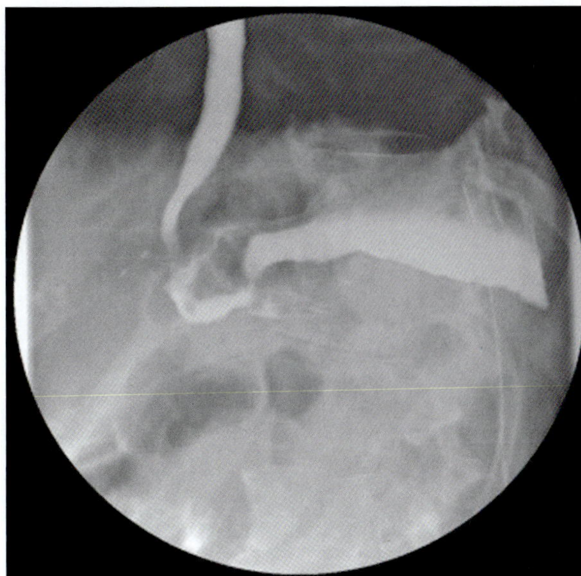

Figure 28-3 Gastrografin esophagram of patient displaying a distal intrathoracic esophageal perforation. Brisk extravasation of contrast can be seen flowing over dome of left hemidiaphragm in pleural space. *(From Freeman RK, van Woerkom JC, Ascioti AJ. Esophageal stent placement for the treatment of iatrogenic intrathoracic esophageal perforation. Ann Thorac Surg. 2007;83:2003-2008.)*

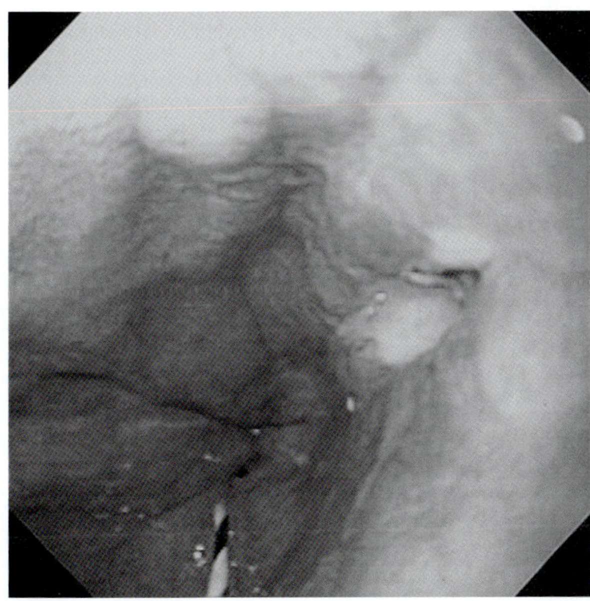

Figure 28-4 Endoscopic finding displaying esophageal perforation recognized on esophagram. *(From Freeman RK, van Woerkom JC, Ascioti AJ. Esophageal stent placement for the treatment of iatrogenic intrathoracic esophageal perforation. Ann Thorac Surg. 2007;83: 2003-2008.)*

were diagnosed more than 24 hours after surgery.[38] Esophageal perforation is associated with prolonged hospitalization and a mortality rate of 20% to 30%.[39] It is therefore imperative that clinical suspicion be high when there is any concern of perforation including post-TEE findings such as pneumothorax, pleural effusions, or postprocedural shortness of breath.[30] Diagnosis can be confirmed endoscopically or radiologically by computed tomography with contrast, upper GI barium swallow studies, and chest radiographs in the upright position (Figs. 28-3 and 28-4).[38]

Probe Mechanical Problems

Mechanical problems can occur with the TEE probe as well. There have been several reported cases of probe tip buckling in which the tip of the TEE probe folded over itself while in the esophagus, leading to difficulty in probe withdrawal. In these cases, all of the TEE operators were experienced and had an uncomplicated introduction.[40] In all reported instances, the probe could be safely removed by manipulation or pushing it into the stomach. The examiner should be wary of signs that may indicate malfunction, such as difficulty in getting images in the absence of a large diaphragmatic hernia, resistance to advancement or withdrawal of the transducer, and finding the rotary control in the maximally flexed position.[41] Inspection of the probe is mandatory, especially when using probes that have been used for more than 300 examinations.[42]

Gastrointestinal Tract Bleeding

Minor mucosal trauma during TEE can result in hematemesis or blood-tinged sputum.[41] This can be recognized from blood in the oropharynx, blood on the TEE probe upon removal from the patient, or from blood return upon suctioning of gastric contents. Norton et al. evaluated the incidence of upper GI hemorrhage in 10,573 patients. They concluded that the risk factors associated with upper GI bleeding due to TEE include previous ulcerative process, advanced age, vasoactive drugs, and failure to use H_2 agonist drugs in the perioperative period.[43] Other studies have reported that extending bypass periods, emergency operations, reoperations,[44] aspirin,[6] and anticoagulant use[45] are other factors associated with an increased risk of GI bleeding.

The issue of anticoagulant use is somewhat debated. In a study of 107 patients on full anticoagulation (intravenous heparin or oral anticoagulation) for thrombotic disease or prosthetic valves, there was no increase in upper GI bleeding after TEE examination.[46] However, there is a report of a patient who underwent TEE while receiving thrombolytic therapy who developed a hemothorax following an esophageal abrasion,[47] and a patient taking Coumadin who developed a supraglottic hematoma requiring tracheostomy post TEE.[45] Although this topic is debated, it is important to take care when dealing with patients who are receiving anticoagulants and undergoing TEE.

Performing TEE on patients with known esophageal varices or undergoing liver transplantation has also been a debated topic because of the potential for esophageal hemorrhage. Spier et al. found on retrospective analysis that TEE without transgastric views can be performed without serious complications in patients with grade 1 or grade 2 esophageal varices who have not had recent hemorrhages.[48] The investigators found no major bleeding complications in any of their patients, even those with histories of prior variceal hemorrhages. This is a change from years before where many clinicians considered esophageal varices to be a contraindication to TEE. It is still prudent, however, to confirm that patients with esophageal varices have a strong clinical indication for TEE.

Other Injuries and Complications in Gastrointestinal Tract and Solid Organs

Intraoperative use of TEE exposes patients to ultrasound waves and pressure from the probe for prolonged periods of time. Greene et al. looked at 50 children undergoing congenital heart surgery with TEE and used flexible esophagoscopy to evaluate their esophagus after removal of the TEE probe.[49] Some 64% (32 of 50) had abnormal results on esophageal examinations (i.e., hematoma, mucosal erosion, and petechiae). It was noted that 20 of the 25 smaller patients (80%) had abnormal results compared with 12 of the 25 larger patients (48%). It has been reported that powerful ultrasound beams (pressure of 1 MPa) can cause vibration of gas-filled structures, leading to hemorrhage and hemolysis.[50] These beams can also produce excessive heat, cavitation, and the ultrasonic activation of gas bodies; this includes the potentially violent collapse of small gas bodies in or near tissue.[51] TEE probes available for clinical use have much lower intensity ($\approx$5 MHz) and are unlikely to cause hemorrhage or harmful side effects. Pressures of up to 60 mmHg generated from the position of the probe (e.g., flexing against the esophagus) can lead to intramural hemorrhage or mucosal tears. It has been suggested that the probe should not be left in the flexed position for extended periods of time.[52]

Splenic laceration has also been reported in two cases using TEE. The first case was a 71-year-old man who went for reoperative coronary artery bypass grafting (CABG) and presented with abdominal distention post bypass. Exploration of the abdomen revealed 1 L of dark red blood and an actively bleeding superficial laceration on the hilar surface of the spleen. There was no other instrumentation in the left upper quadrant, implying that TEE likely caused the trauma. However, the ease of placement and normal function of the orogastric tube led the authors to doubt that TEE was the cause. They noted that no perforation was found on multiple inspections of the stomach, and they believed that manipulation of the probe in the stomach caused traction on the splenic capsule, leading to injury.[53] They hypothesized that simple traction on the gastrosplenic ligament with manipulation of the TEE probe could result in tearing of the fragile splenic capsule. Another case report described a 55-year-old woman undergoing coronary artery bypass and mitral valve repair who presented with significant abdominal distention after an uncomplicated procedure.[54] She was brought back to the operating room after having significant worsening of hemodynamics and an unexpected decline in hemoglobin value, suspect for cardiac tamponade. However, the abdomen was noted to be significantly distended, and exploration revealed brisk bleeding from the splenic hilum. These are isolated events but show that extreme care must be used when operating the TEE probe.

Oftentimes, more than one monitor is placed in the esophagus at any given time. There have been reports of an esophageal stethoscope placed with a TEE probe that became kinked after removal of the TEE probe.[55] Gentle traction and direct laryngoscopy were unable to facilitate retrieval of the probe. Rigid esophagoscopy was performed to retract the stethoscope. Another case described a nasal temperature probe being broken and advanced into the stomach through TEE manipulation.[56] The author suggested proper lubrication to decrease the likelihood of foreign objects being dislodged in the esophagus. Finally, there was a report of an esophageal stethoscope being completely lost in the stomach after cardiac surgery, owing to manipulation of the TEE probe. Multiple endoscopic attempts by a gastroenterologist and finally surgical intervention were required to retrieve the stethoscope.[57]

▣ Respiratory Complications

Although fairly rare, TEE has been reported to cause respiratory complications as well. Although the majority of complications occur in the nonoperative setting, intraoperative TEE has been reported to cause endotracheal malpositioning in 0.03% of cases.[6] This malposition can be potentially disastrous. Endotracheal tube malpositioning due to TEE manipulation is particularly detrimental in the pediatric population. Small changes in endotracheal tube position can lead to inadvertent tracheal extubation or mainstem advancement of the endotracheal tube. The small size of the pediatric airway in relation to the size of the TEE probe can also cause airway compression (Figs. 28-5 and 28-6).[58] Stevenson's 1999 study of 1650 pediatric patients showed that extubation occurred in 0.5% of patients, right mainstem advancement in 0.2%, and airway obstruction in 1%. Airway obstruction can occur by compression of the airway or even compression of the endotracheal tube,[58,59] especially when congenital vascular abnormalities such as double aortic arch and truncus arteriosus coexist.[60]

Multiple cases of airway compression in adults have also been reported. Nakao et al. described a 38-year-old man with a dissecting aneurysm of the ascending aorta and arch who had airway compression due to manipulation of the TEE probe.[61] Arima et al. reported

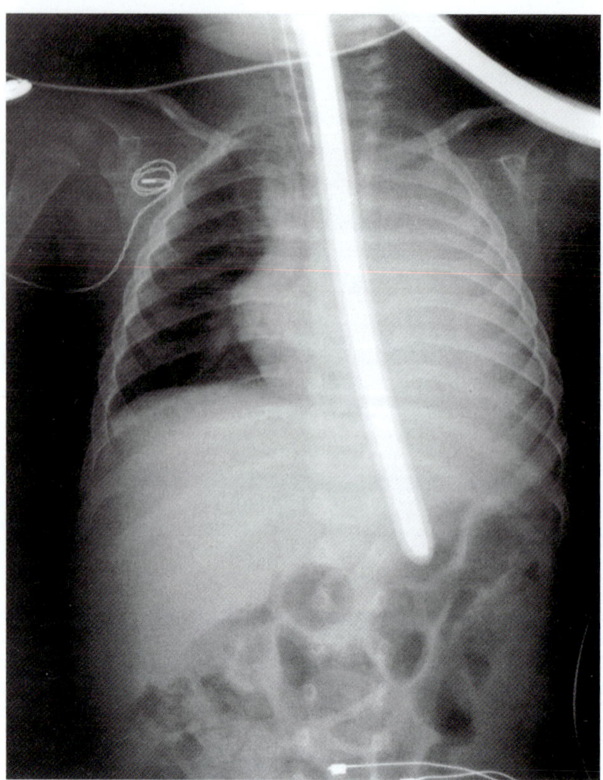

Figure 28-5   Supine anteroposterior portable chest radiograph suggests extrinsic compression of left mainstem bronchus by large-caliber esophageal dilator, resulting in bronchial obstruction and left lung collapse. *(From Everett LL, Spottswood SE. Intraoperative desaturation and unilateral breath sounds during Nissen fundoplication. Anesth Analg. 2000;90: 62-67.)*

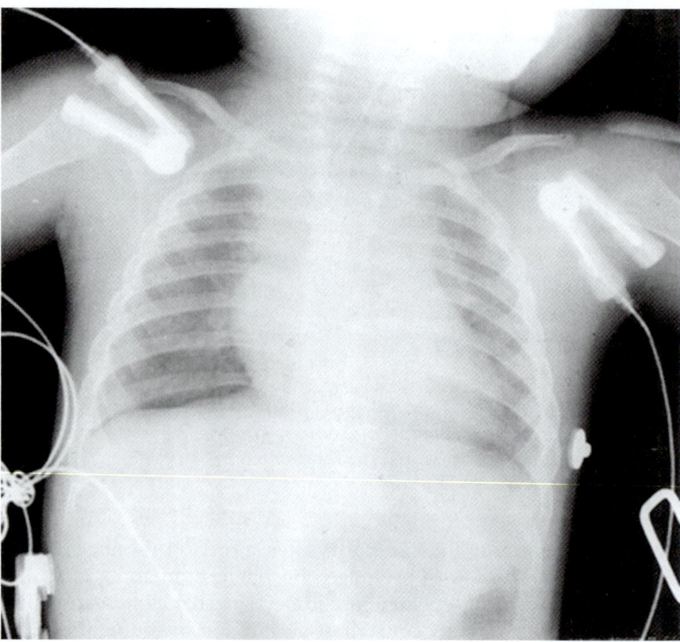

Figure 28-6   Supine anteroposterior portable chest radiograph obtained 8 hours after dilator extraction reveals complete reexpansion of left lung. *(From Everett LL, Spottswood SE. Intraoperative desaturation and unilateral breath sounds during Nissen fundoplication. Anesth Analg. 2000;90: 62-67.)*

airway obstruction during TEE probe placement in a patient with tracheal distortion from an ascending aortic pseudoaneurysm.[62]

In the nonoperative setting, Chan et al. reported mistaken insertion of the TEE probe into the trachea in 4 out of 1500 patients (0.27%). Two of these patients immediately developed stridor and incessant cough, but this can be masked by sedation. One patient in the study who was receiving long-term treatment for bronchial asthma developed severe bronchospasm during the transesophageal examination.[63] Sutton reported a case of transtracheal placement of the TEE probe. He described easy placement of the probe to 26 cm without resistance. Image quality was poor and distal structures were indistinct. The patient was sedated but showed mild coughing, oxygen saturation via pulse oximetry decreased to 90%, and the ventilation pattern showed signs of obstruction without stridor.[64] Other respiratory complications in awake or sedated patients include laryngospasm,[65] posterior pharyngeal wall hematoma,[66] supraglottic hematoma,[67] subglottic stenosis,[68] pulmonary edema,[65] atelectasis,[69] and methemoglobinemia from topicalization of the oropharynx with benzocaine.[70] Recurrent laryngeal nerve injury has also been described in the setting of TEE monitoring for sedated neurosurgical procedures.[71] Kawahito et al., however, did not find a statistically significant difference in the incidence of recurrent laryngeal nerve injury in patients undergoing cardiac surgery.[24] TEE examinations in sedated patients can be associated with a reduction in oxygen saturation. Scriven et al. conducted a study with 150 consecutive patients undergoing TEE and found that oxygen saturation via pulse oximetry fell in 144 of 150 patients (96%).[72] They noted significant hypoxemia (Sao_2 persistently <90%) in 27 patients (18%). Two patients in the significant hypoxemia group developed profound hypoxia (Sao_2 35% and Sao_2 74%). The first patient developed transient apnea and nodal bradycardia, and the second patient became bradypneic. The TEE probe was removed in both cases, and both patients responded to flumazenil and oxygen. Prophylactic oxygen supplementation and arterial oxygen saturation monitoring, for the reasons just described, should be performed on patients undergoing sedation for TEE.

Cardiovascular Effects

TEE placement can also have cardiovascular effects, although they are rare. A European study by Daniel et al. of 10,419 patients reported 3 cases of nonsustained ventricular tachycardia, three cases of transient atrial fibrillation, and 1 case of third-degree atrioventricular block.[47] Most often, the arrhythmia can be terminated by simply removing the offending object, the TEE probe.[41] There is significantly more literature available on cardiovascular complications due to endoscopy than from TEE. Lee et al. described four cases of supraventricular tachycardia, two cases of myocardial infarction, and one case of congestive heart failure in a study of 21,946 endoscopic procedures performed over a 4-year period.[73] Tseng et al. found that in emergent endoscopy for upper GI bleeding, that patients with coronary artery disease (CAD) had a significantly higher incidence of ventricular arrhythmias (42% vs. 16%; $P = .004$) and myocardial ischemia (9 patients vs. 1 patient; $P = .016$) than patients without CAD.[74] Khanderia stated that severely reduced systolic function in conjunction with catecholamines from stimulation and sedation could contribute to heart failure with TEE.[41]

It can be suggested that severely ill patients or patients thought to be at increased risk for heart failure should undergo TEE examinations under general anesthesia. Patients undergoing TEE with sedation only can often cough or retch during the procedure, despite local anesthesia of the oropharynx, and this coughing and retching can increase intrathoracic, central venous, and pulmonary pressures. Fatal pulmonary embolization from a right atrial mass,[75] embolization of a left intracardiac thrombus resulting in stroke,[76] and a progressive aortic dissection with cardiac tamponade[77] have all been reported as a result. Park et al. reported a case of occlusion of the right subclavian artery in an adult patient with a vascular ring after insertion of the TEE probe.

Pediatric patients, probably more so than adults, can have cardiovascular complications from TEE placement. There are reports of compression of a normally positioned[78] or aberrant right subclavian artery,[79] descending aorta,[80] innominate artery,[81] and pulmonary veins in an infant with total anomalous pulmonary venous return.[82,83] Each patient must be evaluated individually, and a plan for TEE must be formed based on the patient's anatomy and comorbidities.

Probe Contamination

The Healthcare Infection Control Practices Advisory Committee (HICPAC) from the Centers for Disease Control and Prevention (CDC) put forth guidelines for disinfection and sterilization in healthcare facilities in 2008.[84] The authors describe a four-step process including cleaning, disinfecting, rinsing, and drying. The U.S. Food and Drug Administration (FDA)-approved high-level disinfectants include 2.4% (and above) glutaraldehyde, 0.55% orthophthalaldehyde (OPA), 0.95% glutaraldehyde with 1.64% phenol/phenate, 7.35% hydrogen peroxide with 0.23% peracetic acid, 1.0% hydrogen peroxide with 0.08% peracetic acid, and 7.5% hydrogen peroxide. Use of these disinfecting solutions has decreased endoscopy-related infection rates but risks causing chemical burns when the rinse process is incomplete. A case report from 2003 reported chemical ulcerations on the lip, tongue, tonsillar pillars, epiglottis, arytenoid region, and esophagus of a patient after undergoing TEE with an improperly rinsed probe that had been cleaned with orthophthalaldehyde.[85] This case highlights the idea that the four-step cleaning process described by the HICPAC must be rigorously followed without deviation to avoid chemical burn injuries.

Infectious Complications

Because many patients undergoing TEE have prosthetic valves or are immunocompromised, infectious complications must be considered. In a study of 140 consecutive patients in London, blood cultures were obtained before and after TEE exams. Positive cultures occurred in 4 (1.4%) of 280 culture bottles before the procedure, 2 (0.7%) of 280 culture bottles immediately after the procedure, and in 2 (0.9%) of 228 late (1 hour later) culture bottles.[86] Bacterial isolates were coagulase-negative staphylococci (5/8), *Propionibacterium* (2/8), and *Moraxella* (1/8). All of the positive blood cultures were considered contaminates. The authors concluded that the incidence of bacteremia related to TEE is very low, and the incidence of blood cultures positive for bacteremia after TEE is indistinguishable from the anticipated contamination rate.[86]

Another study from France of 82 consecutive patients found a single positive blood culture in 2 patients. One patient grew corynebacteria, and the other patient grew *Staphylococcus epidermidis*. Some 15% of patients enrolled in the study were noted to have a transient subfebrile temperature during the first 24 hours, including the two patients with positive blood cultures; none of the patients developed endocarditis after 6 months. These authors concluded that antibiotic prophylaxis prior to TEE is unwarranted.[87]

In 2006, the British Cardiac Society Clinical Practice Committee published guidelines recommending antibiotic prophylaxis routinely for TEE. These recommendations were based on a single case report of a 55-year-old man who underwent TEE for evaluation of bileaflet mitral valve prolapse. A week after TEE he developed anorexia, nausea, lightheadedness, and malaise and subsequently fever and myalgia. At 17 days post TEE he sought medical help, and *Streptococcus sanguis* was grown in both blood cultures.[88] Repeat TEE showed increased nodularity of the flail portion of the posterior mitral leaflet. The patient was treated with a course of antibiotics for 4 weeks. The authors acknowledged in the paper that this case was not conclusively caused by the TEE, but they thought that the temporal relationship was suggestive.

The use of antibiotic therapy before TEE is somewhat controversial. The American Heart Association Guidelines for prevention of bacterial endocarditis states that only patients with the highest risk for infective endocarditis should receive prophylactic antibiotics.[89] Such patients include those who have an artificial heart valve, those who have had a heart valve repaired with an artificial material, those with a history of endocarditis, those with a heart transplant with abnormal valve function, and those with certain congenital heart defects. The Working Party of the British Society of Antimicrobial Chemotherapy published guidelines in 2006 that recommended antibiotic prophylaxis only for high-risk patients undergoing TEE, which included those with previous infective endocarditis, those undergoing cardiac valve replacement surgery, and those with surgically constructed systemic or pulmonary conduits.[90] The evidence points to *not* using antibiotic prophylaxis routinely for TEE, but it is important to use clinical judgment when deciding whether to administer antibiotics. It may be reasonable to consider antibiotics in occasional cases—for example, a patient with a replacement heart valve and evidence of poor oral hygiene in whom the study is being performed for an indication other than suspected endocarditis.[91]

Local Anesthetic Complications

TEE outside the operating room setting is often performed with the help of light sedation and local anesthesia. This method often facilitates placement of the probe into the esophagus and probe manipulation with less patient irritation. Sedation can have the effects discussed previously, but local anesthetics can also have effects, including toxicity, allergic reactions, and methemoglobinemia.

Lidocaine 2% or 4% is the local anesthetic typically used for anesthetizing the oropharynx for TEE probe placement. Lidocaine is rapidly absorbed through mucous membrane surfaces and can lead to local anesthetic toxicity. Case reports exist describing patients who were orally topicalized with lidocaine 10% spray and viscous lidocaine 2% and then became lethargic, disoriented, difficult to arouse, or even had seizure activity.[92,93] Lidocaine levels were drawn, some of which were shown to be markedly high. Lidocaine 10% is rarely if ever used anymore for anesthetizing the oropharynx because of the efficacy of lidocaine 2% or 4% viscous. Benzocaine was also used in the past, but the efficacy of lidocaine and issues with methemoglobinemia have led to less frequent use of this agent.

These local anesthetics are critical in enabling clinicians to comfortably perform TEE on awake patients. Because of the risk of central toxicity it is, however, important to evaluate each patient carefully and potentially decrease the dose empirically in patients with severe liver disease or congestive heart failure.[93] Allergies to local anesthetics are rare but can be life threatening; they are usually associated with ester anesthetics because of the presence of a para-aminobenzoic acid (PABA) metabolite. Amide agents do not undergo this metabolism, but preservative compounds used in the preparation of amide agents can be metabolized to PABA. Patients with known allergy to ester local anesthetics should be treated with a preservative-free amide local anesthetic.[94]

Oral topicalization using local anesthetics has also been reported to have caused methemoglobinemia, a disorder characterized by a higher level of methemoglobin (metHb) in the blood than normal. Methemoglobin has a decreased affinity for oxygen, resulting in a reduced ability to release oxygen to the tissues. This causes a left shift of the hemoglobin dissociation curve. Visually the blood is described as having a chocolate-brown color. Signs and symptoms of methemoglobinemia include shortness of breath, cyanosis, mental status changes, headache, fatigue, dizziness, and even loss of consciousness. Local anesthetics like prilocaine, benzocaine, and articaine have been described as potential causes of methemoglobinemia. A study from the Mayo Clinic including 28,478 TEE procedures reported 19 cases of methemoglobinemia (0.067%) due to benzocaine.[95] All of the patients were cyanotic with low oxygen saturations. Another case report describes a 35-year-old man who presented for TEE to rule out endocarditis.[96] After receiving topical oropharyngeal anesthesia with 20% benzocaine spray, the patient's oxygen saturation dropped to 87% during the procedure, and he did not respond to supplemental oxygen or reversal of sedation. An arterial blood sample revealed chocolate-brown blood with a Pao_2 of 112 mmHg and an oxygen saturation of 97%.

TABLE 28-2   Contraindications to TEE

Absolute Contraindications	Relative Contraindications
Lack of informed consent	Severe cervical arthritis, neck surgery
Lack of clinician experience in TEE placement	Esophageal varices without bleeding
Full stomach	Esophagitis
Perforated viscous	Gastric herniation
Esophageal pathology (stricture, trauma, tumor, scleroderma, Mallory-Weiss tear, diverticulum, fistula)	Symptomatic hiatal hernia
	History of GI surgery
	Recent upper GI bleed
	Prior mediastinal irradiation
	Thoracoabdominal aneurysm
Upper GI bleeding (active)	Barrett esophagus
Recent upper GI surgery	History of dysphagia
Esophagectomy, esophagogastrectomy	Coagulopathy

GI, Gastrointestinal; *TEE,* transesophageal echocardiography.

Contraindications

Increased perioperative use of TEE and demonstration of its benefits have concomitantly increased the number of contraindications to its use (Table 28-2). In 2009, *Miller's Anesthesia* stated that contraindications included previous esophagectomy, severe esophageal obstruction, esophageal perforation, ongoing esophageal hemorrhage, esophageal diverticulum, esophageal varices, esophageal fistula, prior esophageal surgery, history of gastric surgery, mediastinal radiation, and unexplained swallowing difficulties.[97] More recently in 2010, the American Society of Anesthesiologists/Society of Cardiovascular Anesthesiologists Practice Guidelines recommended that TEE *may* be used for patients with oral, esophageal, or gastric disease if the expected benefit outweighs the potential risk, provided the appropriate precautions are applied. These precautions may include considering other imaging modalities (e.g., epicardial echocardiography), obtaining a gastroenterology consultation, limiting the examination, avoiding unnecessary probe manipulation, and using the most experienced operator.[98] To prevent the complications discussed in this chapter, it is critical that physicians use sound clinical judgment when imaging patients using TEE probes.

Summary

TEE is an integral and generally safe modality for diagnosis and monitoring of cardiac function and structural abnormalities. Compared to transthoracic echocardiography (TTE), TEE allows improved proximity to cardiac structures and clearer imaging of cardiac anatomy. Although complications from placement and use of TEE can occur, studies have shown that these events are relatively uncommon. Through awareness of potential complications and judicious use of TEE by properly trained physicians, these complications can be minimized.

REFERENCES

1. Practice Guidelines for Perioperative Transesophageal Echocardiography. *Anesthesiology.* 2010; 112(5):1084-1096.
2. Min J, Spencer K, Furlong K, et al. Clinical features of complications from transesophageal echocardiography: a single-center case series of 10,000 consecutive examinations. *J Am Soc Echocardiogr.* 2005;18:925-929.
3. Khanderia BK, Seward JB, Tajik AJ. Transesophageal echocardiography. *Mayo Clin Proc.* 1994;69: 856-863.
4. Seward JB, Khanderia BK, Oh JK, et al. Critical appraisal of transesophageal echocardiography: limitations, pitfalls, and complications. *J Am Soc Echocardiogr.* 1992;5:288-305.
5. Danieal WG, Erbel R, Kasper W, et al. Safety of transesophageal echocardiography. A multicenter survey of 10, 419 examinations. *Circulation.* 1991;83:817-821.
6. Kallmeyer I, Collard C, Fox J, et al. The safety of intraoperative transesophageal echocardiography: a case series of 7200 cardiac surgical patients. *Anesth Analg.* 2001;92:1126-1130.
7. Lennon MJ, Gibbs NM, Weightman WM, Leber J. Transesophageal echocardiography-related gastrointestinal complications in cardiac surgical patients. *J Cardiothorac Vasc Anesth.* 2005;19(2):141-145.
8. Piercy M, McNicol L, Dinh D, et al. Major complications related to the use of transesophageal echocardiography in cardiac surgery. *J Cardiothorac Vasc Anesth.* 2009;23:62-65.
9. Huang CH, Lu CW, Lin TY, et al. Complications of intraoperative transesophageal echocardiography in adult cardiac surgical patients–experience in two institutions in Taiwan. *J Formos Med Assoc.* 2007;106:92-95.
10. Rafferty T, LaMantia KR, Davis E, et al. Quality assurance for intraoperative transesophageal echocardiography monitoring: a report of 846 procedures. *Anesth Analg.* 1993;76:228-232.
11. Anantharam B, Chahal N, Stephens N, Senior R. Temporo-mandibular joint dislocation: an unusual complication of transesophageal echocardiography. *Eur J Echocardiogr.* 2010;11(2):190-191.

12. Vignon P, Gueret P, Chabernaud JM, et al. Failure and complications of transesophageal echocardiography. Apropos of 1500 consecutive cases. *Arch Mal Coeur Vaiss.* 1993;86:849-855.

13. Na S, Kim CS, Kim JY, Cho JS, Kim KJ. Rigid laryngoscope-assisted insertion of transesophageal echocardiography probe reduces oropharyngeal mucosal injury in anesthetized patients. *Anesthesiology.* 2009 Jan;110(1):38-40.

14. Tam JW, Burwash IG, Ascah KJ, et al. Feasibility and complications of single-plane and biplane versus multiplane transesophageal imaging: a review of 2947 consecutive studies. *Can J Cardiol.* 1997;13:81-84.

15. Mathur SK, Singh P. Transesophageal echocardiography related complications. *Indian J Anesth.* 2009;53(5):567-574.

16. Stevenson JG. Role of intraoperative transesophageal echocardiography during repair of congenital cardiac defects. *Acta Pediatr Suppl.* 1995;410:23-33.

17. Spahn DR, Schmid S, Carrel T, et al. Hypopharynx perforation by a transesophageal echocardiography probe. *Anesthesiology.* 1995;82:581-583.

18. Aviv J, DiTullio M, Jomma SH, et al. Hypopharyngeal perforation near-miss during transesophageal echocardiography. *Laryngoscope.* 2004;114(5):821-826.

19. Takasaki Y. Transient lingual ischemia during anesthesia (case report). *Anesthesia.* 2003;58:717.

20. Tan PH, Lin VC, Chen HS, Hung KC. The effect of transesophageal echocardiography probe insertion on tracheal cuff pressure. *Anaesthesia.* 2011;66(9):791-795.

21. Messina A, Paranicas M, Fiamengo S, et al. Risk of dysphagia after transesophageal echocardiography. *Am J Cardiol.* 1991;67(4):313-314.

22. Hulyalkar AR, Ayd JD. Low risk of gastroesophageal injury associated with transesophageal echocardiography during cardiac surgery. *J Cardiothorac Vasc Anesth.* 1993;7:175-177.

23. Hogue CW, Lappas GD, Creswell LL, et al. Swallowing dysfunction after cardiac operations. *J Thorac Cardiovasc Surg.* 1995;110:517-522.

24. Kawahito S, Kitahata H, Kimura H, et al. Recurrent laryngeal nerve palsy after cardiovascular surgery: relationship to the placement of a transesophageal echocardiographic probe. *J Cardiothorac Vasc Anesth.* 1999;13(5):528-531.

25. Nguyen DT, Wang ZJ, Vedantham V, Badhwar N. Odynophagia after atrial fibrillation ablation. *Circulation.* 2011;123(8):253-254.

26. Chin JH, Lee EH, Choi DK, Choi IC. A modification of the transesophageal echocardiography protocol can reduce post-operative dysphagia following cardiac surgery. *J Int Med Res.* 2011;39(1):96-104.

27. Pong MW, Lin SM, Kao SC, et al. Unusual cause of esophageal perforation during intraoperative transesophageal echocardiographic monitoring for cardiac surgery–a case report. *Acta Anaesthesiol Sin.* 2003;41:155-158.

28. Shapira MY, Hirshberg B, Agid R, et al. Esophageal perforation after transesophageal echocardiogram. *Echocardiography.* 1999;16(2):151-154.

29. Massy SR, Pitsis A, Mehta D, Callaway M. Oesophageal perforation following perioperative transesophageal echocardiography. *Br J Anaesth.* 2000;84(5):643-646.

30. Hilberath J, Oakes D, Shernan S, et al. Comprehensive review–safety of transesophageal echocardiography. *J Am Soc Echocardiogr.* 2010;23(11):1115-1127.

31. Lecharny J, Philip I, Depoix J. Oesophagotracheal perforation after intraoperative transesophageal echocardiography in cardiac surgery. *Br J Anaesth.* 2002;88(4):592-594.

32. Brinkman WT, Shanewise JS, Clements SD, Mansour KA. Transesophageal echocardiography: not an innocuous procedure. *Ann Thorac Surg.* 2001;72:1725-1726.

33. Fernadez FF, Richter A, Freudenberg S, et al. Treatment of endoscopic esophageal perforation. *Surg Endosc.* 1999;13(10):962-966.

34. Urbanowicz J, Kernoff R, Oppenheim G, et al. Transesophageal echocardiography and its potential for esophageal damage. *Anesthesiology.* 1990;72:40-43.

35. Kharasch ED, Sivarajan M. Gastroesophageal perforation after intraoperative transesophageal echocardiography. *Anesthesiology.* 1996;85(2):426-428.

36. O'Shea JP, Southern JF, D'Ambra MN, et al. Effects of prolonged transesophageal echocardiographic imaging and probe manipulation on the esophagus–an echocardiographic-pathologic study. *J Am Coll Cardiol.* 1991;17(6):1426-1429.

37. Ghafoor AU, Schmitz ML, Mayhew J. Esophageal mucosal tear from a transesophageal probe despite preliminary assessment via esophagoscopy in a patient with esophageal disease. *J Cardiothorac Vasc Anesth.* 2004;18:78-79.

38. Côte G, Denault A. Transesophageal echocardiography-related complications. *Can J Anesth.* 2008;55(9):622-647.

39. Lawrence DR, Moxon RE, Fountain SW, et al. Iatrogenic oesophageal perforations: a clinical review. *Ann R Coll Surg Engl.* 1998;80:115-118.

40. Kronzon I, Cziner DG, Katz ES, et al. Buckling of the tip of the transesophageal echocardiography probe: a potentially dangerous technical malfunction. *J Am Soc Echocardiogr.* 1992;5:176-177.

41. Khandheria BK. The transesophageal echocardiographic examination: is it safe? *Echocardiography.* 1994;11(1):55-63.

42. Orihashi K, Sueda T, Matsuura Y, Yamanoue T, Yuge O. Buckling of transesophageal echocardiography probe: a pitfall at insertion in an anesthetized patient. *Hiroshima J Med Sci.* 1993;42:155-157.

43. Norton ID, Pokorny CS, Baird DK, Selby WS. Upper gastrointestinal haemorrhage following coronary artery bypass grafting. *Aust NZ J Med.* 1995;25:297-301.

44. Leitman IM, Paull DE, Barie PS, Isom OW, Shires GT. Intra-abdominal complications of cardiopulmonary bypass operations. *Surg Gynecol Obstet.* 1987;165:251-254.

45. Massa N, Morrison M. Transesophageal echocardiography: an unusual case of iatrogenic laryngeal trauma. *Otolaryngol Head Neck Surg.* 2001;72:2141-2143.

46. Chee TS, Quek SS, Ding ZP, Chua SM. Clinical utility, safety, acceptability and complications of transoesophageal echocardiography (TEE) in 901 patients. *Singapore Med J.* 1995;36:479-483.

47. Daniel WG, Erbel R, Kasper W, et al. Safety of transesophageal echocardiography. A multicenter survey of 10,419 examinations. *Circulation.* 1991;83:817-821.

48. Spier B, Larue S, Teelin T, et al. Review of complications in a series of patients with known gastroesophageal varices undergoing transesophageal echocardiography. *J Am Soc Echocardiogr.* 2009;22:396-400.

49. Greene MA, Alexander JA, Knauf DG, et al. Endoscopic evaluation of the esophagus in infants and children immediately following intraoperative use of transesophageal echocardiography. *Chest.* 1999;116:1247-1250.

50. Baggs R, Penney DP, Cox C, et al. Thresholds for ultrasonically induced lung hemorrhage in neonatal swine. *Ultrasound Med Biol.* 1996;22:119-128.

51. Carstensen EL, Duck FA, Meltzer RS, Schwarz KQ, Keller B. Bioeffects in echocardiography. *Echocardiography.* 1992;9:605-623.

52. Dewhirst WE, Stragant JJ, Fleming BM. Mallory-Weiss tear complicating intraoperative transesophageal echocardiography in a patient undergoing aortic valve replacement. *Anesthesiology.* 1990;73:777-778.

53. Chow MS, Taylor MA, Hanson III CW. Splenic laceration associated with transesophageal echocardiography. *J Cardiothorac Vasc Anesth.* 1998;12:314-316.

54. Olenchock SA, Lukaszczyk JJ, Reed III J, Theman TE. Splenic injury after intraoperative transesophageal echocardiography. *Ann Thorac Surg.* 2001;72:2141-2143.

55. Yascik A, Samra SK. An unusual complication of transesophageal echocardiography. *Anesth Analg.* 1995;81:657-658.

56. Benedict PE, Foley K. Transesophageal echocardiography not without pitfalls. *J Cardiothorac Vasc Anesth.* 1997;11:123.

57. Brook M, Chard PS, Brock-Utmne JG. Gastric foreign body: a potential risk when using transesophageal echo. *Anesth Analg.* 1997;84:1389.

58. Stevenson JG. Incidence of complications in pediatric transesophageal echocardiography: experience in 1650 cases. *J Am Soc Echocardiogr.* 1999;12:527-532.

59. Bezold LI, Pignatelli R, Altman CA, et al. Intraoperative transesophageal echocardiography in congenital heart surgery. The Texas Children's Hospital experience. *Tex Heart Inst J.* 1996;23:108-115.

60. Phoon CK, Bhardwaj N. Airway obstruction caused by transesophageal echocardiography in a patient with double arch and truncus arteriosus. *J Am Soc Echocardiogr.* 1999;12:540.

61. Nakao S, Eguchi T, Ikeda S, et al. Airway obstruction by a transesophageal echocardiography probe in an adult patient with a dissecting aneurysm of the ascending aorta and arch. *J Cardiothorac Vasc Anesth.* 2000;14:186-187.

62. Arima H, Sobue K, Tanaka S, et al. Airway obstruction associated with transesophageal echocardiography in a patient with a giant aortic pseudoaneurysm. *Anesth Analg.* 2002;95:558-560.

63. Chan KL, Cohen GI, Sochowski RA, Baird MG. Complications of transesophageal echocardiography in ambulatory adult patients: analysis of 1500 consecutive examinations. *J Am Soc Echocardiogr.* 1991;4:577-582.

64. Sutton DC. Accidental transtracheal imaging with a transesophageal echocardiography probe. *Anesth Analg.* 1997;85:760-762.

65. Khandheria BK, Seward JB, Bailey KR. Safety of transesophageal echocardiography: experience with 2070 consecutive procedures. *J Am Coll Cardiol.* 1991;17:20A.

66. Saphir JR, Cooper JA, Kerbavez RJ, et al. Upper airway obstruction after transesophageal echocardiography. *J Am Soc Echocardiogr.* 1997;10:977-978.

67. Massa N, Morrison M. Transesophageal echocardiography: an unusual case of iatrogenic laryngeal trauma. *Otolaryngol Head Neck Surg.* 2003;129:602-604.

68. Liu JH, Hartnick CJ, Rutter MJ, et al. Subglottic stenosis associated with transesophageal echocardiography. *Int J Pediatr Otorhinolaryngol.* 2000;55:47-49.

69. Lam J, Neirotti RA, Hardjowijono R, et al. Transesophageal echocardiography with the use of a four-millimeter probe. *J Am Soc Echocardiogr.* 1997;10:499-504.

70. Birchem SK. Benzocaine-induced methemoglobinemia during transesophageal echocardiography. *J Am Osteopath Assoc.* 2005;105:381-384.

71. Practice guidelines for perioperative transesophageal echocardiography. A report by the American Society of Anesthesiologists and the Society of Cardiovascular Anesthesiologists Task Force on Transesophageal Echocardiography. *Anesthesiology.* 1996;84:986-1006.

72. Scriven AJ, Cobbe SM. Hypoxaemia during transesophageal echocardiography. *Br Heart J.* 1994;72:133-135.

73. Lee JG, Leung JW, Cotton PB. Acute cardiovascular complications of endoscopy: prevalence and clinical characteristics. *Dig Dis.* 1995;13:130-135.

74. Tseng PH, Liou JM, Lee YC, et al. Emergency endoscopy for upper gastrointestinal bleeding in patients with coronary artery disease. *Am J Emerg Med.* Sep 2009;27(7):802-806.

75. Cavero MA, Cristobal C, Gonzales M, et al. Fatal pulmonary embolization of a right atrial mass during transesophageal echocardiography. *J Am Soc Echocardiogr.* 1998;11:397-398.

76. Black IW, Cranney GB, Walsh WF, Brender D. Embolization of a left atrial ball thrombus during transesophageal echocardiography. *J Am Soc Echocardiogr.* 1992;5:271-273.

77. Cm Kim, Yu SC, Hong SJ. Cardiac tamponade during transesophageal echocardiography in the patient of circumferential aortic dissection. *J Korean Med Sci.* 1997;12:266-268.

78. Carerj S, Paola TM, Oddo A, Lucisano V, Oreto G. Esophageal duplication cyst: a rare obstacle to transesophageal echocardiography. *Echocardiography.* 1998;15:601-602.

79. Koinig H, Schlemmer M, Keznickl FP. Occlusion of the right subclavian artery after insertion of a transesophageal echocardiography probe in a neonate. *Paediatr Anaesth.* 2003;13:617-619.

80. Lunn RJ, Oliver WC, Hagler DJ, Danielson GK. Aortic compression by transesophageal echocardiographic probe in infants and children undergoing cardiac surgery. *Anesthesiology.* 1992;77:587-590.

81. Janelle GM, Lobato EB, Tang YS. An unusual complication of transesophageal echocardiography. *J Cardiothorac Vasc Anesth.* 1999;13:233-234.

82. Frommelt PC, Stuth EA. Transesophageal echocardiography in total anomalous pulmonary venous drainage: hypotension caused by compression of the pulmonary venous confluence during probe passage. *J Am Soc Echocardiogr.* 1994;7:652-654.

83. Kostolny M, Schreiber C, Henze R, Vogt M, et al. Temporary pulmonary vein stenosis during intraoperative transesophageal echocardiography in total cavopulmonary connection. *Pediatr Cardiol.* 2006;27:134-136.

84. Rutala W, Weber D, et al. *Guideline for disinfection and sterilization in healthcare facilities,* 2008. *Infection Control and Hospital Epidemiology.* 2010;31(2):107-117.

85. Venticinque S, Kashyap V, O'Connell R. Chemical burn injury secondary to intraoperative transesophageal echocardiography. *Anesth Analg.* 2003;97:1260-1261.

86. Melendez LJ, Chan KL, Cheung PK, et al. Incidence of bacteremia in transesophageal echocardiography: a prospective study of 140 consecutive patients. *J Am Coll Cardiol.* 1991;18:1650-1654.

87. Roudaut R, Lartigue MC, Texier-Maugein J, Dallocchio M. Incidence of bacteraemia or fever during transesophageal echocardiography: a prospective study of 82 patients. *Eur Heart J.* 1993;14:936-940.

88. Foster E, Kusumoto FM, Sobol SM, et al. Streptococcal endocarditis temporally related to transesophageal echocardiography. *J Am Soc Echocardiogr.* 1990;427:3424-3427.

89. Wilson W, Taubert K, Gewitz M, et al. AHA Guidelines for Prevention of Infective Endocarditis. *Circulation.* 2007;116:1736-1754.

90. Gould FK, Elliott TS, Foweraker J, et al. Guidelines for the prevention of endocarditis: report of the Working Party of the British Society for Antimicrobial Chemotherapy. *J Antimicrob Chemother.* 2006;57:1035-1042.

91. Chambers JB, Klein JL, Bennett SR, Monaghan MJ, Roxburgh JC. Is antibiotic prophylaxis ever necessary before transoesophageal echocardiography? *Heart.* 2006;92(4):435-436.

92. Sharma S, Rama P, Miller G, Coccio E, Coulter L. Systemic absorption and toxicity from topically administered lidocaine during transesophageal echocardiography. *J Am Soc Echocardiogr.* 1996;9(5):710-711.

93. Wu FL, Razzaghi A, Souney PF. Seizure after lidocaine for bronchoscopy: case report and review of the use of lidocaine in airway anesthesia. *Pharmacotherapy.* 1993;13(1):72-78.

94. Eggleston ST, Lush LW. Understanding allergic reactions to local anesthetics. *Ann Pharmacother.* 1996;30(7):851-857.

95. Kane G, Hoehn S, Behrenbeck T, Mulvagh S. Benzocaine-induced methemoglobinemia based on the Mayo Clinic experience from 28,478 transesophageal echocardiograms: incidence, outcomes, and predisposing factors. *Arch Inter Med.* 2007;167(8):1977-1982.

96. Dhawan S. Methemoglobinemia–a rare complication of transesophageal echocardiography. *Clin Cardiol.* 2009;32(6):E101.

97. Miller RD, Eriksson LI, Fleisher L, et al. eds. *Miller's Anesthesia,* 7th ed. Philadelphia, Pa: Churchill Livingstone; 2009.

98. Practice guidelines for perioperative transesophageal echocardiography. An updated report by the America Society of Anesthesiologists and the Society of Cardiovascular Anesthesiologists Task Force on Transesophageal Echocardiography. *Anesthesiology.* 2010;112:1084-1096.

29

Equipment, Infection Control, and Safety

ROBERT WILLIAMS

Introduction

Transesophageal echocardiography (TEE) systems are state-of-the-art diagnostic equipment that require a large initial investment by a hospital and are also very delicate and costly to maintain. Understanding the procurement and maintenance processes aids clinicians in vendor selection and maximizing the lifespan of this expensive equipment. TEE probes are used invasively on patients, so physicians and technical staff must practice proper infection control technique and follow safety guidelines to minimize risks of patient complications.

Capital Equipment: Funding, Selection and Procurement

Selection and procurement processes for capital medical equipment are complex and dynamic. *Capital equipment* is defined as "nonexpendable" and used to operate a business or provide a service.[1] Institutions have specific definitions in their policies for capital equipment. For example, any item costing more than $500 and/or with a useful life of more than 1 year may be considered capital. TEE systems cost more than $350,000, and prices vary with the choice of technology, probe configurations, and vendor relationships. TEE systems are hospital assets budgeted for and purchased from hospital capital funds, as opposed to being purchased by a physician group(s) within the institution. The rationale for this is that hospitals in the United States are reimbursed for capital expenditures through the federal government's insurance program (i.e., Medicare) at rates set by the Centers for Medicare and Medicaid Services (CMS) payment systems.[2] The Medicare program consists of several parts; the hospital insurance part is known as *Part A*, and the supplemental medical insurance part paying for physician services is known as *Part B*. A portion of capital expenses are reimbursed to hospitals under Medicare Part A, while physician services are reimbursed under Medicare Part B.

TEE vendor selection is best accomplished by a multidisciplinary team that includes expertise from clinicians, administrators, equipment managers, biomedical engineering, purchasing, and the legal departments. The goal of the selection process is to satisfy the needs of clinicians, while determining optimal use of scarce resources. A standard equipment purchasing process includes obtaining bids from multiple manufacturers and organizing a clinical evaluation process. Evaluation and selection of TEE equipment should follow the same process. Criteria for equipment selection include:

- Clinical/technical capabilities
- Training and educational programs offered
- Expected lifespan
- Information technology (IT) considerations
- Cost to purchase a TEE system
- Warranty, preventive maintenance, and repair terms
- Projection of all operating costs
- Quality of service and reputation of vendor

Clinicians suggest vendors for trials of their TEE systems based upon personal experience, information from professional organizations, and/or review of pertinent literature. Equipment selection should be based upon evaluation of the existing system capabilities; promised features may not become available until sometime in the future. Questions to consider regarding options for upgradeability include:

- Are upgrades accomplished by updating software?
- Will additional equipment be necessary?
- What will be the associated costs?
- What are the durability and expected lifespan of the system?

As institutions move to electronic record keeping for all components of the patient's medical record, one must evaluate the IT capabilities of the TEE equipment being considered. File management and image storage options are very important factors. TEE systems should meet digital imaging and communications in medicine (DICOM) specifications. DICOM is the standard for handling, storing, printing, and transmitting medical imaging information developed by the American College of Radiology (ACR) and the National Electrical Manufacturing Association (NEMA).[3] The capability to network wirelessly is also important. The hard drive of the TEE unit should have ample storage and user-friendly features for management of studies, including transfer to portable storage media.

Evaluating Preventive Maintenance Programs and Product Support

Quality of service and preventive maintenance costs, including TEE probe repair or replacement, are important considerations in selecting a vendor. Biomedical engineering and equipment managers are concerned with maintenance schedules and repairs. Expenses for maintenance and repair must be well understood because they are ongoing operational costs that must be forecast in the hospital's operating budget. It is prudent to examine the pros and cons of preventive maintenance agreements. Vendors may offer one plan for maintenance of the ultrasound system and another for service for the TEE probes. As noted in James Carr's white paper on TEE probe care, the majority of service calls generated for TEE systems are related to probe malfunctions because they are delicate and therefore easily damaged.[4] Service agreements for TEE probes may prove cost-effective and should be considered, particularly for large institutions with multiple systems. Vendors usually offer very attractive pricing for service agreements purchased at point of sale (POS). Replacement cost is significant and may exceed $50,000 per probe. For example, a multiple-year service agreement purchased at POS for a TEE probe may be offered at a fraction of the replacement cost. There is a high probability a probe will be damaged or require multiple repairs within the first 5 years of purchase, so this type of service agreement will minimize expenses associated with probe replacement.

Preventive maintenance programs for the ultrasound hardware should also be considered if the institution's biomedical engineering department does not have the resources or expertise to perform planned or emergent maintenance. Replacement parts such as computer hardware, knobs, keyboards, and other components are generally included in maintenance agreements. Costs associated with preventive maintenance agreements are fixed costs. This is advantageous from a budgeting standpoint and will help minimize unexpected expenses.

The quality and reliability of service from the equipment's vendor are of paramount importance. Considerations include the time frame for completing any repairs and the availability of service technicians. Robust maintenance programs will ensure minimal downtime. Questions to consider: Will loaner equipment be available when repairs are needed? What is the anticipated turnaround time for a damaged probe? A rigorous evaluation and comparison of services provided by the manufacturers being considered may be a determining factor in the equipment selection process.

Additional Considerations

Clinical practice may require additional ultrasound transducers that include pediatric TEE and superficial vascular probes, as well as transthoracic probes. Availability of these for procedures such as central line placement in patients who will also undergo TEE studies frees up less specialized ultrasound equipment for other applications.

In addition to clinical capabilities and cost, there are other factors to consider that may influence selection of a particular system. Physical space in operating rooms and procedural areas is frequently limited. The footprint of a system and its portability may be important criteria in the selection process. As examples, Figures 29-1 through 29-3 depict TEE systems from three of the industry's leading vendors: the Philips iE33 XMatrix, the Siemens ACUSON S2000, and G.E. Healthcare's Vivid-e. Photo printers or DVD recorders are options physicians may request. A complete assessment of the user's needs paired with the system's capabilities will determine required accessories.

Administrators set the budget for capital acquisitions based on available resources, and clinicians make recommendations for manufacturer selection after completing clinical evaluations. For best use of available capital resources, the number and configuration of systems to be acquired should be based on current patient volume plus anticipated growth. Financial personnel will oversee bidding strategies and evaluate payment options such as capital leasing. After the purchase has been finalized, appropriate parties will plan for equipment maintenance, schedule education for technical and clinical staff, and attend to other operational issues.

Care of the TEE System

The TEE system requires regular maintenance and care to ensure minimal downtime and repairs.[5] Responsible parties include equipment managers and technicians, biomedical engineering personnel, and clinical users. Following the manufacturer's recommendations for periodic maintenance and hospital equipment protocols for regular

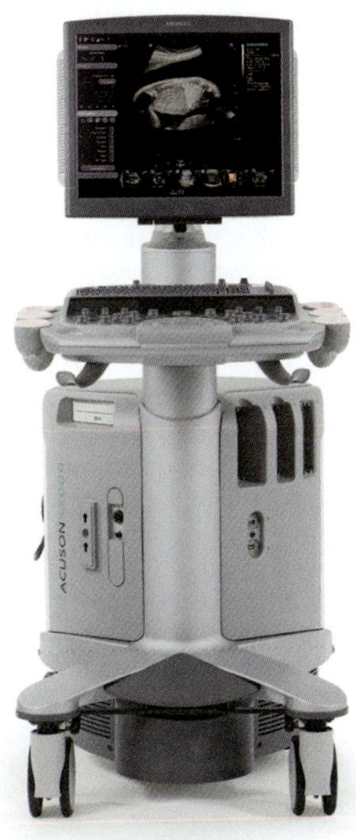

Figure 29-2 Siemens ACUSON S2000 System. *(Reproduced with permission from Siemens Healthcare, Malvern, Pa.)*

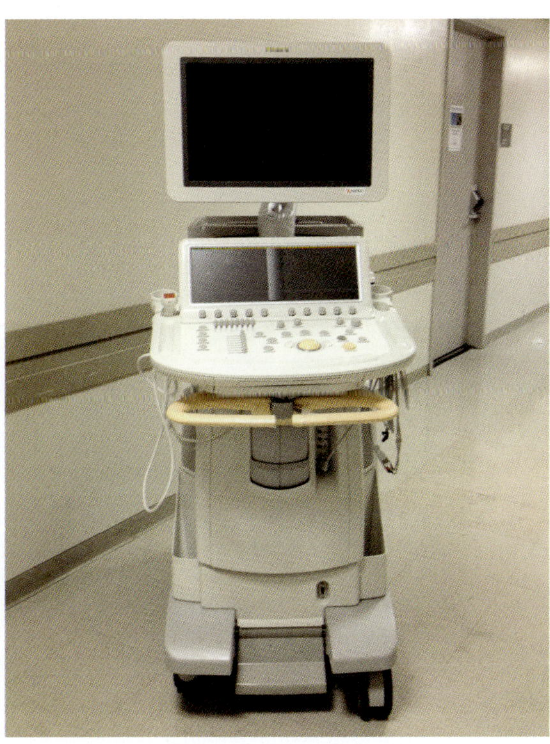

Figure 29-1 Philips iE33 xMatrix System.

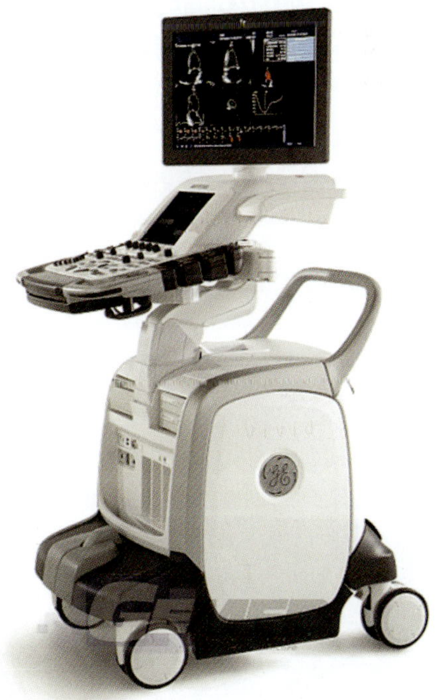

Figure 29-3 G.E. Healthcare's Vivid-e System. *(Reproduced with permission from G.E. Healthcare, Waukesha, Wis.)*

cleaning and probe care ensures minimal system downtime, extends the TEE's lifespan, and ensures continued validity of equipment warranties. Use of cleaning solutions or lubricants not recommended by the manufacturer may damage probes and void the warranty. The clinician using the system will be the first to observe any abnormalities in ultrasound image quality, as well as structural damage to the system and TEE probe. Regular equipment checks should include:

- Inspecting the control panel for broken/missing buttons and knobs
- Inspecting probe connections to the ultrasound unit
- Inspecting probes for cracks, tears, and the like
- Testing the probe's articulation mechanisms
- Monitoring the amount of memory available on the hard drive

Some TEE probes (e.g., those made by Philips) use pin connectors. Bent pin connectors cause imaging or hard drive problems (Fig. 29-4). Other systems (e.g., Siemens) use pinless connectors. Attaching soiled or wet probes may damage the ultrasound machine's computer components. The system's hard drive requires regular maintenance. Completed studies should be periodically transferred to permanent storage devices and deleted from the TEE computer's hard drive. A memory that is full may cause the system to perform slowly or even freeze during a procedure. Probes should be inspected before use to check for damage. Figure 29-5 is an example of a TEE probe with a cracked tip. Figure 29-6 shows a probe with a torn shaft. Such equipment must be removed from service as a safety precaution and then evaluated for repair by appropriate parties.

Tallefer et al. reviewed strategies to avoid TEE probe damage in the operating room.[6] Unique risk factors arise in this cramped environment where many health professionals (anesthesiologists, surgeons, nurses, perfusionists) work in a confined space. These include accidental probe exposure to fluids, impact from falls, or contact with other equipment. Attention to detail in organizing the work area and minimizing clutter are remedies.

During surgical procedures, TEE probes may remain in place for 3 to 5 hours, and damage may occur if the shaft close to the control handle remains kinked for prolonged periods. A solution for this problem is a TEE transducer holder (Fig. 29-7) designed to reduce the risk of kinking and stabilize the control handle while the probe is in use (Civco Medical Instruments, Kalona, Iowa). When not in use, probes should be stored in protective cases or dedicated cabinets, as noted in Figure 29-8. Performing the checks and system maintenance discussed in this section minimizes equipment problems, such as failure during procedures, and reduces potential damage, down time, and associated repair cost.

Infection Control Considerations

TEE studies are invasive procedures performed with reusable probes that require decontamination and disinfection between patients. Poorly executed infection control processes increase the risk of nosocomial infection. To adhere to the age-old medical tenet to "first do no harm," personnel must use proven cleaning and disinfection techniques. Nelson et al. reviewed Spaulding's clear and logical approach to disinfection and sterilization that has become the industry standard.[7] He proposed that medical devices be classified into three groups.

1. *Critical:* devices or instruments that enter normally sterile tissue or the vascular system. Endoscopic instruments and implants are examples. These devices require *sterilization*, defined as destruction of all microbial life.
2. *Semicritical:* devices that come into contact with intact mucous membranes but do not ordinarily penetrate sterile tissue. Endoscopes and laryngoscope blades are examples. Such devices require a minimum of high-level disinfection which destroys vegetative organisms, mycobacteria, viruses, fungal spores, but not all bacterial spores.
3. *Noncritical:* devices that normally do not have direct patient contact or touch only intact skin. Examples are stethoscopes or patient supply carts. These items require low-level disinfection.

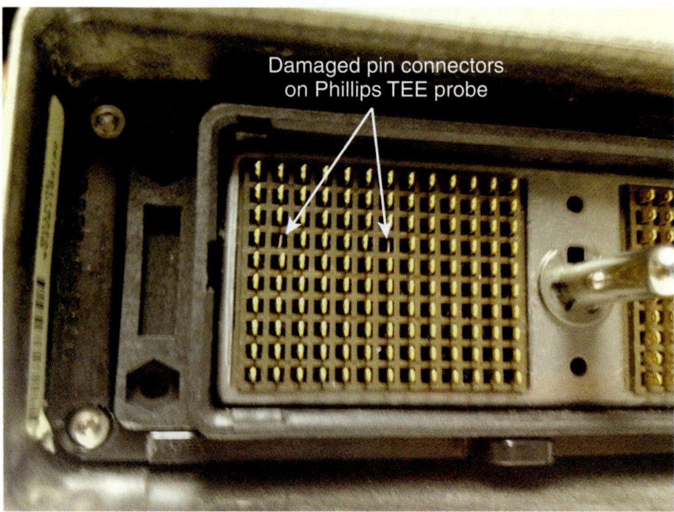

Figure 29-4 Damaged pin connectors on Philips TEE probe.

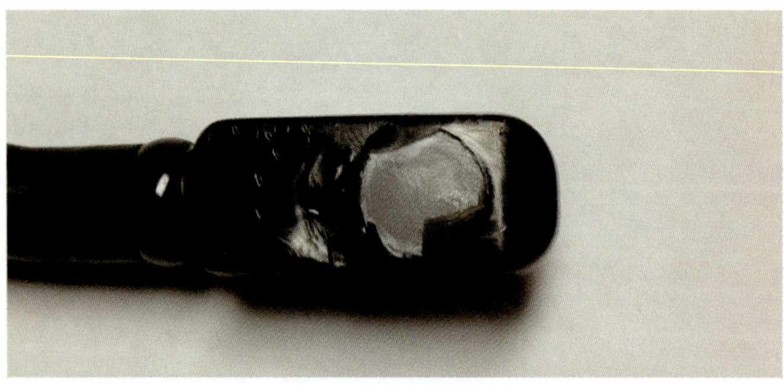

Figure 29-5 Damaged TEE probe tip.

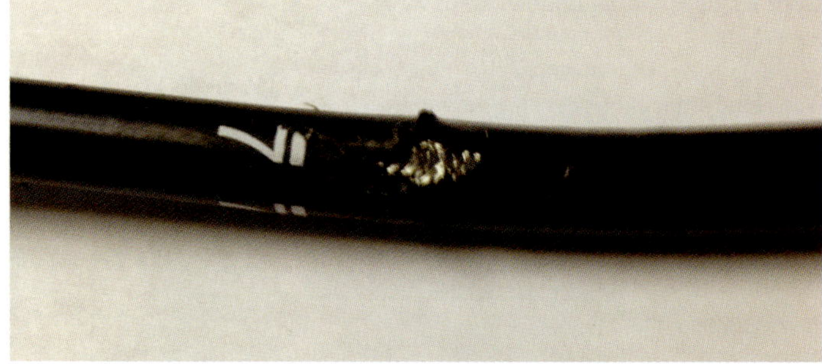

Figure 29-6 Damaged TEE shaft.

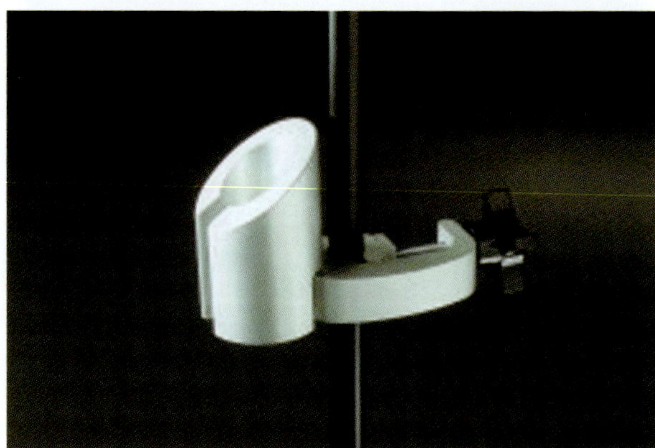

Figure 29-7 Civco TEE pole-mounted holder. *(Reproduced with permission from Civco Medical Solutions, Kalona, Iowa.)*

TEE probes fall into the semicritical device category requiring high-level disinfection. The Centers for Disease Control and Prevention (CDC) guidelines for disinfection of endoscopy equipment have been in place for many years, since many healthcare-associated infections have been traced to contaminated endoscopes.[8] The process for cleaning and disinfection of TEE probes has been adapted from these guidelines, with modifications based on the probe's structure. Unlike an endoscope, the TEE probe has no working channels. This is advantageous from a disinfection standpoint, but sections of the probe are not sealed, cannot be completely immersed in disinfecting solution, and require multiple disinfection methods.[9]

To accomplish proper high-level disinfection, three steps must be followed: clean, disinfect, and rinse. As described in the CDC guidelines, *cleaning* is removal of visible soil (e.g., organic and inorganic material) from objects and surfaces. This is normally accomplished manually using water with detergents or enzymatic products. Thorough cleaning is essential because inorganic and organic materials that remain on instrument surfaces may interfere with the effectiveness of high-level disinfection.

High-level disinfection occurs when the decontaminated instrument is completely covered in solution for a specific time period and/or temperature, depending on the disinfectant used. Unsealed portions of the TEE probe (handle, controls, and connections to the ultrasound system) cannot be submersed in solution (Fig. 29-9), so they must be wiped down with disinfectant wipes following the manufacturer's guidelines. The Association for Professionals in Infection Control and Epidemiology (APIC) recommends the following agents to achieve high level disinfection:

- Glutaraldehyde solutions
- Hydrogen peroxide
- Peracetic acid
- Peracetic acid and hydrogen peroxide mixture
- Orthophalaldehyde

Selection criteria for the best-suited chemical include recommendations from the TEE system's manufacturer and guidelines from the Occupational Safety and Health Administration (OSHA).[10] Exposure to chemical agents may pose health hazards including skin irritation, burns, occupational asthma, and irritation of the eyes and nasal mucosa. Personal protective gear such as safety goggles, plastic aprons, and respirators will protect staff from exposure. A logical choice of chemical disinfectant is one that is minimally toxic and simple to use. For example, glutaraldehyde was first approved for use in the 1960s as an alternative to the highly toxic, irritating, and carcinogenic disinfectant formaldehyde.[11] In 1999, orthophalaldehyde (OPA) was approved by the U.S. Food and Drug Administration (FDA) and offers many advantages: it requires no activation, has a shorter processing time, does not require exposure monitoring, and is not a known eye and nasal passage irritant.[12] For these reasons, OPA is widely used for manual equipment processing.

The third and final step in the manual disinfection process is rinsing. Multiple rinses using sterile or filtered water are recommended to remove residual chemicals. After drying, probes should be stored in dedicated cabinets located in a designated clean room to prevent contamination.

The APIC guidelines call for a designated utility room for equipment processing.[13] Engineering controls for decontamination rooms, such as increased ventilation exchanges or installation of specialized hoods to remove vapors, may be required depending on the chemicals used. There should be separate handwashing and utility sinks, and the utility sink must be large enough to accommodate probe cleaning and rinsing.

Manual Versus Automated Systems

Until recently, manual disinfection systems were the only option for disinfecting TEE probes. The process is labor intensive and requires significant space to accommodate separate tubs for soaking and subsequent rinses. Owing to requirements such as engineering controls, the only suitable space may be located in the institution's central processing department. Transporting soiled probes to a remote area will increase down time and the risk of damage. This practice also reduces efficient use of technical staff. With manual systems, the quality of probe cleaning and disinfection is difficult to monitor and dependent on personnel following guidelines. Chemical solutions require periodic changes and quality control testing to ensure potency of the solution. Documentation of processing is required with both manual and automated systems. Information to be recorded includes the probe's serial number, quality control testing results, time in and out of solution, and room temperature. Technicians may overlook attention to such details while multitasking in the hectic operating room environment. Proper record keeping of equipment reprocessing serves as proof of adherence to infection control standards to accrediting bodies such as The Joint Commission.[14] Inadequate record keeping is a liability to both individual practitioners and institutions in a litigious society. Publication of detailed written policies for both the clinical and technical staff is the key to a safe and functional system for probe disinfection. The staff who perform the disinfection procedures should receive ongoing education, and their competencies in these procedures should be documented.

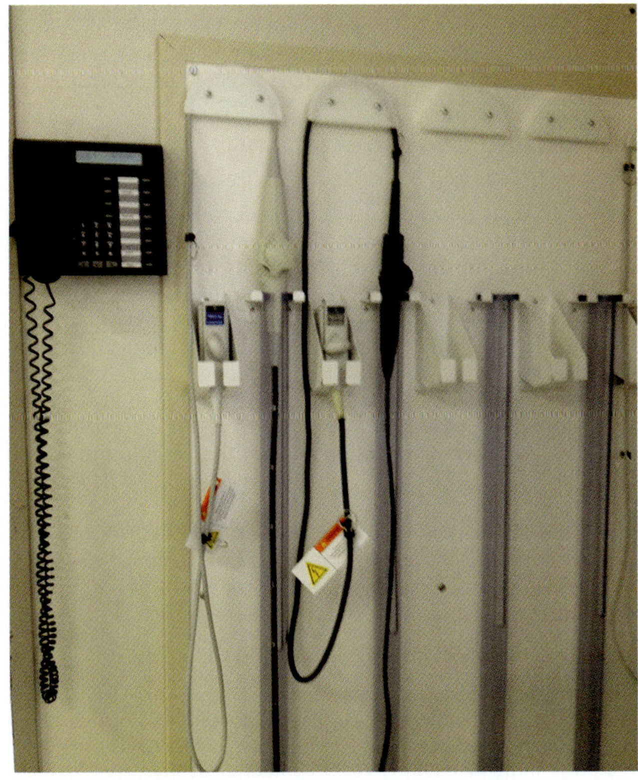

Figure 29-8 Example of proper clean TEE probe storage (PCI Medical).

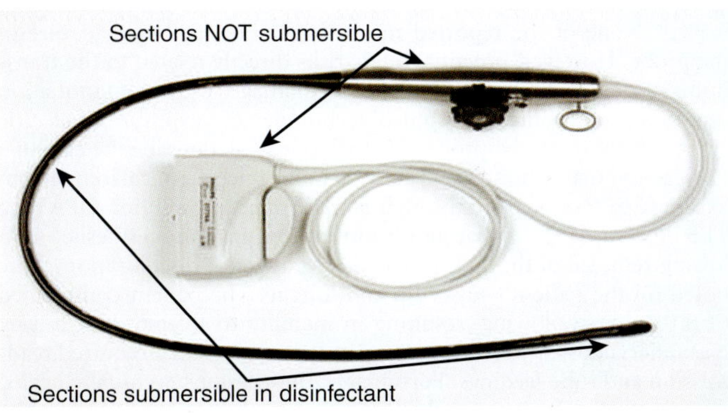

Figure 29-9 Philips TEE probe.

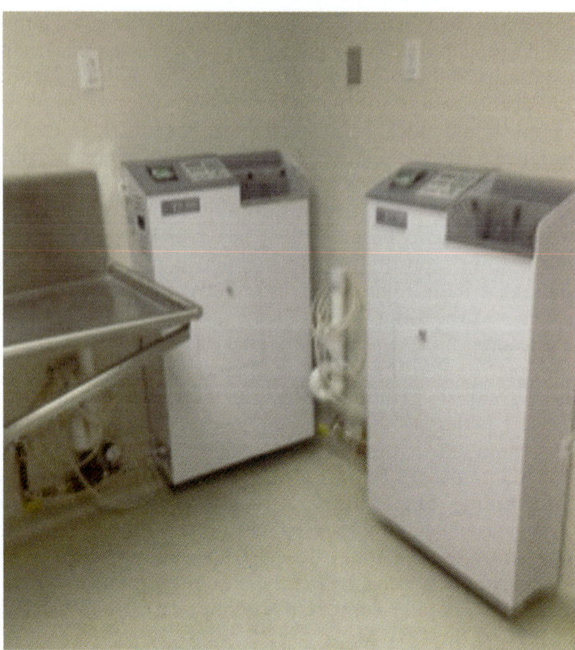

Figure 29-10 CS Medical's TD 100 Automated Processors installed in operating room utility room.

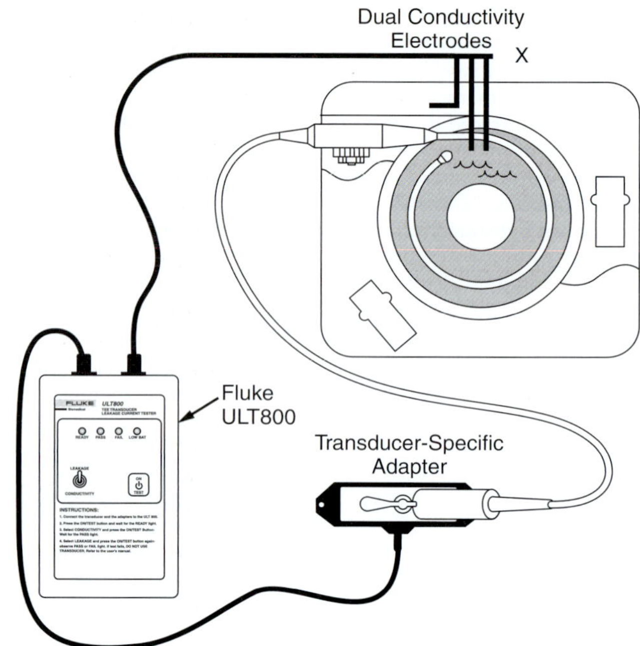

Figure 29-11 Schematic view of Fluke Medical's electrical leakage tester. *(Reproduced with permission from Fluke Biomedical, Everett, Wash.)*

Automated processors are now available to facilitate the disinfection process and streamline record keeping. The first automated TEE disinfector to become commercially available is the TD-100 (CS Medical LLC, Creedmoor, N.C.). The unit is compact and can be installed in a soiled utility room within the operating rooms (Fig. 29-10).[15] After manual cleaning, the probes are disinfected in a 17-minute cycle. The automated process eliminates the accidental prolonged disinfectant soak times that cause probe damage. High-level disinfection is achieved using a glutaraldehyde preparation packaged for single use. The container is pierced inside the machine, thereby minimizing splashes and spills. Air quality monitoring and additional engineering controls are not as stringent because this system has built-in vapor control management. During each disinfection cycle, the unit performs continuous self-diagnostic tests to confirm it is functioning properly. At the end of the cycle, the system produces documentation of processing. The printout includes date, time, disinfectant lot number, cycle status (passed, failed, or aborted), and both operator and probe identification. Printouts should be retained in a log book. These benefits may justify the capital investment of roughly $15,000 per system. Expenses for supplies should be allotted to the operating budget.

Equipment Safety

Complications related to TEE exams are rare. In a study completed in 2001, Kallmeyer et al. reported an intraoperative complication rate of 0.5%.[16] None of the reported morbidities were attributed to care of the probe. However, potential safety risks directly related to the transducer do exist. They include mucosal damage, cross-contamination due to improper infection control technique, and exposure to electric current from damaged probes. Venticinque et al. describe the case of a 72-year-old man who suffered aero-digestive tract chemical injury from exposure to residue from the high-level disinfectant solution OPA on a TEE probe used for cardiac monitoring during general anesthesia.[17] Following removal of the TEE probe, dark gray/black discolorations were noted on the patient's lower lip and tongue. The patient complained of difficulty swallowing, resulting in inability to tolerate oral intake. Nasopharyngoscopy revealed burns and ulcerations that required readmission and tube feedings. Fortunately, these lesions eventually healed after treatment. In this case, the clinicians noted that the normally white depth markers on the TEE probe were stained blue, the same color as

OPA. The manufacturer, Advanced Sterilization Products, recommends three sequential 1-minute immersions in sterile water to rinse the TEE after manual soaking.[18] This case report underscores the importance of following proper infection control technique and the manufacturer's recommendations. In 2006, the Los Angeles County Department of Public Health and Acute Communicable Disease Control investigated an outbreak of *Escherichia coli*, finding positive blood or sputum cultures in nine patients 1 to 4 days after cardiac surgery.[19] They attributed the outbreak to the TEE probe, which tested positive for *E. coli* even after disinfection. Visual inspection revealed cracks on the probe's tip. As discussed earlier, regular inspection of the TEE probe will alert users to obvious damage such as cracks, abrasions, or tears that may harbor dangerous contaminants such as bacteria or chemical disinfectants.

Electrical Leakage Testing

A tiny hole or crack that goes unnoticed can put the next patient at risk for exposure to increased levels of electrical current leakage. To check for leaks from damage that is not clearly visible, the American Society of Echocardiography recommends periodic electrical leak testing.[20] A failed leakage test identifies breaches in the probe's coating or insulation that may not be detected on visual inspection. This process differs from the routine electrical safety testing performed on equipment by biomedical engineers. The test measures the TEE probe's electric current leakage (I) or its impedance (R) while it is not connected to the ultrasound system. Leakage is determined by comparing the impedance of the probe while immersed in a solution such as OPA with the impedance of the solution itself. It is based on Ohm's law, which states that voltage (V) equals current (I) multiplied by impedance (R), or V = IR. Erwine et al. reviewed how Ohm's law is applied to calculate the TEE probe's electrical leakage current.[21] By defining Vs as the test instrument's voltage, Rb as the disinfecting bath's resistance, and Rt as the transducer's insulation barrier resistance, the formula to measure leakage becomes:

$$I = Vs/(Rb + Rt), \text{ or } I = 120/(Rb + Rt)$$

I is inversely related to Rt, such that I is large when Rt is small. A failed test occurs when leakage surpasses a threshold. For example, the ULT2000 analyzer discussed by Erwine et al. has 100 microamps as the upper limit of normal. Figure 29-11 shows the arrangement of the UTL 2000 system, which can be configured with a printer to document leak testing. The probe manufacturer's recommendations must be followed in selecting a leak testing device and testing frequency. Probes that fail the leak test must be removed from service and sent for repair.

Summary

This chapter presents the challenges related to TEE equipment, including an overview of the hospital capital procurement process, analysis of criteria for equipment selection, evaluation of preventive maintenance programs, and methods to take best care of this very expensive diagnostic tool. Strict adherence to infection control practice helps minimize hospital-acquired infections related to inadequate equipment processing. Following the safety recommendations discussed serves a dual purpose: early identification of probe damage and, most importantly, minimizing patient complications and injury.

REFERENCES

1. Hofman E, Maucher D, Hornstein J, Den Ouden R. *Capital Equipment Purchasing: Optimizing the Total Cost of CapEx Sourcing.* Berlin: Springer; 20127–12.
2. Department of Health and Human Services, Centers for Medicare & Medicaid Services. Acute Care Hospital Inpatient Prospective Payment System. *ICN.* Feb 2012;006815.
3. Bigood W, Horii S. PACS Mini Refresher Course, Introduction to the ACR-NEMA DICOM Standard. *Radiographics.* March 1992:345-355.
4. Carr J. On the Proper Care of a Transesophageal Probe. *Sonora Medical Systems.* 2009:Longmont CO.
5. Philips Electronics Technical Publication 4535 61309821 re A. iE33 Ultrasound System. Getting Started Manual. 261-268.
6. Taillefer J, Couture P, Sheridan P, et al. A Comprehensive Strategy to Avoid Trans-esophageal Echocardiography Probe Damage. *Can J Anesth.* May 2002;49(5):500-502.
7. Nelson D, Jarvis R, Rutala W, et al. Multi-society Guideline for Reprocessing Flexible Gastrointestinal Endoscopes. *Infection Control and Hospital Epidemiology.* July 2003:535-535.
8. Rutala W, Weber D, et al. Guideline for Disinfection and Sterilization in Healthcare Facilities, 2008. *Centers for Disease Control and Prevention.* 2008:13-17.
9. Kangala P, Bradley C, Hoffman P, Steeds RP. Guidelines for Transoesophageal Echocardiographic Probe Cleaning and Disinfection form the British Society of Echocardiography. *Eur J Echocardiogr.* 2011(12):i17-i23.
10. U.S. Department of Labor. Occupational Safety and Health Administration. Best Practices for the Safe Use of Glutaraldehyde in Health Care. *OSHA 3258-08N.* 2006:6-30.
11. Stonehill AA, Drop S, Borick PM. Buffered glutaraldehyde–a new chemical sterilizing solution. *Am J Hosp Pharm.* 1963;20:459-465.
12. Rutala W, Weber D. New disinfection and sterilization methods. *Emerg Infect Dis.* 2001;7(2):348-353.
13. Alvarado C, Reicheldefer M. APIC Guideline for Infection Prevention and Control in Flexible Endoscopy. *AJIC Am J Infect Control.* 2000;28:138-155.
14. *The Joint Commission Hospital Accreditation Standards.* Oakbrook, IL: Joint Commission; 2012.
15. C S Medical LLD publication 200486revE. Td-100 TEE Ultrasound Probe Disinfector Operator's Manual.
16. Kallmeyer IJ, Collard CD, Fox JA, et al. The safety of intraoperative transesophageal echocardiography: a case series of 7200 cardiac surgical patients. *Anesth Analg.* 2001;92:1126-1130.
17. Venticinque SG, Kashyap VS, O'Connell RJ. Chemical burn injury secondary to intraoperative transesophageal echocardiography. *Anesth Analg.* 2003;97:1260-1261.
18. Advanced Sterilization Products, Johnson & Johnson Irvine, CA. Cidex OPA High Level Disinfection Solution: Technical Information LC-20390-008 Rev. C: 2004.
19. 2006 Special Studies Report. Transesophageal Echocardiography, Insufficient Cleaning Practices, Lax Equipment Maintenance and Escherichia coli–A Breakdown in Infection Control. Acute Communicable Disease Control Program. Los Angeles Department of Public Health Acute Communicable Disease Control Program: 27-34.
20. Mathew JP, Glas K, Troianos CA, et al. American Society of Echocardiography/Society of Cardiovascular Anesthesiologists recommendations and guidelines for continuous quality improvement in perioperative echocardiography. *J Am Soc Echocardiogr.* 2006;19:1303-1313.
21. Erwine MR. *Are your TEE and Other Types of Invasive" Ultrasound Transducers Safe? BC Group International.* St. Charles: MO; 2009.

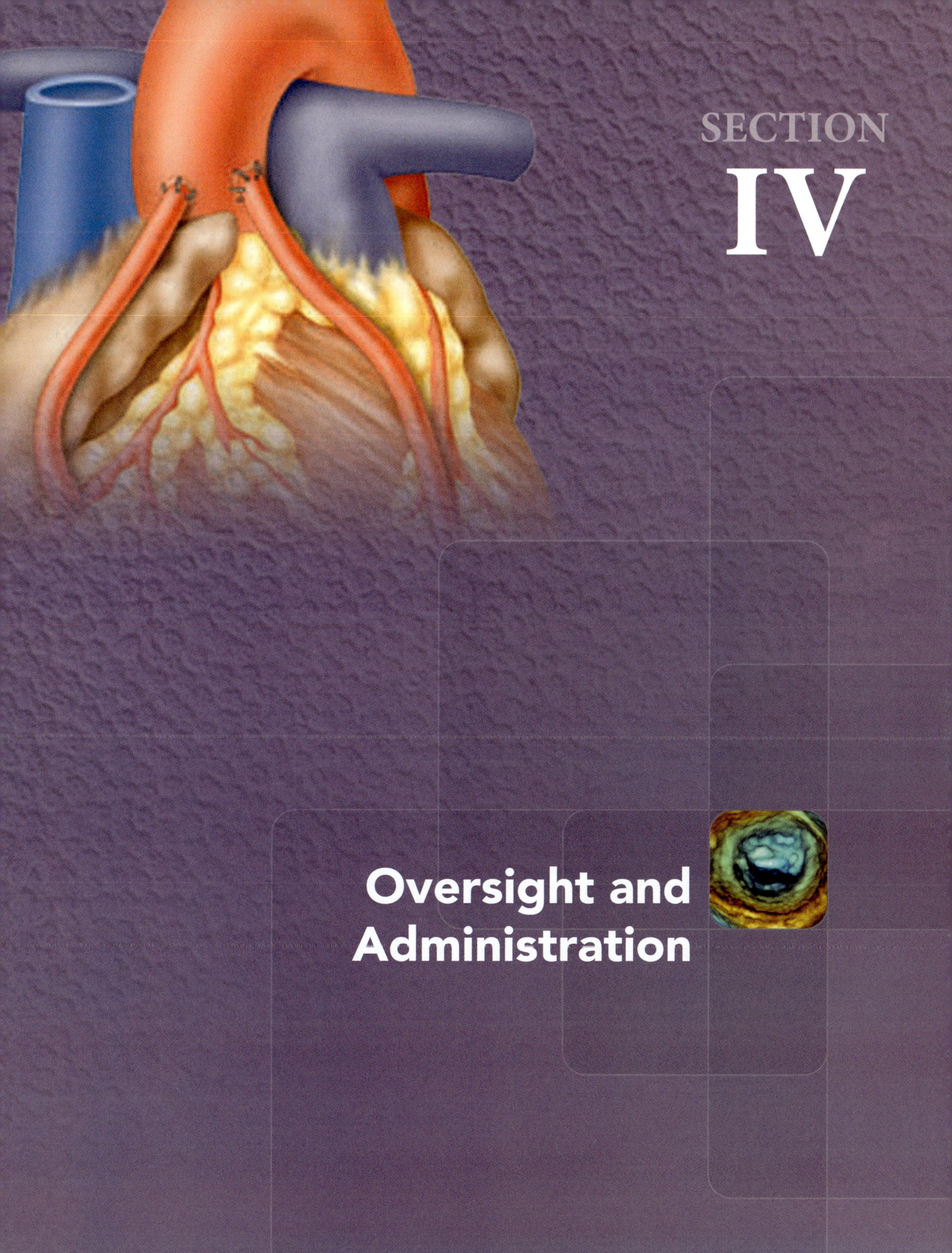
SECTION
IV
Oversight and
Administration

Training and Certification for Transesophageal Echocardiography

W. BRIT SMITH | GREGORY M. JANELLE

The past several decades have seen a surge in ultrasonography use in the field of anesthesiology.[1] Anesthesiologists have increasingly used ultrasound for central venous cannulation and peripheral nerve blockade, which has resulted in increased efficacy and patient safety.[2,3] Use of echocardiography has grown in both the operating room (OR) and intensive care unit (ICU).[4,5] Transesophageal echocardiography (TEE) has transitioned from an adjunctive tool to a required piece of equipment, with utilization by anesthesiologists for perioperative management, and by surgeons for appropriate planning and postprocedure evaluation.[6] Indeed, TEE has become a standard of care for certain cardiac surgical procedures, such as mitral valve repair and transcatheter aortic valve replacement. With increasing use of TEE in the perioperative period, the certification process was developed to ensure that practitioners utilizing this tool are appropriately competent to adequately perform an examination and interpret the findings.

Historical Perspective in the United States

In 1993, the American Society of Anesthesiology (ASA) and the Society of Cardiovascular Anesthesiologists (SCA) created an Ad Hoc Task Force on Practice Parameters for Transesophageal Echocardiography to establish guidelines for the use of TEE in the OR.[7] Beyond recommendations for intraoperative use, the task force also evaluated training guidelines.[8] Previously, the establishment of guidelines for TEE had been developed primarily for cardiologists, while acknowledging the utility of TEE for anesthesiologists regarding intraoperative decision making.[9] The ASA/SCA task force acknowledged that many anesthesiologists used TEE primarily for monitoring and treatment decisions, whereas others used it for diagnostic purposes. It was also recognized that the training and knowledge required for certification varied across institutions.[8] As a result, the American Society of Echocardiography (ASE) and SCA created a task force to establish requisite knowledge and training requirements for individuals seeking to become certified in perioperative TEE.[7] The initial recommendation was published jointly in 1999 by the SCA and ASE (and updated in 2002) regarding the performance of a comprehensive intraoperative TEE.[10,11]

The ASE first developed and administered formal testing of echocardiography for cardiologists (although open to other specialties) in 1996 as the Examination of Special Competence in Adult Echocardiography (ASEeXAM). The SCA independently administered a test of perioperative TEE knowledge in 1998, referred to as the *PTExAM*. With establishment of the National Board of Echocardiography (NBE) through a joint venture between the SCA and ASE, a governing body for testing and certification in echocardiography was formed.[7] Guidelines were established for certification of required knowledge and experience. The first physician TEE certification by the NBE occurred in 2004, with certification lasting for 10 years from the date the knowledge test was passed. A recertification examination (and requirements for qualification) was subsequently developed for those individuals wishing to remain certified in perioperative TEE. Recertification must be undertaken within 8 to 10 years of initial certification and mandates documentation of continued experience in performing and interpreting

perioperative TEE examinations. As of mid 2013, 3310 clinicians currently have Testamur status after having passed the Advanced PTE examination, and 1897 have completed the formal certification process and become Diplomates. Of the latter, 539 have been recertified after 10 years of using TEE in clinical practice (written communication, May 27, 2013, National Board of Echocardiography).

Initially, certification was for advanced TEE clinicians who used the modality primarily for cardiac surgical cases. The utility of perioperative TEE in more than just the realm of cardiac anesthesia led to development of an alternative route for individuals to demonstrate sufficient knowledge in performing a basic examination and using the TEE-derived information to help guide treatment and intraoperative monitoring. The ASA requested that the NBE establish training and certification guidelines for individuals who use TEE in their regular practice, though not necessarily as frequently or to the same degree of diagnostic utilization as advanced PTE diplomats. This led to the first administration of the Basic PTEeXAM in 2010, and development of a certification route for individuals who use TEE in their practice for treatment decisions, but not necessarily for diagnostic purposes. Two hundred and nineteen individuals have passed the Basic PTE examination offered by the NBE since 2010. Seventy-two individuals have completed the formal certification process, of these 57 passed the Basic PTEeXAM, and 15 applicants passed the Advanced PTEeXAM prior to initiating the certification process (written communication, May 27, 2013, National Board of Echocardiography).

Certification

According to the NBE, the stated purpose of TEE certification is fivefold.[12]

- Establish domain of the practice of echocardiography for the purpose of certification.
- Assess the level of knowledge demonstrated by a licensed physician practitioner of echocardiography in a valid manner.
- Enhance the quality of echocardiography and individual professional growth in echocardiography.
- Formally recognize individuals who satisfy the requirements set by the NBE.
- Serve the public by encouraging quality patient care in the practice of echocardiography.

The NBE is the certifying body of echocardiography in several different clinical arenas, including transthoracic echocardiography (TTE), TEE, stress echocardiography, advanced perioperative TEE, and basic perioperative TEE. The NBE board of directors is a multidisciplinary team primarily composed of anesthesiologists and cardiologists.

Physicians wishing to gain certification in perioperative TEE have two options with different levels of training required to attain it. Once certification is attained, they are considered "Diplomates" in TEE.

Basic Certification

According to the NBE, the defined scope of practice for individuals requesting certification in basic TEE is limited to nondiagnostic monitoring within the customary practice of anesthesiology. Although

---

BOX 30-1. PERIOPERATIVE TRANSESOPHAGEAL ECHOCARDIOGRAPHY CERTIFICATION REQUIREMENTS FROM THE NATIONAL BOARD OF ECHOCARDIOGRAPHY

Basic PTE Certification Requirements
- Current unrestricted license to practice medicine
- Board certification in anesthesiology
- Passing the Basic PTEeXAM
- Completed application
- Application fee
- Training in basic perioperative TEE (two pathways are available)
  - *Supervised training pathway:*
    - 150 basic perioperative TEE examinations, of which:
      - 50 basic intraoperative TEE examinations must be personally performed
      - Examinations not personally performed must be reviewed at the institution where the applicant has done his/her 50 personally performed examinations
    - Supervised training must be obtained from an ACGME-accredited or other national agency-accredited anesthesiology residency program, and must be accomplished within a 4-year period of time or less
  - *Practice experience pathway:*
    - At least 150 basic intraoperative TEE examinations within 4 consecutive years immediately preceding application, with no less than 25 in any given year
    - At least 40 hours of AMA category 1 CME devoted to perioperative TEE during time the physician is acquiring the requisite clinical experience in TEE

Advanced PTE Certification Requirements
- Current unrestricted license to practice medicine
- Board certification in an American Board of Medical Specialties, Advisory Board for Osteopathic Specialties, the American Association of Physician Specialists, or Royal College of Physicians and Surgeons of Canada
- Passing the Advanced PTEeXAM
- Completed application
- Application fee
- Training/experience in perioperative care of surgical patients with cardiovascular disease
  - *Fellowship pathway:*
    - Copy of certificate of successful completion of fellowship training (minimum 12 months) dedicated to the perioperative care of surgical patients with cardiovascular disease

- Specific training in advanced TEE under supervision with 300 completed examinations, of which:
  - 150 examinations must be personally performed, interpreted, and reported
  - Non–personally performed examinations must be completed with a supervising physician present for all critical aspects of procedure
  - Examinations done during core residency do not count toward required numbers
- *Practice experience pathway:*
  - Minimum 24 months of clinical experience dedicated to perioperative care of surgical patients with cardiovascular disease, including care personally delivered by applicant to a minimum of 150 patients with cardiovascular disease per year in each of the 2 years preceding application. This pathway is only valid for those who completed an ACGME residency prior to June 30, 2009.
  - Minimum of 300 comprehensive perioperative TEEs within 4 consecutive years, with no less than 50 in any year, which must occur within 10 years preceding the application
    - At least 150 examinations must be intraoperative
    - Must complete an average of 50 examinations for the 4 years preceding application
    - Minimum of 50 hours of AMA category 1 CME devoted to echocardiography obtained during the time the physician is acquiring the required TEE examinations

Recertification in PTE Requirements
- Passing the RePTE
- Must be board certified by the NBE in perioperative TEE
- Current unrestricted license to practice medicine
- Continued maintenance of skills in echocardiography
  - Applicant must have performed and interpreted at least 50 perioperative TEEs per year in 2 of the 3 years preceding application
  - Must have completed 15 hours of AMA category I CME devoted to echocardiography obtained during the 3 years preceding application

ACGME, Accreditation Council for Graduate Medical Education; *AMA,* American Medical Association; *CME,* continuing medical education; *NBE,* National Board of Echocardiography; *PTE,* perioperative transesophageal echocardiography; *TEE,* transesophageal echocardiography.
Adapted from National Board of Echocardiography: http://www.echoboards.org.[17,18,20]

---

diagnoses may be made in emergent situations, findings should be confirmed by an individual with advanced skills in TEE or by other appropriate methods. The areas of anesthesia practice in which TEE is used extensively for treatment decisions include liver transplantation, critical care, and noncardiac surgery in selected operative patients.[13-17] Box 30-1 lists NBE certification requirements.[12]

Advanced Certification

The purpose of advanced perioperative TEE (see Box 30-1)[18] is to utilize the full diagnostic potential of perioperative TEE, including directing perioperative decision making. An anesthesiologist with advanced certification should be able to use the full extent of TEE for diagnostic purposes and aid in surgical planning/assessments, while also being able to formulate treatment plans in real time, based on the echocardiogram. Advanced certification is not exclusively available to cardiac anesthesiologists, but the majority of applicants are from the field of anesthesiology, and maintaining the skills and required perioperative experience for recertification may be difficult for individuals not actively involved in cardiac anesthesiology practice.

The Accreditation Council for Graduate Medical Education (ACGME) did not provide accreditation for fellowship training in adult cardiothoracic anesthesiology until 2007. Completion of advanced perioperative echocardiography education is required during this 1-year fellowship,[19] allowing eligibility for NBE certification once the fellowship is completed and the trainee has passed the PTEeXAM. There is no subspecialty certification in cardiothoracic anesthesiology; however, the prospect of future certification is currently under development.

The fellowship pathway for advanced TEE certification does not specify that training must be accomplished via a cardiothoracic anesthesiology fellowship, but it does require the physician to obtain ACGME fellowship training in the perioperative care of surgical patients with cardiovascular disease. Physicians with critical care fellowship training are currently accepted for advanced TEE certification with the understanding that they must still fulfill all practical requirements.

Because advanced TEE certification was introduced after many anesthesiologists had already incorporated TEE into their practice for years, it was deemed necessary to allow the "grandfathering" of individuals who would not be able to satisfy the current requirements for new trainees. The decision was made to limit advanced TEE certification to (1) only individuals who were fellowship trained in the perioperative care of individuals with cardiac disease and/or (2) those who had completed an ACGME anesthesiology residency prior to June 30, 2009, and satisfied a requisite number of intraoperative TEE examinations and continuing medical education in echocardiography.

Recertification

To maintain their status with the NBE, the recertification examination can be taken by those with "Testamur" status (description follows) and Diplomates of the NBE in their ninth, tenth, or eleventh year surrounding their 10-year anniversary. The requirements to remain certified in TEE are found in Box 30-1.[20]

Testamur Status

A "Testamur" is an individual who has successfully passed the examination of special competence in TEE, but has not supplied the required documentation for certification. Despite a Testamur having displayed adequate knowledge of TEE by passing the PTEeXAM, they are not considered certified in advanced or basic TEE until they have provided proof of their personal TEE experience as required for advanced or basic certification. Individuals who are in the certification process and awaiting approval of their performance-based criteria hold Testamur status until official approval of certification is granted (i.e., Diplomate status).

Certification Outside the United States

In Europe, there has been a collaboration of the European Association of Echocardiography (EAE) and the European Association of Cardiothoracic Anesthesiologists (EACTA) to establish TEE certification. Examination and certification has been carried out by the EAE since 2005, and the stated benefits of TEE certification are as follows:[21]

- *The goals of certification are to protect patients from undergoing transesophageal echocardiographic examinations performed by unqualified persons and to set a European standard for competency and excellence in this field.*
- *Certification in TEE should bring credibility and professional legitimacy to an individual by demonstrating his/her competency getting this certification.*
- *The certification process will identify qualified practitioners of transthoracic echocardiography and should enhance their professional image.*
- *European Certification is designed to test the competency of an individual to be able to perform, interpret, and report routine transesophageal echocardiographic studies unsupervised.*
- *Certification in TEE is not a compulsory or regulatory certificate of competence or excellence. Individuals' rights to report and sign clinical studies in individual countries remain to be defined by National laws and regulations.*
- *Sonographers (technicians) and doctors of all disciplines can apply for certification in TEE.*

The certification process involves two components: (1) a "theoretical" part given as a computer-based written examination and (2) a "practical" part that requires candidates to submit an electronic logbook of 125 personally performed clinical cases (or 75 if already holding certification in TEE). Certification is valid for 5 years, with application for recertification possible after attaining the requisite number of CME credits and maintaining a log of TEEs performed, with a minimum of 50 per year. Currently, certification is held by individuals in multiple countries throughout Europe and the United Kingdom.

The British Society of Echocardiography (BSE) and the Association of Cardiothoracic Anesthetists (ACTA) have also created a joint venture by which individuals may attain TEE certification. The ACTA and BSE recognized developments by the SCA and ASE in establishing certification methods and in 2003 issued a statement regarding the need for developing a certification pathway.[22] Currently, testing is offered yearly, and the process of certification remains under development.

The Australian and New Zealand College of Anaesthetists (ANZCA) does not offer formal certification, but this organization has established recommended training for individuals interested in the practice of TEE.[23]

Why Become Certified?

Beyond the listed goals of the NBE, there are several reasons why individuals should become certified. Certification implies an understanding of an established knowledge base and practical experience. Inter-user variability may be eliminated by ensuring that individuals have mastered TEE, both in performing the examination and interpreting the echocardiogram. Once an echocardiogram has been recorded, anyone with sufficient training should, ideally, be able to review the examination and arrive at the same conclusions as another certified independent practitioner. By ensuring that individuals have the necessary tools to perform and interpret examinations, the ultimate goal of optimizing patient care is attainable.

Credentialing for performing TEE is an institution-dependent decision. An absolute requirement of certification for practitioners who need to use TEE in emergent situations (e.g., cardiac arrest) may not be optimal. Nevertheless, anyone routinely using TEE in their practice could potentially benefit from certification, which would ensure optimal patient care.

It is worth noting that third-party payers in the United States do not differentiate between those certified in TEE and those without certification for payment or reimbursement of TEE-related services.

Barriers to Certification

The requirements for certification set forth by the NBE are potentially unattainable by some physicians, owing to practice limitations; in some cases, a leave of absence would be required to attain the appropriate experience. The absolute number of examinations required for certification, especially for those in the experience pathway, can be limiting. The ability to perform 150 TEE examinations to establish initial certification or 50 examinations a year to maintain certification could restrict participation or diminish interest in establishing or maintaining certification. Even in a high-volume cardiac surgical center, if the work is evenly distributed among multiple cardiac anesthesiologists, it may be difficult to attain the requisite numbers for advanced certification, and noncardiac anesthesiologists may simply not have the opportunity to establish their presence in the cardiovascular OR.

Future of Training/Certification

TEE certification is a fairly new option for physicians. As the requirements for certification evolve and diverse training modalities are being developed, different opportunities for gaining TEE experience may evolve without necessitating direct patient/physician contact. Recently TTE/TEE simulation has been developed and is commercially available (e.g., the HeartWorks Mannikin Simulator, Inventive Medical Ltd., London, England) for use as an adjunct to training. Although the risk to patients from TEE is low,[24] minimizing risks by limiting multiple inexperienced hands on TEE probes could lead to increased utilization of simulation. Simulation may also provide opportunities for certification or maintaining certification for individuals who are unable to attain the requisite number of examinations for initial certification or recertification.

Outside the realm of perioperative TEE, the clinical applications of ultrasound and cardiac ultrasound continue to grow. In many emergency rooms, ICUs, ORs, and inpatient wards, bedside limited echocardiography (BLE) and focused cardiac ultrasound (FCU) continue to gain popularity as a rapid method of assessing unstable patients and patients admitted with heart failure.[25] Effective monitoring of cardiovascular function in conditions such as cardiac arrest or near-arrest is crucial for guiding successful resuscitative efforts. As such, TEE has emerged as one of the preferred cardiac diagnostic and monitoring modalities in these situations; it is less invasive than many other modalities, is immediately accessible, and allows for continuous real-time monitoring of cardiac function. Multiple case reports and case series have demonstrated the benefits of TEE-guided clinical decision making during high-risk procedures and in various emergent clinical scenarios.[26-33]

Although Advanced Circulatory Life Support (ACLS) guidelines are designed to accommodate rescuers with and without advanced medical training, they contain no recommendations for routine use of TEE during cardiopulmonary resuscitation. Similarly, the recently described anesthesiology-specific ACLS (A-ACLS) guidelines do not incorporate TEE into the routine algorithms, despite being designed for medical specialists,[33] although TEE and TTE are frequently utilized for perioperative arrest scenarios at many institutions.

The requisites for certification in basic perioperative TEE remain significantly more arduous than standards for training in multiple other specialties. For example, for established emergency medicine physicians, the training guidelines—as defined by a joint publication from the American College of Emergency Physicians and the American Society of Echocardiography[34]—recommend a 2- or 3-day course to cover all 11 applications of medical ultrasound, with 6 to 8 hours of a skills laboratory and no standardized testing. For a single application course, such as cardiac ultrasound, 3 to 4 hours of didactics are deemed sufficient, with 2 to 4 hours of laboratory training.[34] Similar programs have been adapted for training in trauma surgery fellowships, and the use of miniaturized TEE systems has been proposed for serial monitoring of unstable postsurgical patients.[35,36] Additionally, the American College of Chest Physicians (ACCP) offers 3-day courses for an ACCP Certificate of Completion Critical Care Ultrasonography Program[37] following completion of an online portfolio and passing a final test administered at the annual CHEST conference.

Transesophageal echocardiography appears on both the content outline for the American Board of Anesthesiology (ABA) In-Training Examination[38] and the key words list for the ABA Maintenance of Certification Examination.[39] Proficiency in placement and interpretation of invasive hemodynamic monitors (e.g., pulmonary artery catheters) is presumed by most hospital credentialing committees as part of applicants' ABA board eligibility or certification, despite the absence of objective measurements of competency specific to these monitors. It remains to be seen whether or not specific TEE-related education (and passage of tests for competence in these modules) will be mandated by the ABA for training requirements in accredited anesthesiology residency programs or for maintenance of certification. Like invasive hemodynamic monitoring, skills for hemodynamic TEE assessment could simply be presumed upon completion.

REFERENCES

1. Bennett S. Training guidelines for ultrasound: worldwide trends. *Best Pract Res Clin Anaesthesiol.* 2009;23(3):363-373.
2. Bailey PL, Glance LG, Eaton MP, Parshall B, McIntosh S. A survey of the use of ultrasound during central venous catheterization. *Anesth Analg.* 2007;104(3):491-497.
3. Abrahams MS, Aziz MF, Fu RF, Horn JL. Ultrasound guidance compared with electrical neurostimulation for peripheral nerve block: a systematic review and meta-analysis of randomized controlled trials. *Br J Anaesth.* 2009;102:408-417.
4. Poterack KA. Who uses transesophageal echocardiography in the operating room? *Anesth Analg.* 1995;80(3):454-458.
5. Field LC, Guldan III GJ, Finley AC. Echocardiography in the intensive care unit. *Semin Cardiothoracic Vasc Anesth.* 2011;15(1-2):25-39.
6. American Society of Anesthesiologists and Society of Cardiovascular Anesthesiologists Task Force on Transesophageal Echocardiography. Practice guidelines for perioperative transesophageal echocardiography. *Anesthesiology.* 2010;112(5):1084-1096.
7. Practice guidelines for perioperative transesophageal echocardiography. A report by the American Society of Anesthesiologists and the Society of Cardiovascular Anesthesiologists Task Force on Transesophageal Echocardiography. *Anesthesiology.* 1996;84(4):986-1006.
8. Pearlman AS, Gardin JM, Martin RP, Parisi AF, Popp RL, Quinones MA, Stevenson JG, Schiller NB, Seward JB, Stewart WJ. Guidelines for physician training in transesophageal echocardiography: recommendation of the American Society of Echocardiography Committee for Physician Training in Echocardiography. *J Am Soc Echocardiogr.* 1992;5(2):187-194.
9. Aronson S, Thys DM. Training and certification in perioperative transesophageal echocardiography: a historical perspective. *Anesth Analg.* 2001;93(6):1422-1427.
10. Shanewise JS, Cheung AT, Aronson S, Stewart WJ, Weiss RL, Mark JB, Savage RM, Sears-Rogan P, Matthew JP, Quinones MA, Cahalan MK, Savino JS. ASE/SCA guidelines for performing a comprehensive intraoperative multiplane transesophageal echocardiography examination: recommendations of the American Society of Echocardiography Council for Intraoperative Echocardiography and the Society of Cardiovascular Anesthesiologists Task Force for Certification in Perioperative Transesophageal Echocardiography. *Anesth Analg.* 1999;89(4):870-884.
11. Cahalan MK, Abel A, Goldman M, Pearlman A, Sears-Rogan P, Russell I, Shanewise J, Stewart W, Troianos C. ASE, SCA. American Society of Echocardiography and Society of Cardiovascular Anesthesiologists Task Force Guidelines for Training in Perioperative Echocardiography. *Anesth Analg.* 2002;94(6):1384-1388.
12. Burtenshaw AJ, Isaac JL. The role of trans-oesophageal echocardiography for perioperative cardiovascular monitoring during orthotopic liver transplantation. *Liver Transpl.* 2006;12(11):1577-1583.
13. Wax DB, Torres A, Scher C, Leibowitz AB. Transesophageal echocardiography utilization in high-volume liver transplantation centers in the United States. *J Cardiothorac Vasc Anesth.* 2008;22(6):811-813.
14. Hüttemann E. Transoesophageal echocardiography in critical care. *Minerva Anestesiol.* 2006;72(11):891-913.
15. Colreavy FB, Donovan K, Lee KY, Weekes J. Transoesophageal echocardiography in critically ill patients. *Crit Care Med.* 2002;30(5):989-996.
16. Mahmood F, Christie A, Matyal R. Transesophageal echocardiography and noncardiac surgery. *Semin Cardiothorac Vasc Anesth.* 2008;12(4):265-289.
17. National Board of Echocardiography. Basic PTEeXAMhttp://www.echoboards.org/content/basic-pteexam: Accessed January 29, 2012.
18. National Board of Echocardiography. Advanced PTEeXAM Certificationhttp://www.echoboards.org/content/advanced-pteexam-certification: Accessed January 29, 2012.
19. ACGME Program Requirements for Graduate Medical Education in Adult Cardiothoracic Anesthesiology:Available at http://www.acgme.org/acWebsite/downloads/RRC_progReq/041pr206.pdf: Accessed May 21, 2012.
20. National Board of Echocardiography. RePTE Certificationhttp://www.echoboards.org/content/repte-certification: Accessed January 29, 2012.
21. European Society of Cardiology/European Association of Echocardiography. Adult Transesophageal Echocardiography (TEE)http://www.escardio.org/communities/EAE/accreditation/TEE/Pages/welcome.aspx: Accessed January 29, 2012.
22. Swanevelder J, Chin D, Kneeshaw J, Chambers J, Bennett S, Smith D, Nihovannopoulos P. Accreditation in transoesophageal echocardiography: statement from the Association of Cardiothoracic Anaesthetists and the British Society of Echocardiography Joint TOE Accreditation Committee. *Br J Anaesth.* 2003;91(4):469-472.
23. ANZCA. PS46 Recommendations for Training and Practice of Diagnostic Perioperative Transoesophageal Echocardiography in Adultshttp://www.anzca.edu.au/resources/professional-documents/documents/professional-standards/professional-standards-46.html: (accessed January 29, 2012).
24. Hilberath JN, Oakes DA, Shernan SK, Bulwer BE, D'Ambra MN, Eltzschig HK. Safety of transesophageal echocardiography. *J Am Soc Echocardiogr.* 2010;23(11):1115-1127.
25. Labovitz AJ, Noble VE, Vierig M, Goldstein SA, Jones R, Kort S, Porter TR, Spencer KT, Taval VS, Wei K. Focused cardiac ultrasound in the emergent setting: a consensus statement of the American Society of Echocardiography and the American College of Emergency Physicians. *J Am Soc Echocardiogr.* 2010;23(12):1225-1230.
26. Lin T, Chen Y, Lu C, Wang M. Use of transesophageal echocardiography during cardiac arrest in patients undergoing elective non-cardiac surgery. *Br J Anaesth.* 2006;96(2):167-170.
27. Goins KM, May JM, Hucklenbruch C, Littlewood KE, Groves DS. Unexpected cardiovascular collapse from massive air embolism during endoscopic retrograde cholangiopancreatography. *Acta Anaesthesiol Scand.* 2010;54(3):385-388.
28. Song JE, Chun DH, Shin JH, Park C, Lee JY. Pulmonary thromboembolism after tourniquet inflation under spinal anesthesia – a case report. *Korean J Anesthesiol.* 2010;59(suppl):s82-s85.
29. Newkirk L, Vater Y, Oxorn D, Mulligan M, Conrad E. Intraoperative TEE for the management of pulmonary tumor embolism during chondroblastic osteosarcoma resection. *Can J Anesth.* 2003;50(9):886-890.
30. Ebner FM, Paul A, Peters J, Hartmann M. Venous air embolism and intracardiac thrombus after pressurized fibrin glue during liver surgery. *Br J Anaesth.* 2011;106(2):180-182.
31. Wei J, Yang HS, Tsai SK, Hsiung MC, Chang CY, Ou CH, Chang YC, Lee KC, Sue SH, Chou YP. Emergent bedside real-time three dimensional transesophageal echocardiography in a patient with cardiac arrest following a caesarean section. *Eur J Echocardiogr.* 2010;12(3):E16:Epub 2010 Nov 1.
32. Blavias M. Transesophageal echocardiography during cardiopulmonary arrest in the emergency department. *Resuscitation.* 2008;78(2):135-140.
33. Gabielli A, O'Connor MF, Maccioli GA. Anesthesia Advanced Circulatory Life Support. Monograph by the ASA Committee on Critical Care Medicine: Available at http://search.asahq.org/search?q=acls&site=default_collection&btnG=+Search+&client=asahq_search&output=xml_no_dtd&proxystylesheet=asahq_search&&sort=date%3AD%3AL%3Ad1&oe=UTF-8&ie=UTF-8&ud=1&exclude_apps=1:February 2008. Accessed March 4, 2012.
34. American College of Emergency Physicians. Emergency ultrasound guidelines: 2008: Available at http://www.acep.org:Appendix 3. Accessed January 2012.
35. Wagner CE, Bick JS, Webster BH, Selby JH, Byrne JG. Use of a miniaturized transesophageal echocardiographic probe in the intensive care unit for diagnosis and treatment of a hemodynamically unstable patient after aortic valve replacement. *J Cardiothorac Vasc Anesth.* 2011;26(1):95-97.
36. Costello WT, Billings FTIV, Bick J, Kennedy JD, Wagner CE. Transesophageal echocardiography as a hemodynamic monitor in post operative cardiac surgery patients [abstract A1452]*Programs and abstracts of Anesthesiology 2011.* October 15-19, 2011:Chicago, IL.
37. Ultrasonography. Fundamentals in Critical Care: Available at http://www.chestnet.org/accp/events/ultrasonography-fundamentals-critical-care-2:Accessed March 4, 2012.
38. Outline Content. The Joint Council on Anesthesiology Exminations: Revised September 2009. Available at http://www.theaba.org/pdf/ITEContentOutline.pdf: Accessed May 21, 2012.
39. MOCA Keywords: Available at http://www.theaba.org/pdf/MOCA-Keywords.pdf: Accessed May 21, 2012.

Medical Insurance Claims, Compliance, and Reimbursement for Anesthesiology

DAVID L. REICH | MARIA GALATI

Introduction

In the United States, perioperative transesophageal echocardiography (TEE) is a procedure that is recognized for reimbursement by the Centers for Medicare and Medicaid Services (CMS) and many private medical insurance plans. These insurance plans will reimburse TEE separately from a concomitant anesthetic when it is reasonable and medically necessary, performed by a credentialed provider for diagnostic purposes,* and documented in a compliant manner.

This chapter will discuss the requirements for billing, collection, and compliance with guidelines for the reimbursement of TEE services in the current U.S. healthcare system. While many concepts are applicable to cardiology and intensive care unit settings, this chapter is focused on issues pertinent to anesthesiologists performing TEE in perioperative settings. CMS guidelines will be the primary source used in this discussion, because they often are followed in whole or in part in the payment policies of other insurance plans.

Local Carrier Determinations and Medical Necessity

CMS contracts with agents in the private sector, typically insurance companies, to administer Medicare program services such as physician claims administration. These intermediaries are known as Medicare "carriers." Carriers are regionally based, and although they are charged with following National Coverage Determinations issued by CMS, there is room for local variation in interpreting and applying these guidelines. Carriers publish their own payment guidelines in "local carrier determinations" (LCDs) that define how national Medicare policy is applied within their geographic jurisdiction. Physicians, billing staff, and compliance advisors must consult their specific carrier's LCDs in seeking counsel on reimbursement requirements for TEE; geographic variation in Medicare payment policy is possible.

The LCD (from the National Government Services [NGS] carrier) is paraphrased below as an example of Medicare policy on medical necessity for TEE:[1]

TEE is considered medically necessary when it provides information not available from transthoracic echocardiography (TTE) and when it contributes significantly to decisions in the management and treatment of the patient. Specifically, if TTE is technically inadequate or yields insufficient data about pathology to support a definitive therapeutic decision, TEE may be considered "necessary."

Additionally, TEE is considered superior to TTE in certain cases. Medicare considers TEE appropriate for detecting specific pathophysiologic conditions involving the aorta and the posterior structures of the heart (e.g., left atrium, mitral valve, pulmonary veins, etc.) Carriers will list in their LCDs the medical conditions they deem to be "covered" as indications for TEE (Box 31-1). These indications are derived

from evidence in the medical literature. Inclusion of the appropriate diagnosis codes in support of claims is one essential element for reimbursement of TEE services.

TEE technology is evolving, and there is continual improvement in diagnostic capabilities, especially with the introduction of three-dimensional (3D) TEE, tissue Doppler imaging, and speckle tracking. Medicare recognizes several indications for the use of 3D technology when billed with TEE, including preoperative and intraoperative planning of procedures of the mitral valve and atria, complex repair of congenital heart disease, and for related interventional cardiac procedures. However, not all carriers consider newer applications of TEE such as 3D TEE as "medically necessary." The NGS carrier asserts that the value of 3D TEE in affecting clinical outcomes is not yet proven and therefore is not "medically necessary."[1] Other carriers, such as Wisconsin Physicians Service Insurance Corporation, consider it medically necessary under certain conditions where the referring physician documents the clinical need for 3D imaging in a written request to the interpreting physician, who in turn addresses those clinical issues in the report and maintains a copy of the request.[2] This carrier adds stipulations requiring assignment of eligible diagnosis codes and assurance that equivalent information has not already been provided or could be provided by another procedure.

In summary, medical necessity determinations are a matter of local carrier policy and are subject to many stipulations and requirements that must be in evidence in the claims submission and medical record documentation processes.

Provider Training and Credentialing

The New York City area Medicare carrier revised its LCD on TEE in 2005 to include requirements for provider competence and credentialing as a component of its medical necessity determination.[3] The argument for these changes was that substandard studies led to unnecessary duplication and overutilization of TEE services. Since 2005, training and credentialing requirements have been updated, and providers in this jurisdiction were given until July 1, 2011, to comply with the following levels of competence or face denial of claims for the professional portion of the TEE procedure:

An acceptable level of competence is fulfilled when the interpretation is performed by a physician meeting any one of the following requirements:
- *The physician is board certified in Cardiovascular Diseases or Perioperative Transesophageal Echocardiography (National Board of Echocardiography); or*
- *The physician has Level II training in transesophageal echocardiography (including documentation of the performance of 25 esophageal intubations and 50 supervised interpretations), as defined by the American College of Cardiology/American Heart Association/American College of Physicians Task Force on Clinical Competence in Echocardiography, or the equivalent of Level II training as set forth in that document.*
The submission of claims for transesophageal echocardiography will be considered an attestation that both the technical and professional components of the service were provided within the context of the above stated credentials.[4]

---

*Medicare will *not* pay anesthesiologists for TEE when it is used only for intraoperative monitoring (e.g., CPT 93318). Other insurance plans may have different payment policies.

BOX 31-1. APPROVED INDICATIONS FOR DIAGNOSTIC INTERVENTIONAL AND SURGICAL TEE

1. Guidance during percutaneous cardiac interventions, such as during the creation of shunts, placement of septation devices, valvuloplasty procedures, endomyocardial biopsy, electrophysiologic studies/procedures, placement of septal or atrial appendage occluders, or during percutaneous valve replacement
2. Intraoperative evaluation to assess prosthetic or repaired/reconstructed valve function or the integrity/function of complex congenital heart repairs
3. Intraoperative evaluation to assess the integrity of the cardiopulmonary circulation in patients during lung or heart-lung transplants
4. Intraoperative assessment for presence and/or severity of outflow tract obstruction or presence/repair of an intracardiac shunt
5. Intraoperative assessment of wall motion abnormalities in the case of acute deterioration in the patient's status, once the chest has been closed

Modified from Medicare Carrier: National Government Services, Inc. LCD for Transesophageal Echocardiography L27381: revised 10/17/2011.

Compliant Documentation

Physicians must, with the help of coders and compliance experts, choose the appropriate CPT (Current Procedural Terminology) codes (Table 31-1) and accompanying ICD-9-CM (the *International Classification of Diseases*, 9th revision, Clinical Modification) codes in presenting their TEE claims for reimbursement by insurance plans.[†] However, these claims and the codes chosen must be supported by legible, signed, medical record documentation and must include all of the following elements to evidence compliance:

1. The performing physician's interpretation and written report, including measurements (available upon request)
2. Permanent image storage on digital media or paper (available upon request)
3. Documentation of medical necessity, including:
   - Medical history
   - Physical examination
   - Results of pertinent diagnostic tests or procedures
   - Rationale for repeat testing, as applicable
4. Doppler interrogation should detail the modes used (continuous wave, pulsed wave, and color flow) and provide quantitative and qualitative information.
5. Documentation of the qualifications of personnel involved (available upon request)

Bundling of Reimbursements

Medicare asserts that diagnostic intraoperative TEE procedures performed by the same provider who performed the anesthetic should be billed on the same claim form and may be recognized as a separately reimbursable service. In this case, the modifier 59 is appended to the CPT code to indicate that the TEE is a separate and distinct procedural service (see Table 31-1). If the provider is billing for only the professional portion of the TEE service, the 26 modifier is also used.

In 2003, the CMS Correct Coding Initiative caused rejections of diagnostic intraoperative TEE claims and bundled its reimbursement with that of the anesthetic. It was only after explanation and lobbying by several professional societies that this decision was reversed and TEE for intraoperative diagnostic purposes was again reimbursable under the Medicare program as a separate and distinct service from the anesthetic.

TABLE 31-1	TEE Current Procedural Terminology (CPT) Codes
93312	Echocardiography, transesophageal, real-time with image documentation (2D) (with or without M-mode recording); including probe placement, image acquisition, interpretation and report
93313	Echocardiography, transesophageal, real-time with image documentation (2D) (with or without M-mode recording); placement of transesophageal probe only
93314	Echocardiography, transesophageal, real-time with image documentation (2D) (with or without M-mode recording); image acquisition, interpretation and report only
93315	Transesophageal echocardiography for congenital cardiac anomalies; including probe placement, image acquisition, interpretation and report
93316	Transesophageal echocardiography for congenital cardiac anomalies; placement of transesophageal probe only
93317	Transesophageal echocardiography for congenital cardiac anomalies; image acquisition, interpretation and report only
93318	Echocardiography, transesophageal (TEE) for monitoring purposes, including probe placement, real-time 2D image acquisition and interpretation leading to ongoing (continuous) assessment of (dynamically changing) cardiac pumping function and to therapeutic measures on an immediate time basis
93320	Doppler echocardiography, pulsed wave and/or continuous wave with spectral display (list separately in addition to codes for echocardiographic imaging); complete
93321	Doppler echocardiography, pulsed wave and/or continuous wave with spectral display (list separately in addition to codes for echocardiographic imaging); follow-up or limited study (list separately in addition to codes for echocardiographic imaging)
93325	Doppler echocardiography color flow velocity mapping (list separately in addition to codes for echocardiography)
76376	3D rendering with interpretation and reporting of computed tomography, magnetic resonance imaging, ultrasound, or other tomographic modality; not requiring image postprocessing on an independent workstation
76377	3D rendering with interpretation and reporting of computed tomography, magnetic resonance imaging, ultrasound, or other tomographic modality; requiring image postprocessing on an independent workstation
Modifier 59	Distinct Procedural Service: Under certain circumstances, the physician may need to indicate that a procedure or service was distinct or independent from other services performed on the same day.
Modifier 26	Certain procedures are a combination of professional and technical components. When only the professional component is reported, the service is identified by adding modifier 26 to the procedure code.

2D, Two-dimensional.
From American Medical Association. *CPT 2013 Professional Edition.* Chicago, Ill.: American Medical Association; 2013.

The American Society of Anesthesiologists (ASA) Statement on Transesophageal Echocardiography[5] identifies TEE as a special diagnostic tool providing unique information, outside the scope of standard perioperative anesthetic care, for patients undergoing a variety of surgical interventions. Because of this, they have not incorporated the value of TEE into any of the base valuations of anesthetic management for surgical procedures in the ASA's Relative Value Guide (ASA RVG).

The potential for the bundling of TEE reimbursement into that of the anesthetic is always a concern and becomes more likely as payers scrutinize utilization rates and the growth in expenses. Prudent use of all adjunct technologies with strict adherence to medical necessity guidelines and indications supported by the medical literature is useful in preempting bundling by payers.

Physicians should seek the counsel of certified professional coders and compliance advisors in all matters involving medical claims, coding, and documentation.[‡]

[†]ICD revision 10, already in use internationally, is expected to be in effect in 2014 in the United States.

[‡]CMS also provides a website tailored to physicians seeking information on Medicare claims processing, fees, and policies for reimbursement of anesthesia services at: https://www.cms.gov/Center/Provider-Type/Anesthesiologists-Center.html?redirect=/center/anesth.asp (accessed July 6, 2012).

Contracting for TEE Reimbursement

TEE may also be reimbursable by payers other than Medicare. Private insurance plans also provide coverage for TEE services, and many follow payment policies similar to those of the Medicare program. Physicians and practice managers, however, must be aware of the medical necessity, documentation, billing, and payment policies specific to each insurance plan with which they participate.

In all cases where physicians choose to participate with an insurance plan, the opportunity for negotiating rates of reimbursement for costly and intensive services such as TEE should be considered.

In 2012, the Medicare rate in New York City (Manhattan) for the professional portion of TEE (CPT code 93312-26: TEE, 2D Imaging [with or without M-mode], including probe placement, image acquisition, interpretation and report) was $116.17. Commercial insurance plans often publish their own "standard fee schedules" including rates for TEE. In negotiations for contracts with insurance plans, it is possible to ask for "carve-ups" above the standard fee schedule rates for a subset of codes.

To facilitate such a negotiation, the physician's perspective on TEE is informative and beneficial to discussions between the practice and the insurance plan. Specifically, physicians can educate the parties on the relative risks and benefits to the patient of TEE, and the specialized equipment, training, and skills required in performing the procedure.

Practice administrators can also use the ASA RVG to identify the intensity of work involved in TEE (base value 6 units) versus that of other procedures. This establishes a framework for comparing an insurance plan's fee schedule rates and discussing the possibility of enhanced reimbursement. For example, insurance plans may recognize reimbursement on a per-unit basis for procedures such as the percutaneous placement of arterial lines (CPT 36620). This procedure carries a base unit value of 3—half of that of a TEE procedure. Practice administrators can use this to open a discussion with the insurance plan about the relative work and risk involved in TEE and to argue for a fee that is proportionately higher than that of arterial line placement, for example.

Practices should also work collaboratively with the plans to decide whether contract constructs or operational practicality favor reimbursement of TEE services based on a multiple of the negotiated anesthesia unit value rate or on a flat fee rate per procedure. Either mechanism allows a practice to potentially achieve a rate of reimbursement above that of the insurer's standard fee schedule. Deviation from standard fee schedule rates, however, is not without risk.

Insurance plan representatives who perform contract negotiations are often unaware of the complexity and limitations of their own claims processing systems. Deviations from an insurance plan's standard fee schedule can result in claims adjudication errors, underpayments, and costly claims monitoring and rework. When this process of negotiation for enhanced rates is successful, however, it is possible to glean rates for TEE that are equal to many multiples of the rates paid under the Medicare program.

Monitoring TEE Services and Reimbursement

It is important to monitor all payers to ensure they are properly reimbursing for all services. Scrutiny of reimbursement for TEE services is especially important, given that these procedures are subject to denials or requests for additional documentation supporting medical necessity and compliance with medical record and other payment policy requirements.

Denials of TEE Doppler add-on codes (e.g., 93320-59-26, 93321-59-26, and 93325-26) may also occur when these are billed by an anesthesiologist. Some insurance plans' automated claims systems contain edits that identify Doppler services as procedures performed by radiologists. In this case, the intraoperative TEE may be approved, but the Doppler add-on code will be denied because of a perceived mismatch between the provider type and the procedure type. Clinical necessity denials are also likely for Doppler procedures when test report documentation lacks specificity or if the medical record fails to document clinical support for the examination.

Practices must have the ability to track reimbursement of services by CPT code and payer against the individual payer's contractual and standard fee schedule rates. This may be done as part of real-time posting of payments to patient accounts or by other manual systems of vigilance. Payment verification software products are also available to assist practices in this arduous task. These contract management systems allow for a high degree of customization and detail and provide reporting capabilities that facilitate the filing of appeals with insurance plans. Automated systems are also useful in tracking utilization of TEE services by providers for performance improvement, credentialing, compliance, auditing, and managed care contracting purposes.

Conclusion

TEE is an important procedure, aiding in the diagnosis and treatment of patients undergoing complex surgical interventions and throughout the perioperative period. It may remain a financially viable service to offer if it is utilized according to medical necessity guidelines and continues to be recognized for reimbursement by Medicare and private insurance plans as an intraoperative diagnostic tool separate from the anesthetic service. Practitioners in other nations may use the concepts in this chapter to develop strategies for maximizing the economic benefit of providing TEE services in their own countries.

To ensure success, practices offering TEE services must follow all local and individual insurance plan requirements for provider credentialing, documentation, and reporting of services, and practice on-going monitoring of billing compliance and third-party reimbursement.

REFERENCES

1. National Government Services, Inc. LCD for Transesophageal Echocardiography L27381: revised 10/17/2011. http://www.ngsmedicare.com. Accessed March 2, 2012.
2. Wisconsin Physicians Service Insurance Corporation. LCD for 3D Interpretation and Reporting of Imaging Studies L30729: revision effective 07/16/2012. http://www.cms.gov/medicare-coverage-database/details/lcd-details.aspx?LCDId=30729&ContrId=147&ver=14&ContrVer=1&Date=10%2f24%2f2011&DocID=L30729&bc=iAAAAAgAgAAA&. Accessed July 4, 2012.
3. Empire Medicare Services LCD for Transesophageal Echocardiography L3120: revised 9/06/2005.
4. National Government Services Inc. LCD for Transesophageal Echocardiography L27381: revised 10/17/2011. http://www.ngsmedicare.com. Accessed March 2, 2012.
5. American Society of Anesthesiologists 2012 Relative Value Guide®. Statement on Transesophageal Echocardiography. Last amended on October 21, 2009. Pgs. 51-56.

32

Regulatory, Legal, and Liability Issues Pertaining to Transesophageal Echocardiography

JAMES E. SZALADOS

Disclaimer: The material presented herein is for educational purposes and is not intended as legal advice.

Introduction to the Interface of Law and Medicine

Rules, regulations, and laws become necessary whenever there is an interaction between people who potentially have diverging interests. Optimally, the interests of physicians and their patients are aligned in the mutual goal of a successful diagnostic and therapeutic outcome. Honest communication and consensual therapeutic interactions between patients and their physicians form the basis of good medical care. Disagreements may arise when expectations diverge from perceived outcome. When misperceptions or frank disagreements escalate into conflicts, fair and equitable resolution necessitates a system of rules and procedures for dealing with such conflicts. The legal system is such an "adversarial" process—a process that includes the rights to representation, a fair and impartial hearing, and justice, designed to resolve conflict. The legal system is based on arguments submitted in the context of procedure and rules of evidence; the goal of the legal system is justice, and not the determination of truth.

Since medicine is a profession, the practice of medicine is governed by complex implicit and explicit rules and regulations that share their bases both in ethical theory and principles of morality. The principles of good medical care, inherent in the Hippocratic Oath, form the guiding ethical and legal tenets for professionalism. Physicians must both uphold the interests of the patient and endeavor to "do no harm." Inherent in the professional obligations of physicians is the ethics-based fiduciary duty to act in the best interests of their patients. A fiduciary duty (from the Latin *fiduciarius*, meaning "to hold in trust," and from the root *fides*, meaning "faith") is a legal or ethical relationship of deep confidence and trust between two or more parties. Fiduciary duties arise whenever there is an imbalance of knowledge, training, or experience that puts one party at a relative disadvantage in an agreement for services. In a fiduciary relationship, a party who is in a position of vulnerability and is therefore seeking aid, advice, or protection justifiably vests confidence, good faith, reliance, and trust in another more learned and experienced party. Thus, a fiduciary duty represents, albeit as an aspiration or ideal, the highest standard of professionalism at either equity or law.

Although modern laws are largely based on ethical and moral principles, the legal system has become more complex and less subjective. The rules of modern law are codified as "black-letter law," which embodies the Constitution, federal and state statutes (legislation), and case law (precedent). A parallel system of codes and regulations define the legal processes and procedures that must be strictly adhered to in order to access the judicial system and argue one's point of view. Laws govern all formal interactions between government, institutions, and individuals. Therefore, it is imperative that physicians develop an understanding of basic substantive and procedural law—first, so their practices can be more focused and rewarding, unencumbered by fear of the unknown; second, so they can work proactively to minimize legal risk; third, so they can better communicate with risk managers, attorneys, and insurers; and finally, so physicians can better understand and participate in future legal, legislative, regulatory, and public policy development.[1]

Technology is implicated in medical-legal risk, since no drug or technology is, nor can ever be, completely safe. In addition, early adopters of technology are potentially exposed to unknown product liability risks; late adopters may be criticized for not providing access to state-of-the-art care.

The FDA and Regulation of Medical Devices

The U.S. Food and Drug Administration (FDA) governs all aspects of drugs and medical device regulation in the United States. The FDA has detailed rules and regulations regarding development, approval, marketing, and postmarketing follow-up for medical devices; these largely parallel those for pharmaceuticals. Congressional legislation in the form of the Federal Food, Drug, and Cosmetic Act (FFDCA or FDCA)[2] empowers the FDA as a federal agency with statutory regulatory authority.[3] The Medical Device Amendments Act of 1976 (MDA)[4] expanded the reach of the FFDCA from agriculture and pharmaceuticals to include medical devices.

Within the FFDCA, a *device* is defined as:

any instrument, apparatus, implement, machine, appliance, implant, in vitro reagent or calibrator, software, material, accessory, component part, or related article, intended by the manufacturer to be used, alone or in combination, for humans and for one or more of the specific purposes of (1) diagnosis, prevention, monitoring, treatment or alleviation of disease; (2) diagnosis, monitoring, treatment, alleviation of, or compensation for an injury; (3) investigation, replacement, modification, or support of the anatomy or of a physiological process; (4) supporting or sustaining life; (5) control of conception; (6) disinfection of medical devices; (7) providing information for medical purposes by means of in vitro examination of specimens derived from the human body and which does not achieve its primary intended action in or on the human body by pharmacological, immunological or metabolic means, but which may be assisted in its function by such means.[5]

Thus, medical devices can range from simple tongue depressors to complex computerized imaging equipment and biomedical implants. Under the FFDCA, the distinction between drugs and devices rests in their respective mode of action: drugs effect their intended action through chemical action or via metabolism, whereas devices do not. Devices in turn are classified based upon intended use, potential benefit, approved medical indications for use, and risk. Potential risks associated with devices, in conjunction with potential benefits, are the major factors used in classifying a device on a scale of I to III, where class I devices denote the lowest risk and class III the highest; classification determines the level of FDA controls associated with the manufacture and marketing of the particular device.[6] Transesophageal echocardiography (TEE) equipment is a class II device, an intermediate-risk device, wherein General Controls are insufficient, and methods/standards/ guidance processes and documents must provide assurances of safety and effectiveness.[7]

The intent of the MDA is to provide consumers of medical devices with a reasonable assurance of both safety and efficacy, which together represent the dual statutorily mandated standards upon which the FDA bases its approval of both pharmaceuticals and devices. However, in the case of devices, FDA approval more heavily favors safety over efficacy. The safety profile of any drug or device is a complex interplay between product design, use, and potential for operator error. Courts explicitly recognize that no drug or device is completely safe and that such products are "inherently dangerous."[8]

Medical professionals and consumers naturally expect medical devices to be well manufactured, have comprehensive and accurate labeling and directions for use, and perform reliably in the manner manufacturers intend and advertise. The potential for user or operator error is not considered a threshold issue by the FDA, and it recognizes that operator errors can result from a large number of variables over which the manufacturer has no control (e.g., training and skill of individual operators, patient variability, ergonomics, and the complex clinical environment). However, manufacturers are expected to consider human factor engineering principles during product design and encourage appropriate user education and training so the risk for user errors can be minimized or mitigated.[9]

The formal process whereby the FDA approves a drug or device is highly structured and requires manufacturers to submit data before clinical trials to begin testing in humans. Thereafter, data from carefully controlled clinical trials must be submitted to panels of FDA experts. After premarket approval, medical devices are subject to reporting requirements under the MDA. These requirements include an ongoing obligation for manufacturers to inform the FDA of new device-related clinical investigations, scientific studies, or incidents of patient harm the manufacturer becomes aware of, knows, or should reasonably be aware of. The FDA recognizes that malfunctions and other safety concerns must be reliably communicated to manufacturers so they may consider and potentially take corrective actions based on such reports. Postmarketing surveillance and reporting of adverse events is the process that seeks to ensure that rare adverse events not detected during product development and testing can be followed by the FDA, and that such devices can be subsequently withdrawn from market, modified in subsequent models, or relabeled with additional warnings as the FDA might deem necessary. The FDA's safety-surveillance strategy for medical devices relies on physicians, healthcare institutions, manufacturers, and patients to report medical device failures and complications through the Medical Device Reporting (MDR) system. The process is analogous to the Adverse Event Reporting System (AERS) database, which is the basis for the FDA's postmarketing safety surveillance program for drugs and biological products. The Standards Management Staff (SMS) of the FDA has the responsibility to ensure that evolving medical device standards are published to provide formal notice to designers and manufacturers and thereby facilitate the incorporation of new regulatory standards into product design and manufacture.

Medical device tracking provisions within the FDCA mandate that manufacturers be able to track class II and class III devices through sales and distribution channels to the specific ultimate device users so they can promptly locate and remove specific devices from the clinical arena in the event of any product recall. In 2009, the FDA launched the Sentinel Initiative, a program that integrates the electronic health records (EHRs) of healthcare institutions with FDA databases in order to perform continuous and online postmarketing safety analyses. Since medical devices, in contrast to pharmaceuticals, lacked unique device identifiers (UDIs), the FDA was authorized through the FDCA Amendments Act of 2007 to develop a comprehensive UDI system for medical devices that is expected to soon be integrated with EHRs, as well as administrative and claims databases to identify patients who have been exposed to specific devices and thereby track rare postexposure risks. The UDI project is now under consideration with the Office of Management and Budget (OMB).

With respect to diagnostic ultrasound equipment, FDA regulations governing the output of ultrasound probes are based upon internationally agreed-upon standards developed by a variety of authorities. These include, for example, the International Electrotechnical Commission (IEC), the American Institute of Ultrasound in Medicine (AIUM), and the National Electrical Manufacturers Association (NEMA). For example, NEMA standards are especially material to the issue of safety, and the NEMA Output Display Standard (ODS) specifically address factors such as the thermal (TI) and mechanical indices (MI) for diagnostic ultrasound equipment. In brief, the MI represents an estimate of the maximum amplitude of the acoustic pressure pulse created by the ultrasound beam in tissue and is thus an indicator of risk associated with any potential mechanical bioeffects. The TI represents the ratio of the total acoustic power to that required raising a maximum temperature increase of 1°C in various tissue types. The ALARA ("As Low as Reasonably Achievable") principle[10] would minimize thermal and mechanical output levels from ultrasound devices so as to minimize any potential adverse effects associated with their use. Despite a general consensus that there are no known risks associated with ultrasound imaging per se, there is also a recognition that ultrasound may produce effects on the body such as *cavitation*, whereby ultrasound waves heat tissues slightly and may produce small pockets of gas in body fluids or tissues. The long-term effects of tissue heating and cavitation, especially in fetal tissue, are not presently known with absolute certainty.

Medical Device Defects and Medical Device Malfunctions

Products are marketed with warranties. A warranty can be *express*, where it is explicit and in writing, or it may be *implicit* and implied under the UCC code of commercial law.[11] Strictly speaking, a *warranty* is defined as a legal assurance or promise by a manufacturer that a product is fit for public use as intended, free of defects, and that it meets specifications; a warranty will usually also delineate the rights and obligations of both parties in the event of a dispute. For example, the *warranty of merchantability* is one example of an implied warranty where merchantability requires that goods sold through commerce must reasonably conform to the expectations of the ordinary buyer. The *warranty of fitness* for a particular purpose represents another example of an implied warranty; in this case, a consumer with specific technical requirements reasonably relies on a manufacturer's claim that the goods fit those specific needs. A warranty can be violated when a product does not conform either to reasonable expectations as promised or has inherent defects.

Despite strict standards, a rigid FDA approval process, manufacturing oversight, and postmarketing surveillance, it is a reality that medical devices will sometimes fail, malfunction, or otherwise cause patient harm. Thus, it is inevitable some product recalls will occur under even optimal circumstances; such recalls may result in removal a product from commerce, either voluntarily by the manufacturer[12] or by FDA order[13] and either permanently or temporarily.[14] MDR requirements by manufacturers are mandatory, and failure to report malfunctions can result in punitive damages (as well as render a device misbranded) and rescission of FDA approval. Manufacturers must submit reports to the FDA whenever there are data to suggest a device (1) may have caused or contributed to a death or serious injury or (2) has malfunctioned and that the device or a similar device marketed by the manufacturer or importer would be likely to cause or contribute to a death or serious injury if the malfunction were to recur. Adverse event data are logged by both manufacturers and the FDA. Although physicians and institutions have no absolute legal duty to report, reporting of adverse events and malfunctions are important to prevent future injuries and to trend events—documentation and trending that may later become important in the defense of potential future litigation. In response to MDRs, the FDA may also order product recalls by statutory authority. Recalls conducted at the manufacturer's initiative or at FDA request are both considered voluntary recalls, whereas recalls conducted pursuant to the FDA's statutory authority are considered mandatory recalls.[15]

Product defects are generally categorized as (1) design defects, (2) manufacturing defects, or (3) marketing defects. In the law of products liability, a *design defect* is considered to exist when the defect is inherent in the design of the product. In a products liability case, a plaintiff can establish that a design defect exists only if he or she can establish that an alternative design, albeit hypothetical, would be (1) safer, (2) as economically feasible, and (3) as practical as the original design while retaining the primary purpose.[16] *Manufacturing defects*, on the other hand, are unintended defects occurring during manufacture or assembly. *Marketing defects* are defects that typically pertain to inadequate warnings and/or instructions and are typically exemplified by inadequate or faulty instructions and failures to warn consumers of latent dangers that might be associated with normal use of the product.

Products liability is the field of legal analysis that refers to liability incurred by one or more parties along the chain of commerce of any product. A product liability claim might be based in various grounds such as, for example, negligence, strict liability, misrepresentation, or breach of warranty of fitness. Products liability is generally considered to be a strict liability offense, meaning liability is not predicated on the degree of carefulness used in the design, manufacturing, or marketing of a product. Under strict liability, a manufacturer is liable when it is shown that the product is defective. However, product liability claims are increasingly difficult for plaintiffs to bring against manufacturers of medical devices. Since there is no federal products liability law, the laws governing products liability have been codified in state-specific products liability statutes. Paradoxically, through its ruling in *Reigel v Medtronic*, the U.S. Supreme Court virtually eliminated state product liability claims through its preemption[17] of state tort law claims.[18] After Reigel, medical device manufacturers have been able to use federal patient safety legislation as a shield against claims made under existing state tort laws.

Misrepresentation usually refers to an intentional concealment of defects or potential hazards associated with a product. However, if it can be shown that a reasonable manufacturer should have known that a product defect or hazard existed, a case of negligent (rather than intentional) misrepresentation may be found. Litigation against manufacturers and distributors of medical devices may also be based in allegations that the devices are *adulterated* or *misbranded* under the FFDCA. A device may be determined adulterated or misbranded if it was marketed without FDA approval, not manufactured in accordance with the required manufacturing standards, found to be of inferior quality, or if advertising or labeling is deemed false or misleading.[19]

The Learned Intermediary Doctrine[20] defense provides that manufacturers of prescription drugs and/or medical devices fulfill their duty of care to patients when they provide warnings to physicians regarding their products. This doctrine is grounded in the doctor-patient relationship whereby it is reasonable to expect that the treating physician would be in a better position to warn a patient about pertinent risks than would the manufacturer, since in any decision to prescribe a drug or medical device, there is a professional assessment of risks as balanced against the patient's needs, susceptibilities, and projected benefit. The Doctrine does not obviate a manufacturer's duty to provide adequate warnings, but instead substitutes the medical professional for the patient as the required recipient of the warnings.[21] Therefore, the Doctrine has become another shield to protect manufacturers from liability, since manufacturers are deemed to have discharged their duty under the Doctrine, thereby passing the risks for liability under normal use to the medical professional.

Liability claims may also be predicated in a theory of negligence. *Negligence* is defined as a failure to exercise proper or ordinary care, and a manufacturer might be held liable for negligence if it can be established that a lack of reasonable care in the production, design, or assembly of the manufacturer's product caused a harm. One specific type of negligence action pertaining to medical devices is the "failure to warn" case.[22] The duty to warn arises whenever a manufacturer knows or reasonably should have known of latent dangers associated with

use of its product under normal circumstances.[23] The manufacturer may be found to have had constructive knowledge of latent risks if *by the application of reasonable, developed human skill and foresight* it could have or should have known of such risks. Although the injured party still bears the responsibility to prove that a manufacturer had such actual or constructive knowledge, this evidentiary burden can sometimes be satisfied via documented complaints or prior injuries, reports in relevant scientific or trade literature, recognition of the risks by industry experts, or alerts issued by the FDA or other governmental agencies.

Importance of Practice Guidelines and Society Statements

The promulgation of guidelines, protocols, and pathways represent another potential important driver of medical legal risk. Evidence-based medicine (EBM) emphasizes clinical reasoning that is based on cumulative evidence derived from prior clinical research that is then distilled into guidelines by expert consensus.[24] Practice guidelines represent systematically developed consensus statements intended to assist both practitioner and patients in making rational healthcare decisions in specific clinical circumstances.[25] As the volume and rigor of evidentiary support from meta-analyses accumulates, EBM is ever more widely accepted to at least represent persuasive outlines of best practices that should at least be considered during individualized clinical decision making. Nonetheless, even guidelines are fluid and subject to revision with new developments in medical knowledge, technology, and practice.

Proponents of EBM suggest that adherence to guidelines might bolster a practitioner's medical decision making by demonstrating adherence to an authoritative and widely accepted published statement of standardized care, thereby facilitating administrative review and even potentially reducing legal liability. Although guidelines are colloquially referred to as "standards," they are not truly in themselves legal standards of care. The legal definition for *standard of care* is that physicians employ that level of ordinary skill and care consistent with good medical practice.[26] The appropriateness of a physician's medical care is judged by the testimony of other experts—physicians in the same or a similar field of practice. Despite widespread acceptance of EBM, expert testimony remains the legal basis upon which the appropriateness of medical care is assessed.

EBM standards in the form of guidelines are gradually being successfully admitted into evidence during medical malpractice litigation. In 2006, the New York Court of Appeals decided *Hinlicky v Dreyfuss*,[27] a ruling that addressed the importance of adhering to accepted standards of care as a legal duty. Briefly, in this case a 71-year-old woman underwent a successful carotid endarterectomy but suffered a postoperative myocardial infarction and died 25 days later. The key issue at trial was whether the defendant physician, an anesthesiologist, was negligent in not obtaining a preoperative cardiac evaluation. The plaintiff's cardiology expert asserted that as a "mandatory minimum," the patient should have had a preoperative cardiac stress test. At trial, the defendant anesthesiologist testified at length regarding his deliberate adherence to the American Heart Association (AHA)/American College of Cardiology (ACC) guidelines addressing preoperative testing for patients with cardiac risk factors.[28] The defendant testified that the AHA/ACC guidelines provided him with an algorithm ("a link in the chain of data") on which his decisions regarding preoperative cardiac testing in that particular case were based. The value of the AHA/ACC exhibit was underscored when all defense experts agreed that the algorithm not only "represented the standard of care" but actually represented state of the art medicine. The court subsequently ruled in favor of the physician. The case was appealed, and the momentum of the Hinlicky case continued through the appellate system and reached New York's highest court—the Court of Appeals—where the verdict for the defense was upheld. In its decision, the Court of Appeals recognized that clinical practice guidelines represented systematically developed statements to assist practitioners in decisions; as such, guidelines could be reasonably admitted into evidence for the purpose of illustrating the decision-making steps used in the care of a specific patient.

Importance of State Laws

Individual states have authority to regulate the practice of medicine within their state boundaries through police powers conferred upon them in the Constitution. State laws and regulations regarding the practice of medicine vary significantly, and it is imperative that physicians and other healthcare providers familiarize themselves with the regulations specific to the state in which they practice. State enforcement of regulations related to medical practice is usually delegated to the State Board of Medicine, State Department of Health, Office of Professions, or a similar state agency. The primary responsibilities of State Boards of Medicine are (1) the issuance of licenses to practice medicine, (2) investigation of complaints against licensees, and (3) disciplinary actions. In general, state licensure boards discipline physicians for conduct which is either potentially harmful to public health or conduct involving moral turpitude. Physicians convicted of crimes are uniformly subject to loss of licensure.

Physicians commonly under-appreciate the scope of authority and powers vested in State Boards of Medicine. Lawsuits alleging negligence may subject a physician to liability for plaintiffs' damages both under insurance policy limits and potentially personal financial liability in the case of excess judgment. Medical negligence actions, unless unusually frequent, egregious, or repetitive, are unlikely to result in loss of licensure. On the other hand, State Boards of Medicine can discipline physicians through either licensure sanctions or licensure revocation. Furthermore, although State Boards must adhere to administrative due process, such administrative hearings are typically closed, not bound by legal precedent, limit the introduction of evidence and witnesses, and generally shift the burden of proof to the defendant-physician.

Policies and Procedures Impacting Hospital Practice

Two interrelated administrative processes relating to the practice of medicine by physicians in hospitals as members of the medical staff are (1) peer review and (2) credentialing. *Peer review* refers to a continual process of monitoring and evaluation of the qualifications and skills of individual physicians by their collective colleagues. Peer review occurs through departmental quality improvement and morbidity and mortality reviews, informal observation, and review of external adverse administrative actions.[29] The intent of peer review is to ascertain that the physicians on the medical staff are of the highest quality and help minimize quality-of-care–related litigation against the hospital. The two peer review–related issues that most commonly rise to legal scrutiny under peer review relate to (1) the *confidentiality of peer review* and (2) claims of *restraint of trade* under the guise of peer review.

The Health Care Quality Improvement Act (HCQIA) of 1986[30] established the National Practitioner Data Bank (NPDB) as a national repository and clearinghouse for peer review data regarding physicians. Data that must be reported to the NPDB include (1) settlements without trial and judicial verdicts against or involving a physician;[31] (2) any action by a State Board of Medicine that revokes, suspends, or otherwise restricts a physician's license or censures, reprimands, or places a physician on probation for reasons relating to the physician's professional competence or professional conduct; and (3) any review action by a healthcare entity that completes a professional review action that subsequently adversely affects the clinical privileges of a physician for a period longer than 30 days or involves surrender of a physician's clinical privileges.[32] Since such data are considered material to the due diligence process whereby clinical medical staff privileges are granted or renewed, hospitals are under a duty to query the NPDB both at the time of a physician's initial application for clinical

privileges and then every 2 years thereafter.[33] Thus, peer review is the process that represents the foundation for both (1) the credentialing of providers to ensure that minimum requirements for education, training, and certification have been met and (2) formal internal reviews of adverse clinical events and outcomes.[34] If a hospital or other entity fails to request information on a physician who is later sued for malpractice, it is nonetheless legally on notice regarding the physician's prior history and may be both implicated in the lawsuit and/or held independently liable under a claim of negligent credentialing. In addition to its mandate regarding the NPDB, the HCQIA was also enacted as a means of facilitating the process of peer review and protecting those engaged in candid and objective evaluations of physicians' professional conduct, competence, and abilities. The HCQIA grants limited immunity from liability in suits brought by disciplined physicians for monetary damages to physicians who participate in professional peer review actions.[35] To be granted peer review immunity under the HCQIA, the review action must be (1) in the reasonable belief that the action was in the furtherance of quality health care, (2) after a reasonable effort to obtain the facts of the matter, (3) after notice and hearing procedures are afforded to the physician involved or after such other procedures as are fair to the physician under the circumstances, and (4) in the reasonable belief that the action was warranted by the facts.[36]

Two general circumstances under which legal discovery of otherwise confidential peer review information may be sought are (1) cases of criminal conduct, fraud and abuse, or antitrust actions and (2) in medical negligence cases. In the case where prior training, experience, and outcomes have not been verified through a strict credentialing process, hospitals, departments, and individuals may be liable under a claim of "negligent credentialing." In criminal cases, federal agencies typically have broad reach regarding what they may obtain via their subpoena powers from hospital files; however, in negligence cases, there is significant state-by-state variation regarding the discoverability of confidential peer review materials. Most states have enacted statutory protections whereby the proceedings, minutes, records, and reports of any medical staff committee, utilization review committee, or peer review committee either oral or written, are considered to be privileged communications that may not be disclosed or obtained by legal discovery. However, in New York, for example, the law is explicitly more limited. Although New York law generally immunizes from disclosure all proceedings and records relating to performance of a medical or a quality assurance review function, it nonetheless creates an exception for statements made by any person in attendance at such a medical or quality assurance review meeting who is a party to an action or proceeding the subject matter of which was reviewed at such meeting. Under the New York statute, disclosure may be obtained where the statements were made during a peer review meeting, the peer review meeting concerned the same subject matter as the action, and the statements were made by a defendant in the action.[37] Therefore, physicians must familiarize themselves with the laws regarding the confidentiality of peer review in their own states.

Peer review has also been used to restrain physicians' practices. Physicians whose entry into an established provider market might pose a financial threat to existing providers or practices may be prevented from obtaining medical staff privileges under the guise of peer review. Since administrative decisions regarding peer review and credentialing may be appealed for judicial review, the courts confer an additional level of safeguard aimed to maintain a fair due process. The term *economic credentialing* refers to using economic criteria to determine whether a physician will be granted medical staff membership, privileges, or referrals and is a misuse of the credentialing process to displace existing practitioners and groups from a hospital and replace them with more fiscally desirable medical staff.

In the case of TEE, the credentialing for TEE privileges may cut across the lines of multiple medical specialties such as anesthesiology, cardiology, and radiology. Restriction of TEE credentialing by a dominant specialty within a hospital has been used to prevent credentialing of others. Although strict adherence to a defined credentialing process is important to minimize hospital liability under the negligent credentialing doctrine, inappropriate denial of privileges may conversely result in liability for an unlawful restraint of trade.

Informed Consent

Relatively few medical malpractice claims have been premised solely or specifically on lack of informed consent. However, in those instances in which there is an otherwise valid cause of action based on other elements of medical care, lack of informed consent can further (1) undermine a physician's credibility or professionalism, (2) create an adverse presumption regarding the completeness of the medical record, (3) demonstrate lapses in duty or habit, or (4) suggest a disregard for administrative policies and procedures.[38] It is clear that informed consent is a process that includes discussions between physician, patient, and/or caregiver, and the issue of valid consent extends beyond the signed consent form. It is also recognized that the consent form itself is rebuttable, since patients may claim impaired reading or understanding, coercion, or confusion. Nonetheless, most legal authorities agree that a signed and witnessed consent form continues to have significant persuasive value as demonstrative evidence—an exhibit that can be shown—to the jury and also serves to obviate the need for a physician to continually rely on recollections of discussions that transpired years earlier.

The doctrine of informed consent is premised on the fundamental principles of autonomy[39] and bodily self-determination and thus represents an ethical as well as legal obligation of physicians to share medical decision-making authority with their patients. A fundamental problem with the exercise of one's right of autonomy and self-determination is that informed choice presupposes the (1) availability of information of sufficient scope and quality; (2) comprehension of that information, including the inherent limitations of available data; (3) ability to appreciate the nature of the situation; (4) ability to manipulate the information rationally and to compare the and the relative consequences of competing choices and their associated risks and thereby make a decision that is consistent with one's values or preferences; and (5) ability to communicate one's choice effectively. In another sense, consent may also be viewed as a type of contract that requires the elements of disclosure, consideration, and acceptance, subsequently imposing certain duties and obligations on each party. The result is that legal challenges to the validity of contracts (e.g., fraudulent facts or pretenses, absence of disclosure, duress, lack of capacity, impairment) may each be raised as a challenge to the legal validity of a signed informed consent document. The informed consent document, analogous to a contract, then serves to protect and inform both patient and physician. A patient's consent must be *informed* to be legally effective, requiring the physician to disclose the risks, benefits, and alternatives of the proposed intervention or treatment. *Consent* represents an important example of communication and documentation between patient and physician. However, it is also widely accepted that physicians cannot be expected to communicate everything during the consent process, so less than full disclosure must necessarily suffice. The standards for determining the adequacy of physician disclosure vary significantly from jurisdiction to jurisdiction. Almost half of U.S. states continue to apply a physician-centered standard, referring to that information a "reasonable medical practitioner" would provide in the same or similar circumstances.[40] However, the contemporary trend favors the patient-centered standard, which focuses on the informational needs of a typical patient.[41]

Although the informed consent doctrine is historically grounded in the tort of battery, most courts will treat a lack of medical informed consent as "negligent nondisclosure" and therefore remove consent cases from the criminal realm.[42] In addition, courts generally prosecute the tort of negligence and reserve the more serious tort of battery for cases where (1) the patient gave absolutely no consent to the procedure; (2) the procedure deviated substantially and unjustifiably from that which the patient authorized; (3) the physician disclosed no information at all to the patient; or (4) there was fraudulent concealment, misrepresentation, or other deliberate wrongdoing on the physician's part. Moreover, although it would be theoretically possible

for a state to bring a claim of criminal battery on behalf of an injured patient, such claims are rare and relatively improbable in the absence of severe and egregious conduct. Since battery is not medical malpractice, physicians may not be covered under their medical liability insurance policies against charges of assault and/or battery. Nonetheless, failure to obtain informed consent may have far reaching legal consequences and may even represent professional misconduct under the State Board of Medicine's rules and regulations, thereby exposing the physician who fails to obtain informed consent to licensure sanctions. In addition, federal regulations that define the Medicare Conditions of Participation for Hospitals require that medical records contain a *properly executed informed consent form for the operation…in the patient's chart before surgery, except in emergencies.*

Although express and written consent represents the ideal standard, in emergent clinical situations, there may not be sufficient time for an extended meaningful dialogue about the nature of a planned procedure. In New York, the law limits civil liability for medical treatment rendered without consent to non-emergency treatments and invasive diagnostic procedures. In addition, the doctrine of *implied consent* addresses the relatively common circumstance where the provider could reasonably infer that a patient would have consented to the treatment if he or she could have done so. Implied consent is essentially a matter of the provider's reasonable interpretation of the overall patient's conduct to be consistent with an intention to authorize a procedure, even though express consent to treatment is lacking. For example, in the case where a patient presents to the emergency room and subsequently loses consciousness from a heart attack, consent might be implied from the situational context to suggest that he or she came to the hospital expecting that any necessary and appropriate care be rendered. *Therapeutic privilege* is a somewhat paternalistic doctrine that continues to have force of law in some states; in essence, therapeutic privilege allows the physician to determine that disclosure of risks would pose harm to the patient or leave the patient to harmful choice. Although some state statutes allow physicians to use this discretionary privilege as a defense to an allegation that consent was not obtained, some have argued that a full disclosure may not be mandatory if (1) the patient already knew of the risks, (2) the risk were so obvious it could be reasonably presumed that the patient would have known, (3) the risk was remote, or (4) the risks were unknown.

Competence and *capacity* are frequently used interchangeably to describe the appropriateness of a patient's mental state for complex decision making in the context of ability to provide a meaningful and legally valid consent. Capacity for decision making may be generally considered to be contextual and situational, such as recent treatment with psychoactive substances (e.g., sedatives, analgesics), delusional states such as "ICU psychosis" or abstinence syndromes, acute injury, or metabolic conditions such as disorders of sodium, acid-base, or glucose balance. On the other hand, *competence* more generally refers to a fixed characteristic of a patient, such as age of minority without emancipation or long-term cognitive impairment; most jurisdictions have abandoned this distinction.

Since the risks of any procedure are related in part to the patient's comorbidities, proposed surgery, proposed anesthetic, and skill of the individual providers, it is best that the responsible physician be present for and actively involved in the informed consent process. When a physician chooses to delegate a critically important matter such as consent, in the event of a mishap the patient may raise challenges pertaining to that physician's compassion, caring, and diligence. Furthermore, since supervisory liability rests with the attending physician, it is reasonable that he or she be present for, and also document his or her involvement in, the informed consent process. Ordinarily a hospital does not have a duty to ensure that a patient has given informed consent to a procedure performed by an independent physician; in many institutions specialists are independent physicians who hold exclusive rights to provide services at that institution. Finally, it is noteworthy that since the interests of the hospital and its medical staff may diverge during litigation, specialty physicians may choose not to rely on standard hospital consent forms but instead adopt their own specific consent forms.

Anesthesiologists should carefully consider the implications of informed consent laws as they apply to their own practices. Specific issues that might have to be addressed could include specific departmental policies regarding the use of informed consent, use of an anesthesiology-specific consent form, and consideration of a procedure-specific consent form for invasive procedures.

Scope of Practice and the Anesthesia Care Team

The term *scope of practice* is used to specify the extent of privileges permitted by state law for a given class of allied health provider based on specific criteria like education, training, experience, and special qualifications. There is no defined scope of practice for physicians. Under most if not all state laws, physicians may perform any of the duties associated with the practice of medicine, including those duties that would otherwise fall to allied health support staff. A physician's scope of practice is more defined by national, state, local, and hospital credentialing bodies and tends to be specialty based.

Interpretation of echocardiographic data is not within a sonographer's scope of practice. The American Institute for Ultrasound Medicine (AIUM), in its "Interpretation of Ultrasound Examinations" statement,[43] explicitly endorsed the interpretation of ultrasound studies as the practice of medicine. In its guideline, the AIUM stated that "ultrasound studies shall be supervised and interpreted by a physician with training and experience in the specific area of sonography" and that although a sonographer might, under some circumstances, perform a critical role in helping to extract information essential to the diagnosis, "the rendering of the final diagnosis is the responsibility of the supervising physician."[44] Thus, if a sonographer provides diagnostic interpretations from echocardiographic data, he or she may inadvertently violate state statutes concerning the unauthorized practice of medicine and exceeding one's scope of practice. Legal issues arise when a sonographer renders interpretations independently or when physicians routinely allow or even delegate responsibility for echocardiographic readings to the sonographer. In such instances, the physician may be jointly liable for aiding and abetting the unauthorized practice of medicine.[45] A similar situation might arise if a resident physician, nurse anesthetist, or anesthesiology assistant provides echocardiographic analyses in the operating room.[46] Unauthorized preliminary or final interpretations may also violate various reimbursement rules and policies and even expose the entire care team to malpractice liability if treatment is based on erroneous interpretations.[47] In addition, under Centers for Medicare & Medicaid Services (CMS) rules, certain medical services provided to Medicare and Medicaid patients must occur under the direction of a supervising physician.[48] Patient records must reflect who actually provided the service, and the procedure code on the claim must be consistent with the provider's scope of practice, certification, and/or profession.

Medical Malpractice

A physician-defendant in a case of alleged malpractice should possess at least de minimis understanding about litigation process and procedure to best participate in his or her defense. Medical malpractice represents a type of negligence. Negligence is a tort and is governed under the laws of state-specific civil statutes. To be found liable under any specific cause of action, the court will require that the plaintiff demonstrate each legal element of that particular cause of action.

The civil tort of medical negligence requires the plaintiff to demonstrate that (1) a duty existed, (2) there was a breach in duty, (3) the breach of duty was the actual and proximate cause of the adverse outcome, and (4) ascertainable damages resulted.[49] The standard of proof in a civil action is that of preponderance of the evidence ("more probable than not"). Since medical malpractice, unlike common negligence, is beyond the usual understanding of laypersons, the court requires that the elements of standard of care, breach, and proximate cause be proven through expert testimony. A physician is generally not liable in negligence for errors in judgment; rather, liability can only legitimately be inferred where the treatment rendered clearly falls outside recognized standards of good medical practice.

Duty is created by the physician-patient relationship. Duty requires the physician to adhere to that degree of skill and learning ordinarily possessed and employed by other members of the same profession, who are in good standing, and are engaged in the same type of practice or specialty. In practice, however, the norms of generally accepted medical practice, on the basis of which the standard of care is defined, is difficult to define. The medical literature is replete with controversy, new medications, and technologies, and there is great variation between patients. Nonetheless, the legal standard for a duty is that of a *prudent physician* under *similar circumstances*. Plaintiff and defendant will each introduce expert testimony regarding the applicable standard of care, since there is a gray zone of uncertainty regarding the standard, and only experts are permitted to introduce opinion testimony. Breach of duty must be also be proved by the plaintiff, whose evidentiary burden requires demonstration that the defendant-physician did not act in accordance with the applicable standard of care. The principal types of allegations regarding breach of duty in medical negligence claims include (1) failure to diagnose, (2) failure to treat, (3) inadequate or inappropriate treatment, (4) inadequate supervision or monitoring, and (5) complications or side effects of treatment.

The plaintiff must prove causation by demonstrating that a reasonably close causal connection exists between the negligent act and the resulting injury. The defendant's conduct must be shown to represent a *cause in fact* of the plaintiff's injury, also known as the *actual cause*. In addition, the defendant's conduct must be shown to be the *proximate cause*, or the *legal cause*, of the plaintiff's injury. It is important to note that the concept of legal causation differs from the way physicians refer to medical causation; *legal causation* does not necessarily refer to a single causative factor, nor is it necessarily the major or medically most important cause or even the most immediate cause of the plaintiff's injury. Legal causation considers both *causation-in-fact* and *foreseeability*. Causation-in-fact is often defined using the "but for" test: but for the act or failure to act, the complication or injury would not have occurred. Foreseeability requires that the patient's injuries be a reasonably foreseeable result of the defendant-physician's substandard practice.

Damages describe the actual ascertainable loss or harm suffered by the plaintiff. The term *damages* encompasses claims for compensation by the plaintiff for a range of alleged financial, physical, and emotional injuries. The intent of awarding compensatory damages in a tort action is to "make the plaintiff whole again," which in most medically related injuries is a legal fiction. Since it is impossible to fully alleviate the effects of injuries, public policy demands that redress be made through monetary compensation. There are two types of compensatory damages: special and general. *Special damages* include economic injuries such as subsequent hospital or treatment costs, costs of assistance or custodial care, lost wages, or lost earning capacity. *General* or *non-economic damages* address emotional injuries such as loss of companionship (consortium), mental anguish, grief, pain, and suffering. *Punitive* or *exemplary damages* may also be imposed if the defendant's conduct can be categorized as wanton and willful, reckless, fraudulent, intentional, grossly negligent, or malicious.

Liability may also be premised in the doctrine of "res ipsa loquitur," which literally translates as "the facts speak for themselves." The specific elements of a res ipsa claim vary by state. In New York, a case may be submitted to the jury on the theory of res ipsa only when the plaintiff can establish that (1) the event is one that ordinarily does not occur in the absence of negligence; (2) the event was caused by an agency or instrumentality within the exclusive control of the defendant; and (3) the event cannot have been due to any voluntary action or contribution on the part of the plaintiff.[50] Examples of res ipsa claims include retained instruments or fragments following procedures, positioning injuries, burns, or injuries sustained by patients while sedated or chemically paralyzed under anesthesia. The legal effect of res ipsa loquitur is to create a prima facie case ("valid on its face") of negligence. Res ipsa is especially important to TEE-related injuries, since although TEE is generally accepted to be safe, there may be a greater risk of traumatic damage to the soft tissues in anesthetized patients who cannot complain of pain during probe insertion. Reported complications associated with intraoperative TEE probe placement under general anesthesia include oropharyngeal, esophageal, and gastric trauma, odynophagia, dental injury, aspiration, endotracheal insertion, and endotracheal tube dislodgement—thus leaving the practitioner open to *both* traditional medical negligence and res ipsa claims.

Typically, a physician is covered under a medical malpractice insurance policy that provides insurance coverage for a claim at the time of its accrual. There are two general types of medical malpractice insurance policies. *Occurrence policies* cover incidents that occur during the policy period; the policy in effect at the time of services rendered covers a potential claim based on that service even if it is reported in the future following expiration or discontinuance of that policy. *Claims-made policies* will only cover claims filed during the life of the policy. Since the average malpractice claim is made 1 to 2 years following an incident, a physician may no longer be covered under the policy when a claim is made. Therefore, claims-made policies may require additional purchases of either "nose" or "tail" coverage to maintain coverage during job or insurer-to-insurer transitions. To preserve coverage, and possibly evidence, medical malpractice insurance policies typically require the insured to provide the carrier with prompt notice of any potential claim. Failure to provide such prompt notice might negate the carrier's obligations to defend and/or indemnify. Notification regarding potential claims has its basis in risk management, whereby the funds necessary to either settle or pay on a judgment are encumbered through the potential life of the claim.

The malpractice carrier has two principal obligations to the insured: the duty to defend and the duty to indemnify. To provide a legal defense, an insurance carrier will typically retain knowledgeable and experienced defense counsel and pay the legal fees on behalf of the defendant-physician. The duty to indemnify requires the carrier to pay the amount of a settlement or judgment on a covered claim within the set policy limits.

The party who initiates the lawsuit (plaintiff) must file the claim within a specified period of time, a statutorily defined and state-specific time period known as the *statute of limitations*. A lawsuit is formally commenced when the plaintiff's attorney files a complaint with the court and the clerk of the court issues a summons. Typically, service of the summons is made on the defendant-physician, not on the insurer, and it is important that the physician notify the insurance carrier immediately because the defendant has only a limited period of time during which to answer the complaint. If the answer is not filed by the physician's defense counsel within the statutory time limits, the plaintiff can obtain a default judgment against the defendant-physician, forfeiting the right to contest the matter in court. If the action is not dismissed, then both parties will begin a process of "discovery." *Discovery* relates to the opportunity of each party to obtain relevant information and documents from the parties to the lawsuit. Discovery may include interrogatories; depositions of key parties, support staff, and families; chart reviews; expert reviews; and determination of relevant supporting materials. *Interrogatories* refer to written questions served on parties; *depositions* represent formal oral sworn testimony obtained under oath and transcribed by a court reporter.

At various times during the litigation process, the parties might choose to settle, attempt alternative dispute resolution such as mediation or arbitration, proffer motions for either summary judgment or dismissal, or voluntarily discontinue the action. Settlement prior to trial is generally encouraged by the courts in the interests of judicial efficiency. Medical malpractice cases frequently settle out of court, since there are many potential advantages of doing so: (1) juries are unpredictable; (2) the negative consequences and publicity of a guilty verdict are lessened; (3) defense attorney, expert witness, and court costs are potentially lessened; and (4) the precedential impact of the verdict to future similar cases is eliminated. If the matter proceeds to trial, the court will set a trial date on the "docket," or trial calendar. The defense strategy is often a complex interplay between the facts of the case, credibility of the witnesses, opinions of experts, and personalities of the parties. A party generally has the right to appeal a judgment to at least one higher court, which has the power to affirm, reverse, or modify the judgment of the trial court.

By its very nature, medicine is an area of professional practice wherein the risk of litigation is high. Physicians must understand that a bad outcome does not equate with medical malpractice. Clear, open, and honest communication with patients and families is the best way to prevent a lawsuit. However, when a malpractice lawsuit is filed, the best outcomes occur when physicians choose knowledgeable and experienced defense counsel and participate actively in the defense process.

Medical Error and Disclosure

It is axiomatic that each healthcare practitioner and institution practices his or her profession with a dedication to excellence. Nonetheless, complications occur in the clinical setting related either to progression of disease, medical error, exposure to nosocomial pathogens, or iatrogenic injury. Whenever possible, patient safety optimization strategies should be implemented to streamline routine processes and minimize or mitigate patient harm stemming from potential medical errors.

Recognition that patient harm due to medical error is frequently a system-wide issue has resulted in increased scrutiny by plaintiffs' attorneys of institutional policies and processes. Although in the past, patient harm caused by the negligence of nurses, therapists, and other hospital staff has been frequently imputed to the hospital, there is possibly a more recent trend to also impute physician liability to the hospital. Case law has expanded the scope of a hospital's independent duty of care to its patients. Therefore, it is not uncommon to find a hospital named as codefendant for damages due to care provided by either employed or attending physicians. The typical legal doctrine under which liability is imputed to hospitals is that of *vicarious liability* or *respondeat superior*.[51] In cases of corporate vicarious liability, the hospital may be jointly liable for physicians' negligence or be individually liable under agency theory. It has been held that an acute care hospital has a nondelegable duty to provide non-negligent physician care.

The culture of safety has also resulted in a philosophy of transparency with respect to medical errors. CMS, the Joint Commission, and many state agencies advocate that hospitals develop and adhere to disclosure policies and protocols. In the process of disclosure, patients and/or families are informed early following recognition that an iatrogenic injury or medical error has occurred. Preliminary studies suggest that full disclosure may decrease litigation, but the optimal policy and procedure for such disclosure remains somewhat controversial. Some states have developed so-called safe harbors to protect the information conveyed during a disclosure meeting from discovery during litigation. However, there is wide variation among states in such safe harbor laws.

Honesty and empathy are often appreciated and can substantiate the overall atmosphere of professionalism and caring essential to health care. Disclosure of adverse events may be even be mandatory under state law, regulatory agency rules, or under hospital policy and procedure. However, the process whereby a physician or care team discloses a medical error to a patient or patient's representative should occur only after careful deliberation and consideration. In general, it is a legal tenet that anything said or done may be used against the defendant, and in some cases a disclosure may be treated as an *admission against interest* under evidentiary rules. Also, a disclosure that is perceived to be a confession and is thereafter subsequently admitted into evidence as such can eliminate potential defenses to a malpractice claim. In the case of a lawsuit where an admission or confession eliminates triable issues of fact, the plaintiff may potentially move for summary judgment, leaving only the amount of damages to be determined by the courts or in settlement. Most insurance policies also contain a "cooperation clause," which requires that the insured cooperate fully in the defense of a claim. There is a possibility that engaging in a disclosure meeting might cause the defense of a malpractice claim to be jeopardized, violating the cooperation clause and thereby voiding the policy.

Physician leadership and attending physicians should be aware of the applicable disclosure policy in effect at their institution and be prepared to develop, review, or comply with it. Additionally, although hospital risk-management personnel frequently oversee implementation of the disclosure policy, physicians may need to consider the personal legal ramifications of a disclosure conference and consider prior consultation with an attorney.

Documentation, Coding, and Billing for Services: False Claims Act Implications

The False Claims Act (FCA) was first enacted by Congress in 1863. Initially known as the "Informer's Act," the FCA was designed to combat defense procurement fraud by providing to any private citizen the right to file a civil action against anyone who submitted a false claim for payment to the U.S. government. These civil suits were known by the Latin phrase *qui tam pro domino rege quam pro si ipso in hac parte sequitur*, which in English means "he who sues on behalf of the King as well as for himself." In 1986, Congress once again amended the FCA and importantly revised the prior requirement of a showing of intent, and instead ruled that "no proof of specific intent to defraud" was required and that a defendant will be liable under the FCA if it could be shown that the defendant "knowingly" submitted a false claim. The term *knowingly* was broadly defined[52] to include either actual knowledge of the false information, deliberate ignorance of the truth or falsity of the information, or reckless disregard of the truth or falsity of the information. The FCA applies to any person who knowingly assisted in causing the government to pay claims grounded in fraud or waste. In 2009, the Fraud Enforcement and Recovery Act of 2009[53] (FERA) was signed into law with the intent of further deterring fraud. In 2010, the Patient Protection and Affordable Care Act[54] (PPACA) was signed into law and again further expanded and strengthened the reach of the FCA.[55]

In health care, compliance with the FCA[56] is essential. The importance of compliance is mandated by routine government and third party payer audits of claims, billing patterns, and qui tam complaints. A claim is generally considered false if it seeks money or property to which the claimant is not entitled owing to a violation of a statute, regulation, or contract. Examples of false claims in the healthcare context include claims for unnecessary services, services not rendered or not documented, services upcoded to reflect a higher level of care than was actually rendered, claims misrepresenting the provider of the services, unbundling of services, or submitted in violation of the anti-kickback or Stark statutes. *Unbundling* refers to the practice of charging separately for procedures that were otherwise combined into a single charge. The statute of limitations, or the period of time after a claim is submitted that the government may pursue an FCA case, is within 6 years of the false claim or 3 years from when the government learns of the false claim (but no more than 10 years).

In 2011, the United States recovered more than $2.4 billion in healthcare fraud cases. Since 1986, the United States has recovered more than $21 billion in healthcare fraud cases. Physicians prosecuted under the FCA are subject to a variety of sanctions, including:

1. Criminal sanctions
2. The United States Attorney General may bring a civil action for damages and penalties.
3. The Attorney General may refer the matter to the Secretary of the Department of Health and Human Services (DHHS) for possible administrative penalties and sanctions.
4. The Secretary of DHHS may seek to recover past overpayment in an administrative recoupment proceeding.

The FCA is enforced by the Office of Inspector General (OIG), regional offices of the Assistant U.S. Attorney, and the Federal Bureau of Investigation (FBI). Violators of the FCA are potentially liable for a civil penalty of the FAC for not less than $5500 and not more

than $11,000, plus 3 times the amount of damages for each fraudulent claim;[57] a supervisory period ("Corporate Integrity Agreement"); debarment from Medicare and Medicaid; and/or criminal penalties. Notably, persons prosecuted under the FCA may be independently liable under the Federal Fraud and False Statements criminal statute of unlawfully and knowingly making false statements of material facts to a government agency. Moreover, many states have now enacted their own FCA statutes mirrored after the federal statute. For example, the Office of the Medicaid Inspector General (OMIG) in New York investigates and prosecutes false claims submitted under the Medicaid program. Action may be brought by a private party on behalf of the government under the qui tam or "whistleblower" lawsuit provisions. If the government declines to intervene in the lawsuit, the whistleblower may proceed on his or her own and may receive a portion of the government's recovery if he ultimately prevails. Typically, the whistleblower can receive 25% to 30% of the judgment or settlement.

Compliance with CMS billing and coding requirements in the teaching hospital setting require that the attending physician be physically present and immediately available in order for the teaching physician to submit a claim for reimbursement to CMS. Medicare also makes payments to teaching hospitals under the prospective payment system for the higher indirect operating costs hospitals incur by having graduate medical education (GME) programs. It also supports GME programs in teaching hospitals through claims submitted for the services of attending physicians who involve residents in the care of their patients under Medicare Part B, and therefore a service provided by an unsupervised resident cannot be billed because it would represent a "double reimbursement."[58] CMS defines the general rule to state that:

If a resident participates in a service furnished in a teaching setting, physician fee schedule payment is made only if a teaching physician is present during the key portion of any service or procedure for which payment is sought. In the case of surgical, high-risk, or other complex procedures, the teaching physician must be present during all critical portions of the procedure and immediately available to furnish services during the entire service or procedure….In the case of evaluation and management services, the teaching physician must be present during the portion of the service that determines the level of service billed…. [T]he medical records must document that the teaching physician was present at the time the service is furnished….The presence of the teaching physician during procedures may be demonstrated by the notes in the medical records made by a physician, resident, or nurse. In the case of evaluation and management procedures, the teaching physician must personally document his or her participation in the service in the medical records.[59]

The Secretary of DHHS initiated the Physicians at Teaching Hospitals (PATH) program to review Medicare Part B billings by teaching hospitals with the intent of recovering past overpayments for services rendered.[60] Following a PATH audit of the billings submitted by the University of Pennsylvania Health System, a settlement of over $30 million was made to the government for Medicare claims submitted between 1989 and 1994.

Although the FCA addresses claims for payment for services rendered to Medicare and Medicaid patients, there is a trend for private insurers to also monitor and enforce coding and billing. Furthermore, CMS contracts with local and national private insurers to process claims for Medicare and Medicaid patients on behalf of CMS; in such instances, noncompliant claims submitted to such private insurers are reported for potential enforcement action. Recovery audit contractors (RACs) are additional private entities contracted by CMS to oversee the recovery of overpayments.

Individual compliance with rules and regulations is the cornerstone of any FCA compliance plan.[61] Additionally, a complete, contemporaneous, and accurate medical record is essential in the defense of any claim for reimbursement for services rendered and serves not only to document the analysis and plan of an episode of care for future reference but should document the medical necessity, actual time spent in the encounter, and level of decision making. In the case of intraoperative TEE, the teaching attending anesthesiologist should be immediately available during probe insertion and manipulation and during formal interpretations rendered for the purposes of medical decision making. In the non-teaching setting where cases are performed under the anesthesia care team model, the attending anesthesiologist must be aware that scope of practice regulations affect not only who can do the procedure, but also implicate billing for services performed in the context of limitations on scope of practice.

HIPAA, Privacy, and Medical Information Security

Professional respect for the privacy and confidentiality of medical information is a well-established principle in both medical ethics and health law. Respect for a patient's privacy is essential to ensure trust, maintain physician professionalism and patient dignity, and promote the full communication necessary to the physician-patient relationship. Fiduciary duty imposes a heightened obligation of loyalty, integrity, and devotion and represents the ethical foundation for the privacy of medical information. Moreover, the duty of confidentiality dates to the Hippocratic Oath and was codified in the Principles of Medical Ethics of the AMA and the guiding principles of the Joint Commission. However, all physicians must be familiar with the rules embodied within the Health Insurance Portability and Accountability Act of 1996 (HIPAA).[62] Congress enacted HIPAA[63] for several explicit purposes.

1. Improve portability and continuity of health insurance coverage in the group and individual markets.
2. Combat waste, fraud, and abuse in health insurance and health care delivery.
3. Promote the use of medical savings accounts.
4. Improve access to long-term care services and coverage.
5. Simplify the administration of health insurance, and for other purposes.

HIPAA also contains statutory rules and procedures that regulate medical records privacy, standards for security and electronic healthcare transactions, and standards for data storage and recovery that apply to healthcare providers, health plans, and health data clearinghouses, collectively referred to under HIPAA as *covered entities*. Similar to most federal statutes, HIPAA generally trumps state law unless state laws impose even more stringent requirements.

There are four basic standards under HIPAA: (1) the Electronic Transactions and Code Set Standard, (2) the Privacy Rule, (3) the Security Rule, and (4) the National Identifier requirement. Additionally, DHHS published the Enforcement Rule, which defines the procedural and substantive requirements for civil monetary penalties.

HIPAA's privacy regulations define the circumstances and the procedures under which covered entities may use and disclose protected health information (PHI). *PHI* refers to any individually identifiable health information that is transmitted or maintained in any form or medium. The Privacy Rule states that individually identifiable medical information cannot be disclosed by covered entities without the consent of the individual. However, there are instances where disclosure is permitted without authorization from the individual. For example, disclosure is permitted for treatment, payment, or healthcare operations; for the disclosure of protected information for law enforcement purposes; and, with consent, in medical malpractice litigation.

Penalties for violation of HIPAA provisions are jointly enforced by the Office of Civil Rights, which has the authority to receive and investigate privacy complaints, and the U.S. Department of Justice. Civil monetary penalties for HIPAA violations are $100 per violation to a maximum of $25,000 per year for each violation. However, intentional or malicious disclosures that fall under the category of criminal violations range from $50,000 to $100,000 and up to 5 years in prison for false pretenses. Up to $250,000 and 10 years in prison is the penalty if information is sold for commercial advantage, personal gain, or malicious harm.[64]

Stark and Anti-kickback Statutes

Physicians are under increasing scrutiny by federal and state enforcement agencies with regard to their practice entities' financial structures and relationships with practice partners. The Ethics in Patient Referrals Act (the Stark law)[65] governs physician self-referral for Medicare and Medicaid patients. Physician self-referral is the practice of a physician referring a patient to a medical entity in which he or she has a financial interest—be it ownership, investment, or a structured compensation arrangement—based on the proposition that such arrangements constitute an inherent conflict of interest, given the physician's position to potentially benefit from such a referral.[66] Proponents of Stark suggest that such self-referral arrangements may encourage overutilization of services, creating a captive referral system and limitation of competition, and in turn escalate healthcare costs.

To determine whether the Stark statute applies to a particular arrangement, three questions must be answered.

1. Does this arrangement involve a referral of a Medicare or Medicaid patient by a physician or an immediate family member of a physician?
2. Is the referral for a "designated health service" (DHS)?
3. Is there a financial relationship of any kind between the referring physician or family member and the entity to which the referral is being made?

If the answer to any question is "no," Stark does not apply. If the answers to all three questions are "yes," the next level of inquiry is necessary to determine whether the arrangement falls within a statutory exception. If it does, the Stark law does not apply. If the activity is not a recognized exception[67] under the statute, Stark *does* apply to the situation, and the referral would violate federal law.

The Stark statute applies only to physicians who refer Medicare and Medicaid patients for specific services (DHS) to entities with which they (or an immediate family member) have a "financial relationship." The lists of designated health services and financial relationships addressed by the statute are extraordinarily broad. Initially, Stark applied only to clinical laboratory services reimbursable by Medicare. Stark law revisions subsequently expanded the list of implicated DHS to include, among others, radiology services including magnetic resonance imaging, computerized axial tomography scans, and ultrasound services including echocardiograms and vascular imaging. The elements of DHS implicated in Stark may include the professional as well as the technical or facility component of the fee, depending on the type of service and how it is reimbursed by Medicare. A referral to oneself is not considered a referral if the referring physician personally performs the service regardless of whether the physician bills the programs directly or another entity bills pursuant to an assignment.

Anti-kickback law[68] makes it a felony for anyone to receive any form of payment in return for referring a patient to another for Medicare or Medicaid covered services, including payment in return for purchasing, leasing, or ordering any good, facility, service, or item reimbursed from Medicare or Medicaid funds. Physician-physician and physician-hospital interrelationships may fall under anti-kickback laws. The anti-kickback statute provides criminal penalties for individuals or entities that knowingly and willfully offer, pay, solicit or receive remuneration to induce the referral of business reimbursed by Medicare or Medicaid programs; again, this offense is a felony. The requisite elements necessary to prove a violation of the anti-kickback statute are *scienter* (knowing and willful) and *remuneration* (solicitation, receipt or payment). *Kickbacks* refer to overt or covert payments used to induce referrals. Examples of kickbacks might include discounted office space, rebates or referral-based bonuses, or recruitment packages.

Although the Stark statute pertains only to physician referrals under Medicare and Medicaid, the anti-kickback statute is much broader and affects anyone engaging in business with a federal healthcare program. The Stark statute does not require bad intent; a financial relationship may violate Stark law regardless of intent. In contrast, the anti-kickback statute requires specific intent, and violations may result in criminal actions.

Violations of Stark can result in a range of sanctions such as civil penalties, denial of payments for the services provided in violation of Stark, and exclusion from participation in Medicare, Medicaid, or any other federal healthcare program. Referrals and claims that violate the Stark statute are punishable by a $15,000 civil money penalty per event. Any claim paid as the result of an improper referral is considered to constitute an overpayment and is punishable by a $100,000 civil money penalty. Although the Stark statute does not allow physicians to be compensated in a way that rewards referrals, physicians in a group may share in the overall profits of the group and may be paid a productivity bonus for their own services or services *incident to* their services, so long as certain standards are met. In addition to CMS, many other federal and state agencies have the authority to investigate and refer for prosecution or prosecute cases involving noncompliant physician financial relationships. The offices of the U.S. Attorneys, U.S. Department of Justice, and FBI have authority to investigate and prosecute alleged violations of federal healthcare laws. The DHHS OIG has as its mission the identification and elimination of fraud, waste, and abuse in DHHS programs, as well as the promotion of efficiency and economy in departmental operations.

The terms *medically necessary* or *medical necessity* refer to healthcare services a physician exercising prudent clinical judgment would provide to a patient for the purpose of preventing, evaluating, diagnosing, or treating an illness, injury, disease, or its symptoms. Such services are (1) in accordance with generally accepted standards of medical practice; (2) clinically appropriate in terms of type, frequency, extent, site, and duration and considered effective for the patient's illness, injury, or disease; and (3) not primarily for the convenience of the patient, physician, or other healthcare provider, and not more costly than an alternative service or sequence of services at least as likely to produce equivalent therapeutic or diagnostic results as to the diagnosis or treatment of that patient's illness, injury, or disease. For these purposes, "generally accepted standards of medical practice" means standards based on credible scientific evidence published in peer-reviewed medical literature generally recognized by the relevant medical community or otherwise consistent with the standards set forth in policy issues involving clinical judgment. In the United States, payments for medical goods and services by the CMS are statutorily limited to those items and services deemed to be reasonable and necessary for the diagnosis or treatment of illness or injury or to improve the functioning. On the other hand, in the context of managed care litigation, *medically necessary services* have been defined by the courts as what is medically necessary for a particular patient and therefore an individual assessment of individual need rather than a general determination based upon standard practices.

Under self-referral laws, an anesthesiologist may determine that TEE is indicated in a specific clinical circumstance and perform that intervention him- or herself without necessarily falling outside self-referral laws. However, if there is a referral to another provider or group in return for compensation, self-referral laws may be implicated. Stark may also be implicated where the hospital provides the anesthesiologist or group with the TEE equipment and shares "per click" revenue with the physicians based on its use, or where the equipment is leased to physicians below fair market value to drive usage and hospital referrals. Stark and self-referral laws are highly complex, and whenever there is a sense that a financial arrangement might implicate self-referral laws, consultation with expert legal counsel is imperative to minimize the risk of severe future liability under state and federal laws.

Remote Monitoring and Telemedicine

Telemedicine can be broadly defined as the use of telecommunication technology to interface in real time with and remotely provide medical care to patients in geographically removed locations.[69] A telemedicine system can be as simple as a computer hookup through a webcam or as advanced as remotely controlled robotic surgery.[70] Tele-radiologists and tele-pathologists have long used telecommunication to read radiographs and specimens offline, respectively, for diagnostic or consultation purposes. More recently, medical evaluation and management services have become amenable to patient examination and management in real time using audiovisual communications, digital stethoscopes, and remote access to medical records.

Telemedicine's legal issues fall into three categories: traditional medicolegal issues that are not unique to the telecommunication medium, conflicts in state healthcare laws and regulations, and issues unique to telemedicine. In addition, despite aspirational support by government agencies in the interest of increasing access to specialist care, several challenges to the expansion of telemedicine exist: (1) inadequate technology infrastructure; (2) regulatory distortions, limitations on competition, and fragmented demand; (3) public and private reimbursement policies that do not compensate for telemedicine services; (4) physician licensing and credentialing rules that discourage practicing telemedicine within states and across state and national boundaries; (5) concerns about malpractice liability; and (6) concerns about confidentiality of transmitted patient information.

In telemedicine, the physical location of the patient defines where the care has been delivered and also the jurisdiction of applicable regulations. Thus, although a patient is diagnosed and treated by a physician in another state, the location of the patient, *not* the physician, defines the point of care. Physicians who practice or engage a physician-patient relationship in a state must be licensed and registered in that state. The physician-patient relationship is considered to be as real in the virtual world of telemedicine as it is at the bedside, and state laws explicitly uphold the existence of that relationship even if the service is not billed, reimbursable, or reimbursed. Having engaged in a professional relationship via telemedicine, the physician and provider care team must meet the same standards of care as would be expected in the traditional face-to-face medical care encounter. In addition, the fact that medical advice or treatment was transmitted over electronic media does not change the requirement for documentation and even follow-up care. In telemedicine, as in face-to-face encounters, a medical record must be created and maintained according to prevailing medical record standards.[71] Telemedicine is subject to enhanced confidentiality regulations, and the standards of confidentiality of medical records are legislatively mandated in HIPAA and the Health Information Technology for Economic and Clinical Health (HITECH) Act.[72]

TEE is ideally suited to telemedicine applications so long as a sonographer is available to remotely position the probe. Telemedicine could theoretically expand access to this specialized service in operating rooms and intensive care units that could not normally offer such diagnostic interventions. The potential value of telemedicine to TEE services is enormous. Nonetheless, the legal issues outlined within this chapter apply equally to medical care via tele-sonography.

Summary and Conclusions

The practice of medicine is highly regulated through a plethora of federal legislation, state statutes, and multiple layers of regulations from a variety of governmental and quasi-governmental agencies. The legal and regulatory environment must support rather than detract from a physician's ability to practice good medicine on behalf of his or her patients. Since physicians should devote their time and energy to practicing medicine and keeping current with developments in their chosen field of practice rather than to administration, it is important that physicians partner with skilled administrators and legal counsel to best represent their interests.

REFERENCES

1. Szalados JE. Legal issues in the practice of critical care medicine: a practical approach. *Crit Care Med.* 2007;35(Suppl.):S44-S58.
2. 21 U.S.C. §§307-399.
3. Szalados JE. "Statutory and Regulatory Controls" in Pharmaceutical Law: Regulation of Research, Development, and Marketing. In: Clark ME, ed. BNA Books; 2007:1-120.
4. Pub. L. No. 94-295, 90 Stat. 538 (1976).
5. Generally see 21 C.F.R. 800 – 1299.

6. 21 C.F.R. 860.

7. FDCA § 510(k), 21 U.S.C. § 360(k).

8. Colacicco v. Apotex, Inc., 521 F.3d 253, 257 (3d Cir. 2008) (citing 21 U.S.C. §§ 301-397 (2006))."The FDA is charged with 'promot[ing] the public health by promptly and efficiently reviewing [drug manufacturers'] clinical research and taking appropriate action on the marketing of regulated products in a timely manner' and 'protect[ing] the public health by ensuring that... drugs are safe and effective.'"

9. See eg Venticinque SG, Kashyap VS, O'Connell RJ. Chemical burn injury secondary to intraoperative transesophageal echocardiography. *Anesth Analg.* 2003;97(5):1260-1261.

10. 10 CFR 20.1003

11. The law of products liability is found mainly in common law (state judge-made law) and in the Uniform Commercial Code, Article 2; the key section addressing warranties and products liability are the in §§ 2-314 and 2-315.

12. 21 CFR § 7.40.

13. The FDA may issue a recall order to the manufacturer under 21 CFR § 810, Medical Device Recall Authority.

14. Resnic FS, Normand S- LT. Postmarketing surveillance of medical devices–filling in the gaps. *N Engl J Med.* 2012;366:875-877.

15. Section 518(e) of the FDCA and 21 CFR § 810.13.

16. Restatement (Third) of Torts: Products Liability § 2 1998.

17. U.S. Constitution. Article VI., Clause 2.

18. Riegel v. Medtronic, 128 S. Ct. 999 (U.S., Feb. 20, 2008).

19. United States v. Caputo, 288 F. Supp. 2d 912 (N.D. Ill. 2003). If the intended use of a product changes, manufacturers must obtain Food and Drug Administration approval for the new use so that they can label the product appropriately. 21 C.F.R. § 807.81(a)(3); 21 C.F.R. § 801.4. Including off-label uses in the product's labeling renders it adulterated and promoting off-label uses makes it misbranded. 21 U.S.C.S. §§ 351(f)(1)(B), 352(f). Manufacturing or introducing an adulterated or misbranded product into interstate commerce is prohibited. 21 U.S.C.S. § 331(a-c), (g). Aff'd, United States v. Caputo, 517 F.3d 935 (7th Cir. 2008).

20. Sterling Drug v. Cornish, 370 F.2d 82, 85 (8th Cir. 1966).

21. See Larkin v. Pfizer, Inc., 153 S.W.3d 758, 770 (Ky. 2004) ("[O]nly health-care professionals are in a position to understand the significance of the risks involved and to assess the relative advantages and disadvantages of a given form of prescription-based therapy."); see also Vitanza v. Upjohn Co., 778 A.2d 829, 837 (Conn. 2001); ("The learned intermediary doctrine...is based on the principle that prescribing physicians act as 'learned intermediaries' between a manufacturer and consumer and, therefore, stand in the best position to evaluate a patient's needs and assess the risks and benefits of a particular course of treatment.") (internal citations omitted).

22. See Mason v. SmithKline Beecham Corp. (Mason I), 546 F. Supp. 2d 618, 625 (C.D.Ill. 2008).

23. The standard for judging both design defects and failure-to-warn claims under the Restatement (Third) states that products should be judged according to "foreseeable risks of the harm posed by the product" at the time that the product was manufactured. Restatement (Third) of Torts: Products Liability § 2(b), (c) (1998).

24. Sackett DL, et al. Evidence based medicine: what it is and what it isn't. *BMJ.* 1996;312:71-72.

25. Rosoff AJ. The role of clinical practice guidelines in health care reform. *5 Health Matrix.* 1995;369.

26. See Spensieri v Lasky, 94 NY2d 231, 723 N.E.2d 544, 701 NYS2d 689 (1999); Barrett v Hudson Valley Cardiovascular Assoc., P.C., 91 AD3d 691, 936 NYS2d 304 (2d Dept 2012).

27. Hinlicky v. Dreyfuss 815 N.Y.S.2d 908 (2006).

28. Eagle KA, Berger PB, Calkins H, et al. ACC/AHA guideline update for perioperative cardiovascular evaluation for noncardiac surgery–executive summary: a report of the American College of Cardiology/American Heart Association Task Force on Practice Guidelines (Committee to Update the 1996 Guidelines on Perioperative Cardiovascular Evaluation for Noncardiac Surgery). *J Am Coll Cardiol.* 2002;39:542-553.

29. See JCAHO, Comprehensive Manual on Accreditation, Medical Staff Standard 5.2.

30. Health Care Quality Improvement Act, Pub. L. No. 99-660, 100 Stat. 3784 (codified as amended at 42 U.S.C. §§ 11101–11152 [1999]).

31. 42 U.S.C. § 11131.

32. 42 U.S.C. § 11133(a)(1)(A).

33. 42 U.S.C. § 11135(a)(2).

34. 42 U.S.C.§ 11151(4)(A)(ii).

35. 42 U.S.C.§ 11112, See also Sugarbaker v. SSM Health Care, 190 F.3d 905 (8th Cir. 1999) 'The HCQIA creates a statutory presumption that professional review actions are conducted in accordance with the statutory requirements.' See also 42 U.S.C. § 11137(c)"The HCQIA also contains a separate immunity provision stating that no person or entity shall be held liable in any civil action with respect to any report to the NPDB in the absence of "knowledge of the falsity of the information contained in the report."

36. 42 U.S.C. § 11112(a). See Wayne v. Genesis Med. Ctr., 140 F.3d 1145, 1148 (8th Cir. 1998).

37. N.Y. Pub. Health L. § 2805-m

38. Szalados JE. Informed consent: a legal overview for clinicians. *Curr Rev Clin Anesth.* 2008;29(11):123-131.

39. Schloendorff v. Soc'y of N.Y. Hosp., 105 N.E. 92 (N.Y. 1914).

40. See Tashman v. Gibbs, 556 S.E.2d 772, 777 (Va. 2002).

41. See Canterbury v. Spence, 464 F.2d 772, 784 (D.C. Cir. 1972).

42. See Restatement (Second) of Torts § 18 (2006). Claims for battery may also be brought in criminal proceedings as well as civil proceedings as a tort. Battery in the medical malpractice context is generally considered a tort, rather than a criminal act.

43. American Institute of Ultrasound in Medicine. 'Interpretation of Ultrasound Examinations' March 27, 2010:Available online at http://www.aium.org/publications/viewStatement.aspx?id=15. Link verified February 16, 2012.

44. Dubinsky T. Medical liability and responsibility: the sonographer's expanding role and legal liability. *J Diagn Med Sonography.* 1985;1(6):286.

45. Kisslo J, Millman DS, Adams DB, et al. Interpretation of echocardiographic data: are physicians and sonographers violating the law? *J Am Soc Echocardiogr.* 1988;1:95-99.

46. American Institute of Ultrasound in Medicine. 'Training Guidelines for Physicians Who Evaluate and Interpret Diagnostic Ultrasound Examinations': ; November 5, 2011:Available online at http://www.aium.org/publications/viewStatement.aspx?id=14. Link verified February 16, 2012.

47. Kisslo J, Millman DS, Adams DB, Weiss JL. Interpretation of echocardiographic data: are physicians and sonographers violating the law? *J Am Soc Echocardiogr.* 1988 Jan-Feb;1(1):95-99.

48. Wegman B, Stannard JP, Bal BS. Medical liability of the physician in training. *Clin Orthop Relat Res.* 2012;470(5):1379-1385.

49. See eg. Hytko v. Hennessey, 62 A.D.3d 1081, 879 N.Y.S.2d 595, 598 (3d Dep't 2009) (internal citations omitted); Smith v. Masterson, 353 F. App'x 505, 507–08 (2d Cir. 2009); Keane v. Sloan-Kettering Inst. for Cancer Research, 96 A.D.2d 505, 464 N.Y.S.2d 548, 549 (2d Dep't 1983).

50. Simmons v. Neuman, 50 A.D.3d 666, 667, 855 N.Y.S.2d 189 (2d Dep't 2008) (citations omitted); see also States v. Lourdes Hosp., 100 N.Y.2d 208, 211-12, 792 N.E.2d 151, 762 N.Y.S.2d 1 (2003) (citations omitted); "To rely on the doctrine of res ipsa loquitur, a plaintiff must demonstrate that (1) the injury is of a kind that does not occur in the absence of someone's negligence, (2) the injury is caused by an agency or instrumentality within the exclusive control of the defendants, and (3) the injury is not due to any voluntary action on the part of the injured plaintiff."

51. See Schloendorf v. Society of New York Hospital, 211 N.Y. 125, 105 N.E. 92 (1914) overruled Bing v. Thunig, 2 N.Y.2d 656, 163 N.Y.S.2d 3, 143 N.E.2d 3(1951); Moeller v. Hauser, 237 Minn. 368, 54 N.W.2d 639, 57 A.L.R.2d 364 (1952); Rice v. California Lutheran Hosp., 27 Cal.2d 296, 163 P.2d 860 (1945).

52. 31 U.S.C. § 3729.

53. Fraud Enforcement and Recovery Act of 2009, Pub. L. No. 111-21, 123 Stat. 1617 (May 20, 2009).

54. Patient Protection and Affordable Care Act of 2010, Pub. L. No. 111-148, 124 Stat. 119 (2010).

55. See Affordable Care Act § 6402(f)(2), 124 Stat. at 759; see also United States ex rel. Hutcheson et-al. v. Blackstone Med., Inc., 647 F.3d 377, 389 (1st Cir. 2011).

56. 31 U.S.C. §§ 3729 et seq.

57. CMP Statute (Section 1128A of the Social Security Act) at 42 U.S.C. § 1320a–7a(b)(1).

58. Centers for Medicare and Medicaid Services (CMS). *Medicare Part B Reference Manual. "Teaching Physician's Billing Guide."* March 2003.

59. DOH & DHHS CMS Manual System, Pub 100–04 Medicare Claims Processing. Centers for Medicare & Medicaid Services (CMS)Transmittal 2303, September 14, 2011:Available online at https://www.ouhsc.edu/bc/documents/2011-10-R2303CP-TPrulespartial.pdf.

60. Association of American Medical Colleges. *"Background Paper Physicians at Teaching Hospitals (PATH) Initiative."* October 20, 1997.

61. *Fed Reg.* Feb 23, 1998;63(35):8987-8998.

62. Szalados JE. Health information privacy and HIPAA: The Health Insurance Portability and Accountability Act. *Curr Rev Clin Anesth.* 2004;25(1):3-14.

63. Most of the healthcare delivery provisions of the HIPAA statute, Pub. L. No. 104-191, 110 Stat. 2021 (Aug. 21, 1996), are codified as amendments or additions to the Social Security Act, 42 U.S.C. §§ 1301 et seq.

64. 42 U.S.C. § 1320d-5(a)(1) (2000); 45 C.F.R. § 160.508. A civil penalty may not be imposed for a violation if it is punishable as a criminal offense under 42 U.S.C. § 1320d-6, which is administered by the Department of Justice. 42 U.S.C. § 1320d-5(b)(1); HIPAA Administrative Simplification: Enforcement, 70 Fed. Reg. at 20,237.

65. 42 U.S.C. § 1395 et seq.

66. United States v. Ruttenberg, 625 F.2d 173, 177 (7th Cir. 1980).

67. Medicare and state health care programs: fraud and abuse; safe harbors for protecting health plans. *61 Fed Regist.* Jan. 25, 1996;2122:2124.

68. 42 U.S.C. § 1320a-7b(b).

69. Daly HL. Telemedicine: the invisible legal barriers to the health care of the future. *Ann Health Law.* 2000;9:73-106 (citing Conduct on Medical Education and Hospitals and Council on Medical Service and the American Medical Association, Joint Report, 1994).

70. Mendelsohn LB. A piece of the puzzle: telemedicine as an instrument to facilitate the improvement of healthcare in developing countries?*18 Emory Int Law Rev.* 2004;151:163 see also Hamilton-Piercy M. Cybersurgery: why the united states should embrace this emerging technology. 7 J High Tech Law. 203, 210(2007).

71. NYS DOH. Statements on Telemedicine Board for Professional Medical Conduct. Available online at http://www.health.ny.gov/professionals/doctors/conduct/telemedicine.htm.

72. Title XIII, Div. A, and Title IV, Div. B, of the American Recovery and Reinvestment Act of 2009, Pub. L. No. 111-05, 123 Stat. 115 (Feb. 17, 2009), contain the Health Information Technology for Economic and Clinical Health Act (the HITECH Act).

Note: Page numbers followed by *f* indicate figures, and those followed by *t* refer to tables.